The more you know, the healthier you'll be.

Completely revised and updated!

THE MOST COMPLETE FOOD COUNTER

Third Edition

With more than 7.5 million of their popular *Counter* books in print, the nutrition experts answer all of your questions about healthy eating, food shopping, and eating out.

Now Karen J. Nolan and Jo-Ann Heslin present the ultimate, one-stop encyclopedia of food values, nutrition basics, and advice for eating well.

- The MOST nutrient values—calories plus 12 key nutrients
- The MOST food categories
- The MOST restaurant chains
- The MOST take-out items
- The MOST gluten-free, low-sugar, low-carb, low-fat, vegetarian, ethnic, and organic foods
- The MOST nutrition information—right at your fingertips—to help you make sense of the latest health research, trends, and guidelines

Books by Karen J. Nolan and Jo-Ann Heslin

The Calorie Counter (Sixth Edition)
The Complete Food Counter (Fourth Edition)
The Ultimate Carbohydrate Counter (Third Edition)
The Protein Counter (Third Edition)
The Diabetes Counter (Fourth Edition)
The Most Complete Food Counter (Third Edition)

Books by Annette B. Natow, Jo-Ann Heslin and Karen J. Nolan

The Cholesterol Counter (Seventh Edition)
The Fat Counter (Seventh Edition)
The Healthy Wholefoods Counter

Books by Annette B. Natow and Jo-Ann Heslin

Eating Out Food Counter
The Healthy Heart Food Counter
The Vitamin and Mineral Food Counter

Ebooks by Karen J. Nolan, Jo-Ann Heslin and Annette B. Natow

The Most Complete Food Counter (Second Edition)

Apps by Karen J. Nolan and Jo-Ann Heslin

Your Complete Food Counter
(http://itunes.apple.com/us/app/your-complete-food-counter/id444558777?mt=8)

THE MOST COMPLETE FOOD COUNTER, 3RD EDITION

KAREN J. NOLAN, PH.D., AND JO-ANN HESLIN, M.A., R.D., C.D.N.

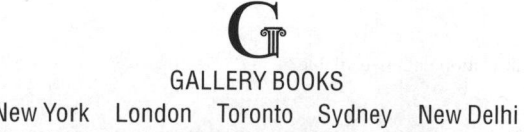

GALLERY BOOKS

New York   London   Toronto   Sydney   New Delhi

Gallery Books
A Division of Simon & Schuster, Inc.
1230 Avenue of the Americas
New York, NY 10020

This Gallery Books trade paperback edition January 2013

GALLERY BOOKS and colophon are registered trademarks of Simon & Schuster, Inc.

For information about special discounts for bulk purchases,
please contact Simon & Schuster Special Sales
at 1-866-506-1949 or business@simonandschuster.com.

The Simon & Schuster Speakers Bureau can bring authors to your live event.
For more information or to book an event contact the Simon & Schuster Speakers Bureau
at 1-866-248-3049 or visit our website at www.simonspeakers.com.

Manufactured in the United States of America

10 9 8 7 6 5 4 3 2 1

Library of Congress Cataloging-in-Publication data is available.

ISBN 978-1-4516-2164-8

To our families,
who support us through every project.

ACKNOWLEDGMENTS

For all her continuous support and help, our agent, Nancy Trichter.

For her suggestions and editing skills, Sara Clemence.

For all her patience, comments, and questions—our favorite reviewer, Jean Schwarsin.

Without the tireless cooperation of the production department at Gallery Books, *The Most Complete Food Counter, 3rd Edition* would never have been completed.

A special thank you to our editor, Emilia Pisani.

We would also like to thank all of our readers for their suggestions and questions. Your input helps us provide you with the most useful information.

CONTENTS

. . . foods, though so numerous and so varied in form, can be reduced to rather simple terms.

Mary Swartz Rose, Ph.D.
Feeding the Family
The Macmillan Company, 1919

INTRODUCTION

Everyone loves to talk about food and everyone has questions about their health.

Just listen to the conversations around you. They almost always turn to food—what's the best choice for lunch, how much cholesterol is in a food, or what the latest health report means to you.

We wrote *The Most Complete Food Counter, 3rd Edition,* to give you answers. It is the *most complete* food and nutrition resource available, listing calories and nutrient values for over 21,000 foods, along with information on how to get enough of or how to limit each nutrient. You'll find out how to personalize your need for every nutrient.

You'll also find information on how to use the latest Dietary Guidelines for Americans. If that isn't comprehensive enough, we've sprinkled the book with **You Should Know** boxes to give you interesting extra information. And we've included a dictionary, "Just the Facts, A to Z," which explains nutrition terms in simple language. Let's say the TV news mentions something about trans fats. Not quite sure what they are? Go to page 50 and you'll learn everything you need to know about this type of fat and what it means to your health.

Let's talk about food—it's fun.
Let's talk about nutrition, too—it's important to your health.

NUTRITION BASICS

Nutrition is the most important environmental factor in good health.
It is something you can control, so choose well and eat well.

Calories, fat, saturated fat, cholesterol, protein, carbohydrate, sugar, fiber, calcium, sodium, potassium, folic acid, and vitamin C—there are a lot of nutrients out there and your body needs them all.

Your body is working all the time, even when you are sleeping. It's walking, breathing, digesting food, pumping blood, fighting infection, growing hair, and on and on. You body needs fuel and building block for all these activities: calories and nutrients, which come from the food you eat.

When it comes to calories, the goal is simple: Eat enough to keep your body running smoothly, but not so many that you gain weight.

Nutrients are a little more complicated. Your body needs different amounts of different kinds. For some—protein, carbohydrate, fiber, calcium, potassium, folic acid, and vitamin C—the goal is to get enough each day for optimum health. For other nutrients—fat, saturated fat, cholesterol, sugar, and sodium—the goal is to limit the amount each day for optimum health.

Meanwhile, different foods contain different assortments of nutrients. Some foods, like meat and cheese, are high in protein. Milk and yogurt have a lot of calcium. Fruits and vegetables are good sources of vitamins and fiber.

Eating a variety of foods ensures that you get all the calories and nutrients you need. That may sound simple but first you have to know which foods are rich in which nutrients. And, which foods are dense in calories and which are not.

That is where *The Most Complete Food Counter, 3rd Edition*, comes in. It shows you how to track all these important nutrients and helps you determine your individual need for each one. It will help you make the best choices.

Counting Calories (cals)

Calories are energy powerhouses found in food.

Every time you eat, you take in calories. All foods, except water, have some. Calories are calories, whether they come from apples or chocolate fudge. Your body is a machine that uses food calories as fuel. When the amount of fuel you take in equals the amount of fuel you need for your body to run, your weight remains constant. There is no extra fuel to store and no deficit to make up. Eat too many calories, and your body uses what it needs and stores the leftover for future use. You see the storage on your thighs, hips, and waist. Eat too few calories, and your body draws on its fuel reserves. Your thighs, hips, and waist get slimmer as the surplus is depleted.

Calories come from the fat, protein, and carbohydrate in foods. Fat has the most calories of the three, more than twice as many as protein and carbohydrate. One teaspoon of fat has 40 calories; a teaspoon of either carbohydrate or protein has only 16 calories.

Over and over studies have shown that if you cut calories, you lose weight. If you eat too many calories—even from healthy foods—you gain weight. It doesn't matter if those calories come from bread, meat, or salad dressing. The key to long-term weight control is to burn as many calories as you eat. In order to do that effectively, you need to know how many calories you need, and how many calories you burn in activity. Then, you can see if the two balance each other out.

CALCULATING CALORIES

To find out how many calories you need each day, you need to do two things. First, how much do you want to weigh? Not your current weight, but your target weight. Second, select an activity factor that fits your current activity level.

1. Your target weight is: _____
2. Your activity factor is: _____
   20 = Very active men
   15 = Moderately active men or very active women
   13 = Inactive men, moderately active women, and people over 55
   10 = Inactive women, repeat dieters, and seriously overweight people
3. Target weight × activity factor = calories needed each day.

For example, if your target weight is 130 pounds and you are a moderately active women (factor 13), you need between 1,600 and 1,700 calories a day.

130 pounds × 13 (activity factor) = 1,690 calories a day

For more information, see CALORIES page 28.

Figuring Out Fat (fat)

Most Americans over the age of 6
eat about 33% of their daily calories as fat.
We are actually doing better eating less fat.

The view that all fats are bad and you should eat less fat is no longer accurate. The more accurate message is:

- All fats are not bad for you.
- The type of fat you eat may be more important than how much fat you eat.
- A moderate fat intake can be healthy.

Don't head for the bacon just yet. Even though the current research suggests that a moderate fat intake may be healthier, no one is suggesting a *high* fat intake is good for you. Eating too much fat can put you at risk for:

- Heart disease
- Stroke
- High blood pressure
- High cholesterol
- Cancer
- Obesity
- Diabetes
- Arthritis
- Gout
- Age-related macular degeneration (ARMD), a leading cause of blindness
- Alzheimer's disease, a leading cause of dementia

- Increased airway inflammation for asthma sufferers

A high fat diet may even disrupt your body's clock. We all operate on a 24-hour circadian cycle that regulates sleeping, waking, fluid balance, body temperature, heart output, oxygen use, and gland functions. Recent research on animals confirmed that a high fat diet disrupts normal circadian rhythms. When the body's clock is disrupted, it throws off our internal signals, including appetite control. Researchers have found that a misaligned body clock can increase the risk for obesity and diabetes. This is another good reason to eat a moderate amount of fat.

Total fat intake should be 20% to 35% of your total calories

If you aim to eat 20% to 25% of your daily calories as fat you will have a low fat intake; 30% to 35% is considered a moderate fat intake. Either can be part of a healthy eating plan.

It is easy to figure out your daily fat requirement. If you regularly eat 1,800 calories a day, you should try to eat between 40 grams (20%) and 70 grams (35%) of fat each day.

After you have decided what percentage of fat you will eat each day, multiply the percentage by your daily calorie intake.

For a low fat diet:

20% × 1,800 calories = 360 fat calories a day

For a moderate fat diet:

35% × 1,800 calories = 630 fat calories a day

To convert fat calories into grams of fat, all you need to know is that 1 gram of fat = 9 calories.

360 fat calories (20%) ÷ 9 = 40 grams of fat
630 fat calories (35%) ÷ 9 = 70 grams of fat

Sorting Out Fats—Choose Wisely

Saturated fats—eat less of this type of fat. Keep portions small.

Meat, whole milk, cheese, cream, regular or premium ice cream, butter, lard, bacon, sour cream, and pastries.

Monounsaturated fats—use these fats to replace some saturated fat.

Olives, olive oil, canola oil, peanuts, peanut oil, almonds, almond oil, avocados, cashews, hazelnuts, macadamia nuts, pine nuts, and pistachios.

Polyunsaturated fats— eat more of these fats.

Safflower oil, sesame oil, soybean oil, soybeans, corn oil, sunflower oil, grapeseed oil, nuts, seeds, soft margarine, wheat germ, flaxseeds, walnuts, walnut oil, herring, mackerel, tuna, trout, sardines, salmon, bluefish, and oysters.

Trans fats—eat as little as possible of these fats.

Pastries, solid shortening, stick margarine, doughnuts, deep-fried foods, processed cheese, and partially hydrogenated oil.

For more information see FATS page 34 and TRANS FAT pages 50–51.

Eating Less Saturated Fat (sat fat)

*Most adults get slightly more than 11% of their daily calories from saturated fat.
We are doing better eating less saturated fat.*

The current Dietary Guidelines for Americans recommends less than 10% of our daily calories from saturated fat, while the American Heart Association and others recommend less than 7% daily. Using common sense and knowing that we currently eat about 11% of our daily calories as saturated fat, a few simple dietary changes would bring us closer to 10%, providing more health benefits.

To set your daily target saturated fat intake, first, determine the number of calories you need to eat each day (see page 3). Next, select the percentage of saturated fat calories you wish to eat.

If you regularly eat 1,800 calories a day, you should eat less than 14 grams (7%) or less than 20 grams (10%) of saturated fat each day.

After you have decided what percentage of saturated fat you want to aim for daily, multiply the percentage times your daily calorie intake.

10% × 1,800 calories = 180 saturated fat calories a day

or

7% × 1,800 calories = 126 saturated fat calories a day

To convert saturated fat calories into grams of fat, all you need to know is that 1 gram of fat = 9 calories.

180 fat calories (10%) ÷ 9 = 20 grams of saturated fat
126 fat calories (7%) ÷ 9 = 14 grams of saturated fat

If for lunch you ordered 2 slices of cheese pizza with 16 grams of saturated fat (see page 486) you would use up more than your total saturated fat amount for the day, if you are aiming for 7%. At 10% you have a few grams left over for the remainder of the day.

SAVING SATURATED FAT

Eat This	Instead of This	Grams of Sat Fat Saved
Low fat cheddar cheese	Regular cheddar cheese	4
Skim milk	Whole milk	4.5
Low fat frozen yogurt	Regular ice cream	6
Bran bagel	Croissant	6.5
Safflower oil	Lard	4
Soft margarine	Butter	5
Extra-lean ground beef	Regular ground beef	4.6
Roasted chicken breast	Fried chicken leg	2.5
Baked fish	Fried fish	2
Sliced roast beef	Bologna	7.5

You don't need to eliminate all saturated fats from your diet, but it is important to limit them. That's easy when it comes to milk, cream, sour cream, and cheese. Simply choose the nonfat or lower fat versions. When it comes to meat, choose leaner cuts and smaller portions. Trim fat and skin from poultry and don't use bacon grease or lard for cooking. When you eat food naturally high in saturated fat—butter, bacon, coconut—keep portions small.

You Should Know—

When you eat less total fat, you automatically eat less saturated fat.

For more information see FATS page 34.

Controlling Cholesterol (chol)

*On average, women eat 225 milligrams
of cholesterol a day;
men eat 307 milligrams daily.*

You get cholesterol every time you eat animal foods—meat, poultry, fish, eggs, milk, yogurt, cheese or butter. Vegetables, fruits, nuts, seeds, cereals, and grains have none. Cholesterol can also be made in the body. In fact, most people make three times more cholesterol than they eat in food.

You Should Know—

It's simple. If a food grows in the ground, it has no cholesterol. If a food has a face, it has cholesterol.

The National Cholesterol Education Program recommends eating no more than 200 milligrams of cholesterol a day. The American Heart Association (AHA) recommends that you limit cholesterol to less than 300 milligrams a day; 200 milligrams if you already have heart disease.

High cholesterol does not cause any symptoms, but it can quietly damage your body, building up on the wall of your arteries. Over time, this buildup can cause the arteries to harden and become narrower, a process called *atherosclerosis*. A blocked artery to the heart can cause a heart attack. A blocked artery to the brain can cause a stroke. The only way you know if your cholesterol level is too high is to have a blood test and find out your number.

You Should Know—

It's wise to fast for at least 8 hours before getting your blood drawn. Eating a high fat meal within 4 hours of a blood test can affect the results by raising blood fats.

Your daily cholesterol intake will be based on the results of your blood test.

Total Blood Cholesterol

Desirable: less than 200 mg/dl
Borderline high: 200 to 239 mg/dl
High: 240 mg/dl or higher

If your total cholesterol level is within the desirable range, limit your cholesterol to less than 300 milligrams a day. If your numbers are up, reduce your daily intake to 200 milligrams a day.

EASY STEPS TO LOWER CHOLESTEROL

- Use liquid vegetable oils—olive, canola, corn, soybean, sunflower, and safflower—instead of butter, lard, shortening or stick margarines.
- Limit servings of meat, poultry, fish, and shellfish to 3- to 4-ounce sized portions.
- Use lean cuts of meat and trim all visible fat.
- Eat poultry without the skin.
- Don't fry in lard or bacon fat.
- Bake, broil, or roast.
- Use more beans and vegetables to make up for smaller servings of meat, fish, and poultry.
- Substitute two egg whites for one egg with yolk.
- Use low fat or nonfat milk, cheese, yogurt, ice cream, and fat free sour cream.
- Use soft margarine instead of stick margarines or butter.

- Use low fat or fat free salad dressings and gravies.
- Eat fiber-rich foods—beans, whole grains, bran, brown rice, dried fruits, fruits, and vegetables.
- Eat more cholesterol-lowering foods—nuts, soyfoods, and antioxidant-rich fruits and vegetables.
- Eat soy, nuts, and flaxseed with natural cholesterol-lowering plant sterols, or foods fortified with plant sterols—margarines, cereal, chocolate, orange juice, and yogurt.
- If your doctor prescribes a cholesterol-lowering medication, take it daily, even when your cholesterol values return to normal.

See also CHOLESTEROL page 29, CHOLESTEROL VALUES page 30, HDL (HIGH DENSITY LIPOPROTEINS) page 38 and LDL (LOW DENSITY LIPOPROTEINS) page 41.

Protein Packs a Punch (prot)

The word protein *comes from the Greek word* protos, *which means of prime importance.*

Your body loses millions of cells each day. They are used up, worn out, rubbed off, and even cut off, like your hair or beard. All those cells—and tissues and substances—contain protein. You need a continuous supply of protein to replace and repair these worn-out cells.

You also lose protein when your body is stressed, physically or mentally. When it's too hot or too cold, you need extra protein. More protein is needed during heavy sweating. Exercise, fever, surgery, injury, infection, and broken bones all increase your need for protein. Even emotional strain, such as losing your job or taking an exam, causes protein loss.

You cannot live without protein because:

- It helps to form the structures of your body: skin, organs, bones, hair, and muscles.
- It provides the raw material to build and repair your body.
- It is part of your immune system—fighting infections and viruses.
- It is a major part of every enzyme in the body.
- It is part of many important hormones.
- It helps to keep the body's fluids stable.
- It transports needed substances and nutrients around the body.
- It helps maintain the body's neutrality—preventing it from becoming too acidic or alkaline—which is essential to life.
- It helps you lose weight and maintain weight loss.
- It offers protection against chronic disease.
- It is a source of energy (calories).

The protein in your body is very similar to the protein found in food. Both are made up of smaller building blocks called *amino acids*. Your body uses amino acids in different combinations to build and repair parts of the body—muscles, glands, skin, bones—just like the letters in the alphabet are used in various combinations to form words. Active tissues—like muscles and glands—contain a lot of protein. Less active tissue—like fat—has far less.

A quick way to estimate your daily protein need is to divide your weight by 2.2. For example, if you weigh 150 pounds, you should be eating approximately 68 grams of protein a day.

$$150 \text{ pounds} \div 2.2 = 68 \text{ grams of protein}$$

Most people eat more than their recommended level of protein daily. On average, men eat slightly over 100 grams of protein a day; women eat 70 grams.

For more information see PROTEINS page 47.

Consider Carbs Carefully (carb)

Most Americans eat half of their daily
calories from carbohydrates.

So, how many carbs should you be eating? The National Academy of Sciences' Recommended Dietary Allowance (RDA) for carbohydrate is at least 130 grams a day. The Food and Drug Administration (FDA) has set 300 grams of carb as the Daily Value (DV) for the nutrition facts panel on food labels, the amount recommended for the "typical" American consumer eating 2,000 calories a day.

You can estimate your individual carb intake by first deciding what amount of carb you want to eat each day. Since most Americans get 50% of their calories from carbs, let's use 50% as an example. If you eat 1,800 calories a day:

50% of 1,800 calories = 900 carb calories a day

To figure out how many grams of carbs to eat each day, you need to know that 1 gram of carb = 4 calories.

900 carb calories per day ÷ 4 = 225 grams of carb a day

Most food professionals consider a low carb diet one in which 40% or less of your daily calories come from carbohydrates. Let's use 40% as an example, if you wish to follow a low carb diet. If you eat 1,800 calories a day:

40% of 1,800 calories = 720 carb calories a day
720 carb calories per day ÷ 4 = 180 grams of carb a day

Both examples more than meet the RDA recommendation of at least 130 grams of carbohydrate a day.

To make good carb choices, choose more foods that are higher in starch and fiber (complex carbs), and fewer foods that are high in sugar (simple carbs). There are exceptions. Milk, yogurt, fruits, and some vegetables have a lot of natural sugar but are also rich in vitamins and minerals.

SORTING OUT CARBOHYDRATE FOODS

Complex Carbs	Simple Carbs
Bagels	*with natural sugar*
Beans	Fruits
Breads	Fruit juice
Cereals	Honey
Corn	Milk
Crackers	Unsweetened yogurt
Grains	
Pasta	*with added sugar*
Peas	Cake
Popcorn	Candy
Potatoes	Cookies
Pretzels	Fruit drinks
Rice	Jellies/jams
Rolls	Gelatin
Squash	Soda
Tortillas	Sweetened yogurt
Vegetables	Sweetened cereal

See also CARBOHYDRATES, page 28.

Be Sensible with Sugar (sugar)

We should all eat less sugar.

Most of us enjoy sweets. Babies are born with a preference for sweets. Anthropologists believe that our ability to taste the difference between sweet and bitter plants may have helped early man survive. Sweet-tasting foods were usually safe to eat. Bitter-tasting foods were often poisonous.

Americans eat more than 23 teaspoons of added sugars each day, almost 400 sugar calories. For some people the amount is even higher. Teenagers eat the most sugar. Studies have shown, over and over, that as sugar intake goes up, vitamin and mineral intake goes down. We should all be eating less sugar, but there is no specific recommendation on how much to eat every day.

The U.S. Dietary Reference Intakes suggest 25% of daily calories from added sugar as the maximum. Obviously, people should eat less. The World Health Organization (WHO) has suggested limiting added sugars to no more than 10% of total calories, though some experts feel this amount is unrealistically low.

In both cases, the recommendations are for added sugar, not for sugars found naturally in fruits, milk, grains, and vegetables.

NATURAL SUGAR VS. ADDED SUGAR

Grains, fruits, vegetables, milk, and plain yogurt all contain sugars. These are *natural* sugars and they come along with the vitamins, minerals, and fiber also found in those foods. In contrast, soda, candy, fruit drinks, cakes, cookies, ice cream, jelly, and syrup offer little more than sweetness and calories. These foods are loaded with *added* sugar.

> ## You Should Know—
>
> *Beware Sugar In A Glass*
> *Research has shown that the calories in sugar-sweetened drinks—soda, fruit drinks, iced tea, energy drinks—do not provide the same satisfaction as calories from food.*
> *And, the more you are offered, the more you drink.*
> *Up to 20% of our daily calories come in liquid form.*

The way foods are currently labeled for sugar—lumping together natural sugar and added sugars—it can be hard to make the best choices.

For example, the nutrition label on a quart of milk tells you that one cup has 14 grams of sugar. The label on fruit punch tells you that one cup has 30 grams of sugar. But the difference in the kind of sugar is significant. All the sugar in milk comes from naturally occurring *lactose* or milk sugar, but almost all the sugar in the fruit punch is added.

How can you tell natural sugars from added sugars? Check the ingredient listing on food labels for the terms below—if any appear, it means sugar has been added to the food. Ingredients are listed in descending order by volume, so the closer sugar is to the beginning of the list, the more sugar is in each serving of food.

SUGAR BY ANY OTHER NAME

Beet juice	Honey
Brown rice syrup	Invert sugar
Brown sugar	Malt syrup
Cane syrup	Maltodextrin
Barley malt	Maple sugar
Corn sweetener	Maple syrup
Corn syrup	Molasses
Crystalline fructose	Muscavado
Dextrose	Raw sugar
Evaporated cane juice	Sorghum
Fruit juice concentrate	Sucrose
Fructose	Sugar in the raw
High fructose corn syrup (HFCS)	Turbinado

You Should Know—

Sorting Out Sugar On Labels
On the nutrition facts panel,
you will see a value for Total Carbohydrate
and right below a value for Sugars.
Sugar is part of the
total carbohydrate value.
If a food has 30 g (grams) of carb
and 28 g of sugar, it is high in sugar.

See also SUGAR pages 49–50.

Add a Little Fiber to Your Life (fiber)

96% of Americans eat too little fiber.

This is one carbohydrate all experts agree on; we need to eat more fiber. We average about 15 grams of fiber a day, far less than we should be eating. The following chart provides daily fiber recommendations. Check to see how much fiber you should be eating each day.

DAILY FIBER RECOMMENDATIONS

Men

19–50 years	*38 grams of fiber*
51 and older	*30 grams of fiber*

Women

19–50 years	*25 grams of fiber*
51–70 years	*21 grams of fiber*
71 and older	*20 grams of fiber*
Pregnant	*28 grams of fiber*

You Should Know—

Age + 5
Children 2 and older should eat
the amount of fiber daily that
equals their age + 5.
For a 5-year-old that would be
at least 10 grams of fiber a day.
(5 years + 5 = 10 grams)

Fiber is found only in plants, either as the woody part (that helps promote regularity) or as gums and mucilages, the sticky part (that helps lower cholesterol). Even though fiber is a carb, your body cannot break it down and use it the way it uses sugar and starch.

Living in your digestive track are trillions of friendly microbes (*probiotics*) that use fiber as their main source of food. These friendly bacteria have been with you since birth, and help protect you against unfriendly bacteria that might make you sick. When you eat enough fiber, your friendly bacteria are well fed and can put up a good fight against harmful bacteria. When you eat too little fiber, unfriendly bacteria can start to take over. Eating enough fiber stimulates your natural resistance against disease and helps to prevent infections.

Slowly start adding fiber-rich foods to your meals:

- Eat whole fruits and vegetables instead of drinking juices.
- Eat the fiber-rich skins of cucumbers, apples, pears, potatoes, and zucchini.
- Eat more berries—blueberries, blackberries, raspberries, strawberries.
- Choose whole grains—brown rice, cornmeal, barley, cracked wheat, rye, and whole wheat.
- Eat beans and lentils a few times a week.
- Eat whole grain or high fiber cereals like oatmeal, oat flakes, bran, and shredded wheat.
- Eat whole wheat bread, bagels, pasta, pretzels, crackers, and rolls.
- Try soybeans in every form—soynuts, tofu, tempeh, edamame.
- Snack on fiber-rich fig newtons, graham crackers, and popcorn.
- Have vegetarian meals a few times a week.
- Eat dried fruits and raisins.
- Sprinkle ground flaxseed, bran, or whole-grain granola onto cereal or yogurt for a healthy crunch.
- Experiment with higher fiber versions of old favorites, like brown rice instead of white, buckwheat noodles instead of spaghetti, or baked sweet potatoes instead of white potatoes.

- Try some of the new fiber-fortified foods, like high fiber cereal bars and breads.

FIBER-FORTIFIED FOODS

The easiest way to tell if extra fiber has been added to a food is to look at the ingredient list. In addition to natural sources of fiber, like whole wheat and oats, you may see inulin, fructan (also called *fructooligoosaccharides* or *FOS*), and methylcellulose listed.

Inulin is a natural fiber found in burdock root, dandelion root, chicory root, onions, leeks, garlic, bananas, asparagus, artichokes, and wheat. Most of the inulin you find added to foods is extracted from chicory or synthesized. Inulin is a *prebiotic*, a fiber that acts as a food for the good bacteria present in your intestines.

FOS is also a prebiotic and has many of the same benefits of inulin. It is considered a safe additive.

Methylcellulose is a synthetic fiber created by chemically altering cellulose (the cell wall of plants). It can be added to foods or used in fiber supplements as a bulking agent to prevent constipation.

See also FIBER page 34, PREBIOTICS page 46, and PROBIOTICS page 46.

Calcium Counts—Get Enough (calci)

Americans drink more soda than milk, the major source of calcium in our diets.

We've all heard that calcium builds strong bones and teeth, and protects us against *osteoporosis* (adult bone thinning), but it does much more than that.

Calcium:
- helps blood clot
- helps nerves work normally
- helps muscles work and the heart beat
- helps lower high blood pressure
- aids in weight loss
- helps prevent midlife weight gain in women
- relieves PMS (premenstrual syndrome)
- protects against complications in pregnancy
- lowers the risk for some cancers
- lowers the risk for periodontal disease, a leading cause of tooth loss
- protects against infertility
- reduces the risk for kidney stones
- may improve memory and mental performance

Calcium may even influence behavior. A study with rats showed that they became frantic on a low-calcium diet but calmed down when they were fed adequate amounts.

Over half of the calcium in the American diet comes from dairy products—milk, cheese, yogurt, and ice cream. A glass of nonfat milk provides more than one-third of your calcium for the day. Calcium-fortified soymilk is the best nondairy source. Other good nondairy sources are canned sardines and salmon with bones, oysters, clams, tofu, molasses, almonds, calcium-fortified foods (orange juice), beans, and dark green leafy vegetables (Chinese cabbage, kale, mustard, and turnip greens). As much as 25% of your daily calcium can come from mineral-rich bottled waters!

The Dietary Reference Intakes (DRIs) for calcium were updated in 2010. The daily requirement is:

Children 1 to 3	700 milligrams
Children 4 to 8	1,000 milligrams
Children 9 to 18	1,300 milligrams
Adults 19 to 50	1,000 milligrams
Men 51 to 70	1,000 milligrams
Women 51 to 70	1,200 milligrams
Adults 71+	1,200 milligrams

There is no additional need for calcium over and above the normal requirement during pregnancy and breastfeeding. Growing children between the ages of 9 and 18 need the most—1,300 milligrams—to help them form strong bones.

You Should Know—

The Winner Is?—Calcium
Depending on your size and weight, your body may contain up to 3 pounds, more than any other mineral.

You Should Know—

Calcium—Not for Women Only
Most women know they need to get enough calcium each day, but recent information shows that the average man over 40 does not get enough calcium daily.

NOT ALL CALCIUM IS CREATED EQUAL

Calcium rich foods can be divided into 3 groups. The groups depend on how efficiently your body absorbs the calcium found in these foods.

- **Excellent sources**—milk, firm tofu, dark green leafy vegetables, broccoli, and canned salmon and sardines with bones
- **Good sources**—ice cream, soft tofu, and light green leafy vegetables
- **Fair to poor sources**—cottage cheese, silken tofu, beans, almonds, and sesame seeds.

Keep in mind that even "poor sources" contribute some calcium to your overall intake and multiple servings add up.

Many people rely on calcium supplements but experts recommend food first, then a supplement to make up any shortfall. In supplements, calcium is always bound to another compound. Different combinations result in different amounts of actual calcium in the supplement. Calcium carbonate contains the largest amount of calcium, 40%. A 500-milligram tablet of calcium carbonate provides approximately 200 milligrams of actual calcium. The chart below will give you an idea of how much calcium is in each dose of the supplement you are taking.

Calcium Supplement	% Calcium
Calcium carbonate	40
Calcium phosphate (tribase)	38
Calcium phosphate (dibase)	31
Calcium citrate	21
Calcium lactate	13
Calcium gluconate	9

You Should Know—

Research has shown that women who get most of their calcium from food have healthier bones than those who rely mainly on calcium supplements. Women who eat good sources of calcium and take a supplement have the best bone density as they age.

See also CALCIUM page 27.

Lighten Up on Sodium (sod)

On average every person in the U.S. over the age of 2 eats 3,400 milligrams of sodium each day. Experts believe that this is too much.

What are the experts recommending?

- The American Heart Association recommends that people eat no more than 1,500 milligrams of sodium a day.
- The 2010 Dietary Guidelines for Americans recommends less than 2,300 milligrams a day and no more than 1,500 milligrams of sodium a day for people over age 51, African-Americans, and those with high blood pressure or kidney disease.
- The Dietary Reference Intakes from the National Academy of Sciences recommends that people eat no more than 2,300 milligrams a day.

Almost all Americans exceed the recommended upper limit of sodium intake (2,300 milligrams) every day. A study done by the Centers for Disease Control and Prevention (CDC) estimated that 69% of all adults belong to an at-risk group that would benefit from keeping their sodium intake down. Nearly 1 in 4 Americans have high blood pressure and middle-aged adults have a 90% chance of developing high blood pressure as they get older.

How are sodium and high blood pressure connected? The sodium in your body fluids causes your body to hold water. Your heart pumps harder to handle the extra fluid. Sodium also appears to stiffen arteries, making them less flexible. Blood pressure goes up as your body tries to pump blood through these less flexible vessels. When salt intake is lowered, the extra fluid is reduced and the arteries become less stiff, so your heart doesn't have to work so hard.

SALT SENSITIVE OR SALT RESISTANT

The sodium story is complicated because not everyone reacts to sodium the same way. Those who are salt sensitive experience high blood pressure when they eat too much sodium, increasing their risk for heart attack and stroke. If they reduce sodium their blood pressure goes down. But there is even more to the story. Those with high blood pressure who are salt sensitive and over 44 will see their blood pressure go down when they eat less salt. For those who are younger and salt sensitive with high blood pressure, they will see a modest but not remarkable drop in blood pressure when they eat less salt.

Salt has little effect on the blood pressure of salt resistant people.

Does that mean that those who are salt resistant can eat all the salt they want? Not really. A high salt intake contributes to kidney disease, may increase the risk for stomach cancer, and increases the risk for osteoporosis (adult bone thinning). Too much salt is simply not healthy.

Giving up salt isn't easy. Many experts believe that healthy adults could do nicely on as little as 500 milligrams of sodium a day. That may be healthy, but would we consider it tasty?

SALT OR SODIUM?

Table salt is actually a mixture of two minerals—sodium and chloride. A teaspoon of salt contains about 2,400 milligrams of sodium and the rest is chloride.

You Should Know—

¼ teaspoon salt = 582 milligrams sodium
½ teaspoon salt = 1,163 milligrams sodium
1 teaspoon salt = 2,325 milligrams sodium
Cutting the sodium in a recipe by half can make a big difference.

When people are told to eat less sodium, their first reaction is to empty the salt shaker and stop adding salt in cooking. Emptying the salt shaker will reduce only a fraction of the sodium most of us eat daily. Your daily sodium intake actually comes from:

- 65% from processed foods
- 25% from restaurant foods
- 10% from salt added in cooking and from the salt shaker

Cutting down on processed foods will make a bigger dent than dumping the salt shaker. What are processed foods? Prepared salad dressing, jarred tomato sauce, canned tuna, marinated fresh meat and poultry, cake mixes, pickles, pretzels, frozen dinners, desserts, canned soup, microwave meals, deli meats, and hot dogs—to name just a few.

We are a population that loves salty foods—in fact, we often reject foods with less sodium. Research has shown that, for some foods, consumers can taste a sodium reduction as small as 8%. When the consumer's traditional brand does not deliver the anticipated taste, the company can lose sales. For this reason, many companies choose to make "silent reductions" in sodium. They simply lower the sodium without touting the change in advertising campaigns. As consumers embrace the newer lower sodium foods, they may change their advertising approach.

It's not that easy to take the salt out of a recipe. Besides enhancing the taste of food, salt is a functional ingredient.
Salt:

- Keeps foods from spoiling by creating a hostile environment for microorganisms to grow. Salted meat and fish kept early humans from starving.
- Adds texture to foods. It strengthens the gluten (a protein) in bread dough, allowing it to rise without tearing and exploding.
- Provides fermentation control so that baked goods rise at a steady rate in the oven.
- Helps to make cheese and sauerkraut.
- Promotes the typical color that develops in ham, bacon, hot dogs, bologna, and sauerkraut.

Despite these challenges, many food companies and restaurant recipe developers are altering products to be lower in sodium.

All these initiatives are good. As the companies and restaurants lower the salt in products, our desire for very salty foods will shift and we will be more interested in eating lower sodium choices. Research has shown that even modest daily sodium reductions, as little as 400 milligrams, can produce health benefits.

TO LIGHTEN UP ON SALT

- Don't add salt to restaurant or take-out foods.
- Eat naturally low sodium foods, like fresh fruits and vegetables, or plain frozen vegetables to complement take-out or prepared entrees.
- Check the nutrition label. Keep snacks and single-serving foods under 400 milligrams a serving; keep main dishes under 600 milligrams a serving.
- Try some low sodium or "no salt added" choices. You might be pleasantly surprised at the taste.
- Fresh salads are naturally low in sodium; just go easy on the dressing, which can be high in sodium.
- Plain frozen vegetables are lower in sodium than sauced and seasoned varieties.
- Almost all frozen vegetables are lower in sodium than canned vegetables.
- Try baldy pretzels and unsalted nuts.
- Rinse canned beans, sauerkraut, vegetables, and tuna to reduce the sodium by almost half.
- Add salt at the table, not when cooking rice, pasta, or hot cereal. People tend to add less salt when eating and more when cooking.
- Use fresh pepper or herbs to flavor food instead of salt.
- When you eat a high salt/sodium choice, balance it with lower sodium choices later in the day.

See also BLOOD PRESSURE (BP) pages 26–27, HIGH BLOOD PRESSURE (HYPERTENSION) pages 38–39, SALT page 47, and SODIUM page 49.

Potassium Matters (potas)

It protects against the damage caused by too much sodium.

Too much sodium may cause high blood pressure. Adequate potassium lowers blood pressure, but it can do more. It may be able to revitalize arteries, big and small, making them more flexible and youthful. As we age, arteries become less elastic, which boosts blood pressure. Keeping vessels supple is key to keeping pressure low.

As the third most abundant mineral in your body, potassium is found inside the fluid of every cell. It's important for the firing of nerves and working of muscles. Potassium allows the heart muscle to relax—the opposite of calcium, which makes it contract.

Americans eat a good deal of processed foods and too few fruits and vegetables, so many fall short on potassium even though it is abundant.

FOODS HIGH IN POTASSIUM

Apricots	Melons
Avocados	Milk
Bananas	Molasses
Broccoli	Nuts
Carrots	Potatoes
Citrus fruits and juices	Raisins
Corn	Spinach
Dried fruits	Tomatoes and
Dried peas and	tomato products
beans	Whole grains
Green leafy vegetables	Yogurt

The Dietary Reference Intake (DRIs) for potassium has been set at 4,700 milligrams daily for adults. Most American eat between 2,000 and 3,000 milligrams of potassium a day. Simply eating more fruits and vegetables would boost our intake.

POTASSIUM—FOOD OR SUPPLEMENT?

If you take a diuretic to control high blood pressure, this type of medication removes water from your body. Along with the water, your body loses potassium. A supplement will help replace what is lost, but a better way to replace the lost potassium is taking your high blood pressure medication with orange juice, an excellent source of potassium. You might also drink a glass of tomato juice, eat a wedge of cantaloupe, or top your morning cereal with a banana, all great potassium sources.

When you replace lost potassium with a food source you not only get potassium but all the other vitamins and minerals in that food, along with fiber and important antioxidants. A potassium supplement is an isolated source of the mineral. It will replace the lost potassium but do little else. It is also easy to take very large amounts of potassium in supplement form, while this is far less likely when eaten in food. Too much potassium can effect kidney function and slow your heart rate.

See also HIGH BLOOD PRESSURE (HYPERTENSION) pages 38–39 and POTASSIUM page 46.

Folic Acid—Vital to Health (folic)

Scientists estimate that 10% of Americans are folate deficient. Others are not deficient but their normal intake is below the desirable level.

Based on this evidence, fortification of bread, cereal, pasta, flour, and rice was begun in 1998. Since the fortification program started, it's estimated that the average American is getting 200 micrograms more folic acid a day, but most are still falling short of their daily need.

The Dietary Reference Intakes (DRIs) for folic acid are:

Children 1 to 3	150 micrograms
Children 4 to 8	200 micrograms
Children 9 to 13	300 micrograms
Men and women 14 and older	400 micrograms
Pregnant	600 micrograms
Breastfeeding	500 micrograms

The UL (tolerable upper limit) for folic acid is set at 1,000 micrograms from fortified foods and supplements. It is hard to take in too much folate from natural food sources.

You Should Know—

Smoking and exposure to second-hand smoke reduce your body's levels of folic acid.

FOLATE OR FOLIC ACID

Both terms refer to the vitamin that is a member of the B vitamin family.

Folate refers to a group of naturally occurring folates found in food. Food sources include green leafy vegetables, orange juice, beans, liver, asparagus, broccoli, sunflower seeds, wheat germ, dried beans, and peanuts.

Folic acid is a more stable synthetic form of folate used in supplements and for food fortification. Fortified sources are enriched bread, pasta, flour, breakfast cereal, and rice. The folic acid used to fortify foods is slightly more absorbable than the form that naturally occurs in foods like spinach.

That doesn't mean you should rely only on fortified foods for your folic acid needs. The natural food sources are also rich in other important nutrients and phytochemical compounds that are needed by your body. Most experts recommend getting folic acid from a variety of sources, food in which it is naturally found, fortified foods, and supplements too, when needed.

WHY IS FOLIC ACID SO IMPORTANT?

Folic acid is important to the formation and maintenance of every cell in your body. The vitamin is involved in making the cell's genetic material. Folic acid also helps to make proteins and new red blood cells. Too little leads to anemia.

Because folic acid helps to make the genetic material of every cell, it's essential to support the healthy growth of an unborn child. Pregnant women who take in too little folic acid have a higher risk of miscarriage and birth defects involving the spinal cord and brain. These organs begin to develop very soon after conception, even before a woman is aware she is pregnant. That's why most experts recommend that women of childbearing age get adequate folic acid but, unfortunately, many still don't. Less than 30% of women reach the daily recommendation of 400 micrograms.

Research has also shown that men with low sperm counts and more fragile sperm have low intakes of folic acid. So when it comes to a healthy pregnancy, adequate folic acid levels are important for both parents.

Adequate folic acid may also offer protection against:

- The risk of heart disease.
- The risk of colon cancer.
- The natural decline in memory that occurs with age.
- Age-related, high-frequency hearing loss that is common as we get older.
- Bone loss in postmenopausal women.
- Having a baby with a cleft lip or a cleft palate.
- The risk of depression.

See also FOLIC ACID page 35 and TOLERABLE UPPER INTAKE LEVEL (UL) page 50.

Vitamin C Saves Cells (vit C)

One-quarter of the world's adults eat chili peppers every day. By weight, they are one of the richest food sources of vitamin C and help protect the heart.

Vitamin C plays a critical role in the formation of *collagen*, the connective tissue that holds together the structures of your body. Lack of vitamin C was the downfall of early ocean explorers. At sea for many months, with no fresh fruits and vegetables, sailors often developed, and died of, scurvy, a deficiency of vitamin C. They suffered from bleeding gums and aching joints because they were unable to make collagen.

Vitamin C is found in most of the tissues throughout your body, but especially in the heart, brain, pancreas, adrenal glands, thymus, lungs, pituitary gland, and lens of the eyes. The retina of the eye, which is part of the central nervous system, needs to be bathed in vitamin C to function correctly. This could have implications for glaucoma, which is caused by the dysfunction of nerve cells in the retina. A vitamin C–rich diet could be protective.

Vitamin C is a powerful antioxidant, helping to minimize free radicals which are renegade oxygen molecules that damage cells. In addition, vitamin C helps the body recycle vitamin E, another antioxidant, for reuse by the body. Iron from plant sources is normally poorly absorbed in the body, but in the presence of vitamin C absorption increases markedly.

The vitamin is found in mainly fruits and vegetables, but Americans eat far too few of them, so we may not be getting enough of this important vitamin daily.

The Dietary Reference Intakes (DRIs) for vitamin C are:

Men 19 and older	90 milligrams
Men who smoke	125 milligrams
Women 19 or older	75 milligrams
Women who smoke	110 milligrams
Pregnant	85 milligrams
Breastfeeding	120 milligrams

Smokers need more vitamin C because smoking produces damaging free radicals and vitamin C is used up when it helps to remove these dangerous substances. Vitamin C is also involved in the systems that break down and clear drugs from the body. Drug use will boost the need for vitamin C.

Vitamin C and the common cold have been linked for decades. The vitamin does help the immune system function properly, which in turn keeps you healthy. Though the evidence is inconclusive, some studies report a slightly lower incidence of colds in people who regularly get enough C. What is conclusive is that vitamin C can shorten a cold's duration and make the symptoms more tolerable. The vitamin has antihistamine properties like those found in common cold medications.

FOODS HIGH IN VITAMIN C

Acerola	Mango
Broccoli	Orange and
Cabbage	orange juice
Cantaloupe	Peppers
Cauliflower	Potatoes
Chili peppers	Strawberries
Grapefruit	Tomatoes
Green leafy	Vitamin C–fortified
vegetables	fruit juice
Kiwi	Watermelon

MEGADOSES OF C

Many people firmly believe that large amounts of vitamin C will keep them healthy. Research, however, has never proven this.

There are a few reasons why you may want to rethink taking large amounts of vitamin C daily. When you take in 100 milligrams of vitamin C, your body absorbs 80 to 90% of the vitamin. As vitamin C intake increases, absorption decreases, with most of the excess being excreted through the urine. So, when you take in very large amounts at one time, the total absorption can be as low as 20%. Some experts also believe that large amounts of vitamin C can reverse its normal protective antioxidant effect. Instead of protecting you from free radical damage, too much vitamin C may promote the formation of free radicals, the exact opposite of what you want.

You Should Know—

Too Much of a Good Thing
May Not Be Good
The best way to get enough vitamin C
each day is by eating fruits and vegetables.
It is hard to overdose on nutrients
by eating food, but it is easy to take
too much as a supplement.

Very large amounts of vitamin C—over 2,000 milligrams daily—may cause nosebleeds, abdominal cramps, and diarrhea. High levels of vitamin C can also cause a false-positive result when testing for diabetes. In people prone to kidney stones, high intakes can cause more stone formation. For people with *hemochromotosis*, a condition that causes excess accumulation of iron in the body, too much vitamin C, which enhances iron absorption, can be a problem. The UL (tolerable upper limit) for vitamin C has been set at 2,000 milligrams daily.

See also ANTIOXIDANTS page 26, TOLERABLE UPPER INTAKE LEVEL (UL) page 50, and VITAMIN C page 52.

UNDERSTANDING THE 2010 DIETARY GUIDELINES FOR AMERICANS

In a nutshell, the Dietary Guidelines:
Help you achieve and maintain a healthy weight
Reduce your risk for disease
and
Keep you healthy

Initiated in 1980 by the U.S. Department of Agriculture (USDA) and the Department of Health and Human Services (DHHS), the dietary guidelines are intended primarily for policymakers. They are designed to promote an optimal eating plan, to prevent diseases, and to set standards for federal programs like the National School Lunch Program. The guidelines allow all government agencies and policymakers to share a common approach when it comes to health and nutrition messages for Americans.

By law, every 5 years, the USDA and DHHS must appoint a committee of experts to review all new scientific information and revise the guidelines. The experts translate the most current scientific information into recommendations for Americans age 2 and older.

The 2010 Dietary Guidelines are the seventh and most complex revision ever released. They include 23 key recommendations and 6 recommendations for specific groups, such as pregnant women. This makes it difficult to distill the message into simple points.

> ### You Should Know—
>
> *Although the Dietary Guidelines for Americans are based on sound scientific information, few Americans are familiar with them. The federal government provided more than $500,000 to develop the 2010 guidelines, but no funding is budgeted to publicize the information to Americans.*

The two major themes of the 2010 Dietary Guidelines are:

1. Balance calories eaten with calories used to manage weight.

- Control total calories eaten each day to manage your weight.
- Enjoy eating but avoid oversized portions—you eat and drink more when served larger portions.

- Increase physical activity and make it part of your daily life; avoid being inactive.
- Those who are already overweight will need to improve eating habits and increase activity.
- Maintain your calorie balance throughout life, using the amount of calories you take in daily.

Weighing too much is the overriding health problem in the U.S. today and a major issue that the Dietary Guidelines needs to address.

2. *Focus on eating nutrient-rich foods.*

- Reduce daily sodium intake to less than 2,300 milligrams a day—eat less processed food, choose more fresh foods.
- Reduce daily sodium intake to less than 1,500 milligrams a day if you are older than 51, are African-American, or have hypertension, diabetes, or chronic kidney disease. This recommendation applies to almost half the U.S. population.
- Eat less solid fat—butter, stick margarine, coconut oil, shortening, and beef, pork, and chicken fat. No more than 10% of your daily calories should be from saturated fat.
- Use more monounsaturated (olive, canola, peanut and almond oil) and polyunsaturated fats (safflower, soybean, corn, sunflower and rapeseed oil). Use more liquid oils and less solid fat.
- Keep your total fat intake between 20% to 35% of your daily calories.
- Eat less than 300 milligrams of cholesterol daily—limit foods from animal sources.
- Eat as little trans fat as possible. Go easy on commercial baked foods (cookies, cakes, donuts, pastries and croissants), shortening, stick margarine, and deep-fried foods (French fries, fried chicken).

- Limit foods made with refined grains, like white bread, to less than 3 servings a day.
- Eat more whole grain choices, which are rich in fiber—make half of your grain choices each day whole grains. Aim for 14 grams of fiber for every 1,000 calories you eat.
- Eat fewer foods with added sugar—candy, soda, sweetened drinks, jelly, syrup, cakes, and cookies.
- Drink water or no-calorie drinks instead of sugary drinks. Soda, energy drinks, and sports drinks make up 36% of Americans added sugar intake while providing few important nutrients.
- Fill your plate half full with fruits and vegetables—eat a wide variety, including dark green, red, and orange choices. Aim for at least 2½ cups each day.
- Eat more beans and peas.
- Drink more fat-free or low fat milk. Use less whole milk. For those who do not drink milk, use calcium-fortified dairy substitutes.
- Use low fat or reduced fat yogurt and cheese.
- Vary your protein choices—eat seafood, lean meat, poultry, eggs, soy products, unsalted nuts and seeds, and peas and beans.
- Eat more fish—aim for 8 ounces weekly.
- Consume alcohol in moderation—1 drink a day for women and 2 drinks for men.

Americans typically are overfed but undernourished—heavy on calories but short on nutrients. The top four nutrients of concern for both adults and children are: potassium, calcium, vitamin D, and fiber.

> ## You Should Know—
>
> *Here are some expected and unexpected sources of:*
>
> *Potassium—Beet greens, orange juice, tomato juice, bananas, sweet potatoes, beans, strawberries, clams, lima beans, halibut, tuna, cod, milk, spinach, soybeans, potatoes, and dry beans*
>
> *Calcium—Milk, calcium processed firm tofu, milk substitutes with added calcium, chocolate milk, yogurt, cheese, sesame seeds, sardines, soybeans, spinach, canned salmon with bones, calcium-fortified orange juice, calcium-fortified breakfast cereals, and blackeyed peas*
>
> *Vitamin D—Salmon, tuna, sardines, herring, cod, beef liver, egg, milk, vitamin D-fortified soymilk, vitamin D-fortified orange juice, and mushrooms*
>
> *Fiber—Beans, bran, artichokes, pears, soybeans, green peas, berries, prunes, figs, apples, pumpkin, green leafy vegetables, bananas, oranges, cooked barley, broccoli, okra, popcorn, and whole grain breads, cereal and pasta*

The 2010 Dietary Guidelines recommendations for specific groups include:

For women who may become pregnant—

- Choose iron-rich foods—lean meat, poultry and seafood. The iron in these foods is more effectively absorbed than the iron in plant sources.
    Choose vitamin C-rich foods that aid in the absorption of iron.
    Eat plant-based sources of iron, too— spinach, white beans, lentils, and iron-fortified breads, cereals and pasta.

- Eat folic acid-fortified foods or take a supplement to ensure adequate intake of 400 micrograms daily.
    Eat foods rich in folate, too—beans and peas, oranges and orange juice, and dark green, leafy vegetables.

For women who are pregnant or breastfeeding—

- Take an iron supplement in addition to eating food sources rich in iron.
- Get 600 micrograms of folic acid daily by eating both natural and fortified food sources, as well as taking a folic acid supplement.
- Eat 8 to 12 ounces of seafood a week from a variety of sources.
    Limit white (albacore) tuna to no more than 6 ounces a week because of its mercury content.
    Do not eat tilefish, shark, swordfish, or king mackerel because of their mercury content.

For those over the age of 50—

- Eat vitamin B_{12}-fortified cereals or take a B_{12} supplement due to decreased absorption as we age.

Few people will be able to apply all of these recommendations to their daily lives. But every positive change you make will have a positive impact on your health.

The 2010 Dietary Guidelines report offered some general tips to help you achieve a healthy eating style.

- Focus on nutrient-dense foods.
- Remember that liquid calories count.
- Cook, or at least assemble, healthy meals.

- Enjoy food, but not too much of it.
- Nutrient needs are met over time, not at one meal or on one day. Make good food choices as often as possible.
- Set up an eating plan that is right for you. Consider your culture, traditions, and preferences, as well as food costs and availability.
- Keep the foods you eat safe.
  - Clean hands, counters, and fruits and vegetables before preparing food or eating.
  - Separate raw, cooked, and ready-to-eat foods when shopping, storing or preparing foods.
  - Cook foods to a safe temperature. Use a food thermometer.
  - Refrigerate foods promptly.
- Make use of information resources available.
  - www.health.gov
  - www.nutrition.gov
  - www.letsmove.gov
  - www.healthypeople.com
  - www.choosemyplate.com

Think of the Dietary Guidelines as just that, guidelines for living a healthier life, not an all-or-nothing rule book.

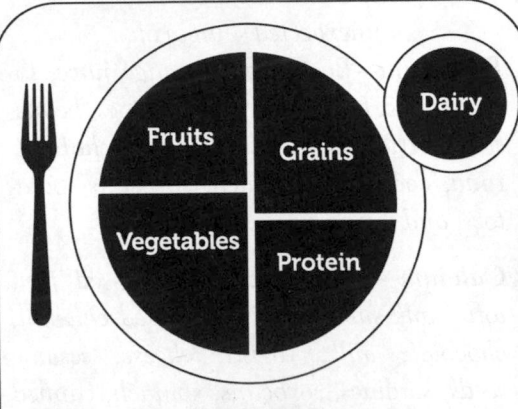

Dishing Up MyPlate

ChooseMyPlate.gov

MyPlate offers a quick visual guide to healthy eating based on the recommendation from the 2010 Dietary Guidelines. It helps you prioritize food choices when you choose your next meal. MyPlate replaces the MyPyramid food guide, which has served as the U.S. food group symbol for the last two decades. We have a long way to go before most dinner plates resemble MyPlate. It is estimated that only 2% of Americans meet the recommendations, which means that less than 7 days a year we eat a meal that resembles MyPlate.

JUST THE FACTS—A TO Z

Science is evolutionary not revolutionary. Information changes as research progresses.

A1C—The test that shows your blood glucose level over the past 2 to 3 months. Normal values are about 5% for people without diabetes. For those with diabetes treatment aims for a value below 7%.

ACADEMY OF NUTRITION AND DIETETICS—Formerly known as the American Dietetic Association, this organization changed its name in early 2012. It is the world's largest organization of food and nutrition professionals, with over 72,000 members. It serves the public by promoting nutrition and health messages. Members must meet minimum education requirements, which include a 4-year college degree. If they are registered dietitians (RDs), they are required to complete an internship, pass a national qualifying exam, and pursue continuing education to maintain their RD status. The Academy's Consumer Hotline (1-800-366-1655) offers food and nutrition information and nationwide referrals to registered dietitians (RDs) who offer nutrition counseling. See also DIETITIAN.

ADIPOSE TISSUE—This is fat tissue. It can accumulate anywhere in the body; too much can be harmful to your health. See also OBESITY.

AFLATOXINS—These are poisons produced by molds found in foods. They can cause cancer and birth defects. Grains and peanuts are most likely to be contaminated, but the USDA monitors these foods for aflatoxin to prevent health problems.

ALCOHOL—Ethyl alcohol (ethanol) is the type found in alcoholic beverages. Vodka, gin, rye, and scotch average 40% to 50% alcohol, wine 10% to 14%, and beer 2% to 4%. Some brands of flavoring (like vanilla), over-the-counter drugs, and herbal extracts also contain alcohol, which must be noted on the label. Excessive use of alcohol contributes to 3 leading causes of death: cirrhosis of the liver, accidents, and suicide. But moderate drinking (1 drink a day for women and 2 drinks a day for men) may have health benefits. One drink is defined as 12 ounces of beer, 5 ounces of wine, 1½ ounces of 80-proof liquor, and 1 ounce of 100-proof liquor. See also PROOF.

AMERICAN DIETETIC ASSOCIATION—See ACADEMY OF NUTRITION AND DIETETICS.

AMINO ACIDS—These are protein fragments that make up larger protein structures. Twenty amino acids are needed in your body. Some are *essential* and can only be supplied by the protein foods you eat, such as eggs, meat, and fish. Others are *nonessential* because they can be made in the body. See also PROTEINS.

ANABOLISM—The process by which simple substances and structures in your body are made into more complex substances and structures. It is also called *constructive metabolism* and is the opposite of *catabolism*. Catabolism plus anabolism equals *metabolism*, which is the process by which your body uses energy. See also CATABOLISM and METABOLISM.

ANOREXIA—A lack of appetite, which can be temporary or may last a long time. It may occur as the side effect of a disease, disease treatment, medication, pain, or a mental disorder. *Anorexia nervosa* is an eating disorder in which a person refuses to maintain a minimal normal weight and has a distorted body image. See also EATING DISORDERS.

ANTIOXIDANTS—Substances, somewhat like a police force, that protect healthy cells against harmful substances called *free radicals*, which damage cells. Free radicals are caused by smoking, air pollution, and sun exposure, and are the by-products of normal body functions. Antioxidants scoop up free radicals and prevent them from damaging cells which might otherwise lead to heart disease and cancer. Fruits, vegetables, nuts, and tea are rich sources. Antioxidant compounds found in foods are quite complex. Some work more efficiently in the body than others. For example, the antioxidant capacity (AOC) of grapes and kiwifruit is higher and works more efficiently in the body than the AOC of plums and blueberries.

APHRODISIACS—Named for Aphrodite, the Greek goddess of love and beauty, this is anything that arouses sexual desire. The list of foods that is thought to increase sex drive is long, including oysters (Casanova is reported to have eaten 50 a day), asparagus, avocados, bananas, figs, ginseng, yohimbe, pomegranates, wild yams, carrots, cucumbers, fertilized duck eggs, cacao beans, caviar, blueberries, and prairie oysters (the testicles of bulls and rams). In studies that measured blood flow to the penis and vagina, men appeared to be turned on by smelling lavender and pumpkin pie. Women were aroused by the scents of Good & Plenty candy and cucumber.

APPETITE—Your desire to eat at a given time. It can be affected by hunger, the taste of food, your social setting, environment, culture, and habits. Appetite can affect when you eat, what you eat, and how much you eat. See also HUNGER, SATIATION, and SATIETY.

AQUACULTURE—Growing salt water and fresh water fish or shellfish under controlled conditions for food. Species typically raised in fish farms include salmon, catfish, tilapia, and cod. If a fish is farm raised it must be stated on the label.

ARTIFICIAL SWEETENERS—See SUGAR SUBSTITUTES.

ATHEROSCLEROSIS—See CARDIOVASCULAR DISEASE.

B VITAMINS—See VITAMINS.

BARIATRICS—The field of medicine that treats obesity and the diseases associated with it.

BETA-CAROTENE—See CAROTENOIDS.

BINGE EATING—Previously called "compulsive eating," this condition is characterized by frequent episodes of eating very large amounts. The person feels a lack of control over their eating behavior. See also EATING DISORDERS.

BLOOD PRESSURE (BP)—This is the force that the blood places against the wall of the blood vessels every time your heart beats. It is measured with a *sphygmomanometer* (blood-pressure machine). The blood pressure during the contraction of the heart is called *systolic* pressure. The pressure when the heart relaxes between beats is the *diastolic* pressure. Blood pressure is reported as systolic over diastolic. A good blood pressure reading for an adult is 120/80 or lower. See also DASH DIET (DIETARY APPROACHES TO STOP HYPERTENSION), HIGH BLOOD PRESSURE, and SODIUM.

BLOOD SUGAR LEVEL (BSL)—The normal level of blood sugar (glucose) is 70 to 110 for adults; 80 to 115 for those over 60; and 60 to 90 for pregnant women. A *fasting blood sugar* is measured after a person has not eaten for 8 to 12 hours. A normal fasting blood sugar level is 100 or below.

BODY IMAGE—This is a person's mental image of their physical appearance. It is the result of many different influences which cause positive or negative feelings about one's body. Body image and self-esteem are closely linked.

BODY MASS INDEX (BMI)—BMI is used to estimate body fat. As BMI goes up, so does the risk for early death and serious illness. To determine your BMI:

1. Multiply your weight in pounds by 700.
2. Divide the result by your height in inches.
3. Divide the result by your height in inches again.

The National Institutes of Health (NIH) recommends that adults aim for a BMI below 25. A BMI of 18.5 to 24.9 is considered normal. A BMI of less than 18.5 is considered underweight. People with BMIs between 25 to 30 are considered overweight. A BMI over 30 is considered obese.

BULIMIA—See EATING DISORDERS.

CACHEXIA—Weakness, extreme weight loss, and severe loss of body tissues as the result of long-standing illness, chronic disease, malnutrition, or terminal illness.

CAFFEINE—This stimulant is found in coffee, tea, soda, cocoa, chocolate, and many over-the-counter medications. It is not addictive, but it is habit forming. Many people can't get going without their morning coffee or cola. Caffeine is absorbed quickly into the body, and its effects can be felt within 30 minutes. It stimulates your brain and heart, increasing work capacity, urination, and stomach acid secretion. For some people, caffeine disrupts sleep, and causes heartburn and stomach upset.

Food	Portion Size	Milligrams of Caffeine
Coffee	1 (8-ounce) cup	110 to 175
Coffee Decaf	1 (8-ounce) cup	3 to 4
Espresso	1 (3-ounce) cup	175
Tea	1 (8-ounce) cup	40 to 120
Iced tea	1 (16-ounce) bottle	10 to 45
Cola drinks	1 (12-ounce) can	40 to 70
Hot chocolate	1 (5-ounce) cup	2 to 20
Chocolate milk	1 (8-ounce) glass	2 to 7
Chocolate candy	1 ounce	1 to 35

You Should Know—

Energy drinks are a major source of caffeine. One can or 1 shot may contain anywhere from 50 to 400 milligrams. Labels rarely provide the caffeine content.

CALCIUM—The most abundant mineral in the body; 99% is found in the bones and teeth and 1% in the blood and tissues, where it helps with blood clotting, muscle contractions, and nerve impulses. See also NUTRITION BASICS pages 12 to 13.

CALORIES—The energy stored in food. Every time you eat, you take in calories. Proteins and carbohydrates have 4 calories per gram, fats have 9, and alcohol has 7. Your body is a machine that uses food calories as fuel. When the amount of fuel you use equals the amount of fuel you burn, your weight remains constant. Eat too many calories and your body uses what it needs and stores the rest. Cut calories and you lose weight. *Discretionary calories* are those calories left over each day, after a person has met his or her daily nutrient need. These calories can be used for any additional foods that a person wants to eat. Discretionary calories are often used on foods that add to the pleasure of eating but have few if any nutrients, such as: sugar, soda, salad dressing, candy, cake, and butter.

You Should Know—

The average woman eats 1,877 calories a day.
The average man eats 2,618 calories a day.

See also EMPTY CALORIES and NUTRITION BASICS pages 2 to 3.

CANCER—A disease that occurs when a cell has lost its normal control mechanisms and has unregulated growth. As cancer cells grow and multiply, they form a mass of cancerous cells that can invade surrounding tissues and spread (metastasize) around the body. See also CARCINOGEN.

CARBOHYDRATE LOADING—The increased amount of carbohydrates a person eats before a major exercise event that lasts continuously for at least 60 to 90 minutes. The extra carbohydrates helps to maximize the amount of *glycogen* (stored carbohydrates) in the muscles to provide extra fuel during exercise. Marathon runners may carb load.

CARBOHYDRATES—One of the major sources of energy (calories) found in food. Carbohydrates are classified by the amount of sugar units in their structure. *Simple* carbohydrates are made up of one or two sugar units. Examples are glucose and fructose, found in honey and fruits. *Complex* carbohydrates are made up of many sugar units and are found in foods with more starch and fiber. Starches can be broken down in your body to provide energy (calories). Fiber cannot be broken down in the body for energy but it does help to promote regularity and offers protection against some diseases. Carbohydrates are the primary source of energy for your brain and central nervous system. Good sources are: bread, pasta, cereal, rice, vegetables, beans, potatoes, milk, and yogurt. See also FIBER, SUGAR and NUTRITION BASICS page 8.

CARCINOGEN—A cancer-causing substance that changes a cell's genetic material. It can be a chemical, virus, radiation, or sunlight. Food often carries carcinogens into the body. See also CANCER.

CARDIOVASCULAR DISEASE (HEART DISEASE)—Diseases of the heart and the blood vessels. In the most common form of heart disease, *atherosclerosis*, arteries leading to the heart become progressively blocked by plaque, impairing blood flow and depriving the heart of oxygen and nutrients. High levels of cholesterol and fats in the blood contribute to this problem. Eating fewer foods high in cholesterol, saturated fat and trans fat, and more foods high in fiber, can help reduce the risk of heart disease.

CARNITINE—See VITAMIN-LIKE COMPOUNDS.

CAROB—It comes from the seedpods of a tree. It is also called St. John's bread and is used in place of chocolate. Candy and other sweet foods made of carob are often found in health food stores. Some think that carob is healthier than chocolate, but there is no evidence to back up this claim.

CAROTENOIDS—A group of pigments that give the deep yellow, orange, and red colors to fruits and vegetables. The major carotenoids are alpha-carotene, beta-carotene, lutein, zeazanthin, cryptoxanthin, and lycopene. Beta-carotene, found in cantaloupe, carrots, and squash, is the most common. The body can convert alpha-carotene and beta-carotene into vitamin A. Researchers think that those who regularly eat carotene-rich fruits and vegetables may be at lower risk for some eye diseases and cancers.

CATABOLISM—The process by which complex substances and structures in the body are broken down into simpler compounds. The breakdown results in the release of energy. It is the opposite of *anabolism*. Catabolism plus anabolism equals metabolism, the process by which your body uses energy. See also ANABOLISM and METABOLISM.

CDC (CENTERS FOR DISEASE CONTROL AND PREVENTION)—Part of U.S. Department of Health and Human Services (USDHHS) that develops techniques for nutritional assessment and whose mission it is to promote health and the quality of life by preventing and controlling disease, injury, and disability. See also USDHHS.

CELIAC DISEASE—A disease that damages the small intestine and interferes with the absorption of nutrients. People with celiac disease cannot tolerate *gluten*, a protein found in wheat, rye, and barley. They need to eat a gluten-free diet. Instead of wheat they can eat flour, bread, pasta, and crackers made of potato, rice, soy, or bean flour. It is estimated that 3 million Americans have celiac disease but only a fraction of those have been diagnosed. See also GLUTEN-FREE DIET.

CERTIFIED DIABETES EDUCATORS (CDEs)—People who specialize in diabetes and can help a person manage their condition. They are health professionals, such as nurses or dietitians, who have had special training in diabetes and have passed an exam given by the National Certification Board of Diabetes Educators.

CHOLESTEROL—A white, waxy, fatlike substance that is part of every cell in your body. Cholesterol insulates nerve cells and helps skin cells retain moisture. It makes up a major part of your brain, and is the main building block for vitamin D and essential hormones such as cortisone, estrogen, progesterone, and testosterone. Having too much cholesterol in your blood is unhealthy. The extra cholesterol can be deposited in your artery walls, narrowing them and interfering with normal blood flow. You take in cholesterol every time you eat animal foods—meat, poultry, fish, eggs, milk, yogurt, cheese, and butter. This type of cholesterol is called *dietary cholesterol*. There is no cholesterol in any food that grows in the ground—vegetables, fruits, nuts, seeds, cereals, and grains. *Serum cholesterol* is the type that travels in your bloodstream. It is a combination of dietary cholesterol and cholesterol that is made in your liver. In fact, most people make 3 times more cholesterol in their body than they eat in food. See also CHOLESTEROL VALUES, HDL (HIGH DENSITY LIPOPROTEINS), LDL (LOW DENSITY LIPOPROTEINS), and NUTRITION BASICS page 6 to 7.

CHOLESTEROL VALUES—Cholesterol values are measured in milligrams per deciliter (mg/dl), the number of milligrams (mg) of cholesterol in 1 deciliter (dl), or slightly less than ½ cup of blood. For example: 210 mg/dl. Your doctor may just give you the number 210 instead of the complete measurement. The National Cholesterol Education Program (NCEP) recommends that adults over age 20 be screened for cholesterol at least once every 5 years. Those with higher than normal readings should be checked more often. At a screening, you'll find out your total cholesterol and you may also find out your HDL cholesterol, LDL cholesterol, and a ratio. Total cholesterol is just that the total amount of cholesterol in a given volume of blood. Levels below 200 lower your risk of heart disease. Desirable levels of LDL cholesterol are less than 100. Levels of HDL cholesterol under 40 are considered too low. Having low LDL and high HDL cholesterol reduces your risk of developing plaques and lowers your risk of heart disease. Your "ratio" is determined by dividing HDL cholesterol into total cholesterol. For example, if your total cholesterol is 200 and your HDL cholesterol is 50, your ratio is 4:1. A ratio below 5:1 is good. The optimum is 3.5:1. See also CHOLESTEROL, HDL (HIGH DENSITY CHOLESTEROL), and LDL (LOW DENSITY CHOLESTEROL).

CHOLINE—See VITAMIN-LIKE COMPOUNDS.

CLA (CONJUGATED LINOLEIC ACID)—A polyunsaturated fatty acid (a building block of fat), found in beef and dairy foods. Research is showing that CLA may have anticancer properties and may help to lower blood cholesterol and triglyceride levels.

COOL—The abbreviation for the mandatory USDA Country-Of-Origin food *Labeling* program, which tells consumers where their food was grown. All fresh and frozen fruits and vegetables, beef, veal, lamb, chicken, goat, pork, wild and farm-raised fish and shellfish, peanuts, pecans, ginseng, and macadamia nuts are officially COOL. Look on the product label or small tag affixed to fresh fruits and vegetables.

CONSTIPATION—The difficult or infrequent passage of stools. Poor nutrition, lack of exercise, and a low fluid intake can all contribute to the problem. Eating well, and including more fiber and adequate fluids, will make stools bulkier and easier to pass. People mistakenly believe that they need to have a bowel movement every day. Three bowel movements or more a week is considered normal.

C-REACTIVE PROTEIN (CRP)—This protein is released in the body in response to injury, infection, or inflammation. The higher the levels of CRP, the greater the risk for a heart attack. Elevated CRP levels are found in those who smoke and are overweight; lower levels are found in those who are physically active.

CRUCIFEROUS VEGETABLES—A group of vegetables with a four-petal flower that resembles a cross or *crucifer*. Broccoli is probably the most well known cruciferous vegetable. It forms a head while growing, as do Brussels sprouts, rapini, green cabbage, cauliflower, parsnips, bok choy, and white turnips, all part of the group. Headless crucifers include dark green leafy vegetables, such as kale and collard greens. These vegetables are not only good sources of vitamin C and other important vitamins and minerals, but they possess powerful anticancer agents.

DASH DIET (DIETARY APPROACHES TO STOP HYPERTENSION)—The DASH eating plan helps to lower high blood pressure by focusing on plant foods instead of animal foods. It is an eating plan low in total fat, saturated fat, and cholesterol, but rich in fruits, vegetables, and low fat dairy products. Combining the DASH diet with low sodium eating can lower blood pressure even more. See also HIGH BLOOD PRESSURE and SODIUM.

DAILY VALUES (DVs)—% Daily Values are used on food labels to help the consumer compare the amount of a nutrient in a serving of food to the amount of that nutrient needed each day. If the %DV for calcium on the nutrition label is 20%, one serving of food contains 20% of the calcium needed by an adult daily. DVs are based on a 2,000 calorie diet; many people eat less and some more. DVs can only be considered as an estimate but they do help a person determine if a food is rich in a certain nutrient or high in something, like cholesterol, that they may wish to limit. Some nutrients—trans fat, sugar, and protein—do not have DVs because there isn't enough information available to set a recommendation.

DEHYDRATION—This word has two meanings: the removal of water from food, such as drying fruit, or the loss of water from the body. When you are mildly dehydrated (3% weight loss), you will experience impaired physical performance and decreased blood volume. At 5% weight loss, you will experience nausea and difficulty concentrating. At 8% weight loss, you will experience dizziness and increased weakness, and have trouble maintaining your body temperature. Weight loss of 10% or greater can be life threatening. It is easy to become mildly or moderately dehydrated after vigorous physical exercise, especially in hot weather. That is one reason why competitive athletes are weighed before and after competitions.

DIABETES—A chronic disease that results in insulin deficiency or insulin resistance, which upsets the body's ability to use the energy (calories) found in foods. Over 24 million Americans have diabetes, but as many as 6 million have not been diagnosed. There are 3 types of diabetes: *type 1*, *type 2*, and *gestational diabetes* (diabetes during pregnancy). Type 1, which accounts for 5% to 10% of all cases, can occur at any age but is most often diagnosed in people under the age of 30. Lifestyle changes, insulin replacement, and diet are the usual ways to handle this condition. Type 2 is the most common form of diabetes. Your risk for this condition goes up if there is a family history, you are overweight, and you do little or no exercise. In the past, it occurred more frequently in older adults. Today, as more and more people gain weight, type 2 diabetes is occurring in all age groups, even children. Lifestyle changes, including weight loss and diet, are the usual ways to handle this condition. Gestational diabetes develops during pregnancy. Although the condition usually disappears at the end of the pregnancy, 20% to 50% of women with gestational diabetes are at risk for type 2 diabetes 5 to 10 years later. The condition is usually managed during pregnancy by diet and, when necessary, insulin therapy. See also CERTIFIED DIABETES EDUCATORS and INSULIN.

DIARRHEA—The passage of frequent, loose, watery stools. Diarrhea can be caused by infections, drugs, stress, and serious medical conditions. High doses of vitamin C, drinking too much apple juice, or eating large amounts of sugar-free candy, cookies or gum sweetened with sorbitol or mannitol can cause diarrhea. It was once believed that eating nothing was the way to stop diarrhea, but the current thinking is to eat anything you'd like except fatty foods. Apples, bananas, rice, cottage cheese, dry toast, crackers, pretzels, and tea, in addition to plain water, are all good choices. Most cases of diarrhea last only a day or two. If diarrhea lasts for more than 2 days, see your doctor.

DIET—The usual foods and drinks a person eats. An *adequate diet* meets all the nutrition requirements for an individual. A *therapeutic diet* is a selection of foods and drinks that will help prevent or treat a condition. Many think of diet as a way to control calories and weight but in actuality that is a *weight control diet*, which can be used to either gain or lose weight.

DIETARY GUIDELINES FOR AMERICANS—The federal government's health and nutrition messages for Americans. By law, the guidelines must be reviewed and revised every 5 years. The seventh edition was released in 2010. Following the guidelines will help reduce your risk for obesity and chronic disease. See also UNDERSTANDING THE 2010 DIETARY GUIDELINES FOR AMERICANS, page 21 to 24.

DIETARY REFERENCE INTAKES (DRIS)—See RECOMMENDED DIETARY ALLOWANCES (RDAS).

DIETARY SUPPLEMENTS—Any substance that is taken to enhance a regular diet in hopes of improving health. A supplement may be in the form of a pill (a vitamin pill), powder (added fiber), a drink (energy drinks), or an herbal supplement. Many dietary supplements are beneficial; others have no scientifically proven value.

DIETITIAN—A person who specializes in the study of food and nutrition as it relates to health. The credential RD stands for registered dietitian, which means that the person has passed a national qualifying exam assuring proficiency in the field. In order to maintain this credential, the person must participate in continuing education so that his or her knowledge remains current. See also ACADEMY OF NUTRITION AND DIETETICS.

DIGESTION—The process of breaking down the foods you eat into nutrients. Food enters your body through the mouth. The stomach churns it like a blender so that it can be broken down further and absorbed in the small intestines. The absorbed nutrients are used to run and maintain your body. The large intestine recycles minerals and water and excretes wastes.

DISORDERED EATING—Any change in a person's normal eating pattern. It can be caused by illness, stress, or an abnormal desire to improve one's appearance. If it persists it can lead to an eating disorder. See also EATING DISORDERS.

DNA (DEOXYRIBONUCLEIC ACID)—The main carrier of genetic information in your body.

DOUBLE-BLIND EXPERIMENT—In this type of study, neither the subjects nor the researchers know which subjects are being given the real treatment and which are receiving a *placebo*. This helps to keeps researchers from reaching a biased conclusion before all the information is collected. See also PLACEBO.

DYSPEPSIA—Also called *indigestion*, this is an uncomfortable feeling of fullness and bloating after eating.

DYSPHAGIA—Difficulty swallowing. It can occur for a number of reasons, such as inflammation, surgery of the throat, or a stroke. Without the ability to swallow, it is difficult to get adequate nutrition.

EATING DISORDERS—These include a wide range of abnormal eating patterns that can endanger health. Three of the main categories are: *anorexia nervosa*, refusing to maintain a minimal normal weight; *bulimia nervosa*, eating in binges and then purging; and *bulimia*, bingeing without purging. Bingeing is the rapid consumption of food in a short period of time where the person feels out of control. Purging is the use of vomiting, laxatives, diuretics, or enemas to rid the body of food. People with anorexia have a distorted body image and restrict their food intake to the point where they suffer severe weight loss. They may also exercise compulsively and use laxatives. They are desperately afraid of gaining weight. Untreated, the condition can result in malnutrition, sterility, damage to vital organs, and even death. People with bulimia nervosa repeatedly and compulsively eat large amounts of food and then may use laxatives, diet pills, or excessive exercise to control their weight. Often their weight is normal or even above normal, making it harder to detect the problem. Binge eating disorder or bulimia without purging is simply the excessive intake of large amounts of food. It usually occurs in people who are overweight or obese and can make the problem become progressively worse. The more they eat, the heavier they become. The heavier they become, the more they binge.

EDEMA—Also called *fluid retention*, it is the buildup of fluid between cells caused by a disruption in the body's normal ability to control fluid. Pregnant women may experience edema of the ankles and feet late in pregnancy.

EDIBLE FLOWERS—Many flowers can be safely eaten, including squash blossoms, roses, pansies, nasturtium, daylilies, sesbania (*see* page 556), marigolds, hibiscus (*see* pages 355–356), sunflowers, tulips, lavender, violets, and jasmine. Broccoli, cauliflower, capers, and saffron are actually edible flowers. Other flowers, such as lilies of the valley, sweet peas,

foxglove, and delphinium, are not edible. Do not eat flowers from florists, nurseries, or garden centers, as these have not been grown as food crops and may contain unsafe amounts of pesticides, manure, or other chemicals.

EMPTY CALORIES—Foods that contain mainly calories and few if any nutrients. Examples are: soda, sugars, syrups, jelly, lard, and shortening. See also CALORIES.

You Should Know—

Trying to Lose Weight?
Cut back on liquid calories. Sweetened drinks—empty calories—make up 20% of our daily calorie intake or close to 300 calories a day.

ENERGY—During the process of digestion and absorption, energy is released from the food you eat and either used or stored by the body. The amount of energy in food is measured in calories. When a person is in energy balance, the amount of energy (calories) eaten equals the amount of energy used. See also CALORIES.

ENZYMES—Substances made in the body that speed up chemical reactions. They help to break down, build up, or change one substance into another. Many enzymes are proteins, while others have a vitamin or mineral attached to the protein. The names of enzymes often begin with the name of the substance they act on and end in *ase*. An example is *lactase*, which breaks down the milk sugar, *lactose*.

EPIDEMIOLOGICAL STUDY—A study that investigates the incidence and distribution of disease in human populations and tries to determine what factors cause the disease.

EXERCISE—See PHYSICAL ACTIVITY.

FASTING BLOOD SUGAR—See BLOOD SUGAR LEVELS.

FAT REPLACERS—Compounds that mimic the taste and functional properties of fat but have fewer calories. Some are made from carbohydrate (Oatrim). Others are proteins that are modified to become thick and smooth, holding water and incorporating air into foods to dilute calories. The last group are based on fats that are not totally digested (Olean). These fat replacers can withstand heat and have most of the functional capabilities of fat for cooking. Few people object to the carb- or protein-based fat replacers but those based in fat are more controversial. Some people suffer diarrhea, gas, and cramping after eating these.

FATS (LIPIDS)—One of the major sources of energy (calories) for your body. Fats provide double the amount of calories (9 calories per gram) as the same amounts of protein or carbohydrate (4 calories per gram). Fats are made up of chains of *fatty acids*. There are 3 types of fatty acids: *saturated, polyunsaturated,* and *monounsaturated*. All food fats are a combination of the different types, but we classify the foods by the dominant fatty acids. Meat, whole milk, cheese, and butter are high in saturated fats. Nuts, vegetables oils, and fish are high in polyunsaturated fats. Olives, olive oil, canola oil, and peanut oil are high in monounsaturated fats. Too much saturated fat puts you at greater risk for heart disease. Too much of any fat may contribute to weight gain. But, some fat is necessary for your body to function. Fat provides energy, carries fat-soluble vitamins into your body, protects and cushions your vital organs, helps to keep you body temperature regulated, and lubricates your tissues. See also CLA (CONJUGATED LINOLEIC ACID), OMEGA-3 FATS, OMEGA-6 FATS, TRANS FAT, VISCERAL FAT, and NUTRITION BASICS pages 3 to 5.

FDA (FOOD AND DRUG ADMINISTRATION)—A federal agency within the U.S. Department of Health and Human Services (USDHHS). The FDA is responsible for nutrition labeling, and the approval and regulation of food additives and drugs. The FDA protects Americans from unsafe or unsanitary foods by watching for fraud, conducting inspections, analyzing food samples, and testing for toxicity, chemical contamination, and pesticide residues. The agency also prevents the transmission of contagious disease by regulating the movement of foods across state lines. See also USDHHS and NUTRITION LABELING.

FETAL ALCOHOL SYNDROME—A set of physical and mental problems seen in infants born to women who drank alcohol during pregnancy. Depending on the time and amount of alcohol consumed, the problems can be moderate to severe. Affected infants can have low birth weight, poor growth, mental retardation, coordination problems, and face, heart, and eye malformations. Small amounts of alcohol can cause problems, for this reason most experts caution pregnant women not to drink.

FIBER—A type of carbohydrate that cannot be broken down in your body for energy (calories). Fiber prevents and relieves constipation, protects against certain cancers, reduces cholesterol, aids in weight control, helps to control diabetes and may even lower the risk for heart disease. See also CARBOHYDRATES and NUTRITION BASICS pages 10 to 11.

You Should Know—

High fiber foods have 5 or more grams of fiber in a serving. A good source of fiber has 2 or more grams of fiber in a serving.

FLOWERS—See EDIBLE FLOWERS.

FOLIC ACID—A B vitamin that is named for its best natural source, green leafy vegetables (*foliage*). The term *folate* refers to a group of closely related substances. The folic acid form is the one used in vitamin supplements and to fortify foods. To make up for Americans and Canadians not getting enough folic acid, in 1998, folic acid supplementation of enriched flour and enriched grain products became mandatory. Too little folate is associated with birth defects. Fortification has helped to reduce this incidence. See also NUTRITION BASICS pages 17 to 18.

FOOD—Anything taken into the body that nourishes, builds or repairs tissues, supplies energy, or helps regulate body processes. Emotional, cultural, social, and religious factors affect what different groups define as acceptable foods to eat.

FOOD ADDITIVE—Any substance added to food during production, processing, storage, or packaging. Additives are regulated to ensure that they are safe to eat.

FOOD ALLERGY & ANAPHYLAXIS NETWORK—A nonprofit group whose main goal is to increase public awareness of food allergies and anaphylaxis, a life-threatening allergic reaction.

FOOD ALLERGY LABELING—In compliance with the Food Allergen Labeling and Consumer Protection Act, all foods with a label sold in the U.S., even imported products, must inform you if the food contains one of the following major food allergens:

- Milk
- Egg
- Fish
- Shellfish—refers only to crab, lobster, or shrimp, which must be declared on the label.

Oysters, clams, mussels, and scallops are not included.
- Tree nuts—the specific type of nut must be declared on the label.
- Wheat
- Peanuts
- Soybeans—soy or soya are acceptable alternative terms for soy-containing ingredients.

These 8 foods account for 90% of all food allergies. A "Contains" statement is required on the label immediately after or next to the ingredient listing. For example: Contains milk, eggs, peanuts. or Contains shrimp.

FOOD FAD—An idea associated with food or a way of eating, which becomes popular for a short time, though it may or may not stand up to scrutiny. A fad is often an exaggerated truth that promises a special result. Many weight loss diets are based on fads.

FOOD IRRADIATION—The treatment of food with a carefully controlled amount of gamma rays, X-rays, or ionizing radiation. This process enhances food quality and safety by reducing spoilage and slowing down ripening. The FDA requires that irradiated foods be specially labeled. These foods are safe to eat and their nutritional value is the same as those that have not been irradiated. See also FDA.

FOOD INSECURITY—The ongoing worry that a person is unable to secure adequate and safe food to eat.

You Should Know—

The U.S. produces enough food to provide every person with 3,900 calories a day. Few of us need anywhere close to that amount daily.

FOOD SECURITY—Access to enough safe food to ensure an active, healthy life.

FOOD LABELS—Required by the Nutrition Labeling and Education Act (NLEA), these labels must provide: a statement of identity for the food; net contents by weight, volume, or measure for the package; name and address of the manufacturer, packager, or distributor; a list of ingredients; and a nutrition facts panel. Canadian labeling requirements are similar to those in the U.S. See also NUTRITION LABELING.

FOOD POISONING—See FOODBORNE DISEASE.

FOODBORNE DISEASE—Many things can contaminate food—bacteria, mold, viruses, and chemicals—resulting in illness for anyone who eats the food. Examples of common foodborne organisms are *salmonella*, *E. coli*, and *campylobacter*.

FORTIFIED—This term refers to the addition of vitamins and minerals to foods. The nutrients were not in the food originally or the nutrients may have been removed or reduced through processing. Apple juice may be fortified with vitamin C. Wheat flour is fortified with folic acid. Table salt is fortified with iodine.

FREE RADICALS—See ANTIOXIDANTS.

FUNCTIONAL FOODS—This term refers to any food or food ingredient that has been modified to provide health benefits beyond the basic nutrients found in a food. Other terms for this category of foods are *designer foods*, *nutraceuticals*, and *pharmafoods*. Some examples of functional foods are calcium-fortified orange juice, energy drinks, and cholesterol-lowering margarine.

GAS (FLATULENCE)—We all produce gas, some more, some less. If you are lucky and expel it as soon as it is produced, you will not experience bloating and discomfort as gas builds up in your intestine. Everyone swallows some air as they eat or drink. Mouth breathers swallow more. Eating slowly with a closed mouth and drinking through a straw can reduce the amount of air swallowed. Chewing gum and drinking carbonated soda or water increases gas. Some swallowed air is expelled by burping. Bacteria in the intestines also ferment undigested food, producing gas. This gas is expelled through the rectum. Beans have a well-deserved reputation as gas producers. Other foods—onions, celery, applesauce, bagels, broccoli, cabbage, bananas, pretzels, cucumbers, or prune juice—cause gas in some people and none in others. If you suffer from uncomfortable gas or belching, keep a record of the foods you ate before a gassy episode to help you figure out which foods cause discomfort.

GASTRIC BYPASS—A procedure designed to divert the normal food intake through the intestines as a way to control weight. The surgery literally *bypasses* part of the digestive tract that would normally absorb nutrients and calories.

GENERALLY RECOGNIZED AS SAFE (GRAS)—A list of food additives that the FDA considers safe and that can be added to food without establishing their safety through experimental studies. Salt, sugar, spices, and vitamins are examples of GRAS substances. A food company can petition the FDA to add new food additives to the GRAS list.

GENETICALLY MODIFIED (GM) FOODS—Foods that have been modified using gene technology to achieve a desired characteristic. A GM tomato can be modified to produce its own pesticide. Cheese can be started with a GM organism that allows it to be kosher (traditional cheese starters come from animal sources). There is a good deal of controversy about the safety of GM food for humans and for the environment. Currently GM foods do not have to be labeled, and a good deal of U.S. produced corn and soy has been genetically modified. It is estimated that 70% of all foods in the supermarket have at least one GM ingredient. GM ingredients are not allowed in organic products.

You Should Know—

Genetically modified foods currently on the market include:

Soy and soy products	*Sugar beets*
Corn and corn products	*(table sugar)*
Canola oil	*Radicchio*
Alfalfa	*Flax*
Tomatoes	*Papaya*
Potatoes	*Squash*
Rice	*Wheat*
Cantaloupe	

GESTATIONAL DIABETES—See DIABETES.

GI TRACT (GASTROINTESTINAL TRACT)—The passageway that food takes through your body. It is like an enormous tunnel beginning at the mouth and ending at the rectum. With all the twists and turns, the average GI tract is 7 times a person's height. It is made up of the mouth, esophagus, stomach, small intestine, large intestine, and rectum. Food must be broken down and absorbed from the GI tract before it can be used by the body.

GLUTEN-FREE DIET—This is a diet that excludes wheat, barley, and rye and food made from these grains because they all contain the protein gluten. Celiac disease is the classic condition that is treated with a gluten-free diet. Experts now believe that there are other conditions that might benefit from not eating gluten, including wheat allergy, dermatitis herpetiformis (celiac disease of the skin), gluten ataxia (effects the brain), and nonceliac gluten senstivity, a condition which seems to be on the rise.

Grains with Gluten	Gluten FREE Grains
Wheat including spelt,	Amaranth
kamut, farro, durum,	Buckwheat
semolina, and bulgur	Corn
Barley	Millet
Rye	Quinoa
Triticale	Rice
Oats*	Sorghum
	Teff
	Wild Rice

*Oats are gluten-free but some gluten-sensitive people may react to them; follow your doctor's advice.

See also CELIAC DISEASE.

GLYCEMIC INDEX—This index ranks food by how quickly it can be converted into glucose and enter the bloodstream. Foods with a high glycemic index—rice, white bread, potatoes—raise blood sugar levels quickly. Foods with a low glycemic index—beans, whole grains, meat, fat—raise blood sugar levels more slowly, either because they are high in fiber that can't be broken down, or because they don't contain any carbohydrates. The theory behind the glycemic index is correct. Some foods do raise blood sugar quickly; others do not. In practice, it's not that simple. The glycemic index considers foods as if they were eaten one at a time. Straight glucose was given a rating of 100 and individual foods were measured against it. White bread has a very high glycemic index. But if you add peanut butter, the glycemic response is lowered because peanut butter, a high fat food, has a low glycemic index. It gets even more complicated. Ripe fruits have a lower glycemic index than unripe fruits. Cooking pasta al dente is fine; overcook it, and its glycemic value goes up. Even sugars vary. Glucose is high on the index, but fructose (fruit sugar) is low. Bottom line: Research into the health effects of the glycemic index is still evolving. Still, eating more foods with a low glycemic index may lower the risk for heart disease and help to control diabetes.

GRAM (G)—This is a standard unit of weight in the metric system. Protein, fat, carbohydrate, fiber, and sugar are measured in grams on food labels. Vitamins and minerals may be measured in milligrams (mg), 1/1,000th of a gram, or in micrograms (mcg), 1/1,000,000th of a gram. A *kilogram* (kg) equals 1,000 grams and is the unit used to measure body weight. One kilogram equals 2.2 pounds.

HEALTH—A state of physical, mental, and emotional well-being. Keys to good health are: eating a balanced and adequate diet, exercising regularly, having a positive outlook on life, drinking moderate amounts of alcohol, drinking adequate water, getting enough sleep, avoiding stress, using minimal medication, and not smoking or using illicit drugs.

HEALTH CLAIMS—A statement on the food label that one or more dietary components in that food can reduce the risk for disease. For example, the package for yogurt, high in calcium, can say: Adequate calcium may reduce the risk for osteoporosis (adult bone thinning). All health claims must be supported by valid scientific evidence. Health claims are monitored and approved by the FDA.

HEART DISEASE—See CARDIOVASCULAR DISEASE.

HEARTBURN—This condition is also known as *acid indigestion* or *gastroesophageal reflux*, a burning sensation felt in the throat or chest near the heart. It has nothing to do with the heart, but the burning sensation can be so strong that it can be mistaken for a heart attack. Heartburn is caused by the back-splashing of food and acid from the stomach onto the delicate tissues of the *esophagus* (connection between the stomach and throat). Overeating, drinking alcohol, smoking, eating fatty or spicy foods, and lying down after eating all increase your risk for heartburn. If heartburn is persistent, it can damage the esophagus.

HEMOCHROMATOSIS—An inherited condition whereby excessive amounts of iron are absorbed and stored in the body. Men are at greater risk for the condition because women naturally lose iron through menstruation and pregnancy.

HDL (HIGH DENSITY LIPOPROTEINS)—About ⅓ of the blood's cholesterol is carried by HDL. Experts believe that HDL cholesterol carries cholesterol away from arteries and back to the liver, where it is broken down and removed from the body. Because this may slow down the growth of plaque (blockage), HDL is referred to as *good* cholesterol. Levels under 40 are considered too low. See also CHOLESTEROL, LDL (LOW DENSITY LIPOPROTEINS), and LIPOPROTEIN.

HIGH BLOOD PRESSURE (HYPERTENSION)—The main symptom of this condition is continued elevation of blood pressure above normal. This means that *systolic blood pres-*

sure (the top number) is 140 or higher and the *diastolic blood pressure* (the bottom number) is 90 or higher. High blood pressure affects 1 in every 4 Americans. Doctors are on the lookout for adults with *prehypertension*, a condition in which blood pressure is mildly elevated, between 120/80 and 139/89. These people are at greater risk for developing high blood pressure in the future. Blood pressure can increase with higher salt intake, alcohol use, smoking, stress, overweight, and lack of exercise. Blood pressure goes down with adequate intakes of potassium, calcium, and magnesium. Losing weight, exercising, and eating well also help to control blood pressure. See also BLOOD PRESSURE, DASH DIET (DIETARY APPROACHES TO STOP HYPERTENSION), and SODIUM.

HIGH FRUCTOSE CORN SYRUP (HFCS)—A sweetener made by converting cornstarch to syrup. It is widely used in foods and beverages. It is simply another from of sugar and is on the GRAS list.

You Should Know—

Many are concerned that HFCS causes more weight gain than other sugars. Research has not proven this is true. Excess sugar calories, from any source, creates weight gain, not specifically HFCS.

See also GENERALLY RECOGNIZED AS SAFE (GRAS).

HOMOCYSTEINE—Elevated levels of this amino acid increase your risk for heart attack and stroke. Blood levels between 6 and 12 are considered normal. Moderate risk is 12 to 30; high risk over 30. Levels below 7 are associated with the lowest risk for heart disease. Homocysteine levels can be reduced by getting adequate amounts of folic acid (a B vitamin), B_6, and B_{12}. Fruits and vegetables, especially green leafy vegetables, are rich in folic acid, as are bread, cereal, and pasta that have been enriched with the vitamin. See also AMINO ACIDS, CARDIOVASCULAR DISEASE, and FOLIC ACID.

HUMAN GENOME PROJECT—An international effort spearheaded by the U.S. National Institutes of Health (NIH) to provide scientists with clues to the genetic variations that are responsible for common illnesses. Understanding the genetics of disease risk will allow researchers to develop treatments and medications that will help people at risk. As this knowledge unfolds, it will have a dramatic impact on how nutrition professionals approach their work. Knowing someone's genotype can allow them to put in place diet and lifestyle changes that can prevent the development of nutrition-related disorders. See also NUTRITIONAL GENOMICS.

HUNGER—The sensation that the body needs food, which reflects your body's drive to fulfill its need for energy and nutrients. Hunger affects when you eat and how much you eat. See also APPETITE, SATIATION, and SATIETY.

HYDROGENATION—A process by which hydrogen atoms are added to a liquid fat to make it solid at room temperature. On food labels you may see this as *hydrogenated vegetable oil* or *partially hydrogenated vegetable oil*. Hydrogenated fats are more stable for deep-frying and work every well in baked goods. But, hydrogenation creates a type of fat, called *trans fat*, that is considered unhealthy. See also TRANS FAT.

HYPER—A prefix meaning above normal or an excess.

- **Hypercholesterolemia**—higher than normal levels of cholesterol in the blood

- **Hyperglycemia**—higher than normal levels of blood sugar
- **Hyperkalemia**—higher than normal levels of potassium
- **Hyperlipidemia**—higher than normal levels of one or more fats in the blood, such as cholesterol or triglycerides
- **Hypertension**—refers to repeated blood pressure readings above 140/90
- **Hypetriglyceridemia**—higher than normal levels of triglyercerides in the blood
- **Hypervitaminosis**—excessive intakes of one or more vitamins at levels that may cause health problems

HYPERTENSION—See HIGH BLOOD PRESSURE.

HYPERVITAMINOSIS—This condition, also called *vitamin toxicity*, happens when the level of a vitamin in the blood or in body tissues is so high that it causes undesirable symptoms. Hypervitaminosis has been associated with high intakes of vitamins A and D. See also VITAMIN.

HYPO—A prefix meaning below normal, a deficiency, or lack of a substance.

- **Hypoglycemia**—lower than normal levels of blood sugar
- **Hypokalemia**—lower than normal levels of potassium

IATROGENIC—This term means caused by a medical treatment or a diagnostic procedure. Iatrogenic malnutrition is an induced nutrition deficiency caused by drug therapy or medical procedures.

IMMUNE SYSTEM—The role of the immune system is to protect the body against foreign invaders such as microbes, cancer cells, and even transplanted organs. The immune system's main job is to recognize enemies of the body, mobilize forces against them, and finally to attack and conquer the enemy. The organs of the immune system include the bone marrow, thymus, lymph nodes, lymphatic vessels, tonsils, adenoids, and spleen.

INDIGESTION—See DYSPEPSIA.

INOSITOL—See VITAMIN-LIKE COMPOUNDS.

INSULIN—A hormone secreted by the pancreas that helps glucose enter cells to be used for energy. Lower levels of insulin or the complete lack of it causes diabetes. About 25% of all people with diabetes are given insulin. The rest control the condition through diet or with diet and medications that stimulate the pancreas to produce more insulin. Because insulin is a protein it would be digested in the GI tract if it were taken by mouth. That is why it must be injected.

IU (INTERNATIONAL UNIT)—A system to measure vitamin activity, used less frequently today.

JOULE—The international unit of energy. One joule = 4.184 calories. See also CALORIES.

JUNK FOOD—A dated term that usually refers to food with little nutrition value, often high in calories, fat, and sugar. See also EMPTY CALORIES.

KILOGRAM—See GRAM.

LACTOSE INTOLERANCE—This occurs when a person cannot digest *lactose*, the main sugar in milk and other dairy foods. They lack the enzyme *lactase*, which breaks down this sugar. When lactose moves through the large intestine (colon) without being digested, it can cause uncomfortable symptoms, including bloating, gas, cramps, diarrhea, and nausea. There is no cure for lactose intolerance but symptoms can be avoided by using smaller portions of regular milk, yogurt, processed cheese, and ice cream, or by avoiding dairy foods and using dairy substitutes such as soymilk. Lactose-free foods are also available, as well as drops and tablets that can help a person better tolerate foods containing lactose.

LDL (LOW DENSITY LIPOPROTEINS)— The main carrier of cholesterol in your body. If too much LDL cholesterol circulates in the blood, it can stick to the walls of the arteries that lead to the heart and brain, making the vessels narrower. Optimum values for LDL cholesterol are under 100. See also CHOLESTEROL, HDL, and LIPOPROTEIN.

LEAN BODY MASS—The parts of the body that have no stored fat—muscle, bone, connective tissue, organs, and water.

LEARN—This acronym stands for: Listen, Explain, Acknowledge, Recommend, and Negotiate. It serves as a guideline to be used in an intervention process. The LEARN technique might be used to counsel a person to lose weight.

LIPIDS—Fat compounds that differ in size and composition. See FATS.

LIPOIC ACID—See VITAMIN-LIKE COMPOUNDS.

LIPOPROTEIN—A combination of fat and protein. An example is cholesterol, a fatlike substance that is coated with a protein so it can travel in your blood, which is mainly water. The combination is a *lipoprotein*. See also HDL (HIGH DENSITY LIPOPROTEINS) and LDL (LOW DENSITY LIPOPROTEINS).

LITER—A liter equals 33.8 fluid ounces, 1.8 ounces more than a quart, which has 32 ounces. Soda and other beverages are sold in liters.

MACRONUTRIENTS—Nutrients needed by the body in large amounts including proteins, fats, and carbohydrates. This group of nutrients provides calories. See also MICRONUTRIENTS.

MAD COW DISEASE (BOVINE SPONGIFORM ENCEPHALOPATHY OR BSE)—A contagious, degenerative, and fatal disease that affects the central nervous system of adult cattle. It was first diagnosed in 1986. Researchers believe that people who eat BSE infected meat are at greater risk of developing a human brain-wasting illness, *variant Creutzfeldt-Jakob disease (vCJD)*.

MALNUTRITION—This can also be called undernutrition or poor nutrition. It results when too few or too many nutrients and calories are consumed, both of which can jeopardize health. Too few nutrients may result in starvation or deficiency diseases, such as scurvy (too little vitamin C). Taking in too many nutrients, like calories, can result in obesity. We rarely think of someone who is overweight as malnourished, but their condition truly is the result of poor nutrition. See also UNDERNUTRITION.

MEDICAL NUTRITION THERAPY (MNT)—The use of nutrition to treat an illness, injury, or condition.

METABOLIC SYNDROME—This condition, also referred to as *prediabetes*, is not a disease but a cluster of symptoms that doubles the risk for heart disease and quadruples the risk for diabetes. Having 3 of the following risk factors classifies a person as having metabolic syndrome.

- Being 30 or more pounds overweight with a waist larger than 42 inches for men and 35 inches for women.

- Having HDL cholesterol of less than 40 for men and less than 50 for women.
- Having triglycerides of 150 or higher after fasting or above 400 without fasting.
- Having blood pressure readings that are consistently above 130/85 or being on high blood pressure medication.
- Having blood sugar readings that are higher than normal but not high enough to be diagnosed with diabetes—100 or higher after fasting or 140 or higher 2 hours after eating.

Many of these risk factors can be eliminated with diet and lifestyle changes.

METABOLISM—The process by which the body extracts energy (calories) from food and makes use of it. Metabolism has 2 parts: *catabolism* and *anabolism*. Catabolism is the breakdown of complex substances, like food, into simpler substances. It results in the release of energy. Anabolism occurs when simple substances are used to build more complex substances. For example, muscles in your body are made from smaller protein fragments. See also ANABOLISM and CATABOLISM.

MICROGRAM (mcg)—See GRAM.

MICRONUTRIENTS—Nutrients needed by the body in small amounts, including vitamins and minerals. This group of nutrients does not provide calories. See also MACRONUTRIENTS.

MILLIGRAM (mg)—See GRAM.

MG/DL—The abbreviation for milligrams per deciliter. Blood cholesterol is measured as mg/dl, the amount of cholesterol in a certain volume of blood. See also CHOLESTEROL VALUES.

MINERALS—Unlike vitamins, minerals cannot be destroyed or have their shape changed by the body. Calcium, for example, is the same whether it is found in seashells, milk, or bones. Minerals are divided into 2 groups: *major* minerals and *trace* minerals. Each day, your body needs 100 milligrams or more of major minerals. Your body needs less than 100 milligrams of trace minerals per day.

Major Minerals	Trace Minerals
Calcium	Chromium
Chloride	Cobalt
Magnesium	Copper
Phosphorous	Fluorine
Potassium	Iodine
Sodium	Iron
Sulfur	Manganese
	Molybdenum
	Selenium
	Zinc

See also CALCIUM, NUTRITION BASICS pages 12 to 13, POTASSIUM, and SODIUM.

MONOUNSATURATED FATS—See FATS.

NATIONAL INSTITUTES OF HEALTH (NIH)—The U.S. Department of Health and Human Services oversees the National Institutes of Health, which is made up of 27 institutes and centers. These institutes and centers conduct or support research, training, and education to promote the health of Americans. They include: National Cancer Institute (NCI), National Eye Institute (NEI), National Heart, Lung, and Blood Institute (NHLBI), National Human Genome Research Institute (NHGRI), National Institute on Aging (NIA), National Institute on Alcohol Abuse and Alcoholism (NIAAA), National Institute of Allergy and Infectious Diseases (NIAID), National Institute of Arthritis and Musculoskeletal and Skin Diseases (NIAMS), National Institute of Biomedical Imaging and Bioengineering

(NIBIB), National Institutes of Child Health and Human Development (NICHD), National Institute on Deafness and Other Communication Disorders (NIDCD), National Institute of Dental and Craniofacial Research (NIDCR), National Institute of Diabetes and Digestive and Kidney Diseases (NIDDK), National Institute on Drug Abuse (NIDA), National Institute of Environmental Health Sciences (NIEHS), National Institute of General Medical Sciences (NIGMS), National Institute of Mental Health (NIMH), National Institute of Neurological Disorders and Stroke (NINDS), National Institute of Nursing Research (NINR), National Library of Medicine (NLM), Center for Information Technology (CIT), Center for Scientific Review (CSR), John F. Fogarty International Center (FIC), National Center for Complementary and Alternative Medicine (NCCAM), National Center for Research Resources (NCRR), and NIH Clinical Center (CC).

NAUSEA—A general feeling of uneasiness which often leads to an urge to vomit. It may be caused by pregnancy, gallbladder disease, food poisoning, a virus, or as the side effect of chemotherapy or medications. See also VOMITING.

NEAT (nonexercise activity thermogenesis)—This is the sum of the energy (calories) used up through spontaneous ordinary movements. It is also referred to as the *fidget factor*—finger tapping, leg jiggling, foot wiggling, or even chewing gum, which burns 10 calories an hour. It may not seem like much, but over time these calories add up. What were once considered nervous habits actually burn calories, sometimes as many as a few hundred a day.

NIGHT EATING SYNDROME (NES)—A type of disordered eating in which there is a pattern of interrupting sleep to eat.

NUTRIENT-DENSE FOOD—Foods that are rich in one or more important nutrients. Citrus fruits are rich in vitamin C; milk is rich in calcium.

NUTRIENTS—For nutrition to be complete and adequate a person must get the right amount of nutrients—carbohydrates, fats, proteins, vitamins, minerals, and water. These nutrients are used by the body to support growth, repair, and normal functioning. Some nutrients are *essential* and must be supplied through the food you eat. Others are *nonessential* because the body can make as much of them as it needs.

NUTRITION—The study of how food and the nutrients found in food affect your body and your health. You truly are what you eat.

NUTRITION LABELING—The *Nutrition Labeling and Education Act (NLEA)* was signed into law in 1994. It requires nutrition information on most packaged foods and allows the use of FDA-approved health claims on labels. The main features of the Nutrition Facts Panel, which must appear on food labels, include:

- Serving size
- Servings per container
- Calories
- Total fat, trans fat, saturated fat
- Cholesterol
- Sodium
- Total carbohydrates, dietary fiber, sugars
- Protein
- Daily Values (DVs), which are standards set by the government based on a diet of 2,000 or 2,500 calories a day. Some values are recommended maximums, such as less than 65 grams of fat, less than 20 grams of saturated fat, less than 300 milligrams of cholesterol, and less than 2400 milligrams of sodium.

Others are recommended minimums, such as 300 grams of carbohydrates and 25 grams of fiber. The Daily Values for a 2,500 calorie diet are slightly higher.

- % Daily Value (%DV) shows how a food fits into your daily eating plan. The %DVs are set for a 2,000 calorie diet. The percentage listed on the label reflects the amount of the daily value found in one serving of food. For example: if the %DV for carbohydrate is 10%, this means 1 serving of that food provides 30 grams of carbohydrate, because the DV for carbohydrates is 300 grams (10% × 300 = 30).
- Vitamins A and C, and the minerals calcium and iron, are required to be listed. Food companies may voluntarily include additional vitamins and minerals on nutrition labels.
- Health claims that have been approved by the FDA.

See also: DAILY VALUES (DVs), FDA, FOOD LABELS, and HEALTH CLAIMS.

NUTRITION SCREENING—A way for a health professional to examine health variables to see if you are at risk for a specific problem. A nutrition screening could target pregnant women, older adults, or those at risk for certain conditions, like heart disease. Once the screening is complete, a level of risk is assigned. Someone at high risk for a condition, such as heart disease, would be taught how to implement positive health behaviors to lower their risk. Someone at moderate or low risk would be re-evaluated periodically.

NUTRITIONAL GENOMICS—Also referred to as *nutrigenomics*, this is the study of how bioactive food components trigger genes. Foods may switch genes on or off. Knowing which foods act on a particular gene variant would allow nutrition professionals to design the optimum healthy diet for each person. See also HUMAN GENOME PROJECT.

OBESITY—Also called *adiposity*, this is a state of malnutrition in which the accumulation of body fat is so excessive that it negatively impacts a person's health. Mild obesity is defined as 20% to 40% over desirable weight or a BMI of 30 to 34.9. Moderate obesity is 60% to 80% over desirable weight or a BMI of 35 to 39.9. Extreme obesity is more than 100% over desirable weight or a BMI over 40. Obesity puts a person at greater risk for heart disease, diabetes, respiratory problems, stroke, joint problems, and some types of cancer. See also BODY MASS INDEX and OVERWEIGHT.

OMEGA-3 FATS—A type of polyunsaturated fat found mainly in fish, shellfish, olive oil, canola oil, flaxseed, and walnuts. We eat less of these fats than we should.

You Should Know—

Among men, the higher the intake of omega-3 fats, the lower the risk of dying from heart disease. People who eat fish at least twice a week are 42% less likely to develop age-related hearing loss.

See also FATS and OMEGA-6 FATS.

OMEGA-6 FATS—A type of polyunsaturated fat found mainly in vegetable oils such as soybean, corn, grapeseed, and safflower oil. See also FATS and OMEGA-3 FATS.

ORAC (OXYGEN RADICAL ABSORBANCE CAPACITY)—This analysis measures the antioxidant capacity of foods. The more free radicals (damaging substances in the body) a food can absorb and deactivate, the higher the ORAC score. Researchers suggest we consume

3,000 to 5,000 ORAC units a day. If you eat the recommended 5 servings of fruits and vegetables a day, it is easy to meet the ORAC recommendation.

ORAC UNITS IN A SERVING

Food	Portion	ORAC Units
Blueberries	1 cup	5,486
Strawberries	1 cup	3,520
Dried cherries	¼ cup	3,060
Spinach, cooked	1 cup	2,268
Broccoli, cooked	1 cup	1,342
Orange juice	8 ounces	1,125
Raisins	¼ cup	1,026
Tangerine	1	900
Cherries, fresh	20	893
Kiwi	1	542

See also ANTIOXIDANTS and FREE RADICALS.

ORGANIC FOODS—Foods grown and processed without pesticides, herbicides, fertilizers, preservatives, irradiation, or genetic engineering. Organic animals are raised without hormones and antibiotics, except for vaccines that prevent animal diseases. Organic labeling requirements were established in the U.S. in 2000. The words *100% organic* or *organic* can be used only on foods that contain at least 95% organic ingredients.

OSTEOPOROSIS—This condition is commonly referred to as *adult bone-thinning*. It occurs when the amount of bone breakdown in the body exceeds the amount of bone formation, resulting in porous bones that are prone to fracture. It usually occurs in people over age 50, especially postmenopausal women. Men and younger adults can also be affected but usually to a lesser degree. The primary prevention is adequate nutrition and calcium early in life to form strong bones. Exercising, not smoking, limiting caffeine intake, and moderate use of alcohol all decrease your risk for osteoporosis.

OVERWEIGHT—Defined as a body mass index of 25 to 25.9, which is 10% to 20% over a person's ideal weight. See also BODY MASS INDEX and OBESITY.

PATHOGEN—An organism that can cause illness.

PH—A numerical scale that measures the acidity or alkalinity of a substance. A pH of 7.0 to 14.0 is alkaline. A pH below 7.0 is acid. Every food has a pH: limes are 2.0, bananas are 4.6, milk is 6.6, and egg whites are 8.0. The pH of your blood is 7.4, or nearly neutral, which is important to your health. Even small changes in the body's pH can be life threatening.

PHYSICAL ACTIVITY—This includes all movement that burns calories and increases your heart rate, such as walking, bicycling, weeding, dancing, swimming, or cleaning the house. Physical activity helps to prevent weight gain and reduces your risk for many health problems. See also SEDENTARY LIFESTYLE.

PHYTOCHEMICALS—Naturally occurring plant substances that help protect your body or lower your risk for disease. More than 900 different phytochemicals have been found in foods. Fruits, vegetables, grains, beans, seeds, soy, and tea are all rich in phytochemicals.

PLACEBO—An inactive substance that appears to be the same as an active substance that is being studied. A placebo is sometimes called a "sugar pill." The *placebo effect* is a physical or emotional change that is the result of the person's expectations and not directly a result of the substance they were given. See also DOUBLE BLIND EXPERIMENT.

PLU (PRODUCT LOOK UP)—Numbers that appear on the tiny sticker on fresh fruit or on plastic bags holding prepackaged produce. Every time you buy a fresh fruit or vegetable, the cashier uses a PLU code to determine the price. They can appear as PLU-4211, #4211 or just 4211. For conventionally grown produce the PLU code consists of 4 numbers (like 4011 for bananas). Organically grown produce has a 5 digit PLU starting with the number 9—94011 for organic bananas. If the produce is genetically modified the 5 digit PLU starts with an 8. PLU codes are only assigned to fresh fruits and vegetables and are used in countries throughout the world. Many predict that PLU codes will be replaced by mini bar codes in the future. See also GENETICALLY MODIFIED (GM) FOODS and ORGANIC FOODS.

POLYUNSATURATED FATS—See FATS.

PORTION SIZE—The amount of food served at one time. Restaurant portion sizes are often larger than those you would typically eat at home. Portion sizes vary widely, whereas serving sizes are standardized. See also SERVING SIZE.

POTASSIUM—This mineral helps to maintain balance in the body and is part of many enzyme reactions. Potassium is stored in body cells, with most of it stored in muscles. The flow of potassium into and out of cells is coupled with the movement of sodium. These two minerals work together to contract muscles, transmit nerve impulses, and regulate blood pressure and heartbeat. Some medications taken to control high blood pressure increase the need for potassium. Eating potassium-rich foods helps to lower blood pressure. See also ENZYMES, MINERALS, and NUTRITION BASICS pages 16 to 17.

PREDIABETES—See METABOLIC SYNDROME.

PREBIOTICS—Food for probiotics that allow them to grow and thrive. Whole grains, onions, bananas, garlic, honey, leeks, and artichokes are natural sources. Prebiotics can also be isolated from natural sources. Inulin and fructo-oligosaccharides (FOS) are two of the most common and will appear on the ingredient list. Prebiotics (food) and probiotics (friendly organisms living in your digestive tract) work together to boost your health from the inside out. See also PROBIOTICS.

PROBIOTICS—An umbrella term for more than 30 different types of bacteria and yeast needed for good health. There are trillions of friendly bacteria, called *flora*, living in your digestive tract. They are one of the first lines of defense against unfriendly invading bacteria that enter the body. Healthy and harmful organisms are constantly jostling for the upper hand. Decreased use of fermented foods and increased use of antibiotics can upset the natural gut flora and give harmful bacteria the chance to grow. Eating extra probiotics can increase the amount of healthy bacteria, which helps control diarrhea, chronic constipation, irritable bowel syndrome, and inflammatory bowel disease. Yogurt, buttermilk, kefir, miso, and sauerkraut are natural sources of probiotics, but many foods such as soymilk, cereal, and granola bars are fortified. Probiotics are nourished by prebiotics. See also PREBIOTICS.

PROOF—This refers to the concentration of ethanol (alcohol) in a liquid. In the U.S., proof is twice the alcohol content. Gin or vodka labeled 80 proof has 40% alcohol. Wine is usually 10% to 14% alcohol, which is 20 to 28 proof. Vanilla flavoring is often alcohol-based, as are many medications. Both will list the percent alcohol on the label; double that number to get the proof. See also ALCOHOL.

PROTEINS—Complex structures made up of smaller building blocks called *amino acids*. Proteins are strung together to make up body parts, such as muscle, blood, skin, and cartilage. Proteins can also provide energy (calories). The body constantly assembles, breaks down and uses protein. The protein foods you eat each day replace what is being used. Good sources of protein include: meat, fish, poultry, dry beans, eggs, nuts, nut butters, seeds, milk, yogurt, cheese, tofu, bread, cereal, rice, and pasta. See also AMINO ACIDS and NUTRITION BASICS pages 7 to 8.

QUACKWATCH—A nonprofit organization (www.quackwatch.com) that attempts to combat health-related frauds, myths, fads, and fallacies.

QUACKERY—In the field of foods and nutrition, quackery refers to false claims about the power of a food or a nutrient to cure or prevent a health problem. The 10 red flags for a food fad or food quackery are:

1. Recommendations that promise a quick fix
2. Claims that sound too good to be true
3. Simplistic conclusions drawn from a complex study
4. Recommendations that are based on a single study
5. The use of vague terms such as cure-all
6. Advertisements that promote something new or a scientific breakthrough
7. Recommendations that ignore the differences between individuals or groups of people
8. Advertisements that do not state any disadvantages to following the advice
9. Lists of good and bad foods
10. Use of questionable publications to promote claims

QUALITY OF LIFE—Defined by the World Health Organization as "a complete state of physical, mental, and social well-being and not merely the absence of disease or infirmity."

RECOMMENDED DIETARY ALLOWANCES (RDAs)—Daily requirements for the nutrients needed by healthy people in all age and sex categories. These recommendations are published periodically by the National Academy of Sciences. Beginning in 1989, the RDAs underwent a comprehensive review and revision, the results of which were published in a series of reports called *Dietary Reference Intakes (DRIs)*.

REGISTERED DIETITIAN (RD)—See DIETITIAN.

REQUIREMENT—In nutrition, this is defined as the lowest continuous level of a nutrient that a person needs to maintain health and prevent a deficiency.

RISK—The possibility that an event may occur. There are numerous risk factors that can affect your health.

SALT—Table salt is made up of two minerals, 40% sodium and 60% chloride. One teaspoon of table salt has slightly more than 2,300 milligrams of sodium. *Kosher* salt and *sea* salt are slightly less salty than table salt because they are less dense and coarser in shape. Most of these coarser salts average between 1,100 and 1,900 milligrams of sodium in a teaspoon. Many cooks prefer coarser salt because they feel it offers more texture and flavor. See also SODIUM.

SATURATED FATS—See FATS and NUTRITION BASICS pages 4 to 5.

SATIATION—The sensation that tells you that you have eaten enough. It affects how much you eat at a given time. See also APPETITE, HUNGER, and SATIETY.

SATIETY—The satisfaction you feel after you have been fed, and how long that satisfaction lasts. It influences the time between meals and the number of times you eat in a day. See also APPETITE, HUNGER, and SATIATION.

SCOVILLE SCALE—A standard test for measuring the heat of peppers. The scale goes from 0 for bell peppers to 2,500 to 10,000 for jalapeños and chipotles, to a four-alarm 100,000 to 350,000 for habanera and Scotch bonnet peppers. All types of peppers are rich in vitamins A and C. The ingredient in hot peppers that stimulates the sensors in the mouth and creates the burning sensation is *capsaicin*. The burn you feel actually activates pain receptors in your mouth, which causes the brain to release endorphins, feel-good chemicals that produce a pleasurable sensation. The result: Your mouth is on fire, but you keep eating. Hot dishes may temporarily speed up your metabolism and help to stimulate the breakdown of fats. These dishes also activate the body's natural cooling system, making you sweat. Capsaicin is part of a family of compounds called *capsaicinoids*, which are used in rub-on creams that treat pain. Spicing food with chilies may also be heart healthy, lowering blood pressure, reducing blood cholesterol, and reducing blood clot formation. Over 25% of the world's population eats hot peppers every day.

SEDENTARY LIFESTYLE—Frequent behaviors that include little or no physical activity, such as excessive TV watching daily. A sedentary lifestyle increases your risk for gaining weight and for serious health problems, such as osteoporosis, heart disease, and diabetes. See also PHYSICAL ACTIVITY.

SERVING SIZE—Most foods have standard serving sizes, such as ½ cup of cooked vegetables, 1 slice of bread, or 8 ounces of milk. These standard serving sizes are used to calculate diets, provide weight control advice, and compare foods. Serving sizes are different from portion sizes, which in the U.S. have increased to the point that most people can no longer recognize the standard serving size of different foods.

WHAT IS A SERVING?

Food	Serving Size
Breads, cereals, high carb foods	
bread	1 slice
roll, bun, or pita pocket	½
crackers	4 to 6
tortilla	1 (6 inches across)
cereal, cooked	½ cup
cereal, ready-to-eat	¾ cup
popcorn	3 cups
Vegetables, fruits	
raw or cooked vegetables	½ cup
raw or cooked leafy greens	1 cup
green peas	½ cup
potato	1 small
French fries	10 pieces
fresh fruit	1 small
banana	½ regular or 1 very small
dried fruit	2 tablespoons
canned fruit	½ cup
juice	½ cup
Milk, yogurt, cheese	
nonfat or low fat milk	1 cup
nonfat or low fat yogurt	1 cup

Milk, yogurt, cheese (cont.)

cheese	1 oz or 1 slice
cottage cheese	½ cup

Meat, poultry, fish

cooked	3 to 4 ounces
egg, cooked	1

Fats

butter or margarine	1 teaspoon
cream cheese	2 tablespoon
salad dressing	2 tablespoons
oil	1 tablespoon

Sugar

sugar or honey	1 teaspoon
syrup	2 tablespoons

See also PORTION SIZE.

SODIUM—This mineral regulates the fluid levels outside and inside of the cells in your body, which in turn affects blood volume, blood pressure, and your body's acidity. The movement of sodium into and out of cells allows other important substances to make this journey, too, helping to transmit nerve impulses and electrical messages vital to your body's minute-by-minute functioning. See also HIGH BLOOD PRESSURE, SALT, and NUTRITION BASICS pages 13 to 16.

STEARIC ACID—This *saturated fatty acid* (a building block of fat) doesn't act like a typical saturated fat; it doesn't raise cholesterol levels. It's found in meats, milk, and some plant foods. This finding suggests that not all saturated fats are bad. See also FATS.

STEROLS—Plant sterols are natural substances that reduce the absorption of cholesterol. They occur naturally or can be added to foods—margarines, orange juice, cereal bars, chocolate, and yogurt. Studies show that getting 2 to 3 grams of plant sterols daily can reduce total cholesterol by 5% to 13% and LDL cholesterol by 6% to 24%.

You Should Know—

Sunflower seeds, pistachios, pumpkin seeds, pine nuts, flaxseed, almonds, macadamia nuts, walnuts, pecans, cashews, peanuts, peanut butter, hazelnuts, and brazil nuts are all rich in natural plant sterols.

SUGAR—Is a simple carbohydrate made up of one sugar molecule (glucose, fructose, and galatose) or two sugar molecules bound together (sucrose, lactose, or maltose). Cereals, grains, fruits, vegetables, milk, and plain yogurt all contain sugar. These are *natural sugar* choices and the sweet foods come packaged with vitamins, minerals and fiber. Soda, candy, fruit drinks, cakes, cookies, ice cream, jelly, and syrup, in contrast, are loaded with *added sugar* and offer little more than sweetness and calories. Choose foods with natural sugars more often and choose foods with added sugars less often.

SOME SURPRISING SUGAR FACTS

- Humans are genetically programmed to like sweets. Amniotic fluid and breast milk are slightly sweet.
- Sugar does not make kids hyper. Contrary to popular beliefs, sugar has a calming effect on the brain and acts as a pain reliever in infants.
- Preschoolers average 14 to 17 teaspoons of added sugar every day, mostly from sweetened drinks, desserts, and soda.
- Sugar is not addictive. Sugar cravings are more likely driven by habits.
- A high sugar intake increases triglyerceride levels and lowers good HDL cholesterol.

- A high sugar, highly refined, carb diet increases the risk for cataracts by almost 30% and increases the risk for age-related macular degeneration (AMD).
- A high sugar intake makes it more difficult for people with diabetes to control blood sugar levels.

See also NUTRITION BASICS page 9 to 10.

SUGAR SUBSTITUTES—Different types of sugar substitutes have been in use for decades. *Sugar alcohols*—sorbitol, mannitol, xylitol, isomalt, lactitol, maltitol, and trehalose—contain some calories but are absorbed very slowly by the body, so they have very little effect on blood sugar. High intakes can cause diarrhea. *Artificial sweeteners*—saccharin, aspartame, acesulfame-K, sucralose, and neotame—don't raise blood sugar and have no calories. Some lose their sweetness when heated, so they cannot be used in cooking.

Artificial Sweetener	Brand Name
Saccharin	Sweet'N Low
	Sweet Twin
	Necta Sweet
Aspartame	Nutrasweet
	Equal
	Sugar Twin
Acesulfame-K	Sunett
	Sweet & Safe
	Sweet One
Sucralose	Splenda
Stevia	Truvia
	PureVia
	SweetLeaf
	OnlySweet

SYMPTOM—An indication of a disease as the person experiences it, in contrast to a sign, which is an indication of a disease that a doctor can evaluate. For example, a headache is a symptom, but high blood pressure is a sign, because a headache can be described but not measured while blood pressure can be measured.

TASTE—Humans have the ability to taste sweet, sour, salty, and bitter flavors through receptors found on the tongue and in the mouth. Scientists have found that humans can also taste *umami*, described as full-bodied, savory, or rich. The umami taste results from the addition of MSG (monosodium glutamate) to foods or by the presence of the amino acid glutamine (also called *glutamate*). Recently, it was found that there are receptors on the tongue for fat. Some people perceive this taste more strongly than others. This may be the reason why certain people crave fatty foods.

TAURINE—See VITAMIN-LIKE COMPOUNDS.

THIRST—A sensation that signals the body needs fluid. Thirst is normally a good guide for fluid needs, except in infants, the sick, and older adults, who may have a diminished sense of thirst. Water is the ideal thirst quencher but all fluids, except alcohol, count toward your daily fluid need. In extreme heat and during excessive sweating, thirst may not always keep up with your body's need for fluid.

TOLERABLE UPPER INTAKE LEVEL (UL)—The highest average amount of a nutrient a person can take without causing a problem. A UL for each nutrient is set based on sex and age. As amounts increase over the UL, the potential for problems increase.

TRANS FAT (TRANS FATTY ACIDS)—A type of fat that is usually made by passing hydrogen gas through vegetable oil, a process called *hydrogenation*, which makes oils harder and more stable. Cutting back or cutting out foods with trans fat is a good idea—eating even small amounts of trans fat raises total cholesterol and lowers HDL, good cholesterol. Trans fat must be listed on the nutrition facts panel. We are eating less today because food manufacturers and restaurants are reformulating recipes to eliminate or cut down on trans fat. There are small amounts of naturally occurring trans fat in meat, butter, milk, cheese, and cabbage. These natural trans fats have a different structure then those artificially produced and they may have health benefits. One natural trans fat, CLA (conjugated linoleic acid), may play a role in preventing cancer, heart disease, and diabetes.

> ### You Should Know—
>
> #### *Labeling Loophole*
> *The value for trans fat listed on the nutrition label includes both artificially produced and natural trans fat. This can be confusing because only artificial trans fat needs to be limited.*

See also CLA (CONJUGATED LINOLEIC ACID) and HYDROGENATION.

TRIGLYCERIDES—The main type of fat found in food, and the major storage form of fat in your body. Triglycerides are transported through the blood to cells where they are burned for energy (calories), or to fat tissues where they are stored for future use. Levels of triglycerides in your blood above 150 mg/dl put you at greater risk for heart disease. Your risk for high triglycerides goes up if you are overweight, do little exercise, drink too much alcohol, eat a high carbohydrate diet, smoke, or have diabetes.

TYPE 1 DIABETES—See DIABETES.

TYPE 2 DIABETES—See DIABETES.

UL—See TOLERABLE UPPER INTAKE LEVEL (UL).

UNDERNUTRITION—Poor health that results from an inadequate nutrition intake over time. It is often associated with poverty, alcoholism, or an eating disorder. See also MALNUTRITION.

UNDERWEIGHT—Describes a person with a BMI below 18.5 or who is 10% or more below the normal weight for a person of that age, sex, and height. A weight 30% below normal or a BMI of 15 or less can be life threatening. See also BODY MASS INDEX.

USDA (UNITED STATES DEPARTMENT OF AGRICULTURE)—This agency is responsible for monitoring the wholesomeness and quality of meat, poultry, and eggs. The USDA has a consumer hotline number at 1-800-535-4555.

USDHHS (UNITED STATES DEPARTMENT OF HEALTH AND HUMAN SERVICES)—This agency is responsible for setting all policies related to human development, and the general health and welfare of all Americans. See also FDA.

URINE—The fluid excreted by the kidneys. Most people make 1,000 to 1,500 milliliters in 24 hours. At night, you make half the amount of urine that you do during the day. The color of urine is a simple way to tell if you are drinking enough fluids. The deeper the yellow, the more likely it is that you are mildly dehydrated. Pale yellow to clear means good hydration. *Urinalysis*, a physical, chemical, and microscopic evaluation of a urine sample, is used to evaluate your health and nutritional status. See also DEHYDRATION and WATER.

VEGETARIAN DIET—A way of eating that excludes some or all animal foods. *Vegans* eat only plant foods. They eat no animal foods and often do not use animal-based products like silk or leather. *Lacto* vegetarians eat plant foods and dairy products. *Lacto-ovo* vegetarians eat plant foods, plus dairy products and eggs. As more people attempt to eat a plant-based diet the definition of vegetarians has broadened to include people who eat a vegetarian diet some or most of the time but not exclusively. *Flexitarians* is a new term used to describe those who are mostly vegetarian but occasionally eat meat. *Pescatarians* eat a plant-based diet but include fish. *Partial vegetarians* or *semi-vegetarians* eat plant foods but no red meat, and may or may not eat chicken, fish, dairy products, and eggs.

VISCERAL FAT—A type of fat that shields and cushions internal organs. When it accumulates in the trunk or belly region, it increases a person's risk for heart disease, diabetes, hypertension, and stroke because it can easily be released into the bloodstream. Fat in other areas of the body, called *subcutaneous* fat, is not so easily released.

VITAMIN—The word comes from the Latin *vita*, meaning *life*. All vitamins are vital to life, even though they are needed by your body in very small amounts. They help absorb, digest, and use the fats, carbohydrates, and proteins found in food. Vitamins do not provide energy (calories) and can be destroyed or have their shape changed. Cooking at high temperatures destroys vitamins. Your body is able to change a vitamin's shape making it easier to use in certain situations. Vitamins are divided into two groups, fat soluble and water soluble. *Fat soluble* vitamins are carried into the body by foods containing fat and are stored in your fat tissues, waiting to be used. *Water soluble* vitamins are absorbed directly into the blood and travel freely around the body in the bloodstream.

Water Soluble	Fat Soluble
Thiamin (B_1)	Vitamin A
Riboflavin (B_2)	Vitamin D
Niacin (B_3)	Vitamin E
Vitamin B_6	Vitamin K
Vitamin B_{12}	
Vitamin C	
Biotin	
Folic acid	
Pantothenic acid	

See also FOLIC ACID, NUTRITION BASICS pages 17 to 20, VITAMIN C, and VITAMIN-LIKE COMPOUNDS.

VITAMIN C—Although most animals make their own vitamin C, humans cannot. We need to get vitamin C through food. The best sources are fruits, vegetables, and fortified drinks. Being pregnant, taking or using drugs, and smoking all increase the need for vitamin C. See also VITAMIN and NUTRITION BASICS pages 18 to 20.

VITAMIN-LIKE COMPOUNDS—These are substances that have properties similar to vitamins but do not fit the definition for a vitamin, which is necessary to life. The lack of it causes a deficiency disease. The body can't make enough of essential vitamins but it can make the vitamin-like compounds that it needs. These include:

- *Choline* helps maintain cell structure and transmits nerve messages. It can be made from an amino acid, *methionine*. When you eat enough protein you are able to make enough choline.
- *Carnitine* helps to deliver needed substances into cells and remove waste from cells. The liver is able to make carnitine from amino acids. Carnitine is also found in dairy foods and meat.

- *Inositol* is found mainly in brain tissue and is part of cell structures. The body can make inositol from glucose. Animal foods also are a good source of inositol.
- *Taurine* is found mainly in muscle, blood, and nerve tissues and helps them to function properly. It is made in the body from amino acids.
- *Lipoic acid* helps the body to use energy and acts as an antioxidant. It can easily be made in the body. Red meat, liver, and brewer's yeast are good food sources.

See also AMINO ACIDS and VITAMIN.

VOMITING—The process of getting rid of or throwing up material from the stomach through the esophagus and out the mouth. It is the body's response to something irritating. It can be caused by too much alcohol or caffeine, an infection, or foodborne illness. Vomiting results in weakness, mild dehydration, and the loss of some important minerals, including sodium, magnesium, and chloride. Prolonged vomiting can lead to nutritional deficiencies and severe dehydration. Do not eat anything immediately after vomiting; just relax and give the digestive tract a chance to rest. After an hour with no further vomiting, try a little water. If this stays down, slowly add other drinks, such as tea or ginger ale. Then try crackers, dry toast, pretzels, bananas, applesauce, plain rice, or plain pasta. Most cases of vomiting last for a very short time. If you vomit profusely or if vomiting continues for more than 24 hours, call your doctor.

WAIST CIRCUMFERENCE—This measurement can be used as a simple tool to determine if a person is overweight. A man with a waist greater than 40 inches and a woman with a waist greater than 35 inches are at increased risk for obesity-related diseases—type 2 diabetes, high cholesterol, high triglycerides, high blood pressure, and heart disease. Fat in the abdominal region is a greater health risk than fat deposits in other regions of the body, such as the thighs and hips.

WATER—A continuous supply of water is one of your most basic nutrition needs. Without water you can survive for less than a week. It makes up 50% to 80% of your body weight. The fluids in your body are found in 2 places—inside your cells and outside your cells. Fluid inside your cells is called *intracellular fluid* and the fluid outside your cells is called *extracellular fluid*. Both types of fluid help your body to function by:

- Giving structure and shape to your cells
- Helping to form structures like protein
- Lubricating for your eyes and joints
- Helping to regulate your body's temperature
- Aiding in digestion and absorption of nutrients
- Transporting nutrients to cells
- Carrying waste products away from cells in urine, stools, and perspiration
- Aiding in your body's chemical reactions

Drinking water and other liquids are your major sources of water but many foods, like fruits and vegetables, are good sources, too. See also WATER REQUIREMENTS.

WATER REQUIREMENTS—Most people believe that they need to drink 8 servings of 8 ounces of water each day. Interestingly, there is no foundation for this recommendation and no scientific evidence to support it. Everyone needs water every day but the amount is based on a person's calorie need—1 milliliter of water for each calorie eaten. If a person needs 1,800 calories a day, they also need 1,800 milliliters of water. Translated into cups: 1 cup = 240 milliliters.

$$1,800 \div 240 = 7.5 \text{ cups per day}$$

These 7½ cups a day don't have to all be water. Solid food contains a good deal of water; you get 3 to 4 cups a day from food. Other liquids like juice and soup count, too. If you drink caffeinated beverages—tea, coffee, soda, energy drinks—you can count half of your intake toward your daily fluid, but not all, since the caffeine acts as a diuretic, causing you to lose some of the water. In many cases, you can meet your fluid requirement without extra water. The exceptions would be during extremely hot weather or heavy exercise, when you need more fluids. Drinking some water each day is a good habit because it is calorie free and contains minerals.

WEIGHT LOSS—The loss of body weight happens when a person decreases food intake and increases their physical activity, or both.

WELLNESS—This defines a lifestyle with appropriate levels of nutrition, exercise, work, and rest to ensure that a person gets the best experience from life.

WHO (WORLD HEALTH ORGANIZATION)—A United Nations organization that aims to eliminate disease on a global scale.

WHOLE GRAINS—The entire grain seed or kernel of a grain, made up of 3 parts: bran, germ, and endosperm. *Bran* is the outer protective layer. It provides fiber and minerals. The *germ* can sprout into a new plant and contains vitamins, minerals and healthy fats. The *endosperm* is rich in protein and starch. It is the warehouse of food the germ would use to sprout and grow if the grain were planted. Eating a whole grain gives you the full benefit of all 3 parts. You should try to eat at least 3 servings of whole grain foods each day.

You Should Know—

One serving of whole grains equals:
1 slice 100% whole grain bread
1 cup whole grain cereal
½ cup cooked whole grain hot cereal
(ex. oatmeal) or pasta
½ cup cooked brown or wild rice
½ cup any type of cooked whole grain
(ex. bulgur, quinoa)
2 cups popcorn

XEROSTOMIA—A condition that occurs when salivary glands in the mouth do not work properly and the mouth becomes very dry. Over 70% of older adults have this condition. It effects taste and puts the person at greater risk for tooth decay and mouth infections.

YEAST—A microscopic, single-cell, fungal plant that can be used to make foods and beverages. *Baker's yeast* is used to make dough rise. *Brewer's yeast* is a bitter-tasting byproduct of the production of beer. It's rich in protein, minerals, and some B vitamins. It can be bought as a nutrition supplement in flake, powder, or tablet form. *Nutritional yeast* is grown especially to be used as a dietary supplement and has a pleasant, nutty cheese flavor. It is rich in B vitamins, particularly folic acid, and rich in protein. Brewer's yeast and nutritional yeast cannot be substituted for baker's yeast in cooking. See also YEAST page 653 for nutrition information.

YOGURT—A fermented milk product that is considered a functional food because it contains benefical bacteria (probiotics) that promote health. It is also lower in lactose (milk sugar) and may be tolerated by those with lactose intolerance who can't drink milk. See also FUNCTIONAL FOODS, LACTOSE INTOLERANCE, and PROBIOTICS.

YO-YO DIETING—This term refers to repeated dieting whereby a person loses weight only to regain most or all of the weight that was lost. They may diet again and again throughout their lifetime, but rarely retain the weight loss for any extended period of time. This up and down weight loss/weight gain syndrome is also called *weight cycling*.

ZEN MACROBIOTIC DIET—This diet is based on the idea that one's health and happiness depends on a proper balance between yin and yang foods. Macrobiotic diets are vegan and stress whole grains, vegetables, beans, sea vegetables, and soups. Extreme forms of this diet are very limiting, relying mostly on brown rice. See also VEGETARIAN DIET.

USING *THE MOST COMPLETE FOOD COUNTER*

The Most Complete Food Counter, 3rd Edition, lists the calories, fat, saturated fat, cholesterol, protein, carbohydrate, sugar, fiber, calcium, sodium, potassium, vitamin C, and folic acid in more than 21,000 foods. These are key nutrients for you to consider when you are choosing foods. Fat, saturated fat, cholesterol, sugar, and sodium are nutrients you may want to limit. You can be more liberal with the others, aiming for moderate amounts of calories, protein, and carbohydrates, and higher amounts of the rest. Recommended intakes for all nutrients listed are described in the chapter called "Nutrition Basics (pages 2 to 20)." There are still other nutrients needed for good health, but when you eat a variety of foods containing the nutrients listed in this counter, you will get these other necessary nutrients along with them.

Now, you can compare the values in your favorite foods and, when necessary, choose substitutes before you go out to shop or eat. This will save you time and help you decide what to buy.

The counter section of the book is divided into two parts: Part One: Brand Name, Nonbranded (Generic), and Take-out Foods (page 61); and Part Two: Restaurant Chains (page 667). Each part lists foods or restaurant chains alphabetically.

In Part One, for each category, you will find nonbranded (generic) foods listed first, in al-phabetical order, followed by an alphabetical listing of brand name foods. The nonbranded listings will help you estimate calorie values when you don't see your favorite. They can also help you to evaluate store brands. Large categories are divided into subcategories, such as canned, fresh, frozen, and ready-to-eat, to make it easier to find what you're looking for. Some categories have *see* and *see also* references, to help you find related items.

Because we eat out so often, we listed more than 900 take-out foods in Part One. These are found in the take-out subcategory in many categories throughout this section. Look there for foods you take out or order in, because these foods are not nutrition labeled.

Most foods are listed alphabetically. But, in some cases, foods are grouped by category. For example, a tuna sandwich is found in the SANDWICH category. Other group categories include:

ALCOHOL DRINKS	Page 63
Includes all alcoholic beverages and mixed drinks except beer and ale, champagne, and wine, which have their own separate categories.	
ASIAN FOOD	Page 77
Includes all types of Asian foods except egg rolls and sushi, which	

are found in the egg rolls and sushi categories.

DELI MEATS/COLD CUTS Page 276

Includes all sandwich meats except chicken, ham, and turkey, which have their own separate categories.

DINNER Page 278

Includes all prepared dinners listed by brand name, except pasta dinners, which are found in the pasta dinners category.

NUTRITION SUPPLEMENTS Page 428

Includes all dieting aids, meal replacements, and drinks, except energy bars and energy drinks, which have their own separate categories.

SANDWICHES Page 535

Includes popular sandwich, calzone, and panini choices.

SNACKS Page 563

Includes a variety of snack items, such as pork rinds and cheese puffs.

SPANISH FOOD Page 595

Includes all types of Spanish and Mexican foods except salsa and tortillas, which have their own separate categories

In Part Two, Restaurant Chains (page 667), 113 national and regional restaurant, coffee, doughnut, frozen yogurt, ice cream, pizza, sandwich, soup, and sushi chains are listed. Brand name foods are required by federal law to have nutrition information on labels, but in most areas of the country restaurants provide this information voluntarily.

With *The Most Complete Food Counter, 3rd Edition,* as your guide, you have at your fingertips the most comprehensive guide to the calories and important nutrients in the foods you eat.

DEFINITIONS

as prep (as prepared): refers to food that has been prepared according to package directions

lean and fat: describes meat with some fat on its edges that is not cut away before cooking, or poultry prepared with skin and fat as purchased

lean only: refers to lean meat that is trimmed of all visible fat, or poultry without skin

not prep (not prepared): refers to food that has not been cooked and may require the addition of other ingredients to prepare

shelf-stable: refers to prepared products found on the supermarket shelf that are not canned or frozen but are packaged and ready-to-eat or are ready to be heated and do not require refrigeration

take-out: describes prepared dishes that you purchase ready-to-eat; those included serve as a guide to the calories, fat, saturated fat, cholesterol, protein, carbohydrate, sugar, fiber, calcium, sodium, potassium, folic acid, and vitamin C values of similar products you may purchase

ABBREVIATIONS

avg	=	average
diam	=	diameter
fl	=	fluid
frzn	=	frozen
g	=	gram
in	=	inch
lb	=	pound
lg	=	large
med	=	medium
mg	=	milligram
oz	=	ounce
pkg	=	package
pt	=	pint
prep	=	prepared
qt	=	quart
reg	=	regular
sec	=	second
serv	=	serving
sm	=	small
sq	=	square
tbsp	=	tablespoon
tr	=	trace
tsp	=	teaspoon
w/	=	with
w/o	=	without
<	=	less than

NOTES

CALS = Calories

PROT = Protein
 All protein values are given in grams (g).

FAT = Fat
 All fat values are given in grams (g).

SAT FAT = Saturated Fat
 All saturated fat values are given in grams (g).

CHOL = Cholesterol
 All cholesterol values are given in
 milligrams (mg).

CARB = Carbohydrate
 All carbohydrate values are given in
 grams (g).

SUGAR = Sugar
 All sugar values are given in grams (g).

FIBER = Fiber
 All fiber values are given in grams (g).

CALCI = Calcium
 All calcium values are given in
 milligrams (mg).

SOD = Sodium
 All sodium values are given in
 milligrams (mg).

POTAS = Potassium
 All potassium values are given in
 milligrams (mg).

FOLIC = Folic Acid
 All folic acid values are given in
 micrograms (mcg).

VIT C = Vitamin C
 All vitamin C values are given in
 milligrams (mg).

tr (trace) = less than 1 gram of fat, saturated fat,
 protein, carbohydrate, sugar, or fiber; less
 than 1 milligrams of cholesterol, calcium,
 sodium, potassium, and vitamin C; and less
 than 1 microgram of folic acid.

— (dash) indicates data was not available.

0 (zero) indicates that there is none of the
 nutrient in that food.

Discrepancies in figures are due to rounding, product reformulation, and reevaluation. Labeling law allows rounding of values. Because much of the data is analysis data, obtained directly from manufacturers, not from labels, in some cases our values may not be exactly the same as label information because they have not been rounded.

PART ONE

BRAND NAME, NONBRANDED (GENERIC) AND TAKE-OUT FOODS

Our Best Eating Advice

Eat less, but enjoy what you eat
Eat lots of fruits and vegetables
Eat whole grains instead of refined carbs (like white bread)
Eat less sugar (but you don't have to give it up)
Eat more good fats like olive oil, fish, and nuts
Eat lean proteins—fish, chicken without the skin, lean beef, pork, and lamb
Enjoy a glass of wine, but not the whole bottle
Move more and move often—find ways to be active throughout the day

FOOD	PORTION	CALS	FAT	SAT FAT	CHOL	PROT	CARB	SUGAR	FIBER	CALCI	SOD	POTAS	FOLIC	VIT C
ABALONE														
breaded & fried	1 serv (3 oz)	162	6	1	80	17	9	tr	tr	50	980	295	6	3
steamed	1 serv (3 oz)	127	3	1	84	17	6	tr	0	31	574	253	5	3
ACAI JUICE														
ARTHUR'S														
Acai Plus	1 bottle (11 oz)	230	5	1	0	2	45	25	5	60	0	680	180	24
BOSSA NOVA														
Acai Juice Blueberry	8 oz	89	0	0	0	0	21	18	0	20	14	—	—	5
Acai Juice Mango	8 oz	89	0	0	0	0	23	16	0	—	14	—	—	2
Acai Juice Original	8 oz	94	0	0	0	0	21	18	0	20	14	—	—	5
Acai Juice Passion Fruit	8 oz	89	0	0	0	0	23	18	0	30	14	—	—	2
Acai Juice Raspberry	8 oz	89	0	0	0	0	23	18	0	40	13	—	—	5
O.N.E.														
Amazon Acai	1 bottle (11 oz)	157	3	1	0	1	32	29	3	66	28	—	—	99
ULTRA LO-GLY														
Acai-Blue	1 bottle (10 oz)	45	0	0	0	0	11	10	0	40	10	—	—	66
ZOLA														
100% Juice	1 box (11 oz)	170	2	1	0	2	30	29	1	40	45	30	—	15
ACEROLA														
fresh	1 (5 g)	2	tr	tr	0	tr	tr	—	tr	1	0	7	1	81
ACEROLA JUICE														
juice	1 cup	56	1	tr	0	1	12	11	1	24	7	235	0	3872
ADZUKI BEANS														
canned sweetened	½ cup	351	tr	tr	0	6	81	—	—	33	323	176	158	0
dried cooked w/o salt	½ cup	147	tr	tr	0	9	28	—	8	32	9	6124	139	0
ARROWHEAD MILLS														
Organic Dried not prep	¼ cup	130	0	0	0	8	26	1	5	20	0	510	—	0
AKEE														
fresh	3.5 oz	223	20	—	0	5	5	—	—	40	—	—	—	26
AGAVE														
(see SYRUP)														
ALCOHOL DRINKS														
(see also BEER AND ALE, CHAMPAGNE, MALT, WINE)														
7&7	1 serv	178	0	0	0	0	19	—	0	4	21	3	—	—
alabama slammer	1 serv	103	tr	0	0	tr	7	—	tr	1	tr	13	2	3
amaretto sour	1 serv	295	tr	tr	0	2	57	—	4	75	98	362	55	98
angel's kiss	1 serv	85	1	1	5	tr	5	—	0	7	4	12	tr	tr
anisette	1 oz	111	0	0	0	—	11	—	0	—	—	—	—	—

FOOD	PORTION	CALS	FAT	SAT FAT	CHOL	PROT	CARB	SUGAR	FIBER	CALCI	SOD	POTAS	FOLIC	VIT C
antifreeze cocktail	1 serv	177	tr	tr	0	1	31	—	tr	20	2	372	56	93
apricot brandy	1 oz	96	0	0	0	—	9	—	0	—	—	—	—	—
apricot sour	1 serv	164	tr	0	0	tr	8	—	tr	3	5	49	4	14
aquavit	1 oz	65	0	0	—	0	0	0	0	—	—	—	—	0
b 52	1 serv	247	4	2	0	1	25	—	0	—	24	7	—	—
b&b	1 serv	75	0	0	0	0	0	0	0	—	tr	—	—	—
bahama breeze	1 serv	70	tr	0	0	tr	9	—	tr	3	2	34	5	6
bahama mama	1 serv	153	tr	tr	0	1	23	—	tr	23	2	207	33	27
bailey's & amaretto	1 serv	184	5	3	0	1	16	—	0	—	29	0	—	—
banana colada	1 serv	376	1	tr	0	2	64	—	3	49	4	736	77	36
bay breeze	1 serv	173	tr	tr	0	1	18	—	tr	17	2	302	19	73
bend me over	1 serv	242	tr	tr	0	1	32	—	tr	18	33	319	47	78
benedictine	1 oz	104	0	0	0	—	11	—	0	—	—	—	—	—
betsy ross	1 serv	206	0	0	0	tr	5	—	0	2	3	44	1	—
black devil	1 serv	220	tr	tr	0	tr	1	—	tr	5	43	6	—	2
black russian	1 serv	184	tr	tr	0	0	12	—	0	—	3	8	—	—
bloody mary	1 serv	150	tr	tr	0	1	5	—	1	11	332	195	21	32
blue whale	1 serv	222	tr	0	0	tr	23	—	0	1	63	18	—	2
bourbon & soda	1 serv (4 oz)	105	0	0	0	0	0	0	0	4	16	2	0	0
bourbon sour	1 serv	166	tr	0	0	tr	8	—	tr	3	5	49	4	14
brandy	2 oz	255	—	—	—	—	—	—	—	—	—	—	—	—
brandy alexander	1 serv	266	6	4	20	1	12	—	0	29	17	48	—	tr
brandy sour	1 serv	164	tr	0	0	tr	8	—	tr	4	5	49	4	14
bushwacker	1 serv	286	5	2	0	tr	27	—	tr	tr	23	18	3	tr
campari	2 oz	245	—	—	—	—	—	—	—	—	—	—	—	—
cherry heering	2 oz	245	—	—	—	—	—	—	—	—	—	—	—	—
coffee liqueur	1 serv (1.5 oz)	175	tr	tr	0	tr	24	24	0	1	4	16	0	0
cognac	1 oz	67	0	0	0	0	tr	0	0	—	—	—	—	0
cosmopolitan martini	1 serv	126	tr	0	0	tr	7	—	tr	2	1	18	1	7
creme de almonde	1 oz	102	—	—	—	—	—	—	—	—	—	—	—	—
creme de banana	1 oz	99	—	—	—	—	—	—	—	—	—	—	—	—
creme de cassis	1 oz	82	—	—	—	—	—	—	—	—	—	—	—	—
creme de menthe	1 serv (1.5 oz)	186	tr	tr	0	0	21	21	0	0	3	0	0	0
curacao liqueur	1 oz	81	0	0	0	—	9	—	0	—	—	—	—	—
daiquiri	1 serv (2 oz)	112	tr	tr	0	tr	4	3	tr	2	3	13	1	1
daiquiri banana	1 serv	277	tr	tr	0	1	32	—	1	4	7	235	11	5
daiquiri frozen	1 serv	393	2	—	—	—	—	—	—	—	—	—	—	—
daiquiri frozen pineapple	1 serv	186	tr	tr	0	1	28	—	2	21	3	365	37	123
dark & stormy	1 serv	64	0	0	0	0	0	0	0	—	tr	1	—	—
doctor pepper	1 serv	95	0	0	0	0	12	—	0	1	1	tr	—	—
drambuie	2 oz	225	—	—	—	—	—	—	—	—	—	—	—	—
fuzzy navel	1 serv	247	tr	tr	0	1	10	—	tr	10	2	188	28	47

FOOD	PORTION	CALS	FAT	SAT FAT	CHOL	PROT	CARB	SUGAR	FIBER	CALCI	SOD	POTAS	FOLIC	VIT C
gibson	1 serv (4 oz)	254	—	—	—	—	—	—	—	—	—	—	—	—
gin	1 serv (1.5 oz)	110	0	0	0	0	0	0	0	0	1	0	0	0
gin & tonic	1 serv (7.5 oz)	171	0	0	0	0	16	—	—	4	10	12	1	1
gin ricky	1 serv	114	tr	0	0	tr	1	—	tr	10	38	20	1	5
grasshopper	1 serv	275	5	3	15	1	26	—	0	22	13	38	1	tr
happy hawaiian	1 serv	434	8	5	0	2	60	—	tr	32	50	266	43	20
harvey wallbanger	1 serv	198	tr	tr	0	1	16	—	tr	17	2	311	47	78
head banger	1 serv	165	0	0	0	0	4	—	0	—	tr	1	—	—
hot buttered rum	1 serv (3 oz)	316	12	8	30	tr	4	4	tr	10	8	10	3	0
hot toddy	1 serv	188	1	tr	0	tr	13	—	5	102	9	33	5	4
hurricane	1 serv	205	tr	0	0	tr	19	—	tr	3	2	43	7	9
kamikaze	1 serv	136	0	0	0	0	2	—	0	—	2	1	—	—
long island iced tea	1 serv	292	tr	0	0	tr	7	—	0	1	33	10	—	1
lynchburg lemonade	1 serv	465	tr	tr	0	tr	85	—	1	11	38	107	15	27
mai tai	1 serv	165	tr	tr	0	tr	17	—	tr	2	51	24	—	1
manhattan	1 serv	171	tr	0	0	tr	3	—	tr	2	9	16	—	—
margarita	1 serv	173	0	0	0	0	11	—	0	—	3	—	—	—
margarita strawberry	1 serv	106	tr	tr	0	tr	11	—	1	11	1	128	13	41
martini	1 serv (3 oz)	206	0	0	0	tr	2	tr	0	1	3	14	0	0
martini apple	1 serv	147	tr	tr	0	tr	4	—	tr	2	2	38	tr	tr
martini rum	1 serv	131	0	0	0	tr	tr	—	tr	1	1	3	—	1
mellow yellow	1 serv	95	0	0	0	0	4	—	0	—	0	0	—	—
mexican grasshopper	1 serv	638	19	12	66	1	52	—	0	42	29	79	2	tr
mint julep	1 serv	136	tr	tr	0	tr	17	—	tr	8	3	19	4	1
mississippi mud	1 serv	496	12	7	45	3	46	—	0	87	46	132	4	1
mudslide	1 serv	566	10	6	0	2	46	—	0	—	65	20	—	—
narragansett	1 serv	168	0	0	0	0	2	—	0	1	5	6	—	—
nutcracker	1 serv	730	10	6	0	2	64	—	0	—	65	20	—	—
old fashioned	1 serv	223	tr	0	0	tr	4	—	tr	1	5	12	—	—
orange crush	1 serv	461	tr	tr	0	0	65	—	tr	8	5	46	1	90
pain killer	1 serv	277	tr	tr	0	1	20	—	tr	26	5	231	38	29
peppermint pattie	1 serv	344	tr	tr	0	tr	37	—	0	1	7	15	—	—
pina colada	1 serv (4.5 oz)	245	3	2	0	1	32	31	tr	11	8	100	17	7
planter's cocktail	1 serv	105	0	0	0	tr	3	—	tr	1	1	19	2	7
planter's punch	1 serv	233	tr	tr	0	2	34	—	4	79	33	447	67	124
presbyterian	1 serv	170	0	0	0	tr	8	—	tr	8	26	5	tr	1
purple passion	1 serv	215	tr	tr	0	tr	22	—	0	11	14	102	6	23
rob roy	1 serv	171	0	0	0	tr	3	—	tr	3	13	15	tr	1
rum	1 serv (1.5 oz)	97	0	0	0	0	0	0	0	0	0	1	0	0
rum boogie	1 serv	134	tr	0	0	tr	12	—	tr	5	3	12	1	3
rum cola	1 serv	209	tr	0	0	tr	21	—	tr	7	8	19	1	4

FOOD	PORTION	CALS	FAT	SAT FAT	CHOL	PROT	CARB	SUGAR	FIBER	CALCI	SOD	POTAS	FOLIC	VIT C
rum highball	1 serv	170	0	0	0	0	11	—	0	4	9	2	—	—
rum punch	1 serv	448	1	tr	0	1	88	—	1	33	12	300	34	217
rum screwdriver	1 serv	166	tr	tr	0	1	16	—	tr	17	2	311	47	78
rum sour	1 serv	156	tr	0	0	tr	8	—	tr	4	5	49	4	14
rum swizzle	1 serv	187	0	0	0	0	15	—	0	9	44	5	—	—
rusty nail	1 serv	159	0	0	0	0	6	—	0	—	tr	1	—	0
sake	1 serv (1 oz)	39	0	0	0	tr	1	0	0	1	1	7	0	0
salty dog	1 serv	210	tr	tr	0	1	19	—	tr	18	3	304	19	71
scotch & soda	1 serv	104	0	0	0	tr	tr	—	tr	10	38	5	tr	1
sea breeze	1 serv	207	tr	tr	0	tr	19	—	tr	8	3	118	6	57
sex on the beach	1 serv	190	tr	tr	0	tr	18	—	tr	4	2	58	—	34
singapore sling	1 serv (4 oz)	115	—	—	—	—	—	—	—	—	—	—	—	—
slippery nipple	1 serv	142	2	2	0	tr	11	—	0	—	16	5	—	—
sloe gin fizz	1 serv (2.5 oz)	132	0	0	0	0	4	—	0	2	1	35	tr	11
snake bite	1 serv	362	0	0	0	0	22	—	0	—	7	2	—	—
southern comfort	1 serv (1.5 oz)	184	—	—	—	—	—	—	—	—	—	—	—	—
tequila	1 serv (1.5 oz)	117	—	—	—	—	—	—	—	—	—	—	—	—
tequila frozen screwdriver	1 serv	159	tr	tr	0	1	17	—	1	16	2	287	39	84
tequila gimlet	1 serv	150	tr	0	0	tr	6	—	1	7	3	21	2	6
tequila sour	1 serv	156	tr	0	0	tr	8	—	tr	3	5	48	4	14
tequila stinger	1 serv	221	tr	0	0	0	14	—	0	—	2	—	—	—
tequila sunrise	1 serv (6.8 oz)	232	tr	tr	0	1	24	—	0	0	120	21	23	41
tom collins	1 serv (7.5 oz)	121	0	0	0	tr	3	—	—	10	39	18	2	4
vermouth cassis	1 serv	97	tr	0	0	tr	5	—	tr	14	54	31	1	4
vodka	1 serv (1.5 oz)	97	0	0	0	0	0	0	0	0	0	0	0	0
vodka gimlet	1 serv	150	tr	0	0	tr	6	—	1	7	3	21	2	6
vodka sour	1 serv	138	tr	0	0	tr	3	—	tr	1	1	17	1	4
vodka stinger	1 serv	378	tr	tr	0	0	28	—	0	—	4	1	—	—
whiskey	1 serv (1.5 oz)	105	0	0	0	0	tr	—	0	0	0	0	0	0
whiskey sour	1 serv (3.5 oz)	162	tr	tr	0	tr	14	14	0	1	65	19	0	2
white russian	1 serv	290	8	5	31	tr	17	—	0	14	12	27	1	tr
zombie	1 serv	235	tr	tr	0	tr	10	—	tr	8	5	129	19	31
ABSOLUT														
Vodka	1 shot (1.5 oz)	98	0	0	0	—	0	—	—	—	—	—	—	—
BACARDI														
Gold Rum	1 shot (1.5 oz)	98	0	0	0	—	0	—	—	—	—	—	—	—
CAPT. MORGAN'S														
Original Spiced Rum	1 shot (1.5 oz)	86	0	0	0	—	0	—	—	—	—	—	—	—
CROWN ROYAL														
Canadian Whiskey	1 shot (1.5 oz)	96	0	0	0	—	0	—	—	—	—	—	—	—

FOOD	PORTION	CALS	FAT	SAT FAT	CHOL	PROT	CARB	SUGAR	FIBER	CALCI	SOD	POTAS	FOLIC	VIT C
JACK DANIEL'S														
Old No.7 Tennessee Whiskey	1 shot (1.5 oz)	98	0	0	0	—	0	—	—	—	—	—	—	—
JOSE CUERVO														
Gold Tequila	1 shot (1.5 oz)	96	0	0	0	—	0	—	—	—	—	—	—	—
SEAGRAM'S														
Gin	1 shot (1.5 oz)	120	0	0	0	—	0	—	—	—	—	—	—	—
SMIRNOFF														
Vodka	1 shot (1.5 oz)	96	0	0	0	—	0	—	—	—	—	—	—	—

ALE
(*see* BEER AND ALE)

ALFALFA
sprouts	½ cup	40	tr	tr	0	1	1	tr	tr	5	1	13	6	1

ALLIGATOR
cooked	3 oz	126	2	—	57	28	0	0	0	—	66	—	—	—

ALLSPICE
ground	1 tsp	5	tr	tr	0	tr	1	—	tr	13	1	20	1	1

ALMONDS
almond butter w/ salt	2 tbsp	203	19	2	0	5	7	2	1	86	144	243	21	tr
almond butter w/o salt	2 tbsp	203	19	2	0	5	7	—	1	86	4	243	21	tr
almond extract	1 tsp	38	tr	—	0	5	—	—	0	—	—	—	—	—
almond paste	¼ cup	260	16	1	0	5	27	21	3	98	5	178	41	tr
chocolate covered	6 pieces (0.6 oz)	102	8	1	1	3	6	3	2	37	8	107	4	0
dry roasted w/ salt	¼ cup	206	18	1	0	8	7	2	4	92	117	257	11	0
dry roasted w/o salt	¼ cup	206	18	1	0	8	7	2	4	92	0	257	11	0
honey roasted	¼ cup	214	18	2	0	7	10	—	5	95	47	202	12	tr
jordan almonds	6 (0.7 oz)	99	4	tr	0	2	14	13	1	21	3	54	3	0
oil roasted w/ salt	¼ cup	238	22	2	0	8	7	2	4	114	133	274	11	0
oil roasted w/o salt	¼ cup	238	22	2	0	8	7	2	4	114	0	274	11	0
praline	17 pieces (1.4 oz)	210	12	1	0	5	21	17	3	60	45	—	—	0
yogurt covered	6 pieces (0.8 oz)	122	8	3	0	3	10	8	1	46	13	104	4	tr
AMERICAN ALMOND														
Marzipan	2 tbsp	130	5	0	0	2	19	17	1	20	0	—	—	0
ARROWHEAD MILLS														
Organic Almond Butter Creamy	2 tbsp	200	17	2	0	7	6	2	4	80	0	—	—	—
BACK TO NATURE														
California Sea Salt Roasted	1 oz	160	14	1	0	6	6	1	3	80	95	—	—	0

FOOD	PORTION	CALS	FAT	SAT FAT	CHOL	PROT	CARB	SUGAR	FIBER	CALCI	SOD	POTAS	FOLIC	VIT C
BARNEY BUTTER														
Almond Butter Crunchy	2 tbsp (1.1 oz)	180	16	2	0	6	7	3	3	80	80	—	—	0
Almond Butter Smooth	2 tbsp (1.1 oz)	180	15	2	0	6	8	3	3	80	100	—	—	0
DIAMOND														
Slivered	¼ cup (1 oz)	170	15	1	0	7	6	1	3	60	0	—	—	0
EDEN														
Tamari	3 tbsp (1 oz)	160	11	1	0	8	8	—	4	60	65	230	—	—
FISHER														
Roasted & Salted	¼ cup (1 oz)	170	15	1	0	6	5	1	3	80	110	—	—	0
FRITO LAY														
Roasted Salted	3 tbsp (1 oz)	190	16	2	0	6	5	1	3	60	170	—	—	0
GODIVA														
Dark Chocolate Almonds	1 pkg (2 oz)	310	24	7	0	8	23	14	5	80	40	—	—	0
JUSTIN'S														
Almond Butter Classic	2 tbsp (1.1 oz)	200	18	2	0	7	6	1	4	80	0	—	—	0
Almond Butter Maple	2 tbsp (1.1 oz)	190	16	2	0	6	8	4	3	80	65	—	—	0
KETTLE														
Butter Salted	2 tbsp	180	17	2	0	5	6	0	2	80	55	—	—	0
Butter Unsalted	2 tbsp	180	17	2	0	5	6	0	2	80	0	—	—	0
LOVE'N BAKE														
Almond Paste	2 tbsp	140	9	1	0	4	13	11	2	40	0	—	—	0
Almond Schmear	2 tbsp	140	8	0	0	4	14	11	2	40	0	—	—	0
Roasted Butter	2 tbsp	180	16	2	0	6	6	1	3	100	55	—	—	0
MAISIE JANE'S														
Almond Butter	1 oz	184	16	2	0	5	6	0	0	80	4	—	—	0
Cappuccino	9 pieces (1.4 oz)	220	15	6	5	4	19	16	2	100	20	—	—	0
Chocolate Toffee	9 pieces (1.4 oz)	210	13	5	5	4	21	19	2	60	45	—	—	0
Coffee Glazed	2 tbsp (1 oz)	150	12	1	0	4	8	3	3	60	15	—	—	0
Cowboy BBQ	2 tbsp (1 oz)	140	11	0	0	4	8	3	3	80	220	—	—	0
Mint Chocolate	9 pieces (1.4 oz)	210	15	7	0	3	20	17	2	60	20	—	—	0
Organic Honey Glazed	2 tbsp (1 oz)	160	14	1	0	6	12	6	4	80	32	—	—	0
Tamari	2 tbsp (1 oz)	160	14	2	0	5	7	1	4	80	60	—	—	0
MRS. MAY'S														
Almond Crunch	1 oz	156	13	1	0	5	8	3	3	60	37	—	—	0
NATURALLY MORE														
Almond Butter	2 tbsp	190	16	2	0	9	8	2	4	0	65	—	232	0

FOOD	PORTION	CALS	FAT	SAT FAT	CHOL	PROT	CARB	SUGAR	FIBER	CALCI	SOD	POTAS	FOLIC	VIT C
NUT HARVEST														
Lightly Roasted	2 tbsp	180	15	2	0	6	6	1	3	60	150	160	—	0
PLANTERS														
Chocolate Lovers Dark Chocolate	11 pieces (1.4 oz)	220	17	6	5	4	18	13	3	40	15	—	—	0
Flavor Grove Chili Lime	1 oz	170	15	1	0	6	6	2	3	60	160	—	—	0
Flavor Grove Sea Salt & Olive Oil	1 oz	170	15	2	0	6	5	1	3	60	190	—	—	0
NUT-rition Bone Health Mix	¼ cup (1.2 oz)	170	10	3	0	4	19	11	2	100	30	160	—	6
Slivered	1 pkg (2 oz)	330	28	2	0	12	11	3	7	150	0	—	—	0
Smoked	1 pkg (1.5 oz)	250	22	2	0	9	8	2	5	100	370	—	—	0
SUNKIST														
Accents Italian Parmesan	1 tbsp	40	4	0	0	1	1	0	0	20	95	—	—	0
Accents Original Oven Roasted	1 tbsp	40	4	0	0	1	1	0	0	20	70	—	—	0
SUNRIDGE FARMS														
Dark Chocolate Cane Sweetened	11 (1.4 oz)	220	16	7	0	4	19	14	3	40	0	—	—	0
ALOE JUICE														
ALO														
Appeal Aloe Vera + Pomelo Pink Grapefruit & Lemon	8 oz	60	0	0	0	0	15	13	0	30	35	—	—	18
Awaken Aloe Vera + Wheatgrass	8 oz	50	0	0	0	0	15	15	0	40	50	—	—	27
Enliven Aloe Vera + 12 Fruits & Vegetables	8 oz	50	0	0	0	0	13	12	0	40	70	—	—	18
Enrich Aloe Vera + Pomegranate & Cranberry	8 oz	70	0	0	0	0	15	13	0	30	35	—	—	18
Exposed Aloe Vera Original	8 oz	60	0	0	0	0	15	13	0	30	45	—	—	18
TROPIKING														
Aloe Vera Juice	8 oz	88	0	0	0	0	22	21	tr	10	5	—	—	1
Aloe Vera Juice & Grape	8 oz	100	0	0	0	0	25	22	1	40	30	—	—	9
Aloe Vera Juice & Pineapple	8 oz	100	0	0	0	0	25	24	1	20	20	—	—	0
Aloe Vera Juice & Pomegranate	8 oz	120	0	0	0	0	30	24	1	40	130	—	—	0

FOOD	PORTION	CALS	FAT	SAT FAT	CHOL	PROT	CARB	SUGAR	FIBER	CALCI	SOD	POTAS	FOLIC	VIT C
AMARANTH														
leaves cooked	½ cup	14	tr	tr	0	1	3	—	—	138	170	423	38	27
uncooked	½ cup (3.4 oz)	365	6	2	0	14	65	—	15	149	20	357	48	4
ARROWHEAD MILLS														
Organic Whole Grain not prep	¼ cup	180	3	1	0	7	31	1	7	—	10	170	—	2
ANCHOVY														
boneless	1 oz	60	3	1	24	8	0	0	0	66	1042	154	4	0
canned in oil drained	1 can (2 oz)	94	4	1	38	13	0	0	0	104	1651	245	6	0
fresh	1 (4 g)	8	tr	tr	3	1	0	0	0	9	147	22	1	0
fresh fillets	3 (0.4 oz)	21	1	—	—	2	tr	—	—	20	—	—	—	0
ARROYABE														
In Olive Oil	1 oz	60	3	1	25	9	0	0	0	60	1370	—	—	0
POLAR														
Rolled Fillets w/ Capers In Olive Oil	7 pieces (0.6 oz)	40	3	0	15	4	0	0	0	40	970	—	—	0
ANGLERFISH														
raw	3.5 oz	72	1	—	—	15	0	0	0	—	109	235	—	—
ANISE														
seed	1 tsp	7	tr	tr	0	tr	1	—	tr	14	0	30	0	tr
ANTELOPE														
roasted	4 oz	215	4	2	127	41	0	0	0	7	304	353	12	0
APPLE														
CANNED														
sliced sweetened	½ cup	68	1	tr	0	tr	17	15	2	4	3	69	0	tr
DOLE														
Squish'ems	1 pkg	80	0	0	0	0	18	17	1	0	0	135	—	60
GLORY														
Fried Apples	½ cup	80	0	0	0	0	21	11	1	0	170	—	—	0
JAKE & AMOS														
Red Spiced Rings	1 (1 oz)	35	0	0	0	0	9	8	0	0	5	—	—	0
POLAR														
Fuji	½ cup	50	0	0	0	0	12	11	2	—	20	—	—	0
DRIED														
chopped	½ cup	104	tr	tr	0	tr	28	24	4	6	37	192	0	1
cooked w/o sugar	½ cup	73	tr	tr	0	tr	20	17	3	4	26	134	0	1
rings	5	78	tr	tr	0	tr	21	18	3	4	28	144	0	1
BARE FRUIT														
Chips Cinnamon	1 pkg (0.6 oz)	43	0	0	0	0	12	10	2	0	15	—	—	1
CHUKAR CHERRIES														
Cherry Apple Slices	10 (1 oz)	110	0	0	0	0	28	24	4	0	0	—	—	0

FOOD	PORTION	CALS	FAT	SAT FAT	CHOL	PROT	CARB	SUGAR	FIBER	CALCI	SOD	POTAS	FOLIC	VIT C
DEL MONTE														
Dried Apples	¼ cup (1.4 oz)	110	0	0	0	1	27	19	3	0	270	190	—	1
FRUIT RIPPLES														
Cinnamon Apple	1 pkg	50	0	0	0	0	13	10	1	—	75	—	—	—
Strawberry Apple	1 pkg	50	0	0	0	0	13	10	1	—	75	—	—	—
MOTT'S														
Snacks Freeze Dried	1 pkg (0.55 oz)	60	0	0	0	0	15	11	3	—	0	—	—	5
MRS. MAY'S														
Fruit Chips	1 pkg	35	0	0	0	0	8	7	1	0	0	—	—	8
NATURE'S ENVY														
Apple Chips Original	1 pkg (0.8 oz)	80	0	0	0	0	20	17	tr	0	20	—	—	0
STONERIDGE ORCHARDS														
Green Wedges	⅓ cup (1.4 oz)	140	0	0	0	0	32	27	1	0	0	—	—	12
SUN-MAID														
Apples	¼ cup (1.4 oz)	120	0	0	0	1	29	22	2	0	135	240	—	1
FRESH														
apple	1 lg	110	tr	tr	0	1	29	22	5	13	2	227	6	10
apple	1 med	72	tr	tr	0	tr	19	14	3	8	1	148	4	6
apple	1 sm	55	tr	tr	0	tr	15	11	3	6	1	113	3	5
candied	1 med (6.5 oz)	234	4	3	0	2	52	42	4	66	103	241	6	7
candied	1 lg (9.8 oz)	357	6	4	6	3	79	64	6	101	157	368	8	10
candied	1 sm (4.9 oz)	179	3	2	0	2	40	32	3	51	79	185	4	5
w/ skin sliced	1 cup	57	tr	tr	0	tr	15	11	3	7	1	118	3	5
w/o skin sliced	1 cup	53	tr	tr	0	tr	14	11	1	6	0	99	0	4
CHIQUITA														
Apple	1 (6.4 oz)	95	0	0	0	0	25	19	4	10	2	134	—	9
Apple Bites w/ Caramel	1 pkg (2.5 oz)	70	0	0	0	0	17	13	2	40	55	—	—	15
Apple Slices	1 pkg (2.2 oz)	30	0	0	0	0	8	5	2	20	0	—	—	15
CRUNCH PAK														
Foodles Apples w/ Raisins & Peanut Butter	1 pkg (5 oz)	260	11	2	35	6	35	24	4	80	105	—	—	132
Grab And Go Apples w/ Peanut Butter	1 pkg	220	14	3	0	7	21	13	4	80	135	—	—	144
Grab And Go Apples w/ Grapes	1 pkg	80	0	0	0	0	19	15	2	60	0	—	—	132
Party Tray Apple-tizer Grand Crunch & Munch	¹⁄₁₀ pkg	150	6	3	15	4	20	12	2	100	240	—	—	48

FOOD	PORTION	CALS	FAT	SAT FAT	CHOL	PROT	CARB	SUGAR	FIBER	CALCI	SOD	POTAS	FOLIC	VIT C
CRUNCH PAK (CONT.)														
Snackers Apples w/ Caramel Dip & Cheese	1 pkg (4.7 oz)	230	11	6	30	7	24	14	2	250	210	—	—	114
Snackers Apples w/ Caramel Dip & Chocolate	1 pkg (4.7 oz)	260	10	5	<5	2	42	31	2	100	50	—	—	114
Snackers Apples w/ Pretzels & Cheese	1 pkg (4.7 oz)	240	10	6	30	8	29	9	2	250	430	—	—	114
Snackers Apples w/ Raisins & Pretzels	1 pkg (4.7 oz)	210	2	0	0	2	51	23	3	60	290	—	—	114
Snackers Apples w/ Grapes & Caramel	1 pkg (4.7 oz)	140	2	0	0	0	29	19	1	60	35	—	—	114
Sweet Apples w/ Yogurt Dip	⅕ pkg	70	0	0	0	0	16	9	1	40	20	—	—	78
DOLE														
Apple	1 med (5.4 oz)	80	0	0	0	0	22	16	4	0	0	—	—	6
EARTHBOUND FARMS														
Organic Slices	1 pkg (2 oz)	30	0	0	0	0	7	5	1	40	0	—	—	78
EASTERN SELECT														
Gala	1 (5.5 oz)	80	0	0	0	0	22	16	5	0	0	170	—	5
GRAPPLE														
Grape Flavored	1 med (6.4 oz)	95	0	0	0	0	25	19	4	10	0	—	—	8
MRS. PRINDABLE'S														
Caramel Triple Chocolate	¼ apple (1.7 oz)	120	6	4	5	1	17	15	1	20	10	—	—	1
Caramel Walnut	¼ apple (2 oz)	160	10	4	5	2	17	15	1	40	15	—	—	1
READY PAC														
Apples w/ Caramel Dip	1 pkg (6 oz)	200	0	0	0	2	52	34	2	40	200	—	—	6
Apples w/ Peanut Butter Dip	1 pkg (5.7 oz)	340	24	5	0	12	28	17	6	40	230	—	—	5
SULLIVAN														
McIntosh	1 (5.4 oz)	80	1	—	0	0	22	20	4	0	0	160	—	4
FROZEN														
sliced w/o sugar	½ cup	42	tr	tr	0	tr	11	—	2	3	3	67	1	tr
REFRIGERATED														
COUNTRY CROCK														
Cinnamon Apples	½ cup (4.4 oz)	130	3	0	0	0	26	22	1	0	200	—	—	1
DOLE														
Fruit Crisp Apple Cinnamon	1 pkg (4 oz)	160	4	0	0	1	29	20	3	0	20	70	—	24
Parfait Apples & Creme	1 pkg (4.3 oz)	130	3	2	0	0	26	20	1	0	10	40	—	15

FOOD	PORTION	CALS	FAT	SAT FAT	CHOL	PROT	CARB	SUGAR	FIBER	CALCI	SOD	POTAS	FOLIC	VIT C
TAKE-OUT														
baked no sugar added	1 (5.6 oz)	90	tr	tr	0	tr	24	18	4	10	2	167	3	6
baked w/ sugar	1 (6 oz)	162	tr	tr	0	tr	42	37	4	10	2	159	3	6
fried apple rings	1 serv (2.7 oz)	91	4	1	0	tr	15	12	2	5	33	73	2	2
scalloped	½ cup (3.3 oz)	90	tr	tr	0	tr	24	20	2	6	1	88	2	3

APPLE JUICE

FOOD	PORTION	CALS	FAT	SAT FAT	CHOL	PROT	CARB	SUGAR	FIBER	CALCI	SOD	POTAS	FOLIC	VIT C
cider	1 cup	117	tr	tr	0	tr	29	27	tr	17	7	295	0	2
juice + vitamin C & calcium	1 cup	117	tr	tr	0	tr	29	27	tr	278	17	312	0	86
mulled cider	1 serv	265	1	tr	0	1	42	—	6	129	12	409	18	37
unsweetened w/o vitamin C	1 cup	117	tr	tr	0	tr	29	27	tr	17	7	295	0	2
AFTER THE FALL														
Organic	8 oz	90	0	0	0	0	22	18	—	0	20	240	—	0
APPLE & EVE														
100% Juice	8 oz	110	0	0	0	1	26	22	—	—	5	—	—	60
BACK TO NATURE														
100% Juice	1 pkg (6 oz)	80	0	0	0	0	21	20	—	—	25	—	—	—
FIZZ ED.														
Green Apple	1 can (8.4 oz)	100	0	0	0	0	25	21	1	—	30	—	—	4
HOOD														
100% Juice	1 cup	120	0	0	0	0	31	31	0	0	5	—	—	72
KEDEM														
100% Juice	8 oz	100	0	0	0	0	24	21	—	—	35	—	—	—
LAND O LAKES														
Juice	1 cup (8 oz)	120	0	0	0	0	29	26	0	20	45	—	—	60
LANGERS														
Diet Cocktail 50% Juice	8 oz	60	0	0	0	0	14	13	—	150	10	95	—	60
MOTT'S														
100% Natural	1 bottle (14 oz)	200	0	0	0	1	48	48	0	40	35	420	—	60
NANTUCKET NECTARS														
100% Juice Pressed Apple	8 oz	120	0	0	0	0	30	26	tr	0	15	—	—	0
Organic Cloudy Apple	8 oz	120	0	0	0	0	29	28	0	0	30	—	—	60
OCEAN SPRAY														
Juice	8 oz	100	0	0	0	0	28	28	—	0	35	240	—	0
OLD ORCHARD														
100% Juice Apple Cider	8 oz	130	0	0	0	0	31	29	—	0	25	280	—	72
R.W. KNUDSEN														
Organic 100% Juice	8 oz	120	0	0	0	tr	30	30	0	100	25	180	—	60

FOOD	PORTION	CALS	FAT	SAT FAT	CHOL	PROT	CARB	SUGAR	FIBER	CALCI	SOD	POTAS	FOLIC	VIT C
SANTA CRUZ														
Organic	8 oz	120	0	0	0	tr	30	30	0	—	25	180	—	5
SMART JUICE														
Organic 100% Juice	8 oz	117	0	0	0	tr	29	27	tr	20	7	295	—	103
SNAPPLE														
100% Juice Green Apple	8 oz	160	0	0	0	0	41	39	—	150	20	310	—	60
Juice Drink Apple	8 oz	110	0	0	0	0	27	27	—	—	5	—	—	—
TASTEE														
Cider 100% Juice	8 oz	120	0	0	0	0	30	30	—	—	60	—	—	4
TREE RIPE														
Organic 100% Juice	6 oz	80	0	0	0	0	21	19	0	20	10	—	0	2
TROPICANA														
Orchard Style	1 bottle (14 oz)	200	0	0	0	tr	50	48	0	0	20	500	—	60
Trop50 Farmstand Apple	8 oz	50	0	0	0	0	12	12	0	0	15	0	—	60
WALNUT ACRES														
Organic Juice	8 oz	110	0	0	0	0	29	27	0	60	0	—	—	—
APPLESAUCE														
sweetened	½ cup	97	tr	tr	0	tr	25	21	2	5	4	78	1	2
unsweetened	½ cup	52	tr	tr	0	tr	14	12	2	4	2	92	1	2
BETH'S FARM KITCHEN														
Chunky	2 tbsp (1 oz)	50	0	0	0	tr	14	11	1	20	0	—	—	2
EDEN														
Organic Apple Cherry	½ cup	70	0	0	0	0	17	12	3	0	10	130	—	0
Organic Apple Strawberry	½ cup	60	0	0	0	0	13	10	2	0	10	105	—	0
GOGO SQUEEZE														
Apple	1 pkg (3.2 oz)	60	1	0	0	0	14	13	1	0	3	—	—	0
Apple Banana	1 pkg (3.2 oz)	60	tr	0	0	0	14	11	1	0	3	—	—	0
Apple Cinnamon	1 pkg (3.2 oz)	50	tr	0	0	0	10	9	1	0	3	—	—	0
Apple Peach	1 pkg (3.2 oz)	60	tr	0	0	0	13	12	1	0	3	—	—	0
MOTT'S														
Healthy Harvest Granny Smith No Sugar Added	1 pkg (3.9 oz)	50	0	0	0	0	13	11	1	—	0	70	—	15
Organic Original	½ cup (4.5 oz)	110	0	0	0	0	27	25	1	—	0	100	—	1
Organic Unsweetened	½ cup (4.3 oz)	50	0	0	0	0	14	—	1	—	0	100	—	1
Single-Serve Cinnamon	1 pkg (4 oz)	100	0	0	0	0	25	23	1	—	0	—	—	12
MUSSELMAN'S														
Unsweetened	1 pkg (4 oz)	50	0	0	0	0	12	8	2	0	20	—	—	0

FOOD	PORTION	CALS	FAT	SAT FAT	CHOL	PROT	CARB	SUGAR	FIBER	CALCI	SOD	POTAS	FOLIC	VIT C
REVOLUTION FOODS														
Organic Unsweetened	1 pkg (4 oz)	50	0	0	0	0	13	10	2	0	5	—	—	1
SANTA CRUZ														
Organic	½ cup (4.5 oz)	60	0	0	0	0	13	11	2	—	20	75	—	18
Organic Apple Apricot	1 pkg (4 oz)	60	0	0	0	0	14	11	2	—	17	65	—	60
Organic Apple Blueberry	1 pkg (4 oz)	60	0	0	0	0	14	11	2	—	17	65	—	60
Organic Apple Cherry	½ cup (4.5 oz)	60	0	0	0	0	15	12	2	—	20	75	—	18

APRICOT JUICE

FOOD	PORTION	CALS	FAT	SAT FAT	CHOL	PROT	CARB	SUGAR	FIBER	CALCI	SOD	POTAS	FOLIC	VIT C
nectar	6 oz	106	tr	tr	0	1	27	26	1	13	6	215	2	1
CERES														
100% Juice	8 oz	130	0	0	0	0	32	28	0	0	15	250	—	60
SANTA CRUZ														
Organic Nectar	8 oz	120	0	0	0	0	29	27	tr	20	35	320	—	6

APRICOTS

FOOD	PORTION	CALS	FAT	SAT FAT	CHOL	PROT	CARB	SUGAR	FIBER	CALCI	SOD	POTAS	FOLIC	VIT C
canned heavy syrup	½ cup	91	tr	tr	0	1	23	20	3	11	4	157	2	3
canned in juice	½ cup	59	tr	tr	0	1	15	13	2	15	5	201	2	6
canned in water	½ cup	33	tr	tr	0	1	8	6	2	10	4	233	2	4
canned light syrup	½ cup	80	tr	tr	0	1	21	19	2	14	5	175	3	3
dried halves	6	51	tr	tr	0	1	13	11	2	12	2	244	2	tr
dried halves cooked w/o sugar	½ cup	106	tr	tr	0	2	28	24	3	24	5	514	4	tr
fresh	1	17	tr	tr	0	tr	4	3	1	5	0	91	3	4
fresh sliced	½ cup	40	tr	tr	0	1	9	8	2	11	1	214	7	8
frozen sweetened	½ cup	119	tr	tr	0	1	30	—	3	12	5	277	2	11
DEL MONTE														
Halves In Heavy Syrup	½ cup (4.5 oz)	100	0	0	0	0	26	25	1	0	10	—	—	5
DOLE														
Fresh	3 (4 oz)	60	1	0	0	0	11	11	1	20	0	—	—	10
ELIZABETH'S NATURAL														
Turkish Dried	5 (1.8 oz)	90	0	0	0	1	22	19	3	40	10	—	—	0
HARVEST BAY														
Dried	5 (1.4 oz)	60	0	0	0	2	15	15	3	40	6	552	—	tr
MARIANI														
Ultimate Dried	¼ cup (1.4 oz)	100	0	0	0	1	24	16	6	20	10	400	—	1
S&W														
Whole In Heavy Syrup	½ cup (4.5 oz)	120	0	0	0	tr	29	28	1	0	10	—	—	1
SUNSWEET														
Dried	¼ cup (1.4 oz)	130	0	0	0	0	36	26	3	20	25	420	—	0

FOOD	PORTION	CALS	FAT	SAT FAT	CHOL	PROT	CARB	SUGAR	FIBER	CALCI	SOD	POTAS	FOLIC	VIT C
ARROWHEAD														
corm boiled	1 med	9	tr	—	0	1	2	—	—	1	2	106	1	0
ARROWROOT														
raw	1 root (1.2 oz)	21	tr	tr	0	1	4	—	tr	2	9	150	112	1
raw root sliced	1 cup	78	tr	tr	0	5	16	—	2	7	31	545	406	2
BOB'S RED MILL														
Starch	¼ cup	110	0	0	0	0	28	0	1	—	0	—	—	—
ARTICHOKE														
CANNED														
hearts in oil	1 serv (3 oz)	100	7	1	0	3	9	1	4	34	73	273	39	8
CENTO														
Hearts Quartered Marinated	2 pieces	20	2	0	0	0	2	—	—	—	80	—	—	6
GERTIE'S FINEST														
Tapenade	2 tbsp	29	3	tr	0	1	2	tr	tr	15	210	—	—	1
NATIVE FOREST														
Organic Hearts Quartered	1 serv (4 oz)	35	0	0	0	2	6	1	4	40	390	—	—	2
POLAR														
Hearts	2	18	0	0	0	2	3	0	2	20	480	—	—	1
Hearts Quartered Marinated	1 oz	25	2	0	0	1	5	0	1	20	90	—	—	2
PROGRESSO														
Hearts	2	30	0	0	0	1	7	2	2	0	400	—	—	2
Hearts Marinated	2 (1.1 oz)	60	5	1	0	0	2	7	0	—	110	—	—	4
REESE														
Cocktail Artichokes Original	½ jar (5 oz)	50	0	0	0	3	9	2	2	40	420	—	—	12
ROLAND														
Hearts	½ cup (4.6 oz)	50	0	0	0	3	9	1	4	40	380	—	—	5
THE GRACIOUS GOURMET														
Artichoke Parmesan Tapenade	2 tbsp (1 oz)	30	2	0	0	1	3	0	tr	20	150	—	—	4
FRESH														
cooked	1 med	60	tr	tr	0	4	13	1	7	54	114	425	61	12
hearts cooked	½ cup	42	tr	tr	0	3	9	1	5	38	80	297	43	8
OCEAN MIST														
Lemon	1 (4.2 oz)	60	0	0	0	4	13	1	6	60	115	—	—	12
FROZEN														
cooked	1 cup	42	tr	tr	0	3	9	1	5	38	80	297	43	8
cooked w/o salt	1 pkg (9 oz)	108	1	0	0	7	22	2	11	50	127	634	286	12
C&W														
Hearts	12 pieces (3 oz)	40	1	0	0	2	7	1	5	40	55	—	—	6

FOOD	PORTION	CALS	FAT	SAT FAT	CHOL	PROT	CARB	SUGAR	FIBER	CALCI	SOD	POTAS	FOLIC	VIT C
TAKE-OUT														
stuffed	1 (8.8 oz)	397	14	3	8	15	54	6	10	259	1037	622	113	17

ASIAN FOOD

(*see also* CURRY, DINNER, EGG ROLLS, SAUCE, SOY SAUCE, SUSHI)

FOOD	PORTION	CALS	FAT	SAT FAT	CHOL	PROT	CARB	SUGAR	FIBER	CALCI	SOD	POTAS	FOLIC	VIT C
CANNED														
chow mein chicken w/o noodles	1 cup	194	8	2	51	20	10	6	2	37	955	403	53	9
LA CHOY														
Chow Mein Beef	1 cup	90	2	1	15	8	11	2	2	40	880	—	—	15
Chow Mein Chicken	1 cup (9.3 oz)	100	3	1	20	8	10	3	2	20	1210	—	—	0
Sweet & Sour Noodles	1 cup	150	2	1	20	6	29	23	5	20	790	—	—	12
Teriyaki Chicken	1 cup (8.6 oz)	120	4	2	20	7	16	7	3	20	1370	—	—	9
FRESH														
wonton wrapper	1 (0.3 oz)	23	tr	tr	1	1	5	—	tr	4	46	7	7	0
NASOYA														
Won Ton Wraps	8 (2.1 oz)	160	1	0	10	6	31	1	1	20	370	—	—	0
FROZEN														
AMY'S														
Asian Noodle Stir Fry	1 pkg	290	7	1	0	9	50	16	4	100	630	—	—	30
Indian Mattar Paneer	1 pkg (10 oz)	320	8	2	5	11	54	8	6	100	780	—	—	18
Indian Palak Paneer	1 pkg (9.9 oz)	270	9	3	5	10	38	5	5	150	680	—	—	15
Indian Paneer Tikka	1 pkg (9.4 oz)	320	18	7	20	8	36	6	5	200	550	—	—	12
Indian Vegetable Korma	1 pkg (9.4 oz)	310	12	4	0	9	41	7	7	60	680	—	—	18
Thai Stir Fry	1 pkg (9.4 oz)	310	11	7	0	8	45	2	5	40	420	—	—	27
CONTESSA														
Chow Mein Chicken w/ Sauce not prep	1¾ cups	320	3	1	25	16	55	10	3	40	1060	—	—	30
Curry Chicken w/ Sauce not prep	1¾ cups	240	8	4	25	12	29	4	2	40	330	—	—	9
Fried Rice Chicken w/ Sauce not prep	1¾ cups	260	4	1	100	17	49	5	4	20	680	—	—	12
General Tsao Shrimp w/ Sauce not prep	1¾ cups	270	4	1	35	10	49	17	4	40	930	—	—	42
Kung Pao Shrimp w/ Sauce not prep	1¾ cups	200	4	1	45	10	30	4	3	60	760	—	—	9
Lo Mein Shrimp w/ Sauce not prep	1¾ cups	250	10	2	35	11	29	11	2	40	830	—	—	15

FOOD	PORTION	CALS	FAT	SAT FAT	CHOL	PROT	CARB	SUGAR	FIBER	CALCI	SOD	POTAS	FOLIC	VIT C
CONTESSA (CONT.)														
Stir-Fry Beef w/ Sauce not prep	1¾ cup	190	3	1	20	13	28	17	4	60	820	—	—	36
Stir-Fry Chicken w/ Sauce not prep	1¾ cups	160	3	1	25	16	18	14	4	60	870	—	—	4
Stir-Fry Shrimp w/ Sauce not prep	1¾ cups	120	3	1	40	9	16	12	2	60	980	—	—	1
Sweet & Sour Shrimp w/ Sauce not prep	1½ cups	180	0	0	50	9	40	12	3	40	430	—	—	21
Tandoori Chicken w/ Sauce not prep	1⅓ cups	200	4	1	30	15	27	2	3	40	660	—	—	12
CRAZY CUIZINE														
Korean Inspired BBQ Chicken	¼ pkg (5 oz)	240	10	2	55	21	16	16	0	0	820	—	—	0
Mandarin Orange Chicken	1 cup (5 oz)	260	7	1	30	13	35	14	0	20	500	—	—	1
Tangerine Beef	1 cup (5 oz)	360	18	6	30	13	38	18	1	0	550	—	—	0
ETHNIC GOURMET														
Bhartha Eggplant	1 pkg (11 oz)	300	9	2	0	8	47	2	10	150	650	—	—	24
Dal Bahaar	1 pkg (11 oz)	360	8	1	0	13	61	5	8	100	500	—	—	0
Kaeng Kari Kai	1 pkg (10 oz)	390	11	4	35	20	54	13	2	40	770	—	—	12
Korma Chicken	1 pkg (10 oz)	340	9	1	40	21	44	4	3	60	720	—	—	12
Korma Vegetable	1 pkg (11 oz)	300	6	1	0	8	52	5	4	60	680	—	—	30
Pad Thai Chicken	1 pkg (10 oz)	410	7	1	25	20	66	22	3	40	830	—	—	12
Pad Thai Shrimp	1 pkg (10 oz)	410	7	1	55	17	70	24	3	60	850	—	—	9
Tandoori Chicken w/ Spinach	1 pkg (10 oz)	170	5	1	30	14	19	4	3	80	840	—	—	12
FRENCH MEADOW BAKERY														
Vegetarian Dal Makhani	1 pkg (12 oz)	370	19	7	20	8	39	2	5	80	340	—	—	9
GLUTINO														
Gluten Free Chicken Pad Thai Peach	1 pkg (7 oz)	370	5	1	75	17	65	10	3	60	890	—	—	2
HEALTHY CHOICE														
Sweet & Sour Chicken	1 pkg (11.9 oz)	420	9	2	20	14	71	25	6	40	480	490	200	6
HELEN'S KITCHEN														
Thai Yellow Curry w/ Tofu Steaks & Vegetables & Basmati Rice	1 pkg (9 oz)	280	5	1	0	12	30	1	2	300	390	—	—	15
JOY OF COOKING														
Lo Mein Vegetable	1 cup (7.7 oz)	220	3	0	15	9	40	6	11	—	870	—	—	—
KAHIKI														
Beef & Broccoli	1 pkg (10.9 oz)	360	10	4	50	23	42	4	2	20	1060	—	—	9

FOOD	PORTION	CALS	FAT	SAT FAT	CHOL	PROT	CARB	SUGAR	FIBER	CALCI	SOD	POTAS	FOLIC	VIT C
KAHIKI (CONT.)														
Chicken Fried Rice	1 pkg (10.9 oz)	460	10	2	85	16	75	2	2	40	1090	—	—	1
General Tso's Chicken	1 pkg (10 oz)	400	10	2	20	12	66	23	2	40	1340	—	—	2
Naturals General Tso's Chicken	1 pkg (10 oz)	330	5	1	35	18	52	24	3	60	1080	—	—	9
Naturals Mandarin Orange Chicken	1 pkg (10 oz)	340	5	1	35	17	58	31	3	40	750	—	—	9
Naturals Szechuan Peppercorn Beef	1 pkg (10 oz)	350	14	5	50	19	35	9	3	40	780	—	—	30
Naturals Teriyaki Mixed Vegetables	1 pkg (10 oz)	260	2	0	0	8	51	18	4	100	750	—	—	9
Sesame Orange Chicken	1 pkg (10.9 oz)	420	12	2	25	15	60	15	2	60	1390	—	—	5
Soothing Lettuce Wraps	4 tbsp (2 oz)	90	4	1	10	5	9	2	1	20	310	—	—	1
Tempura Chicken Nuggets	¾ cup (3.5 oz)	230	14	3	40	13	10	0	0	20	470	—	—	0
Tropical Sweet & Sour Chicken	1 pkg (10.9 oz)	490	11	2	25	14	82	36	4	60	910	—	—	24
LEAN CUISINE														
Cafe Cuisine Chow Fun Beef	1 pkg (9 oz)	320	5	2	20	15	54	18	3	60	520	300	—	6
Cafe Cuisine Sweet & Sour Chicken	1 pkg (10 oz)	300	3	1	30	18	51	16	2	20	490	700	—	27
Cafe Cuisine Thai-Style Chicken	1 pkg (9 oz)	260	4	1	35	21	35	9	0	150	540	750	—	21
Simple Favorites Chicken Chow Mein	1 pkg (9 oz)	240	4	1	25	13	39	3	3	40	550	380	—	4
ORGANIC CLASSICS														
Thai Chicken Curry	1 pkg (10 oz)	420	17	6	40	19	50	4	3	40	510	—	—	36
PURELY ASIAN BRAND														
Broccoli Beef	½ pkg (11 oz)	400	22	5	20	20	32	8	8	80	1390	—	—	18
Mandarin Orange Chicken	½ pkg (12 oz)	450	10	3	35	18	73	47	7	250	1010	—	—	18
Sweet & Sour Chicken	½ pkg (12 oz)	380	11	4	25	13	58	39	5	150	570	—	—	4
SEEDS OF CHANGE														
Asian Stir-Fry Noodles	1 pkg (11 oz)	290	4	1	5	11	55	14	4	40	720	—	—	12
Spicy Peanut Noodles	1 pkg (11 oz)	370	12	5	5	15	53	6	4	100	650	—	—	9

FOOD	PORTION	CALS	FAT	SAT FAT	CHOL	PROT	CARB	SUGAR	FIBER	CALCI	SOD	POTAS	FOLIC	VIT C
SEEDS OF CHANGE (CONT.)														
Teriyaki Stir Fried Rice	1 pkg (11 oz)	340	8	1	5	10	56	15	6	100	650	—	—	9
TANDOOR CHEF														
Chicken Tikka Masala	1 pkg (9.9 oz)	330	22	8	85	21	10	4	1	40	770	—	—	6
TYSON														
Meal Kit Chicken Fried Rice	2½ cups	440	6	2	30	27	69	15	5	40	1810	—	—	0
WEIGHT WATCHERS														
Chicken Teriyaki Stir Fry	1 pkg (11.8 oz)	340	6	1	45	25	49	13	5	60	600	—	—	9
MIX														
ANNIE CHUN'S														
Meal Kit Chow Mein Noodles w/ Peanut Sesame Sauce	⅓ pkg	270	7	1	0	9	42	8	2	0	600	—	—	2
Meal Kit Chow Mein Noodles w/ Teriyaki Sauce	⅓ box	210	1	0	0	8	43	8	2	20	870	—	—	0
Meal Kit Pad Thai Noodles w/ Pad Thai Sauce	⅓ pkg	210	1	0	0	3	48	8	—	0	570	—	—	1
NISSIN														
Chow Mein Chicken as prep	½ pkg (2 oz)	240	9	5	0	6	34	5	2	40	660	—	—	4
Chow Mein Thai Peanut as prep	½ pkg (2 oz)	270	12	4	0	6	35	3	tr	0	780	—	—	0
SHELF-STABLE														
DR. MCDOUGALL'S														
Asian Entree Pad Thai Noodle Gluten Free as prep	1 pkg (2 oz)	200	2	0	0	5	42	2	2	0	480	—	—	1
Asian Entree Spicy Kung Pao Noodle as prep	1 pkg (2 oz)	220	2	0	0	8	42	5	2	20	480	—	—	4
Asian Entree Teriyaki Noodle as prep	1 pkg (2 oz)	200	1	0	0	7	43	8	3	20	480	—	—	1
Asian Entree Thai Peanut Noodles as prep	1 pkg (2 oz)	220	3	0	0	8	40	4	4	20	480	—	—	2
FANTASTIC														
Pad Thai w/ Rice Noodles	1 pkg (7 oz)	400	11	3	0	18	59	7	5	80	680	—	—	5

FOOD	PORTION	CALS	FAT	SAT FAT	CHOL	PROT	CARB	SUGAR	FIBER	CALCI	SOD	POTAS	FOLIC	VIT C
FANTASTIC (CONT.)														
Thai Lemon Grass w/ Rice Noodles	1 pkg (7.4 oz)	340	10	4	0	8	48	4	5	40	690	—	—	5
TAKE-OUT														
beef & broccoli	1 cup	221	12	3	54	18	10	3	3	46	399	436	67	35
beef w/ black bean sauce	1 serv (7 oz)	288	14	5	85	35	6	5	1	32	1373	516	—	—
bo bia roll shrimp	1 (2.5 oz)	82	2	1	15	6	10	1	2	16	49	175	11	8
buddha's delight w/ cellophane noodles fat choi jai	1 serv (7.6 oz)	211	4	1	tr	7	44	3	2	77	772	986	36	59
bun baked red bean	1 (1.1 oz)	102	3	2	8	3	16	—	1	11	54	0	—	—
cha siu bao steamed buns w/ chicken filling	1 (2.3 oz)	160	3	1	15	5	26	4	tr	0	300	—	—	0
chicken masala	1 serv (8 oz)	430	25	9	128	44	8	—	0	69	1165	—	—	0
chicken tandoori	1 serv (4 oz)	156	8	3	49	19	2	—	0	40	480	—	—	—
chicken tikka	1 serv (2.5 oz)	173	8	3	60	24	1	—	1	25	187	230	—	—
chinese garlic chicken	1 cup (5.7 oz)	290	19	5	83	22	8	3	1	21	778	379	10	2
chinese style fried egg noodles w/ seafood &lettuce	1 serv (14 oz)	694	37	14	257	27	63	1	8	196	1563	437	—	14
chow mein beef w/o noodles	1 cup	271	15	4	51	22	12	4	3	37	922	543	51	21
chow mein chicken w/ noodles	1 cup (7.7 oz)	273	14	2	44	19	20	5	2	37	1054	363	53	8
chow mein noodles	1 cup	237	14	2	0	4	26	tr	2	9	198	54	40	0
chow mein pork w/o noodles	1 cup	284	16	4	55	22	12	4	3	46	889	510	44	21
chow mein shrimp w/ noodles	1 cup (7.7 oz)	262	12	2	119	15	24	6	3	99	1274	319	68	9
chow mein shrimp w/o noodles	1 cup	154	5	1	92	16	11	6	2	59	737	394	44	10
chow mein vegetable w/o noodles	1 cup	224	15	2	0	5	16	8	4	40	1014	469	55	38
dim sum deep fried beancurd w/ shrimp	1 (1.1 oz)	77	6	2	9	5	2	—	1	11	133	259	—	0
dim sum deep fried yam	1 (2.4 oz)	201	12	5	3	3	23	—	2	10	794	148	—	0
dim sum meat filled	3 pieces (4 oz)	124	3	1	54	13	11	1	1	20	484	213	22	1

FOOD	PORTION	CALS	FAT	SAT FAT	CHOL	PROT	CARB	SUGAR	FIBER	CALCI	SOD	POTAS	FOLIC	VIT C
dim sum pork hash	1 (1.1 oz)	59	3	1	3	2	5	—	0	2	64	23	13	0
dim sum shrimp	3 (4 oz)	307	16	4	14	10	31	6	2	36	549	222	83	31
dim sum steamed chives & prawns	1 (1.2 oz)	48	2	1	10	3	5	—	1	14	164	61	—	0
egg foo yung beef	1 patty (6 oz)	243	16	4	336	17	7	3	1	54	243	292	54	6
egg foo yung chicken	1 patty (3 oz)	121	8	2	166	8	4	2	1	28	121	141	27	3
egg foo yung pork	1 patty (3 oz)	125	8	2	166	8	4	2	1	28	120	162	26	3
egg foo yung shrimp	1 patty (3 oz)	153	12	3	184	8	3	2	1	36	483	159	20	2
filipino chicken adobo	1 serv (15 oz)	555	26	7	116	33	45	tr	1	56	468	366	15	3
foochow fish ball	1 (1 oz)	36	2	1	6	2	3	0	1	—	163	—	—	—
fried rice	1 cup	333	12	2	103	12	42	2	1	38	834	196	97	3
fried rice beef	1 cup	346	14	3	107	12	42	1	1	38	649	271	22	3
fried rice chicken	1 cup	329	12	2	105	12	42	1	1	38	602	246	143	3
fried rice pork	1 cup	335	13	3	103	12	42	1	1	40	602	269	91	3
fried rice shrimp	1 cup	323	12	2	115	11	42	2	1	44	851	176	97	4
general tsao's chicken	1 cup (5 oz)	296	17	4	66	19	16	5	1	26	844	251	23	12
green beans szechuan style	1 cup	176	12	2	0	4	16	3	6	83	446	424	56	26
indian style fried egg noodles w/ eggs tomato sauce & lime	1 serv (15 oz)	721	31	13	377	29	80	2	8	159	2418	499	—	0
korean spicy shredded chicken	1 serv (5 oz)	258	16	5	30	23	5	5	2	40	816	383	—	—
kung pao beef	1 cup	410	30	8	62	28	9	2	2	21	645	528	31	2
kung pao chicken	1 cup (5.7 oz)	434	31	5	65	29	12	4	2	50	907	428	42	8
kung pao pork	1 cup	460	34	7	60	26	12	4	2	50	862	541	34	8
kung pao shrimp	1 cup (5.7 oz)	345	20	3	191	30	11	3	2	83	791	415	28	4
lemon chicken w/o vegetables	1 serv (6.6 oz)	503	28	7	127	34	26	3	1	42	1327	335	30	6
lo mein beef	1 cup	286	11	3	26	14	31	3	3	36	594	360	94	8
lo mein chicken	1 cup (7 oz)	280	9	2	26	16	33	3	3	36	536	336	90	8
lo mein meatless	1 cup	234	6	1	0	8	38	3	3	36	366	260	116	7
lo mein pork	1 cup	314	14	4	22	13	34	3	3	40	508	346	90	8
lo mein shrimp	1 cup	236	7	1	48	11	33	2	4	46	180	246	92	10
moo goo gai pan chicken	1 cup (7.6 oz)	272	19	4	35	15	12	5	3	130	305	480	43	34
moo shu pork w/o pancake	1 cup	512	46	7	172	19	5	2	1	32	1048	337	21	8
pad thai w/ chicken	1 cup (7 oz)	358	15	3	64	18	39	5	2	38	564	292	34	5
pad thai w/ shrimp	1 cup (7 oz)	314	11	2	186	11	40	6	1	110	1498	244	38	25
pakhoras	1 (2.5 oz)	163	8	3	0	8	16	—	4	35	470	359	—	0

FOOD	PORTION	CALS	FAT	SAT FAT	CHOL	PROT	CARB	SUGAR	FIBER	CALCI	SOD	POTAS	FOLIC	VIT C
paneer pakhora	1 (2.2 oz)	183	13	6	16	8	8	—	2	173	125	147	—	0
peking duck w/ pancakes & seafood sauce	1 serv (14 oz)	1871	121	39	189	39	157	39	5	177	1953	546	—	—
pork w/ chinese cabbage	1 serv (4 oz)	120	8	3	25	11	1	0	1	22	219	202	—	—
sesame seed paste bun	1 (2.5 oz)	220	6	1	0	5	39	12	2	125	53	—	—	0
shrimp chips banh phong tom	6 med	214	14	2	21	3	20	1	tr	15	456	29	1	tr
shrimp w/ lobster sauce	1 cup	298	12	2	259	35	8	2	1	83	1030	420	24	3
shu mai chicken & vegetable dumplings	6 (3.6 oz)	160	5	1	35	10	18	6	1	20	910	—	—	5
sukiyaki beef	1 cup	165	7	3	130	19	6	4	1	68	654	454	62	4
sukiyaki chicken	1 serv (18 oz)	436	8	2	175	71	19	7	4	110	1048	—	—	58
sweet & sour chicken w/o rice	1 cup	670	37	9	169	45	36	4	2	53	1819	441	40	9
sweet & sour pork w/ rice	1 cup	268	6	2	29	13	40	10	2	29	898	315	51	15
sweet & sour pork w/o rice	1 cup	231	8	2	38	15	25	15	2	29	1209	396	9	21
sweet & sour shrimp	1 cup	480	30	4	70	12	46	40	1	46	2020	375	9	6
szechuan chicken	1 cup (5.7 oz)	180	9	2	42	16	9	2	2	28	616	301	16	23
szechuan shrimp & vegetables	1 cup	159	7	1	94	14	10	3	2	62	629	342	24	27
tempura hawaiian fish tofu vegetable	2 cups	285	22	4	200	11	13	9	2	81	430	237	34	4
tempura vegetable	8 pieces	90	6	1	36	2	8	1	1	13	20	96	20	2
teriyaki beef	1 cup	454	19	6	149	51	13	9	tr	27	1386	586	34	16
teriyaki chicken	¾ cup	399	27	6	92	30	7	—	—	39	2190	511	14	tr
teriyaki chicken w/ rice	1 serv (11 oz)	430	6	1	25	19	77	10	1	60	1210	—	—	12
teriyaki shrimp	1 cup	271	3	1	269	39	14	6	1	115	3103	486	16	5
thai style pineapple rice w/ ham & pork floss	1 serv (7.7 oz)	408	14	6	63	13	60	22	6	51	1277	189	—	0
wonton fried meat filled	1 (0.7 oz)	54	3	1	20	3	5	tr	tr	5	111	51	8	tr
wonton meat & shrimp boiled	1 (0.5 oz)	19	1	tr	3	1	2	—	tr	2	48	—	—	—

ASPARAGUS

CANNED

FOOD	PORTION	CALS	FAT	SAT FAT	CHOL	PROT	CARB	SUGAR	FIBER	CALCI	SOD	POTAS	FOLIC	VIT C
spears	1 cup	46	2	tr	0	5	6	3	4	39	695	416	232	45
spears	1	3	tr	tr	0	tr	tr	tr	tr	3	52	31	17	3

FOOD	PORTION	CALS	FAT	SAT FAT	CHOL	PROT	CARB	SUGAR	FIBER	CALCI	SOD	POTAS	FOLIC	VIT C
DEL MONTE														
Spears Extra Long	½ cup	20	0	0	0	2	3	0	1	0	365	—	—	15
GERTIE'S FINEST														
White	1 oz	15	0	0	0	1	3	2	1	20	340	—	—	0
GREEN GIANT														
Spears Extra Long	5 (4.4 oz)	20	0	0	0	2	3	1	1	0	430	—	—	9
MCSWEET														
Pickled Spears	6 (1 oz)	25	0	0	0	0	6	6	0	0	290	—	—	1
NATIVE FOREST														
White	1 serv (4 oz)	20	0	0	0	2	3	1	1	20	550	—	—	21
S&W														
Spears	½ cup (4.4 oz)	20	0	0	0	2	3	0	1	0	365	—	—	15
FRESH														
cooked	½ cup	20	tr	tr	0	2	4	1	2	21	13	202	134	7
spears cooked	4	13	tr	tr	0	1	2	1	1	14	8	134	89	5
spears raw	4	10	tr	tr	0	1	2	1	1	12	1	97	25	3
ALPINE FRESH														
Fresh Green	5 spears (3.3 oz)	20	0	0	0	2	5	2	2	20	0	—	—	6
DOLE														
Spears	5 med (2.8 oz)	15	0	0	0	2	3	2	2	20	0	—	40	4
OCEAN MIST														
Spears	5 (3.3 oz)	25	0	0	0	2	4	2	2	20	0	—	—	9
FROZEN														
cooked	1 pkg (10 oz)	53	1	tr	0	9	6	1	5	53	9	504	396	72
spears cooked	4	11	tr	tr	0	2	1	tr	1	11	2	103	81	15
C&W														
Spears	7 (3 oz)	20	0	0	0	2	3	2	tr	0	0	—	—	9
JOY OF COOKING														
Tender	½ cup (3.3 oz)	70	5	3	10	2	4	1	1	—	210	—	—	—
SEABROOK FARMS														
Spears	7 (2.9 oz)	20	0	0	0	3	3	2	2	0	5	—	—	15
ATEMOYA														
fresh	½ cup	94	1	—	—	1	24	—	—	—	2	314	—	9
AVOCADO														
california mashed	¼ cup	96	9	1	0	1	5	tr	4	7	5	292	51	5
california peeled & pitted	1	289	27	4	0	3	15	1	12	22	14	877	154	15
florida mashed	¼ cup	69	6	1	0	1	5	0	1	6	1	202	20	10
florida peeled & pitted	1	365	31	6	0	7	24	7	17	30	6	1067	106	53
CABILFRUT														
Hass fresh	⅓ med (1.1 oz)	55	3	1	0	tr	3	0	3	0	0	—	—	2
CALAVO														
Fresh	⅓ med (1 oz)	55	5	1	0	tr	3	0	3	0	0	—	—	2

FOOD	PORTION	CALS	FAT	SAT FAT	CHOL	PROT	CARB	SUGAR	FIBER	CALCI	SOD	POTAS	FOLIC	VIT C
CHIQUITA														
Fresh	1 (7 oz)	322	29	4	0	4	17	1	13	20	14	727	—	20
DOLE														
Fresh	⅓ med (1 oz)	50	5	1	0	tr	3	0	2	0	0	—	—	2
EARTHBOUND FARMS														
Organic Fresh	⅓ med (1 oz)	55	5	1	0	1	3	0	3	0	0	—	—	2
MARGARITAVILLE														
Guacamole Zesty Island Garlic	1 oz	40	4	1	0	tr	3	0	2	0	100	—	—	1
SIMPLY AVO														
Hass Avocado Pulp	2 tbsp	50	5	1	0	1	3	1	2	0	0	—	—	2
Hass Halves	⅙ pkg (1.1 oz)	50	5	1	0	1	3	0	2	0	0	—	24	2
WHOLLY GUACAMOLE														
Classic	2 tbsp (1 oz)	60	5	1	0	1	3	0	2	0	90	170	16	1
Organic	2 tbsp	50	5	1	0	1	2	0	2	0	50	190	24	2
Pico De Gallo Style	2 tbsp	40	3	0	0	1	2	0	2	0	85	190	16	2
TAKE-OUT														
guacamole	1 serv (2.2 oz)	105	10	1	0	1	5	1	2	9	187	378	38	7
# BACON														
bacon grease	1 tbsp	116	13	5	12	0	0	0	0	0	19	0	0	0
beef breakfast strips cooked	3 strips	153	12	5	40	11	tr	0	0	3	766	140	3	0
gammon lean & fat grilled	4.2 oz	274	15	—	—	35	0	—	0	11	—	—	—	0
pan fried	3 strips	109	9	3	16	6	tr	—	0	2	303	—	1	0
turkey	2 (0.8 oz)	84	6	6	22	7	1	0	0	2	503	87	2	0
BOAR'S HEAD														
Fully Cooked Slices	3 (0.5 oz)	70	6	2	15	4	0	0	0	—	260	—	—	—
BUTTERBALL														
Turkey Bacon	1 slice (0.5 oz)	25	2	1	10	2	0	0	0	0	135	—	—	0
DIETZ & WATSON														
Gourmet	2 strips (0.5 oz)	70	6	3	15	4	1	1	0	0	250	—	—	0
Pancetta	⅙ pkg (0.5 oz)	50	5	2	10	2	0	0	0	0	230	—	—	0
HORMEL														
Black Label Lower Sodium	2 slices (0.5 oz)	80	7	3	15	5	0	0	0	0	230	—	—	0
Microwave Ready	2 slices (0.5 oz)	80	7	3	20	5	0	0	0	0	300	—	—	0
Real Bits	1 tbsp (7 g)	25	2	1	5	3	0	0	0	0	240	—	—	0
JENNIE-O														
Turkey Bacon	1 slice (0.5 oz)	35	3	1	10	2	0	0	0	20	170	—	—	—
JIMMY DEAN														
Lower Sodium	1 slice (0.3 oz)	50	4	2	10	4	0	0	0	0	105	—	—	0
Original	1 slice (0.3 oz)	50	4	2	10	4	0	0	0	0	230	—	—	0

FOOD	PORTION	CALS	FAT	SAT FAT	CHOL	PROT	CARB	SUGAR	FIBER	CALCI	SOD	POTAS	FOLIC	VIT C
JIMMY DEAN (CONT.)														
Thick Slice	1 slice (0.5 oz)	80	6	2	15	5	0	0	0	0	320	—	—	0
ORGANIC PRAIRIE														
Uncured Hardwood Smoked	2 strips (2 oz)	270	27	10	35	5	1	1	0	0	620	—	—	0
Uncured Turkey	2 strips (1 oz)	40	1	0	25	7	0	0	0	0	160	—	—	0
OSCAR MAYER														
Bacon Bits	1 tbsp (7 g)	25	2	1	5	2	0	0	0	—	170	—	—	1
Fully Cooked	3 slices (0.5 oz)	70	5	2	15	5	0	0	0	—	320	—	—	4
Hardwood Smoked	2 slices (0.5 oz)	70	6	2	15	4	0	0	0	—	290	—	—	4
Lower Sodium	3 slices (0.5 oz)	70	6	3	10	4	0	0	0	—	170	—	—	4
Super Thick Applewood Smoked	0.6 oz	90	7	3	15	5	1	0	—	—	350	—	—	5
Turkey	0.5 oz	35	3	1	15	2	0	0	0	—	180	—	—	4
Turkey Lower Sodium	0.5 oz	35	3	1	15	2	0	0	0	—	135	—	—	4
TYSON														
Hickory Thick Cut	2 pieces (0.8 oz)	140	11	4	25	8	0	0	0	0	380	—	—	0
BACON SUBSTITUTES														
bacon bits meatless	1 tbsp	33	2	tr	0	2	2	0	1	7	124	10	9	tr
meatless	1 strip	16	1	tr	0	1	tr	0	tr	1	73	9	2	0
BOB'S RED MILL														
Bac'Ums	4 tsp	25	1	0	0	3	2	0	0	—	140	—	—	—
LIGHTLIFE														
Organic Tempeh Smokey Strips	3 slices (2 oz)	80	3	1	0	8	6	1	1	—	230	160	—	—
Smart Bacon	2 strips (0.8 oz)	45	2	0	0	6	1	1	1	—	350	80	—	—
MCCORMICK														
Bac'n Pieces	1 tbsp (7 g)	30	1	—	0	3	2	—	0	—	180	—	—	—
WORTHINGTON														
Stripples	2 strips (0.5 oz)	60	5	1	0	2	2	0	tr	0	220	15	—	0
BAGEL														
cinnamon raisin	1 lg (4 in)	244	2	tr	0	9	49	5	2	17	287	132	99	1
cinnamon raisin mini	1	71	tr	tr	0	3	14	2	1	5	84	38	23	tr
egg	1 lg (4.5 in)	364	3	1	31	14	69	—	3	17	662	89	115	1
low carb	1 (4 oz)	216	0	0	10	12	42	0	14	40	360	—	—	0
oat bran	1 lg (4 in)	227	1	tr	0	10	47	1	3	11	451	102	87	tr
onion mini	1 (1.4 oz)	100	0	0	0	4	20	1	1	20	90	—	—	0
plain	1 med (3.5 in)	289	2	tr	0	11	56	—	2	19	561	106	92	0
plain	1 lg (4.5 in)	360	2	tr	0	14	70	—	3	24	700	132	115	0
plain	1 sm (3 in)	190	1	tr	0	7	37	—	2	12	368	70	61	0

FOOD	PORTION	CALS	FAT	SAT FAT	CHOL	PROT	CARB	SUGAR	FIBER	CALCI	SOD	POTAS	FOLIC	VIT C
ENJOY LIFE														
Nut Gluten Free Classic Original	1 (3 oz)	270	7	0	0	5	46	9	3	150	380	—	140	2
FINAGLE A BAGEL														
Cinnamon Raisin	1 (4 oz)	300	1	0	0	8	67	18	5	40	350	—	120	0
Everything	1 (4 oz)	310	3	1	0	9	62	8	5	20	420	—	120	0
Onion	1 (4 oz)	300	1	0	0	9	65	8	4	20	380	—	120	0
Plain	1 (4 oz)	290	1	0	0	8	63	8	4	20	410	—	120	0
Poppy Seed	1 (4 oz)	310	4	1	0	11	60	9	4	20	409	—	120	0
Sesame	1 (4 oz)	310	5	2	0	10	60	8	5	20	380	—	120	0
FRENCH MEADOW BAKERY														
100% Spelt	1 (3.4 oz)	270	2	0	0	11	52	1	8	20	520	—	—	0
Hemp	1 (3.4 oz)	280	8	1	0	19	35	3	13	100	370	—	—	0
Sprouted Cinnamon Raisin	1 (3.5 oz)	270	2	0	0	15	50	11	7	40	270	—	—	6
NATURAL OVENS														
Blueberry	1 (3 oz)	250	2	0	0	11	47	13	5	40	270	—	—	0
Brainy	1 (3 oz)	230	3	0	0	11	40	7	8	60	270	—	—	0
Whole Wheat	1 (3 oz)	230	3	0	0	10	40	7	8	40	260	—	—	0
NEW YORK STYLE														
Crisps Natural Whole Wheat	6	120	6	3	0	4	16	1	2	0	180	—	—	0
Crisps Plain	7	140	6	3	0	3	17	1	1	0	70	—	—	0
PEPPERIDGE FARM														
Bagel Flats Plain	1	100	1	0	0	4	22	3	5	20	120	—	24	0
THOMAS'														
100% Whole Wheat Mini	1 (1.5 oz)	110	1	0	0	5	22	3	3	40	180	—	8	0
Bagel Holes Plain	3 (1.6 oz)	120	1	0	0	4	24	3	1	40	230	—	—	0
Bagel Thins Everything	1 (1.6 oz)	110	1	0	0	5	24	3	5	40	190	—	32	0
Bagelbread Mini Squares 100% Whole Wheat	1 (2 oz)	150	1	0	0	7	30	4	4	60	240	—	—	0
UDI'S														
Gluten Free Plain	1 (3.5 oz)	280	9	1	0	6	43	5	3	20	480	—	—	0
Gluten Free Whole Grain	1 (3.5 oz)	280	9	1	0	7	43	4	3	20	470	—	—	0
BAKING POWDER														
baking powder	1 tsp	2	0	0	0	0	1	0	0	270	488	1	0	0
low sodium	1 tsp	5	tr	tr	0	tr	2	0	tr	217	4	505	0	0
BOB'S RED MILL														
Baking Powder	1 tsp	5	0	0	0	0	1	0	0	—	590	—	—	—
CALUMET														
Double Acting	⅛ tsp	0	0	0	0	0	0	0	0	20	60	—	—	—

FOOD	PORTION	CALS	FAT	SAT FAT	CHOL	PROT	CARB	SUGAR	FIBER	CALCI	SOD	POTAS	FOLIC	VIT C
CLABBER GIRL														
Baking Powder	⅛ tsp (0.6 g)	0	0	0	0	0	tr	—	—	20	65	—	—	—
DAVIS														
Baking Powder	⅛ tsp (0.6 g)	0	0	0	0	0	tr	—	—	20	65	—	—	—
RUMFORD														
Aluminum Free	⅛ tsp (0.6 g)	0	0	0	0	0	tr	—	—	40	55	—	—	—
BAKING SODA														
baking soda	1 tsp	0	0	0	0	0	0	0	0	0	1259	0	0	0
ARM & HAMMER														
Baking Soda	¼ tsp	0	0	0	0	0	0	0	0	—	300	—	—	—
BOB'S RED MILL														
Baking Soda	¼ tsp	0	0	0	0	0	0	0	0	—	270	—	—	—
BALSAM PEAR (BITTER GOURD)														
leafy tips cooked w/o salt	1 cup	20	tr	tr	0	2	4	1	1	24	8	349	51	32
leafy tips raw	1 cup	14	tr	—	0	3	2	—	—	40	5	292	61	42
pods raw sliced	1 cup	16	tr	—	0	1	3	—	3	18	5	275	67	78
pods sliced cooked w/ salt	1 cup	24	tr	—	0	1	5	2	3	11	300	396	63	41
BAMBOO SHOOTS														
canned sliced	½ cup	12	tr	tr	0	1	2	1	1	5	5	52	2	1
fresh sliced cooked w/ salt	½ cup	7	tr	tr	0	1	1	—	1	7	144	320	1	0
raw sliced	½ cup	20	tr	tr	0	2	4	2	2	10	3	402	5	3
LA CHOY														
Bamboo Shoots	½ cup	10	0	0	0	tr	2	0	tr	0	10	—	—	0
POLAR														
Sliced	½ cup	25	0	0	0	1	3	1	2	20	15	—	—	1
BANANA														
baked	1 (4.5 oz)	163	tr	tr	0	2	42	26	4	8	1	463	18	13
banana chips	1 oz	147	10	8	0	1	17	—	2	5	2	152	4	2
fresh	1 med (7 in)	105	tr	tr	0	1	27	14	3	6	1	422	24	10
fresh	1 lg (8 in)	121	tr	tr	0	1	31	17	4	7	1	487	27	12
fresh	1 sm (6 in)	90	tr	tr	0	1	23	12	3	5	1	362	20	9
fresh baby	1 extra sm (<6 in)	72	tr	tr	0	1	19	10	2	4	1	290	16	7
fresh mashed	½ cup	100	tr	tr	0	1	26	14	3	6	1	403	23	10
fresh sliced	1 cup	134	1	tr	0	2	34	18	4	8	2	537	30	13
green fried	1 (3.1 oz)	152	8	1	0	1	21	11	2	4	1	296	9	6
green pickled	½ cup	240	22	3	0	1	11	6	1	8	144	166	7	4
green sliced fried	1 cup	323	18	2	0	2	45	24	5	10	2	628	19	12
powder	1 tbsp	21	tr	tr	0	tr	5	3	1	1	0	92	1	tr
red ripe	1 (7 in)	93	tr	tr	0	1	24	13	3	5	1	372	21	9

FOOD	PORTION	CALS	FAT	SAT FAT	CHOL	PROT	CARB	SUGAR	FIBER	CALCI	SOD	POTAS	FOLIC	VIT C
red ripe sliced	1 cup	134	1	tr	0	2	34	18	4	8	2	537	30	13
whole dried	1 piece (1.2 oz)	130	1	0	0	1	33	22	2	0	0	—	—	0
BOB'S RED MILL														
Chips	25 (1.4 oz)	210	11	1	0	0	26	20	0	—	1	—	—	—
BROTHERS-ALL-NATURAL														
Crisps	1 pkg (0.58 oz)	66	0	0	0	1	16	8	2	0	0	—	—	6
CHIQUITA														
Fresh	1 med (4.1 oz)	105	0	0	0	1	27	14	3	10	1	422	—	10
CRISPY GREEN														
Crispy Bananas	1 pkg (0.5 oz)	55	0	0	0	1	13	8	2	0	0	—	—	6
CRUNCHIES														
Freeze Dried Organic	¼ cup (0.3 oz)	32	0	0	0	tr	9	7	1	0	1	—	—	10
CRUNCHY N' YUMMY														
Organic Freeze Dried	1 pkg (1 oz)	110	0	0	0	1	23	0	tr	5	3	214	—	2
DOLE														
Fresh	1 med (4.4 oz)	110	0	0	0	1	29	15	3	0	0	450	—	12
FRIEDA'S														
Dried	1 piece (1.2 oz)	130	1	0	0	1	33	22	2	0	0	—	—	12
KOPALI														
Organic Dark Chocolate Covered	½ pkg (1 oz)	120	6	4	0	1	19	17	2	10	0	—	—	1
NANA FLAKES														
100% Natural	1 tbsp (0.2 oz)	22	0	0	0	0	6	3	1	—	tr	—	—	—
TREE OF LIFE														
Dried Sweetened	½ cup (1.6 oz)	240	15	13	0	1	27	18	4	0	0	—	—	2
TAKE-OUT														
batter dipped fried	1 sm (4 oz)	266	15	2	17	3	32	9	3	9	103	264	32	5
batter dipped fried sliced	1 cup	335	19	3	22	4	40	12	3	11	129	332	41	6
fried dwarf w/ cheese	1 (1.4 oz)	84	5	1	4	1	10	5	1	30	38	142	5	3
fritter	1 (2.3 oz)	197	5	3	0	1	36	14	2	31	103	218	—	1

BANANA JUICE

FOOD	PORTION	CALS	FAT	SAT FAT	CHOL	PROT	CARB	SUGAR	FIBER	CALCI	SOD	POTAS	FOLIC	VIT C
R.W. KNUDSEN														
Sensible Sippers Organic	1 box (4.23 oz)	35	0	0	0	0	9	8	—	—	5	55	—	—
SNAPPLE														
Juice Drink Go Bananas	8 oz	110	0	0	0	0	28	28	—	—	5	—	—	—

BARBECUE SAUCE

FOOD	PORTION	CALS	FAT	SAT FAT	CHOL	PROT	CARB	SUGAR	FIBER	CALCI	SOD	POTAS	FOLIC	VIT C
barbecue	2 tbsp	52	tr	0	0	0	13	9	tr	4	392	73	1	tr
low sodium	2 tbsp	52	tr	0	0	0	13	9	tr	4	47	73	1	tr

FOOD	PORTION	CALS	FAT	SAT FAT	CHOL	PROT	CARB	SUGAR	FIBER	CALCI	SOD	POTAS	FOLIC	VIT C
ANNIE'S HOMEGROWN														
Organic	2 tbsp (1.2 oz)	45	1	—	—	0	9	5	—	—	240	—	—	—
BEAR-MAN														
Black Bear Boogie	2 tbsp	40	1	0	0	0	8	5	0	0	220	—	—	4
Growlin' Grizzly	2 tbsp	60	1	0	0	1	12	8	tr	20	290	—	—	5
BONE SUCKIN'														
Sauce	2 tbsp	40	0	0	0	0	10	8	0	0	110	—	—	0
CATTLEMEN'S														
Classic	2 tbsp	60	0	0	0	tr	15	10	tr	—	400	—	—	—
Honey	2 tbsp	70	0	0	0	0	17	13	tr	—	370	—	—	—
Smokehouse	2 tbsp	60	0	0	0	tr	14	12	tr	20	490	—	—	—
CHEF HYMIE GRANDE														
Cascabel Express Barbecue Glaze	2 tbsp (1.2 oz)	30	0	0	0	tr	7	5	1	—	15	—	—	6
Polapote Barbecue Glaze	2 tbsp (1.2 oz)	30	0	0	0	tr	7	4	2	—	15	—	—	6
DAVE'S GOURMET														
Badlands BBQ	2 tbsp (1.1 oz)	40	1	—	—	1	8	7	—	0	100	—	—	15
DAVID BURKE														
Flavor Spray Memphis BBQ	2 sprays	0	0	0	0	0	0	0	0	—	10	—	—	—
DAVID'S UNFORGETTABLES														
Balsamic Spicy	2 tbsp (1 oz)	70	5	0	0	0	6	5	0	0	190	—	—	1
JAKE & AMOS														
Apple Butter Barbecue Sauce	2 tbsp (0.5 oz)	30	0	0	0	0	7	7	0	0	15	—	—	0
NATURALLY FRESH														
BBQ	2 tbsp	40	0	0	0	0	10	8	0	—	200	0	—	—
ORGANICVILLE														
Original No Added Sugar	2 tbsp (1 oz)	50	0	0	0	0	13	11	tr	0	200	—	—	2
RIBBER CITY														
Kansas City	2 tbsp (1.1 oz)	40	0	0	0	0	11	9	0	20	210	—	—	0
STEEL'S														
No Sugar Added Gluten Free	2 tbsp (1.3 oz)	24	0	0	0	0	3	3	0	0	200	—	—	0
THE GRACIOUS GOURMET														
Spicy Barbeque Glaze	2 tbsp (1 oz)	35	1	0	0	1	7	6	0	20	300	—	—	2
WALDEN FARMS														
Original Calorie Free	2 tbsp (1 oz)	0	0	0	0	0	0	0	0	0	210	—	—	0
WORLD HARBORS														
Bar-B	2 tbsp (1.2 oz)	70	0	0	0	0	16	14	0	0	540	—	—	0
Buccaneer Blends Fra Diavlo	2 tbsp (1.2 oz)	45	0	0	0	1	11	10	0	0	260	—	—	1

FOOD	PORTION	CALS	FAT	SAT FAT	CHOL	PROT	CARB	SUGAR	FIBER	CALCI	SOD	POTAS	FOLIC	VIT C
WORLD HARBORS (CONT.)														
Buccaneer Blends Honey Mango	2 tbsp (1.3 oz)	60	0	0	0	0	13	12	0	0	260	—	—	2
Buccaneer Blends Sticky Rum	2 tbsp (1.2 oz)	50	0	0	0	0	13	12	0	0	340	—	—	2
BARLEY														
flour	1 cup	511	2	tr	0	16	110	1	15	47	6	457	12	0
pearled cooked	1 cup (5.5 oz)	193	1	tr	0	4	44	tr	6	17	5	146	25	0
pearled uncooked	¼ cup	176	1	tr	0	5	39	tr	8	15	5	140	12	0
ARROWHEAD MILLS														
Organic Pearled not prep	¼ cup	160	1	0	0	5	32	1	8	0	5	200	—	0
ROBINSONS														
Barley Water Lemon as prep	9 oz	48	5	—	—	tr	tr	—	—	—	—	—	—	—
BARRACUDA														
broiled	4 oz	239	14	4	62	27	tr	tr	0	31	480	543	3	4
cooked flaked	1 cup	287	16	4	75	32	1	tr	0	37	575	651	4	5
poached	4 oz	227	11	3	67	29	0	0	0	33	111	496	2	2
TAKE-OUT														
breaded & fried	4 oz	282	17	4	59	26	5	tr	tr	31	432	519	10	2
BARRAMUNDI														
AUSTRALIS														
Barramundi	4 oz	90	2	tr	55	23	0	0	0	20	40	—	—	1
Crispy Asian Sesame Panko	1 piece (4 oz)	240	11	2	30	20	24	2	1	20	270	—	—	1
Lemon Herb Butter	1 piece (6 oz)	170	4	0	70	30	3	2	0	0	600	—	—	2
BASIL														
fresh chopped	2 tbsp	1	tr	tr	0	tr	tr	tr	tr	9	0	15	4	1
ground	1 tsp	4	tr	tr	0	tr	1	tr	1	30	tr	48	4	1
leaves fresh	5	1	tr	tr	0	tr	tr	tr	tr	4	0	7	2	1
DOROT														
Chopped Cube frzn	1 cube (4 g)	5	tr	tr	0	tr	tr	—	tr	—	12	—	—	—
BASS														
breaded baked	4 oz	205	7	1	129	25	10	1	1	121	506	346	18	2
pickled mero en escabeche	2 oz	156	14	2	16	7	tr	tr	tr	7	114	111	2	tr
striped baked	3 oz	105	3	1	88	19	0	0	0	16	75	279	8	0
striped bass farm raised	4 oz	110	3	1	90	20	0	0	0	20	80	—	—	0
BAY LEAF														
crumbled	1 tsp	2	tr	tr	0	tr	tr	tr	tr	15	0	24	2	tr

BEAN SPROUTS

(*see* ALFALFA, SPROUTS)

BEANS

(*see also individual names*)

FOOD	PORTION	CALS	FAT	SAT FAT	CHOL	PROT	CARB	SUGAR	FIBER	CALCI	SOD	POTAS	FOLIC	VIT C
CANNED														
baked beans plain	½ cup	119	tr	tr	0	6	27	—	5	43	428	276	15	0
baked beans vegetarian	½ cup	119	tr	tr	0	6	27	—	5	43	428	276	15	0
baked beans w/ franks	½ cup	184	9	3	8	9	20	—	9	62	557	304	39	3
baked beans w/ pork	½ cup	134	2	1	9	7	25	—	7	67	524	391	46	3
baked beans w/ pork & tomato sauce	½ cup	119	1	tr	9	7	24	7	5	71	553	373	19	4
refried beans	½ cup	134	1	1	—	8	23	—	—	59	534	495	—	8
ALLENS														
Original Baked	½ cup	150	1	0	0	6	29	10	8	40	350	—	—	0
Refried Black Beans No Fat Added	½ cup	120	0	0	0	7	23	1	8	40	500	—	—	1
AMY'S														
Organic Refried	½ cup	140	3	0	0	8	21	1	6	40	440	—	—	4
Organic Refried Light In Sodium	½ cup (4.6 oz)	140	3	0	0	7	21	1	6	40	190	—	—	0
B&M														
Baked Original	½ cup (4.6 oz)	180	3	1	<5	7	31	10	8	60	420	—	—	0
Barbeque Baked	½ cup (4.6 oz)	190	1	0	0	8	39	19	9	80	570	—	—	2
Country Style	½ cup (4.6 oz)	170	1	tr	<5	7	35	15	7	60	720	—	—	0
Vegetarian	½ cup (4.6 oz)	160	1	0	0	7	31	12	8	60	380	—	—	0
BUSH'S														
Boston Recipe	½ cup (4.6 oz)	150	1	0	0	6	31	11	5	80	440	—	—	0
Country Style	½ cup (4.6 oz)	160	1	0	0	6	33	16	5	40	680	—	—	0
Honey	½ cup	160	1	0	0	6	32	14	6	60	540	—	—	0
Maple Cured Bacon	½ cup (4.6 oz)	140	1	0	0	6	28	11	5	60	620	—	—	1
Original	½ cup (4.6 oz)	140	1	0	0	6	29	12	5	40	550	—	—	0
Vegetarian Fat Free	½ cup	130	0	0	0	6	29	12	5	40	550	—	—	0
CAMPBELL'S														
Pork & Beans	½ cup	140	2	1	5	6	25	8	7	40	440	—	—	0
GEBHARDT														
Refried	½ cup	90	2	1	0	6	16	0	4	40	490	—	—	0
Refried Fat Free	½ cup	80	0	0	0	6	17	tr	5	40	500	—	—	0
Refried Jalapeno	½ cup	100	2	1	0	6	17	1	5	40	400	—	—	0

FOOD	PORTION	CALS	FAT	SAT FAT	CHOL	PROT	CARB	SUGAR	FIBER	CALCI	SOD	POTAS	FOLIC	VIT C
GREEN GIANT														
Three Bean Salad	½ cup	80	0	0	0	3	18	10	3	20	470	—	—	0
HORMEL														
Kid's Kitchen Microwave Meals Beans & Wieners	1 pkg (7.7 oz)	310	13	5	30	12	37	14	7	80	780	—	—	0
JAKE & AMOS														
Four Bean Salad	2 tbsp	32	0	0	0	0	8	6	0	—	78	—	—	—
OLD EL PASO														
Refried Fat Free Spicy	½ cup	100	0	0	0	6	18	1	6	40	570	—	—	0
PACE														
Refried Salsa	½ cup	70	0	0	0	4	14	4	4	40	590	—	—	0
READ														
3 Bean Salad	⅓ cup	60	0	0	0	1	13	8	2	20	300	90	—	2
ROSARITA														
Refried	½ cup	120	2	2	0	7	18	tr	6	—	310	—	—	—
Refried Black Beans No Fat	½ cup	110	0	0	0	7	19	0	8	20	320	—	—	1
Refried Fat Free	½ cup	100	0	0	0	7	19	tr	6	40	510	—	—	1
Refried Vegetarian	½ cup	120	2	0	0	7	19	0	7	40	540	—	—	1
VAN CAMP'S														
Baked Beans Homestyle	½ cup	170	1	0	0	7	33	15	6	60	680	—	—	1
Beanee Weenec BBQ	1 can	260	8	3	30	15	35	12	9	150	940	—	—	4
Beanee Weenee Original	1 can	240	8	3	40	14	29	8	8	100	990	—	—	0
Beanee Weence w/ Chili	1 can	240	9	3	45	14	26	2	6	80	990	—	—	0
Pork And Beans	½ cup	110	1	0	0	6	23	7	6	40	390	—	—	0
WAGON MASTER														
Pork & Beans	½ cup	130	1	0	0	7	23	4	9	60	420	—	—	0
FROZEN														
LEAN CUISINE														
Simple Favorites Sante Fe Rice & Beans	1 pkg (10.4 oz)	290	5	2	15	11	50	8	4	200	590	600	—	9
MIX														
FANTASTIC														
Instant Black Beans not prep	⅓ cup	160	2	0	0	10	29	7	7	60	310	—	—	0
Instant Refried Beans not prep	¼ cup	130	2	0	0	7	23	0	8	40	330	—	—	2
TAKE-OUT														
baked beans	½ cup	191	7	2	6	7	27	—	7	77	534	453	61	1

FOOD	PORTION	CALS	FAT	SAT FAT	CHOL	PROT	CARB	SUGAR	FIBER	CALCI	SOD	POTAS	FOLIC	VIT C
barbecue beans	3.5 oz	120	tr	tr	0	4	26	—	—	40	460	—	—	2
frijoles a la charra w/ pork tomatoes & chili peppers	1 cup	341	22	8	27	14	23	2	5	51	719	557	80	9
refried beans	½ cup	43	2	1	2	2	5	—	—	9	104	79	9	0
three bean salad	1 cup	114	5	1	0	4	15	2	5	34	651	252	56	4

BEAR
simmered	3 oz	220	11	3	83	28	0	0	0	4	60	224	5	0

BEAVER
roasted	4 oz	240	8	2	132	39	0	0	0	25	67	456	12	3

BEE POLLEN
bee pollen	1 tsp (5 g)	16	tr	tr	0	1	2	2	tr	4	0	11	0	3
TREE OF LIFE														
Bee Pollen	1 tsp (7 g)	30	1	0	0	tr	3	0	0	<20	30	—	—	tr

BEECHNUTS
dried	1 oz	163	14	2	0	2	10	—	—	0	11	288	32	4

BEEF
(*see also* BEEF DISHES, JERKY, MEATBALLS, VEAL)

CANNED														
corned beef	1 oz	71	4	2	24	8	0	0	0	3	285	39	3	0
HORMEL														
Corned Beef	1 serv (2 oz)	120	6	4	20	15	0	0	0	0	490	—	—	0
Dried Beef	1 oz	50	2	1	25	8	1	1	0	0	1200	—	—	0
LIBBY'S														
Corned Beef	2 oz	120	7	3	40	14	0	0	0	—	490	—	—	—
Potted Meat	¼ cup	120	9	4	40	9	0	0	0	0	410	—	—	0
Roast Beef w/ Gravy	⅔ cup	140	4	2	60	25	3	0	0	0	750	—	—	0
FRESH														
arm pot roast trim 0 fat braised	3.5 oz	297	19	8	95	29	0	0	0	16	47	231	9	0
arm pot roast trim ⅛ in fat braised	3.5 oz	302	19	8	79	30	0	0	0	17	50	242	9	0
beef crumbles 70% lean pan browned	3 oz	230	15	6	75	22	0	0	0	35	82	279	11	0
bottom round roast trim 0 fat braised	4 oz	253	10	4	112	38	0	0	0	9	50	307	11	0
bottom round roast trim 0 fat roasted	3.5 oz	187	8	3	86	27	0	0	0	7	36	223	9	0
bottom round roast trim ½ in fat braised	4 oz	337	22	8	109	22	0	0	0	7	57	325	11	0
bottom round roast trim ⅛ in fat braised	4 oz	280	13	5	86	37	0	0	0	9	49	301	11	0

FOOD	PORTION	CALS	FAT	SAT FAT	CHOL	PROT	CARB	SUGAR	FIBER	CALCI	SOD	POTAS	FOLIC	VIT C
bottom round roast trim ⅛ in fat roasted	4 oz	247	13	5	85	30	0	0	0	7	40	243	9	0
bottom sirloin butt roast trim 0 fat roasted	3.5 oz	182	8	3	71	27	0	0	0	17	55	340	9	0
brisket flat half trim ⅛ in fat braised	3.5 oz	298	19	8	80	29	0	0	0	16	46	227	9	0
brisket flat trim 0 fat braised	3.5 oz	221	9	4	46	32	0	0	0	17	52	254	10	0
brisket point half trim 0 fat braised	3.5 oz	358	29	11	92	24	0	0	0	8	68	233	7	0
brisket point half trim ¼ in fat braised	3.5 oz	404	22	14	92	22	0	0	0	9	65	221	6	0
brisket point half trim ⅛ in fat braised	3.5 oz	349	27	11	92	24	0	0	0	8	69	241	7	0
chuck boston cut roast trim 0 fat roasted	3.5 oz	207	11	4	69	26	0	0	0	7	71	367	9	0
chuck boston cut roast trim ¼ in fat roasted	3.5 oz	242	15	6	75	24	0	0	0	8	67	337	9	0
chuck bottom roast trim 0 fat braised	3.5 oz	334	24	10	104	27	0	0	0	13	65	236	5	0
chuck bottom roast trim ¼ in fat braised	3.5 oz	345	26	10	104	27	0	0	0	13	64	231	5	0
chuck fillet steak trim 0 fat broiled	4 oz	181	6	2	71	29	0	0	0	9	80	332	9	0
chuck top roast trim 0 fat broiled	4 oz	245	13	4	69	29	0	0	0	8	76	339	9	0
club steak trim ½ in fat broiled	4 oz	384	29	12	91	28	0	0	0	10	70	381	8	0
corned beef brisket cooked	3 oz	213	16	5	83	15	tr	0	0	7	964	123	8	0
crosscut shank trim ¼ in fat stewed	1 serv (6.8 oz)	510	28	11	155	60	0	0	0	58	118	784	17	0
delmonico steak trim ¼ in fat broiled	4 oz	409	33	13	95	27	0	0	0	15	70	372	8	0
entrecote steak trim ½ in fat broiled	4 oz	413	33	14	95	27	0	0	0	15	70	369	8	0
eye round roast trim 0 fat roasted	4 oz	190	5	2	61	33	0	0	0	8	43	266	10	0

FOOD	PORTION	CALS	FAT	SAT FAT	CHOL	PROT	CARB	SUGAR	FIBER	CALCI	SOD	POTAS	FOLIC	VIT C
eye round roast trim ¼ in fat roasted	4 oz	283	17	7	82	31	0	0	0	4	67	415	8	0
filet mignon roast trim ¼ in fat roasted	4 oz	376	29	11	97	27	0	0	0	10	63	369	8	0
filet mignon roast trim ⅛ in fat roasted	4 oz	367	28	11	96	27	0	0	0	10	65	375	9	0
filet mignon trim 0 fat broiled	4 oz	247	13	5	95	31	0	0	0	23	63	386	10	0
filet mignon trim ⅛ in fat broiled	4 oz	303	19	8	102	30	0	0	0	22	61	373	9	0
ground 70% lean broiled	3.5 oz	273	18	7	82	25	0	0	0	35	81	275	11	0
ground 75% lean broiled	2.5 oz	195	13	5	62	18	0	0	0	21	55	202	8	0
ground 80% lean broiled	3 oz	234	15	6	77	22	0	0	0	20	64	258	9	0
ground 85% lean pan fried	3 oz	197	12	5	73	21	0	0	0	17	67	297	7	0
ground 90% lean pan fried	3 oz	173	9	4	70	21	0	0	0	13	64	309	7	0
ground 95% lean pan fried	3 oz	139	5	2	65	22	0	0	0	8	60	320	6	0
ground 97% lean irradiated	4 oz	160	8	3	70	22	0	0	0	0	85	—	—	0
ground lowfat w/ carrageenan raw	4 oz	160	7	4	53	20	tr	—	—	—	70	—	—	—
london broil trim 0 fat broiled	3.5 oz	188	8	3	45	28	0	0	0	20	56	339	9	0
london broil trim ¼ in fat broiled	4 oz	260	12	4	95	35	0	0	0	7	68	490	14	0
new york strip steak trim 0 fat broiled	4 oz	219	9	3	66	33	0	0	0	24	67	403	10	0
oxtails cooked	6 pieces (6.3 oz)	472	26	10	191	56	0	0	0	23	419	472	11	0
porterhouse steak trim 0 fat broiled	1 lb	1252	87	33	304	109	0	0	0	32	295	1356	32	0
porterhouse steak trim ¼ in fat broiled	1 lb	1492	117	46	327	102	0	0	0	36	281	1157	32	0
porterhouse steak trim ⅛ in fat broiled	1 lb	1324	99	38	322	107	0	0	0	36	290	1455	32	0
porterhouse steak trim ⅛ in fat broiled	4 oz	337	25	10	80	27	0	0	0	9	73	364	8	0

FOOD	PORTION	CALS	FAT	SAT FAT	CHOL	PROT	CARB	SUGAR	FIBER	CALCI	SOD	POTAS	FOLIC	VIT C
rib eye roast trim ¼ in fat roasted	3.5 oz	365	30	12	85	23	0	0	0	10	64	288	7	0
rib eye steak trim ⅛ in fat broiled	4 oz	221	9	3	81	34	0	0	0	22	70	429	11	0
rib roast trim ¼ in fat roasted	4 oz	406	33	13	95	26	0	0	0	12	71	341	8	0
rib steak trim ¼ in fat broiled	4 oz	388	31	13	93	25	0	0	0	14	71	354	7	0
round tip roast trim 0 fat roasted	4 oz	213	9	3	105	30	0	0	0	7	40	246	9	0
sandwich steaks thinly sliced	1 serv (2 oz)	173	15	6	40	9	0	0	0	7	38	130	4	0
shell steak trim ¼ in fat broiled	4 oz	366	27	11	90	29	0	0	0	10	71	392	8	0
shortribs lean & fat braised	1 serv (7.8 oz)	1060	94	40	212	49	0	0	0	27	113	504	11	0
skirt steak trim 0 fat broiled	4 oz	289	19	8	67	27	0	0	0	12	104	430	8	0
t-bone steak trim 0 fat broiled	4 oz	280	18	7	68	27	0	0	0	6	76	342	8	0
t-bone steak trim ¼ in fat broiled	1 lb	1388	103	40	295	106	0	0	0	32	304	1279	32	0
t-bone steak trim ⅛ in fat broiled	1 lb	804	56	22	178	70	0	0	0	23	489	964	20	0
tip round roast trim ⅛ in fat roasted	4 oz	248	13	5	93	31	0	0	0	7	71	416	9	0
top loin steak boneless trim ⅛ in fat broiled	4 oz	299	19	7	100	30	0	0	0	22	61	372	9	0
top round roast trim 0 fat braised	4 oz	237	7	3	102	40	0	0	0	5	51	374	10	0
top round roast trim ¼ in fat braised	4 oz	281	13	5	102	38	0	0	0	6	51	357	10	0
top round roast trim ¼ in fat roasted	4 oz	265	15	6	93	31	0	0	0	7	71	407	8	0
top round steak trim ¼ in fat pan fried	4 oz	314	17	6	110	37	0	0	0	7	77	533	14	0
top sirloin steak trim ⅛ in fat broiled	4 oz	275	16	6	85	31	0	0	0	23	63	381	9	0
top sirloin steak trim ⅛ in fat pan fried	4 oz	355	24	9	111	33	0	0	0	14	80	460	10	0
tri-tip roast trim 0 fat roasted	3.5 oz	218	12	5	94	26	0	0	0	17	50	308	8	0

FOOD	PORTION	CALS	FAT	SAT FAT	CHOL	PROT	CARB	SUGAR	FIBER	CALCI	SOD	POTAS	FOLIC	VIT C
tri-tip steak trim 0 fat broiled	4 oz	300	17	6	77	34	0	0	0	14	82	495	11	0
DIETZ & WATSON														
Prime Rib Seasoned	3 oz	150	8	3	55	20	0	1	0	0	190	—	—	0
LAURA'S LEAN														
Eye Of Round	4 oz	135	4	2	50	25	0	0	0	—	75	—	—	—
Flank Steak	4 oz	140	5	2	55	—	—	—	—	—	85	—	—	—
Ground Beef 92% Lean	4 oz	160	9	4	60	21	0	0	0	—	70	—	—	—
Ground Beef Patties	1 (4 oz)	160	9	4	60	21	0	0	0	—	70	—	—	—
Ground Round 96% Lean	4 oz	140	5	2	60	24	0	0	0	—	85	—	—	—
Ribeye Steak	4 oz	175	9	4	60	—	—	—	—	—	—	—	—	—
Sirloin Steak	4 oz	145	5	2	65	—	—	—	—	—	70	—	—	—
Sirloin Tip	4 oz	130	4	2	60	24	0	0	0	—	65	—	—	—
Strip Steak	4 oz	150	5	2	55	—	—	—	—	—	70	—	—	—
Tenderloin Filet	4 oz	145	5	2	55	—	—	—	—	—	80	—	—	—
Top Round	4 oz	135	4	2	55	25	0	0	0	—	55	—	—	—
MAVERICK RANCH														
Ground Beef 85% Lean not prep	4 oz	150	17	7	70	22	0	0	0	—	55	—	—	—
Ground Beef 96% Lean not prep	4 oz	130	5	5	60	22	0	0	0	—	75	—	—	—
NY Strip Steak not prep	4 oz	180	10	4	55	22	0	0	0	—	55	—	—	—
Ribeye Steak not prep	4 oz	215	15	6	50	20	0	0	0	—	55	—	—	—
ORGANIC PRAIRIE														
Grass Fed Ground	4 oz	240	17	7	75	21	0	0	0	20	75	—	—	0
RUMBA														
Cheekmeat	4 oz	300	25	10	80	18	0	0	0	20	75	—	—	0
Crosscut Hind Shank	4 oz	190	10	4	45	23	0	0	0	20	70	—	—	0
Marrow Bones	4 oz	290	22	9	75	21	0	0	0	100	0	—	—	0
Oxtail	4 oz	260	21	8	75	21	0	0	0	0	65	—	—	0
Short Ribs	4 oz	400	36	16	70	17	0	0	0	20	56	—	—	0
READY-TO-EAT														
dried beef smoked chopped	1 oz	37	1	1	13	6	1	—	0	2	352	106	2	0
roast beef spread	¼ cup	127	9	4	40	9	2	tr	tr	13	413	148	5	tr
APPLEGATE FARMS														
Organic Roast Beef	2 oz	80	3	1	35	12	0	0	0	0	320	—	—	0

FOOD	PORTION	CALS	FAT	SAT FAT	CHOL	PROT	CARB	SUGAR	FIBER	CALCI	SOD	POTAS	FOLIC	VIT C
BOAR'S HEAD														
Corned Beef Brisket	2 oz	80	4	2	40	12	0	0	0	0	460	—	—	0
Top Round Deluxe	2 oz	80	2	1	30	15	tr	0	0	0	80	—	—	0
Top Round Oven Roasted No Salt Added	2 oz	90	3	2	30	14	0	0	0	0	40	—	—	0
HEALTHY ONES														
Deli Roast Beef	2 oz	70	2	1	0	9	1	1	0	0	480	—	—	0
LAURA'S LEAN														
Beef Pot Roast Au Jus	3 oz	110	4	2	45	17	3	—	—	—	380	—	—	—
OSCAR MAYER														
Slow Roasted Shaved	¼ pkg (1.8 oz)	60	3	1	30	10	0	0	0	—	520	—	—	—
SARA LEE														
Roast Beef Medium or Rare	2 oz	60	2	1	30	11	1	0	0	0	420	—	—	0
TYSON														
Beef Strips Seasoned	1 serv (3 oz)	130	6	2	55	18	1	1	0	0	420	—	—	0
TAKE-OUT														
roast beef rare	2 oz	70	2	1	30	12	0	0	0	—	210	—	—	—
BEEF DISHES														
CANNED														
corned beef hash	3 oz	155	10	5	—	10	9	—	—	11		—	—	—
HORMEL														
Beef Stew	1 pkg (7.5 oz)	150	6	3	25	10	15	2	2	0	890	—	—	1
Corned Beef Hash	1 cup (8.3 oz)	390	24	11	80	21	22	1	2	20	1000	—	—	0
Corned Beef Hash 50% Reduced Fat	1 cup (8.3 oz)	290	12	6	60	21	24	2	2	20	1070	—	—	0
Roast Beef Hash	1 cup (8.3 oz)	390	24	10	70	21	22	1	2	20	790	—	—	0
Roast Beef & Gravy	1 serv (5.8 oz)	130	3	2	40	18	8	1	0	0	740	—	—	0
LIBBY'S														
Corned Beef Hash	1 cup	420	24	11	55	19	33	1	3	20	1230	—	—	0
Hawaiian Corned Beef	2 oz	120	7	3	40	14	0	0	0	—	490	—	—	—
FROZEN														
QUAKER MAID														
Sandwich Steaks Pure Beef	1 serv (1.8 oz)	120	10	4	30	8	0	0	0	0	35	—	—	0
TYSON														
Steak Country Fried	1 (3.2 oz)	310	23	7	25	10	15	1	1	0	710	—	—	0

FOOD	PORTION	CALS	FAT	SAT FAT	CHOL	PROT	CARB	SUGAR	FIBER	CALCI	SOD	POTAS	FOLIC	VIT C
MIX														
HAMBURGER HELPER														
Beef Pasta as prep	1 cup	270	10	4	54	4	24	1	1	60	816	350	40	—
Cheddar Cheese Melt as prep	1 cup	310	12	5	57	3	30	2	tr	100	385	768	60	—
Cheesy Baked Potato as prep	1 cup	310	11	5	57	2	30	2	2	100	816	595	—	—
Chili Cheese as prep	1 cup	340	13	5	57	4	33	4	1	100	720	490	60	—
Double Cheesy Quesadilla as prep	1 cup	350	11	5	57	3	36	2	tr	150	888	455	40	—
Italian Sausage as prep	1 cup	290	10	4	24	4	29	5	1	20	840	385	40	—
Microwave Singles Cheesy Lasagna	1 pkg	210	5	2	5	8	33	6	1	40	580	60	40	—
Philly Cheesesteak as prep	1 cup	320	13	5	57	4	27	2	1	60	768	—	40	—
Salisbury as prep	1 cup	260	10	4	54	4	27	1	1	40	840	350	40	—
Tomato Basil Penne as prep	1 cup	300	10	4	54	4	31	6	1	20	720	350	40	—
REFRIGERATED														
HORMEL														
Beef Tips & Gravy	1 serv (4 oz)	170	8	3	60	21	4	3	1	20	700	—	—	0
LAURA'S LEAN														
Meatloaf w/ Tomato Sauce	1 serv (5 oz)	230	8	4	60	19	27	—	—	—	580	—	—	—
Shredded Beef w/ Barbecue Sauce	1 serv (5 oz)	245	5	2	65	22	27	—	—	—	390	—	—	—
TYSON														
Chuck Roast w/ Vegetables	1 serv (4 oz)	320	21	9	70	18	14	0	2	20	340	—	—	12
Seasoned Meatloaf	1 serv (5 oz)	320	23	10	60	14	16	5	0	20	600	—	—	0
Steak Tips In Bourbon Sauce	1 serv (5 oz)	180	5	2	45	20	12	11	0	40	480	—	—	0
TAKE-OUT														
beef bourguignon	1 cup	339	12	3	85	36	10	3	1	44	124	766	29	4
beef satay + peanut sauce	2 skewers	253	16	8	62	25	6	4	1	15	433	436	15	tr
bool kogi korean marinated beef ribs	4 oz	190	10	4	55	18	6	4	0	20	580	—	—	0
bracciola	1 roll (4.7 oz)	276	14	5	76	27	8	1	1	16	485	494	25	2
bubble & squeak	5 oz	186	13	—	—	2	16	—	3	30	—	—	—	10
bulgogi korean grilled beef	1 serv (5.2 oz)	256	15	5	67	23	5	3	tr	19	834	367	10	3

FOOD	PORTION	CALS	FAT	SAT FAT	CHOL	PROT	CARB	SUGAR	FIBER	CALCI	SOD	POTAS	FOLIC	VIT C
chipped beef on toast	1 slice (5 oz)	226	10	3	22	11	22	7	1	152	715	242	38	0
cornish pasty	1 (8 oz)	847	52	—	—	20	79	—	3	153	—	—	—	0
goulash w/ potatoes	1 cup	298	12	4	66	27	19	3	2	24	437	825	32	18
greek moussaka	1 serv (8.5 oz)	450	33	14	179	24	12	4	1	243	763	423	25	4
irish stew	1 cup (7 oz)	280	16	9	—	23	10	—	—	17	—	—	—	11
kebab indian	1 (5.4 oz)	553	40	—	—	47	2	—	—	62	—	—	—	3
kheema	6.7 oz	781	71	—	—	34	1	—	tr	32	—	—	—	2
koftas	5	280	22	—	—	18	3	—	tr	23	—	—	—	2
meatloaf	1 lg slice (5 oz)	294	17	6	114	23	9	2	1	75	596	396	23	1
pepper steak	1 cup	317	20	4	69	28	5	2	1	28	562	542	26	24
pot roast w/ gravy	1 serv (6 oz)	320	10	4	110	54	4	0	0	40	620	—	—	0
samosa	2 (4 oz)	652	62	—	—	6	20	—	2	37	—	—	—	1
shepherds pie	1 serv (7 oz)	282	16	6	70	16	20	—	2	120	840	500	20	4
sloppy joes	1 serv (9 oz)	398	6	2	67	39	48	5	12	80	88	—	—	53
steak & kidney pie w/ top crust	1 slice (5 oz)	400	26	—	—	21	23	—	1	52	—	—	—	3
stew w/ potatoes & vegetables	1 cup	199	5	1	30	16	22	3	3	35	504	630	35	15
stroganoff	1 cup	394	25	10	69	26	15	2	1	105	1155	527	31	1
swiss steak w/ sauce	1 serv (8 oz)	234	10	2	66	26	8	3	1	36	563	631	23	7
toad in the hole	1 (4.7 oz)	383	29	—	—	10	23	—	1	117	—	—	—	0
BEEFALO														
ground	3.5 oz	171	18	—	20	32	0	0	0	21	80	286	—	—
roasted	3.5 oz	188	6	3	58	31	0	0	0	24	82	459	18	9
t-bone steak	3.5 oz	111	3	—	13	24	0	0	0	52	78	394	—	—
BEER AND ALE														
alcohol free beer	7 fl oz	50	tr	—	—	1	11	5	—	5	3	40	15	—
ale brown	10 oz	77	0	0	0	1	8	—	0	19	—	—	—	0
ale pale	10 oz	88	0	0	0	1	12	—	0	25	—	—	—	0
beer cooler	1 (16 oz)	194	0	0	0	1	34	—	1	—	43	—	—	—
beer light	12 oz can	103	0	0	0	1	6	tr	0	14	14	74	21	0
beer regular	12 oz can	153	0	0	0	2	13	0	0	14	14	96	21	0
black & tan	1 serv (12 oz)	146	0	0	0	1	13	—	1	18	18	89	21	—
black velvet	1 (10 oz)	160	0	0	0	1	8	—	1	—	10	—	—	—
boilermaker	1 serv	216	0	0	0	1	13	—	1	18	18	90	21	—
lager	10 oz	80	0	0	0	1	4	—	0	11	—	—	—	0
lager & black	1 (14 oz)	241	0	0	0	1	39	—	—	—	31	—	—	—
mead	1 serv	250	0	0	0	1	13	—	1	18	18	90	21	—
pilsener lager	7 oz	85	tr	—	—	1	13	2	—	4	4	55	6	—
shandy	1 serv	125	0	0	0	1	12	—	1	16	16	76	18	1
stout	10 oz	102	0	0	0	1	6	—	0	25	—	—	—	0
trojan horse	1 (16 oz)	189	0	0	0	1	35	—	—	—	57	—	—	—

FOOD	PORTION	CALS	FAT	SAT FAT	CHOL	PROT	CARB	SUGAR	FIBER	CALCI	SOD	POTAS	FOLIC	VIT C
AMSTEL														
Light	1 bottle (12 oz)	95	0	0	0	—	5	—	—	—	—	—	—	—
BARD'S														
Gluten Free	1 bottle (12 oz)	155	0	0	0	—	14	—	—	—	—	—	—	—
BECK'S														
Pilsner	1 bottle (12 oz)	138	0	0	0	—	12	—	—	—	—	—	—	—
BUD														
Dry	1 bottle (12 oz)	130	0	0	0	—	8	—	—	—	—	—	—	—
BUDWEISER														
Beer	1 bottle (12 oz)	145	0	0	0	—	11	—	—	—	—	—	—	—
Bud Light	1 bottle (12 oz)	110	0	0	0	—	7	—	—	—	—	—	—	—
COORS														
Lite	1 bottle (12 oz)	104	0	0	0	—	5	—	—	—	—	—	—	—
Non-Alcohol	1 bottle (12 oz)	66	0	0	0	—	15	—	—	—	—	—	—	—
Original	1 bottle (12 oz)	149	0	0	0	—	12	—	—	—	—	—	—	—
Super Dry	1 bottle (12 oz)	149	0	0	0	—	11	—	—	—	—	—	—	—
CORONA														
Extra	1 bottle (12 oz)	149	0	0	0	—	14	—	—	—	—	—	—	—
GUINNESS														
Draft In A Bottle	1 bottle (12 oz)	128	0	0	0	—	11	—	—	—	—	—	—	—
Extra Stout	1 bottle (12 oz)	174	0	0	0	—	12	—	—	—	—	—	—	—
HEINEKEN														
Beer	1 bottle (12 oz)	150	0	0	0	—	12	—	—	—	—	—	—	—
ICEHOUSE														
5.0	1 bottle (12 oz)	149	0	0	0	—	10	—	—	—	—	—	—	—
KEYSTONE														
Light	1 bottle (12 oz)	103	0	0	0	—	5	—	—	—	—	—	—	—
KILARNEY'S														
Red Lager	1 bottle (12 oz)	197	0	0	0	—	23	—	—	—	—	—	—	—
KILLIAN'S														
Beer	1 bottle (12 oz)	163	0	0	0	—	14	—	—	—	—	—	—	—
LABATT														
Blue	1 bottle (12 oz)	127	0	0	0	—	9	—	—	—	—	—	—	—
LOWENBRAU														
Beer	1 bottle (12 oz)	160	0	0	0	—	—	—	—	—	—	—	—	—
MICHELOB														
Porter	1 bottle (12 oz)	196	0	0	0	—	17	—	—	—	—	—	—	—
Ultra	1 bottle (12 oz)	95	0	0	0	1	3	—	—	—	—	—	—	—
MILLER														
Genuine Draft	1 bottle (12 oz)	143	0	0	0	—	13	—	—	—	—	—	—	—
Lite	1 bottle (12 oz)	96	0	0	0	—	3	—	—	—	—	—	—	—
MGD 64	1 bottle (12 oz)	64	0	0	0	—	2	—	—	—	—	—	—	—
O'DOULS														
Non-Alcoholic	1 bottle (12 oz)	65	0	0	0	—	13	—	—	—	—	—	—	—

FOOD	PORTION	CALS	FAT	SAT FAT	CHOL	PROT	CARB	SUGAR	FIBER	CALCI	SOD	POTAS	FOLIC	VIT C
REDBRIDGE														
Gluten Free	1 bottle (12 oz)	160	0	0	0	—	16	—	—	—	—	—	—	—
SIERRA NEVADA														
Porter	1 bottle (12 oz)	194	0	0	0	—	12	—	—	—	—	—	—	—
SMIRNOFF														
Ice	1 bottle (12 oz)	241	0	0	0	—	38	—	—	—	—	—	—	—
WEINHARD'S														
Amber Light	1 bottle (12 oz)	135	0	0	0	—	12	—	—	—	—	—	—	—
Blond Lager	1 bottle (12 oz)	161	0	0	0	—	14	—	—	—	—	—	—	—
Hefeweizen	1 bottle (12 oz)	151	0	0	0	—	12	—	—	—	—	—	—	—
Pale Ale	1 bottle (12 oz)	147	0	0	0	—	13	—	—	—	—	—	—	—

BEET JUICE

FOOD	PORTION	CALS	FAT	SAT FAT	CHOL	PROT	CARB	SUGAR	FIBER	CALCI	SOD	POTAS	FOLIC	VIT C
juice	7 oz	72	0	0	0	2	16	—	—	—	400	484	—	6

BEETS

FOOD	PORTION	CALS	FAT	SAT FAT	CHOL	PROT	CARB	SUGAR	FIBER	CALCI	SOD	POTAS	FOLIC	VIT C
CANNED														
harvard	½ cup	90	tr	tr	0	1	22	—	3	14	199	202	36	3
pickled	½ cup	74	tr	tr	0	1	18	—	3	12	300	168	31	3
sliced	½ cup	37	tr	tr	0	1	9	8	2	22	176	196	36	3
FRESHLIKE														
Pickled Sliced	4 slices (1 oz)	20	0	0	0	0	4	4	0	0	20	—	—	1
GREENWOOD														
Harvard	1 serv (4.4 oz)	100	0	0	0	1	27	19	1	—	370	—	—	—
Pickled	1 oz	25	0	0	0	0	6	5	0	—	100	—	—	—
JAKE & AMOS														
Harvard	1 serv (4 oz)	90	0	0	0	1	23	20	1	—	360	—	—	—
RISE 'N ROLL														
Pickled Baby Beets	3 (1 oz)	30	0	0	0	0	7	7	1	—	140	—	—	—
S&W														
Sliced	½ cup (4.3 oz)	35	0	0	0	1	8	5	2	0	290	—	—	2
Sliced Pickled	1 oz	15	0	0	0	0	4	4	1	0	50	—	—	0
FRESH														
greens cooked w/o salt	½ cup	19	tr	tr	0	2	4	tr	2	82	174	654	10	18
sliced cooked	½ cup	37	tr	tr	0	1	8	7	2	14	65	259	68	3
whole cooked	2 med (3.5 oz)	44	tr	tr	0	2	10	8	2	16	77	305	80	4

BEVERAGES

(*see* ALCOHOL DRINKS, BEER AND ALE, CHAMPAGNE, COFFEE, DRINK MIXERS, ENERGY DRINKS, FRUIT DRINKS, ICED TEA, MALT, MILKSHAKE, SMOOTHIES, SODA, TEA/HERBAL TEA, WATER, WINE, YOGURT DRINKS)

BISCUIT

FROZEN

JIMMY DEAN

FOOD	PORTION	CALS	FAT	SAT FAT	CHOL	PROT	CARB	SUGAR	FIBER	CALCI	SOD	POTAS	FOLIC	VIT C
Snack Size Sausage On A Biscuit	2	400	30	10	40	9	24	4	1	80	650	—	—	1

FOOD	PORTION	CALS	FAT	SAT FAT	CHOL	PROT	CARB	SUGAR	FIBER	CALCI	SOD	POTAS	FOLIC	VIT C
MIX														
plain as prep	1 (2 oz)	190	7	2	2	4	27	—	1	105	541	107	29	tr
BISQUICK														
Heart Smart	⅓ cup (1.4 oz)	140	3	0	0	3	27	3	tr	200	340	45	40	—
KING ARTHUR														
Whole Grain Buttermilk not prep	¼ cup	100	1	0	0	4	19	5	2	100	125	—	—	0
REFRIGERATED														
plain baked	1 (1 oz)	93	4	1	0	2	13	tr	tr	5	325	42	22	0
IMMACULATE BAKING CO.														
Buttermilk	1 (2 oz)	170	7	5	0	4	23	4	0	0	450	—	—	0
PILLSBURY														
Buttermilk	3 (2.2 oz)	150	2	0	0	4	29	4	1	0	570	—	—	0
Flaky Layers	3 (2.2 oz)	160	4	1	0	4	28	4	1	0	550	—	—	0
Grands! Butter Tastin'	1 (2 oz)	190	9	3	0	4	24	5	tr	40	590	—	—	0
Grands! Buttermilk Reduced Fat	1 (2 oz)	170	6	4	0	4	26	4	tr	20	590	—	—	0
Grands! Golden Wheat Reduced Fat	1 (2.1 oz)	180	7	2	0	4	27	6	2	40	590	—	—	0
Grands! Original	1 (2 oz)	190	9	2	0	4	24	5	tr	20	550	—	—	0
Grands! Original Reduced Fat	1 (2 oz)	170	6	3	0	4	26	5	tr	40	600	—	—	0
Perfect Portions Butter Tastin'	1 (1.9 oz)	190	9	3	0	4	23	4	tr	0	440	—	—	0
TAKE-OUT														
buttermilk	1 lg (2.7 oz)	280	13	2	1	5	37	1	1	38	810	172	54	0
oatcakes	2 (4 oz)	115	5	—	—	3	16	—	1	14	—	—	—	0
plain	1 sm (1.2 oz)	127	6	1	0	2	17	tr	1	17	368	78	25	0
tea biscuit	1 (3 oz)	210	3	2	0	5	30	12	1	150	370	—	—	0
w/ egg	1 (4.8 oz)	373	22	5	245	12	32	—	1	82	891	238	57	tr
w/ egg & bacon	1 (5.3 oz)	458	31	8	353	17	29	1	1	189	999	251	60	3
w/ egg & ham	1 (6.7 oz)	442	27	6	300	20	30	2	1	221	1382	319	65	0
w/ egg & sausage	1 (6.3 oz)	581	39	15	302	19	11	1	1	155	1141	320	65	0
w/ egg & steak	1 (5.2 oz)	410	28	9	272	18	21	—	—	138	888	306	56	tr
w/ egg cheese & bacon	1 (5.1 oz)	477	31	11	261	16	33	—	—	164	1260	230	53	2
w/ ham	1 (4 oz)	386	18	11	25	13	44	1	1	160	1433	197	38	tr
w/ sausage	1 (4.4 oz)	485	32	14	35	12	40	1	1	128	1071	198	46	tr

BISON

(*see* BUFFALO)

FOOD	PORTION	CALS	FAT	SAT FAT	CHOL	PROT	CARB	SUGAR	FIBER	CALCI	SOD	POTAS	FOLIC	VIT C
BLACK BEANS														
dried cooked w/o salt	1 cup (6 oz)	227	1	tr	0	15	41	—	15	46	2	611	256	0
ALLENS														
Black Beans	½ cup	100	1	0	0	6	19	1	8	40	400	—	—	0
EDEN														
Organic Refried	½ cup	110	2	0	—	6	18	—	7	40	180	370	—	—
GOYA														
Black Beans	½ cup (4.3 oz)	90	1	0	0	7	19	tr	6	40	460	—	—	0
TREE OF LIFE														
Organic	½ cup (4.6 oz)	130	1	0	0	8	24	1	<6	40	120	—	—	0
BLACKBERRIES														
canned in heavy syrup	½ cup	118	tr	tr	0	2	30	25	4	27	4	127	35	4
fresh	½ cup	31	tr	tr	0	1	7	4	4	21	1	117	18	15
unsweetened frzn	½ cup	48	tr	tr	0	1	12	8	4	22	1	106	26	2
CASCADIAN FARM														
Organic frzn	1 cup	80	1	0	0	1	22	15	7	40	0	200	—	3
DOLE														
Fresh	1 cup (5.1 oz)	60	1	0	0	2	14	7	8	40	0	—	—	30
Marion frzn	1 cup (4.9 oz)	90	0	0	0	2	22	15	7	40	0	—	40	5
OREGON														
In Light Syrup	½ cup	120	0	0	0	1	29	19	6	40	10	170	—	5
BLACKBERRY JUICE														
canned	6 oz	65	1	tr	0	1	13	13	tr	21	2	231	17	19
BLACKEYE PEAS														
CANNED														
cowpeas	1 cup (8.4 oz)	185	1	tr	0	11	33	—	8	48	718	413	122	7
w/pork	1 cup (8.4 oz)	199	4	1	17	7	40	—	8	41	840	427	122	1
DRIED														
catjang cooked w/o salt	1 cup (6 oz)	200	1	tr	0	14	35	—	6	44	32	641	243	1
cooked w/o salt	1 cup (5.8 oz)	160	1	tr	0	5	34	5	8	211	7	690	210	4
FRESH														
cowpeas leafy tips chopped cooked w/o salt	1 cup (1.9 oz)	12	tr	tr	0	2	1	—	—	37	3	186	32	10
FROZEN														
MCKENZIE														
Blackeye Peas	1 serv (2.8 oz)	110	1	0	0	7	18	1	—	—	10	—	—	—
TAKE-OUT														
blackeye peas & pork	1 cup (6.3 oz)	236	5	2	27	24	25	4	8	36	1303	501	252	1

FOOD	PORTION	CALS	FAT	SAT FAT	CHOL	PROT	CARB	SUGAR	FIBER	CALCI	SOD	POTAS	FOLIC	VIT C
frijol de ojo negro guisados	1 cup (9.1 oz)	289	3	1	0	19	49	6	9	91	611	790	322	13
hopping john	1 cup (7.9 oz)	419	20	7	20	11	48	3	6	36	844	311	246	1

BLINTZES

GOLDEN

Cheese	1 (2.1 oz)	80	2	1	15	6	13	5	2	20	135	—	—	0

RATNER'S

Cheese	1 (2.2 oz)	100	2	1	30	5	16	5	0	20	140	—	—	0

TOFUTTI

Mintz's Blintzes Dairy Free	1 (2 oz)	140	5	1	0	3	19	16	2	—	170	—	—	—

TAKE-OUT

cheese	1 (2.7 oz)	160	9	4	65	5	15	4	tr	300	240	—	—	0

BLUEBERRIES

canned in heavy syrup	½ cup	113	tr	tr	0	1	28	26	2	6	4	51	3	1
fresh	1 pt	229	1	tr	0	3	58	40	10	24	4	310	24	39
fresh	½ cup	41	tr	tr	0	1	11	7	2	4	1	56	4	7
frzn unsweetened	½ cup	40	1	tr	0	tr	9	7	2	6	1	42	5	2

COW

Ultimate	¾ cup	70	0	0	0	0	16	3	3	20	0	—	—	2

CHUKAR CHERRIES

Puget Sound Dried	¼ cup	160	0	0	0	tr	38	20	5	0	0	—	—	1
White Chocolate Covered	3 tbsp (1.4 oz)	223	12	7	8	2	26	24	tr	90	33	—	—	0

DE-LITE

Dried Sweetened	1 oz	86	1	tr	0	1	23	19	4	109	4	47	—	22

DOLE

Blueberries frzn	1 cup (4.9 oz)	70	1	0	0	0	17	12	4	20	0	—	—	4
Blueberries frzn	1 pkg (3 oz)	50	1	0	0	0	10	7	2	0	0	—	—	2

EDEN

Organic Dried Wild	¼ cup	150	0	0	0	tr	35	21	5	40	15	300	—	0

EMILY'S

Dark Chocolate Covered	¼ cup (1.4 oz)	170	8	5	0	1	27	22	2	40	0	—	—	2

FRIEDA'S

Dried	¼ cup (1.4 oz)	140	0	0	0	0	33	17	4	0	0	—	—	0

LITEHOUSE

Glaze	3 tbsp	70	0	0	0	0	17	15	0	0	45	—	—	0

MARIE'S

Glaze	2 tbsp	40	0	0	0	0	10	8	0	0	35	—	—	0

OCEAN SPRAY

Fresh	1 cup	85	0	0	0	1	21	15	—	0	1	0	—	14

FOOD	PORTION	CALS	FAT	SAT FAT	CHOL	PROT	CARB	SUGAR	FIBER	CALCI	SOD	POTAS	FOLIC	VIT C
STONERIDGE ORCHARDS														
Organic Dried Wild Whole	⅓ cup (1.4 oz)	130	0	0	0	1	33	29	2	80	0	—	—	9
Whole Dried	⅓ cup (1.4 oz)	130	0	0	0	0	33	31	1	40	15	—	—	4
SUNSWEET														
Dried	¼ cup (1.4 oz)	140	0	0	0	1	33	26	3	60	0	150	—	18
TOP CROP														
Fresh	1 cup (4.9 oz)	80	0	0	0	1	19	9	5	0	0	—	—	9
TREE OF LIFE														
Dried	¼ cup (1.5 oz)	150	0	0	0	4	38	27	4	0	0	—	—	0
BLUEBERRY JUICE														
OCEAN SPRAY														
Diet	8 oz	5	0	0	0	0	2	2	—	0	50	0	—	60
TART IS SMART														
Wild Blueberry Concentrate	0.5 oz	35	0	0	0	0	9	7	1	—	0	69	—	—
WALNUT ACRES														
Organic	8 oz	130	0	0	0	0	31	28	tr	—	15	—	—	1
BLUEFIN														
fillet baked	4.1 oz	186	6	1	88	30	0	0	0	10	90	558	2	tr
BLUEFISH														
fresh baked	3 oz	135	5	1	64	22	0	0	0	8	65	405	2	tr
BOAR														
wild roasted	3 oz	136	4	1	—	24	0	0	0	13	—	—	—	—
NATURAL FRONTIER FOODS														
Wild Boar Steaks	1 (4 oz)	170	8	3	70	25	0	0	0	40	95	—	—	0
BOK CHOY														
(*see* CABBAGE)														
BONITO														
dried	1 oz	50	2	tr	13	8	0	0	0	3	14	88	1	0
fresh	3 oz	117	4	—	—	20	0	0	0	24	—	—	—	0
BORAGE														
fresh chopped	1 cup	19	tr	tr	0	2	3	—	—	83	71	418	12	31
BOTTLED WATER														
(*see* WATER)														
BOYSENBERRIES														
frzn unsweetened	½ cup	33	tr	tr	0	1	8	5	4	18	1	92	42	2
in heavy syrup	½ cup	113	tr	tr	0	1	29	—	3	23	4	115	44	8
BRAINS														
beef pan fried	3 oz	167	13	3	1696	11	0	0	0	8	134	301	5	3
beef simmered	3 oz	123	9	3	2635	10	0	0	0	8	92	207	4	9
lamb braised	3 oz	123	9	2	1737	11	0	0	0	10	114	174	4	10
lamb fried	3 oz	232	19	5	2128	14	0	0	0	18	133	304	6	20

FOOD	PORTION	CALS	FAT	SAT FAT	CHOL	PROT	CARB	SUGAR	FIBER	CALCI	SOD	POTAS	FOLIC	VIT C
pork braised	3 oz	117	8	2	2169	10	0	0	0	8	77	—	3	12
veal braised	3 oz	116	8	2	2635	10	0	0	0	14	133	182	3	11
veal fried	3 oz	181	14	3	1802	12	0	0	0	9	150	401	5	13

BRAN

FOOD	PORTION	CALS	FAT	SAT FAT	CHOL	PROT	CARB	SUGAR	FIBER	CALCI	SOD	POTAS	FOLIC	VIT C
corn	1 cup (2.7 oz)	170	1	tr	0	6	65	—	65	32	5	33	3	0
oat	½ cup (1.6 oz)	116	3	1	0	8	31	—	7	27	2	266	25	0
oat cooked	½ cup (3.8 oz)	44	1	tr	0	4	13	—	3	11	1	101	7	0
rice	½ cup (2.1 oz)	187	12	2	0	8	29	—	12	34	3	786	37	0
wheat	½ cup (2 oz)	63	1	tr	0	5	19	—	12	21	1	343	23	0
BOB'S RED MILL														
Rice Bran	2 tbsp	60	3	1	0	2	8	0	3	—	0	—	—	—
MOTHER'S														
Oat Bran not prep	½ cup (1.4 oz)	150	3	1	0	7	25	1	6	20	0	—	—	0
QUAKER														
Unprocessed	⅓ cup (0.6 oz)	35	1	0	0	3	11	1	8	0	0	250	16	0
TREE OF LIFE														
Oat Bran	½ cup (1.6 oz)	120	4	1	0	3	31	1	7	20	0	—	—	0
Organic Wheat Bran	¼ cup (1.1 oz)	190	18	2	0	4	4	1	2	20	0	—	—	0

BRAZIL NUTS

FOOD	PORTION	CALS	FAT	SAT FAT	CHOL	PROT	CARB	SUGAR	FIBER	CALCI	SOD	POTAS	FOLIC	VIT C
dried unblanched	1 oz	186	19	5	0	4	4	—	—	50	0	170	1	tr

BREAD

FOOD	PORTION	CALS	FAT	SAT FAT	CHOL	PROT	CARB	SUGAR	FIBER	CALCI	SOD	POTAS	FOLIC	VIT C
CANNED														
boston brown	1 slice (1.6 oz)	88	1	tr	0	2	19	5	2	32	284	143	5	0
B&M														
Raisin Brown Bread	½ in slice (2 oz)	130	1	0	0	3	29	16	2	40	380	—	—	0
FROZEN														
CEDARLANE														
Organic Mediterranean Stuffed Focaccia	1 piece (4 oz)	295	10	6	22	13	37	4	1	140	485	—	—	1
CORBI'S														
Chee-Zee Bread Original	½ piece (1.8 oz)	180	8	4	10	6	21	1	1	100	330	—	—	0
KINERET														
Challah Pull Apart	1 piece	140	3	0	0	4	25	2	3	0	220	—	—	0
PEPPERIDGE FARM														
Garlic Toast	1 slice	150	7	3	0	4	18	2	1	0	260	—	—	0
Texas Toast Five Cheese	1 slice	150	7	2	5	5	17	1	2	60	200	—	—	0
Texas Toast Garlic	1 slice	140	7	2	0	3	17	2	tr	0	210	—	—	0
Tuscan Sourdough	2 in slice	170	7	3	0	4	22	1	1	0	310	—	—	0
TANDOOR CHEF														
Tandoori Naan	1 piece (3 oz)	182	2	1	0	4	37	0	3	10	257	—	—	0

FOOD	PORTION	CALS	FAT	SAT FAT	CHOL	PROT	CARB	SUGAR	FIBER	CALCI	SOD	POTAS	FOLIC	VIT C
MIX														
cornbread	1 piece (2 oz)	188	6	2	37	4	29	—	1	44	467	77	33	tr
READY-TO-EAT														
anadama	1 piece (1.1 oz)	87	1	tr	1	2	16	3	1	26	272	100	27	0
baguette whole wheat	2 oz	140	0	0	0	6	29	tr	1	0	360	—	—	0
cassava	1 piece (3.5 oz)	299	1	tr	0	3	71	3	3	31	1187	507	40	29
challah	1 slice (1.4 oz)	115	2	1	20	4	19	1	1	37	197	46	42	0
cinnamon	1 slice (0.9 oz)	69	1	tr	0	2	13	1	1	39	177	26	29	0
cracked wheat	1 slice (1.1 oz)	78	1	tr	0	3	15	—	2	13	161	53	18	0
cuban bread	1 slice (1.1 oz)	83	1	tr	0	3	16	1	1	8	163	29	30	0
french	1 slice (1.1 oz)	88	1	tr	0	3	17	tr	1	24	195	36	47	0
italian	1 loaf (1 lb)	1255	4	1	0	41	256	—	—	77	2656	336	—	0
navajo fry	1 piece	281	10	4	6	6	41	2	—	48	280	65	104	—
oat bran	1 slice (1.1 oz)	71	1	tr	0	3	12	2	1	20	122	44	24	0
oatmeal	1 slice (0.9 oz)	73	1	tr	0	2	13	2	1	18	162	38	17	0
pan criollo	1 piece (0.9 oz)	69	1	tr	0	2	13	tr	tr	6	136	24	25	0
pannetone	1 slice (0.9 oz)	86	2	1	18	2	15	5	1	14	92	51	32	tr
pita	1 lg (2 oz)	165	1	tr	0	5	33	1	1	52	322	72	64	0
pita	1 sm (1 oz)	77	tr	tr	0	3	16	tr	1	24	150	34	30	0
pita whole wheat	1 lg (2.2 oz)	170	2	tr	0	6	35	1	5	10	340	109	22	0
pita whole wheat	1 sm (1 oz)	74	1	tr	0	3	15	tr	2	4	149	48	10	0
pumpernickel	1 slice (0.9 oz)	65	1	tr	0	2	12	tr	2	18	174	54	24	0
raisin	1 slice (1.1 oz)	88	1	tr	0	3	17	2	1	21	125	73	34	0
rye	1 slice (1.1 oz)	83	1	tr	0	3	15	tr	2	23	211	53	35	tr
seven grain	1 slice (1.1 oz)	80	1	tr	0	3	15	3	2	29	456	65	38	tr
wheat berry	1 slice (0.9 oz)	65	1	tr	0	2	12	1	1	26	133	50	23	0
wheat bran	1 slice (1.3 oz)	89	1	tr	0	3	17	3	1	27	175	82	38	0
wheat germ	1 slice (1 oz)	73	1	tr	0	3	14	1	1	25	155	71	33	tr
white cubed	1 cup	93	1	tr	0	3	18	2	1	53	238	35	39	0
whole wheat	1 slice (1 oz)	69	1	tr	0	3	13	6	2	20	148	71	14	0
ALVARADO STREET BAKERY														
Sprouted Soy Crunch	1 slice (1.2 oz)	90	1	0	0	5	15	1	2	0	160	—	—	0
Sprouted Whole Wheat	1 slice	90	1	0	0	4	19	3	3	0	170	—	—	0
ARNOLD														
100% Natural Soft Honey Wheat	2 slices (2 oz)	150	2	0	0	6	28	4	3	100	270	—	40	0
Grains & More Double Omega	1 slice	110	2	0	0	5	19	4	3	60	220	—	16	0
Jewish Rye	1 slice	90	2	0	0	2	17	1	1	40	240	—	24	0
Sandwich Thins Multi-Grain	1 (1.5 oz)	100	1	0	0	4	22	2	5	40	230	—	24	0

FOOD	PORTION	CALS	FAT	SAT FAT	CHOL	PROT	CARB	SUGAR	FIBER	CALCI	SOD	POTAS	FOLIC	VIT C
ARNOLD (CONT.)														
Sandwich Thins Whole Grain White	1 (1.5 oz)	100	1	0	0	4	22	2	5	40	230	—	32	0
Whole Grains 100% Whole Wheat Double Fiber	1 slice	100	2	0	0	4	21	3	5	150	200	—	8	0
Whole Grains 12 Grain	1 slice (1.5 oz)	110	2	0	0	5	21	3	3	40	170	—	24	0
Whole Grains 15 Grain	1 slice	110	2	0	0	5	21	4	3	40	210	—	16	0
Whole Grains 7 Grain	1 slice	110	2	0	0	4	22	4	3	40	190	—	24	0
AUNT GUSSIE'S														
Gluten Free Focaccia Bread Kalamata Olive	1 piece (2.7 oz)	180	2	0	0	3	37	4	4	0	450	—	—	0
Gluten Free Focaccia Bread Rosemary	1 piece (2.7 oz)	180	2	0	0	3	38	4	4	20	420	—	—	1
BAKER'S INN														
9 Grain	1 slice	100	2	0	0	5	18	3	2	150	210	—	32	0
Cracked Wheat	1 slice	100	2	0	0	4	18	3	2	150	190	—	32	0
Honey White Made w/ Whole Grain	1 slice	110	2	0	0	4	19	3	1	150	250	—	32	0
Honey Whole Wheat	1 slice	100	2	0	0	4	19	4	2	150	250	—	32	0
Potato Made w/ Whole Grain	1 slice	100	2	0	0	4	18	3	1	150	220	—	32	0
COMFORT CARE														
Cabin Hearth Whole Wheat	1 oz	170	3	1	0	9	31	7	4	20	0	—	—	0
DAMASCUS														
Roll-Up Flax	1 (2 oz)	110	3	1	0	12	15	1	9	40	360	—	—	0
EARTH GRAINS														
100% Multi-Grain Extra Fiber	1 slice	110	2	0	0	5	19	3	5	150	180	—	40	0
Oat & Nut	1 slice	120	3	1	0	4	20	4	1	100	210	—	40	0
Potato	1 slice	110	1	0	0	4	20	3	tr	100	190	—	40	0
Whole Grain Honey	1 slice	110	2	0	0	5	19	3	2	100	160	—	40	0
Whole Wheat Honey	1 slice	110	2	0	0	5	20	4	5	150	180	—	40	0
ECCE PANIS														
Classic Ciabatta	⅛ loaf (2 oz)	180	2	0	0	6	36	tr	tr	0	340	—	80	0

FOOD	PORTION	CALS	FAT	SAT FAT	CHOL	PROT	CARB	SUGAR	FIBER	CALCI	SOD	POTAS	FOLIC	VIT C
FLATOUT														
Fold It Flatbread 5 Grain Flax	1 (1.7 oz)	100	3	0	0	9	17	1	8	40	420	—	—	0
Fold It Flatbread Traditional Country	1 (1.8 oz)	140	2	0	0	8	24	2	3	40	380	—	—	0
Light Original	1 (2 oz)	90	3	0	0	9	16	0	9	20	320	—	—	0
Light Sundried Tomato	1 (1.9 oz)	90	3	0	0	9	17	tr	9	20	320	—	—	0
Soft & No Crust Garden Spinach	1 (2 oz)	130	2	0	0	7	25	2	3	20	340	—	—	0
The Original	1 (2 oz)	130	2	0	0	7	24	2	3	0	310	—	—	0
Wrap Healthy Grain Harvest Wheat	1 (2 oz)	120	3	0	0	7	23	2	6	0	310	—	—	0
Wrap Healthy Grain Whole Grain White	1 (1.9 oz)	110	2	0	0	8	21	4	7	40	280	—	—	0
Wrap Mini Healthy Grain Harvest Wheat	1 (1 oz)	70	1	0	0	3	13	2	3	0	140	—	—	0
FREIHOFER'S														
100% Whole Wheat	1 slice	90	2	0	0	4	17	3	2	40	160	—	32	0
FRENCH MEADOW BAKERY														
100% Rye Salt Free	1 slice (1.6 oz)	90	0	0	0	2	23	0	3	0	0	—	—	0
100% Spelt	2 slices (2.4 oz)	170	1	0	0	6	33	1	4	0	360	—	—	0
European Sourdough Rye	1 slice (1.7 oz)	90	0	0	0	2	22	0	3	0	220	—	—	0
Gluten Free Multigrain	1 slice (1.8 oz)	150	5	2	0	4	23	0	3	40	230	—	—	6
Hemp	2 slices (2.4 oz)	200	5	1	0	13	24	2	5	100	270	—	—	0
Kamut	2 slices (3 oz)	170	1	0	0	8	31	1	1	0	330	—	—	0
Men's Bread	2 slices (2.4 oz)	200	8	2	0	15	17	1	3	40	250	—	—	0
Our Daily Bread	2 slices (2.4 oz)	160	3	0	0	10	24	1	5	20	240	—	—	0
Sprouted Cinnamon Raisin	1 slice (1.5 oz)	100	1	0	0	2	19	4	3	0	90	—	—	0
Summer	1 slice (1.2 oz)	90	0	0	0	4	17	1	1	0	170	—	—	0
GILLIAN'S FOODS														
Gluten Free Cinnamon Raisin	1 slice (2 oz)	130	1	0	0	5	25	3	2	40	330	—	—	0
KONTOS														
Pocket-Less Pita Whole Wheat	1 (2.8 oz)	210	2	1	0	10	38	4	4	40	510	—	—	0

FOOD	PORTION	CALS	FAT	SAT FAT	CHOL	PROT	CARB	SUGAR	FIBER	CALCI	SOD	POTAS	FOLIC	VIT C
LA TORTILLA FACTORY														
Smart & Delicious Soft Wrap Whole Grain White	1 (2.2 oz)	100	3	0	0	8	23	0	13	80	340	—	—	0
Smart & Delicious Soft Wraps Multi Grain	1 (2.2 oz)	100	4	1	0	9	18	1	12	60	290	—	—	0
Smart & Delicious Soft Wraps Tomato Basil	1 (2.2 oz)	100	3	0	0	9	20	1	12	80	360	—	—	0
Smart & Delicious Soft Wraps Traditional	1 (2.2 oz)	90	3	0	0	8	20	tr	13	80	330	—	—	0
Smart & Delicious Soft Wraps Whole Grain	1 (2.2 oz)	170	4	1	0	6	28	1	5	60	320	—	—	0
LEVY'S														
Real Jewish Rye Everything	1 slice (1.1 oz)	90	2	0	0	3	16	1	tr	60	210	—	24	0
MANNA ORGANICS														
Banana Walnut Hemp	1 slice (2 oz)	140	3	0	0	5	27	12	2	0	5	—	—	1
Carrot Raisin	1 slice (2 oz)	130	0	0	0	5	27	10	5	20	6	—	—	0
Fig Fennel Flax	1 slice (2 oz)	120	2	0	0	4	26	8	5	40	10	—	—	1
Millet Rice	1 slice (2 oz)	130	0	0	0	5	28	9	5	20	10	—	—	0
Whole Rye	1 slice (2 oz)	150	0	0	0	6	32	7	5	20	10	—	—	0
MARTIN'S														
Potato 100% Whole Wheat	1 slice (1.3 oz)	70	1	0	0	6	14	4	4	60	125	—	16	0
MATTHEW'S														
Golden White	1 slice (1.1 oz)	90	1	0	0	3	18	2	tr	0	170	—	8	0
Honey 12 Grain	1 slice (1.1 oz)	80	2	0	0	3	15	3	1	0	140	—	8	0
MRS BAIRD'S														
Acti-Fiber Wheat	2 slices (2.2 oz)	160	3	1	0	5	30	4	4	—	230	—	40	0
Whole Grain Wheat Sugar Free	1 slice (1.1 oz)	70	2	0	0	4	13	0	3	60	130	—	8	0
NATURAL OVENS														
100% Sweet Whole	1 slice	90	2	0	0	4	16	4	4	0	130	—	—	0
Carb Conscious Original	1 slice	80	2	0	0	8	9	1	4	0	120	—	0	0
Healthy Beginnings Better White	1 slice	110	2	0	0	5	20	3	2	100	180	—	—	0
Healthy Beginnings Honey Wheat	1 slice	120	2	0	0	4	21	3	3	40	170	—	—	0

FOOD	PORTION	CALS	FAT	SAT FAT	CHOL	PROT	CARB	SUGAR	FIBER	CALCI	SOD	POTAS	FOLIC	VIT C
NATURAL OVENS (CONT.)														
Hunger Filler Whole Grain	1 slice	100	2	0	0	5	15	2	4	0	100	—	—	0
Organic Plus Whole Grain & Flax	1 slice	120	2	0	0	4	22	3	3	100	160	—	—	0
Whole Grain Oat Nut Crunch	1 slice	100	3	0	0	5	15	2	4	0	110	—	—	0
NATURE'S OWN														
100% Whole Wheat	1 slice	50	1	0	0	4	10	1	2	tr	115	—	16	0
9 Grain	1 slice	120	2	0	0	4	24	4	2	0	190	—	—	0
Hearty Oatmeal	1 slice	100	2	1	0	5	18	3	3	40	170	—	—	0
Wheat Double Fiber	1 slice	50	1	0	0	4	10	1	5	150	150	—	—	0
Wheat Light	2 slices	80	1	0	0	5	19	1	5	80	200	—	40	0
Wheat N' Fiber	1 slice	60	1	0	0	6	7	0	2	40	105	—	—	0
Whole Wheat w/ Organic Flour	1 slice	100	2	0	0	5	21	3	3	40	240	—	—	0
NATURE'S PRIDE														
100% Whole Wheat	1 slice (1.5 oz)	110	1	0	0	5	20	4	3	20	210	—	—	0
100% Whole Wheat Double Fiber	1 slice (1.5 oz)	100	1	0	0	4	20	4	6	20	210	—	—	0
Country Buttermilk	1 slice (1.5 oz)	110	2	0	5	4	21	4	tr	20	190	—	—	0
Healthy Multi-Grain	1 slice (1.5 oz)	110	9	0	0	5	20	4	3	20	190	—	—	0
Honey Wheat	1 slice (1 oz)	70	1	0	0	3	13	3	tr	20	120	—	—	0
Nutty Oat	1 slice (1.5 oz)	110	2	0	0	5	19	4	2	20	150	—	—	0
OROWEAT														
100% Whole Wheat	1 slice (1.3 oz)	100	1	0	0	4	19	4	3	60	210	—	—	0
Country Potato	1 slice (1.3 oz)	100	1	0	0	3	20	3	tr	40	180	—	32	0
Country Whole Grain White	1 slice (1.3 oz)	90	2	1	0	4	17	4	1	200	170	—	60	0
Double Fiber	1 slice (1.3 oz)	70	1	0	0	4	16	2	6	100	160	—	40	0
Honey Fiber Whole Grain	1 slice (1.3 oz)	80	1	0	0	4	18	3	4	150	170	—	60	0
Russian Rye	1 slice (1 oz)	80	1	0	0	3	13	tr	tr	40	200	—	16	0
Seven Grain	1 slice (1.3 oz)	100	1	0	0	3	20	4	2	40	180	—	24	0
Whole Grain & Flax	1 slice (1.3 oz)	100	2	0	0	4	17	3	3	40	180	—	8	0
PEPPERIDGE FARM														
100% Whole Wheat	1 slice	100	2	1	0	5	20	3	4	40	105	—	16	0

FOOD	PORTION	CALS	FAT	SAT FAT	CHOL	PROT	CARB	SUGAR	FIBER	CALCI	SOD	POTAS	FOLIC	VIT C
PEPPERIDGE FARM (CONT.)														
15 Grain Whole Grain	1 slice	100	2	1	0	5	20	3	4	40	115	—	8	0
Ancient Grains	1 slice	100	2	0	0	5	20	3	4	40	120	—	16	0
Cinnamon Swirl	1 slice	80	2	0	0	2	15	4	tr	20	110	—	16	0
Cinnamon Swirl Raisin	1 slice	80	2	0	0	2	15	5	tr	0	100	—	8	0
Deli Swirl	1 slice	80	1	0	0	3	14	tr	1	20	180	—	—	0
Farmhouse Hearty White	1 slice	120	2	1	0	4	22	4	1	40	220	—	40	0
Farmhouse Honey Wheat	1 slice (1.5 oz)	120	2	1	0	4	21	5	2	40	150	—	24	0
Farmhouse Sourdough	1 slice	120	2	1	0	4	22	2	1	20	220	—	60	0
Farmhouse Whole Grain White	1 slice	110	2	1	0	4	21	4	3	100	150	—	60	0
German Dark Wheat	1 slice	100	2	0	0	3	17	2	3	40	130	—	8	0
Goldfish 100% Whole Wheat	2 slices	100	2	1	0	5	21	3	4	60	170	—	40	0
Goldfish Soft White	2 slices	100	1	1	0	3	23	4	4	100	170	—	40	0
Hearty Oatmeal	1 slice	100	2	0	0	4	20	3	4	40	110	—	8	0
Italian w/ Sesame Seeds	1 slice	90	1	0	0	3	15	1	tr	40	130	—	16	0
Jewish Rye Party	5 slices	130	2	0	0	4	25	1	2	60	460	—	24	0
Jewish Rye Seeded	1 slice	80	1	0	0	3	15	1	2	20	170	—	24	0
Light Style Extra Fiber Wheat	1 slice	120	1	0	0	6	26	3	6	80	200	—	24	0
Party Pumpernickel	5 slices	130	2	0	0	5	23	1	3	60	320	—	24	0
Pumpernickel	1 slice	80	1	0	0	3	15	1	1	20	190	—	16	0
Swirl 100% Whole Wheat Cinnamon Swirl w/ Raisins	1 slice	80	1	0	0	3	13	4	2	20	105	—	16	0
ROMAN MEAL														
Muesli	1 slice (1.5 oz)	110	2	0	0	5	19	5	2	40	160	—	8	4
Original Whole Grain	2 slices (2 oz)	130	2	0	0	5	25	5	2	350	250	—	60	2
RUDI'S ORGANIC BAKERY														
100% Whole Wheat	1 slice	100	1	0	0	4	19	2	3	0	150	—	8	0
14 Grain	1 slice	90	1	0	0	4	19	2	4	0	150	—	0	0
Artisan Country French	1 slice	100	1	0	0	4	20	1	tr	0	210	—	8	0

FOOD	PORTION	CALS	FAT	SAT FAT	CHOL	PROT	CARB	SUGAR	FIBER	CALCI	SOD	POTAS	FOLIC	VIT C
RUDI'S ORGANIC BAKERY (CONT.)														
Artisan Rosemary Olive Oil	1 slice	100	1	0	0	3	19	0	tr	0	230	—	8	0
Low Carb Right Choice	1 slice	45	1	0	0	4	7	1	2	0	105	—	8	0
Spelt Ancient Grain	1 slice	120	3	0	0	4	20	3	2	20	170	—	8	1
Whole Grain Apple N Spice	1 slice	110	1	0	0	4	24	6	5	20	190	—	—	0
S. ROSEN'S														
Hawaiian	1 slice	110	2	0	4	3	21	4	0	0	170	—	32	0
Rye Black Bavarian	1 slice	100	2	0	0	3	19	0	1	20	300	—	32	0
SARA LEE														
Soft & Smooth 100% Whole Wheat	1 slice	70	1	0	0	3	12	3	2	100	135	—	16	0
Soft & Smooth Whole Grain White	2 slices	150	2	1	0	6	28	5	3	250	250	—	60	0
SONOMA														
Wraps Organic Multi Grain	1 (2.4 oz)	180	7	1	0	6	27	1	6	50	330	—	—	0
Wraps Organic Wheat	1 (2.4 oz)	190	7	1	0	5	30	2	4	60	380	—	—	0
Wraps Original White Whole Wheat	1 (2.4 oz)	200	5	1	0	6	33	1	4	40	360	—	—	0
STROEHMANN														
Dutch Country Twelve Grain	1 slice	100	2	0	0	4	18	3	2	40	180	—	32	0
Potato	1 slice	100	2	0	0	3	18	3	1	40	170	—	32	0
SUN-MAID														
Raisin Cinnamon Swirl	1 slice (1.2 oz)	100	2	1	5	3	18	8	1	0	130	—	24	0
THE BAKER														
Yoga Bread	1 slice	70	1	0	0	3	13	2	2	20	80	55	—	0
THOMAS'														
Breakfast Original	1 slice	90	1	0	0	4	17	tr	1	80	190	—	—	0
Sahara Pita Pockets Mini Whole Wheat	1 (1 oz)	70	1	0	0	3	13	1	2	60	150	—	—	0
Swirl Cinnamon Raisin	1 slice	120	2	1	0	3	21	9	1	40	160	—	—	0
TUMARO'S														
Deli Style Wraps Cracked Pepper	1 (2.1 oz)	100	3	1	0	9	21	1	12	200	230	—	—	0

FOOD	PORTION	CALS	FAT	SAT FAT	CHOL	PROT	CARB	SUGAR	FIBER	CALCI	SOD	POTAS	FOLIC	VIT C
TUMARO'S (CONT.)														
Deli Style Wraps Everything	1 (2.1 oz)	80	3	0	0	8	17	1	10	200	270	—	—	0
Deli Style Wraps Pumpernickel	1 (2.1 oz)	80	2	0	0	5	19	1	9	100	280	—	—	0
Deli Style Wraps Rye	1 (2.1 oz)	80	2	0	0	5	19	1	9	150	280	—	—	0
Deli Style Wraps Sour Dough	1 (2.1 oz)	80	2	0	0	7	17	1	9	150	430	—	—	0
Wraps Chipotle Chili & Peppers	1 (2.3 oz)	170	2	0	0	4	34	1	2	150	200	—	—	1
Wraps Sun Dried Tomato & Basil	1 (2.3 oz)	170	2	0	0	5	34	2	2	150	210	—	—	1
UDI'S														
Gluten Free Cinnamon Raisin	2 slices (2.1 oz)	160	4	0	0	3	29	10	1	20	220	—	—	0
Gluten Free Whole Grain	2 slices (2 oz)	140	4	0	0	3	22	3	1	20	270	—	—	0
WONDER														
100% Whole Wheat Soft	2 slices (1.6 oz)	110	2	0	0	5	20	3	3	80	220	—	—	0
Classic White	1 slice (1 oz)	70	1	0	0	2	14	2	0	150	150	—	24	0
Light White	1 slice (0.8 oz)	40	0	0	0	2	9	2	2	80	130	—	8	0
Smart White	1 slice (0.9 oz)	50	1	0	0	3	11	2	2	150	115	—	24	0
Texas Toast	1 slice (1.4 oz)	100	1	0	0	3	19	2	tr	150	200	—	40	0
Whole Grain White	2 slices (2 oz)	140	2	1	0	6	25	5	3	400	200	—	60	0
REFRIGERATED														
PILLSBURY														
Italian	⅛ pkg (1.6 oz)	110	2	0	0	4	21	2	tr	0	270	—	—	0
TAKE-OUT														
banana	1 slice (2 oz)	196	6	1	26	3	33	—	1	13	181	80	20	1
chapati as prep w/ fat	1 (1.6 oz)	95	2	1	3	3	18	1	3	10	180	101	11	0
chapati as prep w/o fat	1 (2.5 oz)	141	1	—	—	5	31	—	5	42	—	—	—	0
cornbread	1 piece (2.3 oz)	183	6	1	26	4	27	4	2	130	317	89	47	0
cornstick	1 (1.4 oz)	118	4	1	17	3	18	3	1	83	204	57	30	0
focaccia onion	1 piece (4.6 oz)	282	10	1	0	6	43	2	2	20	536	114	43	2
focaccia rosemary	1 piece (3.5 oz)	251	7	1	0	6	40	1	2	13	535	68	38	tr
focaccia tomato olive	1 piece (4.7 oz)	270	8	1	0	6	42	1	2	31	683	122	39	3
garlic bread	1 slice (1 oz)	96	4	1	0	2	13	tr	1	19	177	32	37	tr
irish soda bread	1 slice (3 oz)	247	4	1	15	6	48	—	2	69	338	226	40	1
italian garlic	1 loaf (11 oz)	990	38	7	0	23	137	1	8	198	1830	327	384	1
naan	1 bread (3.5 oz)	286	9	5	46	7	43	3	2	54	546	107	53	tr

FOOD	PORTION	CALS	FAT	SAT FAT	CHOL	PROT	CARB	SUGAR	FIBER	CALCI	SOD	POTAS	FOLIC	VIT C
papadum fried	1 (6 g)	30	2	1	0	1	2	—	tr	4	125	4	—	0
paratha plain	1 (1.6 oz)	136	5	3	19	3	19	—	2	12	176	71	—	0
poori indian puffed bread	1 piece (1.3 oz)	112	4	2	0	3	16	tr	2	6	226	68	17	tr
zucchini	1 slice (1.4 oz)	150	7	1	26	2	19	10	1	27	115	47	19	1

BREADCRUMBS

FOOD	PORTION	CALS	FAT	SAT FAT	CHOL	PROT	CARB	SUGAR	FIBER	CALCI	SOD	POTAS	FOLIC	VIT C
dry seasoned	¼ cup	115	2	tr	0	4	21	2	2	55	528	69	36	1
fresh	¼ cup	30	tr	tr	0	1	6	tr	tr	17	77	11	12	0
plain	¼ cup	107	1	tr	0	4	19	2	1	49	198	53	29	0
EDWARD & SONS														
Organic Lightly Salted	⅓ cup	110	1	0	0	7	21	2	1	0	110	—	—	0
Organic Panko	⅓ cup	110	1	0	0	2	21	2	1	0	110	—	—	0
GILLIAN'S FOODS														
Plain Gluten Free	¼ cup (1.2 oz)	60	1	0	0	2	14	1	1	20	430	—	—	2
IAN'S														
Panko Italian	¼ cup	70	1	0	0	2	15	1	2	0	137	—	—	0
Panko Original	¼ cup	71	0	0	0	2	15	1	1	0	32	—	—	0
Panko Whole Wheat	¼ cup	70	1	0	0	3	14	1	2	0	23	—	—	0
KIKKOMAN														
Panko	½ cup (1.1 oz)	110	1	0	0	3	24	2	tr	0	40	—	—	0
KRASDALE														
Seasoned	¼ cup	120	2	1	0	4	21	4	2	80	350	—	—	0
PROGRESSO														
Garlic & Herb	¼ cup (1 oz)	110	2	1	0	4	19	2	1	40	520	—	—	0
Italian Style	¼ cup (1 oz)	118	2	1	0	4	20	2	1	40	470	—	—	0
Panko Lemon Pepper	¼ cup (1 oz)	120	5	0	0	2	17	0	tr	0	430	—	—	0
Panko Plain	¼ cup (1 oz)	110	3	0	0	2	19	1	0	0	50	—	—	0
Plain	¼ cup (1 oz)	110	2	1	0	4	20	2	1	40	200	—	—	0
SOUTHERN HOMESTYLE														
Corn Flake Crumbs	2 tbsp	40	0	0	0	1	9	1	0	0	50	—	—	0
Tortilla Crumbs	2 tbsp	40	0	0	0	1	9	1	0	0	50	—	—	0

BREADFRUIT

FOOD	PORTION	CALS	FAT	SAT FAT	CHOL	PROT	CARB	SUGAR	FIBER	CALCI	SOD	POTAS	FOLIC	VIT C
fresh	1 sm (13.5 oz)	396	1	tr	0	4	104	42	19	65	8	1882	54	111
fried	1 cup	379	21	3	0	2	52	21	9	31	3	847	14	39
raw	1 cup	227	1	tr	0	2	60	24	11	37	4	1078	31	64

BREADNUTTREE SEEDS

FOOD	PORTION	CALS	FAT	SAT FAT	CHOL	PROT	CARB	SUGAR	FIBER	CALCI	SOD	POTAS	FOLIC	VIT C
dried	1 oz	104	tr	tr	0	2	23	—	—	27	—	—	13	—

BREADSTICKS

FOOD	PORTION	CALS	FAT	SAT FAT	CHOL	PROT	CARB	SUGAR	FIBER	CALCI	SOD	POTAS	FOLIC	VIT C
plain	1 lg	41	1	tr	0	1	7	tr	tr	2	66	12	16	0
plain	1 sm	21	tr	tr	0	1	3	tr	tr	1	33	6	8	0

FOOD	PORTION	CALS	FAT	SAT FAT	CHOL	PROT	CARB	SUGAR	FIBER	CALCI	SOD	POTAS	FOLIC	VIT C
FATTORIE & PANDEA														
Fornini w/ Sea Salt	5 (1.2 oz)	140	5	1	0	4	21	1	1	20	320	—	—	0
FERRARA														
Slim Thin Torinese Style	6 (0.5 oz)	60	1	0	0	2	11	1	0	0	150	—	—	0
PILLSBURY														
Cornbread Twists	1 (1.4 oz)	140	6	2	0	3	18	4	0	0	340	—	—	0
Original Soft	2 (1.8 oz)	140	3	2	0	4	25	3	tr	0	370	—	—	0
STELLA D'ORO														
Original	1 (0.3 oz)	40	1	0	0	1	6	0	0	0	40	—	—	0
Roasted Garlic	1	45	1	0	0	1	7	0	0	0	80	—	—	0
Sesame	1 (0.4 oz)	50	3	0	0	2	6	0	0	0	50	—	—	0
Sodium Free	1 (0.3 oz)	40	1	0	0	1	6	0	0	0	0	—	—	0

BREAKFAST BARS

(*see* CEREAL BARS, ENERGY BARS)

BROCCOFLOWER

FOOD	PORTION	CALS	FAT	SAT FAT	CHOL	PROT	CARB	SUGAR	FIBER	CALCI	SOD	POTAS	FOLIC	VIT C
fresh flowerets cooked	1 cup (2.9 oz)	26	tr	tr	0	2	5	3	3	26	214	227	34	59
fresh raw	1 cup (2.2 oz)	20	tr	tr	0	2	4	2	2	21	15	192	36	56
head fresh raw	1 lg (18 oz)	158	2	tr	0	15	31	15	16	169	118	1533	291	450

BROCCOLI

FOOD	PORTION	CALS	FAT	SAT FAT	CHOL	PROT	CARB	SUGAR	FIBER	CALCI	SOD	POTAS	FOLIC	VIT C
FRESH														
chinese broccoli (gai lan) cooked	1 cup (3 oz)	19	1	tr	0	1	3	1	2	88	6	230	87	25
cooked w/o salt chopped	½ cup (2.7 oz)	27	tr	tr	0	2	6	1	3	31	32	229	84	51
cooked w/o salt spear 5 in	1 (1.3 oz)	13	tr	tr	0	1	3	1	1	15	15	108	40	24
raab cooked	½ cup (3 oz)	28	tr	tr	0	3	3	1	2	100	48	292	60	31
raw	1 bunch (1.3 lbs)	207	2	tr	0	17	40	10	16	286	201	1921	383	542
raw floweret	1 (0.4 oz)	3	tr	tr	0	tr	1	—	—	5	3	36	8	10
raw flowers	1 cup (2.5 oz)	20	tr	tr	0	2	4	—	—	34	19	231	50	66
raw spear 5 in long	1 (1.1 oz)	11	tr	tr	0	1	2	1	1	15	10	98	20	28
BROCCOSPROUTS														
Broccoli Sprouts	½ cup	16	0	0	0	1	2	—	1	26	3	—	0	20
DOLE														
Broccoli	1 stalk (5.2 oz)	50	1	0	0	4	10	3	4	80	50	470	100	132
Broccoli Slaw	1 cup (3 oz)	25	0	0	0	2	5	2	2	40	25	—	—	72
MANN'S														
Broccoli Wokly	1 serv (3 oz)	25	0	0	0	3	4	2	2	40	25	280	60	78
Broccolini	8 stalks (3 oz)	35	0	0	0	3	6	2	1	60	25	270	—	78

FOOD	PORTION	CALS	FAT	SAT FAT	CHOL	PROT	CARB	SUGAR	FIBER	CALCI	SOD	POTAS	FOLIC	VIT C
OCEAN MIST														
Rapini Broccoli Rabe Chopped Raw	1 cup	9	0	0	0	1	1	0	1	40	13	—	—	8
READY PAC														
Microwave Broccoli Rabe as prep	½ cup (3 oz)	30	0	0	0	3	3	0	2	100	50	—	60	30
FROZEN														
chopped cooked w/o salt	1 cup (6.5 oz)	52	tr	tr	0	6	10	3	6	61	20	261	103	74
spears cooked w/o salt	1 cup (6.5 oz)	52	tr	tr	0	6	10	3	6	94	44	331	55	74
BIRDS EYE														
Broccoli & Cheese Sauce	½ cup	90	5	3	5	3	8	3	1	60	490	—	—	24
Steamfresh Cuts	1 cup (3.1 oz)	30	0	0	0	2	4	2	2	20	20	—	—	30
Steamfresh Florets	1 cup (2.3 oz)	30	0	0	0	1	4	2	2	20	20	—	—	30
C&W														
Broccoli & Cheddar Cheese Sauce	1⅓ cups	70	3	1	5	4	7	3	2	60	370	—	—	36
Florets	1 cup	30	0	0	0	1	4	2	2	20	20	—	—	30
CASCADIAN FARM														
Organic Florets	⅔ cup	20	0	0	0	2	4	2	2	20	20	210	—	24
DR. PRAEGER'S														
Broccoli Bites	2 (2 oz)	110	4	0	0	3	17	2	2	0	220	—	—	2
GREEN GIANT														
Cuts as prep	⅔ cup	25	0	0	0	1	4	2	2	20	20	—	—	30
Pasta Broccoli & Alfredo Sauce as prep	1 cup	210	4	1	<5	9	34	6	3	100	780	—	—	30
Steamers Broccoli & Cheese Sauce as prep	½ cup	45	2	0	0	2	7	3	2	40	380	200	—	30
SEABROOK FARMS														
Broccoli Raab	1 cup (2.9 oz)	25	0	0	0	2	4	tr	2	60	35	—	—	30
SKYY														
Broccoli Bites	3 (2.8 oz)	180	10	3	10	7	16	1	2	250	330	—	—	24
TAKE-OUT														
batter dipped & fried	3 pieces (1.4 oz)	58	4	1	7	1	5	1	1	30	62	108	18	23
w/ cheese sauce	1 cup (8 oz)	242	15	7	32	12	16	5	5	315	426	538	164	94
BROWNIE														
brownie	1 (2 oz)	227	9	2	10	3	36	21	1	16	175	83	26	0
butterscotch	1 (1.2 oz)	151	8	1	20	2	19	12	tr	22	95	69	15	0

FOOD	PORTION	CALS	FAT	SAT FAT	CHOL	PROT	CARB	SUGAR	FIBER	CALCI	SOD	POTAS	FOLIC	VIT C
ARROWHEAD MILLS														
Gluten Free as prep	1	160	8	2	21	1	21	13	tr	0	40	—	—	0
BETTY CROCKER														
Dark Chocolate as prep	1	170	7	1	21	1	25	17	tr	—	100	90	8	—
Fudge Low Fat as prep	1	140	3	1	12	1	28	19	1	—	125	—	8	—
Original Supreme as prep	1	160	6	1	21	1	26	18	tr	—	105	85	8	—
Triple Chunk as prep	1	180	8	2	21	1	25	18	1	—	90	85	8	—
Walnut as prep	1	170	9	1	21	1	22	15	tr	—	90	—	8	—
Warm Delights Hot Fudge	1 pkg (3 oz)	370	12	5	—	5	61	41	3	20	270	—	—	—
BOB'S RED MILL														
Gluten Free as prep	1	140	5	1	0	2	27	17	2	—	180	—	—	—
DUNCAN HINES														
Chocolate Fudge frzn	¹⁄₁₂ pkg (1.4 oz)	170	8	2	20	2	23	16	0	0	85	—	—	0
Dark Chocolate Chunk Mix as prep	¹⁄₁₆ pkg	170	7	2	15	2	25	18	1	20	110	—	—	—
Milk Chocolate Mix as prep	¹⁄₂₀ pkg	180	9	2	25	2	23	16	0	0	75	—	—	0
Peanut Butter Cup Mix as prep	¹⁄₁₆ pkg	170	8	3	15	2	23	16	1	20	105	—	—	—
Turtle Mix as prep	¹⁄₁₆ pkg	160	7	2	15	2	23	15	1	—	115	—	—	—
Walnut Mix as prep	¹⁄₁₆ pkg	180	8	2	15	2	24	16	2	—	115	—	—	—
ERIN BAKER'S														
Organic Bites	1 (1 oz)	100	3	0	5	2	18	10	2	20	70	—	—	0
Organic Bites Double Chocolate Chip	1 (1 oz)	90	2	0	5	2	19	10	2	20	75	—	—	0
FIBER ONE														
Chocolate Peanut Butter	1 (0.89 oz)	90	35	2	0	1	17	7	5	—	110	—	—	—
Chocolate Fudge	1 (0.89 oz)	90	3	2	0	1	18	8	5	—	100	—	—	—
FOODS BY GEORGE														
Gluten Free	¹⁄₉ pkg (1.5 oz)	180	9	1	40	2	24	16	1	20	45	—	—	0
FOXY'S BAKE SHOP														
Milk Chocolate	½ (1.7 oz)	200	11	5	55	3	23	18	0	40	65	—	—	0
White Chocolate	½ (1.7 oz)	200	12	6	0	3	23	18	0	40	70	—	—	0
FRENCH MEADOW BAKERY														
Gluten Free Fudge	1 (2.82 oz)	350	16	2	55	3	48	34	2	20	240	—	—	0

FOOD	PORTION	CALS	FAT	SAT FAT	CHOL	PROT	CARB	SUGAR	FIBER	CALCI	SOD	POTAS	FOLIC	VIT C
GLENNY'S														
100 Calorie 75% Organic	1 (1.45 oz)	100	4	2	—	4	12	11	7	—	85	—	—	—
HERSHEY'S														
Brownie	½ pkg (1.5 oz)	190	9	4	—	2	28	14	1	20	40	—	—	0
JOSEPH'S														
Sugar Free	1 (1.5 oz)	150	7	2	0	2	26	0	1	0	59	—	—	1
SANS SUCRE														
Blondie Mix as prep	⅛ pkg	130	0	0	3	1	25	0	0	0	45	—	—	0
Chocolate Fudge Mix as prep	⅛ pkg	130	3	0	0	1	25	0	tr	0	45	—	—	0
Milk Chocolate Mix as prep	⅛ pkg	130	3	0	0	1	25	1	0	20	50	—	—	0
UNCLE WALLY'S														
Smart Portion	1 (0.9 oz)	80	2	0	10	1	17	11	2	0	75	—	—	0
VITABROWNIE														
Brownie	1 (2 oz)	100	2	1	0	4	25	10	10	200	125	65	200	30
Dark Chocolate Pomegranate	1 (2 oz)	100	2	1	0	3	21	11	6	200	140	160	—	30
BRUSSELS SPROUTS														
CANNED														
JAKE & AMOS														
Pickled Dill Brussels Sprouts	2 tbsp	10	0	0	0	0	1	0	0	—	217	—	—	—
FRESH														
cooked	6 pieces	45	1	tr	0	3	9	2	3	45	26	399	76	78
DOLE														
Brussels Sprouts	4 (2.9 oz)	30	0	0	0	2	6	1	3	40	20	—	60	54
OCEAN MIST														
Brussels Sprouts	4 (2 oz)	40	1	0	0	2	6	2	3	20	25	—	—	72
SELECT GOURMET														
Fresh	½ cup	35	0	0	0	3	8	2	3	40	21	—	—	72
FROZEN														
cooked	1 cup	65	1	tr	0	6	13	3	6	40	23	450	157	71
BIRDS EYE														
Steamfresh Baby	10 (2.9 oz)	45	0	0	0	3	8	2	3	20	15	—	—	54
Steamfresh Singles Baby	1 pkg (3.2 oz)	50	0	0	0	3	9	3	3	20	20	—	—	60
C&W														
Petite	10 (3 oz)	45	0	0	0	3	8	2	3	20	15	—	—	54
GREEN GIANT														
Baby & Butter Sauce as prep	½ cup	60	1	1	<5	3	9	3	3	20	320	—	—	54

FOOD	PORTION	CALS	FAT	SAT FAT	CHOL	PROT	CARB	SUGAR	FIBER	CALCI	SOD	POTAS	FOLIC	VIT C
BUCKWHEAT														
groats roasted cooked	1 cup (6 oz)	155	1	tr	0	7	33	2	5	12	252	148	24	0
groats roasted uncooked	½ cup	292	3	1	0	11	61	—	9	9	1	391	26	0
BOB'S RED MILL														
Organic Kernels	¼ cup	142	1	0	0	5	31	0	3	—	4	—	—	—
WOLFF'S														
Kasha not prep	¼ cup (1.6 oz)	170	1	0	0	6	35	0	2	0	10	220	—	0
BUFFALO														
(*see also* HOT DOG, JERKY, SAUSAGE)														
burger	3 oz	202	13	5	71	20	0	0	0	11	62	290	13	0
chuck braised	4 oz	205	6	2	118	36	0	0	0	7	61	336	22	0
top round steak broiled	3 oz	313	9	4	153	54	0	0	0	9	74	688	34	0
water buffalo roasted	3 oz	111	2	1	52	23	0	0	0	13	48	266	8	—
HIGH PLAINS BISON														
Filet Mignon	4 oz	120	4	2	70	23	1	0	0	0	50	—	—	0
Ground	4 oz	190	11	4	50	20	0	0	0	0	60	—	—	0
Pot Roast	4 oz	150	7	6	70	22	0	0	0	0	85	—	—	0
Ribeye Steak	4 oz	215	14	11	60	21	1	0	0	0	75	—	—	0
Shredded In BBQ Sauce	1 serv (5 oz)	250	3	1	45	22	34	22	0	40	320	—	—	0
Steak Top Sirloin	4 oz	110	3	2	50	25	0	0	0	0	50	—	—	0
Tenderloin Tips	4 oz	120	12	2	70	23	1	0	0	0	50	—	—	0
NATURAL FRONTIER FOODS														
Burgers	1 (5 oz)	170	9	4	55	22	0	0	0	20	85	—	—	0
Ground	4 oz	170	9	4	55	22	0	0	0	20	85	—	—	0
Steaks	1 (4 oz)	160	3	1	75	28	0	0	0	0	75	—	—	0
BULGUR														
cooked	½ cup	76	tr	tr	0	3	17	tr	4	9	5	62	16	0
uncooked	½ cup	239	1	tr	0	9	53	tr	13	25	12	287	19	0
BOB'S RED MILL														
From Soft White Wheat	¼ cup	150	1	0	0	4	32	0	4	—	0	—	—	—
FANTASTIC														
Tabouli Mix not prep	2 tbsp	70	0	0	0	2	15	1	4	20	280	—	—	1
NEAR EAST														
Whole Grain Wheat Pilaf as prep	1 cup	200	4	2	9	7	40	2	8	20	672	—	—	0
TAKE-OUT														
tabbouleh	1 cup	198	15	2	0	3	16	2	4	30	797	250	30	26

FOOD	PORTION	CALS	FAT	SAT FAT	CHOL	PROT	CARB	SUGAR	FIBER	CALCI	SOD	POTAS	FOLIC	VIT C
BURBOT (FISH)														
fresh baked	3 oz	98	1	tr	65	65	0	0	0	54	106	440	—	—
BURDOCK ROOT														
cooked w/o salt	1 cup	110	tr	tr	0	3	26	4	2	61	5	450	25	3
cooked w/o salt	1 root (5.8 oz)	146	tr	tr	0	3	35	6	3	81	7	598	33	4
BUTTER														
clarified butter	¼ cup (1.8 oz)	449	51	32	131	tr	0	0	0	2	1	3	0	0
clarified butter	1 tbsp (0.4 oz)	112	13	8	33	tr	0	0	0	1	0	1	0	0
ghee cow's milk	1 tbsp	126	14	—	39	—	—	—	0	—	0	0	0	0
ghee vegetable oil	1 tbsp	126	14	—	0	—	—	—	0	—	0	0	0	—
honey butter	1 tbsp (0.6 oz)	85	6	4	15	tr	9	9	0	2	42	7	0	tr
honey butter	¼ cup (2.5 oz)	338	23	15	62	tr	36	35	tr	9	168	30	1	tr
light butter whipped salted	1 tbsp (0.3 oz)	48	5	3	10	tr	0	0	0	5	43	7	0	0
stick salted	¼ cup (2 oz)	407	46	29	122	tr	tr	tr	0	14	327	14	2	0
stick salted	1 (4 oz)	810	92	58	243	1	tr	tr	0	27	651	27	3	0
stick salted	1 tbsp (0.5 oz)	102	12	7	31	tr	tr	tr	0	3	82	3	0	0
stick unsalted	¼ cup (2 oz)	407	46	29	122	tr	tr	tr	0	14	6	14	2	0
stick unsalted	1 tbsp (0.5 oz)	102	12	7	31	tr	tr	tr	0	3	2	3	0	0
stick unsalted	1 (4 oz)	810	92	58	243	1	tr	tr	0	27	12	27	3	0
whipped salted	1 tbsp (0.3 oz)	67	8	5	21	tr	tr	tr	0	2	78	2	0	0
whipped salted	¼ cup (1.3 oz)	271	31	19	83	tr	tr	tr	0	9	312	10	1	0
CABOT														
Salted	1 tbsp	100	11	7	30	0	0	0	0	0	90	—	—	0
COUNTRY CROCK														
Spreadable Butter w/ Canola Oil	1 tbsp (0.4 oz)	80	9	4	15	0	0	0	0	—	65	—	—	—
DEERFIELD														
Creamy	1 tbsp	100	11	7	30	0	0	0	0	—	0	—	—	—
EARTH BALANCE														
Butter Blend Unsalted	1 tbsp	100	11	5	0	0	0	0	0	—	0	—	—	4
GOPI														
Pure Ghee	1 tsp (5 g)	35	5	3	12	0	0	0	0	—	0	—	—	—
HORIZON ORGANIC														
European	1 tbsp	100	12	7	30	0	0	0	0	0	0	—	—	0
KAROUN														
Unsalted	1 tbsp (0.5 oz)	100	11	7	30	0	0	0	—	3	0	—	0	0
LAND O LAKES														
Butter Spread Cinnamon Sugar	1 tbsp (0.5 oz)	70	6	3	10	0	4	4	0	0	30	—	—	0
Honey	1 tbsp (0.5 oz)	90	8	4	15	0	4	3	0	0	40	—	—	0
Light Salted	1 tbsp (0.5 oz)	50	6	4	15	0	0	0	0	0	100	—	—	0
Light Whipped Salted	1 tbsp (0.4 oz)	45	5	3	15	0	0	0	0	0	85	—	—	0

FOOD	PORTION	CALS	FAT	SAT FAT	CHOL	PROT	CARB	SUGAR	FIBER	CALCI	SOD	POTAS	FOLIC	VIT C
LAND O LAKES (CONT.)														
Roasted Garlic w/ Oil	1 tbsp (0.5 oz)	90	10	5	20	0	0	0	0	0	110	—	—	0
Salted	1 tbsp (0.5 oz)	100	11	7	30	0	0	0	0	0	95	—	—	0
Spreadable w/ Canola Oil	1 tbsp (0.5 oz)	100	11	5	20	0	0	0	0	0	90	—	—	0
Whipped Salted	1 tbsp (0.2 oz)	50	6	4	15	0	0	0	0	0	50	—	—	0
MOLLY MCBUTTER														
Natural Butter	1 tsp (2 g)	5	0	0	0	0	1	—	0	—	180	0	—	—
ORGANIC VALLEY														
European Style	1 tbsp	110	12	8	25	0	0	0	0	0	0	—	—	0
PLUGRA														
European Style Unsalted	1 tbsp (0.5 oz)	100	11	7	30	0	0	0	0	—	90	—	—	—
STRAUS														
Organic European Style Lightly Salted	1 tbsp (0.5 oz)	110	12	8	30	0	0	0	0	0	45	—	—	0
Organic European Style Sweet Butter	1 tbsp (0.5 oz)	110	12	8	30	0	0	0	0	0	0	—	—	0

BUTTER SUBSTITUTES

FOOD	PORTION	CALS	FAT	SAT FAT	CHOL	PROT	CARB	SUGAR	FIBER	CALCI	SOD	POTAS	FOLIC	VIT C
stick	1 stick	811	91	32	99	1	1	—	—	31	1013	40	2	tr
BUTTER BUDS														
Granules	1 pkg (2 g)	5	0	0	0	0	2	—	—	—	75	—	—	—
SUNSWEET														
Lighter Bake	1 tbsp	35	0	0	0	0	9	5	—	—	0	—	—	—

BUTTERBUR

FOOD	PORTION	CALS	FAT	SAT FAT	CHOL	PROT	CARB	SUGAR	FIBER	CALCI	SOD	POTAS	FOLIC	VIT C
canned fuki chopped	1 cup	3	tr	—	0	tr	tr	—	—	42	5	15	—	15
fresh fuki	1 cup	13	tr	—	0	tr	3	—	—	97	7	616	—	30

BUTTERNUTS

FOOD	PORTION	CALS	FAT	SAT FAT	CHOL	PROT	CARB	SUGAR	FIBER	CALCI	SOD	POTAS	FOLIC	VIT C
dried	1 oz	174	16	tr	0	7	3	—	—	15	0	119	—	—

BUTTERSCOTCH

(*see also* CANDY)

FOOD	PORTION	CALS	FAT	SAT FAT	CHOL	PROT	CARB	SUGAR	FIBER	CALCI	SOD	POTAS	FOLIC	VIT C
E. GUITTARD														
Baking Chips	33 (0.5 oz)	80	5	4	0	tr	10	10	0	20	15	—	—	0
HERSHEY'S														
Chips	1 tbsp (0.5 oz)	80	4	4	—	1	9	9	—	20	35	—	—	0

CABBAGE

(*see also* COLESLAW)

FOOD	PORTION	CALS	FAT	SAT FAT	CHOL	PROT	CARB	SUGAR	FIBER	CALCI	SOD	POTAS	FOLIC	VIT C
chinese bok choy shredded cooked w/o salt	1 cup	20	tr	tr	0	3	3	1	2	158	58	631	70	44

FOOD	PORTION	CALS	FAT	SAT FAT	CHOL	PROT	CARB	SUGAR	FIBER	CALCI	SOD	POTAS	FOLIC	VIT C
chinese pe-tsai shredded cooked w/o salt	1 cup	17	tr	tr	0	2	3	—	2	38	11	268	63	19
green raw shredded	1 cup	19	tr	tr	0	1	4	2	2	28	13	119	30	26
green shredded cooked w/o salt	1 cup	34	tr	tr	0	2	8	4	3	72	12	294	45	56
japanese pickled	½ cup	22	tr	tr	0	1	4	1	2	36	208	640	32	1
red raw shredded	1 cup	22	tr	tr	0	1	5	3	2	32	19	170	13	40
red shredded cooked w/o salt	1 cup	44	tr	tr	0	2	10	5	4	63	42	393	36	52
savoy shredded cooked w/o salt	1 cup	35	tr	tr	0	3	8	—	4	44	35	267	67	24
AUNT NELLIE'S														
Sweet & Sour Red	2 tbsp (1 oz)	20	0	0	0	0	5	4	0	0	110	—	—	1
DOLE														
Shredded Red Fresh	1½ cups (3 oz)	25	0	0	0	1	6	3	2	40	25	—	—	48
GLORY														
Country Cabbage	½ cup	25	0	0	0	1	6	3	1	20	350	—	—	48
READY PAC														
Ready Fixin's Shredded Red	2 cups (3 oz)	25	0	0	0	1	6	3	2	40	25	—	—	48
TAKE-OUT														
coleslaw w/ pineapple & dressing	1 cup (4.6 oz)	194	16	2	8	1	14	10	2	34	124	164	32	28
creamed	1 cup	158	10	3	6	5	13	7	2	140	610	246	28	23
kimchee	1 cup	32	tr	tr	0	2	6	2	2	144	996	380	88	80
stuffed cabbage w/ rice & beef	1 (3.6 oz)	117	5	2	42	9	9	4	1	31	369	283	25	12
sweet & sour red cabbage	4 oz	61	3	—	—	1	8	—	3	43	—	—	—	14
CACAO														
KOPALI														
Organic Dark Chocolate Covered Cacao Nibs	½ pkg (1 oz)	140	10	6	0	2	15	12	2	10	0	—	—	0
NAVITAS NATURALS														
Butter	1 tbsp	120	14	8	0	0	0	0	0	0	0	—	—	0
Nibs	1 oz	130	12	7	0	4	10	0	9	20	0	—	—	0
Powder	1 oz	120	3	2	0	5	18	12	7	40	20	—	—	0
SUNFOOD														
Organic Cacao Beans	1 oz	171	13	8	0	4	8	0	6	0	15	—	—	13

FOOD	PORTION	CALS	FAT	SAT FAT	CHOL	PROT	CARB	SUGAR	FIBER	CALCI	SOD	POTAS	FOLIC	VIT C
SUNFOOD (CONT.)														
Organic Cacao Nibs	1 oz	171	13	8	0	4	8	0	6	0	15	—	—	13
CACTUS														
fresh cooked w/ fat	1 pad (1 oz)	11	1	tr	0	tr	1	tr	1	47	84	56	1	2
fresh cooked w/o fat	1 cup (5.2 oz)	22	tr	tr	0	2	5	2	3	243	399	289	4	8
pricklypear fresh	1 (3.6 oz)	42	1	tr	0	1	10	—	4	58	5	227	6	14
pricklypear fresh	1 cup (5.2 oz)	61	1	tr	0	1	14	—	5	83	7	328	9	21
CAKE														
(*see also* CAKE MIX)														
battenburg cake	1 slice (2 oz)	204	10	—	—	3	28	—	1	48	—	—	—	0
cream puff shell	1 (2.3 oz)	239	17	4	129	6	15	—	—	24	368	64	14	0
crumpet	1 (2.3 oz)	131	1	—	0	4	31	—	2	79	535	61	6	0
dutch honey cake	1 slice (0.8 oz)	70	0	0	0	1	17	8	0	0	25	—	—	0
eccles cake	1 slice (2 oz)	285	16	—	—	2	36	—	1	47	—	—	—	0
madeira cake	1 slice (1 oz)	98	4	—	—	1	15	—	1	11	—	—	—	0
sponge	1 piece (1.3 oz)	110	1	tr	39	2	23	14	tr	27	93	38	18	0
sponge cake desscrt shell	1 (0.8 oz)	70	2	1	20	1	12	7	0	30	150	—	—	0
treacle tart	1 slice (2.5 oz)	258	10	—	—	3	42	—	1	43	—	—	—	0
turnover guava	1 (2.7 oz)	239	13	3	0	3	29	12	3	12	108	164	35	59
AMY'S														
Organic Chocolate	1 slice	170	6	0	0	2	27	16	1	0	130	—	—	0
Toaster Pops Apple	1 (2.1 oz)	150	4	0	0	3	27	10	1	20	110	—	—	0
ATHENS														
Baklava	2 pieces (2 oz)	230	11	2	0	3	30	17	1	20	75	—	—	0
AUNT TRUDY'S														
Organic Baklava Soy Nut	1 (1.8 oz)	190	6	1	0	4	29	17	2	60	60	—	—	0
BALOCCO														
Il Panettone	1 serv (3.5 oz)	380	15	8	120	7	54	27	2	20	75	—	—	0
BELLINO														
Pandoro	1 (2.8 oz)	330	16	10	125	7	39	16	1	10	95	—	—	0
BETTY CROCKER														
Warm Delights Cinnamon Swirl	1 (3.3 oz)	390	10	4	0	4	72	49	1	80	500	—	—	—
COPPENRATH														
Mousse Cake Chocolate	⅛ cake (1.8 oz)	140	7	4	40	3	17	12	2	50	55	—	—	3
Mousse Cake Coconut	⅛ cake (1.8 oz)	140	8	5	45	3	15	11	2	30	50	—	—	2
Mousse Duets Chocolate	1 (3.2 oz)	290	15	9	35	5	32	25	2	60	80	—	—	4

FOOD	PORTION	CALS	FAT	SAT FAT	CHOL	PROT	CARB	SUGAR	FIBER	CALCI	SOD	POTAS	FOLIC	VIT C
COPPENRATH (CONT.)														
Mousse Duets Lemon Chiffon	1 (3.2 oz)	280	16	9	35	3	31	23	tr	40	70	—	—	0
DO GOODIE														
Gluten Free Banana Bread	1 slice (2 oz)	150	4	2	35	2	27	15	2	0	170	—	—	1
Gluten Free Cupcake Chocolate	1	290	14	6	15	2	41	31	1	10	125	—	—	0
Gluten Free Cupcake Vanilla	1	290	14	6	15	2	41	32	0	20	125	—	—	0
EARTH CAFE														
Cheesecake Vegan Blueberry Thrill	1 slice (2 oz)	193	15	6	0	3	12	7	1	60	67	—	—	6
Cheesecake Vegan Coconut Carob	1 slice (2 oz)	206	16	7	0	3	13	8	1	60	61	—	—	5
Cheesecake Vegan Rockin' Raspberry	1 slice (2 oz)	194	15	6	0	3	12	7	2	60	67	—	—	7
EL MONTEREY														
Cheesecake Bites Caramel	1 (2 oz)	180	10	4	15	2	23	9	0	20	150	—	—	0
Cheesecake Bites Raspberry	1 (2 oz)	200	11	5	20	3	21	6	0	40	150	—	—	0
ENTENMANN'S														
Apple Puffs	1 (3 oz)	290	13	6	0	3	41	21	1	20	230	—	—	0
Blackout Iced	⅛ cake (2.2 oz)	210	8	3	30	2	34	23	1	0	230	—		0
Cheese Buns	1 (3 oz)	320	15	6	40	5	42	22	1	40	230	—	—	0
Chocolate Chip Iced	⅛ cake (2.5 oz)	330	18	7	25	2	40	31	tr	40	170	—	—	0
Chocolate Fudge	⅛ cake (2.2 oz)	240	10	4	25	2	37	28	2	40	190	—	—	0
Cinnamon Swirl Buns	1 (3 oz)	320	14	5	35	5	45	21	2	40	230	—	—	0
Coffee Cake Cheese Filled Crumb	⅛ cake (2 oz)	210	10	4	25	4	28	13	tr	20	170	—	—	0
Danish Twist Cheese	⅛ cake (1.9 oz)	220	11	4	20	3	27	14	tr	20	190	—	—	0
Danish Twist Raspberry	⅛ cake (1.8 oz)	210	10	4	15	2	27	14	tr	20	160	—	—	0
Devil's Food Marshmallow Iced	⅛ cake (2.2 oz)	260	12	5	20	2	38	30	tr	40	210	—	—	0
Fudge Iced Golden Cake	⅛ cake (2.2 oz)	260	11	4	25	2	37	28	1	40	150	—	—	0
Lemon Crunch	⅛ cake (3 oz)	320	13	4	45	3	50	35	tr	2	300	—	—	0
Lemon Loaf	⅙ cake (2 oz)	210	10	2	40	2	28	17	0	0	230	—	—	0
Louisiana Crunch	⅛ cake (2.7 oz)	310	13	4	45	3	47	33	tr	100	300	—	—	0

FOOD	PORTION	CALS	FAT	SAT FAT	CHOL	PROT	CARB	SUGAR	FIBER	CALCI	SOD	POTAS	FOLIC	VIT C
ENTENMANN'S (CONT.)														
Utlimate Super Cinnamons	½ bun (2.5 oz)	280	10	4	25	4	41	19	1	20	180	—	—	0
Vanilla Bean Iced	⅛ cake (2.2 oz)	290	17	7	25	1	36	28	0	40	160	—	—	0
FIBER ONE														
Toaster Pastry Blueberry	1 (1.8 oz)	180	4	1	0	3	36	15	5	—	130	100	—	—
Toaster Pastry Chocolate Fudge	1 (1.8 oz)	160	4	2	0	3	35	16	5	—	140	150	—	—
FOODS BY GEORGE														
Gluten Free Crumb Cake	⅑ cake (2.2 oz)	280	14	9	40	2	36	12	tr	60	80	—	—	0
Gluten Free Pound Cake	⅙ cake (2.7 oz)	290	12	8	130	4	35	16	tr	80	190	—	—	0
FRENCH MEADOW BAKERY														
Gluten Free Cupcake Chocolate	1 (2 oz)	220	8	5	20	24	35	27	1	0	240	—	—	0
Gluten Free Cupcake Yellow	1 (2 oz)	230	9	5	20	20	35	28	0	0	230	—	—	0
Vegan Carrot	¼ cake (2.6 oz)	130	0	—	65	2	38	21	1	60	150	—	—	0
GLENNY'S														
Blondie 100 Calorie 75% Organic	1 (1.45 oz)	100	3	1	—	4	12	9	7	—	100	—	—	—
GOURMET PASTRIES														
Baklava Walnut	1 piece (1.8 oz)	240	11	3	5	3	30	18	0	20	100	—	—	0
GUILTLESS GOURMET														
Dessert Bowl Bananas Foster Cake	1 pkg (2 oz)	200	2	1	15	3	42	26	tr	40	250	—	—	0
Dessert Bowl Black Velvet Cake	1 pkg (2 oz)	200	3	2	20	4	42	30	3	40	190	—	—	0
HOSTESS														
100 Calorie Pack Mini Carrot Cake	1 pkg (1.2 oz)	100	3	1	5	2	20	11	4	20	120	—	—	0
100 Calorie Pack Mini Chocolate Cupcakes	1 pkg (1.3 oz)	100	3	2	10	2	22	10	5	80	140	—	—	0
100 Calorie Pack Mini Coffee Cake Cinnamon Streusel	1 pkg (1.2 oz)	100	3	1	10	2	21	7	5	20	135	—	—	0
100 Calorie Pack Mini Golden Cupcakes	1 pkg (1.2 oz)	100	3	1	5	2	20	11	3	80	150	—	—	0

FOOD	PORTION	CALS	FAT	SAT FAT	CHOL	PROT	CARB	SUGAR	FIBER	CALCI	SOD	POTAS	FOLIC	VIT C
HOSTESS (CONT.)														
Cup Cakes Chocolate	1 (1.8 oz)	170	6	3	5	1	30	21	1	100	250	—	—	0
Ho Hos	1	120	6	4	0	1	18	14	0	0	75	—	—	0
Twinkies	1 (1.5 oz)	150	5	3	20	1	27	19	0	20	220	—	—	0
KINERET														
Babka Chocolate	1 piece (1 oz)	100	3	1	10	1	17	9	1	0	55	—	—	0
LANCE														
Honey Bun	1 (3 oz)	320	13	4	0	4	47	13	4	40	200	—	—	0
MRS. FRESHLEY'S														
Golden Cupcakes Creme Filled	1 pkg (1.3 oz)	100	3	2	10	2	24	4	5	10	135	—	—	0
MRS. SMITH'S														
Carrot	⅙ cake (2.9 oz)	300	16	3	30	3	37	27	2	20	320	—	—	0
Cobbler Blackberry	1 serv (4 oz)	260	10	5	0	2	43	20	2	—	250	—	—	—
Singles Heavenly 100 New York Cheesecake	1 (0.9 oz)	100	6	4	25	2	9	6	0	0	75	—	—	0
NATURE'S PATH														
Toaster Pastries Blueberry Organic	1 (1.8 oz)	210	5	2	0	3	40	18	1	20	150	—	—	0
Toaster Pastries Frosted Brown Sugar Maple Cinnamon Organic	1 (1.8 oz)	210	5	3	0	3	39	20	1	20	125	—	—	0
Toaster Pastries Frosted Chocolate Organic	1 (1.8 oz)	210	5	3	0	3	38	18	1	0	130	—	—	0
Toaster Pastries Frosted Strawberry	1 (1.8 oz)	210	4	2	0	3	40	19	1	20	140	—	—	0
NEUMAN'S														
Date Nut Bread	1 oz	90	2	tr	<5	2	17	10	1	0	154	—	—	0
PEPPERIDGE FARM														
Coconut 3 Layer	⅛ cake	240	10	3	20	1	35	25	tr	0	120	—	—	0
German Chocolate 3 Layer	⅛ cake	240	10	3	15	2	34	23	1	20	200	—	—	0
Red Velvet 3 Layer	⅛ cake	230	11	3	20	2	32	25	0	0	80	—	—	0
Turnover Apple	1	260	13	7	0	4	31	11	1	0	230	—	—	0
Turnover Cherry	1	260	13	7	0	4	31	10	1	0	230	—	—	0
PILLSBURY														
Caramel Rolls	1 (1.7 oz)	170	7	2	0	2	24	10	tr	0	320	—	—	0

FOOD	PORTION	CALS	FAT	SAT FAT	CHOL	PROT	CARB	SUGAR	FIBER	CALCI	SOD	POTAS	FOLIC	VIT C
PILLSBURY (CONT.)														
Cinnamon Rolls w/ Icing	1 (3.5 oz)	310	9	2	0	5	54	23	1	20	640	—	—	0
Toaster Strudel	1 (2 oz)	200	9	4	5	3	28	9	1	0	210	—	—	0
Toaster Strudel Blueberry	1 (2 oz)	190	9	4	5	3	26	9	tr	0	190	—	—	0
Toaster Strudel Cream Cheese	1 (2 oz)	200	11	5	10	3	23	8	tr	0	220	—	—	0
Toaster Strudel Raspberry	1 (2 oz)	190	9	4	5	3	26	9	tr	0	190	—	—	0
Toaster Strudel Wildberry	1 (2 oz)	190	9	4	5	3	25	9	tr	0	190	—	—	0
Turnovers Cherry	1 (2 oz)	180	8	2	0	2	24	12	0	0	250	—	—	0
PROSPERITY														
Limoncello	1 serv (3.5 oz)	300	12	6	55	4	43	27	1	40	240	—	—	0
THE FILLO FACTORY														
Organic Apple Strudel	1 (4.4 oz)	290	10	1	0	3	47	15	2	60	110	—	—	0
Organic Apple Turnovers	1 (3 oz)	180	6	1	0	2	30	9	1	40	90	—	—	0
TORTUGA														
Caribbean Rum Golden Original	1 piece (4 oz)	400	19	5	25	4	54	45	2	80	540	—	—	0
WEIGHT WATCHERS														
Lemon Creme	1 (0.9 oz)	80	3	1	25	1	16	8	4	60	85	—	—	0
TAKE-OUT														
angelfood	1 slice (2 oz)	143	tr	tr	0	3	33	17	tr	47	283	75	25	0
apple crisp	1 serv (8.6 oz)	384	8	1	0	4	76	49	4	89	502	192	39	6
apple turnover	1 (6.6 oz)	661	34	7	0	7	83	30	3	13	614	118	78	2
baklava	1 piece (2.7 oz)	334	23	10	35	5	29	10	2	30	253	134	27	1
basbousa namoura	1 piece (1 oz)	60	3	0	0	2	10	10	2	30	144	—	—	—
bean cake	1 cake (1.1 oz)	130	7	1	0	2	16	7	1	3	60	58	20	0
black forest chocolate cherry	1 piece (2.5 oz)	187	9	4	30	2	27	23	1	34	160	118	8	10
boston cream pie	1 slice (3.2 oz)	232	8	2	34	2	39	33	1	21	132	36	13	tr
cannoli w/ cannoli cream	1	369	21	—	—	6	42	28	—	52	—	—	—	0
carrot w/ icing	1 slice (4.7 oz)	543	28	5	80	5	70	52	2	77	245	133	39	1
cheesecake	1 slice (4.5 oz)	410	25	10	86	11	37	28	tr	63	484	116	17	1
cheesecake chocolate	1 slice (4.5 oz)	489	32	15	118	8	49	29	2	72	384	187	38	tr
chinese moon cake	1 (4.8 oz)	458	6	1	69	9	92	49	4	25	119	156	116	tr
cobbler pineapple	1 cup (7.6 oz)	414	10	3	2	4	80	45	2	148	345	171	43	6
coconut mochiko filipino cake	1 piece (2.7 oz)	252	12	10	0	3	35	11	2	55	76	181	8	1
coffeecake iced	1 piece (1.6 oz)	175	8	1	31	3	24	15	1	34	180	52	34	1

FOOD	PORTION	CALS	FAT	SAT FAT	CHOL	PROT	CARB	SUGAR	FIBER	CALCI	SOD	POTAS	FOLIC	VIT C
cream puff custard filled chocolate frosted	1 (3.9 oz)	293	18	5	142	7	27	7	1	71	377	131	48	tr
eclair	1 (3.5 oz)	262	16	4	127	6	24	7	1	63	337	117	43	tr
french apple tart	1 (3.5 oz)	302	15	9	60	4	37	15	2	14	326	93	2	3
fruitcake	1 slice (1.5 oz)	139	4	tr	2	1	26	13	2	14	116	66	9	tr
funnel cake	1 (3.2 oz)	276	14	3	62	7	29	4	1	126	269	152	50	0
gingerbread	1 piece (2.4 oz)	213	7	2	24	3	35	22	1	48	316	167	19	tr
jelly roll	1 slice (1.8 oz)	146	2	1	93	3	28	20	tr	14	92	46	11	2
jelly roll lemon filled	1 slice (3 oz)	210	2	1	35	3	48	29	tr	20	300	—	0	1
napoleon	1 mini (1 oz)	123	9	2	14	2	9	1	tr	13	51	25	10	0
napoleon	1 (3 oz)	348	25	7	39	5	25	4	1	37	144	71	29	tr
panettone	1/12 cake (2.9 oz)	300	12	9	90	6	43	21	2	40	120	—	—	0
petit fours	2 (0.9 oz)	120	7	3	0	1	15	12	0	20	15	—	—	0
pineapple upside down	1 piece (4.2 oz)	387	15	4	27	4	61	41	1	144	385	136	36	2
pound	1 slice (1 oz)	120	5	1	32	2	15	—	—	20	96	28	—	tr
pound fat free	1 slice (2 oz)	160	1	tr	0	3	35	19	1	24	193	62	24	0
pumpkin bread w/ raisins	1 slice (2.1 oz)	178	4	1	26	2	34	22	1	29	151	86	21	1
red velvet cupcake w/ cream cheese frosting	1 sm	272	12	—	63	3	38	—	1	—	178	—	—	—
red velvet w/ cream cheese frosting	1/16 cake	520	24	—	117	6	70	—	1	—	334	—	—	—
sacher torte	1 slice (2.2 oz)	240	11	5	50	4	30	11	4	—	120	—	—	—
sacher torte chocolate + apricot jam	1 serv	430	12	—	—	—	23	—	—	—	—	—	—	—
strawberry shortcake	1 serv (4.1 oz)	211	5	2	109	4	40	35	1	32	112	117	21	27
strudel apple	1 piece (2.2 oz)	175	7	1	4	2	26	16	1	10	172	95	18	1
strudel cheese	1 piece (2.2 oz)	195	8	4	42	6	24	14	tr	91	111	65	20	tr
strudel cherry	1 piece (2.2 oz)	179	6	1	9	3	29	18	1	21	82	99	20	3
strudel pineapple	1 piece (2.2 oz)	159	4	1	10	2	31	22	1	12	88	58	17	3
sweet potato w/ glaze	1 piece (2.7 oz)	275	12	2	40	4	39	26	1	59	285	129	27	5
tiramisu	1 piece (5.1 oz)	409	30	15	171	7	31	17	tr	114	79	211	16	1
tiramisu	1 cake (4.4 lbs)	5732	421	217	2395	101	439	234	3	1602	1107	2953	221	8.3
torte chocolate ganache	1 slice (3.5 oz)	400	26	10	90	7	40	24	6	40	120	—	—	0
trifle w/ cream	6 oz	291	16	—	—	4	34	—	1	119	—	—	—	7
white w/ coconut icing	1 slice (3.9 oz)	399	12	4	1	5	71	64	1	101	318	111	35	tr
zucchini bread	1 slice (1.4 oz)	150	7	1	26	2	19	10	1	27	115	47	19	1

CAKE ICING

FOOD	PORTION	CALS	FAT	SAT FAT	CHOL	PROT	CARB	SUGAR	FIBER	CALCI	SOD	POTAS	FOLIC	VIT C
chocolate	¼ cup	269	7	2	1	1	53	51	1	10	125	92	1	0
vanilla	¼ cup	322	8	2	0	tr	64	62	0	7	152	11	0	0
BETTY CROCKER														
HomeStyle Mix Fluffy White as prep	6 tbsp	100	0	0	0	tr	24	23	—	—	55	30	—	—
Rich & Creamy Butter Cream	2 tbsp (1.3 oz)	140	5	1	0	0	15	19	—	—	70	15	—	—
Rich & Creamy Chocolate	2 tbsp (1.2 oz)	130	5	2	0	0	21	17	tr	—	95	75	—	—
Rich & Creamy Creamy White	2 tbsp (1.2 oz)	140	5	1	0	0	23	20	—	—	70	15	—	—
Rich & Creamy Lemon	2 tbsp (1.2 oz)	140	5	2	0	0	23	19	—	—	70	15	—	—
Rich & Creamy Vanilla	2 tbsp (1.2 oz)	140	5	1	0	0	23	19	—	—	70	15	—	—
Whipped Fluffy White	2 tbsp (0.8 oz)	100	5	2	—	0	15	14	—	—	25	10	—	—
DUNCAN HINES														
Chocolate Butter Cream	2 tbsp (1.2 oz)	140	6	2	0	0	22	20	0	0	90	—	—	0
Chocolate Fudge	2 tbsp (1.2 oz)	130	6	2	0	tr	21	19	0	—	120	—	—	—
Classic Vanilla	2 tbsp	140	6	2	0	0	23	22	0	—	70	—	—	—
Cream Cheese	2 tbsp (1.2 oz)	140	6	2	0	0	23	22	0	—	70	—	—	—
Milk Chocolate	2 tbsp (1.2 oz)	140	6	2	0	0	22	20	0	—	90	—	—	—
MANISCHEWITZ														
Dairy Free Chocolate	2 tbsp (1.2 oz)	138	5	3	0	0	22	19	0	—	95	—	—	—
NATURALLY NORA														
Frosting Mix Chocolate as prep	¹⁄₁₂ pkg	150	7	4	15	1	24	21	0	0	21	—	—	0
Frosting Mix Vanilla as prep	¹⁄₁₂ pkg	170	8	5	21	tr	25	23	0	0	24	—	—	0
PILLSBURY														
Chocolate Fudge Sugar Free	2 tbsp (1 oz)	100	6	2	0	0	16	0	3	—	90	—	—	—
Creamy Supreme Buttercream	2 tbsp (1.2 oz)	150	6	2	0	0	24	22	0	0	70	—	—	0
Creamy Supreme Classic White	2 tbsp (1.2 oz)	150	6	2	6	0	24	0	0	0	70	—	—	0
Creamy Supreme Coconut Pecan	2 tbsp (1.2 oz)	160	10	4	0	1	17	16	tr	0	60	—	—	0
Creamy Supreme Milk Chocolate	2 tbsp (1.2 oz)	140	6	2	0	0	21	19	tr	0	55	—	—	0
Creamy Supreme Vanilla	2 tbsp (1.2 oz)	150	6	2	0	0	24	22	0	0	70	—	—	0

FOOD	PORTION	CALS	FAT	SAT FAT	CHOL	PROT	CARB	SUGAR	FIBER	CALCI	SOD	POTAS	FOLIC	VIT C
PILLSBURY (CONT.)														
Easy Frost Chocolate Fudge	2 tbsp (1.2 oz)	140	6	2	0	0	21	19	tr	0	125	—	—	0
Easy Frost Cream Cheese	2 tbsp (1.2 oz)	150	6	2	0	0	24	22	0	0	80	—	—	0
Easy Frost Vanilla	2 tbsp (1.2 oz)	150	6	2	0	0	24	22	0	0	70	—	—	0
Funfetti Pink Vanilla	2 tbsp (1.2 oz)	140	5	2	0	0	23	22	0	0	65	—	—	0
Vanilla Sugar Free	2 tbsp (1 oz)	100	6	2	0	0	17	0	3	—	60	—	—	—
Whipped Supreme Cream Cheese	1 tbsp (0.8 oz)	100	5	2	0	0	15	14	0	0	20	—	—	0
Whipped Supreme Strawberry	2 tbsp (0.8 oz)	110	5	2	0	0	15	14	0	0	20	—	—	0

CAKE MIX

BETTY CROCKER
FOOD	PORTION	CALS	FAT	SAT FAT	CHOL	PROT	CARB	SUGAR	FIBER	CALCI	SOD	POTAS	FOLIC	VIT C
Gingerbread as prep	1 piece	220	6	2	27	2	39	19	—	40	360	130	32	—
Pineapple Upside Down as prep	⅙ cake	390	13	3	36	2	66	43	—	40	280	70	24	—
Pound Cake as prep	⅛ cake	260	8	3	54	2	45	26	—	40	190	25	40	—
SuperMoist Carrot as prep	¹⁄₁₂ cake	260	12	2	54	1	35	19	—	100	270	25	—	—
SuperMoist Chocolate as prep	¹⁄₁₂ cake	250	11	6	75	2	35	18	1	40	380	105	—	—
SuperMoist Devil's Food as prep	¹⁄₁₂ cake	260	12	2	54	2	35	18	1	40	370	115	—	—
SuperMoist Lemon as prep	¹⁄₁₂ cake	240	9	2	54	1	35	19	—	80	280	20	—	—
SuperMoist Milk Chocolate as prep	¹⁄₁₂ cake	240	9	2	54	2	35	19	tr	80	280	95	—	—
SuperMoist Spice as prep	¹⁄₁₂ cake	270	13	3	54	2	34	19	1	40	370	105	—	—
SuperMoist Vanilla as prep	¹⁄₁₂ cake	230	9	2	54	2	35	18	—	40	300	25	—	—
SuperMoist White as prep	¹⁄₁₂ cake	220	8	2	0	2	35	18	—	40	300	25	—	—
SuperMoist Yellow as prep	¹⁄₁₂ cake	230	9	2	54	1	35	19	—	80	280	20	—	—

BISQUICK
FOOD	PORTION	CALS	FAT	SAT FAT	CHOL	PROT	CARB	SUGAR	FIBER	CALCI	SOD	POTAS	FOLIC	VIT C
Heart Smart	⅓ cup (1.4 oz)	140	3	0	0	3	27	3	tr	200	340	45	40	—

FOOD	PORTION	CALS	FAT	SAT FAT	CHOL	PROT	CARB	SUGAR	FIBER	CALCI	SOD	POTAS	FOLIC	VIT C
DUNCAN HINES														
Angel Food as prep	¹⁄₁₂ cake	140	0	0	0	31	31	23	0	0	280	—	—	9
Cupcake Mix Classic Yellow as prep	1	130	6	2	35	2	17	10	0	0	150	—	—	2
Decadent Carrot as prep	¹⁄₁₂ cake	260	11	3	55	4	37	22	1	60	260	—	—	2
Golden Butter Recipe as prep	¹⁄₁₂ cake	270	14	6	75	3	35	23	0	0	240	—	—	2
Lemon Supreme as prep	¹⁄₁₂ cake	270	12	3	55	3	36	20	—	80	310	—	—	—
Red Velvet as prep	¹⁄₁₂ cake	270	13	3	55	4	35	20	1	60	280	—	—	—
Yellow Classic as prep	¹⁄₁₂ cake	270	12	2	55	3	36	20	—	80	310	—	—	—
KING ARTHUR														
Cinnamon Buns Kit not prep	½ cup	240	1	0	0	6	52	23	3	40	15	—	—	2
NATURALLY NORA														
Cheerful Chocolate as prep	¹⁄₁₂ pkg	300	14	3	39	3	39	21	1	40	168	—	—	0
Sunny Yellow as prep	¹⁄₁₂ pkg	280	12	2	54	2	39	23	tr	40	168	—	—	0
Surprising Stars as prep	¹⁄₁₂ pkg	300	12	2	39	3	42	22	tr	40	168	—	—	0
SANS SUCRE														
Apple Cinnamon Coffee Cake as prep	½ pkg	150	4	0	0	2	30	3	tr	10	150	—	—	0
UNCLE WALLY'S														
Slice 'N Bake Cupcakes Chocolate	1 (2.1 oz)	240	11	5	20	2	32	21	1	20	150	—	—	0

CALZONE

(*see* SANDWICHES)

CANADIAN BACON

FOOD	PORTION	CALS	FAT	SAT FAT	CHOL	PROT	CARB	SUGAR	FIBER	CALCI	SOD	POTAS	FOLIC	VIT C
grilled	2 slices (1.6 oz)	87	4	1	27	11	1	0	0	5	727	183	2	0
APPLEGATE FARMS														
Natural	2 slices (2 oz)	90	4	2	35	12	1	1	0	0	500	—	—	0
BOAR'S HEAD														
Canadian Bacon	2 oz	70	2	1	35	12	1	1	0	0	570	—	—	0
CELEBRITY														
98% Fat Free	3 slices (1.8 oz)	60	1	1	30	10	1	0	0	0	350	—	—	1
DIETZ & WATSON														
Canadian Style	2 oz	70	2	1	30	11	1	1	0	0	490	—	—	0

FOOD	PORTION	CALS	FAT	SAT FAT	CHOL	PROT	CARB	SUGAR	FIBER	CALCI	SOD	POTAS	FOLIC	VIT C
OSCAR MAYER														
Fully Cooked	3 slices (1.9 oz)	60	2	1	30	9	1	1	0	—	480	—	—	12
CANADIAN BACON SUBSTITUTES														
YVES														
Meatless Canadian Bacon	2 slices (2 oz)	80	1	0	0	17	2	tr	0	20	400	220	—	0
CANDY														
butterscotch	1 piece (6 g)	24	tr	tr	1	0	6	—	—	0	3	0	0	0
candied cherries	1 (4 g)	12	tr	tr	0	0	3	—	—	tr	—	—	—	0
candied citron	1 oz	89	tr	—	0	tr	23	—	—	24	82	34	—	—
candied lemon peel	1 oz	90	tr	—	0	tr	23	—	—	—	14	3	—	—
candied orange peel	1 oz	90	tr	—	0	tr	23	—	—	—	14	3	—	—
candied pineapple slice	1 slice (2 oz)	179	tr	tr	0	tr	45	—	—	17	—	—	—	13
candy corn	1 oz	105	0	0	0	tr	27	—	—	2	57	1	—	0
caramels	1 piece (8 g)	31	1	1	1	tr	6	—	—	11	20	17	0	—
caramels chocolate	1 piece (6 g)	22	tr	tr	0	tr	6	—	—	—	—	—	—	—
carob bar	1 (3.1 oz)	453	28	7	—	11	42	—	—	391	—	785	27	—
dark chocolate	1 oz	150	10	6	0	1	16	—	—	7	5	86	—	tr
fondant	1 piece (0.6 oz)	57	0	—	0	0	15	—	—	0	6	3	0	0
fondant chocolate coated	1 piece (0.4 oz)	40	1	1	0	tr	9	—	—	2	3	18	—	—
fondant mint	1 oz	105	0	0	0	tr	27	—	—	2	57	1	—	0
fruit pastilles	1 tube (1.4 oz)	101	0	—	—	2	25	—	—	16	—	—	—	0
fudge brown sugar w/ nuts	1 piece (0.5 oz)	56	1	tr	1	tr	11	—	—	16	14	52	1	tr
fudge chocolate marshmallow	1 piece (0.7 oz)	84	3	2	5	1	14	—	—	9	21	28	0	0
fudge chocolate marshmallow w/ nuts	1 piece (0.8 oz)	96	4	2	5	1	15	—	—	11	21	37	1	tr
fudge chocolate w/ nuts	1 piece (0.7 oz)	81	3	1	3	1	14	—	—	9	11	30	2	tr
fudge peanut butter	1 piece (0.6 oz)	59	1	tr	1	1	13	—	—	7	12	21	2	0
fudge vanilla w/ nuts	1 piece (0.5 oz)	62	2	1	2	tr	11	—	—	7	9	17	2	tr
gumdrops	10 sm (0.4 oz)	135	0	0	0	0	35	—	—	1	15	2	—	—
gumdrops	10 lg (3.8 oz)	420	0	0	0	0	108	—	—	3	48	5	—	—
hard candy	1 oz	106	0	0	0	0	28	—	—	1	11	1	—	—
jelly beans	10 sm (0.4 oz)	40	tr	—	0	0	10	—	—	0	3	4	—	0
jelly beans	10 lg (1 oz)	104	tr	—	0	0	26	—	—	1	7	11	—	0
lollipop	1 (6 g)	22	0	0	0	0	6	—	—	0	2	0	—	—
marzipan	1 oz	128	7	1	0	3	15	—	2	24	5	82	16	tr

FOOD	PORTION	CALS	FAT	SAT FAT	CHOL	PROT	CARB	SUGAR	FIBER	CALCI	SOD	POTAS	FOLIC	VIT C
milk chocolate	1 bar (1.55 oz)	226	14	8	10	3	26	—	—	84	36	169	4	tr
milk chocolate crisp	1 bar (1.45 oz)	203	11	7	8	3	28	—	—	70	59	141	3	tr
milk chocolate w/ almonds	1 bar (1.45 oz)	215	14	7	8	4	22	20	—	92	30	182	—	tr
nougat nut cream	0.5 oz	49	4	—	—	1	8	—	—	2	—	—	—	—
peanut bar	1 (1.4 oz)	209	14	2	—	6	19	—	—	31	91	163	—	—
peanut brittle	1 oz	128	5	1	4	2	20	—	—	8	128	59	20	0
peanuts chocolate covered	1 cup (5.2 oz)	773	50	22	13	19	74	—	—	155	61	748	12	0
peanuts chocolate covered	10 (1.4 oz)	208	13	6	4	5	20	—	—	42	16	201	3	0
praline	1 piece (1.4 oz)	177	10	1	0	1	24	—	—	12	24	82	6	tr
pretzels chocolate covered	1 oz	130	5	2	—	2	20	—	—	21	—	—	—	tr
pretzels chocolate covered	1 (0.4 oz)	50	2	1	—	1	8	—	—	8	10	—	—	tr
sesame crunch	20 pieces (1.2 oz)	181	12	2	0	4	18	—	—	—	—	—	—	—
taffy	1 piece (0.5 oz)	56	1	tr	1	0	14	—	—	0	13	1	0	0
toffee	1 piece (0.4 oz)	65	4	2	13	tr	8	—	—	4	22	6	0	0
truffles	1 piece (0.4 oz)	59	4	3	6	1	5	—	—	19	8	37	0	tr
3 MUSKETEERS														
Bar	1 (2.1 oz)	260	8	5	5	2	46	40	1	20	110	—	—	—
Fun Size	3 bars (1.6 oz)	190	6	4	5	1	34	30	1	20	85	—	—	—
Minis	7 (1.4 oz)	170	5	4	5	1	32	27	1	20	80	—	—	—
Mint	1 bar (1.2 oz)	150	5	4	0	1	26	22	1	0	65	—	—	0
5TH AVENUE														
Bar	1 (2 oz)	260	12	5	—	4	37	28	2	20	120	—	—	0
ALMOND JOY														
Bar	1 (1.6 oz)	220	13	8	—	2	26	20	2	20	50	—	—	0
ANDES														
Dark Chocolate Covered Cherries	2 (1 oz)	110	5	3	0	1	19	15	tr	0	10	—	—	0
Thins Cherry Jubilee	8 pieces (1.3 oz)	200	13	11	0	2	22	20	1	40	20	—	—	1
Thins Creme De Menthe	8 pieces (1.3 oz)	200	13	11	0	2	22	20	tr	40	20	—	—	0
ANNABELLE'S														
Skinny Hunk Chewy Nougat	1 bar (1 oz)	100	1	0	0	0	24	25	0	0	75	—	—	0
BABY RUTH														
Fun Size	2 bars (1.3 oz)	170	8	5	0	2	24	20	tr	20	85	—	—	0
Snack Bars	2 (1.3 oz)	170	8	5	0	2	24	20	tr	20	85	—	—	0
BARTONS														
Cashew Toppers	1 (1 oz)	140	9	3	5	3	14	9	1	40	20	—	—	0

FOOD	PORTION	CALS	FAT	SAT FAT	CHOL	PROT	CARB	SUGAR	FIBER	CALCI	SOD	POTAS	FOLIC	VIT C
BASKIN-ROBBINS														
Soft Candy Mint Chocolate Chip	2 (0.3 oz)	40	1	1	0	tr	7	5	0	—	15	—	—	—
Sugar Free Hard Candy Cookies 'N Cream	4 (0.6 oz)	40	1	1	0	0	15	0	—	—	10	—	—	—
BENECOL														
Smart Chews Caramel	1 piece	20	0	0	0	0	4	3	—	—	15	—	—	—
BENEDETTO														
Cubetti Mini Caramel Crunch Protein 1st	5 pieces (1.7 oz)	178	5	—	—	19	17	4	1	—	—	—	—	—
Cupola Mini Mint Protein 1st	5 pieces (1.7 oz)	122	3	—	—	11	15	3	2	—	—	—	—	—
BETTY CROCKER														
Fruit Gushers Rockin' Blue Raspberry	1 pkg (0.9 oz)	90	1	0	0	0	20	13	—	—	45	—	—	6
BLOW POP														
Regular	1 (0.6 oz)	60	0	0	0	0	16	12	0	150	0	—	—	0
BRACH'S														
Candy Corn	19 (1.4 oz)	140	0	0	0	0	36	32	—	—	70	—	—	—
Mellowcreme Pumpkins	6 pieces (1.5 oz)	150	0	0	0	0	38	33	—	—	80	—	—	—
BREATH SAVERS														
Peppermint	1 (1.8 g)	5	0	0	0	0	2	0	—	—	—	—	—	0
BUBBLE CHOCOLATE														
Dark Chocolate	1 bar (1.41 oz)	200	15	9	0	2	22	15	3	20	0	—	—	0
Milk Chocolate	1 bar (1.41 oz)	220	15	9	10	3	21	20	tr	80	30	—	—	1
BUTTERFINGER														
Crisp Bar	1 (2.1 oz)	270	11	6	0	3	43	29	1	20	135	—	—	0
Original Bar	1 (2.1 oz)	270	11	6	0	4	43	29	1	20	135	—	—	0
Snackerz	1 pkg (1.3 oz)	170	8	4	0	2	23	15	2	100	80	—	—	0
CADBURY														
Caramello	1 (1.6 oz)	220	10	6	10	3	29	25	tr	80	45	—	—	0
Dairy Milk	7 blocks (1.4 oz)	200	11	7	10	3	23	22	tr	80	40	—	—	0
Milk Chocolate Fruit & Nut	10 blocks (1.4 oz)	200	10	5	5	4	24	22	1	80	30	—	—	0
Milk Chocolate Roast Almond	7 blocks (1.4 oz)	210	13	6	10	4	21	19	1	80	35	—	—	0
Royal Dark	7 blocks (1.4 oz)	170	12	8	<5	2	23	20	3	0	—	—	—	0
CELLA'S														
Milk Chocolate Covered Cherries	2 (1 oz)	120	5	2	5	1	20	16	1	40	20	—	—	0

FOOD	PORTION	CALS	FAT	SAT FAT	CHOL	PROT	CARB	SUGAR	FIBER	CALCI	SOD	POTAS	FOLIC	VIT C
CHARGERS														
Chocolate Covered Espresso Beans	1 pkg (0.5 oz)	60	3	2	0	1	9	7	tr	20	0	—	—	0
CHARLESTON CHEWS														
Chocolate	1 bar (1.9 oz)	230	6	5	0	2	43	30	1	40	30	—	—	0
Vanilla	1 bar (1.9 oz)	230	8	5	0	2	44	30	0	40	30	—	—	0
CHARMS														
Fluffy Stuff Cotton Candy	1 pkg (0.6 oz)	70	0	0	0	0	17	17	0	0	0	—	—	0
Sour Balls	1 (5 g)	20	0	0	0	0	5	3	0	0	0	—	—	0
Squares	2 pieces	20	0	0	0	0	6	4	0	0	0	—	—	0
CHEW-ETS														
Peanut Chews Original Dark	3 pieces	170	9	4	0	3	22	16	2	20	55	—	—	0
CHOWARD'S														
Mints All Flavors	3 (5 g)	20	0	0	0	0	5	5	0	0	0	—	—	0
CHUAO CHOCOLATIER														
Choco Pod Banana	1 (0.4 oz)	50	3	2	—	tr	6	5	—	0	10	—	—	0
Choco Pod Passion	1 (0.4 oz)	50	4	2	—	0	5	5	—	—	0	—	—	—
COCO														
Brain Truffles Orange	1 (0.5 oz)	56	3	2	2	0	7	5	1	—	6	—	200	78
Preggers Truffles Dark Chocolate	1 (0.5 oz)	56	3	2	2	0	7	5	1	—	6	—	200	—
COFFEE SPOONS														
Flavored	1 (0.6 oz)	90	5	5	0	1	11	9	1	0	15	—	—	0
COOMBS FAMILY FARMS														
Maple Candy	6 pieces (1.5 oz)	160	0	0	0	0	42	40	0	—	5	—	—	—
CRISPY CAT														
Roasted Peanut	1 bar (1 oz)	220	10	3	0	4	29	14	2	20	125	—	—	0
DARE														
RealFruit Gummies All Flavors	8 pieces (1.4 oz)	120	0	0	0	2	28	19	0	0	5	—	—	0
DOTS														
Gumdrops Fruit	11 (1.4 oz)	130	0	0	0	0	33	21	—	—	15	—	—	—
DOVE														
Dark Chocolate Cranberry Almond	⅓ pkg (1.2 oz)	170	10	6	5	2	20	16	2	20	10	—	—	0
Milk Chocolate Roasted Almond	⅓ bar (1.2 oz)	180	12	6	5	3	18	16	1	40	20	—	—	0

FOOD	PORTION	CALS	FAT	SAT FAT	CHOL	PROT	CARB	SUGAR	FIBER	CALCI	SOD	POTAS	FOLIC	VIT C
E. GUITTARD														
Bar Quevedo Bittersweet 65% Cacao	1 (2 oz)	290	23	13	0	3	29	20	5	20	0	—	—	0
Bar Sur Del Lago Bittersweet 65% Cacao	1 (2 oz)	290	23	13	0	3	29	20	5	20	0	—	—	0
ELMER CHOCOLATES														
Assorted	5 (2 oz)	240	10	6	0	1	41	35	1	20	35	—	—	0
EMILY'S														
Espresso Beans Dark Chocolate Covered	26 (1.4 oz)	220	19	9	<5	2	24	21	3	0	20	—	—	0
ENJOY LIFE														
Boom Choco Boom Dark Chocolate Dairy Nut Soy Free	1 bar (1.4 oz)	200	15	9	0	2	22	17	3	0	0	—	—	0
EQUAL EXCHANGE														
Organic Chocolate Espresso Bean	1 bar (1.4 oz)	216	15	9	0	2	22	17	3	20	2	—	—	0
Organic Milk Chocolate	1 bar (1.4 oz)	230	16	9	12	4	19	12	1	100	40	—	—	1
Organic Very Dark Chocolate	1 bar (1.4 oz)	220	17	10	0	3	18	11	5	20	5	—	—	0
ETHEL'S														
Truffles Assorted	4	200	14	6	15	2	17	9	1	20	30	—	—	0
FERRERO														
Rocher	3 pieces (1.3 oz)	220	16	5	0	3	16	15	1	40	15	—	—	0
Rondnoir	3 pieces (1.4 oz)	220	14	7	<5	3	21	16	2	20	25	—	—	0
FROOTIES														
Chewy Candy Fruit Flavored	12 pieces (1.3 oz)	104	3	0	0	0	29	21	0	20	20	—	—	0
GHIRARDELLI														
Luxe Milk Chocolate	4 sq (1.5 oz)	220	13	8	10	3	26	24	tr	80	30	—	—	1
Squares Milk Chocolate w/ Caramel Filling	3 (1.6 oz)	220	12	7	10	2	27	24	tr	80	60	—	—	0
Squares Mint Indulgence	3 (1.6 oz)	210	11	6	0	1	30	26	2	20	0	—	—	0
Squares 60% Cacao Dark Chocolate	4 (1.5 oz)	220	17	10	0	2	23	23	3	20	0	—	—	0

FOOD	PORTION	CALS	FAT	SAT FAT	CHOL	PROT	CARB	SUGAR	FIBER	CALCI	SOD	POTAS	FOLIC	VIT C
GHIRARDELLI (CONT.)														
Squares 60% Cacao Dark Chocolate w/ Caramel	3 (1.6 oz)	220	15	8	5	2	25	18	3	20	35	—	—	0
GIMME														
Dark Chocolate Omega 3	1 pkg (1 oz)	130	7	4	0	2	19	14	2	0	10	—	—	0
Dark Chocolate Probiotics	1 pkg (1 oz)	130	7	4	0	1	20	14	2	0	5	—	—	0
Milk Chocolate Calcium	1 pkg (1 oz)	120	7	4	0	1	18	14	1	600	30	—	—	0
GODIVA														
Assorted Milk Chocolate	4 pieces (1.4 oz)	190	12	7	5	2	22	19	1	60	40	—	—	0
Gems Truffles Milk Chocolate	4 (1.5 oz)	200	13	8	15	2	20	18	tr	60	30	—	—	0
Truffles Assorted	2 pieces (1.4 oz)	210	13	8	10	3	20	17	2	40	20	—	—	0
GOOD & PLENTY														
Licorice	33 (1.4 oz)	140	0	0	0	tr	35	25	—	0	120	—	—	0
GREEN & BLACK'S														
Organic Chocolate Fairtrade Maya Gold	1 bar (3.5 oz)	526	34	21	—	7	48	43	8	—	14	—	—	—
Organic Dark Chocolate	1 bar (3.5 oz)	551	41	24	—	9	36	29	12	—	16	—	—	—
Organic Dark Chocolate Mint	1 bar (3.5 oz)	478	27	17	—	7	51	44	9	—	42	—	—	—
Organic Dark Chocolate w/ Hazelnuts & Currants	1 bar (3.5 oz)	513	34	17	—	8	45	40	9	—	16	—	—	—
Organic Milk Chocolate	1 bar (3.5 oz)	523	30	18	—	10	54	48	4	—	65	—	—	—
Organic Milk Chocolate Caramel	1 bar (3.5 oz)	495	26	16	—	8	56	53	3	—	15	—	—	—
Organic Milk Chocolate Raisins & Hazelnuts	1 bar (3.5 oz)	556	37	19	—	9	47	42	3	—	58	—	—	—
Organic Milk Chocolate Whole Almonds	1 bar (3.5 oz)	578	42	17	—	12	38	35	5	—	71	—	—	—
Organic White Chocolate	1 bar (3.5 oz)	573	37	22	—	7	54	51	tr	—	81	—	—	—

FOOD	PORTION	CALS	FAT	SAT FAT	CHOL	PROT	CARB	SUGAR	FIBER	CALCI	SOD	POTAS	FOLIC	VIT C
GUYLIAN														
Twists Milk Chocolate Truffle	5 pieces (1.2 oz)	230	19	11	10	2	15	14	1	60	20	—	—	0
Twists Original Praline	4 pieces (1.2 oz)	200	13	6	10	3	19	17	1	80	20	—	—	1
HAMMOND'S														
Root Beer Drops	3 (0.6 oz)	60	0	0	0	0	14	12	0	—	5	—	—	—
HEATH														
Bar	1 (1.4 oz)	210	13	7	10	1	24	23	tr	20	135	—	—	0
HERSHEY'S														
Bar Milk Chocolate w/ Almonds	1 (1.4 oz)	210	14	6	10	4	21	19	2	80	25	—	—	0
Bar Special Dark	1 (1.4 oz)	180	12	8	<5	2	25	21	3	0	15	—	—	0
Bliss Dark Chocolate Bar	1 (1.3 oz)	160	12	7	<5	2	21	17	3	0	10	—	—	0
Bliss Milk Chocolate	6 (1.5 oz)	210	14	9	5	3	24	22	1	80	40	—	—	0
Bliss Milk Chocolate Meltaway	6 (1.5 oz)	220	15	10	5	3	24	33	1	80	65	—	—	0
Bliss Milk Chocolate Raspberry Meltaway	6 (1.5 oz)	220	14	9	5	3	24	23	tr	80	55	—	—	0
Cacao Reserve 35% Cacao Milk Chocolate w/ Hazelnuts	3 sq (1.3 oz)	220	15	7	10	3	18	16	1	60	25	—	—	0
Kisses Cherry Cordial	9 (1.5 oz)	180	7	5	5	2	30	26	—	40	25	—	—	0
Kisses Hugs	9 (1.4 oz)	210	12	7	10	3	23	21	—	100	45	—	—	0
Kisses Milk Chocolate	9 (1.4 oz)	200	12	7	10	3	25	23	1	80	35	—	—	0
Kisses Special Dark	9 (1.4 oz)	180	12	8	<5	2	25	21	3	0	15	—	—	0
Milk Chocolate Bar	1 (1.5 oz)	210	13	8	10	3	26	24	1	80	35	—	—	0
Milk Chocolate w/ Almonds Bar	1 (1.5 oz)	210	13	7	5	3	25	22	2	40	50	—	—	0
Miniatures Special Dark	5 (1.4 oz)	190	13	7	<5	3	24	18	3	0	25	—	—	0
Nuggets Milk Chocolate	4 (1.4 oz)	200	12	7	10	3	25	23	1	80	35	—	—	0
Nuggets Milk Chocolate w/ Almonds	4 (1.3 oz)	200	13	6	10	4	20	17	2	80	25	—	—	0
Pieces All Flavors	51 (1.4 oz)	190	9	7	—	4	25	21	1	0	75	—	—	0

FOOD	PORTION	CALS	FAT	SAT FAT	CHOL	PROT	CARB	SUGAR	FIBER	CALCI	SOD	POTAS	FOLIC	VIT C
HERSHEY'S (CONT.)														
Pot Of Gold Assorted Milk & Dark Chocolate	4 (1.4 oz)	200	12	7	5	2	25	22	1	40	55	—	—	0
ICE BREAKERS														
Coolmint	1 (0.8 g)	0	0	0	0	0	tr	—	—	—	—	—	—	0
JAY'S														
Cotton Candy	1 pkg (2 oz)	220	0	0	0	3	56	56	—	—	0	—	—	—
JELLY BELLY														
Jelly Beans	1 pkg (0.75 oz)	80	0	0	0	0	20	15	—	—	10	—	—	—
Cocktail Classics Peas & Carrots	49 (1.4 oz)	140	0	0	0	0	37	29	—	—	0	—	—	—
JER'S														
Balls Peanut Butter Chocolate	1 piece (0.5 oz)	80	5	2	0	2	8	6	—	—	25	—	—	—
Original IncrediBar Peanut Butter	1 (1.8 oz)	210	12	6	0	6	21	16	2	20	65	—	—	0
JOLLY RANCHER														
Gummies	9 (1.1 oz)	120	0	0	0	2	28	22	—	0	35	—	—	1
Original Assortment	3 (0.5 oz)	50	0	0	0	0	13	7	—	—	20	—	—	0
JUNIOR														
Caramels	1 box (1.4 oz)	170	3	3	0	1	35	32	tr	0	30	—	—	0
Mints	1 box (1.4 oz)	170	3	3	0	1	35	32	tr	0	30	—	—	0
KITKAT														
Bar	1 (1.5 oz)	210	11	7	<5	3	28	22	tr	60	30	—	—	0
KOPALI														
Organic Dark Chocolate Covered Espresso Beans	½ pkg (1 oz)	120	7	4	0	1	17	15	2	10	0	—	—	0
LANCE														
Chewz Strawberry	1 pkg (1.1 oz)	120	1	—	—	0	28	26	—	0	0	—	—	0
Peanut Bar	1 (2.3 oz)	340	19	3	0	13	29	19	3	0	100	—	—	0
LET'S DO ORGANIC														
Black Licorice Bars	1 (0.9 oz)	80	0	0	0	1	20	11	tr	0	20	—	—	0
Black Licorice Chews	8 (1.4 oz)	130	0	0	0	2	30	18	tr	0	30	—	—	0
Gummi Bears	1 pkg (0.9 oz)	80	0	0	0	0	22	18	0	0	15	—	—	0
LIFESAVERS														
Variety	4 pieces	60	0	0	0	0	16	13	—	—	0	—	—	—
LINDT														
Lindor Truffles 60% Extra Dark	3 pieces (1.3 oz)	210	19	13	<5	2	15	11	tr	20	0	—	—	0

FOOD	PORTION	CALS	FAT	SAT FAT	CHOL	PROT	CARB	SUGAR	FIBER	CALCI	SOD	POTAS	FOLIC	VIT C
LINDT (CONT.)														
Lindor Truffles Swiss Dark Chocolate	3 (1.4 oz)	240	18	14	<5	2	17	16	2	20	10	—	—	0
Petits Desserts Assorted	4 (1.3 oz)	210	15	8	10	2	20	17	tr	60	15	—	—	0
LOVE CANDY														
Dark Chocolate	1 bar (1.5 oz)	190	11	6	20	2	21	15	1	20	55	—	—	0
Milk Chocolate	1 bar (1.5 oz)	200	11	6	25	1	22	15	tr	40	65	—	—	0
Yogurt Supreme	1 bar (1.5 oz)	190	11	7	20	1	23	7	tr	20	60	—	—	0
MAMA'S GOODIES														
Butter Nut Crunch Almond	1 piece (1.33 oz)	220	15	4	10	3	20	18	1	—	30	—	—	—
Butter Nut Crunch Macadamia & Coconut	1 piece (1.33 oz)	220	17	5	10	1	20	18	1	—	30	—	—	—
Butter Nut Crunch Sesame Seed	1 piece (1.33 oz)	220	14	4	10	2	20	18	1	—	30	—	—	—
MAMBA														
Fruit Flavor	6 (0.9 oz)	170	3	2	0	0	36	19	0	0	0	—	—	0
Sour	6 (0.9 oz)	100	2	1	0	0	22	11	0	0	20	—	—	0
MAPLE GROVE FARMS														
Maple	5 pieces (1.5 oz)	160	0	0	0	0	42	37	—	40	0	—	—	—
MIKE & IKE														
All Flavors	1 pkg (2 oz)	200	0	0	0	0	50	—	—	—	—	—	—	—
MILK DUDS														
Chocolate	13 (1.4 oz)	170	6	4	—	1	28	20	—	40	100	—	—	0
MILKFULS														
Candy	6 (1.4 oz)	170	3	2	5	tr	35	23	0	40	10	—	—	5
MILKY WAY														
Fun Size	2 bars (1.2 oz)	150	6	4	5	1	24	20	0	40	55	—	—	—
Milk Chocolate Covered Caramels	5 (1.5 oz)	200	8	6	10	2	30	26	0	60	120	—	—	—
MOUNDS														
Bar	1 (1.7 oz)	230	13	10	—	2	29	21	3	0	55	—	—	0
MR. GOODBAR														
Bar	1 (1.7 oz)	250	17	7	<5	5	26	23	2	40	65	—	—	0
NECCO														
Banana Splits	4 (1.4 oz)	150	2	1	0	0	36	21	0	0	55	—	—	0
Clark Junior Bar	1 (0.5 oz)	60	3	1	0	1	10	8	0	0	20	—	—	0
Conversation Hearts Tiny	40 (1.4 oz)	160	0	0	0	0	39	38	0	0	0	—	—	0
Double Dipped Peanuts	15 (1.4 oz)	200	11	6	0	3	25	22	1	20	25	—	—	0

FOOD	PORTION	CALS	FAT	SAT FAT	CHOL	PROT	CARB	SUGAR	FIBER	CALCI	SOD	POTAS	FOLIC	VIT C
NECCO (CONT.)														
Junior Assorted Wafers	1 roll (0.5 oz)	50	0	0	0	0	13	12	—	—	0	—	—	—
Mary Janes	5 (1.4 oz)	160	4	1	0	1	32	20	0	20	65	—	—	0
Mint Juleps	4 (1.4 oz)	150	2	1	0	0	36	21	0	0	55	—	—	0
Nonpareils	10 (1.4 oz)	190	9	5	0	1	29	23	0	0	0	—	—	0
Squirrel Nut Caramel	5 (1.6 oz)	170	3	1	0	1	37	25	0	20	70	—	—	0
NESTLE														
Crunch Stix	1 (0.6 oz)	90	5	4	0	tr	12	9	0	0	30	—	—	0
NEWMAN'S OWN														
Organic Chocolate Sweet Dark	½ bar (1.4 oz)	200	13	7	0	2	24	20	2	—	0	—	—	—
Organic Chocolate Sweet Dark Orange	½ bar (1.4 oz)	200	13	8	0	2	24	20	2	—	0	—	—	—
Organic Milk Chocolate	½ bar (1.4 oz)	210	13	7	9	3	22	20	1	—	34	—	—	—
NIBMOR														
Organic Vegan Dark Chocolate	½ bar (1.1 oz)	120	7	4	0	1	13	8	2	0	20	—	—	0
Organic Vegan Dark Chocolate	½ bar (1.1 oz)	130	8	4	0	2	12	7	3	0	45	—	—	0
Organic Vegan Dark Chocolate w/ Cacao Nibs	½ bar (1.1 oz)	120	7	4	0	2	14	7	3	0	45	—	—	0
Organic Vegan Dark Chocolate w/ Crispy Brown Rice	½ bar (1 oz)	110	7	4	0	1	13	7	2	0	45	—	—	0
PANDA														
Licorice Cherry	1 bar (1.1 oz)	100	0	0	0	1	24	14	0	0	65	—	—	0
PAYDAY														
Peanut Caramel	1 (1.8 oz)	240	13	3	—	7	27	21	2	40	120	—	—	0
POT OF GOLD														
Nut Assortment	4 (1.4 oz)	210	13	7	<5	3	23	20	2	40	40	—	—	0
Pecan Caramel Clusters	4 (1.4 oz)	200	12	7	<5	2	23	21	1	40	60	—	—	0
Truffle Assortment	3 (1.5 oz)	200	9	6	5	2	27	23	1	20	20	—	—	0
PURE FUN														
Organic Vegan Barrels Of Fun Root Beer Float	2 (0.5 oz)	60	0	0	0	0	13	3	0	0	10	—	—	0
Organic Vegan Candy Canes	1 (0.5 oz)	62	0	0	0	0	14	3	1	0	0	—	—	0

FOOD	PORTION	CALS	FAT	SAT FAT	CHOL	PROT	CARB	SUGAR	FIBER	CALCI	SOD	POTAS	FOLIC	VIT C
PURE FUN (CONT.)														
Organic Vegan Chocolate Meltdowns All Flavors	3 (0.6 oz)	70	0	0	0	0	16	4	0	0	10	—	—	0
Organic Vegan Citrus Slices All Flavors	3 (0.6 oz)	60	0	0	0	0	15	3	0	0	10	—	—	0
Organic Vegan Cotton Candy All Flavors	¼ pkg (0.5 oz)	60	0	0	0	0	15	15	0	0	0	—	—	0
Organic Vegan Jaw Boulders All Flavors	2 (0.5 oz)	58	0	0	0	0	13	3	0	0	8	—	—	0
Organic Vegan Pure Pops All Flavors	3 (0.6 oz)	60	0	0	0	0	15	3	0	0	10	—	—	0
RAISINETS														
Candy	¼ cup (1.6 oz)	190	8	5	5	2	32	28	1	40	15	—	—	0
REESE'S														
Crispy Crunchy Bar	1 (1.7 oz)	250	14	5	<5	5	29	22	2	20	85	—	—	0
FastBreak	1 (2 oz)	260	12	5	—	5	35	30	2	20	190	—	—	0
NutRageous	1 (1.8 oz)	260	16	5	—	6	28	22	2	20	100	—	—	0
Peanut Butter Cups Miniatures Dark Chocolate	5 (1.5 oz)	220	14	6	<5	4	24	20	2	0	120	—	—	0
Pieces Peanut Butter	1 pkg (1.5 oz)	210	10	8	—	5	26	24	1	20	85	—	—	0
REESESTICKS														
Wafer Bar Chocolate & Peanut Butter	1 (1.5 oz)	210	13	5	—	4	23	17	1	20	130	—	—	0
RICOCHET														
Coffee Shots Sugar Free	5 (3 g)	10	0	0	0	0	2	—	—	—	0	—	—	—
RIESEN														
Candy	4 (1.3 oz)	170	4	0	0	1	28	15	0	20	15	—	—	0
RITTER SPORT														
Bar Cappuccino	1 (3.5 oz)	574	39	25	18	6	50	48	2	235	77	—	—	1
Bar Chocolate Marzipan	1 (3.5 oz)	484	27	13	tr	6	53	52	5	69	16	—	—	1
Bar Chocolate & Cornflakes	1 (3.5 oz)	525	29	—	9	6	59	50	2	149	184	—	—	—
Bar Chocolate Butter Biscuit	1 (3.5 oz)	556	35	16	15	7	53	51	2	213	148	—	—	3
Bar Dark Chocolate	1 (3.5 oz)	525	33	21	tr	5	51	49	7	52	20	—	—	tr

FOOD	PORTION	CALS	FAT	SAT FAT	CHOL	PROT	CARB	SUGAR	FIBER	CALCI	SOD	POTAS	FOLIC	VIT C
RITTER SPORT (CONT.)														
Bar Milk Chocolate	1 (3.5 oz)	533	31	20	11	7	57	56	3	203	99	—	—	3
Bar Mousse Au Chocolat	1 (3.5 oz)	544	36	22	9	5	48	46	7	92	15	—	—	4
Bar White Chocolate Whole Hazelnuts	1 (3.5 oz)	562	38	18	20	7	48	44	2	189	114	—	—	2
ROLO														
Chewy Caramels In Milk Chocolate	3 pkg (1.7 oz)	220	10	7	5	2	33	29	—	60	80	—	—	0
RUSSELL STOVER														
All Dark Assorted	2 pieces (1.2 oz)	150	7	4	<5	1	23	18	1	20	45	—	—	0
Assorted Chocolates	2 pieces (1.1 oz)	160	7	4	5	1	22	18	1	20	45	—	—	0
Private Reserve Triple Chocolate Mousse	3 pieces (1.3 oz)	220	17	12	<5	2	19	15	2	40	15	—	—	0
Private Reserve Vanilla Bean Brulee	3 pieces (1.3 oz)	180	13	8	<5	3	19	13	3	60	25	—	—	0
SCHARFFEN BERGER														
Semisweet 60% Cacao	1 bar (2 oz)	320	20	13	0	4	32	24	tr	20	0	—	—	0
SEE'S														
Assorted Chocolates	2 (1.2 oz)	160	9	5	10	2	20	16	tr	20	40	—	—	0
Nuts & Chews	3 (1.6 oz)	240	16	6	10	4	25	18	2	60	50	—	—	0
Soft Centers	2 (1.4 oz)	170	9	5	10	1	25	22	tr	20	40	—	—	1
SENCHA NATURALS														
Green Tea Mints All Flavors	3	5	0	0	0	0	1	0	0	—	—	—	—	—
SHAMAN CHOCOLATES														
Organic Extra Dark Chocolate 82% Cacao	½ bar (1 oz)	158	14	9	0	2	7	1	4	0	0	—	—	0
Organic Milk Chocolate w/ Macadamia Nuts & Hawaiian Pink Sea Salt	½ bar (1 oz)	91	1	1	0	1	13	13	2	0	773	—	—	1
SKINNY COW														
Heavenly Crisp Bar	1 (0.8 oz)	110	4	0	0	1	14	9	1	20	40	—	—	0
SKITTLES														
Original Fruit	1 pkg (2.2 oz)	250	3	3	0	0	56	47	0	—	10	—	—	30

FOOD	PORTION	CALS	FAT	SAT FAT	CHOL	PROT	CARB	SUGAR	FIBER	CALCI	SOD	POTAS	FOLIC	VIT C
SKITTLES (CONT.)														
Sour	1 pkg (1.8 oz)	200	0	0	0	0	44	37	0	—	5	—	—	27
SKOR														
Toffee & Milk Chocolate	1 (1.4 oz)	200	12	7	20	1	25	24	tr	20	130	—	—	0
SLIM-FAST														
Protein Snack Chews Peanut Butter	1 pkg (0.9 oz)	100	4	1	0	6	12	5	0	200	90	—	60	9
SMILE CHOCOLATIERS														
Choclatea Ginger Tea Milk Chocolate 37% Cacao	½ bar (1.5 oz)	230	15	9	10	3	23	21	1	80	30	—	—	0
Choclatea Herbal Chai Tea Dark Chocolate 64% Cacao	½ bar (1.5 oz)	220	17	10	0	2	22	15	5	0	0	—	—	0
Choclatea Pistachio Green Tea White Chocolate	½ bar (1.5 oz)	240	16	10	10	5	22	22	1	100	0	—	—	0
Choclatea Pomegranate White Tea Very Dark Chocolate 72% Cacao	½ bar (1.5 oz)	220	16	10	0	3	16	14	2	0	5	—	—	0
Choclatea White Tea Very Dark Chocolate 72% Cacao	½ bar (1.5 oz)	220	17	10	0	2	22	15	5	0	0	—	—	0
SOUR PATCH														
Kids Soft & Chewy	1 pkg (1 oz)	100	0	0	0	0	25	17	—	—	20	—	—	—
STARBUCKS														
Truffles Caffe Mocha	3 (1.3 oz)	200	14	8	10	3	19	17	1	60	35	—	—	0
SUGAR BABIES														
Candy	30 pieces (1.5 oz)	180	2	0	0	0	41	32	0	20	40	—	—	0
Chocolate	19 pieces (1.4 oz)	180	5	2	5	1	33	26	0	40	35	—	—	0
SUGAR DADDY														
Pop	1 lg (1.7 oz)	200	3	1	0	1	43	29	0	20	65	—	—	0
SUNRIDGE FARMS														
Rainbow Drops Milk Chocolate	¼ cup (1.4 oz)	170	10	6	5	2	21	19	1	40	15	—	—	0
SURF SWEETS														
Gummy Bears	16 (1.4 oz)	130	0	0	0	3	30	19	0	0	15	—	—	60

FOOD	PORTION	CALS	FAT	SAT FAT	CHOL	PROT	CARB	SUGAR	FIBER	CALCI	SOD	POTAS	FOLIC	VIT C
SURF SWEETS (CONT.)														
Gummy Worms	4 (1.4 oz)	130	0	0	0	3	30	19	0	0	15	—	—	60
Jelly Beans	31 (1.4 oz)	140	0	0	0	0	34	29	0	0	35	—	—	60
Sour Worms	8 (1.4 oz)	130	0	0	0	0	32	23	1	0	140	—	—	60
SYMPHONY														
Almonds & Toffee	1 (1.5 oz)	220	14	8	10	4	23	22	tr	80	65	—	—	0
TAKE 5														
Original	1 pkg (1.5 oz)	200	11	5	—	4	25	18	1	20	180	—	—	0
TERRA NOSTRA														
Organic Bar Creamy Milk Raisins & Pecans	4 sections (1.2 oz)	180	11	6	5	2	18	17	1	60	20	—	—	0
Organic Bar Vegan Intense Dark	4 sections (1.2 oz)	180	12	7	0	2	15	9	4	0	0	—	—	0
Organic Bar Vegan Ricemilk Choco	4 sections (1.2 oz)	190	14	8	0	tr	18	16	0	0	30	—	—	0
Organic Bar Vegan Robust Dark Raisins & Pecans	4 sections (1.2 oz)	170	11	6	0	2	16	14	3	0	0	—	—	0
THORNTONS														
Chocolates Summer Collection	1	65	4	—	—	1	7	—	—	—	—	—	—	—
TOBLERONE														
Bittersweet w/ Honey & Almond Nougat	⅓ bar (1.2 oz)	170	9	5	5	1	20	16	2	0	5	—	—	0
Milk Chocolate w/ Honey & Almond Nougat	⅓ bar (1.2 oz)	170	9	5	10	2	21	18	1	40	15	—	—	0
White w/ Honey & Almond Nougat	⅓ bar (1.2 oz)	180	10	6	5	2	20	20	1	60	30	—	—	0
TOFFIFAY														
Candy	5 (1.4 oz)	200	11	5	<5	2	25	18	1	80	50	—	—	0
TOOTSIE ROLL														
Midgees	6	140	3	1	0	0	28	20	0	20	10	—	—	0
Pops	1 (0.6 oz)	60	0	0	0	0	15	10	0	0	0	—	—	0
Pops Caramel Apple	1 (0.6 oz)	60	1	0	0	0	15	11	0	0	15	—	—	0
TRUFFULLS														
Chocolate Caramel Gluten Free	1 (1.13 oz)	120	4	3	0	8	17	9	5	40	80	—	—	0
Chocolate Mint Gluten Free	1 (1.13 oz)	120	4	3	10	8	17	8	5	20	70	—	—	0
TWIX														
Fun Size	1 (0.6 oz)	80	4	3	0	1	10	8	0	—	70	—	—	—

FOOD	PORTION	CALS	FAT	SAT FAT	CHOL	PROT	CARB	SUGAR	FIBER	CALCI	SOD	POTAS	FOLIC	VIT C
TWIZZLERS														
Licorice	4 (1.6 oz)	150	1	—	—	1	35	18	—	0	210	—	—	0
Strawberry	4 (1.6 oz)	160	1	—	—	1	36	19	—	0	95	—	—	0
WERTHER'S														
Caramel Milk Chocolate	6 (1.3 oz)	230	16	10	10	2	18	17	0	60	50	—	—	0
Original	3 (0.5 oz)	60	1	1	<5	0	13	11	0	0	60	—	—	0
Original Sugar Free	5 (0.5 oz)	40	1	1	<5	0	14	0	0	0	55	—	—	0
WHITMAN'S														
Assorted Chocolates	4 pieces (1.5 oz)	210	10	6	5	2	29	23	1	40	55	—	—	0
WHOPPERS														
Malted Milk Balls	18 (1.4 oz)	190	7	7	—	1	31	26	—	80	115	—	—	0
WOLFGANG														
Blueberries Dipped In Dark Chocolate	2 (0.7 oz)	80	4	3	0	0	13	12	tr	0	10	—	—	0
Cranberries Dipped In Dark Chocolate	2 (1 oz)	130	6	4	0	1	18	16	1	0	10	—	—	0
Raspberries Dipped In Dark Chocolate	2 (1.1 oz)	130	6	4	0	1	21	19	1	0	5	—	—	0
WONKA EXCEPTIONALS														
Bar Chocolate Waterfall	4 sq (1.4 oz)	210	13	8	5	2	23	22	tr	60	30	—	—	0
Bar Domed Dark Chocolate	4 sq (1.4 oz)	200	13	8	5	2	24	19	3	20	0	—	—	0
Fruit Jellies All Flavors	14 (1.5 oz)	130	0	0	0	0	34	26	—	—	0	—	—	—
Fruit Marvels All Flavors	10 (1.4 oz)	140	0	0	0	0	34	30	—	—	0	—	—	—
YORK														
Peppermint Patty	1 (1.4 oz)	140	3	2	—	tr	31	25	tr	0	10	—	—	0
YOUNG & SMYLIE														
Licorice Black	11 (1.5 oz)	140	2	1	—	tr	32	19	—	0	190	—	—	0
Licorice Strawberry	11 (1.5 oz)	150	2	1	—	1	33	20	—	0	30	—	—	0
ZAGNUT														
Peanut Butter & Coconut	3 (1.5 oz)	200	8	3	—	3	31	22	1	0	90	—	—	0
ZERO														
Bar	1 (1.8 oz)	230	8	5	—	3	37	31	—	60	115	—	—	0
CANTALOUPE														
balls frzn	10 (4.7 oz)	46	tr	tr	0	1	11	11	1	12	22	360	27	47

FOOD	PORTION	CALS	FAT	SAT FAT	CHOL	PROT	CARB	SUGAR	FIBER	CALCI	SOD	POTAS	FOLIC	VIT C
dried	3.5 pieces (1.4 oz)	140	0	0	0	0	34	32	1	40	110	—	—	0
fresh cubed	1 cup (5.6 oz)	54	tr	tr	0	1	13	13	1	14	26	473	34	59
melon large	⅛ (3.6 oz)	35	1	tr	0	1	8	8	1	9	16	272	21	37
melon med	⅛ (2.4 oz)	23	tr	tr	0	1	6	5	1	6	11	184	14	25
melon sm	⅛ (1.9 oz)	19	tr	tr	0	tr	4	4	1	5	9	147	12	20
nectar	1 cup (8.8 oz)	155	tr	tr	0	1	39	39	1	12	20	240	10	26
CHIQUITA														
Fresh Cup Up	1 cup (6.2 oz)	60	0	0	0	1	16	14	2	20	28	473	—	65
CRISPY GREEN														
Freeze-dried	1 pkg (0.35 oz)	40	0	0	0	1	8	7	1	10	0	—	—	11
DOLE														
Fresh	¼ med (4.7 oz)	45	0	0	0	1	11	11	1	20	20	360	40	48
CAPERS														
capers	1 tbsp	2	tr	tr	0	tr	tr	tr	tr	3	255	3	2	tr
CARAWAY														
seed	1 tbsp	22	1	tr	0	1	3	tr	3	46	1	91	1	1
CARDAMOM														
ground	1 tsp	6	tr	tr	0	tr	1	—	1	8	0	22	—	tr
CARDOON														
fresh cooked w/o salt	1 serv (3.5 oz)	22	tr	tr	0	1	5	—	2	72	176	392	22	2
fresh shredded	1 cup (6.2 oz)	30	tr	tr	0	1	7	—	3	125	303	712	121	4
OCEAN MIST														
Cardone Fresh Shredded	1 cup (6.2 oz)	36	tr	tr	0	1	9	0	3	120	303	—	—	4
CARIBOU														
roasted	3 oz	142	4	1	93	25	0	0	0	19	51	264	4	3
CARISSA														
fresh	1	12	tr	—	0	tr	3	—	—	2	1	52	—	8
CAROB														
carob mix	3 tsp	45	0	0	0	tr	11	—	—	—	12	—	—	0
carob mix as prep w/ whole milk	9 oz	195	8	5	33	8	23	—	—	291	132	370	12	2
flour	1 tbsp	14	tr	tr	0	tr	7	—	—	28	3	66	2	0
flour	1 cup	185	1	tr	0	5	92	—	—	359	36	852	30	tr
BOB'S RED MILL														
Powder Toasted	2 tsp	25	0	0	0	1	11	7	2	—	5	—	—	—
TREE OF LIFE														
Chips Malt Sweetened	50 (0.5 oz)	70	4	4	0	1	9	1	1	0	5	—	—	0
CARP														
fresh cooked	1 fillet (6 oz)	276	12	2	143	39	0	0	0	89	107	726	—	3
fresh cooked	3 oz	138	6	1	72	19	0	0	0	44	54	363	—	1

FOOD	PORTION	CALS	FAT	SAT FAT	CHOL	PROT	CARB	SUGAR	FIBER	CALCI	SOD	POTAS	FOLIC	VIT C
fresh raw	3 oz	108	5	1	56	15	0	0	0	15	42	283	—	1
roe raw	1 oz	37	tr	—	103	7	tr	—	—	—	—	—	—	4
roe salted in olive oil	2 tbsp (1 oz)	40	—	—	100	—	6	—	0	0	1400	—	—	—

CARROT JUICE

FOOD	PORTION	CALS	FAT	SAT FAT	CHOL	PROT	CARB	SUGAR	FIBER	CALCI	SOD	POTAS	FOLIC	VIT C
canned	6 oz	73	tr	tr	0	2	17	—	—	44	54	538	7	16
HOLLYWOOD														
100% Juice	1 can (12 oz)	120	1	—	0	2	27	14	1	60	250	930	—	—
LAKEWOOD														
Organic	6 oz	73	0	0	0	2	17	8	2	60	45	467	32	24
ODWALLA														
100% Juice	8 oz	70	0	0	0	2	15	13	1	40	160	520	—	0

CARROTS

FOOD	PORTION	CALS	FAT	SAT FAT	CHOL	PROT	CARB	SUGAR	FIBER	CALCI	SOD	POTAS	FOLIC	VIT C
CANNED														
slices	½ cup	17	tr	tr	0	tr	4	—	1	19	176	131	7	2
slices low sodium	½ cup	17	tr	tr	0	tr	4	—	1	19	31	131	7	2
ALLENS														
Tiny Sliced	½ cup (4.5 oz)	45	0	0	0	1	11	3	3	40	180	—	—	4
DEL MONTE														
Savory Sides Honey Glazed	½ cup	70	0	0	0	1	18	12	tr	40	440	—	—	6
S&W														
Julienne	½ cup (1.3 oz)	35	0	0	0	0	8	5	3	20	300	—	—	4
FRESH														
baby raw	1 (0.5 oz)	6	tr	tr	0	tr	1	—	—	3	5	42	5	1
raw	1 (2.5 oz)	31	tr	tr	0	1	7	—	2	19	25	233	10	7
raw shredded	½ cup	24	tr	tr	0	1	6	—	2	15	19	178	8	5
slices cooked	½ cup	35	tr	tr	0	1	8	—	—	24	52	177	11	2
CHIQUITA														
Carrot Bites w/ Ranch Dressing	1 pkg (2.5 oz)	50	3	0	5	1	7	5	2	20	150	—	—	5
CRUNCH PAK														
Baby Carrots w/ Ranch Dressing	⅓ pkg	50	3	0	<5	1	7	5	2	20	160	—	—	4
DOLE														
Mini Cut	11 (3 oz)	30	0	0	0	1	8	4	2	20	60	—	—	4
EARTHBOUND FARMS														
Organic Tops On	1 (2.7 oz)	35	0	0	0	1	8	5	2	20	40	—	—	6
Organic w/ Organic Ranch Dip	1 pkg (2.2 oz)	90	8	1	5	1	5	3	1	20	180	—	—	4
READY PAC														
Baby Carrots	7 (3 oz)	40	0	0	0	1	9	5	2	20	45	—	—	6
FROZEN														
slices cooked	½ cup	26	tr	tr	0	1	6	—	—	21	43	115	8	2

FOOD	PORTION	CALS	FAT	SAT FAT	CHOL	PROT	CARB	SUGAR	FIBER	CALCI	SOD	POTAS	FOLIC	VIT C
BIRDS EYE														
Steam & Serve Carrots & Cranberries	1 cup	130	5	3	10	1	20	15	3	40	230	—	—	2
C&W														
Whole Baby	⅔ cup	35	0	0	0	tr	7	5	2	20	60	—	—	1
GREEN GIANT														
Honey Glazed	1 cup	90	3	1	0	1	15	11	3	20	190	—	—	2
JOY OF COOKING														
Bite Size	½ cup (3.3 oz)	70	3	1	5	1	12	3	2	—	115	—	—	—
CASABA														
cubed	1 cup (6 oz)	46	tr	tr	0	2	11	10	2	19	15	309	14	37
melon fresh	¼ (14 oz)	115	tr	tr	0	5	27	23	4	45	37	746	33	89
CASHEW JUICE														
O.N.E.														
Cashew Fruit	1 bottle (11 oz)	140	0	0	0	tr	34	33	1	51	20	—	—	89
CASHEWS														
cashew butter w/o salt	1 tbsp	94	8	2	0	3	4	—	—	7	2	87	11	0
dry roasted w/ salt	18 nuts (1 oz)	160	13	3	0	4	9	—	1	13	180	160	16	—
dry roasted w/ salt	1 oz	163	13	3	0	4	9	—	—	13	213	160	20	0
oil roasted w/ salt	1 oz	163	14	3	0	5	8	—	—	12	209	151	19	0
oil roasted w/o salt	1 oz	163	14	3	0	5	8	—	—	12	5	151	19	0
ARROWHEAD MILLS														
Organic Cashew Butter	2 tbsp	160	13	3	0	4	9	2	tr	—	0	—	—	—
BACK TO NATURE														
Jumbo Sea Salt Roasted	1 oz	160	13	2	0	5	9	2	1	0	100	—	—	0
FRITO LAY														
Whole Salted	3 tbsp	180	15	3	0	4	8	2	1	0	120	—	—	0
KETTLE														
Butter Creamy Unsalted	2 tbsp	160	14	3	0	5	8	0	1	20	0	—	—	0
LANCE														
Cashews	1 pkg (1.5 oz)	270	22	5	0	8	11	4	3	0	230	—	—	0
NAVITAS NATURALS														
Cashews	1 oz	160	12	2	0	5	9	2	1	20	0	—	—	0
NUT HARVEST														
Whole Sea Salted	2 tbsp (1 oz)	170	13	3	0	4	9	2	1	0	150	—	24	0
PEELED SNACKS														
Nut Picks Cashew Later	1 pkg (1 oz)	180	14	3	0	4	9	2	tr	—	120	—	—	—

FOOD	PORTION	CALS	FAT	SAT FAT	CHOL	PROT	CARB	SUGAR	FIBER	CALCI	SOD	POTAS	FOLIC	VIT C
PLANTERS														
Chocolate Lovers Milk Chocolate	10 pieces (1.5 oz)	230	16	7	5	5	20	15	1	60	25	—	—	0
Halves & Pieces	1 oz	160	13	3	0	5	9	2	1	0	150	—	—	0
Halves & Pieces Lightly Salted	1 oz	160	13	3	0	5	9	2	1	0	60	—	—	0
Whole Honey Roasted	1 oz	150	11	2	0	4	11	5	1	0	120	—	—	0
SUNFOOD														
Organic	1 oz	164	12	2	0	5	9	2	1	10	3	—	—	0
TREE OF LIFE														
Cashew Butter Creamy	2 tbsp	180	15	3	—	4	9	2	1	20	0	—	—	—
YUMNUTS														
Chili Lime	¼ cup (1 oz)	170	13	2	0	6	7	2	3	0	110	180	—	0
Chocolate	¼ cup (1 oz)	160	11	2	0	4	12	6	2	0	10	160	—	0
Honey	¼ cup (1 oz)	170	12	3	0	5	10	6	1	0	0	160	—	0
Toasted Coconut	½ cup (1 oz)	170	13	4	0	5	9	4	2	0	0	150	—	0
CASSAVA														
diced cooked w/o fat	1 cup (4.6 oz)	213	tr	tr	0	2	51	2	2	20	257	323	24	18
root raw	1 (14.3 oz)	653	1	tr	0	6	155	7	7	65	57	1106	97	84
TAKE-OUT														
fritter crab meat stuffed	1 (4.4 oz)	341	16	4	45	12	38	7	2	154	680	557	42	22
CATFISH														
channel breaded & fried	3 oz	194	11	3	69	15	7	—	—	37	238	289	—	0
wolffish atlantic baked	3 oz	105	3	tr	50	19	0	0	0	—	93	—	—	—
SIMMONS														
Farm Raised	4 oz	140	6	2	50	17	0	0	0	0	40	—	—	0
CAULIFLOWER														
flowerets fresh	1 (0.5 oz)	3	tr	tr	0	tr	1	tr	tr	3	4	39	7	6
flowerets fresh cooked w/o salt	3 (2 oz)	12	tr	tr	0	1	2	1	1	9	8	77	24	24
fresh	1 cup	25	tr	tr	0	2	5	2	3	22	30	303	57	46
fresh cooked w/o salt	1 cup	29	1	tr	0	2	5	3	3	20	19	176	55	55
fresh head small	1 (9.2 oz)	66	tr	tr	0	5	14	6	7	58	80	803	151	123
frzn cooked w/o salt	1 cup	34	tr	tr	0	3	7	2	5	31	32	250	74	56
green fresh	1 cup	20	tr	tr	0	2	4	2	2	21	15	192	36	57
green fresh small head	1 (11.4 oz)	101	1	tr	0	10	20	10	10	107	75	975	185	286

FOOD	PORTION	CALS	FAT	SAT FAT	CHOL	PROT	CARB	SUGAR	FIBER	CALCI	SOD	POTAS	FOLIC	VIT C
pickled	¼ cup	14	tr	tr	0	tr	3	2	1	7	60	64	8	9
pickled chow chow	¼ cup	74	1	tr	0	1	16	15	1	14	323	122	3	4
BIRDS EYE														
Steamfresh Garlic Cauliflower	1 cup (2.4 oz)	40	2	0	0	1	5	2	1	20	330	—	—	21
DOLE														
Fresh	1 cup (3.4 oz)	25	0	0	0	2	5	2	2	20	30	—	60	42
JAKE & AMOS														
Sweet Pickled Hot Cauliflower	1 tbsp	40	0	0	0	0	10	8	0	—	70	—	—	—
MANN'S														
Cauliettes Fresh	1 serv (3 oz)	20	0	0	0	2	4	2	2	20	25	260	48	42
TAKE-OUT														
batter dipped fried	1 piece (0.9 oz)	55	4	1	4	1	4	tr	1	11	48	52	11	6
batter dipped fried	1 cup	178	13	3	14	3	12	1	2	37	156	169	36	20
w/ cheese sauce	1 cup	249	18	8	36	12	12	6	3	315	440	319	68	59

CAVIAR

FOOD	PORTION	CALS	FAT	SAT FAT	CHOL	PROT	CARB	SUGAR	FIBER	CALCI	SOD	POTAS	FOLIC	VIT C
black or red	2 tbsp	81	6	1	188	8	1	0	0	88	480	58	16	0

CELERY

FOOD	PORTION	CALS	FAT	SAT FAT	CHOL	PROT	CARB	SUGAR	FIBER	CALCI	SOD	POTAS	FOLIC	VIT C
fresh	1 lg stalk (2.2 oz)	9	tr	tr	0	tr	2	1	1	26	51	166	23	2
pickled	½ cup	10	tr	tr	0	tr	2	1	1	26	192	159	16	2
raw diced	½ cup	8	tr	tr	0	tr	2	1	1	24	48	156	22	2
seed	1 tsp	1	tr	tr	0	tr	tr	—	tr	8	0	28	2	tr
strips	1 cup	17	tr	tr	0	1	4	2	2	50	99	322	45	4
DOLE														
Hearts	2 stalks (4 oz)	15	0	0	0	tr	3	0	2	40	90	—	40	4
EARTHBOUND FARMS														
Organic Hearts	2 stalks (3.9 oz)	20	0	0	0	1	5	0	2	40	100	—	—	9
READY PAC														
Sticks	5 (3 oz)	10	0	0	0	1	3	1	1	40	70	—	—	2
TAKE-OUT														
creamed	½ cup	87	6	1	3	3	7	4	1	87	383	256	18	4
stir fried	½ cup	30	2	tr	0	1	3	2	1	32	238	213	16	5
stuffed w/ cheese	1 (5 inch)	38	3	2	10	1	1	tr	tr	34	84	71	9	1

CELERY JUICE

FOOD	PORTION	CALS	FAT	SAT FAT	CHOL	PROT	CARB	SUGAR	FIBER	CALCI	SOD	POTAS	FOLIC	VIT C
juice	1 cup	42	tr	tr	0	2	9	6	4	99	215	670	52	14

CELERY ROOT

FOOD	PORTION	CALS	FAT	SAT FAT	CHOL	PROT	CARB	SUGAR	FIBER	CALCI	SOD	POTAS	FOLIC	VIT C
fresh cooked w/o salt	1 cup (5.4 oz)	42	tr	—	0	1	9	—	2	40	95	268	5	6
fresh cut up	1 cup (5.5 oz)	66	tr	tr	0	2	14	3	3	67	156	468	12	13

CELTUCE

FOOD	PORTION	CALS	FAT	SAT FAT	CHOL	PROT	CARB	SUGAR	FIBER	CALCI	SOD	POTAS	FOLIC	VIT C
raw	3.5 oz	22	tr	—	0	1	4	—	—	39	11	330	—	20

CEREAL

FOOD	PORTION	CALS	FAT	SAT FAT	CHOL	PROT	CARB	SUGAR	FIBER	CALCI	SOD	POTAS	FOLIC	VIT C
bran flakes	¾ cup	90	1	tr	0	4	22	—	—	14	264	180	—	0
corn flakes	1¼ cups	110	tr	tr	0	2	24	—	—	1	351	26	—	15
farina as prep w/ water	¾ cup	88	tr	tr	0	2	19	—	2	4	0	23	40	0
granola	½ cup	285	15	3	0	9	32	—	6	45	15	328	53	1
oatmeal instant as prep w/ water	1 cup (8.2 oz)	138	2	tr	0	6	24	—	4	215	377	131	199	0
oatmeal regular & quick as prep w/ water	¾ cup (6.1 oz)	149	2	tr	0	5	19	—	3	14	2	98	7	0
oatmeal regular & quick not prep	⅓ cup (0.9 oz)	104	2	tr	0	4	18	—	3	14	1	95	9	0
puffed rice	1 cup	56	tr	tr	0	1	13	—	tr	1	0	16	3	0
puffed wheat	1 cup	44	tr	tr	0	2	10	—	1	3	0	42	4	0
shredded mini wheats	1 cup	107	1	tr	0	3	24	—	3	11	3	108	14	0
shredded wheat rectangular	1 biscuit (0.8 oz)	85	tr	tr	0	3	19	—	2	10	0	77	12	0
ALPEN														
High Fibre	1 serv (1.6 oz)	154	3	tr	—	4	28	11	tr	—	tr	—	—	—
No Sugar Added	1 serv (1.6 oz)	158	2	tr	—	5	29	7	4	—	tr	—	—	—
ALTI PLANO GOLD														
Instant Quinoa Hot Cereal Spiced Apple Raisin	1 pkg	160	2	0	0	3	35	12	5	—	110	—	—	—
Instant Quinoa Organic Hot Cereal Oaxacan Chocolate	1 pkg	170	3	0	0	6	30	9	5	—	120	—	—	—
AMY'S														
Bowls Organic Cream Of Rice	1 pkg (8.9 oz)	170	1	0	0	2	39	8	2	20	220	—	—	0
Bowls Organic Multigrain	1 pkg (8.9 oz)	190	2	0	0	4	40	12	5	20	300	—	—	0
ANNIE'S HOMEGROWN														
Bunny O's Honey	¾ cup (1 oz)	110	1	0	0	2	25	7	1	100	90	—	60	6
Bunny O's Organic	¾ cup (1 oz)	120	2	0	0	2	24	2	1	100	110	—	60	6
ARROWHEAD MILLS														
Organic Amaranth Flakes	1 cup	140	2	2	0	4	26	4	3	—	0	120	—	18
Organic Kamut Flakes	1 cup	120	1	1	0	4	25	2	2	20	70	135	—	—
Organic Multigrain Flakes	1 cup	170	2	0	0	5	33	3	3	20	180	180	—	15

FOOD	PORTION	CALS	FAT	SAT FAT	CHOL	PROT	CARB	SUGAR	FIBER	CALCI	SOD	POTAS	FOLIC	VIT C
ARROWHEAD MILLS (CONT.)														
Organic Nature O's	1 cup	130	2	1	0	4	25	1	2	0	0	85	—	—
Organic Puffed Corn	1 cup	60	1	0	0	2	12	0	2	—	5	50	—	—
Organic Puffed Millet	1 cup	60	1	0	0	2	11	0	1	0	0	65	—	0
Organic Puffed Wheat	1 cup	60	0	0	0	3	12	0	2	—	0	55	—	0
Organic Rice Flakes Sweetened	1 cup	180	1	0	0	3	40	8	1	—	190	85	—	21
Organic Shredded Wheat	1 cup	190	1	0	0	7	38	—	6	20	5	150	—	0
Organic Spelt Flakes	1 cup	120	1	0	0	4	24	3	3	—	100	135	—	—
BACK TO NATURE														
Granola Apple Blueberry	½ cup (1.8 oz)	200	3	0	0	6	39	13	4	0	10	—	—	1
Granola Chocolate Delight	½ cup (1.75 oz)	220	6	2	0	5	37	13	4	0	5	160	—	01
Granola Classic	½ cup (1.8 oz)	200	3	1	0	6	39	12	4	20	0	—	—	0
Granola Sunflower & Pumpkin Seed	½ cup (1.6 oz)	290	7	1	0	6	31	11	4	20	140	170	—	0
Granola To Go Ginger Roasted Almonds w/ Flax Seed	1 serv (1.5 oz)	190	7	1	0	5	29	10	4	40	20	—	—	0
Granola To Go Wild Blueberry Walnut w/ Flax Seed	1 serv (1.5 oz)	190	6	1	0	5	30	11	4	20	20	—	—	0
BAKERY ON MAIN														
Granola Apple Cinnamon Walnut	½ cup (2 oz)	240	12	1	0	6	29	9	4	40	20	—	—	0
Granola Fiber Power Cinnamon Raisin	½ cup (2 oz)	230	6	1	0	7	40	9	9	40	50	—	—	0
Granola Maple Raisin Almond	½ cup (2 oz)	240	12	1	0	6	30	12	4	60	20	—	—	0
Granola Super Fruit & Nut	½ cup (2 oz)	250	13	3	0	6	29	20	4	40	20	—	—	0
BARBARA'S BAKERY														
Alpen No Sugar Added	⅔ cup	200	3	0	0	7	40	7	4	60	30	250	200	15
Organic Breakfast O's Fruit Juice Sweetened	1 cup	120	2	0	0	4	22	1	3	0	125	80	—	0

FOOD	PORTION	CALS	FAT	SAT FAT	CHOL	PROT	CARB	SUGAR	FIBER	CALCI	SOD	POTAS	FOLIC	VIT C
BARBARA'S BAKERY (CONT.)														
Organic Brown Rice Crisps Fruit Juice Sweetened	1 cup (1 oz)	120	1	0	0	2	25	1	1	0	95	95	—	0
Organic Corn Flakes Fruit Juice Sweetened	1 cup	110	1	0	0	2	25	3	1	0	140	100	—	0
Organic Wild Puffs Fruity Punch	1 cup	110	1	0	0	2	26	9	1	40	55	95	200	15
Organic Ultima High Fiber	½ cup	90	1	0	0	3	24	5	8	0	130	185	—	0
Organic Ultima Pomegranate	½ cup	100	1	0	0	3	24	5	5	0	85	150	—	60
Puffins Honey Rice Gluten Free	¾ cup (1 oz)	120	1	0	0	2	25	6	3	100	80	65	—	9
Puffins Multigrain Gluten Free	¾ cup (1 oz)	110	0	0	0	2	25	6	3	250	80	65	—	15
Puffins Originals	¾ cup (0.9 oz)	90	1	0	0	2	23	5	5	0	190	85	—	6
Shredded Oats Bite Size	1¼ cups (2 oz)	220	3	1	0	6	46	12	5	20	260	230	—	21
Shredded Wheat	2 biscuits (1.4 oz)	140	1	0	0	4	31	0	5	20	0	160	16	0
BASIC 4														
Whole Grain	1 cup (1.9 oz)	200	2	1	0	4	43	14	3	250	320	160	100	6
BEAR NAKED														
Cranberry Raisin	⅔ cup (2 oz)	210	5	1	0	5	41	15	4	0	140	—	—	0
Fit Vanilla Almond Crunch	¼ cup (1.1 oz)	120	3	0	0	4	22	4	2	0	10	—	—	0
Granola Fruit And Nut	¼ cup (1.1 oz)	140	7	2	0	3	17	6	2	0	0	—	—	0
Granola Heavenly Chocolate	¼ cup (1.1 oz)	130	4	1	0	3	21	7	2	0	10	—	—	0
Peak Flax Oats And Honey w/ Blueberries	¼ cup (1.1 oz)	130	4	1	0	3	22	7	2	0	0	—	—	0
BETTER BALANCE														
Protein Cereal All Flavors Gluten Free	1 oz	100	2	0	0	9	15	3	3	40	140	—	—	0
BOB'S RED MILL														
Farina Creamy Brown Rice not prep	¼ cup	150	1	0	0	3	32	0	2	—	5	—	—	—
Muesli Old Country	¼ cup	110	3	0	0	4	21	5	4	—	0	—	—	—
Natural Granola No Fat	½ cup	180	3	0	0	5	35	8	4	—	10	—	—	—

FOOD	PORTION	CALS	FAT	SAT FAT	CHOL	PROT	CARB	SUGAR	FIBER	CALCI	SOD	POTAS	FOLIC	VIT C
BOB'S RED MILL (CONT.)														
Organic Right Stuff Hot Cereal 6 Grain not prep	¼ cup	140	2	0	0	6	27	0	4	—	0	—	—	—
Rolled Oats Gluten Free not prep	½ cup	160	3	1	0	7	27	1	4	—	0	—	—	—
BOO BERRY														
Cereal	3 cup (1.2 oz)	130	1	0	0	1	28	12	1	100	190	35	100	6
BREADY BREK														
Original	1 serv (1 oz)	108	3	tr	—	4	18	tr	2	400	tr	—	51	—
CASCADIAN FARM														
Organic Clifford Crunch	1 cup	100	1	0	0	2	25	6	5	100	160	85	100	6
Organic Granola Oats & Honey	⅔ cup (1.9 oz)	230	6	1	0	5	42	14	3	20	110	140	—	0
CHAPPAQUA CRUNCH														
Original Granola	⅓ cup	115	2	1	0	4	20	4	3	20	0	—	—	—
Simply Granola w/ Raisins	⅓ cup	120	2	1	0	4	22	6	3	20	15	—	—	1
Simply Granola w/ Raspberries	⅓ cup	110	2	5	0	4	21	4	3	20	0	—	—	1
CHEERIOS														
Apple Cinnamon	¾ cup (1 oz)	120	2	0	0	2	24	11	2	100	135	65	200	6
Banana Nut	¾ cup (1 oz)	120	1	0	0	1	26	12	0	60	180	—	100	6
Chocolate	¾ cup (1 oz)	100	1	0	0	1	23	9	1	100	170	60	200	15
Honey Nut	¾ cup (1 oz)	110	2	0	0	2	22	9	2	100	190	115	200	6
MultiGrain	1 cup (1 oz)	110	1	0	0	2	23	6	3	100	160	85	400	15
Whole Grain Oat	1 cup (1 oz)	100	2	0	0	3	20	1	3	100	160	170	200	6
Yogurt Burst Strawberry	¾ cup (1 oz)	120	2	1	0	2	24	9	2	100	180	65	200	6
CHEX														
Chocolate	¾ cup (1.1 oz)	130	3	1	0	1	26	8	tr	100	240	55	200	6
Corn Gluten Free	1 cup (1.2 oz)	120	1	0	0	2	26	3	1	100	290	50	200	6
Multi-Bran	¾ cup (1.6 oz)	160	2	0	0	3	39	10	6	100	310	190	400	6
Rice Gluten Free	1 cup (0.9 oz)	100	0	0	0	2	23	2	tr	100	240	45	200	6
Wheat	¾ cups (1.6 oz)	160	2	0	0	5	38	5	5	100	340	170	400	6
CHIA GOODNESS														
Apple Almond Cinnamon	2 tbsp (1 oz)	130	6	1	0	4	16	4	4	80	125	190	—	2
Cranberry Ginger	2 tbsp (1 oz)	130	7	1	0	4	16	3	4	60	120	190	—	2
Original	2 tbsp (1 oz)	140	8	1	0	6	14	0	5	90	125	200	—	2
CINNAMON TOAST CRUNCH														
Cinnamon Sugar	¾ cup (1.1 oz)	130	3	1	0	1	25	10	1	100	220	45	100	6
COCOA PUFFS														
Cereal	¾ cup (1 oz)	100	2	0	0	1	23	11	2	100	150	70	100	6

FOOD	PORTION	CALS	FAT	SAT FAT	CHOL	PROT	CARB	SUGAR	FIBER	CALCI	SOD	POTAS	FOLIC	VIT C
COOKIE CRISP														
Cereal	¾ cup (0.9 oz)	100	1	0	0	1	22	10	1	100	150	40	100	6
COUNT CHOCULA														
Cereal	¾ cup (0.9 oz)	110	1	0	0	1	23	12	1	100	160	55	100	6
COUNTRY CHOICE ORGANIC														
Multigrain Hot Cereal not prep	½ cup	130	1	0	0	5	29	0	5	0	0	—	—	0
Oats Old Fashioned not prep	½ cup	150	3	1	0	5	27	1	4	0	0	—	—	0
Oats Quick not prep	½ cup	150	3	1	0	5	27	1	4	0	0	—	—	0
DORSET CEREALS														
Berries & Cherries	½ cup	150	1	1	<5	4	40	23	3	0	5	—	—	0
Simply Delicious Muesli	½ cup	200	5	1	<5	6	37	7	4	0	15	—	—	0
Super Cranberry Cherry & Almond	½ cup	200	5	1	<5	5	39	17	4	0	90	—	—	0
DR. MCDOUGALL'S														
Organic Instant Oatmeal	1 pkg (1 oz)	120	2	0	0	4	21	0	3	—	40	—	—	—
Organic Maple 4 Grain	1 pkg (2.6 oz)	260	3	0	0	8	52	16	6	—	260	—	—	—
EARTHBOUND FARMS														
Organic Granola Maple Almond	½ cup	260	14	2	0	6	31	11	4	40	0	—	—	0
ENJOY LIFE														
Allergen Gluten Free Granola Cinnamon	½ cup	160	3	0	0	3	31	8	5	350	10	—	140	6
ENVIROKIDZ														
Amazon Frosted Flakes Organic	⅔ cup (1.1 oz)	120	0	0	0	2	26	6	2	0	115	—	—	0
Koala Crisp Organic	¾ cup (1.1 oz)	110	1	0	0	2	25	11	2	0	100	—	—	0
Panda Puffs Organic	¾ cup (1.1 oz)	130	3	0	0	2	24	7	2	0	130	—	—	0
EREWHON														
Aztec Crunchy Corn & Amaranth	1 cup (1 oz)	110	0	0	0	2	26	1	1	0	70	—	—	0
Barley Plus not prep	¼ cups (1.6 oz)	170	1	0	0	5	37	0	4	0	0	—	—	0
Brown Rice Cream not prep	¼ cup (1.6 oz)	170	1	0	0	5	36	0	1	20	30	—	—	0
Cocoa Crispy Brown Rice	1 cup (1.8 oz)	200	2	0	0	3	44	11	1	0	190	—	—	0

FOOD	PORTION	CALS	FAT	SAT FAT	CHOL	PROT	CARB	SUGAR	FIBER	CALCI	SOD	POTAS	FOLIC	VIT C
EREWHON (CONT.)														
Crispy Brown Rice No Salt Added	1 cup (1 oz)	110	0	0	0	2	25	1	1	20	10	—	—	1
Crispy Brown Rice Original	1 cup (1 oz)	110	0	0	0	2	25	1	1	20	180	—	—	1
Organic Instant Oatmeal Apple Cinnamon not prep	1 pkg (1.2 oz)	130	2	1	0	5	24	4	3	20	100	—	—	—
Organic Instant Oatmeal w/ Oat Bran	1 pkg (1.8 oz)	130	3	1	0	6	25	tr	4	20	0	—	—	—
Rice Twice	¾ cup (1 oz)	120	0	0	0	2	26	8	0	0	60	—	—	0
ERIN BAKER'S														
Granola Fruit & Nut	½ cup (1.6 oz)	190	8	2	0	5	25	10	4	20	0	—	—	4
Granola Oatmeal Raisin	½ cup (1.6 oz)	180	6	1	0	4	30	11	4	0	0	—	—	0
Granola Ultra Protein Power Crunch	½ cup (1.6 oz)	200	6	1	0	8	25	6	4	40	75	—	—	5
FANTASTIC														
Oatmeal Big Cup Apple Cinnamon	1 pkg	270	4	1	0	8	54	17	6	—	320	—	—	—
Oatmeal Big Cup Maple Raisin 3 Grain	1 pkg	270	2	0	0	7	60	22	8	40	310	—	—	0
FARINA														
Original as prep	1 cup	120	0	0	0	3	22	0	tr	100	0	—	40	0
FEED														
Granola Apple A Day	¼ cup (1 oz)	130	3	0	0	3	23	6	3	20	40	—	—	0
Granola Bittersweet'ness	¼ cup (1 oz)	130	4	1	0	3	22	5	3	20	40	—	—	0
Granola Raisin Nut	¼ cup (1 oz)	130	4	0	0	3	20	6	2	20	35	—	—	0
Sweet Mango	¼ cup (1 oz)	120	3	0	0	3	23	5	3	20	15	—	—	1
FIBER ONE														
Caramel Delight	1 cup (1.8 oz)	180	3	1	0	3	41	11	9	100	230	130	100	6
Frosted Shredded Wheat	1 cup (2.1 oz)	200	1	0	0	5	50	12	9	0	0	190	100	—
Honey Clusters	1 cup (1.8 oz)	160	2	0	0	3	44	6	13	100	230	180	100	0
Original	½ cup (1 oz)	60	1	0	0	2	25	0	14	100	105	180	100	6
Raisin Bran Clusters	1 cup (2 oz)	170	1	0	0	4	45	13	11	100	260	330	100	0
GLUCERNA														
Crunchy Flakes 'N Raisins	1 bowl (1.6 oz)	140	1	0	0	4	36	13	6	20	270	260	100	0

FOOD	PORTION	CALS	FAT	SAT FAT	CHOL	PROT	CARB	SUGAR	FIBER	CALCI	SOD	POTAS	FOLIC	VIT C
GLUCERNA (CONT.)														
Crunchy Flakes 'N Strawberries	1 bowl (1.5 oz)	150	1	0	0	4	37	9	7	20	320	240	100	6
GLUTENFREEDA														
Granola Apple Almond Honey	¼ cup (1 oz)	150	11	1	0	3	10	7	2	20	45	—	—	0
Oatmeal Instant as prep	1 pkg (1.8 oz)	190	3	1	0	8	34	1	5	20	0	—	—	0
GLUTINO														
Gluten Free Apple Cinnamon	½ cup	120	2	0	0	1	24	10	1	0	180	—	—	0
Gluten Free Honey Nut	½ cup	130	3	tr	0	2	24	8	1	20	150	—	—	0
GOLDEN GRAHAMS														
Cereal	¾ cup (1.1 oz)	120	1	0	0	2	26	11	1	100	270	60	100	6
GRANDY OATS														
Organic Granola Classic	½ cup	252	14	2	0	8	27	6	5	30	75	—	—	1
Organic Granola Low Fat Cranberry Chew	½ cup	191	1	0	0	5	41	17	3	<10	53	—	—	4
Organic Granola Mainely Maple	½ cup	204	7	tr	0	6	31	9	4	40	109	—	—	1
HEALTH VALLEY														
Empower	1 cup	200	3	0	0	6	42	11	6	500	170	240	—	60
Granola Low Fat Tropical Fruit	⅔ cup	180	1	0	0	5	43	10	6	20	90	—	—	2
Heart Wise	1 cup	200	3	0	0	11	37	11	5	500	140	220	—	48
Organic Cherry Lemon Blast Ems	¾ cup	120	1	0	0	2	25	7	2	40	90	—	—	27
Organic Golden Flax	¾ cup	190	3	0	0	6	38	9	6	60	80	—	—	0
Organic Multigrain Apple Cinnamon Square Ems	1¼ cups	210	3	0	0	5	44	12	8	40	125	180	—	48
Organic Oat Bran O's	¾ cup	100	0	0	0	3	23	14	3	0	90	—	—	0
Rice Crunch-Ems	1 cup	110	0	0	0	4	26	2	2	—	150	—	—	—
HONEST FOODS														
Granola Planks Maple Almond Crunch	½ bar (2 oz)	250	10	1	0	6	37	19	5	40	150	170	24	0
KAIA FOODS														
Organic Granola Buckwheat Cinnamon Raisin	½ cup (2 oz)	230	10	2	0	6	34	12	6	40	30	—	—	0

FOOD	PORTION	CALS	FAT	SAT FAT	CHOL	PROT	CARB	SUGAR	FIBER	CALCI	SOD	POTAS	FOLIC	VIT C
KAIA FOODS (CONT.)														
Organic Granola Buckwheat Cocoa Bliss	½ cup (2 oz)	220	8	2	0	6	35	14	5	40	35	—	—	0
KASHI														
7 Whole Grain Flakes	1 cup	180	1	0	0	6	41	5	6	0	150	160	—	0
7 Whole Grain Honey Puffs	1 cup	120	1	0	0	3	25	6	2	0	6	80	—	0
7 Whole Grain Nuggets	½ cup	210	2	0	0	7	47	3	7	20	260	—	—	0
7 Whole Grain Pilaf as prep	½ cup	170	3	0	0	6	30	0	6	20	15	—	—	0
GoLean	1 cup	140	1	0	0	13	30	6	10	60	85	480	—	0
GoLean Crunch!	1 cup	190	3	0	0	9	36	13	8	40	95	300	—	0
GoLean Crunch Honey Almond Flax	1 cup	200	5	0	0	9	34	12	8	0	140	270	—	0
GoLean Instant Hot Cereal Creamy Truly Vanilla	1 pkg	150	2	0	0	9	25	6	7	0	100	250	—	0
GoLean Instant Hot Cereal Hearty Honey & Cinnamon	1 pkg	150	2	0	0	8	26	7	5	0	100	210	—	0
Good Friends	1 cup	170	2	0	0	5	43	9	12	20	130	—	—	0
Granola Mountain Medley	½ cup	220	7	1	0	6	37	12	6	0	10	140	—	0
Heart To Heart Instant Oatmeal Golden Brown Maple	1 pkg	160	2	0	0	4	33	12	5	100	100	260	400	30
Heart To Heart Instant Oatmeal Raisin Spice	1 pkg	150	2	0	0	3	33	16	4	100	100	230	400	30
Heart To Heart Oat Flakes & Blueberry Clusters	1¼ cups	200	3	1	0	6	42	12	4	0	130	160	400	30
Heart To Heart Toasted Oat	¾ cup	110	2	0	0	4	25	5	5	0	90	100	400	30
Honey Sunshine	¾ cup (1.1 oz)	100	2	0	0	2	25	6	6	0	135	70	—	0
Mighty Bites All Flavors	1 cup	110	2	0	0	5	23	5	3	150	160	110	100	15
Organic Promise Autumn Wheat	1 cup	190	1	0	0	5	45	7	6	0	0	180	—	0

FOOD	PORTION	CALS	FAT	SAT FAT	CHOL	PROT	CARB	SUGAR	FIBER	CALCI	SOD	POTAS	FOLIC	VIT C
KASHI (CONT.)														
Organic Promise Cinnamon Harvest	1 cup	190	1	0	0	4	44	9	5	0	0	170	—	0
Organic Promise Strawberry Fields	1 cup	120	0	0	0	2	28	9	1	0	200	40	—	2
Vive Probiotic Digestive Wellness	1¼ cups	170	3	1	0	4	43	10	12	200	60	25	—	0
KELLOGG'S														
Corn Pops	1 box (1 oz)	110	0	0	0	1	24	9	3	0	105	—	80	4
Cracklin' Oat Bran	¾ cup	200	7	3	0	4	35	15	6	20	150	220	100	15
Crispix	1 cup	110	0	0	0	2	25	3	tr	0	210	35	280	6
Raisin Bran	1 cup (2.1 oz)	190	1	0	0	5	46	17	7	20	250	320	100	0
Smart Start Antioxidants	1 cup	190	1	0	0	3	43	14	3	0	280	90	400	15
KIX														
Corn Puffs	1¼ cups (1 oz)	110	1	0	0	2	25	3	3	150	190	60	200	6
Honey	1¼ cups (1.1 oz)	120	1	0	0	2	28	6	3	150	190	75	200	6
LOVE CRUNCH														
Carrot Cake Organic	¼ cup (1.1 oz)	130	4	1	0	2	23	8	2	20	45	95	—	1
Dark Chocolate & Red Berries Organic	¼ cup (1.1 oz)	140	6	1	0	2	20	6	2	0	55	105	—	1
LUCKY CHARMS														
Swirled	¾ cup (1 oz)	110	1	0	0	2	22	11	1	100	190	45	200	6
LUNDBERG														
Purely Organic Hot'n Creamy Rice	⅓ cup	190	2	0	0	4	43	0	3	0	0	190	—	0
MALT-O-MEAL														
Apple Zings	1 cup (1.2 oz)	130	1	0	0	1	30	16	1	100	150	35	200	6
Chocolate not prep	3 tbsp (1.2 oz)	130	0	0	0	4	27	7	1	100	0	85	400	0
Coco Roos	¾ cup (1 oz)	120	2	0	0	1	26	15	tr	100	135	75	200	6
Crispy Rice	1¼ cups (1.2 oz)	130	0	0	0	2	29	3	0	0	300	40	400	6
Golden Puffs	¾ cup (1 oz)	110	0	0	0	2	24	15	0	0	65	45	200	6
Honey Nut Scooters	1 cup (1 oz)	110	2	0	0	2	24	10	2	100	210	125	200	6
Mateys Marshmallow	1 cup (1 oz)	120	1	0	0	2	25	13	1	100	200	60	200	6
Original Creamy Hot Wheat not prep	3 tbsp (1.2 oz)	130	0	0	0	4	27	0	1	100	0	35	0	0
Original not prep	3 tbsp (1.2 oz)	130	1	0	0	5	27	0	1	100	0	40	400	0

FOOD	PORTION	CALS	FAT	SAT FAT	CHOL	PROT	CARB	SUGAR	FIBER	CALCI	SOD	POTAS	FOLIC	VIT C
MALT-O-MEAL (CONT.)														
Tootie Fruities	1 cup (1.1 oz)	130	1	0	0	2	28	15	1	100	150	35	200	6
MCCANN'S														
Irish Oatmeal Instant Apples & Cinnamon not prep	1 pkg (1.2 oz)	130	2	0	0	3	27	12	3	100	170	—	80	0
Irish Oatmeal Instant Maple & Brown Sugar not prep	1 pkg (1.5 oz)	160	2	0	0	4	32	13	3	100	240	—	80	1
Irish Oatmeal Instant Regular not prep	1 pkg (1 oz)	100	2	0	0	4	18	1	3	100	80	—	—	0
Irish Oatmeal Quick Cooking not prep	½ cup (1.4 oz)	150	2	0	0	4	26	0	4	0	0	—	—	0
Irish Oatmeal Steel Cut not prep	¼ cup (1.4 oz)	150	2	0	0	4	26	0	4	0	0	—	—	0
MOM'S BEST NATURALS														
Blue Pom Wheat-fuls	1 cup (1.9 oz)	210	1	0	0	5	45	11	6	20	10	180	16	—
Honey Grahams	¾ cup (1 oz)	130	3	1	0	1	25	10	1	100	270	50	0	0
Mallow Oats	1 cup (1 oz)	120	1	0	0	2	24	13	1	100	200	60	8	—
Raisin Bran	1 cup (2.1 oz)	230	2	0	0	5	49	20	6	20	340	380	0	—
MOTHER'S														
Barley Hot Cereal not prep	⅓ cup (1.7 oz)	160	1	0	0	5	37	0	5	0	0	115	—	0
Peanut Butter Bumpers	1 cup (1.2 oz)	130	3	1	0	3	26	10	1	0	260	100	—	0
Rolled Oats not prep	½ cup (1.4 oz)	150	3	1	0	5	27	1	4	0	0	—	—	0
Toasted Oat Bran	¾ cup (1.1 oz)	120	2	0	0	4	24	5	3	20	200	160	—	0
NAKED GRANOLA														
Taste Of Seattle Nights	½ pkg (1.2 oz)	110	6	2	0	4	12	5	5	20	—	—	—	1
NATURAL OVENS														
Great Granola	½ cup	250	9	2	0	6	38	8	3	40	10	—	0	0
NATURE'S PATH														
Corn Flakes Organic	¾ cup (1.1 oz)	110	0	0	0	2	24	3	2	0	150	—	—	0
Granola Hemp Plus Organic	¾ cup (1.9 oz)	260	10	2	0	6	36	10	5	20	45	180	—	0
Granola Peanut Butter Organic	¾ cup (1.9 oz)	260	11	2	0	7	35	9	4	20	75	160	—	0

FOOD	PORTION	CALS	FAT	SAT FAT	CHOL	PROT	CARB	SUGAR	FIBER	CALCI	SOD	POTAS	FOLIC	VIT C
NATURE'S PATH (CONT.)														
Granola Pumpkin Flax Plus Organic	¾ cup (1.9 oz)	260	10	2	0	6	37	10	5	20	45	—	—	0
Heritage Crunch Organic	¾ cup (1.9 oz)	230	3	1	0	6	44	6	6	20	210	—	—	0
Instant Oatmeal Flax Plus Organic	1 pkg (1.8 oz)	210	3	1	0	6	38	10	5	20	140	160	—	0
Instant Oatmeal Maple Nut Organic	1 pkg (1.8 oz)	210	4	1	0	5	38	11	4	20	100	—	—	0
Instant Oatmeal Optimum Cranberry Ginger Organic	1 pkg (1.4 oz)	150	2	0	0	5	30	10	3	20	160	110	—	0
Instant Oatmeal Original Organic	1 pkg (1.8 oz)	210	4	1	0	7	37	0	6	20	160	—	—	0
Kamut Puffs Organic	1 cup (0.5 oz)	50	0	0	0	2	11	0	2	0	0	—	—	0
Maple Pecan Crunch Flax Plus Organic	¾ cup (1.9 oz)	220	7	1	0	6	38	10	5	20	190	230	—	0
Millet Rice Flakes Organic	¾ cup (1.1 oz)	120	2	0	0	4	22	4	3	20	115	—	—	0
Optimum Blueberry Cinnamon Organic	1 cup (1.9 oz)	200	3	0	0	9	38	9	7	20	230	—	—	1
Optimum Cranberry Ginger Organic	¾ cup (1.9 oz)	190	3	0	0	5	41	13	8	20	95	—	—	0
Red Berry Crunch Flax Plus Organic	¾ cup (1.9 oz)	210	4	1	0	6	39	10	5	20	160	230	—	9
Rice Puffs Organic	1 cup (0.5 oz)	50	0	0	0	1	14	0	1	0	0	—	—	0
Shredded Oaty Bites Organic	¾ cup (1.1 oz)	110	2	0	0	3	23	5	2	0	115	—	—	0
NATURE'S PLUS														
Instant Oatmeal Hemp Plus Organic	1 pkg (1.4 oz)	160	3	0	0	5	30	6	4	20	105	—	—	0
NEW MORNING														
Cocoa Crispy Rice	¾ cup (1 oz)	120	1	0	0	2	26	10	1	0	100	—	—	0
Oatios Original	1 cup (1 oz)	110	2	0	0	5	22	2	3	0	125	—	—	0
NEWMAN'S OWN														
Sweet Enough Honey Flax Flakes	¾ cup	100	1	0	0	3	24	8	4	0	80	35	200	15

FOOD	PORTION	CALS	FAT	SAT FAT	CHOL	PROT	CARB	SUGAR	FIBER	CALCI	SOD	POTAS	FOLIC	VIT C
NEWMAN'S OWN (CONT.)														
Sweet Enough Honey Nut O's	¾ cup	110	2	0	0	3	22	7	2	0	170	60	200	15
Sweet Enough Wheat Puffs	¾ cup	100	1	0	0	3	22	8	1	0	45	55	200	15
OATMEAL CRISP														
Crunchy Almond	1 cup (2.1 oz)	240	5	1	0	6	47	16	4	40	130	410	32	0
POST														
100% Bran	½ cup (0.8 oz)	80	1	0	0	4	22	7	9	200	0	—	—	0
Bran Flakes	1 cup	100	1	0	0	3	24	5	5	0	220	—	—	0
Cocoa Pebbles	¾ cup (1 oz)	110	2	1	0	1	26	11	3	0	180	—	—	0
Golden Crisp	¾ cup (1 oz)	110	0	0	0	1	25	14	1	0	25	—	—	0
Grape-Nuts	½ cup (2 oz)	200	1	0	0	6	48	5	7	20	290	230	200	0
Grape-Nuts Trail Mix Crunch	1 cup (1.7 oz)	170	2	0	0	4	37	9	5	0	210	—	—	0
Grape-Nuts O's	1 cup (1 oz)	120	0	0	0	2	28	11	2	0	140	—	—	0
Great Grains Raisins Dates & Pecans	¾ cup (2 oz)	200	4	0	0	4	40	14	5	0	160	210	100	0
Honey Bunches Of Oats	1 cup (1.8 oz)	200	2	0	0	3	42	14	2	0	200	120	100	0
Honey Bunches Of Oats Almonds	¾ cup (1.1 oz)	120	3	0	0	2	26	6	2	0	135	70	200	0
Honey Bunches Of Oats Peaches	1 cup	120	2	0	0	2	26	8	2	0	135	—	—	0
Honeycomb	1⅓ cups (1 oz)	120	1	0	0	2	28	10	3	0	170	—	—	0
LiveActive Mixed Berry Crunch	1 cup	190	2	0	0	4	43	12	7	0	250	—	—	0
LiveActive Nut Harvest Crunch	1 cup	220	6	1	0	5	39	8	8	20	270	—	—	0
Oreo O's	1 cup	110	2	1	0	1	22	13	1	0	90	—	—	0
Raisin Bran	1 cup (2 oz)	190	1	0	0	4	46	19	8	20	300	330	200	0
Selects Blueberry Morning	2 oz	220	3	0	0	3	45	16	2	20	280	—	—	0
Selects Cranberry Almond Crunch	¾ cup (1.8 oz)	200	3	0	0	4	40	14	3	0	115	125	100	0
Shredded Wheat Frosted	2 oz	180	1	0	0	4	43	12	5	0	0	—	—	0
Shredded Wheat 'N Bran	2 oz	200	1	0	0	6	49	1	8	20	0	—	—	0
Shredded Wheat Original	2 biscuits (1.6 oz)	160	1	0	0	5	37	0	6	20	0	180	16	0
Shredded Wheat Spoon Size	1 cup (1.7 oz)	170	1	0	0	6	40	0	6	20	0	190	—	0
Toasties Corn Flakes	1 cup (1 oz)	100	0	0	0	2	24	2	1	0	260	—	—	0

FOOD	PORTION	CALS	FAT	SAT FAT	CHOL	PROT	CARB	SUGAR	FIBER	CALCI	SOD	POTAS	FOLIC	VIT C
QUAKER														
Instant Oatmeal Apples & Cinnamon	1 pkg (1.2 oz)	130	2	1	0	3	27	9	3	100	160	115	—	0
Instant Oatmeal Cinnamon & Spice	1 pkg	170	2	1	0	4	35	15	3	100	250	—	80	0
Instant Oatmeal Cinnamon Roll	1 pkg	160	2	1	0	4	33	13	3	100	240	—	80	0
Instant Oatmeal Mixed Berry	1 pkg	190	3	1	0	4	39	16	3	100	250	130	80	0
Instant Oatmeal Express Baked Apple	1 pkg	200	3	1	0	4	42	19	4	100	320	—	80	0
Instant Oatmeal For Kids Dinosaur Eggs	1 pkg	190	4	2	0	4	37	14	3	100	260	—	80	0
Instant Oatmeal Lower Sugar Maple & Brown Sugar	1 pkg	120	2	0	0	4	24	4	3	100	290	—	80	0
Instant Oatmeal Maple Brown Sugar w/ Pecans	1 pkg	160	4	1	0	4	30	9	4	0	75	125	8	0
Instant Oatmeal Nutrition For Women Golden Brown Sugar	1 pkg	170	2	1	0	5	32	12	3	500	330	140	140	0
Instant Oatmeal Organic Regular	1 pkg	100	2	1	0	4	19	0	3	0	0	100	8	0
Instant Oatmeal Regular	1 pkg	100	2	0	0	4	19	0	3	100	80	105	80	0
Instant Oatmeal Simple Harvest Multigrain Maple Brown Sugar w/ Pecans	1 pkg (1.48 oz)	160	4	1	0	4	30	9	4	0	75	125	8	0
Instant Oatmeal Strawberries & Cream	1 pkg	130	3	1	0	3	27	12	2	100	190	—	80	0
Instant Oatmeal Supreme Apple Raisin	1 pkg	150	2	0	0	4	32	13	3	100	290	—	80	0
Instant Oatmeal Supreme Cinnamon Pecan	1 pkg	180	4	1	0	4	33	14	3	100	290	—	80	0
Instant Oatmeal Take Heart Golden Maple	1 pkg	160	3	1	0	4	33	9	5	100	110	350	400	30

FOOD	PORTION	CALS	FAT	SAT FAT	CHOL	PROT	CARB	SUGAR	FIBER	CALCI	SOD	POTAS	FOLIC	VIT C
QUAKER (CONT.)														
Instant Oatmeal Weight Control Banana Bread	1 pkg	160	3	1	0	7	29	1	6	100	260	150	80	0
Oat Bran Hot Cereal not prep	½ cup	150	3	1	0	7	25	1	6	20	0	—	—	0
Oatmeal Squares	1 cup (2 oz)	210	3	1	0	6	44	9	5	100	190	200	400	6
RALSTON														
Corn Flakes	1 cup (1 oz)	100	0	0	0	2	24	2	tr	0	200	25	100	15
Raisin Bran	1 cup (2 oz)	190	1	0	0	4	46	19	7	20	350	340	100	0
READY BREK														
Chocolate	1 serv (1 oz)	108	2	1	—	3	19	7	2	400	tr	—	51	—
REESE'S														
Puffs	¾ cup (1 oz)	120	3	1	0	2	22	10	1	100	160	65	100	6
RICE KRISPIES														
Roasted Rice	1¼ cups (1.2 oz)	130	0	0	0	2	29	4	tr	0	220	30	100	15
ROMAN MEAL														
Cream Of Rye not prep	⅓ cup (1.4 oz)	130	0	0	0	6	27	2	6	20	0	—	24	0
Elements Cranberry Passion	1 cup (1.6 oz)	160	3	0	0	5	33	9	5	20	120	340	8	1
Hot Cereal not prep	⅓ cup (1.3 oz)	120	2	0	0	6	26	1	6	20	0	—	8	0
SILHOUETTE SOLUTION														
Oatmeal Cinnamon Apple	1 pkg. (1.39 oz)	150	2	2	15	15	17	4	4	60	310	135	—	0
SIMPLI														
Instant Oatmeal Apricot Gluten Free	1 pkg (1.7 oz)	170	3	0	0	5	30	10	4	20	200	—	—	0
Instant Oatmeal Plain Gluten Free	1 pkg (1.4 oz)	150	3	0	0	5	27	0	4	20	140	—	—	0
SKINNER'S														
Raisin Bran	1 cup (1.9 oz)	170	1	0	0	6	41	13	7	0	85	—	—	0
SOUTH BEACH														
Crunch Strawberry Harvest	1 cup	170	2	0	0	7	37	9	8	—	290	—	—	—
Crunch Vanilla Almond	1 cup	180	4	0	0	8	35	8	8	—	280	—	—	—
Granola Clusters Cherry Almond	1 pkg (1 oz)	130	4	1	0	6	18	6	6	—	55	—	—	—
Granola Clusters Mixed Berry	1 pkg (1 oz)	130	4	1	0	6	18	6	6	—	55	—	—	—
SPECIAL K														
Cereal	1 box (0.8 oz)	90	0	0	0	5	17	3	tr	0	170	—	280	15

FOOD	PORTION	CALS	FAT	SAT FAT	CHOL	PROT	CARB	SUGAR	FIBER	CALCI	SOD	POTAS	FOLIC	VIT C
STARK SISTERS														
Granola Lo-Fat Raspberry Blueberry	½ cup	230	7	1	0	4	38	16	4	40	0	—	—	1
Granola Nutty Maple	½ cup	250	11	3	0	6	32	9	4	40	5	—	—	0
Granola Original Maple Almond	½ cup	240	10	1	0	6	33	7	5	40	0	—	—	0
SUNBELT														
Granola Low Fat Cinnamon & Raisins	½ cup	250	3	1	0	4	52	20	3	20	90	—	—	0
TOTAL														
Cinnamon Crunch	1 cup (1.8 oz)	190	3	0	0	4	40	9	4	1000	200	120	400	60
Raisin Bran	1 cup (1.9 oz)	160	1	0	0	3	40	17	5	1000	230	280	400	0
Whole Grain	¾ cup (1 oz)	100	1	0	0	2	23	5	3	1000	190	90	400	60
TRIX														
Swirls	1 cup (1.1 oz)	120	2	0	0	1	28	11	1	100	190	50	100	6
UDI'S														
Gluten Free Granola Au Naturel	¼ cup (1.1 oz)	120	4	0	0	3	19	5	3	0	0	—	—	0
UNCLE SAM														
Mixed Berries	1 cup (1.9 oz)	190	4	1	0	7	39	2	10	40	130	250	—	6
Original	¾ cup (1.9 oz)	190	5	1	0	7	38	tr	10	40	135	250	—	1
WEETABIX														
Crunchy Bran	1 serv (1.4 oz)	122	1	tr	—	5	23	6	8	136	tr	—	100	—
Multigrain	1 serv (1.3 oz)	127	1	tr	—	4	26	2	4	—	tr	—	64	—
Oatibix Bites	1 serv (1.4 oz)	148	3	tr	—	4	27	6	4	—	tr	—	68	—
Oatibix Flakes	1 serv (1 oz)	114	2	tr	—	3	22	tr	2	—	tr	—	51	—
Organic	2 biscuits (1.2 oz)	120	1	0	0	4	28	2	4	0	130	120	200	15
Organic Crispy Flakes	¾ cup	110	1	0	0	3	24	4	4	10	180	150	200	15
WHEATENA														
Toasted Wheat	⅓ cup	160	1	0	0	5	33	0	5	200	0	220	—	0
WHEATIES														
Cereal	¾ cup (1 oz)	100	1	0	0	3	22	4	3	20	190	95	200	6
YOGACTIVE														
Probiotic High Fiber Wheat Strawberry Raspberry	⅔ cup	160	3	3	0	5	29	8	6	40	115	230	80	5
Probiotic Kiwi	⅔ cup	120	2	2	25	3	23	7	1	20	150	105	8	9
Probiotic Strawberry	⅔ cup	130	2	2	30	3	25	7	1	20	170	65	16	0

FOOD	PORTION	CALS	FAT	SAT FAT	CHOL	PROT	CARB	SUGAR	FIBER	CALCI	SOD	POTAS	FOLIC	VIT C
YOGACTIVE (CONT.)														
Probiotic Strawberry Dark Chocolate	⅔ cup	130	3	2	0	3	26	9	2	20	170	100	8	0
YOGI														
Granola Crisps Baked Cinnamon Raisin	½ cup	120	3	0	0	3	21	5	2	20	50	—	—	0
Granola Crisps Fresh Strawberry Crunch	½ cup	120	3	0	0	3	21	4	2	0	50	—	—	0
Granola Crisps Mountain Blueberry Flax	½ cup	110	3	0	0	3	21	5	2	0	50	—	—	0

CEREAL BARS

(*see also* ENERGY BARS, FRUIT AND NUT BARS)

FOOD	PORTION	CALS	FAT	SAT FAT	CHOL	PROT	CARB	SUGAR	FIBER	CALCI	SOD	POTAS	FOLIC	VIT C
ALPEN														
Fruit & Nut	1	109	2	tr	—	2	20	9	1	—	tr	—	—	—
Light Chocolate & Fudge	1	63	1	1	—	1	11	5	5	—	tr	—	—	—
Raspberry & Yogurt	1	120	3	2	—	2	22	11	1	—	tr	—	—	—
ANNIE'S HOMEGROWN														
Organic Peanut Butter	1 (1 oz)	120	5	1	0	3	17	5	1	0	50	—	—	0
ARISTO														
Acai Blueberry Lime	1 (1.3 oz)	130	4	1	5	3	22	6	3	40	40	—	—	9
Pomegranate & Cranberry	1 (1.3 oz)	140	5	1	5	3	21	6	3	150	40	—	—	9
ATTUNE														
Wellness Yogurt & Granola Lemon Creme	1 (1.4 oz)	180	7	3	0	5	24	12	2	200	60	—	—	0
Wellness Yogurt & Granola Strawberry Bliss	1 (1.4 oz)	180	7	3	0	5	24	12	5	200	60	—	—	1
BAKERY ON MAIN														
Granola Gluten Free Extreme Trail Mix	1 (1.3 oz)	140	5	1	0	3	23	7	1	40	120	—	—	0
Granola Gluten Free Peanut Butter Chocolate Chip	1 (1.2 oz)	140	5	1	0	2	24	7	1	40	85	—	—	0
BARBARA'S BAKERY														
Fruit & Yogurt Cherry Apple	1	150	3	0	0	3	29	15	1	250	125	—	40	6

FOOD	PORTION	CALS	FAT	SAT FAT	CHOL	PROT	CARB	SUGAR	FIBER	CALCI	SOD	POTAS	FOLIC	VIT C
BARBARA'S BAKERY (CONT.)														
Nature's Choice Blueberry	1 (1.3 oz)	150	2	0	0	2	29	15	2	0	85	—	—	0
Organic Crunchy Granola Cinnamon Crisp	2 (1.5 oz)	190	8	1	0	4	27	10	3	40	10	—	—	0
BEAR NAKED														
Grain-ola Tropical Fruit	1 (2 oz)	220	7	2	0	3	38	18	4	0	60	—	—	0
CASCADIAN FARM														
Organic Chewy Granola Fruit & Nut	1 (1.2 oz)	140	4	1	0	2	24	11	1	—	110	130	—	—
CHEERIOS														
Honey Nut	1 (1.4 oz)	160	4	2	0	3	28	14	1	250	120	115	200	9
CINNAMON TOAST CRUNCH														
Milk 'N Cereal	1 (1.6 oz)	180	4	2	0	3	33	16	1	250	150	110	200	9
CORAZONAS														
Oatmeal Squares Banana Walnut	1 (1.8 oz)	190	6	1	0	6	27	13	5	200	105	—	120	30
Oatmeal Squares Chocolate Chip	1 (1.8 oz)	190	6	1	0	6	28	13	5	200	110	—	120	30
Oatmeal Squares Cranberry Flax	1 (1.8 oz)	180	5	1	0	6	28	14	6	200	110	—	120	30
COUNTRY CHOICE ORGANIC														
Oatmeal Squares Apple Cinnamon	1 (2 oz)	210	3	1	0	4	41	16	1	100	190	—	—	0
Oatmeal Squares Maple	1 (2 oz)	210	3	1	0	4	41	14	4	100	180	—	—	0
EARNEST EATS														
Almond Trail Mix	1 (1.94 oz)	210	9	1	0	6	31	14	1	40	190	190	16	—
Choco Peanut Butter	1 (1.94 oz)	230	10	2	0	6	32	14	4	40	190	120	16	—
Cran Lemon Zest	1 (1.94 oz)	210	9	1	0	5	32	14	4	40	180	190	16	—
ENJOY LIFE														
Allergen Gluten Free Caramel Apple	1 (1 oz)	110	3	0	0	2	21	8	2	150	95	—	140	0
ENVIROKIDZ														
Crispy Rice Cheeth Berry Organic	1 (1 oz)	110	3	0	0	1	21	7	1	0	70	—	—	1
Crispy Rice Lemur Peanut Choco Drizzle Organic	1 (1 oz)	120	5	1	0	2	18	8	1	0	50	—	—	0
Crispy Rice Panda Peanut Butter	1 (1 oz)	110	3	0	0	2	20	7	1	0	65	—	—	0

FOOD	PORTION	CALS	FAT	SAT FAT	CHOL	PROT	CARB	SUGAR	FIBER	CALCI	SOD	POTAS	FOLIC	VIT C
FIBER ONE														
Chocolate Caramel & Pretzel	1 (0.8 oz)	90	2	2	0	tr	17	5	5	—	90	—	—	—
Oats & Caramel	1 (1.4 oz)	140	4	2	0	2	30	9	9	100	105	—	—	—
Oats & Chocolate	1 (1.4 oz)	140	4	2	0	2	29	10	9	100	95	—	—	—
Oats & Peanut Butter	1 (1.4 oz)	150	5	2	0	3	28	9	9	100	110	—	—	—
FRUITION														
Blueberry	1 (1.7 oz)	160	2	0	0	3	34	21	4	20	20	—	—	0
Cran-Raspberry	1 (1.7 oz)	160	2	0	0	3	34	22	4	20	20	—	—	0
Lemon	1 (1.7 oz)	160	3	0	0	3	34	19	4	40	10	—	—	0
FULLBAR														
Cocoa Chip	1 (1.59 oz)	160	3	1	0	4	31	13	4	20	95	—	—	0
Fit Chewy Brownie	1 (1.76 oz)	180	4	1	0	15	24	10	5	40	170	—	—	0
Fit Toffee Crunch	1 (1.76 oz)	180	5	2	0	15	24	10	5	20	250	—	—	0
Peanut Butter Crunch	1 (1.59 oz)	170	5	1	0	6	27	9	4	20	95	—	—	0
GLENNY'S														
Organic Muesli Chocolate Chip	1 (1.6 oz)	170	3	1	0	3	34	15	3	—	50	—	—	—
Organic Muesli Raisins & Dates	1 (1.6 oz)	170	3	1	0	3	34	15	3	—	50	—	—	—
Slim Carb Bars Brownie Cheesecake	1 (1.3 oz)	130	3	2	—	12	19	2	1	—	180	—	—	—
Slim-1 w/ Acai Very Berry Blast	1 (1.1 oz)	100	3	2	—	2	21	8	2	—	40	—	—	—
Slim-1 w/ Green Tea Double Fudge	1 (1.1 oz)	100	3	2	—	3	20	8	2	—	90	—	—	—
GLUTINO														
Gluten Free Breakfast Bar Apple	1 (1.4 oz)	120	1	0	0	2	25	17	3	20	10	—	—	15
Gluten Free Breakfast Bar Chocolate	1 (1.4 oz)	110	1	1	0	2	25	17	4	40	10	—	—	24
Gluten Free Organic Chocolate & Peanut	1 (1 oz)	110	3	1	0	2	19	8	1	0	50	—	—	0
Gluten Free Organic Wildberry	1 (1 oz)	100	1	0	0	1	21	8	1	0	65	—	—	0
GNU														
Flavor & Fiber Banana Walnut	1 (1.6 oz)	140	4	0	0	4	30	8	12	60	40	—	—	0

FOOD	PORTION	CALS	FAT	SAT FAT	CHOL	PROT	CARB	SUGAR	FIBER	CALCI	SOD	POTAS	FOLIC	VIT C
GNU (CONT.)														
Flavor & Fiber Chocolate Brownie Bar	1 (1.6 oz)	140	4	1	0	4	30	9	12	60	30	—	—	0
Flavor & Fiber Cinnamon Raisin	1 (1.6 oz)	130	3	0	0	3	32	11	12	60	30	—	—	0
Flavor & Fiber Expresso Chip	1 (1.6 oz)	140	4	1	0	4	30	8	12	60	35	—	—	0
Flavor & Fiber Lemon Ginger	1 (1.6 oz)	130	4	0	0	3	32	10	12	60	35	—	—	0
Flavor & Fiber Orange Cranberry	1 (1.6 oz)	130	3	0	0	3	32	11	12	60	35	—	—	0
Flavor & Fiber Peanut Butter	1 (1.6 oz)	140	5	1	0	4	30	7	12	60	95	—	—	0
HEALTH VALLEY														
Cafe Creations Cinnamon Danish	1 (1.4 oz)	130	3	0	0	2	27	17	2	20	80	—	—	—
Date Almond Low Fat	1 (1.5 oz)	150	3	1	0	1	32	15	tr	20	25	—	—	0
Granola Chocolate Chip Low Fat	1 (1.5 oz)	160	3	1	0	2	32	13	1	20	20	—	—	0
Granola Moist & Chewy Dutch Apple	1 (1 oz)	100	2	1	0	1	20	10	tr	20	10	—	—	5
Granola Trail Mix Cranberries Nuts & Yogurt Chips	1 (1.2 oz)	140	4	1	0	3	23	12	1	20	100	—	—	0
Organic Fig Cobbler	1 (1.4 oz)	130	3	0	0	2	26	14	2	20	80	—	—	0
Organic Raspberry Tarts	1 (1.4 oz)	150	3	0	0	2	30	16	tr	20	95	—	—	—
Organic Strawberry Cobbler	1 (1.3 oz)	130	3	0	0	2	26	14	1	0	85	—	—	1
Peanut Butter & Grape	1 (1.3 oz)	130	3	0	0	2	26	16	1	20	140	—	—	—
HERSHEY'S														
Sweet & Salty Granola Bar Reese's w/ Chocolate	1 (1.2 oz)	160	9	2	—	4	18	8	1	20	170	—	—	0
Sweet & Salty Granola Bar w/ Pretzels	1 (1.2 oz)	140	5	2	—	3	22	8	1	0	240	—	—	0

FOOD	PORTION	CALS	FAT	SAT FAT	CHOL	PROT	CARB	SUGAR	FIBER	CALCI	SOD	POTAS	FOLIC	VIT C
HONEST FOODS														
Cran Lemon Zest	1 (2.2 oz)	240	9	1	0	6	35	17	4	40	150	190	—	0
Farmer's Trail Mix	1 (2.2 oz)	240	9	1	0	6	35	17	4	40	150	190	—	0
JUNGLE GRUB														
Berry Bamboozle w/ Vanilla Icing Gluten Free	1 (0.9 oz)	100	4	1	0	4	14	8	1	150	55	—	—	12
Chocolate Chip Cookie Dough w/ Chocolate Coating Gluten Free	1 (0.9 oz)	100	4	1	0	4	13	8	4	200	60	—	—	12
Peanut Butter Groove w/ Vanilla Icing Gluten Free	1 (0.9 oz)	100	4	1	0	4	13	8	1	150	140	—	—	12
KARDEA														
Lemon Ginger	1 (1.34 oz)	140	5	1	0	7	20	8	7	—	75	120	—	6
KASHI														
TLC Chewy Granola Dark Mocha Almond	1 (1.2 oz)	130	4	1	0	6	21	6	4	0	90	—	—	0
TLC Chewy Granola Honey Almond Flax	1 (1.2 oz)	140	5	1	0	5	19	5	4	0	115	90	—	0
TLC Soft Baked Apple Spice	1 (1.2 oz)	110	3	0	0	2	21	9	3	0	105	—	—	0
TLC Soft Baked Blackberry Graham	1 (1.2 oz)	110	1	0	0	2	21	9	3	0	125	—	—	0
TLC Soft Baked Ripe Strawberry	1 (1.2 oz)	110	3	0	0	2	21	9	3	0	105	—	—	0
KELLOGG'S														
FiberPlus Antioxidants Berry Yogurt Crunch	1 box (1.4 oz)	130	1	0	0	3	32	9	8	0	150	—	100	9
FiberPlus Antioxidants Chocolate Chip	1 (1.2 oz)	120	4	2	0	2	26	7	9	100	55	—	—	0
FiberPlus Antioxidants Chocolatey Peanut Butter	1 (1.2 oz)	130	5	3	0	3	24	7	9	100	95	—	—	0
FiberPlus Antioxidants Dark Chocolate Almond	1 (1.2 oz)	130	5	3	0	2	24	7	9	100	50	—	—	0
Nutri-Grain Yogurt Vanilla	1	140	3	1	0	1	26	14	tr	200	105	—	40	0

FOOD	PORTION	CALS	FAT	SAT FAT	CHOL	PROT	CARB	SUGAR	FIBER	CALCI	SOD	POTAS	FOLIC	VIT C
KELLOGG'S (CONT.)														
Snack Bites	1 pkg (0.8 oz)	90	2	1	0	1	18	7	tr	0	125	—	60	4
Special K Snack Bar Chocolate Peanut	1 (0.9 oz)	110	4	2	0	4	15	11	1	60	60	—	40	12
KERIBAR														
Vegan Apple Peanut Butter	1 (1.4 oz)	140	6	1	0	6	21	10	5	40	115	—	—	0
Vegan Cherry Almond	1 (1.4 oz)	140	6	1	0	8	21	10	5	60	75	—	—	0
Vegan Strawberry Chocolate Chip	1 (1.4 oz)	130	5	1	0	6	23	12	5	40	85	—	—	0
KIND														
Peanut Butter Dark Chocolate + Protein	1 (1.4 oz)	180	12	4	0	7	17	11	2	40	65	150	—	0
KRAFT														
MilkBite Chocolate	1 (1.2 oz)	140	6	3	10	5	18	10	3	300	75	—	—	0
MilkBite Mixed Berry	1 (1.2 oz)	140	5	3	15	5	18	10	3	300	65	—	—	0
MilkBite Oatmeal Raisin	1 (1.2 oz)	130	5	3	15	5	18	10	3	300	65	—	—	0
MilkBite Peanut Butter	1 (1.2 oz)	140	6	3	10	5	17	8	3	300	60	—	—	0
MilkBite Strawberry	1 (1.2 oz)	140	5	3	15	5	18	10	3	300	65	—	—	0
LEAN BODY														
Hi-Protein Granola Peanuts 'N Chocolate	1 (2.8 oz)	340	11	2	0	20	39	13	4	50	580	300	—	0
NATURAL OVENS														
Great Granola Mixed Fruit	1 (1.4 oz)	150	3	0	0	4	27	15	2	20	140	—	0	0
NATURE VALLEY														
Chewy Granola Blueberry Yogurt	1	140	4	2	0	2	26	13	1	100	130	—	—	0
Chewy Granola Lemon Yogurt	1	140	4	2	0	2	26	13	1	100	130	—	—	0
Chewy Granola Vanilla Yogurt	1	140	4	2	0	2	26	13	1	100	130	—	—	0
Chewy Trail Mix Fruit & Nut	1 (1.2 oz)	140	4	1	0	3	25	13	2	—	65	—	—	—
Crunchy Granola Peanut Butter	2 (1.5 oz)	190	7	1	0	5	28	11	2	—	180	—	—	—
Oats 'N Honey	2 (1.5 oz)	190	6	1	0	4	29	12	2	—	160	—	—	—

FOOD	PORTION	CALS	FAT	SAT FAT	CHOL	PROT	CARB	SUGAR	FIBER	CALCI	SOD	POTAS	FOLIC	VIT C
NATURE VALLEY (CONT.)														
Protein Chewy Peanut Almond & Dark Chocolate	1 (1.4 oz)	190	12	4	0	10	14	6	5	40	180	—	—	—
Protein Chewy Peanut Butter Dark Chocolate	1 (1.4 oz)	190	12	4	0	10	14	6	5	20	170	—	—	—
Sweet & Salty Granola Almond	1 (1.2 oz)	160	7	2	0	3	22	12	2	20	150	—	—	—
Sweet & Salty Granola Peanut	1	170	9	3	0	4	19	11	2	—	150	—	—	—
NATURE'S PATH														
Granola Bar Apple Pie Crunch Chia Plus Organic	2 (1.4 oz)	190	8	1	0	3	27	8	3	0	120	—	—	0
Granola Bar Honey Oat Crunch Flax Plus Organic	2 (1.4 oz)	190	7	1	0	3	28	9	3	0	60	115	—	0
Granola Bar Peanut Choco Organic	1 (1.2 oz)	150	6	2	0	3	22	11	2	20	125	80	—	0
Granola Bar Pumpkin-N-Spice Organic	1 (1.2 oz)	140	4	1	0	3	23	10	2	20	80	65	—	0
Granola Bar Sunny Hemp Organic	1 (1.2 oz)	140	4	1	0	3	24	11	3	20	90	100	—	0
NUTRI-GRAIN														
Apple Cinnamon	1 (1.3 oz)	120	3	1	0	2	24	12	3	200	110	—	40	0
PLANTERS														
Nut-rition Antioxidant Almonds Blueberries & Dark Chocolate	1 (1.2 oz)	160	8	2	0	5	18	9	2	40	130	—	—	0
Nut-rition Bone Health Honey Roasted Peanuts Cashews & Almonds	1 (1.2 oz)	160	9	2	0	5	18	8	2	100	150	—	—	6
Nut-rition Energy Honey Roasted Peanuts Almonds & Chocolate	1 (1.2 oz)	170	9	2	0	5	17	10	2	40	170	—	—	0
Nut-rition Heart Healthy Cranberry Almond Peanut	1 (1.2 oz)	160	8	1	0	5	19	9	3	20	130	—	—	0

FOOD	PORTION	CALS	FAT	SAT FAT	CHOL	PROT	CARB	SUGAR	FIBER	CALCI	SOD	POTAS	FOLIC	VIT C
POST														
Honey Bunches Of Oats Banana Nut	1 (1.2 oz)	140	4	2	0	2	24	11	1	100	115	—	—	0
Honey Bunches Of Oats Oatmeal Raisin	1 (1.2 oz)	130	3	0	0	2	25	9	2	300	105	—	—	0
PROBAR														
Cran-Lemon Twister	1 (3 oz)	360	16	2	0	9	49	28	7	80	55	—	—	4
Kettle Corn	1 (3 oz)	390	20	4	0	10	47	17	8	60	170	—	—	0
Koka Moka	1 (3 oz)	360	18	4	0	9	47	21	7	8	55	—	—	4
Old School PB&J	1 (3 oz)	370	17	2	0	9	48	20	6	80	55	260	16	4
Superfood Slam	1 (3 oz)	380	19	5	0	11	46	17	7	80	50	—	—	6
QUAKER														
Breakfast Bar Apple Crisp	1 (1.3 oz)	130	3	1	0	1	27	9	1	200	90	—	100	6
Breakfast Bar Iced Raspberry	1 (1.3 oz)	130	3	1	0	1	26	16	1	200	100	—	100	—
Breakfast Bites Iced Raspberry	1 pkg (1.3 oz)	130	3	1	0	1	28	9	3	200	75	—	100	6
Breakfast Bites Strawberry	1 pkg (1.3 oz)	130	3	1	0	1	27	8	2	200	90	—	100	6
Chewy Chocolate Chip	1 (0.8 oz)	100	3	2	0	1	18	7	1	80	75	—	—	—
Chewy Cookies & Cream	1 (0.8 oz)	90	3	1	0	1	18	5	2	100	85	—	—	—
Chewy 90 Calorie Cinnamon Sugar	1 (1 oz)	90	2	0	0	1	19	6	1	80	80	—	—	—
Chewy 90 Calorie Honey Nut	1 (0.8 oz)	90	2	0	0	1	19	6	1	80	80	—	—	—
Chewy Dipps Peanut Butter	1 (1 oz)	150	7	4	0	3	18	12	1	20	105	—	—	—
Chewy Granola w/ Protein Peanut Butter & Chocolate	1 (1 oz)	110	3	1	0	5	18	7	1	0	140	—	—	0
Chewy Low Fat S'mores	1 (1 oz)	110	2	1	0	1	22	10	1	100	70	—	—	—
Crunchy Granola Oats & Berries	1 (1 oz)	130	4	1	0	2	23	8	1	0	125	—	—	6
Oatmeal To Go Oatmeal Raisin	1 (2.1 oz)	220	4	1	15	4	43	19	5	200	240	160	80	0
Oatmeal To Go Raspberry Streusel	1 (2.1 oz)	220	4	1	15	4	43	19	5	200	220	125	80	0

FOOD	PORTION	CALS	FAT	SAT FAT	CHOL	PROT	CARB	SUGAR	FIBER	CALCI	SOD	POTAS	FOLIC	VIT C
QUAKER (CONT.)														
Q-Smart Cranberry Vanilla Almond	1 (1 oz)	120	6	2	0	10	9	1	2	100	106	—	40	6
Trail Mix Cranberry Raisin & Almond	1 (1.2 oz)	150	5	1	0	2	24	10	1	0	50	—	—	0
REVOLUTION FOODS														
Jammy Sammy Apple Cinnamon & Oatmeal	1 (1 oz)	100	2	0	0	1	21	10	1	0	50	—	—	0
Organic Jammy Sammy PB & Grape	1 (1 oz)	110	3	0	0	2	19	10	1	0	55	—	—	0
Organic Jammy Sammy PB & Strawberry	1 (1 oz)	110	3	0	0	2	19	10	1	0	55	—	—	5
RISE BAR														
Breakfast Crunchy Cranberry Apple	1 (1.4 oz)	160	7	1	0	3	25	19	3	20	40	35	—	1
Breakfast Crunchy Cashew Almond	1 (1.4 oz)	190	12	2	0	5	19	11	3	0	25	100	—	0
ROMAN MEAL														
Whole Grain & Fruit	1 (2 oz)	190	2	0	0	4	43	21	6	20	240	300	80	2
SILHOUETTE SOLUTION														
Blueberry Pomegranate	1 (1.3 oz)	130	3	2	5	15	14	7	3	200	180	110	—	0
Peanut Passion	1 (1.3 oz)	130	4	2	5	15	14	5	3	200	180	140	—	0
SOUTH BEACH														
Fiber Fit Granola Mocha	1 (1.2 oz)	120	4	3	0	2	25	7	9	—	125	—	—	—
Fiber Fit Granola S'Mores	1 (1.2 oz)	120	4	3	0	2	25	7	9	—	125	—	—	—
SWEET & SAVORY														
Cocoa Pistachio	1 (3 oz)	390	22	5	0	11	42	17	7	80	190	—	—	0
TASTY														
Carrot Cake	1 (1.2 oz)	110	2	0	0	2	24	14	3	20	80	—	40	0
Pumpkin Pie	1 (1.2 oz)	120	3	0	0	2	25	15	3	20	85	—	40	0
WEETABIX														
Oaty Chocolate	1	67	2	1	—	2	12	3	6	—	tr	—	—	—
Weetos	1	88	3	1	—	1	14	8	tr	—	tr	—	—	—
WINGS OF NATURE														
Organic Almond Raisin	1 (1.4 oz)	170	11	2	0	5	17	12	3	40	15	—	—	0
Organic Cafe Mocha Coffee	1 (1.2 oz)	153	9	3	0	3	18	9	3	17	26	—	—	0

FOOD	PORTION	CALS	FAT	SAT FAT	CHOL	PROT	CARB	SUGAR	FIBER	CALCI	SOD	POTAS	FOLIC	VIT C
WINGS OF NATURE (CONT.)														
Organic Cranberry Crunch	1 (1.4 oz)	170	10	2	0	5	18	9	2	20	20	—	—	0
Organic Espresso Coffee	1 (1.4 oz)	180	10	3	0	3	21	12	2	20	25	—	—	0
YOTTA														
Apple Cinnamon	1 (1.2 oz)	120	1	0	0	2	25	11	2	20	40	—	—	12
Cherry	1 (1.2 oz)	120	1	0	0	2	26	11	1	20	40	—	—	15
Orange	1 (1.2 oz)	120	1	0	0	2	26	11	2	20	45	—	—	12
ZONE PERFECT														
Cookie Dough Chocolate Chip	1 (1.58 oz)	180	5	3	30	10	24	18	tr	100	170	85	60	27
Cookie Dough Oatmeal Raisin	1 (1.58 oz)	170	4	2	20	10	25	16	tr	100	180	105	60	27
Cookie Dough Peanut Butter	1 (1.58 oz)	190	7	3	20	10	22	16	1	100	200	115	60	27
Sweet & Salty Cashew Pretzel	1 (1.58 oz)	200	7	3	<5	10	23	14	1	100	300	115	80	24
Sweet & Salty Trail Mix	1 (1.58 oz)	200	8	3	<5	10	21	12	1	100	270	140	80	24
CHAMPAGNE														
champagne	1 serv (3.5 oz)	84	0	0	0	tr	3	1	0	9	5	73	1	0
mimosa	1 serv	117	tr	tr	0	1	12	—	tr	10	1	186	28	47
punch	1 serv (4 oz)	73	tr	tr	0	tr	8	6	0	9	6	95	6	3
sekt german champagne	1 serv (3.5 oz)	84	0	0	0	tr	5	—	—	—	—	—	—	—
CHAYOTE														
fresh cooked	1 cup	38	1	—	0	1	8	—	—	21	1	276	—	13
raw	1 (7 oz)	49	1	—	0	2	11	—	—	39	8	305	—	22
raw cut up	1 cup	32	tr	—	0	1	7	—	—	25	198	34	—	15
DOLE														
Fresh cooked	½ cup (2.8 oz)	17	0	0	0	1	4	0	2	0	3	138	—	8
CHEESE														

CHEESE

(*see also* CHEESE DISHES, CHEESE SUBSTITUTES, COTTAGE CHEESE, CREAM CHEESE, CREAM CHEESE SUBSTITUTES, NEUFCHATEL)

FOOD	PORTION	CALS	FAT	SAT FAT	CHOL	PROT	CARB	SUGAR	FIBER	CALCI	SOD	POTAS	FOLIC	VIT C
american	1 oz	93	7	4	18	6	2	—	—	163	337	79	—	0
american cheese spread	1 oz	82	6	4	16	5	2	—	—	159	381	69	2	0
beaufort	1 oz	115	9	6	34	8	tr	tr	0	297	128	33	1	0
bel paese	1 oz	112	9	—	—	7	0	0	0	173	—	—	—	—
blue	1 oz	100	8	6	21	6	1	—	—	150	396	73	10	0
blue crumbled	1 cup (4.7 oz)	477	39	25	102	29	3	—	—	712	1884	346	49	0
bocconcini smoked	1 oz	90	6	4	25	6	1	0	0	100	90	—	—	0
brick	1 oz	105	8	5	27	7	1	—	—	191	159	38	6	0
brie	1 oz	95	8	—	28	8	tr	—	—	52	178	43	18	0

FOOD	PORTION	CALS	FAT	SAT FAT	CHOL	PROT	CARB	SUGAR	FIBER	CALCI	SOD	POTAS	FOLIC	VIT C
cacio di roma sheep's milk cheese	1 oz	130	10	6	30	8	0	0	0	300	170	—	—	—
caerphilly	1.4 oz	150	13	—	—	9	0	—	0	220	—	—	—	tr
camembert	1 oz	85	7	4	20	6	tr	—	—	110	239	53	18	0
cantal	1 oz	105	9	6	26	7	tr	tr	0	277	269	39	6	0
caraway	1 oz	107	8	—	—	7	1	—	—	191	196	—	—	0
chabichou	1 oz	95	8	5	23	6	tr	tr	0	86	189	69	36	0
chaource	1 oz	83	7	4	20	5	tr	tr	0	111	230	27	27	0
cheddar	1 oz	114	9	6	30	7	tr	—	—	204	176	28	5	0
cheddar low sodium	1 oz	113	9	6	28	7	1	—	—	200	6	32	5	0
cheddar lowfat	1 oz	49	2	1	6	9	1	—	—	118	174	19	3	0
cheddar reduced fat	1.4 oz	104	6	—	—	13	0	—	0	336	—	—	—	tr
cheddar shredded	1 cup	455	37	24	119	28	1	—	—	815	701	111	21	0
cheshire	1 oz	110	9	—	29	7	1	—	—	182	198	27	—	0
cheshire reduced fat	1.4 oz	108	6	—	—	13	tr	—	0	260	—	—	—	tr
colby	1 oz	112	9	6	27	7	1	—	—	194	171	36	—	0
colby low sodium	1 oz	113	9	6	28	7	1	—	—	200	6	32	5	0
colby lowfat	1 oz	49	2	1	6	9	1	—	—	118	174	19	3	0
comte	1 oz	114	9	5	34	8	tr	tr	0	251	105	34	1	0
coulommiers	1 oz	88	7	5	23	6	tr	tr	0	70	195	46	19	0
crottin	1 oz	105	9	6	23	6	tr	tr	0	33	133	83	—	0
derby	1.4 oz	161	14	—	—	10	0	—	0	272	—	—	—	tr
edam reduced fat	1.4 oz	92	4	—	—	13	tr	—	0	—	—	—	—	tr
emmentaler	1 oz	115	9	—	26	8	tr	—	—	291	129	31	tr	tr
feta	1 oz	75	6	4	25	4	1	—	—	140	316	18	—	0
fontina	1 oz	110	9	5	33	7	tr	—	—	156	—	—	—	0
frais	1.6 oz	51	3	—	—	3	3	—	0	40	—	—	—	tr
gjetost	1 oz	132	8	5	—	3	12	—	—	113	170	—	1	0
gloucester double	1.4 oz	162	14	—	—	10	0	—	0	264	—	—	—	tr
goat fresh	1 oz	23	2	1	5	1	tr	tr	0	31	18	—	—	—
goat hard	1 oz	128	10	7	30	9	1	—	—	254	98	14	—	—
gorgonzola	1 oz	107	9	—	—	5	tr	—	—	175	—	—	tr	—
gouda	1 oz	101	8	5	32	7	1	—	—	198	232	34	6	0
grana padano parmesan shaved	1 tbsp	20	2	1	5	2	0	0	0	60	45	—	—	0
gruyere	1 oz	117	9	5	31	8	tr	—	—	287	95	23	3	0
lancashire	1.4 oz	149	12	—	—	9	0	—	0	224	—	—	—	tr
leicester	1.4 oz	160	14	—	—	10	0	—	0	264	—	—	—	tr
limburger	1 oz	93	8	5	26	8	tr	—	—	141	227	36	16	0
lymeswold	1.4 oz	170	16	—	—	6	tr	—	0	108	—	—	—	tr
maroilles	1 oz	97	8	5	26	6	tr	tr	0	229	300	37	3	0

FOOD	PORTION	CALS	FAT	SAT FAT	CHOL	PROT	CARB	SUGAR	FIBER	CALCI	SOD	POTAS	FOLIC	VIT C
monterey	1 oz	106	9	—	—	7	tr	—	—	212	152	23	—	0
morbier	1 oz	99	8	5	23	7	tr	tr	0	217	283	29	6	0
mozzarella	1 oz	80	6	4	22	6	1	—	—	147	106	19	1	0
mozzarella fresh	1 oz	80	6	4	20	6	tr	0	0	150	160	—	—	0
mozzarella part skim	1 oz	72	5	3	16	7	1	—	—	183	132	24	2	0
muenster	1 oz	104	9	5	27	7	tr	—	—	203	178	38	3	0
parmesan grated	1 tbsp	23	2	1	4	2	tr	—	—	69	93	5	tr	0
parmesan hard	1 oz	111	7	5	19	10	1	—	—	336	454	26	2	0
picodon	1 oz	99	8	5	23	6	tr	tr	0	29	—	—	—	0
pimento	1 oz	106	9	6	27	6	tr	—	—	174	405	46	2	—
pont l'eveque	1 oz	86	7	4	20	6	tr	tr	0	134	191	39	3	0
port du salut	1 oz	100	8	5	35	7	tr	—	—	184	151	—	5	0
provolone	1 oz	100	8	5	20	7	1	—	—	214	248	39	3	0
pyrenees	1 oz	101	8	5	26	6	tr	tr	0	181	235	19	7	0
quark 20% fat	1 oz	33	1	—	5	4	1	—	—	24	10	25	tr	tr
quark 40% fat	1 oz	48	3	—	11	3	1	—	—	27	10	23	—	1
quark made w/ skim milk	1 oz	22	tr	—	tr	4	1	—	—	26	11	27	tr	tr
queso anejo	1 oz	106	9	5	30	6	1	—	—	193	321	25	0	0
queso asadero	1 oz	101	8	5	30	6	1	—	—	188	186	25	2	0
queso chihuahua	1 oz	106	8	5	30	6	2	—	—	185	175	15	1	0
queso fresco	1 oz	41	2	—	—	4	1	—	0	194	—	—	—	0
queso manchego	1 oz	107	8	—	27	8	tr	—	0	237	341	57	6	—
queso panela	1 oz	74	5	—	—	6	1	—	0	195	—	—	—	0
raclette	1 oz	102	8	5	26	7	tr	tr	0	157	217	32	15	0
reblochon	1 oz	88	7	5	23	6	tr	tr	0	179	240	54	7	0
ricotta part skim	½ cup (4.4 oz)	171	10	6	38	14	6	—	—	337	155	155	—	0
ricotta whole milk	½ cup (4.4 oz)	216	16	10	63	14	4	—	—	257	104	130	—	0
romadur 40% fat	1 oz	83	6	—	—	7	tr	—	—	115	—	—	—	—
romano	1 oz	110	8	—	29	9	1	—	—	302	340	—	2	0
roquefort	1 oz	105	9	5	26	6	1	—	—	188	513	26	14	0
rouy	1 oz	95	8	5	23	7	tr	tr	0	143	138	21	—	0
saint marcellin	1 oz	94	8	5	23	5	tr	tr	0	49	171	53	38	0
saint nectaire	1 oz	97	8	5	23	6	tr	tr	0	169	169	36	6	0
saint paulin	1 oz	85	6	4	20	7	tr	tr	0	223	174	23	6	0
sainte maure	1 oz	99	8	5	23	6	tr	tr	0	51	411	—	—	0
selles sur cher	1 oz	93	8	5	20	5	tr	tr	0	28	181	—	—	0
stilton blue	1.4 oz	164	14	—	—	9	0	—	0	128	—	—	—	tr
stilton white	1.4 oz	145	13	—	—	8	0	—	0	100	—	—	—	tr
swiss	1 oz	107	8	5	26	8	1	—	—	272	74	31	2	0
swiss processed	1 oz	95	7	5	24	7	1	—	—	219	388	61	—	0
tilsit	1 oz	96	7	5	29	7	1	—	—	198	213	18	—	0
tome	1 oz	92	7	5	23	6	tr	tr	0	115	231	22	6	0

FOOD	PORTION	CALS	FAT	SAT FAT	CHOL	PROT	CARB	SUGAR	FIBER	CALCI	SOD	POTAS	FOLIC	VIT C
triple creme	1 oz	113	11	7	34	3	tr	tr	0	28	86	46	3	tr
vacherin	1 oz	92	8	5	23	5	tr	tr	0	200	129	34	3	0
wensleydale	1.4 oz	151	13	—	—	9	0	—	0	224	—	—	—	tr
whey cheese	1 oz	126	8	5	—	4	9	0	0	97	146	—	—	1
yogurt cheese	1 oz	80	7	3	15	6	0	0	0	350	60	—	—	—
ALPINE LACE														
Reduced Fat Provolone	1 slice (0.8 oz)	70	5	3	10	6	1	0	0	200	135	—	—	0
Reduced Fat Swiss	1 slice (0.8 oz)	70	5	3	15	7	1	1	0	250	95	—	—	0
Reduced Fat White American	1 slice (0.8 oz)	70	5	3	15	5	1	1	0	150	310	—	—	0
Reduced Sodium Muenster	1 slice (0.8 oz)	90	7	5	15	6	0	0	0	150	110	—	—	0
APPLEGATE FARMS														
Organic Cheddar Milk	1 slice (0.7 oz)	85	6	4	20	5	0	0	0	150	130	—	—	0
Organic Muenster Kase	1 slice (0.8 oz)	85	7	4	20	5	0	0	0	150	130	—	—	0
Yogurt Cheese w/ Probiotics	1 slice (0.7 oz)	80	6	4	15	5	tr	0	—	150	105	—	—	0
ATHENOS														
Blue Crumbled	¼ pkg (1.1 oz)	110	9	6	30	7	2	0	1	150	430	—	—	0
Feta Black Peppercorn	1 oz	80	6	4	20	5	1	0	0	80	330	—	—	0
Feta Crumbled Garlic & Herb	⅕ pkg (1.2 oz)	90	7	4	25	6	2	0	1	80	400	—	—	0
Gorgonzola Crumbled	2 tbsp (1.1 oz)	110	9	6	30	7	2	0	1	150	400	—	—	0
BEL GIOIOSO														
Mozzarella Fresh	1 in cube (1 oz)	80	6	4	20	5	0	0	0	150	85	—	—	0
BOAR'S HEAD														
American	1 oz	100	9	6	25	6	1	0	0	150	380	—	—	0
American 25% Lower Sodium 25% Lower Fat	1 oz	90	6	5	20	6	1	0	0	150	300	—	—	0
Cheddar Sharp	1 oz	110	9	5	30	7	tr	0	0	200	190	—	—	0
Cream Havarti	1 oz	110	10	7	35	6	0	0	0	200	210	—	—	0
Creamy Blue	1 oz	90	8	5	30	6	0	0	0	150	310	—	—	0
Double Gloucester Yellow	1 oz	110	10	6	35	7	0	0	0	200	200	—	—	0
Edam	1 oz	90	7	5	20	7	0	0	0	250	280	—	—	0
Gouda	1 oz	110	9	5	30	6	0	0	0	200	280	—	—	0
Imported Swiss	1 oz	110	8	5	20	8	tr	0	0	300	70	—	—	0
Longhorn Colby	1 oz	110	9	5	30	7	tr	0	0	200	170	—	—	0
Monterey Jack	1 oz	100	9	6	25	6	0	0	0	200	180	—	—	0
Mozzarella	1 oz	90	7	5	20	6	1	0	0	150	150	—	—	0

FOOD	PORTION	CALS	FAT	SAT FAT	CHOL	PROT	CARB	SUGAR	FIBER	CALCI	SOD	POTAS	FOLIC	VIT C
Muenster	1 oz	100	8	5	25	6	0	0	0	200	180	—	—	0
Muenster Low Sodium	1 oz	100	8	5	20	6	0	0	0	200	75	—	—	0
Provolone 42% Lower Sodium	1 oz	100	8	5	20	7	1	0	0	200	140	—	—	0
Provolone Picante Sharp	1 oz	100	8	5	25	7	1	0	0	200	250	—	—	0
Swiss No Salt Added	1 oz	110	8	5	25	8	tr	0	0	250	10	—	—	0
CABOT														
Cheddar Extra Sharp	1 oz	110	9	6	30	7	tr	0	0	200	180	—	—	0
Cheddar Horseradish	1 oz	110	9	6	30	7	tr	0	0	200	180	—	—	0
Cheddar Tomato Basil	1 oz	110	9	6	30	7	tr	0	0	200	180	—	—	0
Cheddar Light 50% Reduced Fat	1 oz	70	5	3	15	8	tr	0	0	200	170	—	—	0
Cheddar Light 50% Reduced Fat Omega-3	1 oz	70	5	3	15	8	tr	0	0	200	170	—	—	0
Cheddar Light 75% Reduced Fat	1 oz	60	3	2	10	9	tr	0	0	200	200	—	—	0
Cheddar Shake	2 tsp	25	2	1	5	1	1	1	0	40	220	—	—	0
Monterey Jack	1 oz	110	9	6	30	7	tr	0	0	200	170	—	—	0
Pepper Jack 50% Reduced Fat	1 oz	70	5	3	15	8	tr	0	0	200	170	—	—	—
Swiss Slices	1 (1 oz)	110	8	5	25	8	1	0	0	250	60	—	—	0
CONNOISSEUR														
Asiago Spread	1 tbsp	90	7	4	20	5	2	2	0	150	240	—	—	0
Brie Spread	2 tbsp	90	7	4	25	4	2	2	0	150	250	—	—	0
Gorgonzola Spread	1 tbsp	90	7	5	20	5	2	2	0	150	340	—	—	0
Wheel Asiago Pesto	2 tbsp	90	6	4	20	5	4	4	0	150	240	—	—	0
Wheel Swiss Bacon	2 tbsp	90	7	4	25	5	2	2	0	150	260	—	—	0
CRACKER BARREL														
Fontina	1 slice (0.7 oz)	80	7	4	15	6	tr	0	0	150	230	—	—	0
Sharp Cheddar 2% Milk	1 oz	90	6	4	20	7	tr	0	0	200	240	—	—	0
CRYSTAL FARMS														
American Singles	1 slice (0.7 oz)	70	5	2	15	4	2	1	0	100	340	—	—	0
American Singles 2%	1 slice (0.7 oz)	50	3	2	10	4	2	1	0	250	340	—	—	0
American Singles Fat Free	1 slice (0.7 oz)	30	0	0	<5	5	2	2	0	150	360	—	—	0

FOOD	PORTION	CALS	FAT	SAT FAT	CHOL	PROT	CARB	SUGAR	FIBER	CALCI	SOD	POTAS	FOLIC	VIT C
CRYSTAL FARMS (CONT.)														
Deli Slices Muenster	1 slice (0.8 oz)	80	7	4	16	6	0	0	0	150	200	—	—	0
Deli Slices Swiss	1 slice (0.7 oz)	80	6	4	20	6	0	0	0	200	50	—	—	0
Marble Jack	1 oz	110	9	6	30	6	tr	0	0	200	180	—	—	0
Pepper Jack	1 oz	110	9	6	30	6	tr	0	0	200	200	—	—	0
Shredded Mexican 4 Cheese	¼ cup	100	8	5	25	67	tr	0	0	200	170	—	—	0
Shredded Mozzarella	¼ cup	80	6	4	20	7	tr	0	0	200	180	—	—	0
Shredded Pizza Blend	¼ cup	100	8	5	25	7	tr	0	0	200	180	—	—	0
Shredded Sharp Cheddar	¼ cup	110	9	6	30	6	tr	0	0	200	180	—	—	0
DIETZ & WATSON														
Aalsbruk Edam	1 oz	90	7	5	25	6	1	0	0	200	180	—	—	0
American Yellow	1 slice (1 oz)	110	8	9	10	6	0	0	0	200	370	—	—	1
Cheddar Sharp	1 oz	110	9	5	28	6	1	1	0	200	270	—	—	0
Danish Blue	1 oz	100	12	5	15	6	0	0	0	150	310	—	—	0
Danish Havarti	1 oz	110	9	5	28	6	1	1	0	200	270	—	—	0
Gorgonzola	1 oz	100	8	6	20	6	0	0	0	150	390	—	—	0
Muenster	1 slice (0.7 oz)	75	6	4	19	5	0	0	0	150	203	—	—	0
DIGIORNO														
Shredded Three Cheese Parmesan Romano & Asiago	¼ cup (1 oz)	110	8	5	25	9	1	0	0	250	270	—	—	0
DRAGONE														
Mozzarella Whole Milk	1 oz	90	7	5	20	6	tr	0	0	150	170	—	—	0
Parmesan Wedge	1 oz	100	7	4	20	9	tr	tr	0	300	390	—	—	0
Ricotta Part Skim	¼ cup (2.2 oz)	90	6	4	30	6	4	3	0	100	85	—	—	0
EASY CHEESE														
American	2 tbsp (1.1 oz)	90	6	3	20	5	2	1	0	200	410	—	—	0
Cheddar	2 tbsp (1.1 oz)	90	6	3	20	5	2	1	0	200	410	—	—	0
FINLANDIA														
Baby Muenster	1 oz	100	8	5	20	7	0	0	0	250	160	—	—	0
Double Gloucester Deli Slices	1 slice (0.8 oz)	83	7	4	23	5	1	0	0	140	115	—	—	0
Gouda Deli Slices	1 slice (0.8 oz)	79	6	4	15	6	0	0	0	180	132	—	—	0
Havarti Deli Slices	1 slice (0.8 oz)	86	7	4	18	6	0	0	0	170	132	—	—	0
Muenster Deli Slices	1 slice (0.8 oz)	86	7	4	19	6	0	0	0	170	132	—	—	0
Swiss Deli Slices	1 slice (0.8 oz)	86	7	4	16	6	0	0	0	240	62	—	—	0
Swiss Light Deli Slices	1 slice (0.8 oz)	57	3	2	8	7	0	0	0	220	110	—	—	0
Viola	2 tbsp (1 oz)	87	8	5	19	3	1	1	0	110	280	—	—	0

FOOD	PORTION	CALS	FAT	SAT FAT	CHOL	PROT	CARB	SUGAR	FIBER	CALCI	SOD	POTAS	FOLIC	VIT C
FRESH MADE														
Farmers Cheese Nonfat	2 tbsp	15	0	0	3	5	1	0	0	30	10	—	—	0
FRIENDSHIP														
Farmer	2 tbsp (1 oz)	50	3	2	10	5	0	0	0	0	120	—	—	—
Farmer No Salt Added	2 tbsp (1 oz)	50	3	2	10	5	0	0	0	0	10	—	—	—
FRIGO														
Mozzarella Part Skim	1 oz	80	6	4	15	7	tr	0	0	100	210	—	—	0
Parmesan Shredded	¼ cup (1 oz)	100	7	4	20	9	1	1	tr	100	430	—	—	0
Ricotta Whole Milk	¼ cup (2.2 oz)	110	8	5	35	7	2	2	0	100	150	—	—	0
Romano Shredded	¼ cup (1 oz)	100	7	5	20	8	1	tr	tr	100	460	—	—	0
GRANA PADANO														
PDO Cheese	1 oz	120	8	5	12	—	10	0	0	400	170	—	—	0
HANS ALL NATURAL														
Spread Cheddar & Jalapeno	2 tbsp (1 oz)	90	7	4	20	5	3	3	0	150	240	—	—	0
Spread Swiss Cheese & Almonds	2 tbsp (1 oz)	90	7	4	20	5	3	3	0	150	200	—	—	0
HAOLAM														
Cheddar Sliced	1 slice (1 oz)	114	9	5	28	7	1	0	0	200	181	—	—	0
HORIZON ORGANIC														
American	1 slice (0.7 oz)	60	5	4	15	4	1	1	0	100	250	—	—	0
Cheddar	1 oz	110	9	5	30	7	tr	0	0	200	180	—	—	0
Monterey Jack	1 oz	100	8	5	30	7	0	0	0	200	170	—	—	0
Shred Mexican	¼ cup	110	9	5	30	7	tr	0	0	200	180	—	—	0
Shred Parmesan	1 tbsp	20	2	1	5	2	0	0	0	60	70	—	—	0
Slice Provolone	1 slice (0.7 oz)	70	6	4	15	5	0	0	0	150	140	—	—	0
Sticks Colby	1 (1 oz)	110	9	5	30	7	tr	0	0	200	180	—	—	0
String Mozzarella	1 stick (1 oz)	80	5	3	15	8	tr	0	0	200	170	—	—	0
J.L. KRAFT														
Spreadable Feta & Spinach	2 tbsp	80	7	4	25	3	1	tr	0	40	160	—	—	1
KAROUN														
Ackawi	1 oz	110	8	5	10	6	0	0	0	200	180	—	—	0
Ani	1 in cube (1 oz)	110	8	5	10	6	0	0	0	200	180	—	—	0
Labne Kefir	2 tbsp (1 oz)	80	5	3	20	2	2	1	0	60	25	—	—	0
Paneer	1 oz	90	7	5	25	6	1	1	0	200	5	—	—	0
KRAFT														
Crumbles Three Cheese	¼ cup (1 oz)	110	9	5	25	6	tr	0	0	200	190	—	—	0

FOOD	PORTION	CALS	FAT	SAT FAT	CHOL	PROT	CARB	SUGAR	FIBER	CALCI	SOD	POTAS	FOLIC	VIT C
KRAFT (CONT.)														
LiveActive 2% Milk Marbled Colby & Monterey Jack	1 stick (1 oz)	90	6	4	20	8	tr	0	0	200	240	—	—	0
LiveActive Cheddar Cheese Sticks	1 (1 oz)	120	10	6	30	6	0	0	0	200	180	—	—	0
LiveActive Colby & Monterey Jack Cubes	7 (1 oz)	110	9	6	30	7	tr	0	0	200	200	—	—	0
LiveActive Mozzarella Sticks	1 (1 oz)	80	5	3	15	8	tr	0	0	200	200	—	—	0
Shredded Mexican Style Cheddar & Monterey Jack	¼ cup	110	9	5	25	6	1	0	0	200	190	—	—	0
Singles 2% Milk Pepperjack	1 slice (0.7 oz)	45	3	2	10	4	2	0	0	200	330	—	—	0
Swiss Extra Thin Slices	1 (0.6 oz)	60	5	3	15	4	0	0	0	150	25	—	—	0
LAND O LAKES														
American	1 slice (0.7 oz)	70	5	3	15	4	2	1	0	200	280	—	—	0
Chedarella	1 oz	110	9	6	25	7	0	0	0	200	190	—	—	0
Cheddar	1 oz	110	9	6	30	7	0	0	0	200	190	—	—	0
Snack 'N Cheese To Go Cheddar Mild	1 serv (0.7 oz)	80	7	5	20	7	0	0	0	150	140	—	—	0
Snack 'N Cheese To Go Cheddar Mild Reduced Fat	1 serv (0.5 oz)	60	5	3	15	5	0	0	0	150	115	—	—	0
Snack 'N Cheese To Go Co-Jack	1 serv (0.7 oz)	80	7	5	20	5	0	0	0	150	140	—	—	0
Snack 'N Cheese To Go Co-Jack Reduced Fat	1 serv (0.7 oz)	60	5	3	15	5	0	0	0	150	120	—	—	0
Swiss	1 oz	110	8	5	25	8	1	1	0	250	115	—	—	0
LAUGHING COW														
Blue Light	1 wedge (0.7 oz)	35	2	1	5	2	2	1	0	60	230	—	—	0
Creamy Swiss Light	1 wedge (0.7 oz)	35	2	1	<5	2	1	1	0	80	210	—	—	0
Creamy Swiss Original	1 wedge (0.7 oz)	50	4	3	10	2	1	1	0	80	210	—	—	0
French Onion Light	1 wedge (0.7 oz)	35	2	1	<5	2	1	1	0	80	210	—	—	0
Garlic & Herb Light	1 wedge (0.7 oz)	35	2	1	<5	2	1	1	0	80	210	—	—	0

FOOD	PORTION	CALS	FAT	SAT FAT	CHOL	PROT	CARB	SUGAR	FIBER	CALCI	SOD	POTAS	FOLIC	VIT C
LAUGHING COW (CONT.)														
Mozzarella Sun-Dried Tomato & Basil Light	1 wedge (0.7 oz)	35	2	1	5	2	2	1	0	60	220	—	—	0
Queso Fresco & Chipotle Light	1 wedge (0.7 oz)	35	2	1	5	2	2	1	0	60	240	—	—	0
LIFEWAY														
Farmer	2 tbsp (1.1 oz)	40	2	1	6	3	4	4	—	100	10	—	—	0
Farmer Lite	2 tbsp (1.1 oz)	25	1	1	<5	3	2	1	—	100	10	—	—	0
Sweet Kiss Spread Peach	1 oz	50	2	1	<5	3	6	6	—	40	10	—	—	0
Sweet Kiss Spread Raisins	1 oz	45	1	1	<5	3	6	6	—	40	10	—	—	0
MOLLY MCBUTTER														
Natural Cheese	1 tsp (2 g)	5	0	0	0	0	1	—	0	—	125	0	—	—
ORGANIC VALLEY														
Blue Crumbles	1 oz	100	8	5	25	6	1	0	0	150	380	—	—	0
Cheddar Mild	1 oz	110	9	6	30	7	0	0	0	200	170	—	—	0
Feta	1 oz	60	4	3	10	5	tr	0	0	100	430	—	—	0
Monterey Jack Shredded	¼ cup	80	5	4	15	8	1	0	0	200	180	—	—	0
Muenster	1 slice (0.7 oz)	80	6	4	20	5	0	0	0	150	160	—	—	0
Provolone	1 slice (0.7 oz)	70	6	4	15	5	0	0	0	150	190	—	—	0
Swiss	1 oz	110	9	6	25	7	0	0	0	200	125	—	—	0
PIZZA ZING														
Spicy Hot Cheese Shake	2 tsp	15	1	1	5	2	0	0	0	50	86	—	—	0
POLLY-O														
Mozzarella Shredded	¼ cup	90	7	4	20	6	tr	0	0	200	190	—	—	0
ROSENBORG														
Danish Camembert	1 oz	80	7	4	23	5	0	0	0	200	168	—	—	0
ROUGE ET NOIR														
Breakfast	1 oz	90	7	5	25	6	0	0	0	80	210	—	—	0
Brie Garlic	1 oz	90	7	5	30	6	0	0	0	80	210	—	—	0
Brie Pesto	1 oz	90	7	5	30	6	0	0	0	80	210	—	—	0
Brie Tomato Basil	1 oz	90	7	5	30	6	0	0	0	80	210	—	—	0
Brie Triple Creme	1 oz	110	10	7	30	4	0	0	0	100	160	—	—	0
Camembert	1 oz	90	7	5	30	6	0	0	0	80	210	—	—	0
Le Petit Bleu	1 oz	110	10	7	30	4	0	0	0	100	160	—	—	0
Le Petit Chevre	1 oz	90	6	4	20	5	0	0	0	100	210	—	—	0
Marin French Blue	1 oz	110	10	7	30	4	0	0	0	100	160	—	—	0
Marin French Gold	1 oz	110	10	7	30	4	0	0	0	100	160	—	—	0
Schlosskranz	1 oz	85	7	5	30	5	0	0	0	80	390	—	—	0

FOOD	PORTION	CALS	FAT	SAT FAT	CHOL	PROT	CARB	SUGAR	FIBER	CALCI	SOD	POTAS	FOLIC	VIT C
SALADENA														
Goat Crumbles	¼ cup	80	7	4	30	5	tr	0	0	20	110	—	—	0
SAP SAGO														
Fat Free Cheese Grated	1 tsp	10	0	0	0	2	0	0	0	60	136	—	—	0
SARGENTO														
4 Cheese Italian Shredded	¼ cup	80	5	3	15	8	1	0	0	200	220	—	—	0
4 Cheese Mexican Reduced Fat Shredded	¼ cup (1 oz)	80	6	4	15	8	1	0	0	250	190	—	—	0
American Burger	1 slice (0.7 oz)	70	6	4	20	4	tr	0	0	150	240	—	—	0
Bistro Blends Shredded Italian Pasta Cheese	¼ cup (1 oz)	90	6	4	15	7	2	0	0	200	310	—	—	0
Blue Crumbled	¼ cup (1 oz)	100	8	5	25	6	1	0	0	150	380	—	—	0
Cheddar Chipotle Shredded	¼ cup	100	8	5	15	6	1	0	0	200	190	—	—	0
Cheddar Chipotle Sticks	1 (0.7 oz)	80	6	4	0	5	1	0	0	150	150	—	—	0
Cheddar Mild Cubes	7 (1 oz)	120	10	8	30	7	tr	0	0	200	190	—	—	0
Cheddar Mild Shredded Reduced Sodium	¼ cup (1 oz)	110	9	5	25	7	1	0	0	200	135	20	—	0
Cheddar White Vermont Sharp	1 slice (0.7 oz)	80	7	4	20	5	0	0	0	150	125	—	—	0
Cheddar White Vermont Sharp Shredded	¼ cup (1 oz)	110	9	5	25	7	1	0	0	200	190	—	—	0
Cheese Dips Cheddar & Buttery Pretzels	1 pkg (3.8 oz)	360	16	5	15	9	47	5	2	150	1430	—	—	0
Cheese Dips Cheddar & Tortilla Chips	1 pkg (3 oz)	320	21	6	15	7	26	4	1	200	880	—	—	0
Colby-Jack Sticks Reduced Sodium	1 (0.7 oz)	80	7	5	20	5	tr	0	0	150	105	15	—	0
Jarlsberg	1 slice (0.8 oz)	80	6	4	15	6	tr	0	0	200	110	—	—	0
Monterey Jack Shredded	¼ cup (1 oz)	110	9	5	30	7	1	0	0	200	190	—	—	0
Mozzarella Reduced Fat Shredded	¼ cup (1 oz)	80	5	2	10	8	tr	0	0	200	200	—	—	0
Mozzarella Shredded	¼ cup (1 oz)	80	6	4	15	7	1	0	0	200	190	—	—	0
Muenster	1 slice (0.7 oz)	80	6	4	20	5	tr	0	0	150	135	—	—	0

FOOD	PORTION	CALS	FAT	SAT FAT	CHOL	PROT	CARB	SUGAR	FIBER	CALCI	SOD	POTAS	FOLIC	VIT C
SARGENTO (CONT.)														
Nacho & Taco Shredded	¼ cup (1 oz)	110	9	5	30	7	1	0	0	200	200	—	—	0
Parmesan Grated	2 tsp (5 g)	25	2	1	5	2	0	0	0	60	80	—	—	0
Parmesan Shredded	2 tsp	20	2	1	<5	2	0	0	0	40	55	—	—	0
Pepper Jack Reduced Sodium	1 slice (0.7 oz)	70	6	4	15	4	0	0	0	150	90	20	—	0
Provolone	1 slice (0.7 oz)	70	5	4	15	5	0	0	0	150	125	—	—	0
Provolone Reduced Sodium	1 slice (0.7 oz)	70	5	4	15	5	0	0	0	150	100	20	—	0
Ricotta Fat Free	¼ cup	50	0	0	10	5	5	2	0	100	65	—	—	0
Ricotta Light	¼ cup	60	3	2	15	5	3	3	0	100	55	—	—	0
Ricotta Whole Milk	¼ cup	90	8	4	25	7	3	3	0	150	75	—	—	0
String Light	1 piece (0.7 oz)	50	3	2	10	6	1	0	0	150	160	—	—	0
String Reduced Sodium	1 (0.7 oz)	60	4	3	10	6	tr	0	0	150	110	15	—	0
Swiss Reduced Fat	1 slice (0.7 oz)	60	4	2	15	7	1	0	0	250	30	20	—	0
Swiss Shredded	¼ cup (1 oz)	110	8	5	25	8	tr	0	0	300	60	—	—	0
Swiss Thick Slice	1 slice (1 oz)	110	8	5	25	8	1	0	0	300	60	—	—	0
Swiss Thin Sliced	1 slice (0.6 oz)	70	5	3	20	5	0	0	0	200	40	—	—	0
SMART BALANCE														
Creamy Cheddar Slices	1 (0.7 oz)	40	2	1	<5	4	2	2	0	100	290	60	—	0
Fat Free Lactose Free Slices	1 (0.7 oz)	40	2	1	<5	4	2	2	0	100	290	60	—	0
SORRENTO														
Mozzarella Fresh	1 oz	90	6	4	30	5	0	0	0	100	130	—	—	0
STELLA														
3 Cheese Italian Shredded	¼ cup	100	7	4	25	8	1	tr	tr	300	410	—	—	0
Asiago Wedge	1 oz	110	9	6	30	6	tr	tr	0	200	280	—	—	0
Gorgonzola Wedge	1 oz	100	9	6	25	6	tr	0	0	150	390	—	—	0
Kasseri Wedge	1 oz	110	9	6	30	6	tr	tr	0	200	280	—	—	0
THE GREEK GODS														
Kefir Cheese	2 tbsp (1 oz)	80	5	3	20	2	2	1	0	60	25	—	—	0
TREASURE CAVE														
Blue Cheese Crumbled	¼ cup (1 oz)	100	8	5	20	6	tr	—	—	150	400	—	—	—
Feta Crumbled	¼ cup (1 oz)	80	6	4	20	5	1	0	tr	60	320	—	—	2
Gorgonzola Crumbled	¼ cup (1 oz)	100	8	5	20	6	tr	—	—	150	310	—	—	—
WEIGHT WATCHERS														
String Light	1 stick (0.8 oz)	50	3	1	5	6	tr	0	0	150	150	—	—	0

FOOD	PORTION	CALS	FAT	SAT FAT	CHOL	PROT	CARB	SUGAR	FIBER	CALCI	SOD	POTAS	FOLIC	VIT C
WHOLESOME VALLEY														
Organic American	1 slice (0.7 oz)	50	4	3	10	3	tr	0	0	100	210	—	—	0
YANNI														
Grilling Cheese Original	1 oz	80	7	5	25	6	0	0	0	200	180	—	—	0

CHEESE DISHES

FOOD	PORTION	CALS	FAT	SAT FAT	CHOL	PROT	CARB	SUGAR	FIBER	CALCI	SOD	POTAS	FOLIC	VIT C
ALEXIA														
Cheddar Bites	3 (1.2 oz)	110	6	3	15	4	8	0	0	100	160	—	—	0
Mozzarella Stix	2 pieces (1.3 oz)	120	6	3	10	5	10	1	1	100	230	35	—	0
BANQUET														
Mozzarella Nuggets	7	270	16	8	35	10	21	tr	tr	150	570	—	—	0
FARM RICH														
Cheese Sticks	2 (2 oz)	170	9	4	15	8	14	1	0	200	370	—	—	0
Mozzarella Sticks Marinara Stuffed	2 (2.3 oz)	160	8	3	10	6	14	2	1	150	410	—	—	1
Mozzarella Bites	4 (1.8 oz)	150	6	3	10	8	13	4	1	150	320	—	—	0
STOUFFER'S														
Welsh Rarebit	¼ pkg (2.5 oz)	140	10	6	20	6	6	2	0	200	270	—	—	0
THE FILLO FACTORY														
Tyropita Cheese Fillo Appetizers	3 (3 oz)	230	14	8	40	7	19	2	0	150	310	—	—	1
TAKE-OUT														
fondue	½ cup (3.8 oz)	247	15	9	49	15	4	—	—	514	142	113	5	0
fried mozzarella sticks	3 (4.6 oz)	503	32	16	107	33	20	2	1	855	759	168	28	0
souffle	1 serv (7 oz)	504	38	17	370	23	18	5	1	446	848	274	38	tr
welsh rarebit	1 slice	228	16	—	—	8	14	—	1	204	—	—	—	tr

CHEESE SUBSTITUTES

FOOD	PORTION	CALS	FAT	SAT FAT	CHOL	PROT	CARB	SUGAR	FIBER	CALCI	SOD	POTAS	FOLIC	VIT C
mozzarella	1 oz	70	3	1	0	3	7	—	—	173	194	129	3	0
soya cheese	1.4 oz	128	11	—	—	7	tr	—	0	180	—	—	—	0
DAIYA														
Cheddar Style Shreds	¼ cup (1 oz)	90	6	2	0	1	7	0	1	0	250	—	—	0
Mozzarella Style Shreds	¼ cup (1 oz)	90	6	2	0	1	7	0	1	0	280	—	—	0
PLAYFOOD														
Cheesey Cheese	1 oz	60	5	1	0	2	4	0	1	60	190	—	—	0
RICE														
American Flavor	1 slice (0.7 oz)	50	3	1	0	4	tr	0	0	200	230	—	—	0
American Flavor Vegan	1 slice (0.7 oz)	45	3	1	0	1	0	0	0	200	130	—	—	0
Shreds Mozzarella Flavor	⅓ cup (1 oz)	70	4	1	0	6	3	0	0	300	370	—	—	0

FOOD	PORTION	CALS	FAT	SAT FAT	CHOL	PROT	CARB	SUGAR	FIBER	CALCI	SOD	POTAS	FOLIC	VIT C
SHEESE														
Blue Style	1 oz	100	8	5	0	4	3	0	0	30	340	—	—	0
Cheddar Style Medium	1 oz	100	8	5	0	4	3	0	0	30	340	—	—	0
Creamy Mexican	2 tbsp	80	7	3	0	2	2	0	0	0	140	—	—	0
Creamy Original	2 tbsp	80	7	3	0	2	2	0	0	0	140	—	—	0
SUPER STIX														
Mozzarella Flavor	1 (1 oz)	70	5	0	0	6	0	0	0	350	370	—	100	2
TOFUTTI														
Better Ricotta Milk Free	¼ cup (2.2 oz)	100	7	4	0	2	8	0	1	—	150	—	—	—
Soy American	1 slice (0.7 oz)	80	6	3	0	2	2	—	0	—	290	—	—	—
Soy Mozzarella	1 slice (0.7 oz)	80	6	3	0	2	2	—	0	—	290	—	—	—
VEGAN GOURMET														
Cheese Alternative Cheddar	1 oz	50	4	1	0	2	2	0	2	40	200	—	—	0
Cheese Alternative Monterey Jack	1 oz	70	7	1	0	1	2	0	2	40	150	—	—	0
Cheese Alternative Mozzarella	1 oz	70	8	1	0	1	1	0	1	40	120	—	—	0
Cheese Alternative Nacho	1 oz	45	4	1	0	2	2	0	2	40	210	—	—	0
VEGGIE														
American Flavor	1 slice (0.6 oz)	40	3	0	0	3	tr	0	0	200	220	—	40	1
Grated Parmesan Flavor	2 tsp	15	1	0	0	2	0	0	0	60	90	—	16	0
Pepper Jack Flavor	1 oz	60	4	0	0	6	2	0	0	250	390	—	100	1
Shreds Cheddar Flavor	1 oz	70	4	0	0	6	0	0	0	300	260	—	120	2
VEGGY														
Mozzarella Flavor	1 slice (0.7 oz)	40	3	0	0	4	tr	0	0	200	230	—	—	0
CHERIMOYA														
fresh	1	515	2	—	0	7	131	—	—	126	—	—	—	49
CHERRIES														
CANNED														
maraschino	1 (4 g)	7	tr	tr	0	tr	2	2	tr	2	0	1	0	0
maraschino	¼ cup (1.4 oz)	66	tr	tr	0	tr	17	16	1	22	2	8	0	0
sour in heavy syrup	½ cup	116	tr	tr	0	1	30	28	1	13	9	119	10	3
sour in light syrup	½ cup	94	tr	tr	0	1	24	—	1	13	9	120	10	3
sour water packed	½ cup	44	tr	tr	0	1	11	9	1	13	9	120	10	3
sweet juice pack	½ cup	68	tr	tr	0	1	17	15	2	18	4	164	5	3
sweet pitted in heavy syrup	½ cup	105	tr	tr	0	1	27	25	2	11	4	183	5	5
sweet water pack	½ cup	57	tr	tr	0	1	15	13	2	14	1	162	5	3

FOOD	PORTION	CALS	FAT	SAT FAT	CHOL	PROT	CARB	SUGAR	FIBER	CALCI	SOD	POTAS	FOLIC	VIT C
CHUKAR CHERRIES														
Cherry Jubilee Dessert Sauce	1 tbsp	40	0	0	0	0	10	8	tr	0	0	—	—	1
DEL MONTE														
Sweet Dark Pitted In Heavy Syrup	½ cup (4.2 oz)	100	0	0	0	tr	24	24	tr	0	10	—	—	4
JAKE & AMOS														
Brandied Sweet	½ cup (4.4 oz)	90	0	0	0	1	22	10	2	20	9	—	—	2
S&W														
Sliced	½ cup (4.7 oz)	140	0	0	0	1	34	26	1	0	10	—	—	1
THE GRACIOUS GOURMET														
Spiced Sour Cherry Spread	1 tbsp(0.5 oz)	15	0	0	0	0	4	3	0	0	25	—	—	0
DRIED														
bing unsulfured	¼ cup	130	0	0	0	0	31	21	2	20	10	—	—	0
montmorency tart pitted	⅓ cup	160	1	0	0	2	36	24	2	20	0	—	—	0
rainier unsulfured	⅓ cup	140	1	0	0	1	32	30	2	20	0	—	—	6
tart	½ cup	200	1	0	0	2	49	41	2	20	0	—	—	0
yogurt covered	¼ cup	170	6	6	0	1	29	22	5	40	20	—	—	0
BOB'S RED MILL														
Tart	⅓ cup	140	0	0	0	1	33	18	11	—	0	—	—	—
CHUKAR CHERRIES														
Bing	3 tbsp	130	1	0	0	1	33	29	3	20	10	—	—	5
Bing Chocolate Covered	3 tbsp (1.4 oz)	180	9	5	0	2	24	19	2	60	20	—	—	5
Cabernet Dark Chocolate Covered	2 tbsp (1.5 oz)	180	9	5	<5	2	26	17	3	40	10	—	—	5
Columbia River Tart	⅓ cup	120	1	0	0	2	36	24	2	20	0	—	—	0
Rainier	3 tbsp	130	1	0	0	tr	33	29	3	20	10	—	—	12
Totally Tart	⅓ cup	140	1	0	0	1	33	16	3	60	0	—	—	0
DE-LITE														
Tart	1 oz	95	tr	0	0	1	23	22	1	10	14	103	—	2
EDEN														
Montmorency	¼ cup	140	0	0	0	0	36	31	3	40	15	350	—	—
EMILY'S														
Dark Chocolate Covered	11 (1.4 oz)	180	9	6	0	1	27	23	2	40	0	—	—	0
FRIEDA'S														
Bing	¼ cup (1.4 oz)	120	0	0	0	2	26	17	3	20	5	—	—	0
PEELED SNACKS														
Fruit Picks Cherry-Go-Round	1 pkg (1.5 oz)	130	0	0	0	2	30	24	4	20	0	—	—	12

FOOD	PORTION	CALS	FAT	SAT FAT	CHOL	PROT	CARB	SUGAR	FIBER	CALCI	SOD	POTAS	FOLIC	VIT C
RAISINETS														
Dark & Milk Chocolate	¼ cup (1.6 oz)	200	8	5	5	1	32	28	2	20	5	—	—	0
STONERIDGE ORCHARDS														
Bing	⅓ cup (1.4 oz)	130	0	0	0	1	32	31	1	0	10	—	—	4
Organic Montmorency Whole	⅓ cup (1.4 oz)	135	1	—	0	0	33	27	2	20	12	—	—	0
SUNSWEET														
Cherries	¼ cup (1.4 oz)	100	0	0	0	1	30	22	2	20	5	115	—	0
FRESH														
sour	1 cup	52	tr	tr	0	1	13	9	2	16	3	178	8	10
sour pitted	1 cup	78	tr	tr	0	2	19	13	3	25	5	268	12	16
sweet	20	86	1	tr	0	1	22	17	3	18	0	302	5	10
CHIQUITA														
Cherries	1 cup (4.8 oz)	87	0	0	0	1	22	18	3	20	0	306	—	9
DOLE														
Cherries	1 cup (4.9 oz)	90	0	0	0	1	22	18	3	20	0	—	—	9
DOMEX SUPERFRESH GROWERS														
Rainier	21 (5 oz)	90	0	0	0	1	19	16	3	20	0	270	—	6
FROZEN														
sour unsweetened	½ cup	36	tr	tr	0	1	9	7	1	10	1	96	4	1
sweet sweetened	½ cup	115	tr	tr	0	2	29	26	3	16	1	258	5	1
DOLE														
Dark Sweet	1 cup (4.9 oz)	90	0	0	0	1	22	18	3	0	0	—	—	9
CHERRY JUICE														
tart cherry concentrate	1 cup	140	0	0	0	1	34	27	0	20	25	—	—	0
CHERIBUNDI														
Skinny Cherry	8 oz	90	0	0	0	0	23	17	—	20	5	260	—	0
Tart Cherry	8 oz	130	0	0	0	1	32	28	—	20	5	290	—	0
Whey Cherry	8 oz	160	0	0	0	8	30	27	—	20	20	280	400	0
FROOSE														
Cheerful Cherry	1 box (4.2 oz)	80	0	0	0	0	18	8	3	0	10	70	—	15
HP														
Tart Montmorency Concentrate	1 oz	80	0	0	0	tr	19	15	0	—	15	202	—	—
OLD ORCHARD														
Very Cherre 100% Tart Cherry Juice	8 oz	130	0	0	0	0	31	21	—	30	45	245	—	60
SANTA CRUZ														
Organic 100% Juice Red Tart	8 oz	120	0	0	0	0	30	30	0	—	25	310	—	—

FOOD	PORTION	CALS	FAT	SAT FAT	CHOL	PROT	CARB	SUGAR	FIBER	CALCI	SOD	POTAS	FOLIC	VIT C
SMART JUICE														
Organic 100% Juice Tart Cherry	8 oz	140	0	0	0	1	32	24	1	20	20	410	—	9
TART IS SMART														
Tart Cherry Concentrate	1 oz	80	0	0	0	1	19	15	0	—	15	202	—	—
CHERVIL														
seed	1 tsp	1	tr	—	0	tr	tr	—	—	8	tr	28	—	—
CHESTNUTS														
chinese steamed	3 (1 oz)	43	tr	tr	0	1	10	—	—	3	1	87	13	7
creme de marrons	1 oz	73	tr	tr	0	1	18	10	1	4	1	49	9	0
japanese roasted	1 oz	57	tr	tr	0	1	13	—	—	10	5	121	17	8
ready-to-eat vacuum packed	5 (1 oz)	40	0	0	0	tr	8	0	0	0	10	—	—	0
roasted	3 (1 oz)	70	1	tr	0	1	15	3	1	8	1	168	20	7
GEFEN														
Whole Roasted & Peeled	¼ cup (1.4 oz)	52	0	0	0	1	11	11	1	10	1	—	—	8
MATIZ														
Organic	7–8	86	1	0	0	2	17	12	5	20	0	—	—	0
CHEWING GUM														
bubble gum	1 block	20	tr	tr	0	0	5	5	tr	0	0	0	0	0
stick	1 piece	7	tr	tr	0	0	2	2	tr	0	0	0	0	0
sugarless	1 piece	5	tr	tr	0	0	2	0	0	0	0	0	0	0
BUBBLE YUM														
Original	1 piece (8 g)	25	0	0	0	0	6	5	—	0	—	—	—	0
Sugarless	1 piece (5 g)	10	0	0	0	0	3	—	—	—	—	—	—	0
CHOWARD'S														
Scented Gum	3 pieces	10	0	0	0	0	3	3	0	0	0	—	—	0
DUBBLE BUBBLE														
Gumball	1 piece	10	0	0	0	0	2	2	0	0	0	—	—	0
EXTRA														
Sugar Free All Flavors	1 piece	5	0	0	0	0	2	0	—	—	0	—	—	—
FLARE														
Warming Cinnamon	1 piece	5	0	0	0	0	2	0	—	—	0	—	—	—
ORBIT														
Sugarfree Citrusmint	1 piece	<5	0	0	0	0	1	0	—	—	0	—	—	—
White Melon Breeze	2 pieces	5	0	0	0	0	2	0	0	—	0	—	—	—
STRIDE														
All Flavors	1 piece (1.9 g)	<5	0	0	0	0	1	0	—	—	0	—	—	—
Spark	1 piece (1.9 g)	5	0	0	0	0	1	0	—	—	0	—	—	—

FOOD	PORTION	CALS	FAT	SAT FAT	CHOL	PROT	CARB	SUGAR	FIBER	CALCI	SOD	POTAS	FOLIC	VIT C
TRIDENT														
Extra Care	1 piece	<5	0	0	0	0	1	0	—	—	0	—	—	—
White Peppermint	2 pieces (3 g)	5	0	0	0	0	2	0	—	—	0	—	—	—
VITAMINGUM														
Fresh Sugar Free All Flavors	1 piece (3 g)	5	0	0	0	0	2	0	—	—	0	—	40	6
Sport Bubblegum	1 piece (6 g)	15	0	0	0	0	4	4	—	—	10	—	100	15
WINTERFRESH														
Gum	1 stick	10	0	0	0	0	2	2	—	—	0	—	—	—
CHIA SEEDS														
dried	1 oz	134	7	3	0	5	14	—	—	150	—	—	—	—
HEALTH WARRIOR														
Chia Bar Peanut Butter Chocolate	1 (0.9 oz)	100	5	1	0	3	15	4	3	40	35	—	—	1
Chia Seeds	1 tbsp (0.5 oz)	60	5	—	—	3	6	—	6	110	—	—	—	—
TRUROOTS														
Chia	1 tbsp (0.4 oz)	55	9	0	0	2	5	—	6	70	2	—	—	0
CHICKEN														
(*see also* CHICKEN DISHES, CHICKEN SUBSTITUTES, DINNER, HOT DOG, MEATBALLS)														
CANNED														
chicken spread	1 serv (2 oz)	88	10	2	31	10	2	tr	tr	9	404	59	2	0
meat drained	1 can (5 oz)	230	10	3	62	32	1	0	0	18	169	191	2	0
w/ broth	½ can (2.5 oz)	117	6	2	—	15	0	0	0	10	357	98	—	1
HORMEL														
Chunk White & Dark	2 oz	70	3	1	45	10	0	0	0	0	250	—	—	0
Premium Chunk Breast	2 oz	60	2	1	40	12	0	0	0	0	250	—	—	0
SWANSON														
Chunk Breast In Water	2 oz	50	1	0	25	9	1	0	0	0	300	—	—	0
TYSON														
Premium Chunk	½ can (2 oz)	60	3	1	30	10	0	0	0	0	200	—	—	0
Premium Chunk Breast	½ can (2 oz)	60	1	0	30	13	0	0	0	0	200	—	—	0
VALLEY FRESH														
Chunk White	2 oz	70	1	0	25	15	0	0	0	0	180	—	—	0
White & Dark Chunk	2 oz	80	2	1	50	15	0	0	0	0	130	—	—	0
FRESH														
back w/ skin roasted bones removed	1 (3.7 oz)	318	22	6	93	28	0	0	0	22	92	223	6	0
back w/o skin roasted bones removed	1 (2.8 oz)	191	11	3	72	23	0	0	0	19	77	190	6	0

FOOD	PORTION	CALS	FAT	SAT FAT	CHOL	PROT	CARB	SUGAR	FIBER	CALCI	SOD	POTAS	FOLIC	VIT C
breast roasted diced	1 cup (5 oz)	231	5	1	119	43	0	0	0	21	104	358	8	0
breast w/ skin battered fried bones removed	½ breast (4.9 oz)	364	18	5	119	35	13	0	tr	28	385	281	21	0
breast w/ skin floured fried bones removed	1 (3.4 oz)	218	9	2	87	31	2	—	tr	16	74	254	6	0
breast w/ skin roasted bones removed	½ breast (3.4 oz)	193	8	2	82	29	0	0	0	14	70	240	4	0
breast w/ skin stewed bones removed	½ breast (3.9 oz)	202	8	2	82	30	0	0	0	14	68	196	3	0
breast w/o skin fried bones removed	½ breast (3 oz)	161	4	1	78	29	tr	0	0	14	68	237	3	0
breast w/o skin roasted bones removed	½ breast (3 oz)	142	3	1	73	27	0	0	0	13	64	220	3	0
breast w/o skin stewed bones removed	1 (3.3 oz)	143	3	1	73	28	0	0	0	12	60	178	3	0
broiler/fryer w/ skin roasted bones removed	½ (10.5 oz)	715	41	11	263	82	0	0	0	45	245	667	15	0
capon meat & skin roasted bones removed	½ (1.4 lbs)	1459	74	21	548	184	0	0	0	89	312	1624	38	0
cornish hen w/ skin roasted	1 (9 oz)	668	47	13	337	57	0	0	0	33	164	630	5	1
cornish hen w/ skin roasted	½ (4.5 oz)	335	23	7	169	29	0	0	0	17	83	316	3	1
cornish hen w/o skin roasted	½ (4 oz)	147	4	1	117	26	0	0	0	14	69	275	2	1
cornish hen w/o skin roasted	1 (7.7 oz)	295	9	2	233	51	0	0	0	29	139	550	2	1
dark meat w/o skin roasted diced	1 cup (5 oz)	287	14	4	130	38	0	0	0	21	130	336	11	0
drumstick w/ skin battered floured & fried bones removed	1 (1.7 oz)	120	7	2	44	13	1	—	0	6	44	112	5	0
drumstick w/ skin battered fried bones removed	1 (2.5 oz)	193	11	3	62	16	6	—	tr	12	194	134	13	0
drumstick w/ skin roasted bones removed	1 (1.8 oz)	112	6	2	47	14	0	0	0	6	47	119	4	0

FOOD	PORTION	CALS	FAT	SAT FAT	CHOL	PROT	CARB	SUGAR	FIBER	CALCI	SOD	POTAS	FOLIC	VIT C
drumstick w/ skin stewed bones removed	1 (2 oz)	116	6	2	47	14	0	0	0	6	43	105	4	0
drumstick w/o skin fried bones removed	1 (1.5 oz)	82	3	1	39	12	0	0	0	5	40	105	4	0
drumstick w/o skin roasted bones removed	1 (1.5 oz)	76	2	1	41	12	0	0	0	5	42	108	4	0
drumstick w/o skin stewed bones removed	1 (1.6 oz)	78	3	1	40	13	0	0	0	5	37	92	4	0
feet cooked	1 (1.2 oz)	73	5	1	29	7	tr	0	0	30	23	11	29	0
ground crumbled fried	3 oz	161	9	3	91	20	0	0	0	7	64	575	2	0
ground patty cooked	1 med (2.1 oz)	142	8	2	52	16	0	0	0	9	242	133	3	0
ground patty cooked	1 lg (2.8 oz)	190	11	3	70	22	0	0	0	12	323	177	4	0
ground patty cooked	1 sm (1.7 oz)	114	6	2	42	13	0	0	0	7	194	106	2	0
meat & skin stewed bones removed	¼ chicken (4.6 oz)	372	25	7	103	35	0	0	0	17	95	238	7	0
neck w/ skin battered fried	1 (1.8 oz)	172	12	3	47	10	5	—	—	16	144	79	8	0
neck w/ skin fried	1 (1.3 oz)	120	9	2	34	9	2	—	—	11	30	65	4	0
neck w/ skin simmered	1 (1.3 oz)	94	7	2	27	7	0	0	0	10	20	41	1	0
roaster meat & skin roasted bones removed	¼ chicken (8.4 oz)	535	32	9	182	58	0	0	0	29	175	506	12	0
skin battered fried from ½ chicken	6.7 oz	749	55	14	141	20	44	—	—	49	1104	142	76	0
skin floured fried from ½ chicken	2 oz	281	24	7	41	11	5	—	—	8	30	70	18	0
skin roasted from ½ chicken	2 oz	254	23	6	46	11	0	0	0	8	36	76	1	0
skin stewed from ½ chicken	2.5 oz	261	24	7	45	11	0	0	0	9	40	84	1	0
tail cooked	1 (1 oz)	84	5	1	25	7	3	0	tr	6	85	54	5	0
thigh w/ skin battered & fried bones removed	1 (3 oz)	238	14	4	80	19	8	—	tr	15	248	165	16	0
thigh w/ skin floured fried bones removed	1 (2.2 oz)	162	9	3	60	17	2	—	tr	9	55	147	7	0

FOOD	PORTION	CALS	FAT	SAT FAT	CHOL	PROT	CARB	SUGAR	FIBER	CALCI	SOD	POTAS	FOLIC	VIT C
thigh w/ skin roasted bones removed	1 (2.2 oz)	153	10	3	58	16	0	0	0	7	52	138	4	0
thigh w/ skin stewed bones removed	1 (2.4 oz)	158	10	3	57	16	0	0	0	7	48	116	4	0
thigh w/o skin fried bones removed	1 (1.8 oz)	113	5	1	53	15	1	—	0	7	49	135	5	0
thigh w/o skin roasted bones removed	1 (1.8 oz)	109	6	2	49	13	0	0	0	6	46	124	4	0
thigh w/o skin stewed bones removed	1 (1.9 oz)	107	5	1	50	14	0	0	0	6	41	101	4	0
wing w/ skin battered fried bones removed	1 (1.7 oz)	159	11	3	39	10	5	—	tr	10	157	68	9	0
wing w/ skin floured fried bones removed	1 (1.1 oz)	103	7	2	26	8	1	—	0	5	25	57	1	0
wing w/ skin roasted bones removed	1 (1.4 oz)	100	7	2	28	9	0	0	0	5	27	56	1	0
wing w/o skin fried bones removed	1 (0.7 oz)	42	2	1	17	6	0	0	0	3	18	42	1	0
wing w/o skin roasted bones removed	1 (0.7 oz)	43	2	tr	18	6	0	0	0	3	19	44	1	0
wing w/o skin stewed bones removed	1 (0.8 oz)	43	2	tr	18	7	0	0	0	3	18	37	1	0
COLEMAN														
Organic Breast Boneless Skinless	4 oz	120	2	0	65	26	0	0	0	0	75	—	—	1
Organic Drumsticks	4 oz	180	10	3	90	22	0	0	0	0	95	—	—	2
FOSTER FARMS														
Back & Necks	4 oz	340	31	—	100	16	0	0	0	—	70	—	—	1
Breast Skinless Boneless	4 oz	120	2	—	65	26	0	0	0	—	75	—	—	1
Drumsticks not prep	1 (2.8 oz)	130	7	—	65	15	0	0	0	—	65	—	—	2
Ground not prep	4 oz	210	14	—	93	20	0	0	0	—	90	—	—	2
Party Wings	5 (3.8 oz)	230	17	—	80	19	0	0	0	—	75	—	—	—
Thighs	1 (4.6 oz)	270	20	—	110	22	0	0	0	—	95	—	—	2
PERDUE														
Boneless Skinless Breasts cooked	3 oz	110	1	0	70	25	0	0	0	0	30	—	—	0

FOOD	PORTION	CALS	FAT	SAT FAT	CHOL	PROT	CARB	SUGAR	FIBER	CALCI	SOD	POTAS	FOLIC	VIT C
PERDUE (CONT.)														
Breast Boneless Herb & Pepper	1 piece (4.8 oz)	140	2	0	80	29	0	0	0	20	330	—	—	4
Breast Boneless Roasted Garlic w/ White Wine	1 piece (4.8 oz)	110	2	0	80	29	1	0	—	0	520	—	—	1
Breast Boneless Skinless cooked	3 oz	100	1	0	65	23	0	0	0	0	25	—	—	0
Breast Perfect Portions Boneless Skinless	1 (4.8 oz)	130	2	0	80	19	0	0	—	0	350	—	—	1
Ground cooked	3 oz	170	11	4	125	18	0	0	0	40	50	—	—	0
Ground Breast cooked	3 oz	80	1	0	55	19	0	0	0	0	60	—	—	0
Oven Ready Cornish Hen Seasoned	4 oz	160	10	3	75	16	1	0	—	20	420	—	—	1
Oven Ready Roaster Bone-In Breast	4 oz	140	7	2	75	20	1	0	0	20	410	—	—	0
Oven Ready Roaster Seasoned	4 oz	210	15	5	70	17	1	1	—	20	430	—	—	0
Oven Stuffer Drumstick	1 (3.6 oz)	190	11	3	125	25	0	0	0	0	85	—	—	0
Patties cooked	1 (3 oz)	170	11	4	130	19	0	0	0	0	75	—	—	0
Thigh Filets Boneless Skinless	4 oz	150	8	2	110	22	0	0	0	0	85	—	—	2
Thighs Tender & Tasty Boneless Skinless cooked	3 oz	150	9	4	90	17	0	0	0	0	380	—	—	1
Whole Dark Meat cooked	3 oz	210	15	5	100	18	0	0	0	0	60	—	—	0
Whole White Meat cooked	3 oz	170	9	3	80	21	0	0	0	0	50	—	—	0
Whole Chicken Tender & Tasty cooked	3 oz	150	8	3	110	20	0	0	0	0	280	—	—	6
Wingettes cooked	3 oz	170	10	3	135	20	0	0	0	20	250	—	—	6
Wings cooked	3 oz	170	10	3	135	20	0	0	0	20	250	—	—	6
ROCKY														
The Range Chicken Whole	4 oz	240	17	5	100	21	0	0	0	0	80	—	—	0
ROSIE														
Organic Breast Boneless Skinless	4 oz	120	2	0	65	26	0	0	0	0	75	—	—	1
TYSON														
Breasts Boneless Skinless	4 oz	110	3	1	65	23	0	0	0	0	180	—	—	0

FOOD	PORTION	CALS	FAT	SAT FAT	CHOL	PROT	CARB	SUGAR	FIBER	CALCI	SOD	POTAS	FOLIC	VIT C
TYSON (CONT.)														
Cornish Hen	1 serv (4 oz)	200	14	4	130	19	0	0	0	0	65	—	—	0
Drumsticks	4 oz	150	9	3	95	18	0	0	0	0	180	—	—	0
Thigh Cutlets Boneless Skinless	4 oz	130	7	2	90	18	0	0	0	0	160	—	—	0
Whole Cut Up	4 oz	220	16	5	80	19	0	0	0	0	170	—	—	0
Wings	4 oz	220	17	5	105	17	0	0	0	0	190	—	—	0
FROZEN														
breast roll roasted	2 oz	75	4	1	22	8	1	tr	0	3	494	181	2	0
fajita strips	1 (0.3 oz)	13	1	tr	8	2	tr	0	0	1	75	27	2	0
patty cooked	1 (3.5 oz)	287	20	4	43	15	13	0	tr	19	532	261	7	0
BANQUET														
Wings Hot & Spicy	¼ pkg (3 oz)	260	17	5	55	19	8	0	5	20	320	—	—	0
BARBER														
Buffalo Fingers	1 (3.3 oz)	160	4	1	35	15	18	0	tr	0	380	—	—	0
Nuggets 4 Cheese Stuffed	3 (3 oz)	230	16	3	45	14	9	1	tr	80	570	—	—	1
Nuggets Cheddar & Bacon Stuffed	3 (3 oz)	240	17	4	45	14	8	1	tr	60	520	—	—	1
Potato Chip Sticks	2 pieces (4.5 oz)	350	24	4	60	18	16	0	tr	20	950	—	—	1
BELL & EVANS														
Breaded Breast Nuggets	1 serv (4 oz)	220	9	2	45	21	13	2	1	0	380	—	—	0
Breasts Grilled	1 (2.75 oz)	90	1	0	50	21	1	0	0	0	320	—	—	1
Breasts Grilled Buffalo Style	1 (3 oz)	110	1	1	65	24	0	1	0	0	340	—	—	0
Burgers	1 (4 oz)	160	6	2	95	31	3	0	0	0	140	—	—	0
Chicken Tenders Gluten Free	1 serv (4 oz)	180	6	1	45	19	12	0	1	40	440	—	—	1
Wings Honey Barbeque	3 (4.6 oz)	160	8	2	80	17	6	6	0	40	27	—	—	0
COLEMAN														
Breast Nuggets Gluten Free	6 (2.7 oz)	130	6	1	30	12	10	1	0	0	380	—	—	1
Breast Strips	6 (2.7 oz)	130	3	0	30	13	14	1	1	0	250	—	—	0
HEALTH IS WEALTH														
Nuggets	4 (3 oz)	130	4	1	35	13	11	0	0	0	230	—	—	0
IAN'S														
Fingers	3 pieces	190	8	2	40	15	14	1	0	0	460	—	—	1
Nuggets	5 pieces	190	8	2	40	15	14	1	0	0	250	—	—	3
Nuggets Allergy Free	5 pieces	190	8	2	40	15	14	1	0	0	250	—	—	4
Patties	1 (3.4 oz)	220	9	2	40	18	16	1	0	0	300	—	—	1

FOOD	PORTION	CALS	FAT	SAT FAT	CHOL	PROT	CARB	SUGAR	FIBER	CALCI	SOD	POTAS	FOLIC	VIT C
ORGANIC PRAIRIE														
Breast Boneless Skinless	4 oz	150	2	1	90	32	1	1	tr	0	160	—	—	1
Ground	4 oz	200	12	3	95	21	1	—	—	20	90	—	—	0
PERDUE														
Breast Chunks Breaded BBQ Glazed	3 oz	190	8	3	25	11	17	9	—	20	630	—	—	2
Breast Chunks Breaded General Tso's Glazed	3 oz	190	8	3	25	12	16	10	—	20	610	—	—	1
Breast Chunks Breaded Honey BBQ Glazed	3 oz	180	8	3	55	12	17	1	—	0	520	—	—	0
Breast Chunks Breaded Honey Dijon Glazed	3 oz	200	11	2	30	12	16	3	—	20	600	—	—	0
Simply Smart Grilled Chicken Strips	3 oz	110	3	1	55	21	1	0	—	0	340	—	—	0
Simply Smart Lightly Breaded Chicken Strips	3 oz	140	5	1	40	17	6	0	—	0	400	—	—	0
Simply Smart Roasted Chicken Chunks	3 oz	120	2	0	45	23	2	1	—	0	420	—	—	0
TYSON														
Any'tizers Barbeque Style Wings	3 (3.2 oz)	200	13	4	110	19	7	7	0	0	380	—	—	0
Any'tizers Homestyle Chicken Fries	7 (3.2 oz)	230	11	3	25	13	19	0	1	0	590	—	—	0
Any'tizers Popcorn Chicken	6 (2.8 oz)	220	10	2	25	12	19	1	1	0	670	—	—	0
Breast Pattie	1 (2.6 oz)	180	11	3	25	10	12	1	1	0	300	—	—	0
Cordon Bleu	1 piece (5.9 oz)	380	24	8	80	22	20	6	1	100	790	—	—	0
Diced Strips	1 serv (3 oz)	90	1	0	45	20	0	0	0	0	250	—	—	0
Kiev	1 piece (5.9 oz)	480	37	17	150	17	19	6	1	20	420	—	—	0
WEAVER														
Breast Nuggets	4 (2.8 oz)	190	11	2	20	10	13	0	1	20	500	—	—	0
Breast Strips	2 (2.7 oz)	190	12	3	15	10	10	0	0	40	520	—	—	0
Patties Breast	1 (2.9 oz)	200	11	3	20	11	13	0	1	20	530	—	—	0
Popcorn Chicken	12 pieces (2.9 oz)	200	10	2	20	9	19	0	1	20	520	—	—	0
Wings Buffalo Style	3 (2.9 oz)	160	10	2	90	13	3	0	0	0	520	—	—	0

FOOD	PORTION	CALS	FAT	SAT FAT	CHOL	PROT	CARB	SUGAR	FIBER	CALCI	SOD	POTAS	FOLIC	VIT C
READY-TO-EAT														
APPLEGATE FARMS														
Organic Roasted	2 oz	60	2	1	30	10	1	1	0	0	580	—	—	0
BOAR'S HEAD														
Breast Hickory Smoked	2 oz	60	1	0	35	13	0	0	0	0	360	—	—	0
Breast Oven Roasted	2 oz	60	1	0	35	13	0	0	0	0	350	—	—	0
BUTTERBALL														
Breast Oven Roasted Thin Sliced	4 slices (2 oz)	50	1	0	20	11	1	0	0	0	480	—	—	0
Breast Strips Oven Roasted	½ pkg (3 oz)	90	2	1	60	18	1	—	—	—	760	—	—	—
CARL BUDDIG														
Chicken Sliced	2 oz	85	5	—	—	10	1	—	—	—	—	—	—	—
DIETZ & WATSON														
Breast Southern Fried	3 slices (1.9 oz)	70	2	1	30	11	1	1	0	0	390	—	—	0
FOSTER FARMS														
Breast Strips Grilled	3 oz	110	3	—	45	19	2	0	0	—	550	—	—	—
Cutlets Breaded	3 oz	180	8	2	35	13	14	tr	0	0	490	—	—	0
HEALTHY ONES														
Oven Roasted 97% Fat Free	4 slices (2 oz)	60	2	1	25	9	2	tr	0	0	410	—	—	0
HORMEL														
Natural Choice Carved Breast Grilled	½ pkg (2 oz)	60	1	1	35	12	0	0	0	0	230	—	—	0
OSCAR MAYER														
Breast Oven Roasted Thin Sliced	⅓ pkg (2 oz)	60	2	1	30	10	1	1	0	0	710	—	—	0
Breast Strips Breaded	½ pkg (3 oz)	170	6	1	30	15	14	—	—	—	800	—	—	—
Breast Strips Grilled	½ pkg (3 oz)	110	3	1	55	19	1	—	—	—	770	—	—	—
PERDUE														
Breast Bites Popcorn Breaded	12 (3 oz)	190	12	3	30	10	14	1	—	20	580	—	—	0
Breast Strips Breaded Original	2 (2.6 oz)	160	10	3	25	9	12	1	—	0	500	—	—	0
Cutlets Breaded Original	1 (3 oz)	200	13	3	45	10	13	0	—	20	450	—	—	0
Nuggets Original	5 (2.9 oz)	200	13	3	45	10	13	0	—	20	450	—	—	0

FOOD	PORTION	CALS	FAT	SAT FAT	CHOL	PROT	CARB	SUGAR	FIBER	CALCI	SOD	POTAS	FOLIC	VIT C
PERDUE (CONT.)														
Nuggets w/ Whole Grain Breading	4 (2.8 oz)	160	8	2	30	11	13	1	—	0	450	—	—	0
Short Cuts Carved Chicken Breast Original Roasted	½ cup (2.5 oz)	90	2	1	60	16	1	—	—	—	460	—	—	1
Short Cuts Chicken Breast Grilled	½ cup (2.5 oz)	90	2	1	60	16	1	0	—	0	460	—	—	1
SARA LEE														
Breast Oven Roasted	4 slices (2 oz)	45	1	0	25	10	0	0	0	0	430	—	—	0
TYSON														
Chicken Strips Fajita	1 serv (3 oz)	110	2	1	60	19	3	0	0	0	450	—	—	0
Honey Roasted Breast	2 slices (1.6 oz)	50	1	0	15	8	3	2	0	0	530	—	—	0
Hot Wings Buffalo Style	4	220	15	4	110	20	1	0	0	0	560	—	—	0
Roasted Whole Chicken Lemon Pepper	1 serv (3 oz)	120	6	2	75	17	1	1	0	0	510	—	—	0
Salad Kit Chunk Chicken	1 pkg (3.4 oz)	210	9	2	50	18	15	3	1	0	640	—	—	0
TAKE-OUT														
chicken tenders	4 (2.2 oz)	180	10	2	31	11	11	1	tr	9	445	167	10	1

CHICKEN DISHES

FROZEN

BANQUET

FOOD	PORTION	CALS	FAT	SAT FAT	CHOL	PROT	CARB	SUGAR	FIBER	CALCI	SOD	POTAS	FOLIC	VIT C
Boneless Popcorn Chicken	11 pieces	180	9	3	20	8	18	tr	tr	0	510	—	—	0
Wings Honey BBQ	¼ pkg (3 oz)	270	17	5	65	17	12	tr	5	20	520	—	—	0
BARBER														
Broccoli & Cheese Reduced Fat	1 piece (5.5 oz)	250	13	3	55	25	11	1	tr	150	610	—	—	12
Cordon Bleu	1 piece (6 oz)	370	23	7	95	28	14	1	0	150	840	—	—	1
Cordon Bleu Reduced Fat	1 piece (5.5 oz)	260	13	4	75	27	11	1	0	100	700	—	—	1
Creme Brie & Apple	1 piece (6 oz)	350	21	5	90	25	18	8	tr	150	830	—	—	1
Kiev	1 piece (6 oz)	430	29	11	110	27	15	1	tr	40	720	—	—	1
Mashed Potato Stuffed	1 piece (6 oz)	340	18	8	85	21	21	2	tr	20	630	—	—	6
Skinless Breast Stuffed	1 piece (6 oz)	280	11	3	45	21	24	1	tr	20	860	—	—	2

FOOD	PORTION	CALS	FAT	SAT FAT	CHOL	PROT	CARB	SUGAR	FIBER	CALCI	SOD	POTAS	FOLIC	VIT C
CRAZY CUIZINE														
Teriyaki Chicken	1 cup (5 oz)	240	8	2	45	19	23	21	3	0	620	—	—	0
MIX														
CHICKEN HELPER														
Asian Chicken Fried Rice as prep	1 cup	250	8	2	117	3	22	1	1	40	552	245	40	—
Classic Creamy Chicken & Noodles as prep	1 cup	280	8	3	60	3	24	1	tr	100	744	350	40	—
Jambalaya as prep	1 cup	280	8	2	57	3	15	tr	1	60	816	280	40	—
REFRIGERATED														
TYSON														
Chicken Breast Medallions In White Wine & Garlic Sauce	1 serv (5 oz)	140	6	2	45	19	3	0	1	20	500	—	—	0
VENTERA														
Rollatini w/ Rice Stuffing & Marsala Wine Sauce	1 serv + sauce (6 oz)	230	10	5	70	24	9	2	0	40	590	—	—	0
TAKE-OUT														
arroz con pollo	1 serv (16 oz)	579	14	7	126	48	62	3	2	260	1433	—	—	67
barbecued pulled chicken	1 serv (9 oz)	312	2	1	147	36	37	27	2	90	794	—	—	2
boneless breast w/ apple stuffing	1 serv (5 oz)	260	9	2	80	32	10	2	1	30	250	—	—	1
breast & wing breaded & fried	2 pieces (5.7 oz)	494	30	8	148	36	20	—	—	60	975	566	29	0
buffalo wing + sauce	2 (1.7 oz)	147	10	3	39	12	tr	tr	0	7	97	88	1	tr
cacciatore breast + sauce	1 serv (5.9 oz)	323	18	4	88	29	9	3	1	42	422	463	15	8
cacciatore drumstick + sauce	1 serv (3.2 oz)	172	9	2	47	15	5	2	1	22	225	247	8	4
cacciatore thigh + sauce	1 serv (3.8 oz)	204	11	3	56	18	6	2	1	27	268	293	10	5
cacciatore wing + sauce	1 serv (2.1 oz)	113	6	2	31	10	3	1	tr	15	148	132	5	3
chicharrones de pollo	3 (2.6 oz)	289	18	4	58	16	14	tr	1	14	898	158	25	4
chicken & dumplings	1 cup (8.6 oz)	368	19	5	88	26	22	1	1	127	920	293	39	0
chicken & noodles in cream sauce	1 cup (8 oz)	323	11	3	76	22	32	5	1	128	706	276	90	tr
chicken a la king	1 cup (8.5 oz)	465	34	12	190	24	16	4	1	149	880	429	34	6

FOOD	PORTION	CALS	FAT	SAT FAT	CHOL	PROT	CARB	SUGAR	FIBER	CALCI	SOD	POTAS	FOLIC	VIT C
chicken cordon bleu + sauce	1 roll (8 oz)	504	29	15	188	44	11	1	1	197	598	472	21	1
chicken meatloaf	1 lg slice (5 oz)	243	9	3	122	29	11	3	1	73	658	312	29	5
chicken paprikash	1½ cups	296	10	—	90	—	—	—	—	99	—	—	—	—
chicken pie w/ top crust	1 slice (5.6 oz)	472	31	—	—	19	32	—	1	122	—	—	—	0
chicken satay + peanut sauce	2 skewers	239	12	6	64	27	6	4	1	24	439	346	12	tr
chicken breast parmigiana	1 serv (5.8 oz)	278	14	5	119	25	13	3	1	161	684	393	24	3
chicken creole w/o rice	1 cup (8.6 oz)	187	4	1	69	29	8	5	2	52	598	662	17	24
chicken kiev breast meat	1 serv (9 oz)	653	34	16	276	72	11	1	1	59	975	611	23	0
chicken salad white meat	1 serv (4 oz)	300	21	2	85	28	1	0	0	0	450	—	—	0
creamed chicken	1 cup (8.5 oz)	388	23	6	87	30	14	8	tr	186	641	436	24	tr
croquette	1 (2.2 oz)	159	9	2	28	10	8	2	tr	45	239	126	11	1
curry	1 cup (8.3 oz)	288	16	3	83	27	9	5	2	40	1187	588	21	12
curry breast half + sauce	1 (7 oz)	244	14	3	70	23	8	4	2	34	1006	498	18	10
curry drumstick + sauce	1 (3.7 oz)	129	7	1	37	12	4	2	1	18	533	264	10	6
curry thigh + sauce	1 (4.4 oz)	154	9	2	44	14	5	3	1	21	634	314	11	7
curry wing + sauce	1 (2.4 oz)	84	5	1	24	8	3	1	1	12	347	172	6	4
drumstick & thigh breaded & fried	2 pieces (5.2 oz)	431	27	7	166	30	16	—	—	36	755	445	25	0
fricassee	1 cup (8.6 oz)	322	18	5	85	29	8	tr	tr	20	695	295	22	0
groundnut stew hkatenkwan	1 serv (15.7 oz)	576	40	10	116	38	18	3	4	79	1009	973	51	21
jamaican jerk wings	4 wings (9.9 oz)	709	51	14	172	57	3	tr	tr	51	1045	402	10	4
jambalaya w/ sausage & rice	1 cup (8.6 oz)	393	21	6	98	26	23	2	1	46	488	412	49	6
kobete turkish chicken w/ pastry	1 serv	513	13	4	71	—	—	—	—	—	551	—	—	—
rotisserie seasoned breast w/ skin	1 serv (3.5 oz)	184	8	2	96	27	0	0	0	15	347	289	11	0
rotisserie seasoned breast w/o skin	1 serv (3.5 oz)	148	3	1	89	29	0	0	0	14	314	296	11	0
rotisserie seasoned thigh w/ skin	1 serv (3.5 oz)	233	16	4	132	23	0	0	0	15	345	260	12	0
rotisserie seasoned thigh w/o skin	1 serv (3.5 oz)	196	11	3	130	24	0	0	0	13	337	264	12	0
sancocho de pollo dominican chicken stew	1 serv	702	30	8	195	71	34	4	1	72	653	1324	52	49

FOOD	PORTION	CALS	FAT	SAT FAT	CHOL	PROT	CARB	SUGAR	FIBER	CALCI	SOD	POTAS	FOLIC	VIT C
stew	1 cup (8.8 oz)	176	5	1	43	15	19	4	3	40	496	580	30	12
tandoori chicken breast	1 serv	260	13	—	—	—	5	—	—	—	—	—	—	—
tandoori chicken leg & thigh	1 serv	300	17	—	—	—	6	—	—	—	—	—	—	—
tetrazzini	1 cup (8.6 oz)	369	18	6	49	20	29	2	2	130	669	204	59	5

CHICKEN SUBSTITUTES

CHICKEN FREE CHICKEN

FOOD	PORTION	CALS	FAT	SAT FAT	CHOL	PROT	CARB	SUGAR	FIBER	CALCI	SOD	POTAS	FOLIC	VIT C
Country Smoked	2 oz	80	2	0	0	11	5	1	0	80	245	—	—	1

GARDEIN

FOOD	PORTION	CALS	FAT	SAT FAT	CHOL	PROT	CARB	SUGAR	FIBER	CALCI	SOD	POTAS	FOLIC	VIT C
Buffalo Wings	1 serv (3.5 oz)	120	3	0	0	16	8	1	2	100	630	—	—	1
Chick'n Filets	1 (3.5 oz)	120	2	0	0	20	7	1	2	40	470	—	—	0
Chick'n Scallopini	1 piece (2.5 oz)	90	2	0	0	14	4	0	2	80	330	—	—	0
Crispy Fingers	2 (3.2 oz)	160	5	1	0	16	12	1	2	80	430	—	—	1
Crispy Tenders	1 (1.8 oz)	90	2	0	0	9	9	0	1	40	260	—	—	0
Tuscan Breasts	1 (5.3 oz)	150	3	0	0	22	11	1	3	150	550	—	—	2

GARDENBURGER

FOOD	PORTION	CALS	FAT	SAT FAT	CHOL	PROT	CARB	SUGAR	FIBER	CALCI	SOD	POTAS	FOLIC	VIT C
Chik'n Grill	1 (2.5 oz)	100	3	0	0	13	5	0	5	40	360	—	—	0

HEALTH IS WEALTH

FOOD	PORTION	CALS	FAT	SAT FAT	CHOL	PROT	CARB	SUGAR	FIBER	CALCI	SOD	POTAS	FOLIC	VIT C
Chicken-Free Nuggets	3 pieces (2.9 oz)	120	2	0	0	14	14	0	2	60	450	—	—	0

LIGHTLIFE

FOOD	PORTION	CALS	FAT	SAT FAT	CHOL	PROT	CARB	SUGAR	FIBER	CALCI	SOD	POTAS	FOLIC	VIT C
Smart Menu Chick'n Nuggets	4 pieces	220	11	2	0	14	16	1	2	—	520	130	—	—
Smart Menu Chick'n Patties	1 patty	160	7	1	0	11	14	0	2	—	540	110	—	—

LOMA LINDA

FOOD	PORTION	CALS	FAT	SAT FAT	CHOL	PROT	CARB	SUGAR	FIBER	CALCI	SOD	POTAS	FOLIC	VIT C
Fried Chik'n w/ Gravy	2 pieces (2.8 oz)	150	10	2	0	12	5	0	2	20	430	70	—	0

MORNINGSTAR FARMS

FOOD	PORTION	CALS	FAT	SAT FAT	CHOL	PROT	CARB	SUGAR	FIBER	CALCI	SOD	POTAS	FOLIC	VIT C
Chik'n Roasted Herb	1 pattie (2.2 oz)	110	3	1	0	13	9	1	2	20	380	210	—	0
Meal Starters Chik'n Strips	12 pieces (3 oz)	140	4	1	0	23	6	1	1	40	510	110	—	0

QUORN

FOOD	PORTION	CALS	FAT	SAT FAT	CHOL	PROT	CARB	SUGAR	FIBER	CALCI	SOD	POTAS	FOLIC	VIT C
Naked Cutlet	1 (2.4 oz)	80	3	1	5	11	5	0	2	50	420	—	—	0

VEAT

FOOD	PORTION	CALS	FAT	SAT FAT	CHOL	PROT	CARB	SUGAR	FIBER	CALCI	SOD	POTAS	FOLIC	VIT C
Chick'n Free Nuggets	1 serv (2.5 oz)	140	5	0	0	21	5	2	2	100	690	—	—	2
Vegetarian Breast	1 (1.8 oz)	90	3	1	0	11	5	1	tr	60	280	—	—	0

VEGGIE PATCH

FOOD	PORTION	CALS	FAT	SAT FAT	CHOL	PROT	CARB	SUGAR	FIBER	CALCI	SOD	POTAS	FOLIC	VIT C
Chick'n Nuggets	4 (2.7 oz)	170	7	1	0	9	20	1	2	200	440	310	16	0

VIANA

FOOD	PORTION	CALS	FAT	SAT FAT	CHOL	PROT	CARB	SUGAR	FIBER	CALCI	SOD	POTAS	FOLIC	VIT C
Veggie Chickin Fillets	1 (3.7 oz)	260	14	3	0	29	8	5	4	60	890	—	—	0

FOOD	PORTION	CALS	FAT	SAT FAT	CHOL	PROT	CARB	SUGAR	FIBER	CALCI	SOD	POTAS	FOLIC	VIT C
VIANA (CONT.)														
Veggie Chickin Nuggets	3 pieces (2.6 oz)	200	12	2	0	16	8	1	2	40	590	—	—	0
WORTHINGTON														
FriChik Original	2 pieces (3.2 oz)	140	8	1	0	12	3	0	1	20	430	90	—	0
Meatless Chicken Style	1 slice (2 oz)	90	5	1	0	9	2	0	1	100	240	240	—	0
YVES														
Meatless Smoked Chicken Slices	4 (2.2 oz)	100	2	0	0	14	5	1	0	20	460	220	—	18
CHICKPEAS														
CANNED														
chickpeas	1 cup	285	3	tr	0	12	54	—	—	78	718	413	160	9
ALLENS														
Garbanzo Beans	½ cup	120	3	0	0	5	19	0	8	20	330	—	—	0
EDEN														
Organic Garbanzo	½ cup	130	1	0	0	7	23	tr	5	60	30	250	—	—
GREEN GIANT														
Garbanzo Beans	½ cup	100	2	0	0	5	17	2	4	20	430	—	—	0
PROGRESSO														
Chick Peas	½ cup (4.6 oz)	120	3	0	0	5	20	3	5	40	280	—	—	0
DRIED														
cooked	1 cup	269	4	tr	0	15	45	—	—	80	11	477	282	2
ARROWHEAD MILLS														
Organic Dried Chickpeas not prep	¼ cup	160	3	0	0	9	27	5	8	40	10	390	–	2
FROZEN														
TANDOOR CHEF														
Channa Masala	½ pkg (5 oz)	190	9	1	5	5	22	6	7	60	640	—	—	2
CHICORY														
endive fresh chopped	½ cup	4	tr	tr	0	tr	1	—	—	13	6	79	36	2
greens raw chopped	½ cup	21	tr	tr	0	2	4	—	—	90	41	378	—	22
root raw	1 (2.1 oz)	44	tr	tr	0	1	11	—	—	25	30	174	—	3
roots raw cut up	½ cup (1.6 oz)	33	tr	tr	0	1	8	—	—	18	23	131	—	2
witloof head raw	1 (1.9 oz)	9	tr	tr	0	tr	2	—	—	10	1	112	20	2
witloof raw	½ cup (1.6 oz)	8	tr	tr	0	tr	2	—	—	9	1	95	17	1
CHILI														
powder	1 tbsp	24	1	tr	0	1	4	1	3	21	76	144	8	5
AHH!GOURMET														
Wriggly Sambal Chili Sauce Paste	4 tbsp	170	9	1	32	7	15	11	4	103	391	—	—	tr

FOOD	PORTION	CALS	FAT	SAT FAT	CHOL	PROT	CARB	SUGAR	FIBER	CALCI	SOD	POTAS	FOLIC	VIT C
ALLERGAROO														
Gluten Free Chili Mac	1 pkg (8 oz)	240	4	1	0	5	50	8	3	40	700	—	—	9
AMY'S														
Organic Black Bean Medium	1 cup	200	2	0	0	13	31	3	15	80	680	—	—	18
Whole Meals Chili & Cornbread	1 pkg	340	6	3	10	11	59	14	10	100	680	—	—	15
COMFORT CARE														
Vegetarian White	1 cup (8 oz)	150	2	0	0	11	26	4	5	100	310	—	—	18
DENNISON'S														
Con Carne	1 cup	350	15	7	40	22	31	2	11	60	970	—	—	0
Fat Free w/ Beans	1 cup	210	2	1	60	20	29	2	8	40	1020	—	—	2
Turkey	1 cup	210	3	2	45	16	29	3	7	100	850	—	—	4
Vegetarian	1 cup	190	2	0	0	9	34	6	9	100	800	—	—	0
DYNASTY														
Thai Chili Garlic Paste	1 tsp (5 g)	0	0	0	0	0	0	0	0	—	40	—	—	9
FANTASTIC														
3 Bean	1 pkg (8 oz)	180	4	0	0	10	28	5	5	100	680	—	—	6
Vegetarian Mix not prep	¼ cup	100	1	0	0	8	17	4	4	60	480	—	—	5
FRONTERA														
Chili Mix Chipotle Black Bean	½ cup (4.2 oz)	60	1	0	0	3	12	3	3	40	910	—	—	9
Chili Starter Green Chile White Bean	½ cup (4.4 oz)	80	2	0	0	3	14	2	4	40	450	—	—	12
HEALTH VALLEY														
Chunky Spicy Vegetarian No Salt Added	1 cup	150	1	0	0	9	31	5	10	100	75	—	—	18
Vegetarian Spicy	1 cup	150	1	0	0	9	31	5	10	100	480	—	—	18
HEINZ														
Chili Sauce	1 tbsp (0.6 oz)	20	0	0	0	0	5	3	0	0	230	—	—	0
HIGH PLAINS BISON														
Campfire Chili	1 cup (8 oz)	190	6	3	100	15	18	8	6	80	720	—	—	12
HORMEL														
Chili Mac	1 pkg (9.9 oz)	270	7	3	30	17	34	10	6	100	980	—	—	4
Chili No Beans	1 pkg (7.3 oz)	190	8	4	35	14	16	3	2	20	860	—	—	0
Chili No Beans Less Sodium	1 serv (8.3 oz)	220	9	4	40	16	18	3	3	40	710	—	—	0
Chili w/ Beans	1 serv (8.7 oz)	260	7	3	30	16	33	5	7	60	1200	—	—	0
Chili w/ Beans Less Sodium	1 serv (8.7 oz)	260	7	3	30	16	33	5	7	60	880	—	—	0

FOOD	PORTION	CALS	FAT	SAT FAT	CHOL	PROT	CARB	SUGAR	FIBER	CALCI	SOD	POTAS	FOLIC	VIT C
HORMEL (CONT.)														
Turkey Chili w/ Beans	1 serv (8.7 oz)	210	3	1	45	17	28	6	6	80	1250	—	—	0
Vegetarian Chili w/ Beans	1 serv (8.7 oz)	190	1	0	0	11	35	6	10	60	780	—	—	0
LIGHTLIFE														
Smart Chili	1 pkg	200	0	0	0	14	34	8	12	—	1120	870	—	—
MASTER CHILI														
Chipotle Chicken No Bean	1 serv (8.3 oz)	230	10	4	95	18	18	7	3	20	990	—	—	2
Roasted Tomato w/ Bean	1 serv (8.7 oz)	210	6	2	25	14	25	7	7	40	990	—	—	0
MCILHENNY														
Original Recipe	½ cup	50	1	0	0	2	10	5	3	80	610	—	—	2
MEALS TO LIVE														
White Chicken Chili Relleno w/ Ranchero Sauce	1 pkg (9 oz)	210	5	2	25	15	20	10	4	—	480	—	—	258
MIMI'S GOURMET														
Organic Vegan Gluten Free 3 Bean w/ Rice	1 pkg (11.5 oz)	270	6	1	0	10	46	9	10	150	670	—	—	36
Organic Vegan Gluten Free Black Bean & Corn	1 pkg (10.5 oz)	250	6	1	0	10	40	9	11	150	680	—	—	42
Organic Vegan Gluten Free White Bean	1 pkg (10.5 oz)	230	6	1	0	10	35	11	9	150	660	—	—	42
SPICE HUNTER														
Powder Blend Salt Free	¼ tsp	0	0	0	0	0	0	0	0	—	0	—	—	—
STAGG														
Turkey Ranchero w/ Beans	1 cup	240	3	1	35	22	31	6	6	60	880	—	—	4
THAI KITCHEN														
Roasted Red Chili Paste	1 tbsp (0.5 oz)	50	3	0	5	1	6	4	0	20	180	—	—	1
TRUITT BROTHERS														
Beef Natural Shredded	1 cup (9.4 oz)	240	5	2	25	16	32	4	7	100	1110	—	—	4
Vegetarian	1 cup (9.4 oz)	220	2	0	0	11	42	5	10	80	920	—	—	1
WORTHINGTON														
Vegetarian	1 cup	280	10	2	0	24	25	3	8	40	1130	330	—	0
TAKE-OUT														
chiles rellenos cheese filled	1 (5 oz)	365	30	13	167	17	8	5	1	399	496	376	29	111

FOOD	PORTION	CALS	FAT	SAT FAT	CHOL	PROT	CARB	SUGAR	FIBER	CALCI	SOD	POTAS	FOLIC	VIT C
chili con carne w/ beans	1 cup	264	11	4	53	21	22	6	7	74	1275	693	43	11
chili con carne w/ beans & chicken	1 cup (8.9 oz)	218	7	2	53	19	19	6	6	69	945	643	30	10
con carne w/ beans & rice	1 cup	298	9	4	28	11	45	2	7	82	1172	598	90	3
vegetarian con carne	1 cup	272	7	1	0	19	35	7	11	64	1090	917	155	13

CHILI PEPPER

(*see* PEPPERS)

CHINESE FOOD

(*see* ASIAN FOOD)

CHINESE PRESERVING MELON

FOOD	PORTION	CALS	FAT	SAT FAT	CHOL	PROT	CARB	SUGAR	FIBER	CALCI	SOD	POTAS	FOLIC	VIT C
cooked	½ cup	11	tr	tr	0	tr	3	—	—	16	93	5	—	9

CHIPS

(*see also* SNACKS)

FOOD	PORTION	CALS	FAT	SAT FAT	CHOL	PROT	CARB	SUGAR	FIBER	CALCI	SOD	POTAS	FOLIC	VIT C
apple chips	10 (0.8 oz)	101	5	tr	0	tr	16	14	2	3	22	100	0	tr
banana	1 oz	147	10	8	0	1	17	10	2	5	2	152	4	2
carrot	28 (1 oz)	95	tr	tr	0	2	22	11	7	59	77	711	15	4
corn	1 oz	147	8	1	0	2	18	tr	2	46	175	38	4	0
plantain	1 oz	158	10	2	—	tr	16	—	1	2	111	198	10	—
potato salted	1 oz	155	11	3	0	2	14	tr	1	7	149	466	21	5
potato sticks	½ cup (0.6 oz)	94	6	2	0	1	10	tr	1	3	45	223	7	9
potato sticks	1 pkg (1 oz)	148	10	3	0	2	15	tr	1	3	45	223	7	9
potato unsalted	1 oz	152	10	3	0	2	15	tr	1	7	2	361	13	9
potato unsalted reduced fat	1 oz	138	6	1	0	2	19	tr	2	6	2	494	3	7
shrimp	4 lg (1.4 oz)	219	14	4	33	3	20	1	tr	27	551	13	2	tr
shrimp	4 sm (0.4 oz)	56	4	1	8	1	5	tr	tr	7	142	3	0	tr
shrimp	4 med (0.9 oz)	141	9	2	21	2	13	tr	tr	17	355	8	1	tr
soy	1 oz	107	2	0	0	8	15	1	1	48	239	0	68	0
sweet potato	1 oz	141	7	1	0	1	18	2	1	20	10	262	10	0
taro	10 (0.8 oz)	115	6	1	0	1	16	1	2	14	79	174	5	1
tortilla lowfat baked	1 oz	118	2	tr	0	3	23	tr	2	45	119	77	5	tr
tortilla lowfat unsalted	1 oz	118	2	tr	0	3	23	tr	2	45	4	77	5	tr
tortilla white corn	1 oz	139	7	1	0	2	19	tr	2	49	119	61	6	0
tortilla yellow corn	1 oz	139	6	1	0	2	19	tr	1	27	80	62	—	—
BACHMAN														
Corn Jumbo Chipitos	16 (1 oz)	150	8	2	0	1	18	0	2	40	170	—	—	0
Potato Golden Ridges	22 (1 oz)	160	10	3	<5	2	15	—	0	0	140	—	—	15
Tortilla Black Bean	1 oz	140	7	1	0	2	18	—	3	40	135	—	—	0

FOOD	PORTION	CALS	FAT	SAT FAT	CHOL	PROT	CARB	SUGAR	FIBER	CALCI	SOD	POTAS	FOLIC	VIT C
BACHMAN (CONT.)														
Tortilla Restaurant Style	11 (1 oz)	140	6	1	0	2	19	0	2	40	50	—	—	0
Tortilla Toasted Sweet Potato	11 (1 oz)	130	5	1	0	2	20	2	3	40	70	—	—	6
BEANFIELDS														
Bean & Rice Naturally Unsalted	⅙ pkg (1 oz)	140	6	0	0	4	18	0	3	40	5	—	—	0
Bean & Rice Pico De Gallo	⅙ pkg (1 oz)	140	6	0	0	4	18	0	4	40	190	—	—	0
Bean & Rice Sea Salt	⅙ pkg (1 oz)	140	6	0	0	4	18	0	4	40	140	—	—	0
Bean & Rice Sea Salt & Pepper	⅙ pkg (1 oz)	140	6	0	0	4	18	0	4	40	160	—	—	0
BEANITOS														
Pinto Bean & Flax	10 (1 oz)	150	8	1	0	4	14	0	5	20	190	—	—	0
BETTER BALANCE														
Protein Chips Gluten Free All Flavors	1 oz	110	4	0	0	10	14	0	3	40	230	—	—	0
BETTY CROCKER														
Potato Kettle Cooked Lightly Salted	1 oz	120	5	1	0	2	15	0	1	0	105	—	—	9
BOULDER CANYON														
Potato 50% Reduced Salt	14 (1 oz)	150	8	1	0	2	17	0	2	0	68	—	—	6
Potato Sour Cream & Chive	14 (1 oz)	150	8	1	0	2	15	1	2	0	205	—	—	9
Potato Spinach & Artichoke	14 (1 oz)	150	8	1	0	2	17	0	2	20	334	—	—	6
BROTHERS-ALL-NATURAL														
Potato Crisps Fresh Onion & Fresh Garlic	1 pkg	45	0	0	0	1	10	0	1	0	250	—	—	0
Potato Crisps Original w/ Sea Salt	1 pkg	45	0	0	0	1	10	0	1	0	280	—	—	1
BUFFALO NICKEL WINGERS														
Potato Level 1: No Bull Barbecue	25 (1 oz)	120	4	0	0	1	19	2	1	0	350	—	—	0
Potato Level 3: Nacho Chiliehanga	25 (1 oz)	120	4	0	0	1	19	1	1	0	420	—	—	0
Potato Level 5: Fiery Buffalo Bleu	25 (1 oz)	120	4	0	0	1	19	1	1	0	420	—	—	0

FOOD	PORTION	CALS	FAT	SAT FAT	CHOL	PROT	CARB	SUGAR	FIBER	CALCI	SOD	POTAS	FOLIC	VIT C
BURGER KING														
Potato Flame Broiled	16 (1 oz)	150	8	1	0	1	19	1	1	0	170	—	—	0
Potato Ketchup & Fries	16 (1 oz)	150	8	1	0	1	19	1	1	0	240	—	—	0
BUTTERFIELD														
Potato Sticks Shoestring	1 pkg (1.7 oz)	250	15	5	0	3	26	0	3	20	150	—	—	15
CORAZONAS														
Potato Lightly Salted	1 oz	130	6	1	0	3	18	0	2	0	90	—	—	6
Potato Parmesan Peppercorn	1 oz	140	6	1	0	2	18	tr	2	0	160	—	—	6
Potato Spicy Rio Habanero	1 oz	130	6	1	0	2	18	1	2	0	120	—	—	6
Tortilla Lightly Salted	14 (1 oz)	140	7	1	0	2	18	0	3	20	75	—	—	0
Tortilla Squeeze Of Lime	14 (1 oz)	140	7	1	0	2	17	0	3	20	170	—	—	0
DEEP RIVER SNACKS														
Potato Baked Fries Sweet Maui Onion	1 oz	135	5	1	0	3	19	2	1	30	235	—	—	2
Potato Kettle Cooked Asian Sweet & Spicy	1 oz	150	8	2	0	2	15	3	1	0	160	—	—	6
Potato Kettle Cooked Original Salted	1 oz	150	8	2	0	2	16	0	1	0	110	—	—	6
Potato Kettle Cooked Rosemary & Olive Oil	1 oz	150	8	2	0	2	16	1	1	0	180	—	—	6
Potato Kettle Cooked Salt & Vinegar	1 oz	150	8	2	0	2	15	0	1	0	240	—	—	6
Potato Zesty Jalapeno	1 oz	150	8	2	0	2	15	0	1	0	240	—	—	6
DORITOS														
Tortilla Flamas	11 (1 oz)	140	8	1	0	2	16	0	1	0	200	—	—	0
Tortilla Nacho Cheese	11 (1 oz)	150	8	2	0	2	17	1	1	0	210	—	—	0
Tortilla Spicy Nacho	12 (1 oz)	140	7	1	0	2	19	1	1	20	210	—	—	0
Tortilla Toasted Corn	13 (1 oz)	140	7	1	0	2	18	0	1	40	120	—	—	0

FOOD	PORTION	CALS	FAT	SAT FAT	CHOL	PROT	CARB	SUGAR	FIBER	CALCI	SOD	POTAS	FOLIC	VIT C
EDEN														
Vegetable	25	130	4	2	0	tr	24	2	0	0	260	35	—	0
Wasabi	25	130	4	2	0	tr	24	2	0	0	260	35	—	0
FLAT EARTH														
Baked Fruit Crisps Apple Cinnamon Grove	14 (1 oz)	130	5	1	0	1	21	6	2	20	35	105	—	6
Baked Fruit Crisps Peach Mango Paradise	14 (1 oz)	130	5	1	0	1	21	7	1	20	35	95	—	6
Baked Fruit Crisps Wild Berry Patch	14 (1 oz)	130	5	1	0	1	21	6	1	20	40	100	—	6
Baked Veggie Crisps Farmland Cheddar	14 (1 oz)	130	5	1	0	2	19	3	2	20	190	170	—	6
Baked Veggie Crisps Garlic & Herb Field	14 (1 oz)	130	5	1	0	2	19	3	2	20	190	170	—	6
Baked Veggie Crisps Tangy Tomato Ranch	14 (1 oz)	130	5	1	0	2	19	3	2	20	210	180	—	6
FOODSHOULDTASTEGOOD														
Tortilla Buffalo	10 (1 oz)	130	6	1	0	2	18	1	3	20	270	—	—	0
Tortilla Chocolate Gluten Free	1 pkg (1 oz)	140	7	1	0	2	19	4	3	20	80	—	—	0
Tortilla Multigrain Gluten Free	1 pkg (1 oz)	140	7	1	0	3	18	2	3	20	80	—	—	0
Tortilla Sweet Potato Gluten Free	10 (1 oz)	130	6	1	0	2	18	2	3	20	80	—	—	0
FRENCH'S														
Potato Sticks Barbecue	¾ cup	160	10	5	0	2	16	2	1	40	190	—	—	0
Potato Sticks Cheddar	¾ cup	170	12	5	0	2	14	tr	tr	150	200	—	—	0
Potato Sticks Original	¾ cup	190	12	5	0	2	16	0	1	80	190	—	—	0
FRITOS														
Corn Lightly Salted	1 oz	160	10	2	0	2	16	0	1	20	80	—	—	0
Corn Original	32 (1 oz)	160	10	2	0	2	15	tr	1	20	170	—	—	0
Corn Scoops	10 (1 oz)	160	10	2	0	2	16	0	1	40	110	—	—	0
FRONTERA														
Tortilla Blue Corn	⅑ pkg (1 oz)	130	5	1	0	2	20	0	2	40	75	—	—	0
Tortilla Thick & Crunchy	⅑ pkg (1 oz)	130	5	1	0	2	20	0	2	40	75	—	—	1

FOOD	PORTION	CALS	FAT	SAT FAT	CHOL	PROT	CARB	SUGAR	FIBER	CALCI	SOD	POTAS	FOLIC	VIT C
GLENNY'S														
Organic Soy Barbeque	1 oz	110	3	0	—	8	13	3	3	—	350	—	—	—
Organic Soy Creamy Ranch	1 oz	110	3	0	—	9	12	1	3	—	300	—	—	—
Soy Crisps Apple Cinnamon	½ pkg (0.6 oz)	70	2	0	—	5	10	2	2	—	90	—	—	—
Soy Crisps Caramel	½ pkg (1.3 oz)	70	2	0	0	5	9	2	1	—	125	—	—	—
Soy Crisps Low Fat Lightly Salted	½ pkg (0.6 oz)	70	1	0	—	5	9	1	2	—	170	—	—	—
Soy Crisps No Salt	½ pkg (0.6 oz)	70	1	0	—	5	9	1	2	—	100	—	—	—
Soy Crisps Salt & Pepper	½ pkg (0.6 oz)	70	1	0	—	5	9	1	2	—	190	—	—	—
Soy Crisps White Cheddar	½ pkg (0.6 oz)	70	2	0	—	5	9	1	2	—	180	—	—	—
Spud Delites Sea Salt	1 pkg (1.1 oz)	100	1	0	—	2	21	0	1	—	270	—	—	—
Veggie Fries	½ pkg (0.6 oz)	70	1	0	0	1	13	0	0	—	120	—	—	—
Zen Health Tortilla Crisps Original	1 oz	110	3	0	0	9	12	0	tr	—	250	—	—	—
GUILTLESS GOURMET														
Tortilla Blue Corn	18 (1 oz)	120	3	0	0	3	23	0	2	40	250	—	—	0
Tortilla Chili Lime	18 (1 oz)	120	3	0	0	2	19	0	2	0	150	—	—	0
Tortilla Chipotle	18 (1 oz)	123	3	0	0	2	22	1	2	60	250	—	—	0
Tortilla Yellow Corn	18 (1 oz)	120	3	0	0	2	22	0	2	0	250	—	—	0
Tortilla Yellow Corn Unsalted	18 (1 oz)	120	2	0	0	3	22	1	2	60	26	—	—	0
HIPPIE CHIPS														
Baked Potato Chive-Talkin' Sour Cream	1 pkg (0.7 oz)	90	3	0	0	2	14	1	tr	20	300	—	—	1
Baked Potato Haight AshBerry Jalapeno	1 pkg (0.7 oz)	90	3	0	0	1	15	2	tr	0	310	—	—	1
Baked Potato Memphis Blues Barbecue	1 pkg (0.7 oz)	90	3	0	0	1	15	2	tr	0	310	—	—	1
Baked Potato Sea Of Love Salt	1 pkg (1 oz)	125	4	0	0	2	21	0	1	0	280	—	—	2
Baked Potato Woodstock Ranch	1 pkg (0.7 oz)	90	3	0	0	2	14	1	tr	20	300	—	—	1
JAY'S														
Potato	1 oz	150	10	2	0	2	14	0	1	0	190	—	—	5

FOOD	PORTION	CALS	FAT	SAT FAT	CHOL	PROT	CARB	SUGAR	FIBER	CALCI	SOD	POTAS	FOLIC	VIT C
KETTLE														
Bakes Potato Aged White Cheddar	1 oz	120	3	1	0	3	20	1	2	20	170	430	—	9
Bakes Potato Hickory Honey Barbeque	1 oz	120	3	0	0	3	21	0	2	0	160	420	—	9
Bakes Potato Lightly Salted	1 oz	120	3	0	0	3	21	0	2	0	115	450	—	9
Krinkle Cut Potato Barbeque	1 oz	150	9	1	0	2	16	1	2	150	170	420	—	0
Krinkle Cut Potato Dill & Sour Cream	1 oz	150	9	1	0	2	16	1	2	20	170	420	—	9
Krinkle Cut Potato Lightly Salted	1 oz	150	9	1	0	2	15	0	2	0	115	430	—	9
Krinkle Cut Potato Salt & Fresh Ground Pepper	1 oz	150	9	1	0	2	16	0	2	0	200	420	—	9
Organic Tortilla Blue Corn	1 oz	140	6	1	0	3	18	0	2	40	80	25	—	0
Organic Tortilla Brown Rice & Black Bean w/ Garlic & Onions	1 oz	120	6	1	0	3	16	0	2	150	85	20	—	0
Organic Tortilla Fire Roasted Chili	1 oz	140	7	1	0	3	18	0	2	60	150	5	—	1
Organic Tortilla Five Grain Yellow Corn	1 oz	140	6	1	0	2	18	0	2	40	80	35	—	0
Organic Tortilla Lightly Salted Yellow Corn	1 oz	140	6	1	0	2	19	0	2	40	80	25	—	0
Organic Tortilla Little Dippers	1 oz	140	6	1	0	2	19	0	2	40	80	25	—	0
Organic Tortilla Sesame Blue Moons	1 oz	150	8	1	0	3	18	0	2	30	80	25	—	0
Potato Cheddar Beer	1 oz	150	9	1	0	2	15	2	1	0	180	430	—	9
Potato Honey Dijon	1 oz	150	9	1	0	2	16	1	1	0	150	410	—	9
Potato Sea Salt & Vinegar	1 oz	150	9	1	0	2	16	0	1	0	160	410	—	9
Potato Spicy Thai	1 oz	150	9	1	0	2	15	2	1	0	180	430	—	9
Potato Unsalted	1 oz	150	9	1	0	2	15	0	2	0	0	430	—	9
Potato Yogurt & Green Onion	1 oz	150	9	1	0	2	15	0	1	20	190	430	—	9

FOOD	PORTION	CALS	FAT	SAT FAT	CHOL	PROT	CARB	SUGAR	FIBER	CALCI	SOD	POTAS	FOLIC	VIT C
LATE JULY														
Organic Multigrain Dude Ranch	13 (1 oz)	120	5	1	0	2	17	0	2	20	190	—	—	1
Organic Multigrain Mild Green Mojo	13 (1 oz)	110	5	0	0	2	17	1	2	20	210	—	—	0
LAY'S														
Potato Balsamic Sweet Onion	15 (1 oz)	160	10	1	0	2	16	2	1	0	160	320	—	6
Potato Chipotle Ranch	15 (1 oz)	160	10	1	0	2	15	1	1	20	170	340	—	6
Potato Classic	15 (1 oz)	160	10	1	0	2	15	tr	1	0	170	350	—	6
Potato Garden Tomato & Basil	15 (1 oz)	160	10	1	0	2	16	2	1	20	170	420	—	6
Potato Kettle Cooked Crinkle Cut Spice Rubbed BBQ	15 (1 oz)	140	8	1	0	2	17	2	1	0	130	350	—	6
Potato Kettle Cooked Original	16 (1 oz)	160	9	1	0	2	16	tr	1	0	90	370	—	6
Potato Kettle Cooked Spicy Cayenne & Cheese	16 (1 oz)	150	9	1	0	2	16	1	1	0	140	350	—	6
Potato Lightly Salted	15 (1 oz)	160	10	1	0	2	16	tr	1	0	85	350	—	6
Potato Original Baked	15 (1 oz)	120	2	0	0	2	23	2	2	0	135	270	—	2
Potato Stax Sour Cream & Onion	12 (1 oz)	150	9	3	0	2	17	1	1	0	190	—	—	1
Potato Sweet Southern Heat Barbecue	15 (1 oz)	160	10	1	0	2	16	2	1	0	150	310	—	6
Potato Wavy Original	11 (1 oz)	160	10	1	0	2	15	tr	1	0	140	340	—	6
LITTLE WINGS														
Multi Grain Hot Buffalo Wing w/ Bleu Cheese Drizzle	1 pkg (0.5 oz)	60	3	1	0	1	10	2	2	100	200	—	—	0
LUNDBERG														
Rice Chips Original Sea Salt	1 oz	140	7	1	0	2	18	0	tr	0	110	35	—	0
Rice Chips Sesame Seaweed	1 oz	140	7	1	0	2	18	0	tr	0	90	35	—	0
Rice Chips Wasabi	1 oz	140	6	1	0	2	18	1	1	20	210	—	—	1

FOOD	PORTION	CALS	FAT	SAT FAT	CHOL	PROT	CARB	SUGAR	FIBER	CALCI	SOD	POTAS	FOLIC	VIT C
MADHOUSE MUNCHIES														
Potato Sea Salt	16	150	9	1	0	2	16	0	1	0	80	—	—	6
Potato Sea Salt & Vinegar	16	150	9	1	0	2	16	0	2	0	130	—	—	6
Tortilla White	9	140	6	0	0	2	19	0	1	0	110	—	—	0
MARGARITAVILLE														
Tortilla Sea Salt	1 oz	140	7	1	0	2	16	0	0	40	90	—	—	0
MAUI STYLE														
Potato	14 (1 oz)	150	9	1	0	2	16	tr	1	0	140	360	—	0
Shrimp Chips	1 oz	150	8	1	0	0	18	0	tr	0	280	—	—	0
MEDITERRANEAN SNACKS														
Baked Lentil Cucumber Dill	22 (1 oz)	110	3	0	0	4	19	1	3	60	210	—	—	0
Baked Lentil Roasted Pepper	22 (1 oz)	110	3	0	0	4	19	2	3	40	190	—	—	9
Baked Lentil Sea Salt	22 (1 oz)	110	3	0	0	4	19	0	3	60	180	—	—	0
Multi Grain Original	16 (1 oz)	130	6	1	0	2	17	2	1	0	225	—	—	0
Veggie Medley Original	28 (1 oz)	130	7	1	0	1	15	1	1	0	250	—	—	12
MEXI-SNAX														
Tortilla Multi-Grain Blue	15 (1 oz)	140	7	1	0	2	17	0	2	40	110	—	—	0
Tortilla Pico De Gallo	15 (1 oz)	140	7	0	0	2	18	0	2	20	185	—	—	0
Tortilla Salted	15 (1 oz)	140	7	1	0	2	18	0	2	20	70	—	—	0
Tortilla Tamari	15 (1 oz)	130	6	0	0	2	17	0	2	20	170	—	—	0
MICHAEL SEASON'S														
Popped Black Bean Nacho	17 (1 oz)	120	4	0	0	4	20	1	3	40	135	—	—	1
Popped Black Bean Red Pepper	17 (1 oz)	120	4	0	0	4	20	1	3	40	140	—	—	9
Popped Black Bean Sea Salt	17 (1 oz)	120	4	0	0	4	20	1	3	40	130	—	—	0
Potato Kettle Style Reduced Fat	18	130	6	1	0	2	18	1	1	0	240	—	—	6
Potato Reduced Fat	20	140	7	1	0	2	17	0	1	0	130	—	—	9
Potato Reduced Fat Unsalted	20	140	7	1	0	2	17	0	1	0	10	—	—	9
Potato Crisps Thin Baked Low Fat	14	120	2	0	0	2	23	2	2	40	180	—	—	2
POORE BROTHERS														
Original	14 (1 oz)	140	9	3	0	2	15	tr	1	0	180	—	—	9
Salt & Vinegar	15 (1 oz)	150	9	3	0	2	15	1	1	0	470	—	—	9
Sweet Maui Onion	14 (1 oz)	140	9	3	0	2	15	2	1	0	247	—	—	9

FOOD	PORTION	CALS	FAT	SAT FAT	CHOL	PROT	CARB	SUGAR	FIBER	CALCI	SOD	POTAS	FOLIC	VIT C
POPCHIPS														
Potato Barbeque	19 (1 oz)	120	4	0	0	1	20	2	1	20	250	—	—	1
Potato Cheddar	20 (1 oz)	120	4	1	0	2	20	1	1	20	290	—	—	1
Potato Original	22 (1 oz)	120	4	0	0	1	20	0	1	20	280	—	—	0
Potato Parmesan Garlic	20 (1 oz)	120	4	0	0	2	20	1	1	20	310	—	—	0
Potato Salt & Pepper	11 (0.4 oz)	50	2	0	0	1	8	0	1	0	120	—	—	0
Potato Sea Salt & Vinegar	20 (1 oz)	120	4	0	0	1	20	1	1	20	290	—	—	1
Potato Sour Cream & Onion	20 (1 oz)	120	4	1	0	2	20	2	1	20	290	—	—	1
PRINGLES														
Jalapeno	15 (1 oz)	150	10	3	0	1	14	1	tr	0	190	—	—	4
Loaded Baked Potato	15 (1 oz)	150	10	3	0	1	14	1	tr	0	170	—	—	4
Minis Cheddar Cheese	1 pkg	120	7	2	0	1	12	1	tr	—	220	—	—	4
Minis Original	1 pkg	120	7	2	0	1	13	—	tr	—	140	—	—	4
Original	14 (1 oz)	160	11	3	0	1	14	1	tr	0	170	—	—	4
Pizza	15 (1 oz)	150	10	3	0	1	14	1	tr	20	190	—	—	4
Select Cinnamon Sweet Potato	28 (1 oz)	150	9	2	0	1	16	3	1	20	15	—	—	2
Select Parmesan Garlic	28 (1 oz)	140	9	2	0	1	15	1	tr	20	180	—	—	4
Snack Stacks Original	1 pkg	140	10	3	0	1	12	0	tr	—	150	—	—	4
REVOLUTION FOODS														
Organic Popalongs Whole Grains Cheesy Cheese	16 (0.7 oz)	90	3	1	5	2	14	1	1	20	210	—	—	0
Organic Popalongs Whole Grains Original	16 (0.7 oz)	100	3	0	0	2	15	1	1	0	200	—	—	0
Organic Popalongs Whole Grains Simply Cinnamon	16 (0.7 oz)	100	3	0	0	1	16	3	1	0	85	—	—	0
RHYTHM														
Crispy Kale Bombay Curry	½ pkg (1 oz)	101	2	0	0	4	11	2	2	60	189	—	—	47
Crispy Kale Kool Ranch	½ pkg (1 oz)	100	5	1	0	6	10	1	2	60	190	—	—	48
Crispy Kale Zesty Nacho	½ pkg (1 oz)	106	5	1	0	5	12	2	2	60	187	—	—	70
ROBERT'S AMERICAN GOURMET														
Soy Crisps Country Barbecue	1 oz	130	4	1	0	7	15	3	3	40	280	—	—	0

FOOD	PORTION	CALS	FAT	SAT FAT	CHOL	PROT	CARB	SUGAR	FIBER	CALCI	SOD	POTAS	FOLIC	VIT C
RUFFLES														
Baked Original Potato	9 (1 oz)	120	3	0	0	2	22	1	2	0	135	250	—	0
Original Potato	12 (1 oz)	160	10	1	0	2	15	tr	1	0	160	340	—	6
Reduced Fat Potato	13 (1 oz)	140	7	1	0	2	18	0	1	0	180	310	—	6
Reduced Fat Sea Salted Potato	1 oz	140	7	1	0	2	17	0	1	0	160	—	—	6
SALBA SMART														
Organic Blue Corn Omega-3 Enriched	1 oz	104	6	1	0	2	19	0	4	40	75	—	—	0
SANTITAS														
Tortilla Triangles White Corn	9 (1 oz)	140	6	1	0	2	19	0	2	20	115	—	—	0
Tortilla Triangles Yellow Corn	9 (1 oz)	140	6	1	0	2	19	0	2	20	110	—	—	0
SENECA														
Crispy Apple Apple Pie Ala Mode	12 (1 oz)	140	7	1	0	0	20	12	2	0	40	85	—	18
Crispy Apple Caramel	12 (1 oz)	140	7	1	0	0	20	12	2	0	15	85	—	18
Crispy Apple Cinnamon	14 (1 oz)	150	7	1	0	1	18	8	4	40	30	—	—	0
Crispy Apple Original	12 (1 oz)	140	7	1	0	0	20	12	2	0	15	—	—	18
Crispy Apple Sour Apple	12 (1 oz)	150	9	1	0	0	18	9	3	0	10	85	—	18
SENSIBLE PORTIONS														
Garden Veggie Sea Salt	1 pkg (0.5 oz)	70	4	1	0	1	8	tr	tr	0	140	—	—	6
SIMPLY 7														
Hummus Chips Sea Salt	30 (1 oz)	130	5	1	0	2	19	2	tr	40	290	—	—	0
Lentil Chips Sea Salt	31 (1 oz)	140	6	0	0	3	18	0	tr	0	350	—	—	0
SNIKIDDY														
Fries Potato Bold Buffalo Gluten Free	1 oz	130	5	1	0	2	20	2	1	40	180	—	—	2
Fries Potato Classic Ketchup Gluten Free	1 oz	130	5	0	0	2	21	21	1	20	190	—	—	1
Fries Potato Original Gluten Free	1 oz	130	5	0	0	2	20	1	1	20	190	—	—	1

FOOD	PORTION	CALS	FAT	SAT FAT	CHOL	PROT	CARB	SUGAR	FIBER	CALCI	SOD	POTAS	FOLIC	VIT C
SNIKIDDY (CONT.)														
Fries Potato Southwest Cheddar Gluten Free	1 oz	130	5	1	0	2	20	2	1	40	180	—	—	2
SNYDER'S OF HANOVER														
Kosher Dill	1 oz	140	6	2	0	2	20	1	4	0	360	—	—	9
MultiGrain Sunflower	1 oz	140	6	1	0	2	20	2	2	0	190	—	—	0
MultiGrain Sunflower Southwestern Cheddar	1 oz	140	6	1	0	2	20	2	2	0	190	—	—	9
MultiGrain Tortilla Lightly Salted	1 oz	130	5	0	0	2	20	2	3	0	110	—	—	0
MultiGrain Tortilla Strips Flaxseed Gold	1 oz	140	6	1	0	2	18	1	2	40	230	—	—	9
Organic Veggie Crisps	1 oz	140	7	1	0	1	18	0	2	0	290	—	—	0
Potato Original	1 oz	150	7	2	0	2	19	0	3	0	90	—	—	9
Sweet Potato Baked	1 oz	110	2	0	0	1	23	4	1	40	310	—	—	0
Tortilla Gluten Free MultiGrain	10 (1 oz)	150	7	1	0	2	19	2	3	40	80	—	—	0
Tortilla White Corn	1 oz	140	5	0	0	2	23	0	2	0	110	—	—	0
STACY'S														
Bagel Chips Everything	12 (1 oz)	130	4	1	0	4	19	1	1	20	320	—	—	0
Pita Chips Cinnamon Sugar	1 oz	140	5	1	0	3	20	6	1	0	115	—	—	0
Soy Thin Chips Sticky Bun	18 (1 oz)	130	5	1	0	6	15	3	3	20	180	—	—	0
SUNCHIPS														
Multigrain French Onion	15 (1 oz)	140	6	1	0	2	18	3	3	0	150	75	—	0
Multigrain Original	16 (1 oz)	140	6	1	0	2	19	2	3	0	120	—	—	0
T.G.I. FRIDAY'S														
Potato Cheese Pizza	16 (1 oz)	160	9	2	0	2	17	1	1	0	190	—	—	0
TATER SKINS														
Cheddar Bacon	16 (1 oz)	150	8	1	0	1	19	1	1	0	170	—	—	0
Original	16 (1 oz)	150	8	1	0	1	19	1	1	0	170	—	—	0

FOOD	PORTION	CALS	FAT	SAT FAT	CHOL	PROT	CARB	SUGAR	FIBER	CALCI	SOD	POTAS	FOLIC	VIT C
TERRA														
Exotic Vegetable Original	14 (1 oz)	150	9	1	0	7	16	3	3	20	150	—	—	5
Exotic Vegetable Zesty Tomato	14 (1 oz)	150	9	1	0	1	16	3	3	20	190	—	—	5
Kettles Potato Sea Salt & Pepper	15 (1 oz)	140	6	1	0	2	18	tr	tr	20	65	—	—	15
Parsnip Chips	12 (1 oz)	150	10	1	0	2	13	0	5	60	50	—	—	5
Potato Au Natural	18 (1 oz)	150	9	1	0	2	15	0	2	0	0	—	—	4
Potato Blues	1 oz	130	6	1	0	2	19	0	3	0	115	—	—	0
Potato Golds Original	1 oz	130	5	1	0	2	19	0	0	20	80	—	—	0
Potato Potpourri	1 oz	140	7	1	0	2	17	2	4	0	110	—	—	4
Potato Red Bliss	1 oz	140	7	1	0	1	18	0	2	0	110	—	—	0
Potato Frites Sea Salt & Vinegar	1 oz	150	8	1	0	2	18	7	3	0	200	—	—	2
Stix Original Exotic Vegetable	1 oz	150	9	1	0	1	16	3	3	20	110	—	—	5
Sweet Potato	17 (1 oz)	160	11	1	0	1	15	3	3	20	10	—	—	6
Sweets & Beets	16 (1 oz)	150	9	1	0	2	15	0	1	20	5	—	—	5
Taro	1 oz	140	6	1	0	1	19	1	4	0	110	—	—	2
THE WHOLE EARTH														
Tortilla Really Seedy Multigrain	9 (1 oz)	140	9	1	0	2	14	1	2	20	150	—	—	0
THUNDER														
Potato Buffalo Wing w/ Blue Cheese	22 (1 oz)	150	8	2	0	1	16	tr	tr	0	280	—	—	9
TOSTITOS														
Tortilla Baked Scoops	14 (1 oz)	120	3	1	0	2	22	0	2	20	140	—	—	0
Tortilla Bite Size Rounds	24 (1 oz)	140	7	1	0	2	18	0	2	20	110	—	—	0
Tortilla Multigrain	8 (1 oz)	150	7	1	0	2	19	tr	2	20	110	—	—	0
Tortilla Scoops	12 (1 oz)	140	7	1	0	2	19	0	2	20	120	—	—	0
UMPQUA INDIAN FOODS														
Nana Crisps	⅓ pkg (1 oz)	120	6	0	0	0	15	3	tr	20	0	—	—	9
Veggie	¼ pkg (1 oz)	120	6	0	0	1	18	2	2	20	55	—	—	5
UTZ														
Pita Natural w/ Sea Salt	1 oz	120	5	1	0	3	18	1	tr	20	140	—	—	0
Potato	20 (1 oz)	150	9	2	0	2	14	0	1	0	95	370	—	9
Potato Baked	1 oz	110	2	0	0	2	23	2	2	40	170	—	—	2
Potato BBQ	20 (1 oz)	150	10	3	0	2	14	1	1	0	200	—	—	6
Potato Grandma Kettle	1 oz	140	8	3	5	2	14	0	1	0	120	—	—	9

FOOD	PORTION	CALS	FAT	SAT FAT	CHOL	PROT	CARB	SUGAR	FIBER	CALCI	SOD	POTAS	FOLIC	VIT C
UTZ (CONT.)														
Potato Homestyle Kettle	1 oz	140	8	2	0	2	14	0	1	0	120	—	—	9
Potato Kettle Classics	20 (1 oz)	150	9	2	0	2	15	0	1	0	120	—	—	9
Potato Mystic Kettle	1 oz	150	9	2	0	2	15	0	1	0	120	—	—	9
Potato Mystic Kettle Reduced Fat	1 oz	130	6	2	0	2	18	0	1	0	120	—	—	6
Potato Natural Lightly Salted Kettle	1 oz	140	8	1	0	2	15	0	1	0	95	—	—	9
Potato No Salt Added	20 (1 oz)	150	9	2	0	2	14	0	1	0	5	370	—	9
Potato Onion & Garlic	1 oz	150	9	2	0	2	14	tr	1	0	180	—	—	6
Potato Ripple	20 (1 oz)	150	10	3	0	2	14	0	1	0	95	370	—	9
Sweet Potato Kettle Classics	20 (1 oz)	150	9	2	0	1	16	3	2	20	65	—	—	11
Tortilla Baked	10	120	2	1	0	2	23	0	1	20	125	—	—	0
Tortilla Organic Yellow Corn	1 oz	140	6	1	0	2	19	0	2	20	100	—	—	0
Vegetable Natural Exotic Medley	1 oz	160	10	1	0	2	15	2	2	20	110	—	—	6
WANT'EMS														
Wonton Asian BBQ	16 (1 oz)	140	8	1	0	2	16	tr	1	0	210	—	—	0
Wonton Original	16 (1 oz)	140	8	1	0	2	16	0	1	0	100	—	—	0
WISE														
Potato	1 pkg (1 oz)	150	10	3	0	2	14	0	1	0	190	—	—	6
YOGACHIPS														
Organic Apple Chips Peach	1 pkg (0.35 oz)	35	0	0	0	0	9	7	tr	0	7	—	—	0
ZAPP'S														
Potato Cajun Dill	1 oz	150	8	2	0	2	17	0	1	0	180	—	—	5
Potato No Salt	1 oz	150	9	2	0	2	18	0	1	0	0	—	—	6
Potato Original	1 oz	150	8	2	0	2	17	0	1	0	50	—	—	5
Potato Sizzlin Steak	1 oz	150	8	2	0	2	17	tr	1	0	270	—	—	5
Sweet Potato Lightly Salted	1 oz	150	8	1	0	1	17	6	1	40	30	—	—	0
CHITTERLINGS														
pork cooked	3 oz	258	24	9	122	9	0	0	0	23	33	—	3	0

FOOD	PORTION	CALS	FAT	SAT FAT	CHOL	PROT	CARB	SUGAR	FIBER	CALCI	SOD	POTAS	FOLIC	VIT C
CHIVES														
freeze-dried	1 tbsp	1	tr	tr	0	tr	tr	—	—	2	—	6	—	1
fresh chopped	1 tbsp	1	tr	tr	0	tr	tr	—	—	3	0	9	3	2
fresh chopped	1 tsp	0	tr	tr	0	tr	tr	—	—	1	0	3	1	1
CHOCOLATE														

CHOCOLATE

(*see also* CANDY, CHOCOLATE SPREAD, CHOCOLATE SYRUP, COCOA, HOT CHOCOLATE, ICE CREAM TOPPINGS, MILK DRINKS)

FOOD	PORTION	CALS	FAT	SAT FAT	CHOL	PROT	CARB	SUGAR	FIBER	CALCI	SOD	POTAS	FOLIC	VIT C
BAKING														
baking	1 oz	145	15	9	0	3	8	—	—	22	1	235	—	0
grated unsweetened	¼ cup	165	17	11	0	4	10	tr	6	99	8	274	9	0
liquid unsweetened	1 oz	134	14	7	0	3	10	0	5	15	3	331	5	0
mexican baking	1 sq (0.7 oz)	85	3	2	0	1	15	14	1	7	1	79	1	0
squares unsweetened	1 sq (1 oz)	145	15	9	0	4	9	tr	5	59	7	241	8	0
BAKER'S														
Semi-Sweet	0.5 oz	70	5	3	0	1	8	6	1	0	0	—	—	0
Unsweetened	0.5 oz	70	7	5	0	2	4	0	2	0	0	—	—	0
White	0.5 oz	80	5	3	0	1	9	9	0	20	10	—	—	0
HERSHEY'S														
Unsweetened Block	1 (0.5 oz)	70	7	5	—	2	4	—	2	0		—		0
CHIPS														
milk chocolate	1 cup (6 oz)	862	52	31	38	12	100	—	—	321	138	646	14	1
semisweet	60 pieces (1 oz)	136	9	5	0	1	18	—	—	9	3	104	1	0
semisweet	1 cup (6 oz)	804	50	30	0	7	106	—	—	54	19	614	4	0
E. GUITTARD														
Cappuccino	30 (0.5 oz)	80	5	5	0	tr	9	9	0	20	15	—	—	0
Milk Chocolate	12 (0.5 oz)	80	5	3	5	1	9	9	0	20	10	—	—	0
Semisweet	30 (0.5 oz)	70	4	3	0	tr	10	8	tr	0	0	—	—	0
GHIRARDELLI														
Semi-Sweet	32 (0.5 oz)	70	5	3	0	1	10	8	tr	0	0	—	—	0
HERSHEY'S														
Milk Chocolate	1 tbsp (0.5 oz)	70	5	3	<5	1	9	8	1	20	10	—	—	0
Premier White	1 tbsp (0.5 oz)	80	4	4	—	1	9	9	—	20	30	—	—	0
Semi-Sweet	1 tbsp (0.5 oz)	70	4	3	—	tr	10	8	tr	0	—	—	—	0
Special Dark	1 tbsp (0.5 oz)	70	5	3	—	tr	9	8	1	0	5	—	—	0
Sugar Free	1 tbsp (0.5 oz)	70	5	3	—	tr	9	—	1	0	—	—	—	0
MIX														
drink mix powder	2–3 heaping tsp	75	1	tr	0	1	20	—	—	8	45	128	—	tr
drink mix powder as prep w/ whole milk	9 oz	226	9	5	33	9	31	—	—	300	165	498	12	3

FOOD	PORTION	CALS	FAT	SAT FAT	CHOL	PROT	CARB	SUGAR	FIBER	CALCI	SOD	POTAS	FOLIC	VIT C
NESQUIK														
Chocolate Powder	2 tbsp (0.6 oz)	60	1	0	0	tr	14	13	tr	100	30	—	—	6
Chocolate Powder No Sugar Added	2 tbsp (0.4 oz)	35	1	1	0	1	7	3	1	100	70	—	—	6
SUNFOOD														
Organic Powder	2 tbsp (1 oz)	120	4	2	0	6	15	0	9	48	6	—	—	—

CHOCOLATE MILK

(*see* MILK DRINKS)

CHOCOLATE SPREAD

FOOD	PORTION	CALS	FAT	SAT FAT	CHOL	PROT	CARB	SUGAR	FIBER	CALCI	SOD	POTAS	FOLIC	VIT C
LOVE'N BAKE														
Chocolate Schmear	2 tbsp	140	8	0	0	4	14	11	2	40	0	—	—	0

CHOCOLATE SYRUP

FOOD	PORTION	CALS	FAT	SAT FAT	CHOL	PROT	CARB	SUGAR	FIBER	CALCI	SOD	POTAS	FOLIC	VIT C
chocolate fudge	1 tbsp (0.7 oz)	73	3	1	—	1	12	—	—	21	27	45	—	—
chocolate fudge	1 cup (11.9 oz)	1176	46	19	—	15	200	—	—	340	442	731	—	—
syrup	1 cup	653	3	2	0	6	177	—	—	42	287	672	12	1
syrup	2 tbsp	82	tr	tr	0	1	22	—	—	5	36	84	2	tr
syrup as prep w/ whole milk	1 cup (9.9 oz)	254	8	5	25	9	36	32	1	251	133	409	14	0
HERSHEY'S														
Lite	2 tbsp (1.2 oz)	45	0	0	0	0	11	10	tr	0	70	—	—	0
Sugar Free	2 tbsp (1.1 oz)	15	0	0	0	tr	5	—	tr	0	120	—	—	0
Sundae Syrup Double Chocolate	2 tbsp (1.3 oz)	100	0	0	0	tr	24	21	1	0	15	—	—	0
Syrup	2 tbsp (1.4 oz)	100	0	0	0	tr	24	20	1	0	15	—	—	0
NESQUIK														
Calcium Fortified	2 tbsp (1.3 oz)	100	0	0	0	0	25	23	tr	100	55	—	—	0
SANTA CRUZ														
Organic	2 tbsp	110	0	0	0	1	27	25	tr	—	0	—	—	0
STEEL'S														
No Sugar Added Fat Free	2 tbsp (1 oz)	50	0	0	0	1	17	0	0	0	10	—	—	0
U-BET														
Original	2 tbsp (1.4 oz)	128	0	0	0	1	29	23	—	—	35	—	—	—

CHUTNEY

FOOD	PORTION	CALS	FAT	SAT FAT	CHOL	PROT	CARB	SUGAR	FIBER	CALCI	SOD	POTAS	FOLIC	VIT C
apple	1.2 oz	68	0	—	—	tr	18	—	1	9	—	—	—	1
coconut	2 oz	87	9	7	0	1	1	1	3	8	217	123	—	0
fresh mint	2 oz	18	0	0	0	1	3	3	1	14	432	93	—	4
mango	¼ cup (2 oz)	227	5	1	0	2	43	16	10	36	—	253	—	46
tomato	1 oz	90	7	1	6	1	6	6	2	26	269	248	—	5
BETH'S FARM KITCHEN														
Blazing Tomato	2 tbsp (1 oz)	25	0	0	0	0	6	5	0	0	10	—	—	5

FOOD	PORTION	CALS	FAT	SAT FAT	CHOL	PROT	CARB	SUGAR	FIBER	CALCI	SOD	POTAS	FOLIC	VIT C
CHUKAR CHERRIES														
Curried Cherry	1 tbsp	30	0	0	0	0	8	7	tr	0	85	—	—	1
PATAK'S														
Major Grey	1 tbsp	60	0	0	0	0	14	14	0	0	290	—	—	0
Mango Hot	1 tbsp	60	0	0	0	0	14	14	0	0	300	—	—	0
Mango Sweet	1 tbsp	60	1	0	0	0	14	14	0	0	310	—	—	0
ROBERT ROTHCHILD FARM														
Hot Peach & Apple	2 tbsp	45	0	0	0	0	12	9	tr	0	35	—	—	2
SCHOOL HOUSE KITCHEN														
Bardshar	1 oz	80	0	0	0	0	20	19	1	0	240	—	—	4
THE GRACIOUS GOURMET														
Mango Pineapple	2 tbsp (1 oz)	45	1	0	0	0	9	7	0	0	5	—	—	0
WILD THYMES FARM														
Apricot Cranberry Walnut	1 tbsp	16	0	0	0	tr	4	3	tr	0	0	—	—	5
Plum Currant Ginger	1 tsp	20	0	0	0	tr	5	4	tr	10	1	—	—	1
CILANTRO														
fresh	¼ cup	1	tr	tr	0	tr	tr	tr	tr	3	2	21	2	1
fresh	1 tsp (2 g)	<1	tr	0	0	tr	tr	—	tr	1	1	8	1	1
fresh sprigs	5 (5 g)	1	tr	tr	0	tr	tr	tr	tr	4	3	29	3	2
DOROT														
Chopped Cube frzn	1 cube (4 g)	5	tr	tr	0	tr	tr	—	tr	—	17	—	—	—
CINNAMON														
cinnamon sugar	1 tsp	16	tr	tr	0	tr	4	4	tr	3	0	1	0	tr
ground	1 tsp	6	tr	tr	0	tr	2	tr	1	26	0	11	0	tr
sticks	0.5 oz	39	tr	tr	—	1	8	0	3	175	4	—	—	4
MCCORMICK														
Grinder Cinnamon Sugar	1 tsp (3.5 g)	10	0	0	0	0	2	—	0	—	0	—	—	—
CISCO														
raw	3 oz	84	2	tr	—	16	0	0	0	—	47	301	—	—
smoked	1 oz	50	3	tr	9	5	0	0	0	7	135	82	1	—
CLAMS														
CANNED														
liquid only	1 cup	6	tr	—	—	1	tr	—	—	31	516	—	—	—
liquid only	3 oz	2	tr	—	—	tr	tr	—	—	11	183	—	—	—
meat only	1 cup	236	3	tr	107	41	8	—	—	148	179	1005	158	—
meat only	3 oz	126	2	tr	57	22	4	—	—	78	95	534	—	—
CHICKEN OF THE SEA														
Chopped	¼ cup	30	0	0	12	5	2	0	0	0	370	—	—	0
Whole Baby	¼ cup	30	0	0	10	6	1	0	0	0	290	—	—	0

FOOD	PORTION	CALS	FAT	SAT FAT	CHOL	PROT	CARB	SUGAR	FIBER	CALCI	SOD	POTAS	FOLIC	VIT C
POLAR														
Baby	¼ cup	30	0	0	20	5	3	0	0	20	280	—	—	5
FRESH														
cooked	20 sm	133	2	tr	60	23	5	—	—	83	100	565	—	—
cooked	3 oz	126	2	tr	57	22	4	—	—	78	95	534	—	—
raw	20 sm (6.3 oz)	133	2	tr	60	23	5	—	—	83	100	565	—	—
raw	9 lg (6.3 oz)	133	2	tr	60	23	5	—	—	83	100	565	—	—
raw	3 oz	63	1	tr	29	11	2	—	—	39	47	267	—	—
FROZEN														
MRS. PAUL'S														
Fried	18 (3 oz)	270	13	3	20	9	29	3	1	0	690	—	—	0
SEAPAK														
Oven Crunchy Strips	1 serv (3 oz)	250	14	2	15	7	24	0	0	0	420	—	—	0
TAKE-OUT														
breaded & fried	20 sm	379	21	5	115	27	19	—	—	119	684	612	—	—

CLEMENTINES

FOOD	PORTION	CALS	FAT	SAT FAT	CHOL	PROT	CARB	SUGAR	FIBER	CALCI	SOD	POTAS	FOLIC	VIT C
CUTIES														
Fresh	2 (6 oz)	80	1	0	0	1	17	13	4	40	0	400	60	174
DISNEY GARDEN														
Clementines	1	35	0	0	0	1	9	7	1	20	1	—	—	36

CLOVES

FOOD	PORTION	CALS	FAT	SAT FAT	CHOL	PROT	CARB	SUGAR	FIBER	CALCI	SOD	POTAS	FOLIC	VIT C
ground	1 tsp	7	tr	tr	0	tr	1	tr	1	14	5	23	2	2

COCOA

(*see also* HOT CHOCOLATE)

FOOD	PORTION	CALS	FAT	SAT FAT	CHOL	PROT	CARB	SUGAR	FIBER	CALCI	SOD	POTAS	FOLIC	VIT C
cocoa butter	1 tbsp	120	14	8	0	0	0	0	0	0	0	0	0	0
powder unsweetened	1 tbsp	12	1	tr	0	1	3	tr	2	7	1	82	2	0
COCOAVIA														
Beverage Mix Dark Chocolate	1 pkg (0.28 oz)	30	1	—	—	1	5	—	1	—	90	—	—	—
HERSHEY'S														
Cocoa	1 tbsp (5 g)	10	1	—	—	tr	3	—	2	0	—	—	—	0
HONEST COCOANOVA														
Cherry Cacao	8 oz	50	0	0	0	0	13	13	—	—	5	—	—	—

COCONUT

FOOD	PORTION	CALS	FAT	SAT FAT	CHOL	PROT	CARB	SUGAR	FIBER	CALCI	SOD	POTAS	FOLIC	VIT C
dried sweetened shredded	¼ cup	116	8	7	0	1	11	10	1	3	61	78	2	tr
dried toasted	1 oz	168	13	12	0	2	13	—	—	8	10	157	3	tr
dried unsweetened	1 oz	187	18	16	0	2	7	2	5	7	10	154	3	tr
fresh from 1 coconut	14 oz	1405	133	118	0	13	60	25	36	56	79	1413	103	13
fresh shredded	¼ cup	71	7	6	0	1	3	1	2	3	4	71	5	1

FOOD	PORTION	CALS	FAT	SAT FAT	CHOL	PROT	CARB	SUGAR	FIBER	CALCI	SOD	POTAS	FOLIC	VIT C
BAKER'S														
Angel Flake Sweetened	0.5 oz	70	5	5	0	1	6	5	1	0	40	—	—	0
BOB'S RED MILL														
Shredded	3 tbsp	120	11	10	0	1	4	1	2	—	5	—	—	—
LET'S DO ORGANIC														
Organic Reduced Fat Shredded	1 can (0.5 oz)	70	6	5	0	1	4	0	2	0	0	—	—	0
Shredded	3 tbsp (0.5 oz)	110	10	9	0	1	4	1	2	0	5	—	—	0
MOUNDS														
Sweetened Flakes	2 tbsp (0.5 oz)	70	5	4	—	tr	6	5	1	0	35	—	—	0
PROSPERITY														
Organic Coconut Flax Butter Garlic & Onion	1 tbsp	140	15	9	0	0	0	0	0	0	0	—	—	0
COCONUT JUICE														
coconut water fresh	½ cup	23	tr	tr	0	1	4	3	1	29	126	300	4	3
creamed sweetened canned	½ cup	264	12	11	0	1	39	38	tr	3	27	75	10	0
milk canned	½ cup	276	29	25	0	3	7	4	3	19	18	316	19	3
COCO KING														
Roasted w/ Pulp	1 can (11.75 oz)	130	0	0	0	1	29	26	1	40	80	—	—	0
W/ Pulp	1 can (11.85 oz)	130	2	1	0	0	30	28	—	40	60	—	—	12
COCOZONA														
Coconut Water	1 bottle (14.5 oz)	70	0	0	0	0	18	16	0	40	220	—	—	5
GOYA														
Coconut Water	1 can (11.8 oz)	120	1	0	0	0	29	22	tr	80	130	—	—	0
LET'S DO ORGANIC														
Creamed	1 oz	220	19	17	0	4	8	2	6	0	10	—	—	0
Milk	¼ cup	100	11	10	0	1	2	1	0	0	5	—	—	0
O.N.E.														
Natural Coconut Water	1 box (11 oz)	60	0	0	0	1	15	14	0	40	60	670	—	—
THAI KITCHEN														
Coconut Milk	⅓ cup (2.8 oz)	140	14	12	0	1	3	1	0	0	20	—	—	0
Lite Coconut Milk	2 oz	45	4	3	0	0	1	1	0	20	0	—	—	0
ZICO														
Coconut Water All Flavors	1 pkg (11 oz)	60	0	0	0	1	15	14	0	40	60	670	—	—
COD														
atlantic canned	3 oz	89	1	tr	47	19	0	0	0	18	185	449	—	1
atlantic canned	1 can (11 oz)	327	3	1	171	71	0	0	0	66	680	1647	—	1
atlantic dried	3 oz	246	2	tr	129	53	0	0	0	136	5973	1239	—	3

FOOD	PORTION	CALS	FAT	SAT FAT	CHOL	PROT	CARB	SUGAR	FIBER	CALCI	SOD	POTAS	FOLIC	VIT C
atlantic fresh cooked	1 fillet (6.3 oz)	189	2	tr	99	41	0	0	0	25	141	440	—	2
atlantic fresh cooked	3 oz	89	1	tr	47	19	0	0	0	12	66	208	—	1
atlantic fresh raw	3 oz	70	1	tr	37	15	0	0	0	13	46	351	—	1
pacific fresh baked	3 oz	95	1	tr	43	21	0	0	0	8	82	465	—	—
roe canned	1 oz	34	1	—	—	6	tr	—	—	4	—	—	—	—
roe tarama	3.5 oz	547	55	—	—	8	6	tr	—	29	600	111	—	—
MRS. PAUL'S														
Filets Lightly Breaded	1 (4 oz)	220	11	5	40	12	17	4	1	0	430	—	—	0
TAKE-OUT														
roe baked w/ butter & lemon juice	1 oz	36	1	—	—	6	tr	—	—	43	21	38	—	—

COFFEE

(*see also* COFFEE BEVERAGES, COFFEE SUBSTITUTES)

FOOD	PORTION	CALS	FAT	SAT FAT	CHOL	PROT	CARB	SUGAR	FIBER	CALCI	SOD	POTAS	FOLIC	VIT C
INSTANT														
decaffeinated as prep	8 oz	2	0	0	0	tr	0	0	0	5	5	128	0	0
decaffeinated powder	1 rounded tsp	4	0	0	0	tr	1	0	0	3	0	63	0	0
regular powder	1 rounded tsp	4	tr	tr	0	tr	1	0	0	3	64	319	0	0
REGULAR														
brewed	8 oz	2	tr	tr	0	tr	0	0	0	5	5	116	5	0
roasted beans	1 oz	64	4	—	—	4	18	—	2	42	—	—	—	—
SPAVA														
Calm Decaffeinated	1 cup	0	0	0	0	0	0	0	0	—	0	—	80	—

COFFEE BEVERAGES

FOOD	PORTION	CALS	FAT	SAT FAT	CHOL	PROT	CARB	SUGAR	FIBER	CALCI	SOD	POTAS	FOLIC	VIT C
CAFE SEPIA														
House Blend	1 bottle (6.2 oz)	80	0	0	5	2	15	14	0	60	70	—	—	0
Mocha	1 bottle (6.2 oz)	70	0	0	0	1	14	14	0	40	40	—	—	—
CINNABON														
Lattes All Flavors	1 can (9.5 oz)	190	5	—	15	4	32	30	1	200	260	—	—	2
CLICK														
Espresso Protein Drink as prep	2 scoops (1.1 oz)	120	2	0	<5	15	12	7	tr	250	115	290	80	18
EMMI														
Caffe Latte Cappuccino	1 pkg	140	4	2	15	6	20	19	0	200	150	370	—	2
Caffe Latte Vanilla	1 pkg (7.7 oz)	140	4	2	15	6	20	19	0	200	150	370	—	2
FROID														
Original or French Vanilla	1 bottle (11 oz)	180	3	—	10	6	34	31	1	200	260	—	—	0

FOOD	PORTION	CALS	FAT	SAT FAT	CHOL	PROT	CARB	SUGAR	FIBER	CALCI	SOD	POTAS	FOLIC	VIT C
GENERAL FOODS														
International Coffees Vanilla Bean Latte	1 serv	60	2	2	—	0	12	9	—	—	50	—	—	—
GODIVA														
Latte French Vanilla	1 bottle (12 oz)	200	4	3	15	6	36	35	0	200	140	—	—	0
Mocha Dark Chocolate	1 bottle (16 oz)	200	4	3	15	6	37	35	1	200	160	—	—	0
HEALTH IS WEALTH														
Nutriccino Vitamin Infused All Flavors	1 bottle (9.5 oz)	190	3	2	10	4	37	31	0	100	260	—	400	60
Vitamin Coffee Ener-G Infused Vanilla Latte	1 bottle (9.5 oz)	190	3	2	10	4	37	31	0	100	260	—	400	60
ICED 'SPRESSO														
Ultra Light American Vanilla	1 bottle (9.5 oz)	90	3	—	10	6	11	8	0	200	180	—	—	0
Ultra Light Espresso Latte	1 bottle (9.5 oz)	70	0	0	0	6	11	8	0	250	190	—	—	0
N.O. BREW														
Iced Coffee not prep	1 serv (2.6 oz)	10	0	0	0	0	1	0	0	0	0	—	—	0
O.N.E.														
Coffee Fruit	1 bottle (11 oz)	107	1	—	0	tr	26	25	1	19	10	—	—	570
POMX														
Iced Cafe Au Lait	1 bottle (10.5 oz)	170	3	2	15	7	29	20	0	250	130	—	—	0
Iced Cafe Vanilla	1 bottle (10.5 oz)	180	0	0	0	11	43	28	0	350	130	—	—	0
SEATTLE'S BEST COFFEE														
Iced Latte	1 can (9.5 oz)	130	2	2	10	3	25	23	0	100	50	—	—	0
Iced Latte Vanilla	1 can (9.5 oz)	130	2	2	0	3	25	24	0	100	50	—	—	0
Iced Mocha	1 can (9.5 oz)	130	2	2	10	3	24	24	0	100	95	—	—	0
SHOCK														
Triple Latte	1 can (8 oz)	125	2	—	—	4	27	27	0	30	125	—	—	0
STARBUCKS														
DoubleShot	1 (6.5 oz)	140	6	—	20	4	18	17	—	150	70	—	—	—
WOLFGANG PUCK														
Culinary Iced All Flavors	1 bottle (8.5 oz)	120	3	2	10	3	23	21	—	100	150	—	—	—
TAKE-OUT														
cafe amaretto w/ alcohol	1 serv	192	9	6	33	1	15	—	0	25	14	197	1	tr
cafe au lait	1 cup (8 oz)	77	4	3	17	4	6	7	—	148	62	249	6	1
cafe brulot	1 cup	48	0	0	0	tr	3	3	—	2	2	64	tr	0

FOOD	PORTION	CALS	FAT	SAT FAT	CHOL	PROT	CARB	SUGAR	FIBER	CALCI	SOD	POTAS	FOLIC	VIT C
cafe brulot w/ alcohol	1 serv	130	tr	tr	0	1	16	—	3	55	4	162	12	24
cappuccino	1 cup (8 oz)	77	4	3	17	4	6	7	—	148	62	249	6	1
coffee con leche	1 cup (6 oz)	104	4	2	10	3	16	17	0	103	36	171	6	0
cuban coffee w/ rum & creme de cacao	1 (9 oz)	112	2	—	—	3	6	—	0	—	—	—	—	—
dutch coffee w/ gin	1 (7 oz)	181	10	—	29	1	6	5	0	—	19	—	—	—
espresso	1 cup (4 oz)	2	tr	tr	0	tr	0	0	0	2	17	138	1	tr
french coffee w/ orange liqueur & kahlua	1 (8 oz)	232	10	—	29	1	24	—	0	—	—	—	—	—
irish coffee	1 serv (8 oz)	209	11	6	38	1	5	4	0	19	13	89	4	tr
italian coffee w/ strega	1 (7 oz)	163	10	—	—	1	12	10	0	—	19	—	—	—
latte w/ skim milk	1 serv (13 oz)	88	tr	tr	4	8	12	11	0	304	128	470	13	2
latte w/ whole milk	1 serv (14 oz)	143	6	3	20	9	15	14	0	310	126	555	12	tr
mocha	1 serv (17 oz)	403	9	5	29	11	69	54	2	335	199	739	15	1
puerto rican coffee w/ rum & kahlua	1 (8 oz)	166	10	—	29	1	9	—	0	—	—	—	—	—
turkish	1 cup (4 oz)	50	1	0	0	tr	12	12	0	1	1	53	2	0

COFFEE SUBSTITUTES

PIXIE

FOOD	PORTION	CALS	FAT	SAT FAT	CHOL	PROT	CARB	SUGAR	FIBER	CALCI	SOD	POTAS	FOLIC	VIT C
Mate Latte Chai	½ cup (4 oz)	80	0	0	0	0	18	17	tr	20	5	—	—	0
Mate Latte Dark Roast	½ cup (4 oz)	70	0	0	0	0	16	13	tr	20	0	—	—	0
Mate Latte Mocha	½ cup (4 oz)	70	0	0	0	0	18	16	0	0	0	—	—	0
Mate Latte Original	½ cup (4 oz)	70	0	0	0	0	17	15	0	0	0	—	—	0

COFFEE WHITENERS

BAILEYS

FOOD	PORTION	CALS	FAT	SAT FAT	CHOL	PROT	CARB	SUGAR	FIBER	CALCI	SOD	POTAS	FOLIC	VIT C
Caramel	1 tbsp (0.5 oz)	40	2	1	0	0	6	5	0	0	0	—	—	0
French Vanilla	1 tbsp (0.5 oz)	40	2	1	5	0	6	5	0	0	0	—	—	0
Hazelnut	1 tbsp (0.5 oz)	35	2	1	5	0	5	5	0	0	5	—	—	0
Original Irish Cream	1 tbsp (0.5 oz)	40	2	1	5	0	5	5	0	0	5	—	—	0

FARMLAND

FOOD	PORTION	CALS	FAT	SAT FAT	CHOL	PROT	CARB	SUGAR	FIBER	CALCI	SOD	POTAS	FOLIC	VIT C
Nondairy Creamer	2 tbsp	40	3	2	15	1	2	1	0	40	15	—	—	0

HOOD

FOOD	PORTION	CALS	FAT	SAT FAT	CHOL	PROT	CARB	SUGAR	FIBER	CALCI	SOD	POTAS	FOLIC	VIT C
Country Creamer Non Dairy	1 tbsp	20	2	0	0	0	2	0	0	0	0	—	—	0

INTERNATIONAL DELIGHT

FOOD	PORTION	CALS	FAT	SAT FAT	CHOL	PROT	CARB	SUGAR	FIBER	CALCI	SOD	POTAS	FOLIC	VIT C
Amaretto	1 tbsp (0.5 oz)	40	2	1	0	0	7	6	0	0	5	—	—	0
Caramel Macchiato	1 tbsp (0.5 oz)	40	2	1	0	0	7	6	0	0	5	—	—	0

FOOD	PORTION	CALS	FAT	SAT FAT	CHOL	PROT	CARB	SUGAR	FIBER	CALCI	SOD	POTAS	FOLIC	VIT C
INTERNATIONAL DELIGHT (CONT.)														
Caribbean Cinnamon Creme	1 tbsp (0.5 oz)	45	2	1	0	0	6	6	0	0	5	—	—	0
Dark Chocolate Cream	1 tbsp (0.5 oz)	35	2	1	5	0	6	6	0	0	0	—	—	0
English Almond Toffee	1 tbsp (0.5 oz)	45	2	1	0	0	6	6	0	0	5	—	—	0
French Vanilla	1 tbsp (0.5 oz)	45	2	1	0	0	6	6	0	0	5	—	—	0
French Vanilla Fat Free	1 tbsp (0.5 oz)	30	0	0	0	0	7	5	0	0	0	—	—	0
French Vanilla Sugar Free	1 tbsp (0.5 oz)	20	2	1	0	0	1	0	0	0	0	—	—	0
Irish Creme	1 tbsp (0.5 oz)	40	2	1	0	0	7	6	0	0	5	—	—	0
Vanilla Caramel Cream	1 tbsp (0.5 oz)	35	2	1	5	0	6	6	0	0	0	—	—	0
Vanilla Latte	1 tbsp (0.5 oz)	40	2	1	0	0	7	6	0	0	5	—	—	0
SILK														
French Vanilla	1 tbsp (0.5 oz)	20	1	0	0	0	3	3	0	0	10	—	—	0
Original	1 tbsp (0.5 oz)	15	1	0	0	0	1	1	0	0	10	—	—	0
WILDWOOD														
Soymilk Creamer Plain	1 tbsp	15	2	0	0	0	1	1	0	0	0	0	0	0
COLESLAW														
DOLE														
Classic Coleslaw	1½ cups (3 oz)	20	0	0	0	1	5	3	2	40	20	—	—	24
Kit Creamy Coleslaw as prep	1½ cups (3.5 oz)	100	6	1	20	1	12	9	2	40	200	—	—	27
FRESH EXPRESS														
3 Color Deli	1½ cups	20	0	0	0	1	5	3	2	40	15	—	0	27
Kit w/ Sweet & Creamy Dressing as prep	1 cup	120	8	1	5	1	12	10	2	40	135	—	0	40
Old Fashioned	2 cups	25	0	0	0	1	5	3	2	40	15	—	—	24
MANN'S														
Broccoli Cole Slaw w/o Dressing	1 serv (3 oz)	25	0	0	0	2	5	2	3	40	25	270	52	66
READY PAC														
Coleslaw	1½ cups (3 oz)	20	0	0	0	1	5	3	2	40	20	—	—	27
Coleslaw Mix as prep	1 cup (3.5 oz)	130	9	2	5	1	13	11	2	40	160	—	—	24
TAKE-OUT														
coleslaw w/ dressing	¾ cup	147	11	2	5	1	13	—	—	34	267	177	39	8
vinegar & oil coleslaw	3.5 oz	150	9	1	0	1	16	—	—	20	480	—	—	30

FOOD	PORTION	CALS	FAT	SAT FAT	CHOL	PROT	CARB	SUGAR	FIBER	CALCI	SOD	POTAS	FOLIC	VIT C
COLLARDS														
fresh cooked	½ cup	17	tr	—	0	1	4	—	—	15	10	84	4	8
frzn chopped cooked	½ cup	31	tr	—	0	3	6	—	—	179	42	214	65	23
raw chopped	½ cup	6	tr	—	0	tr	1	—	—	5	4	30	2	4
ALLENS														
Seasoned Southern Style	½ cup (4.1 oz)	35	0	0	0	2	6	3	2	200	930	—	—	12
GLORY														
Green Fresh	2 cups	25	0	0	0	2	5	0	3	100	15	—	—	27
Seasoned canned	½ cup	35	0	0	0	2	5	1	2	80	490	—	—	12
Sensibly Seasoned canned	½ cup	20	0	0	0	2	4	1	2	100	240	—	—	12
SEABROOK FARMS														
Chopped Greens frzn	½ cup (3.1 oz)	30	0	0	0	2	2	1	2	80	20	—	—	15
COOKIES														
MIX														
chocolate chip	1 (0.56 oz)	79	4	1	7	1	10	—	—	7	47	34	—	0
oatmeal	1 (0.6 oz)	74	3	1	7	1	10	—	tr	5	75	30	—	—
oatmeal raisin	1 (0.6 oz)	74	3	1	7	1	10	—	tr	5	75	30	—	—
BETTY CROCKER														
Caramelita Bars as prep	1	190	8	4	9	2	28	17	1	—	115	50	8	—
Chocolate Chip as prep	2	170	8	5	27	1	21	13	tr	—	105	45	8	—
Oatmeal as prep	2	160	7	4	27	2	22	11	tr	—	105	35	8	—
Peanut Butter as prep	2	150	7	1	12	2	20	12	—	—	140	—	8	—
Reese's Dessert Bar Mix No Bake as prep	1	180	10	4	12	2	20	13	1	—	125	—	—	—
Sugar as prep	2	160	8	4	27	1	21	12	0	—	80	15	16	—
Sunkist Lemon Bars as prep	1	140	4	1	39	tr	24	17	—	—	80	10	8	—
Turtle Cookie Bars as prep	1	180	8	4	9	2	27	16	tr	—	140	40	16	—
DUNCAN HINES														
Chocolate Chip as prep	2 (1.1 oz)	180	9	3	10	1	23	14	0	0	85	—	—	0
KING ARTHUR														
Chocolate Chip Whole Grain not prep	2 tbsp	90	3	2	0	2	16	10	1	20	35	—	—	0
READY-TO-EAT														
animal crackers	11 (1 oz)	126	4	1	—	2	21	—	—	12	112	28	4	0

FOOD	PORTION	CALS	FAT	SAT FAT	CHOL	PROT	CARB	SUGAR	FIBER	CALCI	SOD	POTAS	FOLIC	VIT C
animal crackers	1 box (2.4 oz)	299	9	4	11	4	51	—	—	11	274	57	22	tr
animal crackers	1 (2.5 g)	11	tr	tr	—	tr	2	—	—	1	10	2	0	0
australian anzac biscuit	1	98	3	1	0	1	17	—	1	11	59	—	—	—
butter	1 (5 g)	23	1	1	—	tr	3	—	tr	1	18	6	0	0
chocolate chip	1 box (1.9 oz)	233	12	5	12	3	36	—	—	20	188	82	16	tr
chocolate chip	1 (0.4 oz)	48	2	1	—	1	7	—	tr	2	32	14	1	0
chocolate chip low sugar low sodium	1 (0.24 oz)	31	1	1	0	tr	5	—	—	—	1	14	—	0
chocolate chip lowfat	1 (0.25 oz)	45	2	tr	0	1	7	—	—	2	38	12	—	—
chocolate chip soft-type	1 (0.5 oz)	69	4	1	0	1	9	—	tr	2	49	14	1	0
chocolate w/ creme filling	1 (0.35 oz)	47	2	tr	—	1	7	—	tr	3	36	18	0	0
chocolate w/ creme filling chocolate coated	1 (0.60 oz)	82	5	1	—	1	11	—	—	6	55	41	—	—
chocolate w/ creme filling sugar free low sodium	1 (0.35 oz)	46	2	1	—	1	7	—	—	—	24	29	—	—
chocolate w/ extra creme filling	1 (0.46 oz)	65	3	1	—	1	9	—	—	3	64	16	—	0
chocolate wafer	1 (0.2 oz)	26	1	tr	0	tr	4	—	—	2	35	13	—	—
cream cheese	1 (1.1 oz)	141	9	6	25	2	14	6	tr	12	53	24	4	0
digestive biscuits plain	2	141	7	—	—	2	21	—	1	28	—	—	—	0
fig bars	1 (0.56 oz)	56	1	tr	—	1	11	—	1	10	56	33	2	—
fortune	1 (0.28 oz)	30	tr	tr	—	tr	7	—	tr	1	22	3	1	0
fudge	1 (0.73 oz)	73	1	tr	—	1	17	—	tr	7	40	29	—	—
gingersnaps	1 (0.24 oz)	29	1	tr	0	tr	5	—	—	5	48	24	—	0
graham	1 sq (0.24 oz)	30	1	tr	0	1	5	—	—	2	42	9	1	0
graham chocolate covered	1 (0.49 oz)	68	3	2	0	1	9	—	—	8	41	29	—	0
graham honey	1 (0.24 oz)	30	1	tr	0	1	5	—	tr	2	42	9	1	0
hermits	1 (1 oz)	117	5	2	23	2	18	10	1	16	54	76	5	tr
jumbles coconut	1 (1 oz)	121	7	5	26	1	13	7	1	5	19	31	4	tr
ladyfingers	1 (0.38 oz)	40	1	tr	40	1	7	—	—	5	16	12	4	tr
macaroons	1 (0.8 oz)	97	3	3	0	1	17	—	—	12	59	38	1	0
madeleines	1 (0.8 oz)	86	5	3	46	2	10	5	tr	7	34	17	5	tr
marshmallow chocolate coated	1 (0.46 oz)	55	2	1	—	1	9	—	—	6	22	24	—	—
marshmallow pie chocolate coated	1 (1.4 oz)	165	7	2	—	2	26	—	—	18	66	72	—	—
molasses	1 (0.5 oz)	65	2	tr	0	1	11	—	—	11	69	52	—	0

FOOD	PORTION	CALS	FAT	SAT FAT	CHOL	PROT	CARB	SUGAR	FIBER	CALCI	SOD	POTAS	FOLIC	VIT C
neapolitan tri-color cookie	1 (0.6 oz)	79	5	2	17	1	8	5	tr	12	10	36	4	tr
oatmeal	1 (0.6 oz)	81	3	1	0	1	12	—	1	7	69	26	—	—
oatmeal soft-type	1 (0.5 oz)	61	2	tr	—	1	10	—	tr	13	52	20	—	—
oatmeal raisin	1 (0.6 oz)	81	3	1	0	1	12	—	1	7	69	26	—	—
oatmeal raisin low sugar no sodium	1 (0.24 oz)	31	1	1	0	tr	5	—	—	—	1	12	—	—
oatmeal raisin soft-type	1 (0.5 oz)	61	2	tr	—	1	10	—	tr	13	52	20	—	—
peanut butter sandwich	1 (0.5 oz)	67	3	1	0	1	9	—	—	7	52	27	—	0
peanut butter sandwich sugar free low sodium	1 (0.35 oz)	54	3	1	—	1	5	—	—	—	41	29	—	0
peanut butter soft-type	1 (0.5 oz)	69	4	1	0	1	9	—	tr	2	50	16	1	0
pinenut cookies	1 (1.1 oz)	134	9	1	0	4	11	8	1	29	11	130	7	tr
raisin soft-type	1 (0.5 oz)	60	2	1	0	1	10	—	—	7	51	21	—	—
reginette queen's biscuit	1 (0.8 oz)	86	3	1	tr	2	13	4	tr	27	83	32	8	tr
shortbread	1 (0.28 oz)	40	2	tr	2	1	5	—	—	3	36	8	—	0
shortbread pecan	1 (0.49 oz)	79	5	1	5	1	8	—	tr	4	39	10	—	—
spritz	1 (0.4 oz)	42	2	1	6	1	6	3	tr	4	9	11	2	tr
sugar	1 (0.52 oz)	72	3	1	8	1	10	—	—	3	53	9	—	—
sugar low sugar sodium free	1 (0.24 oz)	30	1	tr	0	1	5	—	—	—	0	7	—	0
sugar wafers w/ creme filling	1 (0.12 oz)	18	1	tr	0	tr	3	—	—	1	5	2	—	0
sugar wafers w/ creme filling sugar free sodium free	1 (0.14 oz)	20	1	tr	0	tr	3	—	—	2	0	2	0	0
toll house original	1 (0.8 oz)	105	6	2	15	2	13	9	tr	15	57	57	4	tr
vanilla sandwich	1 (0.35 oz)	48	2	tr	0	tr	7	—	tr	3	35	9	0	0
vanilla wafers	1 (0.21 oz)	28	1	tr	—	tr	4	—	—	2	18	6	—	—
zeppole	1 (0.8 oz)	78	6	2	24	1	6	4	tr	3	14	9	3	0
6 HOUR ENERGY														
Almond Cranberry Chocolate Chunk	½ (1.25 oz)	100	6	2	0	4	12	5	5	—	—	—	—	—
ABC														
Vegan Colossal Chocolate Chip	1 (2.1 oz)	240	7	3	0	3	41	20	1	0	190	—	—	0
Vegan Double Chocolate Decadence	1 (2.1 oz)	240	8	3	0	3	39	21	2	20	120	—	—	0

FOOD	PORTION	CALS	FAT	SAT FAT	CHOL	PROT	CARB	SUGAR	FIBER	CALCI	SOD	POTAS	FOLIC	VIT C
ABC (CONT.)														
Vegan Luscious Lemon Poppyseed	1 (2.1 oz)	240	7	2	0	3	40	17	0	20	125	—	—	0
Vegan Mac The Chip	1 (2.1 oz)	250	10	4	0	4	35	20	3	20	200	—	—	0
Vegan Peanut Butter Chocolate Chip	1 (2.1 oz)	240	8	3	0	4	39	17	1	20	160	—	—	0
Vegan Phenomenal Pumpkin Spice	1 (2.1 oz)	220	7	2	0	4	39	18	3	20	115	—	—	1
ALMOND JOY														
Cookies	2 (1 oz)	140	8	4	—	2	17	12	tr	20	60	—	—	0
ALMONDINA														
BranTreats w/ Cinnamon	4 (1 oz)	127	3	tr	0	3	22	9	2	20	11	91	—	0
Gingerspice	4 (1 oz)	137	4	tr	0	3	22	9	1	20	10	79	—	0
Sesame	4 (1 oz)	138	5	1	0	3	21	8	2	80	10	69	—	0
The Original	4 (1 oz)	133	4	tr	0	3	22	10	1	20	9	88	—	0
The Original Chocolate Dipped	2	130	5	2	0	3	16	13	4	30	15	—	—	0
ANNA'S														
Almond Cinnamon	6 (1 oz)	140	7	3	0	2	18	5	1	20	150	—	—	0
Cappuccino	6 (1 oz)	140	7	3	0	2	18	6	2	0	150	—	—	0
Chocolate Mint	6 (1 oz)	140	5	2	0	2	20	14	1	0	150	—	—	0
Orange	6 (1 oz)	140	7	3	0	2	19	6	3	0	150	—	—	0
Vanilla Chocolate Chip	6 (1 oz)	140	6	2	0	1	20	8	0	0	140	—	—	0
ANNIE'S HOMEGROWN														
Bunny Ginger Gluten Free	29 (1 oz)	130	4	2	0	2	21	8	1	20	55	—	—	0
Bunny Gluten Free	27 (1 oz)	120	4	2	0	2	22	9	1	0	90	—	—	0
Bunny Grahams Chocolate	27 (1 oz)	130	5	0	0	2	21	9	2	200	75	—	—	0
Bunny Grahams Honey	28 (1 oz)	140	5	0	0	2	22	7	2	200	150	—	—	0
ARCHWAY														
Coconut Macaroon	2 (1.3 oz)	160	8	7	0	1	22	16	2	0	85	—	—	0
Frosty Lemon	1 (0.9 oz)	110	5	2	0	1	18	10	0	20	105	—	—	0
Fruit Filled Raspberry	1 (0.8 oz)	90	3	1	0	1	15	7	0	0	75	—	—	0

FOOD	PORTION	CALS	FAT	SAT FAT	CHOL	PROT	CARB	SUGAR	FIBER	CALCI	SOD	POTAS	FOLIC	VIT C
ARICO														
Gluten Free Casein Free Almond Cranberry	1 bar (1.4 oz)	140	6	2	25	3	22	10	4	250	120	—	—	0
Gluten Free Casein Free Double Chocolate	1 (0.9 oz)	100	5	2	15	2	15	7	3	150	70	—	—	0
Gluten Free Casein Free Lemon Ginger	1 (0.9 oz)	90	4	1	15	2	15	6	3	150	85	—	—	0
Gluten Free Casein Free Peanut Butter	1 bar (1.4 oz)	160	7	2	25	5	19	3	4	250	140	—	—	0
ARROWROOT														
Biscuit	1 (5 g)	20	1	0	0	0	4	1	0	0	15	—	—	0
AUNT GUSSIE'S														
Biscotti Almond	1 (0.8 oz)	110	6	0	15	2	13	5	1	20	10	—	—	0
Biscotti Almond Sugar Free	2 (1 oz)	150	10	5	20	2	14	3	1	0	40	—	—	0
Biscotti Cinnamon Raisin No Sugar Added	1 (0.8 oz)	110	6	1	15	2	14	2	1	20	10	—	—	0
Biscotti Italian w/ Olive Oil	2 (1.2 oz)	160	5	1	25	3	25	13	1	20	30	—	—	0
Coconut Crisp	2 (1.1 oz)	170	9	6	20	2	18	9	1	20	65	—	—	0
Latte Sugar Free	1 (0.9 oz)	110	6	3	15	2	18	0	0	0	15	—	—	0
Lemon Sugar Free	3 (1.2 oz)	160	9	5	30	2	22	0	1	20	55	—	—	0
Mexican Wedding Cakes	3 (1.2 oz)	160	10	5	20	2	19	8	1	0	45	—	—	0
Snickerdoodle	2 (1.1 oz)	180	12	6	25	2	16	4	1	0	45	—	—	0
Vanilla Spritz Sugar Free Gluten Free	2 (0.9 oz)	110	5	3	25	0	17	0	0	0	15	—	—	0
BACK TO NATURE														
Granola Cranberry Pecan	1 (1.1 oz)	130	6	1	0	2	20	10	2	0	105	—	—	0
Granola Honey Nut	1 (1.1 oz)	140	7	1	0	3	18	8	2	0	105	—	—	0
BAHLSEN														
Delice	6 (1.1 oz)	150	8	5	0	2	19	6	tr	0	135	—	—	0
Deloba	5 (1.2 oz)	170	8	5	<5	2	23	12	tr	0	100	—	—	0
Hannover Waffeln	6 (1.1 oz)	180	10	6	0	2	19	7	0	20	50	—	—	0
Hit Cocoa Creme Filling	2 (1 oz)	150	8	4	<5	2	18	8	1	0	70	—	—	0
Hit Creme Filling	2 (1 oz)	140	7	4	<5	1	19	9	1	0	70	—	—	0
Waffeletten	4 (1 oz)	160	9	7	5	2	18	10	1	20	55	—	—	0

FOOD	PORTION	CALS	FAT	SAT FAT	CHOL	PROT	CARB	SUGAR	FIBER	CALCI	SOD	POTAS	FOLIC	VIT C
BARBARA'S BAKERY														
Fig Bars Traditional	1	60	1	0	0	0	14	8	—	0	20	—	—	5
Fig Bars Wheat Free	1	60	0	0	0	0	13	8	1	0	25	—	—	5
Organic 100 Calorie Mini Ginger	1 pkg (0.9 oz)	100	2	1	5	1	19	9	—	0	150	—	—	0
Snackimals Chocolate Chip	10 (1 oz)	120	4	0	0	1	19	8	0	0	80	—	—	0
Snackimals Wheat Free Oatmeal	10	120	5	0	0	1	17	6	1	40	130	—	—	0
BARNUM'S														
Animal Crackers	10 (1 oz)	120	4	1	0	2	22	7	1	100	140	—	—	0
BARRY'S BAKERY														
French Twists Wild Raspberry	2 (0.5 oz)	60	2	1	0	0	9	4	0	0	25	—	—	0
BEAR NAKED														
Granola Soft Baked Fruit & Nut	1 (1 oz)	130	6	2	0	2	18	9	2	0	40	—	—	0
BOLANDS														
Custard Creams	1	62	3	2	—	1	8	4	tr	—	25	—	—	—
BREAKTIME														
Ginger	4 (1 oz)	130	4	1	0	2	23	10	0	0	100	—	—	0
Oatmeal	4 (1 oz)	130	4	1	0	2	22	9	tr	0	190	—	—	0
BRENT & SAM'S														
Chocolate Chip	2 (0.8 oz)	110	6	3	5	1	15	10	1	0	90	—	—	0
BROWN & HALEY														
Almond Roca	6 (1 oz)	110	4	2	5	1	19	10	0	0	105	—	—	0
BROWN BUTTER COOKIE														
Brown Butter Sea Salt	1 (0.7 oz)	94	5	3	14	1	11	6	0	10	41	—	—	0
BUZZ STRONG'S														
Real Coffee	1 (1.2 oz)	150	7	4	10	2	22	13	1	20	125	—	—	0
CAMEO														
Sandwich Creme	2 (1 oz)	130	5	1	0	1	21	10	0	—	105	—	—	—
CAVEMAN COOKIES														
Alpine	2 (1 oz)	150	9	1	0	3	16	14	2	20	0	—	—	1
Original	2 (1 oz)	130	7	1	0	3	15	13	1	20	0	—	—	0
Tropical	2 (1 oz)	140	10	3	0	3	13	10	2	20	0	—	—	0
CHIPS AHOY!														
Chocolate Chip	1 pkg (1.4 oz)	190	9	3	0	2	27	13	1	—	140	—	—	—
Mini	1 pkg (1.2 oz)	170	8	3	0	2	24	10	1	0	115	—	—	0
Reduced Fat	1 pkg (1.1 oz)	140	5	2	0	2	23	11	1	0	150	—	—	0

FOOD	PORTION	CALS	FAT	SAT FAT	CHOL	PROT	CARB	SUGAR	FIBER	CALCI	SOD	POTAS	FOLIC	VIT C
COMFORT CARE														
Cabin Hearth Chocolate Chip	1 (2 oz)	250	11	6	15	3	38	23	1	0	230	—	—	0
Cabin Hearth Oatmeal Peach	1 (2 oz)	200	7	4	15	3	31	17	3	20	220	—	—	0
Cabin Hearth Oatmeal Raisin	1 (2 oz)	200	7	2	15	3	31	17	3	20	220	—	—	0
COUNTRY CHOICE ORGANIC														
Fit Kids Snackin' Grahams Chocolate	18 (1 oz)	110	3	1	0	2	20	7	2	100	115	—	—	0
Oatmeal Chocolate Chip	1 (0.8 oz)	100	4	1	5	1	15	8	1	0	60	—	—	0
Oatmeal Raisin	1 (0.8 oz)	100	3	1	5	1	16	9	1	0	65	—	—	0
DARE														
Lemon Creme	1 (0.7 oz)	100	4	1	0	tr	14	7	0	0	70	—	—	0
Maple Leaf Creme	1 (0.6 oz)	80	4	1	0	tr	12	6	0	0	60	—	—	0
DELACRE														
Royal Moments Milk Chocolate Biscuits	2 (0.9 oz)	130	6	4	33	2	18	11	0	0	30	—	—	0
DICAMILLO														
Biscotti DiPrato	5 (1 oz)	130	4	0	15	3	21	12	tr	20	130	—	24	0
DIVVIES														
Chocolate Chip Vegan	1	130	7	3	0	1	17	11	tr	0	105	—	—	0
Oatmeal Raisin Vegan	1	120	5	1	0	1	17	8	tr	0	35	—	—	0
DO GOODIE														
Gluten Free Chocolate Chip	1	140	7	5	20	1	18	11	1	20	115	—	—	0
Gluten Free Oatmeal Raisin	1	120	4	2	15	1	21	13	1	20	60	—	—	0
EARTHBOUND FARMS														
Organic Ginger Snaps	2	120	6	4	20	2	18	8	0	40	70	—	—	0
EMILY'S														
Fortune Dark Chocolate Covered	2 (1.4 oz)	140	6	4	0	2	23	15	2	0	0	—	—	0
Graham Cracker Milk Chocolate Covered	1 (1 oz)	150	9	5	<5	2	17	13	tr	40	45	—	—	—
ENJOY LIFE														
Allergen Gluten Free Gingerbread Spice	2 (1 oz)	100	4	0	0	1	19	10	2	20	120	—	—	0

FOOD	PORTION	CALS	FAT	SAT FAT	CHOL	PROT	CARB	SUGAR	FIBER	CALCI	SOD	POTAS	FOLIC	VIT C
ENJOY LIFE (CONT.)														
Allergen Gluten Free No Oats Oatmeal	2 (1 oz)	120	4	0	0	1	21	10	1	20	50	—	—	0
Allergen Gluten Free Snickerdoodle	2 (1 oz)	130	5	0	0	1	21	14	2	20	110	—	—	0
Snack Bar Sunbutter Crunch	1 (1 oz)	140	5	1	0	3	20	4	3	100	110	—	140	0
ENTENMANN'S														
Original Chocolate Chip	3 (1 oz)	140	7	3	<5	1	20	11	tr	0	90	—	—	0
Soft Baked Chocolate Chunk	1 (1.3 oz)	190	9	5	15	2	25	13	0	0	140	—	—	0
ERIN BAKER'S														
Breakfast Banana Toasted Flax	1 (3 oz)	300	5	1	0	6	55	12	6	40	250	—	—	1
Breakfast Banana Walnut	1 (3 oz)	300	8	1	0	7	52	17	5	40	240	—	—	1
Breakfast Caramel Apple	1 (3 oz)	280	4	1	0	6	55	21	5	40	240	—	—	2
Breakfast Double Chocolate Chunk	1 (3 oz)	300	6	1	0	7	53	19	6	20	230	—	—	1
Breakfast Oatmeal Raisin	1 (3 oz)	290	5	0	0	6	55	22	5	40	230	—	—	1
Breakfast Mini Fruit & Nut	1 (1 oz)	100	3	0	0	2	17	7	2	20	75	—	—	0
Breakfast Vegan Chocolate Chip	1 (3 oz)	310	6	2	0	6	57	22	6	40	250	—	—	1
Organic Breakfast Mini Peanut Butter	1 (1 oz)	110	3	0	0	3	16	7	2	20	115	—	—	0
FAUCHON														
Assorted Chocolate	4 (2 oz)	330	15	10	55	4	34	16	5	0	165	—	—	0
FOODS BY GEORGE														
Gluten Free Biscotti	1 (0.8 oz)	90	5	0	0	2	11	6	1	20	25	—	—	0
FOX'S														
Golden Crunch Creams	1	75	4	2	—	1	9	6	tr	—	200	—	—	—
FRENCH MEADOW BAKERY														
Coconutty Macaroons	2 (1.1 oz)	150	8	7	5	2	17	11	1	40	85	—	—	0

FOOD	PORTION	CALS	FAT	SAT FAT	CHOL	PROT	CARB	SUGAR	FIBER	CALCI	SOD	POTAS	FOLIC	VIT C
FRENCH MEADOW BAKERY (CONT.)														
Gluten Free Chocolate Chip	1 (2.1 oz)	320	16	8	25	1	43	23	1	40	260	—	—	0
Rhubarb Bar	1 (2.7 oz)	250	11	7	30	3	34	18	1	80	80	—	—	0
Vegan Peanut Butter Bliss	2 (1.2 oz)	150	7	3	0	2	19	3	1	20	260	—	—	0
GAK'S SNACKS														
Organic Brownie Chip	1 (1 oz)	130	5	1	0	2	20	11	1	0	115	—	—	0
Organic Chocolate Chip	1 (1 oz)	140	6	1	0	1	21	11	1	0	95	—	—	0
Organic Oatmeal	1 (1 oz)	120	4	0	0	2	19	9	2	0	75	—	—	0
GAMESA														
Animalitos	14 (1 oz)	110	1	0	0	2	25	7	tr	0	160	—	60	0
Emperador Vanilla Creme Sandwich	2 (0.9 oz)	120	4	1	<5	2	19	9	0	0	75	—	32	0
Hawaianas Coconut	3 (1 oz)	130	4	1	0	2	22	9	tr	0	115	—	40	0
Sugar Wafers Chocolate	3 (1.2 oz)	160	7	2	0	1	23	15	0	0	30	—	—	0
GINGER SNAPS														
Cookies	4 (1 oz)	120	3	0	0	1	23	11	0	20	190	—	—	0
GIRL SCOUT														
Do-si-dos	2 (0.8 oz)	110	5	2	0	2	16	7	tr	0	70	—	—	0
Dulce De Leche	4 (1 oz)	160	8	4	0	1	20	9	0	0	70	—	—	0
Peanut Butter Sandwich	3 (1.2 oz)	160	6	3	0	2	26	8	tr	0	135	—	—	0
Samoas	2 (1 oz)	140	7	5	0	1	19	10	1	0	55	—	—	0
Savannah Smiles	5 (1 oz)	140	5	2	0	1	23	10	0	0	125	—	—	0
Shout Outs!	4 (0.9 oz)	130	5	2	0	2	18	8	tr	20	130	—	—	0
Tagalongs	2 (0.9 oz)	140	9	5	0	2	13	8	tr	0	95	—	—	0
Thank U Berry Munch	2 (0.9 oz)	120	5	2	0	1	18	7	tr	0	75	—	—	0
Thin Mints	4 (1.1 oz)	160	8	5	0	1	22	10	tr	0	120	—	—	0
Trefoils	5 (1.2 oz)	160	8	3	0	2	22	7	tr	0	115	—	—	0
GLUTEN-FREE PANTRY														
Gluten Free Buckwheat Raisin	1 (1 oz)	140	6	3	5	1	21	9	1	0	135	—	—	0
Gluten Free Chocolate Chunk	1 (1 oz)	140	8	4	5	1	19	8	1	0	120	—	—	0
GLUTENFREEDA														
Kookies Sugar	1	142	7	4	33	1	19	11	0	10	97	—	—	0
GLUTINO														
Gluten Free Wafers Chocolate	4	160	8	5	5	1	19	14	3	40	25	—	—	0

FOOD	PORTION	CALS	FAT	SAT FAT	CHOL	PROT	CARB	SUGAR	FIBER	CALCI	SOD	POTAS	FOLIC	VIT C
GLUTINO (CONT.)														
Gluten Free Wafers Lemon	3	150	6	4	0	0	24	15	0	0	25	—	—	0
GOTTENA														
Exquisit	5	170	10	9	0	2	19	6	1	0	25	—	—	0
GOURMET PASTRIES														
Kourabiethes Butter Almond	1 (1.1 oz)	150	9	5	25	2	15	5	1	0	110	—	—	0
Phoenicia Honey & Spice	1 (1.3 oz)	140	5	2	0	2	20	12	0	0	60	—	—	1
GRANDMA'S														
Chocolate Brownie	1 (1.4 oz)	190	8	3	<5	2	27	14	2	0	135	95	—	0
Peanut Butter	1 (1.2 oz)	170	9	3	<5	4	19	10	2	0	160	—	—	0
Vanilla Creme Sandwich	5 (1.4 oz)	190	9	3	<5	2	27	12	tr	20	120	—	—	0
HEALTH VALLEY														
Mini Mint Chocolate Chip	4 (1 oz)	120	6	2	5	1	16	7	1	—	125	—	—	—
Oatmeal Raisin	1 (0.8 oz)	90	4	0	0	2	14	8	1	150	50	—	—	—
Raisin Oatmeal Low Fat	3	110	2	0	0	2	23	13	1	20	105	—	—	—
White Chocolate Chunk	1 (1 oz)	140	7	3	10	1	17	10	0	—	150	—	—	—
HEALTHY HANDFULS														
Organic Crocodile Cookies	1 pkg (1 oz)	130	5	0	0	2	20	7	7	20	75	—	—	0
Organic Koala Krackers	1 pkg (1 oz)	120	4	2	5	2	21	7	2	0	35	—	—	0
HOME FREE														
Organic Chocolate Chip	1 (1 oz)	140	6	1	0	1	21	11	1	0	95	—	—	0
Organic Oatmeal	1 (1 oz)	120	4	0	0	2	19	9	2	0	75	—	—	0
HONEY MAID														
Grahams Honey	1 (1.1 oz)	130	4	1	0	2	24	8	1	0	180	—	—	0
Grahams Honey Low Fat	1 (1.1 oz)	120	2	0	0	2	25	8	1	150	190	—	—	0
JACOB'S														
Oat Crumbles Chocolate & Pecan	1	107	6	3	—	1	13	7	1	—	40	—	—	—
JOSEPH'S														
Almond Sugar Free	4	100	5	1	0	1	13	0	1	0	20	—	—	0
Chocolate Chip Sugar Free	4	95	5	1	0	1	13	0	1	0	40	—	—	1

FOOD	PORTION	CALS	FAT	SAT FAT	CHOL	PROT	CARB	SUGAR	FIBER	CALCI	SOD	POTAS	FOLIC	VIT C
JOSEPH'S (CONT.)														
Oatmeal Chocolate Chip w/ Pecans Sugar Free	4	100	6	1	0	1	14	0	1	0	40	—	—	0
Peanut Butter Sugar Free	4	95	5	1	0	1	14	0	0	0	40	—	—	0
JOVIAL														
Checkerboard Organic	2 (0.9)	120	6	3	20	3	15	6	1	20	70	—	—	0
Chocolate Cream Filled Organic	2 (1.1 oz)	160	7	3	15	2	20	9	1	40	75	—	—	0
Crispy Cocoa Organic	3 (1 oz)	140	6	3	0	3	18	6	1	20	80	—	—	0
Fig Fruit Filled Organic	2 (1.1 oz)	130	4	2	5	1	23	12	1	40	65	—	—	0
Ginger Spice Organic	2 (1.1 oz)	150	6	3	25	3	21	7	1	20	80	—	—	0
Vanilla Cream Filled Organic	2 (1.1 oz)	160	7	3	15	2	21	10	1	20	75	—	—	0
JULES DESTROOPER														
Butter Crisp	2 (0.9 oz)	120	4	3	15	2	19	11	tr	10	75	—	—	0
KASHI														
TLC Happy Trail Mix	1 (1 oz)	130	5	1	0	2	21	7	4	0	80	—	—	0
TLC Oatmeal Dark Chocolate	1 (1 oz)	130	5	2	0	2	21	8	3	0	70	—	—	0
TLC Oatmeal Raisin Flax	1 (1 oz)	130	5	1	0	2	20	8	4	0	75	—	—	0
KAY'S NATURALS														
Protein + Cookie Bites All Flavors Gluten Free	1 oz	110	3	0	0	10	15	3	3	40	336	—	—	0
KEDEM														
Tea Biscuits Chocolate	2 (0.3 oz)	32	1	tr	0	1	6	2	tr	0	29	—	—	0
Tea Biscuits Vanilla	2 (0.3 oz)	32	1	tr	0	1	6	2	tr	0	29	—	—	0
KEEBLER														
100 Calorie Right Bites Fudge Shoppe Fudge Grahams	1 pkg (0.7 oz)	100	4	3	0	1	15	7	tr	0	70	—	—	0
100 Calorie Right Bites Sandies Shortbread	1 pkg (0.7 oz)	100	3	1	0	1	17	7	tr	0	90	—	—	0
Animal Crackers Frosted	8	150	7	5	0	1	22	13	tr	0	80	—	—	0

FOOD	PORTION	CALS	FAT	SAT FAT	CHOL	PROT	CARB	SUGAR	FIBER	CALCI	SOD	POTAS	FOLIC	VIT C
KEEBLER (CONT.)														
Chips Deluxe Chocolate Lovers	1	90	5	2	0	tr	10	5	0	—	65	—	—	0
Chips Deluxe Coconut	2	150	9	4	0	2	18	9	1	0	90	—	—	0
Chips Deluxe Fudge Stripes	1	100	6	3	0	1	13	8	tr	—	60	—	—	—
Chips Deluxe Original	1 pkg (2 oz)	300	16	4	0	3	37	18	1	—	180	—	—	—
Chocolate Dip & Cookie Sticks	1 pkg (1 oz)	130	6	2	0	1	18	12	tr	20	65	—	—	0
Danish Wedding	4	130	6	3	0	1	18	10	tr	—	70	—	—	0
Dipping Delights Cheesecake	1	90	4	2	0	<2	13	8	0	0	50	—	—	0
E.L. Fudge Original	1	90	4	2	<5	1	13	6	tr	0	50	—	—	0
Fudge Shoppe Fudge Stripes	3	150	7	5	0	1	21	10	tr	—	110	—	—	0
Fudge Shoppe Grasshoppers	4	140	7	5	0	1	19	11	tr	—	75	—	—	0
Fudge Shoppe Mint Creme Filled	2	160	9	5	0	tr	20	14	tr	0	65	—	—	0
Graham Honey	8 (1 oz)	110	2	0	0	2	22	7	tr	—	150	—	—	—
Graham Original	8 (1 oz)	130	4	1	0	2	22	7	tr	—	160	—	—	—
Oatmeal Country Style	2	130	6	2	0	2	18	8	1	—	115	—	—	—
Sandies Drops Butter Pecan	4	140	7	4	0	1	18	10	tr	—	60	—	—	0
Sandies Fudge Drops	4 (1 oz)	140	7	4	0	1	18	9	tr	0	60	—	—	0
Sandies Pecan Shortbread Reduced Fat	1	80	4	1	0	tr	11	4	0	—	65	—	—	—
Scooby-Doo Graham Sticks	9	130	4	1	0	2	21	8	tr	—	120	—	—	—
S'mores Snack	1 pkg (0.8 oz)	110	6	3	0	1	14	10	0	20	40	—	—	0
Soft Batch Chocolate Chip	1	80	4	2	0	tr	11	6	tr	—	55	—	—	0
Vanilla Wafers	8	140	6	2	0	1	21	9	tr	—	120	—	—	—
Vienna Fingers	2 (1.1 oz)	150	6	2	0	1	23	10	tr	0	95	—	—	0
Vienna Fingers Reduced Fat	2 (1.1 oz)	140	5	2	0	1	24	12	tr	0	115	—	—	0
KHAYA														
Krunchi Orange & Chocolate	5 (1.53 oz)	240	12	6	21	3	29	14	2	30	14	—	—	0
Shortbread Grapeseed	13 (1.15 oz)	193	10	6	26	tr	27	6	tr	0	64	—	—	0

FOOD	PORTION	CALS	FAT	SAT FAT	CHOL	PROT	CARB	SUGAR	FIBER	CALCI	SOD	POTAS	FOLIC	VIT C
KHAYA (CONT.)														
Shortbread Orange Rooibos	13 (1.15 oz)	259	14	8	36	tr	36	8	tr	4	88	—	—	0
LA CHOY														
Fortune	4 (1 oz)	110	0	0	0	2	25	9	0	0	10	—	—	0
LANCE														
Oatmeal Creme	1 (2.5 oz)	300	12	3	0	3	45	26	2	20	300	—	—	0
Van-O-Lunch	1 pkg (1.6 oz)	230	10	3	0	3	34	14	0	0	140	—	—	0
LATE JULY														
Organic Mini Sandwich Milk Chocolate	10 (1 oz)	130	6	3	0	2	19	8	1	100	85	35	—	0
Organic Mini Sandwich White Chocolate	10 (1 oz)	140	7	3	0	2	18	9	1	100	85	60	—	0
LEAN BODY														
Cookie Bar Hi-Protein S'Mores	1 (3.2 oz)	360	13	3	60	30	30	13	2	50	310	—	—	0
LIZ LOVELY														
Vegan Cowboy	½ cookie (1.3 oz)	190	9	2	0	3	24	13	2	0	90	—	—	0
Vegan Cowgirl	½ cookie (1.5 oz)	210	9	2	0	2	30	18	0	0	130	—	—	0
Vegan Ginger Snapdragons	½ cookie (1.5 oz)	190	7	0	0	2	29	14	0	0	230	—	—	0
LOACKER														
Quadratini Dark Chocolate	9 (1.1 oz)	160	8	6	0	2	20	9	2	20	25	—	—	0
LORNA DOONE														
Shortbread	4 (1 oz)	140	7	2	0	1	20	6	0	0	150	—	—	0
LU														
Le Chocolatier	3 (1 oz)	150	9	7	0	1	17	12	1	0	5	—	—	0
Le Fondant	4 (1.1 oz)	170	10	9	0	2	19	9	1	0	5	—	—	0
Le Petit Beurre	4 (1.2 oz)	140	4	2	5	3	24	8	tr	0	230	—	—	0
Petit Ecolier Dark Chocolate	2 (0.9 oz)	130	6	4	5	1	17	9	1	0	50	—	—	0
Petit Ecolier Milk Chocolate	2 (0.9 oz)	130	6	4	5	2	17	10	tr	20	55	—	—	0
Pim's Orange	2 (0.9 oz)	100	3	2	10	tr	17	14	0	0	35	—	—	0
Shortbread	2 (1 oz)	140	8	5	25	1	16	5	tr	20	95	—	—	0
LUCY'S														
Chocolate Chip Gluten Free Vegan	3	130	5	2	0	2	20	12	2	—	170	—	—	—

FOOD	PORTION	CALS	FAT	SAT FAT	CHOL	PROT	CARB	SUGAR	FIBER	CALCI	SOD	POTAS	FOLIC	VIT C
LUCY'S (CONT.)														
Cinnamon Thin Gluten Free Vegan	3	130	5	2	0	2	21	13	1	—	180	—	—	—
Oatmeal Gluten Free Vegan	3	120	5	1	0	2	18	9	1	—	170	—	—	—
Sugar Gluten Free Vegan	3	130	5	2	0	2	21	13	1	—	180	—	—	—
LUNA														
Berry Pomegranate	1 (1.4 oz)	140	3	0	0	3	27	11	4	250	100	105	200	30
Peanut Butter Chocolate	1 (1.4 oz)	150	6	1	0	4	23	10	3	250	170	115	200	30
M&M'S														
Milk Chocolate	1 pkg (1.15 oz)	150	5	1	5	2	22	11	1	200	110	—	—	1
MALLOMARS														
Cookies	2 (0.9 oz)	120	5	3	0	1	18	12	1	0	40	—	—	0
MARKET DAY														
Chocolate Chip Peanut Free	1 (1 oz)	150	9	3	10	1	17	9	0	20	65	—	—	0
MAUNA LOA														
Macadamia Nut Chocolate Chip	4 (1 oz)	150	9	2	—	1	17	5	<1	0	80	—	—	0
MISS MERINGUE														
Meringue Chocolate	1 pkg (1 oz)	100	0	0	0	2	24	23	1	0	20	—	—	0
MONTANA MONSTER MUNCHIES														
Original	½ (1.4 oz)	177	9	4	22	4	21	14	2	10	33	—	—	0
Raisin	½ (1.4 oz)	172	9	4	21	3	22	14	2	10	32	—	—	0
MOONPIE														
Mini All Flavors	1 pkg (1.2 oz)	130	4	3	0	2	23	11	2	0	110	—	—	0
MRS. FIELDS														
Cookie Dough Snacks Brownie Chocolate Chip	7 (1 oz)	120	3	0	5	tr	18	10	0	0	80	—	—	0
Cookie Dough Snacks Chocolate Chip	7 (1 oz)	120	4	2	<5	1	19	12	tr	0	55	—	—	0
MURRAY'S														
Sugar Free Chocolate Sandwich	3 (1 oz)	130	7	3	0	1	19	0	1	0	55	—	—	0
Sugar Free Chocolate Chip	3 (1.1 oz)	160	9	4	<5	2	20	0	1	0	130	—	—	0
Sugar Free Fudge Dipped Grahams	4 (1 oz)	150	8	6	0	2	19	0	1	0	80	—	—	0
Sugar Free Ginger Snap	7 (1.1 oz)	130	5	2	0	2	23	0	2	0	115	—	—	0

FOOD	PORTION	CALS	FAT	SAT FAT	CHOL	PROT	CARB	SUGAR	FIBER	CALCI	SOD	POTAS	FOLIC	VIT C
MURRAY'S (CONT.)														
Sugar Free Oatmeal	3 (1.1 oz)	140	7	3	0	2	21	0	3	0	130	—	—	0
Sugar Free Shortbread	8 (1 oz)	130	5	2	0	2	21	0	2	0	140	—	—	0
NABISCO														
100 Calorie Pack Alpha-Bits Mini	1 pkg	100	3	2	0	1	16	6	0	0	120	15	—	0
100 Calorie Pack Barnum's Animal Choco	1 pkg	100	3	0	0	1	17	6	tr	0	115	40	—	0
100 Calorie Pack Lorna Doone	1 pkg	100	3	2	0	1	16	6	0	0	120	—	—	0
100 Calorie Pack Teddy Grahams Mini Cinnamon	1 pkg	100	3	0	0	1	16	4	1	100	115	35	—	0
Grahams Original	8 (1.1 oz)	130	3	1	0	2	24	7	1	20	190	75	—	0
NAIRN'S														
Oat Fruit & Cinnamon	2 (0.7 oz)	85	3	1	0	2	15	4	2	10	50	—	—	1
Oat Stem Ginger	2 (0.7 oz)	87	3	1	0	2	14	4	1	10	60	—	—	0
NANA'S														
No Gluten Berry Vanilla	1 bar (1.2 oz)	130	4	0	0	1	22	7	tr	20	135	55	—	1
No Gluten Chocolate	1 (3.5 oz)	360	12	0	0	4	62	20	2	40	380	—	—	2
No Gluten Ginger	1 (3.5 oz)	360	10	0	0	4	64	48	2	40	170	—	—	2
No Gluten Nana Banana	1 bar (1.2 oz)	130	5	0	0	1	23	7	0	20	130	50	—	1
No Wheat Oatmeal Raisin	1 (3.5 oz)	280	10	0	0	6	46	18	6	80	150	—	—	0
Vegan Chocolate Chip	1 (4 oz)	320	14	2	0	6	48	20	6	80	210	—	—	2
Vegan Peanut Butter	1 (4 oz)	360	16	1	0	8	46	18	4	40	220	—	—	2
Vegan Sunflower	1 (3.5 oz)	380	14	2	0	8	60	26	6	40	360	—	—	0
NAPOLITANKE														
Lemon Orange	4 (0.7 oz)	108	6	1	—	1	13	7	—	0	12	—	—	0
Mocca	4 (0.7 oz)	101	5	1	—	1	13	7	—	3	27	—	—	0
NATURAL OVENS														
Oatmeal Raisin	1 (1.3 oz)	120	4	1	0	2	20	10	2	0	50	—	0	0
NEW MORNING														
Honey Grahams	2 (1 oz)	130	3	0	0	3	24	8	1	0	180	—	—	0
NEW YORK STYLE														
Biscotti Almond	3 (1 oz)	130	5	1	25	3	20	12	1	20	35	—	—	0

FOOD	PORTION	CALS	FAT	SAT FAT	CHOL	PROT	CARB	SUGAR	FIBER	CALCI	SOD	POTAS	FOLIC	VIT C
NEWTONS														
Fig	2 (1.1 oz)	110	2	0	0	1	22	12	1	20	125	—	—	0
Fig 100% Whole Grain	2 (1.3 oz)	130	3	1	0	1	26	15	3	100	135	—	—	0
Fig Fat Free	2 (1 oz)	90	0	0	0	1	22	12	1	20	125	65	—	0
Fruit Thins Cranberry Citrus Oat	3 (1 oz)	140	5	1	0	2	22	7	1	0	95	40	—	0
Raspberry	2 (1 oz)	100	2	0	0	1	21	13	0	0	110	—	—	0
NILLA WAFERS														
Cookies	1 oz	140	6	2	0	1	21	11	0	20	115	—	—	0
Reduced Fat	1 oz	110	2	0	0	1	24	12	0	20	110	—	—	0
NONNI'S														
Biscotti Limone	1 (0.8 oz)	110	5	2	20	2	17	9	0	20	75	—	—	0
Biscotti Original	1 (0.7 oz)	90	3	1	20	2	14	7	0	0	65	—	—	0
Biscotti Triple Cioccolati	1 (1.3 oz)	170	7	3	25	4	25	14	2	20	100	—	—	0
NUTRABALANCE														
High Fibre	1 (0.7 oz)	90	4	1	0	1	13	6	3	0	85	—	—	0
NUTTER BUTTER														
Bites	1 pkg (1.2 oz)	170	7	2	0	3	24	10	1	0	135	—	—	0
Sandwich Cookie	1 (1 oz)	130	6	1	0	2	19	8	1	20	110	—	—	0
OREO														
Cakesters Mini Golden 100 Calorie Pack	1 pkg (0.8 oz)	100	5	1	0	1	15	10	0	0	65	—	—	0
Double Stuff	1 (1 oz)	140	7	3	0	1	21	13	1	0	120	—	—	0
Golden Chocolate Creme	3 (1.2 oz)	170	7	2	0	2	25	12	tr	0	135	25	—	0
Reduced Fat	3 (1.2 oz)	150	5	1	0	1	27	14	1	20	160	60	—	0
Sandwich Cookie	2 (1.2 oz)	160	7	2	0	2	25	14	1	0	190	—	—	0
ORION														
Choco Pie	1 (1 oz)	120	5	2	<5	1	19	10	tr	0	65	—	—	0
PEPPERIDGE FARM														
Bordeaux	4	130	5	4	10	2	19	12	tr	0	95	—	—	0
Brussels	3	150	7	4	5	2	20	11	1	0	65	—	—	0
Butter Chessmen	3	120	5	3	20	2	18	5	tr	0	80	—	—	0
Chesapeake Dark Chocolate Pecan	1 (0.9 oz)	130	6	4	<5	1	17	10	0	0	60	—	—	0
Geneva	3	160	9	4	0	2	19	8	1	0	95	—	—	0
Homestyle Gingerman	4	130	4	2	10	1	22	13	tr	0	90	—	—	0
Homestyle Lemon	4	160	8	3	5	2	21	8	0	0	105	—	—	0
Homestyle Sugar	3	150	7	3	10	2	21	11	tr	0	65	—	—	0

FOOD	PORTION	CALS	FAT	SAT FAT	CHOL	PROT	CARB	SUGAR	FIBER	CALCI	SOD	POTAS	FOLIC	VIT C
PEPPERIDGE FARM (CONT.)														
Lexington Crispy Milk Chocolate Toffee Almond	1	130	7	3	10	1	17	10	1	0	90	—	—	0
Maui Crispy Milk Chocolate Coconut Almond	1	130	7	4	5	1	17	9	1	0	70	—	—	0
Milano	3	180	10	5	10	2	21	11	tr	0	80	—	—	0
Milano Melts Chocolate Creme	2	140	7	2	<5	2	18	11	1	0	45	—	—	0
Milano Melts Dark Classic Creme	2	140	7	2	<5	1	18	11	1	0	45	—	—	0
Pirouettes Chocolate Hazelnut	2	120	4	2	0	1	19	10	0	0	60	—	—	0
Sausalito Milk Chocolate Macadamia Nut	1	130	6	4	<5	1	17	10	0	0	60	—	—	0
Soft Baked Mystic Sugar	1 (1.1 oz)	140	5	2	10	2	22	9	1	0	100	—	—	0
Soft Baked Sanibel Snickerdoodle	1	140	5	2	10	2	22	9	tr	0	100	—	—	0
Soft Baked Santa Cruz Oatmeal Raisin	1	130	5	2	<5	2	23	13	2	0	90	—	—	0
Tahiti	2	170	10	6	5	2	17	8	2	0	40	—	—	0
Tim Tam Chocolate Creme	2	190	10	5	<5	2	24	18	tr	20	65	—	—	0
Verona Strawberry	3	140	5	3	15	2	22	9	tr	0	55	—	—	0
PIROUETTE														
Sandwich Vanilla Creamed	3 (1.1 oz)	133	4	2	0	1	22	7	0	100	34	—	—	0
POLAR														
Fortune	2	56	0	0	0	2	12	6	0	10	47	—	—	0
Q.BEL														
Wafer Rolls Dark Chocolate	1 pkg (0.9 oz)	120	6	4	0	1	18	13	1	0	25	—	—	0
Wafer Rolls Milk Chocolate	1 pkg (0.9 oz)	130	6	4	0	2	18	13	tr	20	35	—	—	0
QUAKER														
Breakfast Cookie Oatmeal Raisin	1	180	5	2	0	3	33	15	5	300	200	—	—	0
RUGER														
Wafers Vanilla	3 (1 oz)	160	9	8	5	1	20	15	0	<20	25	—	—	tr

FOOD	PORTION	CALS	FAT	SAT FAT	CHOL	PROT	CARB	SUGAR	FIBER	CALCI	SOD	POTAS	FOLIC	VIT C
SIMPLY SHARI'S														
Gluten Free Almond Shortbread	2 (1 oz)	120	6	4	15	1	15	7	0	0	75	—	—	0
Gluten Free Chocolate Chip	2 (1 oz)	120	6	3	10	1	17	9	1	0	55	—	—	0
Gluten Free Fudge Brownies	2 (1 oz)	130	7	4	10	1	16	10	1	0	70	—	—	0
Gluten Free Shortbread	2 (1 oz)	130	6	4	15	1	17	8	0	0	85	—	—	0
SNACKWELL'S														
Cookie Cakes Chocolate Mint	1 (0.6 oz)	50	1	0	0	1	12	7	0	0	40	—	—	0
Devil's Food Fat Free	1 (0.5 oz)	50	0	0	0	1	12	7	0	0	25	—	—	0
Sugar Free Lemon Creme	2 (1.1 oz)	130	6	2	0	1	23	0	2	0	135	—	—	0
Sugar Free Shortbread	2 (1 oz)	130	6	2	5	2	21	0	2	0	140	—	—	0
SNIKIDDY														
Cherry Oaties	1 pkg (0.8 oz)	110	4	1	0	2	17	6	1	20	115	—	—	1
SOUTH BEACH														
Fiber Fit Double Chocolate Chunk	1 pkg (0.8 oz)	100	5	2	0	1	17	5	5	—	85	—	—	—
Fiber Fit Oatmeal Chocolate Chunk	1 pkg (0.8 oz)	100	5	2	0	1	17	5	5	—	80	—	—	—
Wafer Sticke Dark Chocolate Hazelnut Creme	1 pkg	100	6	3	0	5	10	tr	3	—	70	—	—	—
Wafer Sticke Dark Chocolate Peanut Butter	1 pkg	100	6	3	0	5	10	1	3	—	75	—	—	—
STARBUCKS														
Almond Roca Buttercrunch Toffee	6 (1 oz)	110	4	2	5	1	19	10	0	0	105	—	—	0
Biscotti Chocolate Hazelnut	1 (0.9 oz)	100	5	2	20	2	14	7	1	20	70	—	—	0
Madeleines Petite French Cakes	3 (1.8 oz)	230	11	6	70	19	32	19	tr	0	100	—	—	0
White Chocolate & Raspberry	2 (0.9 oz)	120	6	2	0	1	15	8	tr	20	85	—	—	0
STELLA D'ORO														
100 Calorie Pack Breakfast Treats Original	1 pkg (0.8 oz)	100	2	1	15	2	19	6	1	10	96	—	—	0

FOOD	PORTION	CALS	FAT	SAT FAT	CHOL	PROT	CARB	SUGAR	FIBER	CALCI	SOD	POTAS	FOLIC	VIT C
STELLA D'ORO (CONT.)														
Almond Delight	1 (1 oz)	150	8	4	10	2	18	7	tr	0	85	—	—	0
Angelica Goodies	1 (0.7 oz)	90	3	1	10	1	15	5	0	0	45	—	—	0
Anginetti	4 (1.1 oz)	130	3	1	25	1	25	21	0	20	5	—	—	0
Biscotti Almond	1 (0.7 oz)	90	4	2	5	2	15	8	1	0	40	—	—	0
Biscotti French Vanilla	1 (0.7 oz)	90	3	2	5	1	15	7	0	0	50	—	—	0
Breakfast Treats Chocolate	1 (0.9 oz)	110	4	2	20	1	19	10	tr	0	70	—	—	0
Breakfast Treats Original	1 (0.7 oz)	90	3	2	20	1	14	6	0	100	65	—	—	0
Coffee Treats Almond Toast	2 (0.9 oz)	100	2	0	25	2	20	9	tr	20	90	—	—	0
Coffee Treats Angel Wings	3 (1 oz)	160	10	5	0	2	16	5	0	0	90	—	—	0
Coffee Treats Anisette Sponge	2 (0.9 oz)	90	1	0	40	2	18	8	0	20	80	—	—	0
Coffee Treats Anisette Toast	3 (1.2 oz)	130	1	0	35	2	27	13	tr	20	110	—	—	0
Coffee Treats Roman Egg Biscuits	1 (1.1 oz)	130	5	2	15	3	19	7	0	40	125	—	—	0
Egg Jumbo	3 (1.2 oz)	120	2	0	50	2	25	13	0	0	85	—	—	0
Lady Stella	3 (1 oz)	130	5	3	<5	1	19	8	tr	0	60	—	—	0
Margherite	2 (1 oz)	130	5	2	20	2	20	7	0	0	85	—	—	0
Swiss Fudge	3 (1.2 oz)	170	9	5	<5	2	22	12	tr	0	80	—	—	0
TEDDY GRAHAMS														
Chocolate	24 (1.1 oz)	130	5	1	0	2	22	8	2	100	160	—	—	0
Honey	24 (1 oz)	130	4	1	0	2	23	7	1	100	150	—	—	0
TEMPTATIONS														
Chocolate Alps	1 bar (1.6 oz)	170	7	0	0	2	28	12	1	0	130	—	—	0
Chocolate Mocha	1 bar (1.6 oz)	170	6	5	0	2	27	11	1	0	130	—	—	0
No Gluten Chocolate Rush	1 bar (1.6 oz)	170	9	7	0	1	25	10	1	0	90	—	—	0
TITAN														
High Protein Chocolate Chip	1 (1.4 oz)	150	6	3	10	10	15	5	3	20	150	—	—	0
High Protein Oatmeal Raisin	1 (1.4 oz)	150	5	3	10	10	15	5	2	20	190	—	—	0
High Protein Peanut Butter	1 (1.4 oz)	150	5	3	5	10	17	5	2	20	200	—	—	0
VOORTMAN														
Chinese Almond	1 (0.9 oz)	130	7	2	0	1	16	7	0	—	—	—	—	—
Coconut Delight	1 (0.6 oz)	90	6	4	0	1	10	5	tr	—	tr	—	—	—
Dutch Creme	1 (0.8 oz)	110	4	1	0	1	16	8	0	—	60	—	—	—
Fudge Swirl	1 (0.6 oz)	80	4	1	0	1	10	4	0	—	30	—	—	—

FOOD	PORTION	CALS	FAT	SAT FAT	CHOL	PROT	CARB	SUGAR	FIBER	CALCI	SOD	POTAS	FOLIC	VIT C
VOORTMAN (CONT.)														
Gingerboy	1 (0.7 oz)	100	4	1	0	1	15	7	0	—	90	—	—	—
Maple Leaf	1 (0.6 oz)	90	4	1	0	1	13	7	0	—	tr	—	—	—
Molasses	1 (1 oz)	110	3	1	0	2	20	10	tr	—	80	—	—	—
Peanut Delight	1 (0.9 oz)	130	7	2	0	2	15	6	tr	—	90	—	—	—
Shortbread	1 (0.6 oz)	90	5	1	0	1	12	4	0	0	40	—	—	0
Sugar Free Chocolate Chip	1 (0.7 oz)	80	5	2	0	1	13	0	0	—	50	—	—	—
Sugar Free Lemon Wafers	3 (1 oz)	130	8	2	0	0	17	0	0	—	40	—	—	—
Sugar Free Oatmeal	1 (0.7 oz)	70	4	1	0	1	10	0	tr	0	50	—	—	0
Sugar Free Vanilla Creme	2 (0.7 oz)	100	6	2	0	1	13	0	0	—	40	—	—	—
Sugar Free Wafers Peanut Butter	4 (1 oz)	150	8	2	0	2	17	0	0	—	50	—	—	—
Sugar Free Wafers Vanilla	3 (1 oz)	130	8	2	0	0	17	0	0	—	40	—	—	—
Turnover Blueberry	1 (0.9 oz)	110	4	2	0	1	18	9	tr	—	60	—	—	—
Turnover Cherry	1 (0.9 oz)	110	4	2	0	1	18	9	tr	—	50	—	—	—
Turnover Strawberry	1 (0.9 oz)	110	4	2	0	1	18	9	tr	—	60	—	—	—
Wafer Chocolate Covered	1 (0.7 oz)	100	5	2	0	tr	13	9	0	—	15	—	—	—
Wafer Vanilla	3 (1 oz)	140	7	2	0	1	20	12	0	—	25	—	—	—
Wafers Mini Chocolate	5 (1 oz)	130	6	2	0	tr	19	11	0	—	20	—	—	—
WALKERS														
Shortbread Chocolate Chip	2 (1 oz)	140	8	5	20	1	17	7	tr	20	80	—	—	0
Shortbread Rounds	1 (0.6 oz)	90	5	3	15	tr	10	3	0	0	50	—	—	0
WHIPPET														
Original	2 (1.2 oz)	150	5	3	0	1	24	16	1	0	50	—	—	0
WORLD OF GRAINS														
Apple Cinnamon	1 pkg	130	4	2	5	3	21	9	3	—	85	—	—	—
Cranberry	1 pkg	130	4	2	5	3	21	9	3	—	85	—	—	—
Multigrain	1 pkg	130	5	2	5	3	21	6	3	—	100	—	—	—
WOW														
Chocolate Brownie	1 (1.4 oz)	161	9	5	38	2	20	15	1	20	59	—	—	0
Chocolate Chip Gluten Free	1 (1.4 oz)	170	8	5	31	1	25	14	1	0	128	—	—	0
Lemon Burst Gluten Free	1 (1.4 oz)	180	8	5	35	1	24	10	tr	20	160	—	—	0
Peanut Butter	1 (1.4 oz)	170	10	3	25	4	21	12	1	30	171	—	—	0

FOOD	PORTION	CALS	FAT	SAT FAT	CHOL	PROT	CARB	SUGAR	FIBER	CALCI	SOD	POTAS	FOLIC	VIT C
ZWIEBACK														
Toast	1 (8 g)	35	1	0	0	1	6	1	0	—	10	—	—	—
REFRIGERATED														
chocolate chip	1 (0.42 oz)	59	3	1	3	1	8	—	—	3	28	24	—	0
chocolate chip dough	1 oz	126	6	2	7	1	17	—	—	7	59	51	—	0
oatmeal	1 (0.4 oz)	56	3	1	3	1	8	—	—	4	39	20	—	—
oatmeal raisin	1 (0.4 oz)	56	3	1	3	1	8	—	—	4	39	20	—	—
peanut butter	1 (0.4 oz)	60	3	1	4	1	7	—	—	13	52	41	—	0
peanut butter dough	1 oz	130	7	2	8	2	15	—	—	29	112	87	—	0
sugar	1 (0.42 oz)	58	3	1	4	1	8	—	—	11	56	20	—	0
sugar dough	1 oz	124	6	2	8	1	17	—	—	23	120	42	—	0
PILLSBURY														
Chocolate Chip	2 (1.3 oz)	170	9	3	10	2	22	14	tr	0	125	—	—	0
Gingerbread	2 (1.1 oz)	170	7	2	10	1	18	9	0	0	105	—	—	0
Oatmeal Chocolate Chip	2 (1.3 oz)	170	8	3	10	2	23	14	1	0	95	—	—	0
Peanut Butter	2 (1 oz)	130	6	2	5	2	16	9	0	0	135	—	—	0
S'Mores	2 (1.3 oz)	160	7	2	5	1	23	25	tr	0	120	—	—	0
Sugar	2 (1.3 oz)	170	9	3	10	2	22	12	0	0	100	—	—	0
TAKE-OUT														
biscotti w/ nuts chocolate dipped	1 (1.3 oz)	117	6	3	18	2	16	11	1	10	33	—	—	1
black & white	1 lg (3 oz)	302	9	5	58	4	52	31	1	32	72	68	11	tr
finikia	1 (1.2 oz)	171	5	5	27	2	16	5	1	8	26	26	6	tr
koulourakia butter cookie twist	1 (0.9 oz)	113	6	3	32	2	14	5	tr	15	59	16	5	0
linzer tart	1 (2.4 oz)	280	14	4	40	2	34	12	0	20	130	—	—	1
# CORIANDER														
leaf dried	1 tsp	2	tr	tr	0	tr	tr	tr	tr	7	1	27	2	3
leaf fresh	¼ cup	1	tr	—	0	tr	tr	—	—	4	1	22	—	—
seed	1 tsp	5	tr	tr	0	tr	1	—	1	13	1	23	0	tr
# CORN														
CANNED														
cream style	½ cup	93	1	tr	0	2	23	—	—	4	365	172	57	6
w/ red & green peppers	½ cup	86	1	tr	0	3	21	—	—	5	396	174	—	10
white	½ cup	66	1	tr	0	2	15	—	—	—	—	—	—	—
yellow	½ cup	66	1	tr	0	2	15	—	1	—	—	—	—	—
DEL MONTE														
Cream Style Sweet Corn	½ cup (4.4 oz)	70	1	0	0	1	14	6	4	0	300	130	—	0
Savory Sides In Butter Sauce	½ cup	90	3	1	5	2	14	5	tr	0	530	—	—	5

FOOD	PORTION	CALS	FAT	SAT FAT	CHOL	PROT	CARB	SUGAR	FIBER	CALCI	SOD	POTAS	FOLIC	VIT C
DEL MONTE (CONT.)														
Savory Sides Santa Fe	½ cup	70	1	0	0	3	16	1	1	0	510	—	—	9
Whole Kernel	½ cup (4.4 oz)	60	1	0	0	2	13	6	3	0	300	170	—	0
GREEN GIANT														
Mexicorn	½ cup (3.3 oz)	90	1	—	0	2	19	6	1	0	270	—	—	4
Super Sweet Yellow & White	⅓ cup (2.6 oz)	60	1	0	0	2	12	3	1	0	200	—	—	2
Whole Kernel	½ cup (4.3 oz)	90	1	0	0	2	20	6	1	0	320	—	—	2
JAKE & AMOS														
Pickled Dill Baby Corn	2 tbsp	5	0	0	0	0	1	0	0	—	217	—	—	—
ORCHIDS														
Whole Young Spears	½ cup (4.6 oz)	25	0	0	0	2	4	1	2	0	280	—	—	1
DRIED														
CRUNCHIES														
Freeze Dried Corn Snack	⅓ cup (1 oz)	130	7	1	0	2	19	0	4	0	85	—	—	0
Freeze Dried Sweet Buttered	½ cup (1 oz)	100	2	0	0	3	21	5	3	0	210	—	—	6
SUNRICH NATURALS														
Toasted Corn Cool Ranch	1 pkg (1 oz)	100	2	tr	1	3	20	1	1	10	280	—	—	1
FRESH														
white cooked	½ cup	89	1	tr	0	3	21	—	—	2	14	204	38	5
white raw	½ cup	66	1	tr	0	2	15	—	—	2	12	208	35	5
yellow cooked	1 ear (2.7 oz)	83	1	tr	0	3	19	—	—	2	13	192	36	5
yellow cooked	½ cup	89	1	tr	0	3	21	—	—	2	14	204	38	5
yellow raw	½ cup	66	1	tr	0	2	15	—	—	2	12	208	35	5
yellow raw	1 ear (3 oz)	77	1	tr	0	3	17	—	—	2	14	243	41	6
FROZEN														
cooked	½ cup	67	tr	tr	0	2	17	—	—	2	4	114	19	2
on the cob cooked	1 ear (2.2 oz)	59	tr	tr	0	2	14	—	—	2	3	158	19	3
BIRDS EYE														
Steamfresh Singles Super Sweet	1 pkg (3.2 oz)	80	1	0	0	3	14	6	2	0	0	—	—	6
Steamfresh Southwestern	⅔ cup (2.9 oz)	90	2	0	0	2	16	5	1	0	260	—	—	6
Steamfresh Sweet Mini Corn On The Cob	1 (3 oz)	90	1	0	0	3	19	5	1	0	0	—	—	5
C&W														
Cheddar Bacon	½ cup	130	5	2	10	4	18	9	3	40	210	—	—	2

FOOD	PORTION	CALS	FAT	SAT FAT	CHOL	PROT	CARB	SUGAR	FIBER	CALCI	SOD	POTAS	FOLIC	VIT C
C&W (CONT.)														
Early Harvest Supersweet Petite	⅔ cup	70	1	0	0	3	14	6	2	0	0	—	—	6
Salsa Corn	1 cup	90	1	0	0	3	17	7	3	20	250	—	—	12
GLORY														
Savory Accents Fried Corn	½ cup	110	2	1	0	3	24	7	2	20	470	—	—	5
GREEN GIANT														
Cream Style	½ cup	110	1	0	0	2	24	7	2	0	320	—	—	4
Nibblers On-The-Cob	1 (2.1 oz)	70	1	0	0	2	14	2	1	0	5	—	—	2
HEALTH IS WEALTH														
Creamed	½ pkg (4.5 oz)	110	2	1	5	4	23	7	1	20	40	—	—	2
STOUFFER'S														
Souffle	½ pkg (6 oz)	150	5	1	65	5	22	8	2	60	490	—	—	0
TAKE-OUT														
fritters	1 (1 oz)	62	2	tr	12	2	9	—	1	21	126	47	3	1
on the cob w/ butter cooked	1 ear	155	3	2	6	4	32	—	—	5	30	360	44	7
scalloped	1 cup	257	11	3	152	10	34	11	3	92	666	417	54	6

CORN CHIPS

(*see* CHIPS)

CORNISH HEN

(*see* CHICKEN)

CORNMEAL

FOOD	PORTION	CALS	FAT	SAT FAT	CHOL	PROT	CARB	SUGAR	FIBER	CALCI	SOD	POTAS	FOLIC	VIT C
cornmeal mush as prep w/ water	1 cup	223	1	tr	0	5	47	tr	5	12	523	98	98	0
cornmeal yellow	½ cup (2.2 oz)	236	1	tr	0	4	52	tr	1	1	1	57	30	0
whole grain blue	½ cup (1.9 oz)	201	3	—	0	5	41	0	5	3	3	210	—	—
yellow self-rising	½ cup (3 oz)	296	2	tr	0	7	62	—	5	254	1121	176	224	0
INDIAN HEAD														
Stone Ground	¼ cup	100	1	—	0	3	20	0	2	—	0	—	40	—
MARTHA WHITE														
White Self Rising	3 tbsp (1.1 oz)	100	1	0	0	2	22	0	2	0	440	—	40	0
White Enriched	3 tbsp (1.2 oz)	120	1	0	0	3	24	0	2	—	0	—	60	—
Yellow Self Rising	3 tbsp (1.1 oz)	110	1	0	0	2	22	0	2	40	460	—	40	0
QUAKER														
Instant Original not prep	1 pkg (1 oz)	100	0	0	0	2	22	0	1	100	310	—	40	—
Quick Grits not prep	¼ cup (1.3 oz)	130	1	—	0	3	29	0	2	—	0	—	40	—
TAKE-OUT														
corn pone	1 piece (2.1 oz)	128	3	1	0	2	23	tr	2	70	275	87	5	0
fritter puerto rican style	1 (1.4 oz)	109	7	2	8	3	8	tr	1	59	223	27	16	0

FOOD	PORTION	CALS	FAT	SAT FAT	CHOL	PROT	CARB	SUGAR	FIBER	CALCI	SOD	POTAS	FOLIC	VIT C
harina de maize con coco	½ cup	383	27	24	0	4	36	21	4	18	287	320	41	3
harina de maize con leche	1 cup	295	7	4	25	8	51	32	7	234	300	306	45	1
hush puppies	1 (0.8 oz)	74	3	tr	10	2	10	tr	1	61	147	32	20	0
johnnycake	1 piece (1.7 oz)	134	4	1	35	4	21	4	2	51	432	105	56	tr

CORNSTARCH

FOOD	PORTION	CALS	FAT	SAT FAT	CHOL	PROT	CARB	SUGAR	FIBER	CALCI	SOD	POTAS	FOLIC	VIT C
cornstarch	¼ cup (1.1 oz)	122	tr	tr	0	tr	29	0	tr	1	3	1	0	0
cornstarch	1 tbsp (0.3 oz)	34	0	0	0	tr	8	0	tr	0	1	0	0	0
ARGO														
Cornstarch	1 tbsp (0.3 oz)	30	0	0	0	0	7	—	—	—	0	—	—	—
BOB'S RED MILL														
Cornstarch	1 tbsp	30	0	0	0	0	7	0	0	—	0	—	—	—
CLABBER GIRL														
Cornstarch Calcium Fortified	1 tbsp (0.4 oz)	35	0	0	0	0	8	—	—	150	0	—	—	—
RUMFORD														
Cornstarch Calcium Fortified	1 tbsp (0.4 oz)	35	0	0	0	0	8	—	—	150	0	—	—	—

COTTAGE CHEESE

FOOD	PORTION	CALS	FAT	SAT FAT	CHOL	PROT	CARB	SUGAR	FIBER	CALCI	SOD	POTAS	FOLIC	VIT C
creamed large curd	½ cup (4 oz)	110	5	2	19	13	4	3	0	93	410	117	14	0
creamed small curd	½ cup (3.7 oz)	103	5	2	18	12	4	3	0	87	382	109	13	0
dry curd	½ cup (2.5 oz)	52	tr	tr	5	8	5	1	0	62	239	99	7	0
lowfat 1%	½ cup (4 oz)	81	1	1	5	14	3	3	0	69	459	97	14	0
lowfat 1% lactose reduced	½ cup (4 oz)	84	1	1	5	14	4	3	1	60	250	98	14	0
AXELROD														
Lowfat 1%	½ cup (4 oz)	90	2	1	15	14	6	4	0	80	480	—	—	0
BREAKSTONE'S														
2% Low Fat Small Curd	½ cup (4.4 oz)	100	3	2	15	12	6	4	0	150	370	—	—	0
4% Fat Small Curd	½ cup (4.4 oz)	120	5	3	25	12	6	5	0	150	390	—	—	0
LiveActive Mixed Berries	1 pkg (4 oz)	120	2	1	10	8	18	0	3	100	310	—	—	1
CABOT														
Cottage Cheese	½ cup	100	5	3	15	13	4	4	0	100	400	—	—	0
No Fat	½ cup	70	0	0	5	13	5	4	0	100	410	—	—	0
FRIENDSHIP														
1% Lowfat	½ cup	90	1	1	5	16	3	3	0	100	360	—	—	—
1% Lowfat No Salt Added	½ cup	90	1	1	0	16	4	3	1	100	50	—	—	—

FOOD	PORTION	CALS	FAT	SAT FAT	CHOL	PROT	CARB	SUGAR	FIBER	CALCI	SOD	POTAS	FOLIC	VIT C
FRIENDSHIP (CONT.)														
1% Lowfat Whipped	½ cup	90	1	1	5	16	3	3	0	100	360	—	—	—
2% Digestive Health	½ cup	90	3	2	10	14	5	2	3	100	360	—	—	—
2% Pot Style	½ cup	90	3	2	10	15	3	2	0	80	400	—	—	—
4% California Style	½ cup	110	5	3	20	15	3	2	1	80	380	—	—	—
Nonfat	½ cup	80	0	0	0	15	4	4	0	100	380	—	—	—
HOOD														
4% Fat w/ Pineapple	½ cup	130	4	2	20	10	15	13	0	80	320	—	—	2
Fat Free	½ cup	80	0	0	10	14	6	5	0	100	410	—	—	0
Low Fat	½ cup	90	1	1	15	14	5	4	0	100	440	—	—	0
Low Fat No Salt Added	½ cup	90	1	1	15	14	6	5	0	80	55	—	—	0
Low Fat w/ Peaches	½ cup	110	1	1	10	10	18	16	0	80	310	—	—	6
HORIZON ORGANIC														
Lowfat	½ cup	100	3	2	15	13	4	3	0	150	390	—	—	0
Regular	½ cup	120	5	3	20	13	4	3	0	150	390	—	—	0
KNUDSEN														
LiveActive Pineapple	1 pkg (4 oz)	110	2	1	10	8	17	0	3	100	310	—	—	4
LACTAID														
Lowfat	½ cup (4 oz)	80	1	1	10	12	7	3	0	100	380	130	—	0
LAND O LAKES														
1% Lowfat	½ cup (4 oz)	90	2	1	10	13	5	3	0	80	460	—	—	0
2% Lowfat	½ cup (3.7 oz)	100	3	2	15	13	5	3	0	80	480	—	—	0
Cottage Cheese	½ cup (3.7 oz)	110	5	3	20	11	5	4	0	80	410	—	—	0
Fat Free	½ cup (4 oz)	80	0	0	0	14	6	4	0	100	380	—	—	0
LIGHT N'LIVELY														
Lowfat	½ cup	80	2	1	10	12	6	5	0	200	420	—	—	0
NANCY'S														
Organic Lowfat	½ cup	80	1	1	5	14	3	3	0	60	304	—	—	0
ORGANIC VALLEY														
Low Fat	½ cup	100	2	2	10	15	4	tr	0	80	450	—	—	0
COTTONSEED														
kernels roasted	1 tbsp	51	4	1	0	3	2	—	—	10	3	135	—	1
COUSCOUS														
cooked	1 cup (5.5 oz)	176	tr	tr	0	6	36	—	2	13	8	91	24	0
dry	1 cup (6.1 oz)	650	1	tr	0	22	134	—	9	42	17	287	35	0
BOB'S RED MILL														
Pearl not prep	⅓ cup (2 oz)	210	1	0	0	7	43	0	0	0	0	—	—	0

FOOD	PORTION	CALS	FAT	SAT FAT	CHOL	PROT	CARB	SUGAR	FIBER	CALCI	SOD	POTAS	FOLIC	VIT C
BOB'S RED MILL (CONT.)														
Pearl Tricolor not prep	⅓ cup (2 oz)	210	1	0	0	6	44	0	0	0	5	—	—	0
Pearl Whole Wheat not prep	⅓ cup (2 oz)	190	1	0	0	7	38	0	5	0	0	—	—	0
MARRAKESH EXPRESS														
Mango Salsa as prep	1 cup	190	0	0	0	7	38	8	1	20	380	—	—	0
Mushroom as prep	1 cup	190	1	0	0	8	39	2	1	0	600	—	—	0
Plain as prep	1 cup	270	0	0	0	10	57	2	2	0	10	—	—	0
NEAR EAST														
Mediterranean Curry as prep	1 cup	220	4	1	0	8	40	2	3	20	552	—	—	1
Original Plain as prep	1 cup	190	2	0	0	7	37	1	3	0	0	—	—	0
Parmesan as prep	1 cup	220	4	2	9	8	39	3	2	60	600	—	—	0
Toasted Pine Nut as prep	1 cup	230	5	1	0	8	39	2	2	20	510	—	—	0
Wild Mushroom & Herb as prep	1 cup	230	4	3	9	8	40	1	3	20	624	—	—	1
RICE SELECT														
All Varieties not prep	¼ cup	150	0	0	0	4	31	—	—	—	0	—	—	—
CRAB														
CANNED														
blue	½ cup	67	1	tr	60	14	0	0	0	68	225	252	29	2
blue drained	1 can (6.5 oz)	124	2	tr	111	26	0	0	0	126	416	468	54	3
ACE OF DIAMONDS														
Fancy w/ Leg Meat	¼ cup (2 oz)	40	0	0	50	7	2	1	0	60	400	—	—	0
CHICKEN OF THE SEA														
Fancy	⅓ can (2 oz)	40	0	0	50	7	2	0	0	60	400	—	—	0
Jumbo Lump	⅓ can (2 oz)	35	1	0	50	7	1	1	0	20	400	—	—	0
POLAR														
Claw Meat	¼ cup (2 oz)	37	0	0	53	10	1	1	0	100	393	—	—	0
Jumbo Lump Meat	¼ cup (2 oz)	39	1	0	52	8	0	0	0	20	304	—	—	0
WILD PLANET														
Dungeness	2 oz	62	1	tr	142	12	tr	—	—	500	321	—	—	0
FRESH														
alaska king meat only steamed	3 oz	82	1	tr	45	16	0	0	0	50	911	223	43	7
blue cooked flaked	1 cup (4 oz)	120	2	tr	118	24	0	0	0	123	329	382	60	4
dungeness steamed	3 oz	94	1	tr	65	19	1	—	0	50	321	347	36	3
queen steamed	3 oz	98	1	tr	60	20	0	0	0	28	587	170	36	6
DOCKSIDE CLASSICS														
Crabcakes	1 (2.5 oz)	150	11	2	25	7	7	1	0	20	380	—	—	3

FOOD	PORTION	CALS	FAT	SAT FAT	CHOL	PROT	CARB	SUGAR	FIBER	CALCI	SOD	POTAS	FOLIC	VIT C
FROZEN														
MAMA BELLE'S														
Crab Cakes Maryland Style	1 (2 oz)	100	5	1	70	9	4	1	0	40	340	—	—	2
MRS. PAUL'S														
Deviled Crab Cakes	1 (3 oz)	220	12	2	60	20	12	tr	3	80	320	—	—	4
SEAPAK														
Maryland Style Crab Cakes + Sauce	1 (4 oz)	240	13	2	55	11	19	3	1	80	830	—	—	15
TAKE-OUT														
alaska king leg steamed	1 leg (4.7 oz)	130	2	tr	71	26	0	0	0	79	1436	351	68	10
baked	1 (3.8 oz)	160	2	tr	184	29	4	—	—	415	550	598	20	3
cakes	2 (4.2 oz)	186	9	2	180	24	1	—	0	126	396	389	64	3
crab imperial	1 crab (6.8 oz)	289	15	3	242	30	6	3	0	182	782	508	80	10
crab salad	1 serv (5.5 oz)	285	21	3	109	21	3	1	1	120	736	402	62	4
crab thermidor	1 serv (6.4 oz)	456	37	22	313	22	8	tr	tr	185	664	401	37	2
deviled	1 serv (4.5 oz)	254	13	3	126	17	17	6	1	110	825	355	56	9
dungeness steamed	1 crab (4.5 oz)	140	2	tr	97	28	1	—	0	75	480	518	53	5
empanada de jueyes	1 (4.4 oz)	341	16	4	45	12	38	7	2	154	680	557	42	22
fried crab puffs	4 (3.2 oz)	323	18	10	85	10	30	tr	1	52	792	147	47	0
kenagi korean crab cooked	1 serv (3 oz)	71	tr	—	—	16	0	0	0	60	204	170	—	0
salmorejo de jueyes (in tomato sauce)	1 serv (4.5 oz)	215	14	2	99	20	3	1	tr	109	785	404	52	9
soft-shell breaded & fried	1 med (2.3 oz)	216	13	3	79	13	11	1	1	76	353	207	43	1
taco de jueyes	1 (4.2 oz)	266	14	5	79	16	18	1	2	160	800	317	47	11
CRACKER CRUMBS														
cracker meal	1 cup	440	2	tr	0	11	93	tr	3	26	32	132	156	0
graham cracker crumbs	1 cup	355	8	1	0	6	65	26	2	20	508	113	39	0
HONEY MAID														
Graham Cracker Crumbs	2½ tbsp (0.6 oz)	70	2	0	0	1	13	4	0	0	95	—	—	0
KEEBLER														
Graham	¼ cup	93	2	0	0	1	17	4	1	—	187	—	—	—
CRACKERS														
melba toast round	1	12	tr	tr	0	tr	2	tr	tr	3	25	6	4	0
oyster cracker	¼ cup	48	1	tr	0	1	8	tr	tr	8	121	17	16	0
saltines	1	13	tr	tr	0	tr	2	tr	tr	2	32	5	4	0

FOOD	PORTION	CALS	FAT	SAT FAT	CHOL	PROT	CARB	SUGAR	FIBER	CALCI	SOD	POTAS	FOLIC	VIT C
water biscuits	3	92	3	—	—	2	16	—	1	25	—	—	—	0
zwieback	1 oz	107	1	—	—	3	21	—	1	12	75	46	—	—
34 DEGREES														
Crispbread Sesame	19 (1.1 oz)	140	3	0	0	5	26	1	1	60	360	—	—	0
Whole Grain	9 (0.5 oz)	35	0	0	0	1	7	0	1	0	110	—	—	0
ANNIE'S HOMEGROWN														
Cheddar Bunnies Original	50 (1 oz)	140	6	1	0	3	19	1	0	0	230	—	—	0
AUNT GUSSIE'S														
Cracker Flats Spelt Cinnamon Raisin	1 (1 oz)	100	2	0	0	3	19	5	1	0	40	—	—	0
Cracker Flats Spelt Everything	1 (0.8 oz)	60	2	0	0	2	12	0	2	20	80	—	—	1
BACK TO NATURE														
Poppy Thyme	17 (1 oz)	130	4	1	0	2	21	2	1	20	270	65	—	0
Rice Thin Sesame Ginger	16	120	3	0	0	2	23	0	0	0	180	—	—	0
Sesame Tarragon	17 (1 oz)	130	5	1	0	2	21	2	1	0	270	65	—	0
BARBARA'S BAKERY														
Rite Rounds Lite Original	5 (0.5 oz)	60	2	0	0	1	11	tr	—	0	200	—	—	0
Wheatines Original	4	60	1	0	0	1	11	1	tr	0	80	—	—	0
BETTER CHEDDARS														
Original	1.1 oz	160	8	2	5	3	18	0	1	20	360	—	—	0
BLUE DIAMOND														
Nut-Thins Almond Country Ranch	16 (1 oz)	130	4	0	0	3	22	1	tr	20	220	—	—	0
BRAN CRISPBREAD														
GG Scandinavian	1 (0.4 oz)	12	0	0	0	1	7	0	5	20	30	—	—	0
BREMNER WAFERS														
Cracked Wheat	7 (0.5 oz)	70	2	0	0	2	11	0	0	0	100	—	—	0
Original	7 (0.5 oz)	70	2	0	0	2	11	0	0	0	105	—	—	0
Soup & Chili Crackers	50 (0.5 oz)	60	2	0	0	2	11	0	0	0	110	—	—	0
BRETON														
Garden Vegetable	4 (0.7 oz)	100	4	3	0	1	13	1	1	0	160	—	—	0
Minis Cheddar Cheese	20 (0.7 oz)	100	5	3	5	3	13	1	1	40	240	—	—	0
BROWN RICE SNAPS														
Cheddar	6	60	1	0	0	1	12	tr	tr	0	40	—	—	0
Original Tamari Seaweed	9	60	0	0	0	1	12	0	tr	0	120	10	—	0
Unsalted Plain	8	60	0	0	0	1	13	tr	tr	0	0	—	—	0

FOOD	PORTION	CALS	FAT	SAT FAT	CHOL	PROT	CARB	SUGAR	FIBER	CALCI	SOD	POTAS	FOLIC	VIT C
CHEESE NIPS														
Cheddar	1 pkg (1.2 oz)	170	7	2	0	3	22	0	1	0	400	—	—	0
CHEEZ-IT														
Crackers	13 (1 oz)	150	8	2	0	3	17	0	tr	40	230	—	—	0
CHICKEN IN A BISKIT														
Original	1.1 oz	160	8	2	0	2	19	2	1	0	300	—	—	0
DAELIA'S														
Biscuits For Cheese Almond w/ Raisins	4 (1 oz)	133	4	tr	0	3	22	10	1	20	9	88	—	0
Biscuits For Cheese Hazelnut w/ Figs	4 (1 oz)	133	5	0	0	3	20	9	1	10	10	93	—	0
DARE														
Crackers	3 (0.5 oz)	70	4	2	0	1	9	tr	0	0	70	—	—	0
Original	4 (0.7 oz)	90	4	3	0	2	13	1	1	0	170	—	—	0
Reduced Fat & Salt	5 (0.7 oz)	80	2	tr	0	3	16	2	1	80	105	—	—	0
DR. KRACKER														
Flatbread Klassic Seed	1 (1 oz)	120	5	1	0	6	13	0	4	30	220	—	—	0
Flatbread Pumpkin Seed Cheddar	1 (1 oz)	120	5	2	<5	5	12	0	4	50	220	—	—	0
Flatbread Seeded Spelt	1 (1 oz)	120	6	1	0	5	12	0	4	30	200	—	—	0
Flatbread Seedlander	1 (1 oz)	120	5	2	0	5	15	2	3	10	220	—	—	0
Flatbread Spelt Sunflower Cheddar	1 (1 oz)	120	6	2	<5	5	12	0	4	50	220	—	—	0
Krispy Grahams	5 (1 oz)	110	3	1	4	2	17	6	2	10	120	—	—	0
EDEN														
Brown Rice	8 (1.1 oz)	120	2	0	0	3	22	tr	2	20	230	110	—	0
FLATOUT														
Edge On Baked Flatbread Four Cheese	15 (1 oz)	130	5	1	0	6	15	1	5	20	290	—	—	0
Edge On Baked Flatbread Garlic Herb	15 (1 oz)	120	4	0	0	6	16	1	5	20	330	—	—	0
GLUTINO														
Gluten Free	4 (0.5 oz)	70	2	1	5	tr	12	tr	0	0	120	—	—	0
Gluten Free Rusks	2 (0.7 oz)	80	2	1	0	0	15	1	2	0	140	—	—	0
GRAINSFIRST														
Autumn Harvest	7 (1.1 oz)	140	7	2	0	3	16	2	3	40	410	—	—	0

FOOD	PORTION	CALS	FAT	SAT FAT	CHOL	PROT	CARB	SUGAR	FIBER	CALCI	SOD	POTAS	FOLIC	VIT C
GRISSOL														
Crispy Baguettes Garden Herb	8 (1 oz)	110	2	tr	0	3	19	2	1	0	210	—	—	0
HEALTH VALLEY														
Organic Bruschetta Vegetable	4	70	3	0	0	1	10	1	0	—	210	—	—	1
Organic Cracked Pepper	4	70	3	0	0	1	10	1	0	—	190	—	—	—
Organic Cracker Stix Garlic Herb	8	70	3	0	0	1	9	1	tr	20	210	—	—	1
Organic Whole Wheat	4	70	3	0	0	2	9	1	1	—	170	—	—	—
HEALTHY HANDFULS														
Lucky Duckies Cheddar Cheese	1 pkg (1 oz)	100	4	1	0	2	14	0	1	20	180	—	—	0
JACOB'S														
Table Cracker Bran	1	33	1	1	—	1	5	tr	tr	—	37	—	—	—
KASHI														
Heart To Heart Whole Grain	7 (1 oz)	120	4	0	0	3	22	0	4	0	85	—	100	15
TLC Natural Ranch	15 (1 oz)	130	3	0	0	4	22	1	2	20	200	—	—	0
TLC Original 7 Grain	15 (1 oz)	130	3	0	0	3	22	3	2	20	160	—	—	0
TLC Party Mediterranean Bruschetta	4	120	4	1	0	3	18	3	3	20	140	—	—	0
TLC Snack Fire Roasted Vegetable	5	130	4	0	0	3	21	2	2	20	210	—	—	0
TLC Toasted Asiago	15 (1.1 oz)	130	4	1	0	3	21	2	2	0	200	—	—	0
KEEBLER														
Club Multi-Grain	4	70	3	1	0	1	10	2	tr	0	150	—	—	0
Club Original	4 (0.5 oz)	70	3	1	0	1	9	1	tr	0	125	—	—	0
Club Reduced Fat	5	70	3	1	0	1	12	2	tr	0	190	—	—	0
Club Snack Sticks	12	130	6	1	0	1	19	2	tr	0	320	—	—	0
Puffed Original	24	140	6	1	0	2	20	3	1	—	310	—	—	0
Sandwich Cheese & Peanut Butter	1 pkg (1.4 oz)	200	10	2	0	4	23	4	1	—	400	—	—	—
Sandwich Toast & Peanut Butter	1 pkg (1.4 oz)	200	10	2	0	4	23	4	1	—	410	—	—	—
Sandwich Wheat & Cheddar	1 pkg (1.3 oz)	190	10	3	<5	2	23	5	tr	—	370	—	—	—
Toasteds Harvest Wheat	16	130	6	1	0	2	20	3	1	—	260	—	—	0

FOOD	PORTION	CALS	FAT	SAT FAT	CHOL	PROT	CARB	SUGAR	FIBER	CALCI	SOD	POTAS	FOLIC	VIT C
KEEBLER (CONT.)														
Toasteds Sesame	5	80	4	1	0	1	10	1	tr	—	140	—	—	—
Toasteds Wheat	5	80	4	1	0	1	10	1	tr	—	160	—	—	—
Town House Bistro	2	80	3	1	0	1	11	1	tr	—	130	—	—	0
Town House FlipSides Original	5	70	4	1	0	1	10	1	tr	0	200	—	—	0
Town House Original	5 (0.5 oz)	80	5	1	0	tr	10	1	tr	0	130	—	—	0
Town House Reduced Fat	6	60	2	1	0	tr	11	1	tr	—	160	—	—	—
Town House Reduced Sodium	5	80	5	1	0	tr	10	1	tr	—	80	—	—	—
Town House Toppers	3	70	3	1	0	1	9	1	0	—	135	—	—	—
Wheatables 33% Less Fat	19	140	4	1	0	2	22	5	1	—	320	—	—	—
Wheatables Original	17	140	6	2	0	2	20	4	1	—	340	—	—	—
Zesta Saltine Fat Free	5	60	0	0	0	1	13	0	tr	—	280	—	—	0
Zesta Saltine Original	5	60	2	0	0	1	11	0	tr	—	200	—	—	—
KELLOGG'S														
All Bran Garlic Herb	18 (1 oz)	120	6	1	0	3	19	3	5	20	330	—	—	0
Special K Cracker Chips Southwest Ranch	27 (1 oz)	110	3	1	0	2	22	1	3	20	230	170	—	0
KIM'S MAGIC POP														
Onion	1 (5 g)	15	0	0	0	0	3	0	0	0	25	—	—	0
KITCHEN TABLE BAKERS														
Aged Parmesan	3	80	6	4	15	7	tr	0	0	200	150	—	—	0
Everything	3	80	6	4	15	7	tr	0	0	200	150	—	—	0
Garlic	3	80	6	4	15	6	tr	0	0	200	150	—	—	0
Jalapeno	3	80	6	4	15	6	2	0	1	150	150	—	—	0
LANCE														
Captain Wafers	4	70	3	0	0	1	9	1	0	0	105	—	—	0
Nekot	1 pkg (1.7 oz)	240	11	3	0	7	30	13	1	0	150	—	—	0
Nipchee	1 pkg (1.4 oz)	190	11	2	<5	4	22	3	1	40	340	—	—	0
Peanut Butter On Wheat	1 pkg (1.4 oz)	200	9	2	0	4	21	4	1	40	250	—	—	0
Toastchee	1 pkg (1.5 oz)	220	11	2	<5	5	23	3	2	0	430	—	—	1
Toastchee Reduced Fat	1 pkg (1.4 oz)	180	7	2	0	6	23	2	2	20	230	—	—	0

FOOD	PORTION	CALS	FAT	SAT FAT	CHOL	PROT	CARB	SUGAR	FIBER	CALCI	SOD	POTAS	FOLIC	VIT C
LARZARONI														
Bruschette w/ Olives	9 (1.1 oz)	140	5	3	0	4	21	tr	1	—	350	—	—	—
MARY'S GONE CRACKERS														
Wheat Free Gluten Free Black Pepper	13 (1 oz)	140	5	1	0	3	21	0	3	40	180	160	—	0
Wheat Free Gluten Free Onion	13 (1 oz)	140	5	1	0	3	21	0	3	40	190	190	—	0
Wheat Free Gluten Free Original Seed	13 (1 oz)	140	5	1	0	3	21	0	3	40	190	160	—	0
MEDITERRANEAN CRACKERS														
Feta & Oregano	3 (0.6 oz)	91	5	3	0	2	11	1	0	0	90	—	—	0
MEDITERRANEAN SNACKS														
Lentil Cracked Pepper Gluten Free	18 (1 oz)	110	3	0	0	5	16	2	1	40	200	—	—	0
Lentil Sea Salt Gluten Free	18 (1 oz)	110	3	0	0	5	16	2	1	40	100	—	—	0
NABISCO														
Garden Harvest Apple Cinnamon	16 (1 oz)	120	3	0	0	2	22	6	3	0	65	100	—	1
Garden Harvest Banana	16 (1 oz)	120	3	0	0	2	22	8	3	0	60	160	—	4
Garden Harvest Tomato Basil	16 (1 oz)	120	4	0	0	2	20	2	3	20	220	180	—	2
Garden Harvest Vegetable Medley	16 (1 oz)	120	4	0	0	2	20	2	3	20	240	170	—	2
Vegetable Thins	21 (1 oz)	150	7	2	0	2	20	2	tr	40	330	—	—	0
Wheat	4	90	4	0	0	2	12	1	tr	0	160	—	—	0
NAIRN'S														
Oatcake Fine	2 (0.5 oz)	70	3	1	0	2	10	0	1	10	110	—	—	0
Oatcake Rough	2 (0.8 oz)	91	4	1	0	2	14	tr	2	10	160	—	—	0
NEW YORK STYLE														
Crispini Seeds & Spice	6	120	4	1	0	4	19	0	tr	0	190	—	—	0
Panetini Original	2	80	4	2	0	2	10	0	0	0	90	—	—	0
Panetini Three Cheese	2	80	5	2	0	2	9	1	0	0	150	—	—	0
Pita Chips Garlic	7	130	5	3	0	3	17	1	1	0	440	—	—	0
Pita Chips Natural Whole Wheat	7	120	5	3	0	3	17	1	3	0	350	—	—	0

FOOD	PORTION	CALS	FAT	SAT FAT	CHOL	PROT	CARB	SUGAR	FIBER	CALCI	SOD	POTAS	FOLIC	VIT C
NONNI'S														
Panetini Roasted Garlic	5 (1 oz)	120	4	1	0	4	19	1	tr	20	300	50	—	1
Panetini Sun Dried Tomato Basil	5 (1 oz)	120	4	1	0	4	17	1	tr	20	170	55	—	2
ORKNEY														
Oatcakes Thin	4 (1.8 oz)	227	12	3	—	6	25	tr	3	—	600	—	—	—
PEPPERIDGE FARM														
Baked Naturals Cheese Crisps Four Cheese Medley	20	140	5	1	<5	3	19	3	1	60	270	—	—	0
Baked Naturals Cracker Chips Simply Multigrain	27	140	4	1	0	1	24	3	2	20	210	—	—	0
Baked Naturals Cracker Chips Simply Cheddar	27	130	4	1	0	2	24	4	2	20	250	—	—	0
Baked Naturals Cracker Chips Simply Potato	26	140	5	1	0	1	22	3	2	20	240	—	—	0
Baked Naturals Wheat Crisps Toasted Wheat	17	140	5	1	0	2	21	5	2	20	240	—	—	0
Golden Butter	2	35	1	0	0	1	5	tr	0	0	50	—	—	0
Goldfish Cheddar	55	140	5	1	<5	4	20	tr	tr	40	250	—	—	0
Goldfish Colors	55	140	5	1	<5	3	20	tr	1	20	240	—	—	0
Goldfish Original	55	150	6	1	0	3	20	tr	tr	20	230	—	—	0
Goldfish Pretzel	43	130	3	1	0	3	24	tr	tr	0	430	—	—	0
Goldfish w/ Whole Grain Cheddar	55 (1.1 oz)	140	5	1	<5	4	19	tr	2	40	250	—	—	0
Harvest Wheat	2	50	2	0	0	1	7	2	tr	0	85	—	—	0
Pretzel Thins Simply Pretzel	11	110	0	0	0	2	21	2	1	0	340	—	—	0
Snack Sticks Toasted Sesame	12	140	5	1	0	4	20	1	2	60	290	—	—	0
PREMIUM														
Saltines Fat Free	5 (0.5 oz)	60	0	0	0	1	12	0	0	20	170	—	—	0
Saltines Low Sodium	5 (0.5 oz)	80	2	0	0	1	11	0	0	20	25	—	—	0
Saltines Multigrain	5 (0.5 oz)	60	2	0	0	1	10	0	tr	0	170	—	—	0
Saltines Original	5 (0.5 oz)	60	2	0	0	1	11	0	0	0	190	—	—	0
RITZ														
Bites Cheese	13 (1 oz)	150	9	3	0	2	17	4	0	60	250	90	—	0
Hint Of Salt	0.5 oz	80	4	1	0	1	10	1	0	0	35	—	—	0
Original	0.5 oz	80	5	1	0	1	10	1	0	20	135	—	—	0

FOOD	PORTION	CALS	FAT	SAT FAT	CHOL	PROT	CARB	SUGAR	FIBER	CALCI	SOD	POTAS	FOLIC	VIT C
RITZ (CONT.)														
Reduced Fat	5 (0.5 oz)	70	2	0	0	1	11	1	0	20	160	15	—	0
Roasted Vegetable	5 (0.5 oz)	80	4	1	0	1	10	1	0	20	150	—	—	1
SOCIABLES														
Original	0.5 oz	70	4	1	0	1	9	1	0	20	140	—	—	0
SPECIAL K														
Cracker Chips Cheddar	27 (1 oz)	110	3	1	0	2	22	1	3	20	230	170	—	0
SUNRIDGE FARMS														
Japanese Rice	¼ cup (1 oz)	110	0	0	0	2	26	2	0	0	220	—	—	0
SUZIE'S														
Flatbreads Garlic Salt	1 oz	70	1	0	0	2	15	1	0	0	190	—	—	0
TRISCUIT														
Fire Roasted Tomato	1 oz	120	4	1	0	3	20	0	3	0	150	—	—	0
Garden Herb	1 oz	120	4	1	0	3	20	0	3	0	125	—	—	0
Hint Of Salt	1 oz	130	5	1	0	3	19	0	3	0	50	—	—	0
Original	1 oz	120	5	1	0	3	19	0	3	0	180	—	—	0
Reduced Fat	1 oz	120	3	1	0	3	21	0	3	0	160	—	—	0
Rosemary & Olive Oil	1 oz	120	4	1	0	3	20	0	3	0	135	—	—	0
Thin Crisps Original	1 oz	130	5	1	0	3	21	0	3	0	180	—	—	0
Thin Crisps Quattro Formaggio	1.1 oz	140	5	1	0	3	22	1	3	0	160	—	—	0
TRUE NORTH														
Peanut Crunches	¼ cup (1 oz)	150	8	2	0	5	13	5	4	0	130	—	8	0
Pistachio Crisps	12 (1 oz)	140	7	1	0	5	15	4	2	80	240	—	—	0
UTZ														
Cheese Peanut Butter	6	200	10	2	<5	4	21	3	2	0	390	—	—	1
VEGETABLE THINS														
Original	21 (1.1 oz)	150	7	2	0	2	19	2	1	40	320	—	—	0
VINTA														
Original	3 (0.7 oz)	100	5	1	0	2	12	2	1	20	180	—	—	0
WASA														
Hearty	1 (0.5 oz)	45	0	0	0	1	11	0	2	0	70	—	—	0
Light Rye	2 (0.6 oz)	60	0	0	0	2	14	0	3	0	70	—	—	0
Multi Grain	1 (0.5 oz)	45	0	0	0	2	10	0	2	0	80	—	—	0
Sourdough	1 (0.4 oz)	35	0	0	0	1	9	0	2	0	45	—	—	0
Whole Grain	1 (0.4 oz)	40	0	0	0	1	10	0	2	0	50	—	—	0
Whole Wheat	1 (0.5 oz)	50	1	0	0	2	10	tr	1	0	70	—	—	0
WATER CRACKERS														
Original	6 (0.5 oz)	60	2	1	0	2	11	0	0	0	120	—	—	0

FOOD	PORTION	CALS	FAT	SAT FAT	CHOL	PROT	CARB	SUGAR	FIBER	CALCI	SOD	POTAS	FOLIC	VIT C
WELLABY'S														
Cheese Ups Classic Cheese Gluten Free	1 cup (1 oz)	122	5	3	15	4	18	0	tr	200	320	—	—	0
Cheese Ups Parmesan	1 cup (1 oz)	122	5	3	15	4	18	0	tr	200	320	—	—	0
Feta Oregano & Olive Oil Gluten Free	8 (1.1 oz)	130	59	3	15	4	19	1	1	100	130	—	—	0
Original Cheese Mini Gluten Free	8 (1.1 oz)	130	5	3	15	4	19	1	1	100	130	—	—	0
WESTMINSTER														
Oyster	1 pkg (0.5 oz)	66	2	tr	0	1	11	0	0	0	60	—	—	0
WHEAT THINS														
100% Whole Grain	1 oz	140	6	1	0	2	21	3	2	20	290	—	—	0
Low Sodium	1.1 oz	150	6	1	0	2	22	4	1	0	80	—	—	0
Original	16 (1.1 oz)	140	5	1	0	2	22	4	2	20	230	—	—	0
Reduced Fat	1 oz	130	4	1	0	3	21	3	1	20	260	—	—	0
WHEATSWORTH														
Crackers	5 (0.5 oz)	80	4	1	0	2	10	1	1	0	180	—	—	0
CRANBERRIES														
cranberry orange relish	¼ cup	118	tr	tr	0	tr	31	28	2	11	1	52	4	14
dried	½ cup	85	tr	tr	0	tr	23	18	2	3	1	11	0	tr
fresh chopped	1 cup	13	tr	tr	0	tr	3	1	1	2	1	23	2	4
fresh whole	1 cup	11	tr	tr	0	tr	3	1	1	2	1	23	0	4
sauce	¼ cup	109	tr	tr	0	tr	27	26	1	3	20	18	1	1
sauce	1 slice (2 oz)	86	tr	tr	0	tr	22	22	1	2	17	15	1	1
CHUKAR CHERRIES														
North Cove Dried	¼ cup	100	0	0	0	0	24	22	2	0	0	—	—	0
CRAISINS														
Blueberry	⅓ cup	140	0	0	0	0	34	26	—	0	0	0	—	0
Cherry	⅓ cup	130	0	0	0	0	33	26	—	0	0	0	—	0
Dried Cranberries	⅓ cup	130	0	0	0	0	33	26	—	0	0	0	—	0
Orange	⅓ cup	130	0	0	0	0	33	27	—	0	0	0	—	0
DE-LITE														
Dried Sweetened	1 oz	92	tr	tr	0	tr	23	15	1	2	3	—	—	tr
DOLE														
Fresh Whole	1 cup (3.3 oz)	45	0	0	0	0	12	4	4	0	0	—	—	12
EARTHBOUND FARMS														
Organic Dried	⅓ cup	130	0	0	0	0	34	27	2	0	2	—	—	2
EDEN														
Organic Dried	⅓ cup	140	1	0	0	0	33	25	2	20	20	115	—	0

FOOD	PORTION	CALS	FAT	SAT FAT	CHOL	PROT	CARB	SUGAR	FIBER	CALCI	SOD	POTAS	FOLIC	VIT C
EMILY'S														
Milk Chocolate Covered	¼ cup (1.4 oz)	180	10	6	<5	tr	24	23	2	0	0	—	—	—
FOOL														
Cranberry Spread	1 tbsp	30	0	0	0	0	7	6	1	—	0	—	—	—
FRIEDA'S														
Dried	⅓ cup (1.4 oz)	110	1	0	0	0	28	26	2	0	3	—	—	0
FRUITACEUTICALS														
OmegaCrans Dried	¼ cup	91	1	0	0	0	22	20	1	0	0	—	—	2
MARIANI														
Dried Sweetened	⅓ cup	130	0	0	0	0	35	30	2	0	0	20	—	0
NEWMAN'S OWN														
Organic Dried	¼ cup	130	0	0	0	0	34	31	2	—	0	—	—	—
OCEAN SPRAY														
Fresh	2 oz	30	0	0	0	—	6	2	—	0	0	0	—	12
Jellied Sauce	¼ cup (2.5 oz)	110	0	0	0	0	25	21	tr	—	10	—	—	—
Whole Berry Sauce	¼ cup (2.5 oz)	110	0	0	0	0	25	22	1	—	10	—	—	—
S&W														
Sauce Jellied	¼ cup (2.5 oz)	100	0	0	0	0	26	17	1	0	35	—		0
Sauce Whole Berry	¼ cup (2.5 oz)	100	0	0	0	0	26	17	1	0	35	—		0
SARABETH'S														
Relish	1 tbsp (0.7 oz)	45	0	0	0	0	36	31	3	—	0	—	—	1
STONERIDGE ORCHARDS														
Dried	⅓ cup (¼ oz)	140	0	0	0	0	33	26	2	40	10	—	—	4
SUN-MAID														
Dried Cape Cod	⅓ cup (1.4 oz)	130	0	0	0	0	33	27	2	0	0	45	—	2
SUNSWEET														
Dried	⅓ cup (1.4 oz)	140	0	0	0	0	35	29	2	0	0	25	—	0
TREE OF LIFE														
Organic Jellied	¼ cup (2.5 oz)	100	0	0	0	0	26	17	1	0	35	—	—	0
TRUITT BROTHERS														
Sauce Orchard Medley	⅓ cup (2.7 oz)	90	0	0	0	0	24	—	2	0	25	—	—	15
WILD THYMES FARM														
Cranberry Fig Sauce	1 tsp	19	0	0	0	tr	5	4	tr	0	0	—	—	1
Original Cranberry Sauce	1 tbsp	21	0	0	0	0	5	5	tr	0	0	—	—	1
CRANBERRY BEANS														
canned	½ cup	108	tr	tr	0	7	20	—	8	44	432	338	100	1
dried cooked w/o salt	½ cup	120	tr	tr	0	8	22	—	9	44	1	342	183	0

FOOD	PORTION	CALS	FAT	SAT FAT	CHOL	PROT	CARB	SUGAR	FIBER	CALCI	SOD	POTAS	FOLIC	VIT C
GOYA														
Roman Beans Dried not prep	¼ cup (1.4 oz)	80	0	0	0	8	24	2	13	40	15	—	—	0
CRANBERRY JUICE														
cranberry juice cocktail low calorie w/ vitamin C	8 oz	46	tr	0	0	tr	11	11	0	22	7	60	0	77
cranberry juice cocktail w/ vitamin C	8 oz	137	tr	tr	0	0	34	30	0	8	5	35	0	107
unsweetened	8 oz	116	tr	tr	0	1	31	31	tr	20	5	195	3	24
APPLE & EVE														
100% Juice	8 oz	130	0	0	0	0	32	30	—	100	20	—	—	60
LAKEWOOD														
Organic	6 oz	50	0	0	0	1	12	8	1	10	4	120	4	15
Organic Light	6 oz	45	0	0	0	1	18	12	1	40	3	125	4	15
NANTUCKET NECTARS														
Cranberry Cocktail	8 oz	130	0	0	0	0	33	32	0	0	25	—	—	60
NORTHLAND														
100% Juice No Sugar Added	8 oz	130	0	0	0	0	33	29	—	—	35	230	—	60
OCEAN SPRAY														
100% Juice Cranberry Blend	8 oz	140	0	0	0	0	36	36	—	0	35	50	—	60
Cocktail	8 oz	120	0	0	0	0	30	30	—	—	35	30	—	60
Cocktail Light	8 oz	40	0	0	0	0	10	10	—	0	75	65	—	0
Diet	8 oz	5	0	0	0	0	2	2	—	0	50	0	—	0
White Cocktail Light	8 oz	40	0	0	0	0	10	10	—	0	75	30	—	60
White Cranberry	8 oz	110	0	0	0	0	27	27	—	0	50	30	—	60
White Cranberry Strawberry	8 oz	110	0	0	0	0	27	27	—	—	50	30	—	60
OLD ORCHARD														
Cranberry Naturals Classic Cranberry	8 oz	80	0	0	0	0	18	18	—	20	25	35	—	0
SANTA CRUZ														
Organic Nectar	8 oz	110	0	0	0	tr	27	26	0	20	25	75	—	1
SSIPS														
Cocktail	1 box (7 oz)	110	0	0	0	0	28	25	—	—	0	35	—	60
CRAYFISH														
cooked	3 oz	97	1	tr	151	20	0	0	0	26	58	298	—	3
raw	3 oz	76	1	tr	118	16	0	0	0	20	45	233	—	3
raw	8	24	tr	tr	37	5	0	0	0	6	14	74	—	1

CREM

(*see also* WHIPPED TOPPINGS)

FOOD	PORTION	CALS	FAT	SAT FAT	CHOL	PROT	CARB	SUGAR	FIBER	CALCI	SOD	POTAS	FOLIC	VIT C
clotted cream	2 tbsp (1 oz)	164	18	—	48	tr	1	—	0	10	18	15	2	0
creme fraiche	2 tbsp (1 oz)	100	11	—	40	1	1	—	0	20	10	—	—	0
half & half	1 tbsp (0.5 oz)	20	2	1	6	tr	1	tr	0	16	6	20	0	tr
half & half	¼ cup (2.1 oz)	79	7	4	22	2	3	tr	0	64	25	79	2	1
half & half	1 pkg (0.5 oz)	20	2	1	6	tr	1	tr	0	16	6	20	0	tr
half & half fat free	4 oz	67	2	1	6	3	10	6	0	109	164	235	5	1
heavy whipping	1 tbsp (0.5 oz)	52	6	3	21	tr	tr	tr	0	10	6	11	1	tr
heavy whipping	½ cup (4.2 oz)	411	44	27	163	2	3	tr	0	77	45	89	5	1
heavy whipping whipped	½ cup (2.1 oz)	207	22	14	82	1	2	tr	0	39	23	45	2	tr
light coffee	½ cup (4.2 oz)	234	23	14	79	3	4	tr	0	115	48	146	6	2
light coffee	1 tbsp (0.5 oz)	29	3	2	10	tr	1	tr	0	14	6	18	0	tr
light coffee	1 pkg (0.4 oz)	22	2	1	7	tr	tr	tr	0	11	4	14	0	tr
whipped pressurized can	4 tbsp (0.4 oz)	31	3	2	9	tr	2	1	0	12	16	18	0	0
whipped pressurized can	½ cup (1 oz)	77	7	4	23	1	4	2	0	30	39	44	1	0
CABOT														
Whipped	2 tbsp	15	2	1	<.5	0	1	1	0	0	0	—	—	0
HOOD														
Half & Half	2 tbsp	40	4	2	15	1	1	1	0	40	20	—	—	0
Light	1 tbsp	30	3	2	10	1	tr	tr	0	0	10		—	0
Simply Smart Fat Free Half & Half	2 tbsp	15	0	0	<5	tr	2	2	0	40	30	—	—	0
Whipping Cream	1 tbsp	45	5	3	20	0	tr	1	0	0	5	—	—	0
HORIZON ORGANIC														
Half & Half	2 tbsp	35	3	2	10	1	1	1	0	40	15	—	—	0
Heavy Whipping	1 tbsp	50	5	4	20	0	0	0	0	0	10	—	—	0
LACTAID														
Half & Half	2 tbsp (1 oz)	40	3	2	15	tr	1	1	0	40	20	—	—	0
LAND O LAKES														
Aerosol Whipped Light Cream	2 tbsp (0.2 oz)	20	2	1	5	0	1	1	0	0	0	—	—	0
Half & Half	2 tbsp (1.1 oz)	35	4	2	10	tr	1	1	0	0	15	—	—	0
Half & Half Fat Free	2 tbsp (1.1 oz)	20	0	0	0	1	3	2	0	40	30	—	—	0
Heavy Whipping	1 tbsp (0.5 oz)	50	5	4	20	0	0	0	0	0	5	—	—	0
ORGANIC VALLEY														
Half & Half	2 tbsp (1 oz)	40	4	2	10	tr	1	1	0	40	10	—	—	0
STRAUS														
Organic Half And Half	2 tbsp (1 oz)	35	3	2	15	1	1	1	0	40	15	—	—	0

FOOD	PORTION	CALS	FAT	SAT FAT	CHOL	PROT	CARB	SUGAR	FIBER	CALCI	SOD	POTAS	FOLIC	VIT C
CREAM CHEESE														
cream cheese	1 pkg (3 oz)	297	30	19	93	6	2	—	—	68	251	101	11	0
cream cheese	1 oz	99	10	6	31	2	1	—	—	23	84	34	4	0
BOAR'S HEAD														
Cream Cheese	2 tbsp (1 oz)	100	10	7	30	2	2	2	0	20	100	—	—	0
CONNOISSEUR														
Wheel Mango Peach	2 tbsp	110	7	5	20	1	10	5	0	20	110	—	—	0
Wheel Wild Blueberry	2 tbsp	100	7	5	20	1	9	6	0	20	120	—	—	0
EARTH BALANCE														
Brick	2 tbsp	80	6	3	0	3	2	2	0	60	105	—	—	0
Tub	2 tbsp	80	6	3	15	3	2	2	0	60	105	—	—	0
HORIZON ORGANIC														
Reduced Fat	2 tbsp	70	7	4	25	2	2	tr	0	20	100	—	—	0
LIFEWAY														
Whipped	2 tbsp	80	8	5	25	2	1	1	0	20	75	—	—	0
NANCY'S														
Organic	2 tbsp	95	9	6	35	1	2	2	0	50	35	—	—	0
ORGANIC VALLEY														
Cream Cheese	1 oz	100	10	6	35	2	1	tr	0	20	105	—	—	0
Soft	2 tbsp	90	9	6	25	1	2	2	0	20	140	—	—	0
PHILADELPHIA														
⅓ Less Fat	2 tbsp (1.1 oz)	70	6	4	20	2	2	2	0	40	140	—	—	0
Original	1 in cube (1 oz)	100	9	6	35	2	1	tr	0	20	105	—	—	0
Whipped	2 tbsp	60	6	4	20	1	1	tr	0	0	90	—	—	0
CREAM CHEESE SUBSTITUTES														
TOFUTTI														
Better Than Cream Cheese All Flavors	2 tbsp (1 oz)	60	5	2	0	1	2	0	0	—	120	—	—	—
VEGAN GOURMET														
Alternative Cream Cheese	2 tbsp (1 oz)	90	8	4	0	2	3	0	2	20	130	—	—	1
CREAM OF TARTAR														
cream of tartar	1 tsp	8	0	0	0	0	2	0	0	0	2	495	0	0
CREPES														
basic crepe unfilled	1 (7 in)	112	6	2	78	4	11	2	tr	46	142	80	21	0
EKIZIAN														
Chickpea Crepe	1 (7 in) (1.5 oz)	212	13	2	2	7	16	3	3	39	514	244	121	tr
FRIEDA'S														
Ready-To-Use	1 (0.5 oz)	30	1	0	5	1	5	2	0	0	50	—	—	0
TANDOOR CHEF														
Masala Dosa	1 (3 oz)	162	6	2	0	5	22	1	2	40	520	—	—	2

FOOD	PORTION	CALS	FAT	SAT FAT	CHOL	PROT	CARB	SUGAR	FIBER	CALCI	SOD	POTAS	FOLIC	VIT C
CROAKER														
atlantic breaded & fried	3 oz	188	11	3	71	15	6	—	—	27	296	289	—	—
atlantic raw	3 oz	89	3	1	52	15	0	0	0	13	47	293	—	—
CROCODILE														
cooked	3 oz	78	1	—	—	17	0	0	0	9	—	—	—	0
CROISSANT														
apple	1 (2 oz)	145	5	3	18	4	21	—	1	17	156	51	32	tr
butter	1 lg (2.4 oz)	272	14	8	45	5	31	8	2	25	498	79	59	tr
butter mini	1 (1 oz)	114	6	3	19	2	13	3	1	10	208	33	25	tr
cheese	1 (1.5 oz)	174	9	4	24	4	20	5	1	22	233	55	31	tr
chocolate	1 (2 oz)	237	14	8	34	5	25	6	2	25	383	108	47	tr
TAKE-OUT														
w/ egg & cheese	1 (4.5 oz)	368	25	14	216	13	24	—	—	244	551	174	47	tr
w/ egg & sausage	1 (5 oz)	497	34	15	237	16	31	8	2	50	878	207	68	1
w/ egg cheese & bacon	1 (4.1 oz)	385	24	12	253	16	25	8	1	131	806	205	59	2
w/ egg cheese & ham	1 (5.1 oz)	402	24	12	264	21	25	8	1	132	1092	272	60	2
w/ egg cheese & sausage	1 (5.6 oz)	539	39	17	280	20	26	8	1	135	1045	261	59	2
w/ ham & cheese	1 (4 oz)	338	20	12	64	15	25	4	1	164	836	233	45	0
CROUTONS														
plain	1 cup (1 oz)	122	2	tr	0	4	22	—	2	23	209	37	7	0
seasoned	1 cup (1.4 oz)	186	7	2	—	4	25	—	2	38	495	72	16	—
CHATHAM VILLAGE														
Cheese & Garlic	2 tbsp (7 g)	40	3	0	0	1	3	0	0	0	60	—	—	0
EDWARD & SONS														
Organic Lightly Salted	2 tbsp	30	1	0	0	tr	5	0	0	0	25	—	—	0
FRESH GOURMET														
Butter & Garlic	7 (7 g)	35	2	0	0	1	4	0	0	0	80	—	—	0
Cheese & Garlic	12 (0.5 oz)	70	3	0	0	1	9	0	0	0	115	—	—	0
Classic Caesar	6 (7 g)	35	2	0	0	1	4	0	0	0	75	—	—	0
Cornbread Sweet Butter	½ cup (1 oz)	110	1	0	0	3	22	2	1	40	260	—	—	12
Country Ranch	6 (7 g)	35	2	0	0	1	4	0	—	0	75	—	—	0
Fat Free Garlic Caesar	12 (7 g)	30	0	0	0	1	5	0	0	0	45	—	—	0
Italian Seasoned	6 (7 g)	35	2	0	0	1	4	0	0	0	70	—	—	0
Organic Seasoned	5 (7 g)	30	2	0	0	1	4	0	0	0	70	—	—	0
PEPPERIDGE FARM														
Seasoned	6	30	1	0	0	tr	5	tr	tr	0	75	—	—	0
Zesty Italian	6	30	1	0	0	tr	5	tr	tr	0	55	—	—	0

FOOD	PORTION	CALS	FAT	SAT FAT	CHOL	PROT	CARB	SUGAR	FIBER	CALCI	SOD	POTAS	FOLIC	VIT C
CUCUMBER														
fresh peeled	1 med (7 oz)	24	tr	tr	0	1	4	3	1	28	4	273	28	6
fresh sliced	1 cup	14	tr	tr	0	1	3	2	1	17	2	162	17	4
fresh w/ peel sliced	½ cup	34	tr	tr	0	tr	2	1	tr	8	1	76	4	2
TAKE-OUT														
cucumber & onion salad w/ vinegar	1 cup	52	tr	tr	0	1	12	8	1	22	375	196	10	4
cucumber raita	1 serv (3.3 oz)	40	3	2	6	2	3	3	1	82	233	152	—	2
cucumber salad w/ oil & vinegar	1 cup	183	15	2	0	1	11	8	1	21	329	176	10	4
cucumber salad w/ sour cream dressing	1 cup	68	6	3	12	1	3	2	1	45	16	184	17	4
kimchee	½ cup (1.8 oz)	36	2	tr	0	tr	4	3	tr	10	173	79	6	6
tzatziki	½ cup (3.4 oz)	72	6	1	5	2	4	3	1	59	197	146	10	3
CUMIN														
seed	1 tsp (2 g)	8	tr	tr	0	tr	1	tr	tr	20	4	38	0	tr
seed	1 tbsp (6 g)	22	1	tr	0	1	3	tr	1	56	10	107	1	tr
CURRANT JUICE														
black currant nectar	7 oz	110	0	—	—	tr	26	—	—	30	10	196	tr	60
red currant nectar	7 oz	108	tr	—	—	tr	26	—	—	14	tr	220	tr	12
CURRANTC														
Black Currant Juice	8 oz	130	0	0	0	1	32	28	0	20	10	159	—	108
FRUCTAL														
Black Currant	1 bottle (6.75 oz)	102	0	0	0	0	25	24	1	20	1	—	—	0
GOODBELLY														
Black Currant Probiotic Drink	8 oz	120	0	0	0	tr	31	27	0	20	30	120	—	60
CURRANTS														
black fresh	½ cup	36	tr	tr	0	1	9	—	—	31	1	180	—	101
zante dried	½ cup	204	tr	tr	0	3	53	—	—	62	6	642	7	3
SUN-MAID														
Zante	¼ cup (1.4 oz)	120	0	0	0	1	30	28	2	20	10	300	—	0
CURRY														
curry powder	1 tsp	7	tr	tr	0	tr	1	tr	1	10	1	31	3	tr
curry sauce mix as prep	1 cup	120	6	1	0	3	14	—	—	50	1142	99	3	1
curry sauce mix as prep w/ milk	1 cup	270	15	6	35	11	26	—	—	485	1276	—	—	—
paste	1 tube (6 oz)	465	36	12	16	7	30	13	12	245	4394	698	—	6

FOOD	PORTION	CALS	FAT	SAT FAT	CHOL	PROT	CARB	SUGAR	FIBER	CALCI	SOD	POTAS	FOLIC	VIT C
ETHNIC GOURMET														
Gujarati Vegetable Curry	1 pkg (10 oz)	380	11	5	0	8	63	17	4	60	540	—	—	30
Malay Chicken Curry	1 pkg (10 oz)	410	11	5	35	18	59	15	2	40	530	—	—	12
Simmer Sauce Bombay Curry	4 oz	70	3	0	0	2	10	6	2	60	540	—	—	9
FORTUN'S														
Finishing Sauce Mulligatawny Curry	¼ cup (2 oz)	60	2	0	5	1	10	7	1	20	370	—	—	2
FRENCH MEADOW BAKERY														
Fragrant Chicken Curry	1 pkg (12 oz)	280	5	2	65	28	36	2	3	60	590	—	—	5
HELEN'S KITCHEN														
Indian Curry w/ Tofu Steaks & Rice	1 pkg (9 oz)	300	8	1	0	14	63	4	5	300	300	—	—	15
KIKKOMAN														
Sauce Thai Red Curry	¼ cup (2.2 oz)	90	6	4	0	1	7	4	0	20	500	—	—	0
Sauce Thai Yellow Curry	¼ cup (2.2 oz)	90	6	4	0	1	6	4	0	20	510	—	—	0
KNORR														
Curry Sauce Indian Madras	1 oz	30	2	2	5	tr	2	—	—	—	140	—	—	—
Curry Sauce Thai	1 oz	35	3	2	0	tr	3	—	—	—	90	—	—	—
PATAK'S														
Curry Paste Biryani	2 tbsp	180	16	2	0	1	6	0	3	0	890	—	—	0
Garam Masala Paste	2 tsp	130	12	1	0	1	4	1	0	0	1080	—	—	0
Tandoori Paste	2 tbsp	30	1	0	0	1	5	2	1	0	800	—	—	0
Vegetable Curry w/ Rice Rich Creamy Coconut	1 pkg	400	18	10	10	6	54	8	5	20	990	—	—	0
Vegetable Curry w/ Rice Rich Tomato & Onion	1 pkg (10.5 oz)	290	6	1	0	6	53	8	5	20	900	—	—	0
Vegetable Curry w/ Rice Tangy Lemon & Cilantro	1 pkg	300	7	2	0	5	54	8	5	40	1020	—	—	0
Vindaloo Paste	2 tbsp	160	16	1	0	1	4	0	0	0	1020	—	—	0
SO-YAH!														
Creamy Coconut Curry	1 pkg (10 oz)	190	10	7	0	4	21	8	5	100	850	—	—	0

FOOD	PORTION	CALS	FAT	SAT FAT	CHOL	PROT	CARB	SUGAR	FIBER	CALCI	SOD	POTAS	FOLIC	VIT C
SO-YAH! (CONT.)														
Red Vindaloo Curry	1 pkg (10 oz)	150	4	1	0	3	24	11	8	100	710	—	—	0
SPICE HUNTER														
Curry Seasoning Salt Free	¼ tsp	0	0	0	0	0	0	0	0	—	0	—	—	—
TANDOOR CHEF														
Chicken Curry	1 pkg (9.9 oz)	330	19	4	90	30	8	3	1	60	910	—	—	9
Kofta Curry	½ pkg (5 oz)	100	7	1	0	1	6	2	1	20	400	—	—	5
TASTYBITE														
Green Curry Vegetables & Jasmine Rice	1 pkg (12 oz)	320	10	6	0	6	52	2	2	10	530	—	—	3
Yellow Curry Vegetables & Jasmine Rice	1 pkg (12 oz)	380	13	8	0	7	61	4	3	40	440	—	—	3
THAI KITCHEN														
Green Curry Paste	1 tbsp (0.5 oz)	15	0	0	0	0	3	1	0	20	510	—	—	15
Red Curry Paste	1 tbsp (0.5 oz)	15	0	0	0	0	3	1	0	20	390	—	—	1
TAKE-OUT														
beef curry	1 cup	432	31	7	68	27	14	6	3	35	1293	953	19	16
beef kurma	1 serv (10 oz)	611	47	26	114	41	6	3	6	228	589	751	—	—
chicken curry ½ breast	1 serv	160	9	2	45	15	6	3	1	22	624	321	10	7
chicken curry boneless	1 serv (6.2 oz)	219	12	2	62	20	8	4	2	30	857	441	14	9
chicken curry leg & thigh	1 serv	180	10	2	51	17	7	3	1	25	702	361	12	7
chickpea curry	1 serv (8.3 oz)	305	15	8	12	18	23	1	15	220	1206	910	—	0
eggplant curry	1 serv (8 oz)	241	19	9	0	4	12	—	5	55	1009	—	—	—
lamb curry	1 cup	257	14	4	90	28	4	1	1	38	496	493	28	1
mixed vegetable curry	1 serv (7.7 oz)	398	33	—	—	4	22	—	—	86	—	—	—	26
pea & potato curry	1 serv (7 oz)	284	22	—	—	5	19	—	6	56	—	—	—	12
pork vandaloo curry	1 serv	620	47	—	—	—	3	—	—	—	—	—	—	—
potato curry	1 serv (5.5 oz)	791	60	14	12	29	35	5	14	139	668	876	—	0
sambhar dhal curry	1 serv (10 oz)	177	7	4	0	8	21	—	8	54	1314	—	—	—
shrimp curry	1 cup (8.3 oz)	276	14	4	250	25	13	8	1	304	1239	295	28	5
CUSK														
fillet baked	3 oz	106	1	—	50	23	0	0	0	12	38	477	—	—
CUSTARD														
MIX														
egg custard as prep w/ 2% milk	1 serv (3.5 oz)	112	3	1	49	4	18	5	0	146	87	214	8	tr

FOOD	PORTION	CALS	FAT	SAT FAT	CHOL	PROT	CARB	SUGAR	FIBER	CALCI	SOD	POTAS	FOLIC	VIT C
egg custard as prep w/ whole milk	1 serv (3.5 oz)	122	4	2	51	4	18	5	0	139	84	207	9	tr
flan as prep w/ 2% milk	1 serv (3.5 oz)	103	2	1	7	3	19	—	0	113	113	163	4	1
flan as prep w/ whole milk	1 serv (3.5 oz)	113	3	2	12	3	19	—	0	111	112	160	4	1
READY-TO-EAT														
KOZY SHACK														
Custard	1 pkg (4 oz)	130	3	2	15	7	19	17	0	137	90	160	—	1
SIGNATURE														
Flan Coffee	1 pkg (4.5 oz)	340	12	7	175	11	48	47	0	300	140	—	—	2
Flan Vanilla	1 pkg (4.5 oz)	350	13	7	185	11	49	49	0	350	150	—	—	2
TAKE-OUT														
baked	½ cup (5 oz)	147	6	3	118	7	16	16	0	151	86	209	14	0
flan	½ cup (5.4 oz)	222	6	3	138	7	35	35	0	127	81	181	14	0
flan de calabaza	1 serv (3.5 oz)	225	10	2	112	5	30	22	tr	38	342	186	24	3
flan de coco	½ cup (4.3 oz)	345	13	8	145	10	49	49	tr	247	163	358	17	1
flan de pina	1 serv (4.2 oz)	186	5	2	222	7	28	27	tr	36	74	148	25	5
flan de pini	½ cup (4.6 oz)	202	6	2	240	7	31	29	tr	39	81	160	27	6
puerto rican corn custard	½ cup (4.9 oz)	553	34	30	0	5	65	51	5	27	882	557	43	7
tocino del cielo heaven's delight	1 cup	856	21	7	967	14	156	154	0	106	48	114	85	0
zabaglione	½ cup (2 oz)	135	5	2	213	3	13	—	0	23	9	16	24	0
CUTTLEFISH														
steamed	3 oz	134	1	tr	190	28	1	—	—	153	632	542	—	7
DANDELION GREENS														
fresh cooked	½ cup	17	tr	—	0	1	3	—	—	73	23	121	—	9
raw chopped	½ cup	13	tr	—	0	1	3	—	—	52	21	111	—	10
DANISH PASTRY														
READY-TO-EAT														
ENTENMANN'S														
Pecan Danish Ring	⅛ ring (1.9 oz)	240	14	4	15	3	24	11	1	40	150	—	—	0
TAKE-OUT														
cheese	1 (2.5 oz)	266	16	5	11	6	26	5	1	25	320	70	43	tr
cinnamon	1 (5 oz)	572	32	8	30	10	63	28	2	101	527	178	97	tr
fruit	1 (5 oz)	527	27	7	162	8	68	39	3	65	503	118	67	6
lemon	1 (2.5 oz)	263	13	2	28	4	34	—	1	33	251	59	11	3
raisin nut	1 (2.3 oz)	280	16	4	30	5	30	17	1	61	236	62	54	1
DATES														
deglet noor chopped	¼ cup (1.3 oz)	104	tr	tr	0	1	28	23	3	14	1	241	7	tr
deglet noor dried	1 (7 g)	20	tr	tr	0	tr	5	5	1	3	0	47	1	0
jujube dried	1 oz	75	tr	—	—	1	19	—	2	18	2	149	—	4

FOOD	PORTION	CALS	FAT	SAT FAT	CHOL	PROT	CARB	SUGAR	FIBER	CALCI	SOD	POTAS	FOLIC	VIT C
jujube fresh	1 oz	30	tr	—	0	tr	7	—	—	9	1	80	—	17
jujube preserved in sugar	1 oz	91	tr	—	—	tr	22	—	—	7	2	18	tr	tr
medjool	1 (0.8 oz)	66	tr	—	0	tr	18	16	2	15	0	167	4	0
BARD VALLEY GROWERS														
Medjool	1	63	0	0	0	1	17	—	2	—	0	143	—	—
BOB'S RED MILL														
Dried Crumbles	⅓ cup	130	0	0	0	1	33	27	4	—	15	—	—	—
DOLE														
California Chopped	¼ cup (1.4 oz)	120	0	0	0	1	31	26	3	20	0	240	—	0
EARTHBOUND FARMS														
Organic Dried	6 (1.4 oz)	120	0	0	0	1	31	29	3	20	0	—	—	0
FRIEDA'S														
Medjool	2 to 3 (1.4 oz)	120	0	0	0	1	31	29	3	20	0	—	—	0
SUNDATE														
Fancy Medjool	3 (1.4 oz)	120	0	0	0	1	31	25	3	0	0	170	—	0
SUN-MAID														
Pitted	¼ cup (1.4 oz)	110	0	0	0	1	30	21	4	20	0	250	—	0
TREE OF LIFE														
Deglet Noor Pitted	5 (1.5 oz)	120	0	0	0	1	31	28	3	20	0	—	—	0
Organic Medjool	5 (1.5 oz)	120	0	0	0	1	31	28	3	20	0	—	—	0

DEER

(*see* JERKY, VENISON)

DELI MEATS/COLD CUTS

(*see also* BEEF, CHICKEN, HAM, MEAT SUBSTITUTES, TURKEY)

FOOD	PORTION	CALS	FAT	SAT FAT	CHOL	PROT	CARB	SUGAR	FIBER	CALCI	SOD	POTAS	FOLIC	VIT C
barbecue loaf pork & beef	1 slice (0.8 oz)	40	2	1	9	4	1	—	0	13	307	76	2	0
beerwurst beef	2 oz	155	13	5	35	8	2	0	1	15	410	137	3	tr
berliner pork & beef	1 slice (0.8 oz)	53	4	1	11	4	1	1	0	3	298	65	1	0
blood sausage	1 slice (0.9 oz)	95	9	3	30	4	tr	tr	0	2	170	10	1	0
bologna beef	1 slice (1 oz)	88	8	3	16	3	1	0	0	9	302	48	3	4
bologna beef & pork low fat	1 slice (1 oz)	64	5	2	11	3	1	0	0	3	310	44	1	0
bologna beef lowfat	1 slice (1 oz)	57	4	2	12	3	1	0	0	3	330	41	1	tr
bologna beef reduced sodium	1 slice (1 oz)	88	8	3	16	3	1	0	0	3	191	43	1	0
bologna beef & pork	1 slice (1 oz)	87	7	3	17	4	2	1	0	24	209	89	2	tr
braunschweiger pork	1 slice (1 oz)	92	8	3	50	4	1	0	0	3	325	56	12	0
corned beef brisket	2 oz	90	5	2	35	11	0	0	0	—	370	—	—	12

FOOD	PORTION	CALS	FAT	SAT FAT	CHOL	PROT	CARB	SUGAR	FIBER	CALCI	SOD	POTAS	FOLIC	VIT C
dutch brand loaf pork & beef	1 slice (1.3 oz)	104	9	3	23	5	1	0	tr	3	401	82	5	1
headcheese pork	1 slice (1.6 oz)	71	5	2	31	6	0	0	0	7	374	14	1	0
honey loaf pork & beef	1 slice (1 oz)	35	1	tr	10	4	1	0	0	5	370	96	2	8
lebanon bologna beef	2 slices (1 oz)	105	6	2	31	11	tr	0	0	11	783	188	3	1
mortadella beef & pork	1 slice (0.5 oz)	47	4	1	8	2	tr	0	0	3	187	24	0	0
olive loaf pork	2 slices (2 oz)	134	9	3	22	7	5	0	0	62	846	169	1	0
pastrami beef	1 slice (1 oz)	41	2	1	19	6	tr	tr	tr	3	248	66	2	tr
peppered loaf pork & beef	1 slice (1 oz)	41	2	1	13	5	1	0	0	15	426	110	1	0
pepperoni pork & beef	15 slices (1 oz)	135	12	5	34	6	1	tr	tr	6	519	91	2	tr
picnic loaf pork & beef	1 slice (1 oz)	65	5	2	11	4	1	—	0	13	326	75	1	0
salami cooked beef & pork	1 slice (0.8 oz)	58	5	2	15	3	1	0	0	3	245	46	0	0
salami hard pork	3 slices (0.9 oz)	14	8	3	27	6	1	0	0	2	543	102	1	0
salami hard pork & beef less sodium	1 slice (1 oz)	113	9	3	26	4	2	2	tr	27	177	389	2	tr
sandwich spread pork & beef	¼ cup	141	10	4	23	5	7	0	tr	7	608	66	1	0
summer sausage thuringer cervelat	2 oz	203	17	6	41	10	2	tr	0	5	728	146	1	9
APPLEGATE FARMS														
Organic Genoa Salami Sliced	1 oz	100	7	4	25	7	0	0	0	0	400	—	—	0
BOAR'S HEAD														
Abruzzese Hot & Sweet	1 oz	100	8	3	25	8	tr	0	0	0	540	—	—	0
Braunschweiger Lite	2 oz	120	8	5	50	9	1	0	0	0	450	—	—	0
Capocollo Hot & Sweet	1 oz	80	5	2	25	7	0	0	0	0	590	—	—	0
Dutch Loaf	2 oz	150	12	5	25	7	2	2	0	0	610	—	—	0
Liverwurst Smoked	2 oz	170	15	6	45	8	1	1	0	0	620	—	—	0
Mortadella	2 oz	160	14	5	30	9	0	0	0	0	560	—	—	0
Olive Loaf	2 oz	130	12	5	20	6	tr	tr	0	20	630	—	—	0
Pastrami	2 oz	70	3	1	30	12	1	0	0	0	580	—	—	0
Pickle & Pepper Loaf	2 oz	150	13	7	30	6	2	1	0	0	500	—	—	0
Prosciutto	1 oz	60	3	1	15	8	0	0	0	0	750	—	—	0
Salami Beef	2 oz	120	9	3	25	10	0	0	0	0	470	—	—	0
Salami Cooked	2 oz	130	11	5	40	8	0	0	0	0	550	—	—	0

FOOD	PORTION	CALS	FAT	SAT FAT	CHOL	PROT	CARB	SUGAR	FIBER	CALCI	SOD	POTAS	FOLIC	VIT C
BOAR'S HEAD (CONT.)														
Salami Hard	1 oz	110	9	4	30	6	tr	0	0	0	490	—	—	0
Sopressata Hot & Sweet	1 oz	100	7	3	25	8	0	0	0	0	540	—	—	0
Spiced Ham	2 oz	120	10	5	30	7	1	0	0	0	570	—	—	0
BUTTERBALL														
Turkey Bologna	1 slice (1 oz)	60	5	2	15	3	3	—	—	20	300	—	—	—
Turkey Ham	1 slice (1 oz)	35	2	1	10	4	1	—	—	—	340	—	—	—
CARL BUDDIG														
Beef	2 oz	90	5	—	—	10	1	—	—	—	—	—	—	—
Corned Beef	2 oz	90	5	—	—	10	1	—	—	—	—	—	—	—
DIETZ & WATSON														
Bologna Beef	3 slices (1.9 oz)	170	14	6	35	7	3	2	0	0	490	—	—	0
Mortadella	2 oz	150	14	5	30	19	2	0	0	0	560	—	—	0
Sopressata	1 oz	90	7	3	24	8	1	0	0	0	500	—	—	0
FOSTER FARMS														
Bologna Chicken	1 slice (1 oz)	60	5	—	25	4	tr	0	0	20	280	—	—	—
HEALTHY ONES														
Pastrami 97% Fat Free	4 slices (2 oz)	60	2	1	25	10	3	0	0	0	450	—	—	0
HIGH PLAINS BISON														
Pastrami	3 oz	80	2	1	25	14	0	0	0	100	1280	—	—	0
OSCAR MAYER														
Salami Beef	3 slices (1.8 oz)	150	13	6	40	8	1	0	0	0	640	—	—	0
SARA LEE														
Corned Beef	1 slice (2 oz)	50	2	1	25	8	1	0	0	0	600	—	—	15
Pastrami	2 slices (1.6 oz)	60	3	1	25	9	0	0	0	0	380	—	—	0
Salami Genoa	4 slices (1 oz)	110	10	4	35	6	1	0	0	0	390	—	—	0
Salami Hard	4 slices (1 oz)	120	11	4	40	6	0	0	0	0	410	—	—	0
WELLSHIRE														
Salami Genoa	1 oz	100	8	2	30	8	1	0	0	0	530	—	—	0
Salami Hard	1 oz	100	8	2	30	8	1	0	0	0	530	—	—	0
Sopressata Sliced	1 oz	100	8	2	30	8	1	0	0	0	530	—	—	0
DILL														
seed	1 tsp	6	tr	tr	0	tr	1	—	tr	32	0	25	0	tr
sprigs fresh	5 (0.3 oz)	0	tr	tr	0	tr	tr	—	—	2	1	7	2	1
weed dry	1 tbsp	8	tr	tr	0	1	2	—	tr	55	6	103	—	2
DINNER														

DINNER

(*see also* ASIAN FOOD, CURRY, PASTA DINNERS, POT PIE, SPANISH FOOD)

FOOD	PORTION	CALS	FAT	SAT FAT	CHOL	PROT	CARB	SUGAR	FIBER	CALCI	SOD	POTAS	FOLIC	VIT C
A LA CARTE														
Stuffed Zucchini w/ Barley Risotto Chicken Stuffing in Tomato Sauce	1 serv (5 oz)	140	7	3	25	6	14	3	2	40	280	—	—	12

FOOD	PORTION	CALS	FAT	SAT FAT	CHOL	PROT	CARB	SUGAR	FIBER	CALCI	SOD	POTAS	FOLIC	VIT C
AMY'S														
Country Dinner Vegetable Salisbury Steak	1 pkg (10.9 oz)	380	16	7	30	12	50	7	7	200	680	—	—	9
BANQUET														
Boneless Pork Ribs	1 pkg	370	17	6	30	6	47	10	4	60	710	—	—	0
Chicken Fingers	1 pkg	460	15	4	20	13	69	32	11	150	730	—	—	1
Corn Dog Meal	1 pkg	470	18	4	35	11	68	25	8	60	730	—	—	0
Crock Pot Classics Chicken & Dumplings	⅔ cup	200	8	3	35	10	21	4	6	20	940	—	—	0
Crock Pot Classics Hearty Beef & Vegetables	⅔ cup	140	6	3	35	12	15	4	4	40	620	—	—	0
Crock Pot Classics Meatballs In Stroganoff Sauce	⅔ cup	300	14	5	45	14	29	3	5	40	800	—	—	0
Fish Sticks	1 pkg	360	13	3	25	13	46	14	3	80	600	—	—	0
Fried Beef Steak	1 pkg	390	19	6	35	14	41	5	3	0	1040	—	—	5
Meatloaf	1 pkg	300	15	6	35	14	28	tr	5	20	820	—	—	0
Original Fried Chicken	1 pkg	380	20	5	30	14	35	3	5	80	930	—	—	0
Salisbury Steak	1 pkg	300	16	6	25	14	25	2	5	20	1090	—	—	0
Swedish Meatballs	1 pkg	430	23	10	90	20	35	0	5	80	950	—	—	0
Turkey	1 pkg	200	8	2	30	14	27	3	5	40	980	—	—	2
BETTY CROCKER														
Complete Meals Chicken & Buttermilk Biscuits	⅕ pkg (5.4 oz)	280	11	4	15	9	37	3	2	60	950	—	40	0
Complete Meals Stroganoff	⅕ pkg (5 oz)	200	5	1	15	10	30	3	1	40	760	—	60	—
BIRDS EYE														
Steamfresh Meals For Two Asian Chicken Vegetable Medley	½ pkg (11.9 oz)	290	6	1	50	20	36	13	10	80	1290	—	—	24
Steamfresh Meals For Two Grilled Chicken Marinara	½ pkg (11.9 oz)	360	10	3	30	21	45	9	4	100	1030	—	—	21
Steamfresh Meals For Two Sweet & Spicy Chicken	½ pkg (11.9 oz)	370	10	2	35	20	53	8	4	60	930	—	—	1
Voila! Pasta Primavera w/ Chicken	1⅔ cups	250	3	0	10	14	42	2	7	40	1130	—	—	9

FOOD	PORTION	CALS	FAT	SAT FAT	CHOL	PROT	CARB	SUGAR	FIBER	CALCI	SOD	POTAS	FOLIC	VIT C
BIRDS EYE (CONT.)														
Voila! Shrimp Scampi	1¾ cups	190	3	1	60	11	31	4	3	40	540	—	—	15
Voila! Southwestern Chicken	2 cups	250	6	3	30	14	32	7	2	100	640	—	—	21
C&W														
Stir Fry Feast Pot Sticker + Sauce	2 cups	200	4	1	15	10	30	8	4	60	1200	—	—	36
Stir Fry Feast Ultimate + Sauce	1½ cups	190	5	1	30	11	25	9	3	40	1350	—	—	15
CAMPBELL'S														
Supper Bakes Cheesy Chicken w/ Pasta	⅙ pkg	170	4	2	5	6	28	3	1	60	840	—	—	0
Supper Bakes Garlic Chicken w/ Pasta	⅙ pkg	220	2	1	<5	9	42	2	2	100	760	—	—	0
Supper Bakes Savory Pork Chops w/ Herb Stuffing	⅙ box	160	2	1	<5	5	30	4	1	40	780	—	—	0
Supper Bakes Traditional Roast Chicken w/ Stuffing	⅙ pkg	160	3	1	<5	5	29	3	2	40	740	—	—	0
CANDLE CAFE														
Ginger Miso Stir Fry	1 pkg (9 oz)	200	6	1	0	9	27	9	4	40	840	—	—	5
Seitan Piccata w/ Lemon Caper Sauce	1 pkg (9 oz)	210	4	1	0	12	32	6	4	60	920	—	—	1
CONTESSA														
Beef Goulash not prep	1¾ cups	210	5	2	50	12	32	9	3	40	850	—	—	15
Chicken Alfredo not prep	1¾ cups	330	18	10	70	15	28	3	2	100	660	—	—	24
Chicken Cacciatore not prep	1¾ cups	230	7	2	35	14	24	5	6	40	810	—	—	36
FANTASTIC														
Ginger Shiitake w/ Rice Noodles	1 pkg (7.4 oz)	340	10	2	0	8	58	3	4	80	690	—	—	5
FRENCH MEADOW BAKERY														
Garlic Ginger Chicken	1 pkg (12 oz)	310	5	0	60	24	42	9	3	40	880	—	—	2
GARDEIN														
Burgundy Trio	1 pkg	230	4	0	0	22	26	3	4	150	700	—	—	15
Thai Trio	1 pkg	250	8	3	0	19	25	2	3	100	750	—	—	12

FOOD	PORTION	CALS	FAT	SAT FAT	CHOL	PROT	CARB	SUGAR	FIBER	CALCI	SOD	POTAS	FOLIC	VIT C
GLORY														
Savory Singles Chicken & Dumplings	1 pkg	290	8	3	75	16	40	1	6	60	1400	—	—	1
Savory Singles Chicken Smoked Sausage & Rice Casserole	1 pkg	440	18	5	60	18	49	3	1	60	1390	—	—	1
Savory Singles Ham & Sausage Jambalaya	1 pkg	400	18	6	50	17	42	4	2	60	1320	—	—	12
Savory Singles Turkey & Gravy w/ Cornbread Stuffing	1 pkg	440	18	4	30	18	49	9	2	60	1380	—	—	2
GLUTEN FREE CAFE														
Lemon Basil Chicken	1 pkg (9.2 oz)	340	11	5	55	18	42	1	3	350	720	—	140	4
GLUTINO														
Gluten Free Chicken Pomodoro w/ Brown Rice & Vegetables	1 pkg (9.1 oz)	190	3	0	15	11	33	6	3	40	910	—	—	18
Gluten Free Chicken Ranchero w/ Brown Rice	1 pkg (9.1 oz)	180	2	0	20	14	30	5	4	40	790	—	—	27
GREEN GIANT														
Create A Meal Stir Fry Sweet & Sour as prep	1 cup	280	7	1	54	2	36	29	3	40	528	—	—	24
Skillet Meal Chicken Teriyaki as prep	1½ cups	240	1	0	20	13	46	8	3	40	780	—	—	30
HEALTHY CHOICE														
Bacon & Smokey Cheddar Chicken	1 pkg (8.6 oz)	240	6	3	45	17	28	2	3	100	560	500	120	24
Beef Tips Portabello	1 pkg (11.2 oz)	270	6	2	45	18	34	12	6	40	520	630	32	21
Country Breaded Chicken	1 pkg (10.6 oz)	340	9	2	30	14	52	15	6	40	560	520	80	21
Fire Roasted Tomato Chicken	1 pkg (11.6 oz)	310	5	2	35	19	46	18	6	60	500	490	120	30
Fresh Mixers Creamy Roasted Garlic Chicken	1 pkg (7.4 oz)	310	6	2	10	15	50	3	6	40	600	540	—	2

FOOD	PORTION	CALS	FAT	SAT FAT	CHOL	PROT	CARB	SUGAR	FIBER	CALCI	SOD	POTAS	FOLIC	VIT C
HEALTHY CHOICE (CONT.)														
Fresh Mixers Steak Portobello	1 pkg (7.5 oz)	290	6	2	15	16	42	4	5	40	600	900	—	0
Fresh Mixers Sweet Hickory BBQ Chicken	1 pkg (7.9 oz)	370	3	1	35	16	70	16	5	20	600	650	—	0
Grilled Chicken Monterey	1 pkg (10.9 oz)	320	8	3	40	19	43	12	6	100	560	560	160	21
Lemon Pepper Fish	1 pkg (10.6 oz)	300	5	1	25	14	49	15	5	40	360	480	140	24
Lunch Steamers Garlic Herb Shrimp	1 pkg (8.5 oz)	260	7	2	30	11	37	8	5	40	600	240	80	4
Lunch Steamers Lemon Herb Chicken	1 pkg (8.7 oz)	210	4	1	25	15	29	2	4	40	510	490	80	5
Lunch Steamers Rosemary Chicken & Sweet Potatoes	1 pkg (8.9 oz)	170	3	1	30	12	23	10	5	40	500	690	60	2
Pineapple Chicken	1 pkg (9 oz)	380	7	1	10	9	71	29	4	80	190	400	60	15
Portabella Spinach Parmesan	1 pkg (9.3 oz)	270	7	3	10	12	39	3	5	150	580	290	40	1
Salisbury Steak	1 pkg (8 oz)	170	5	2	30	13	18	2	4	80	500	510	80	2
Spicy Caribbean Chicken	1 pkg (8.5 oz)	310	2	1	20	15	56	16	5	60	260	510	100	15
Turkey Breast & Cranberries	1 pkg (10.7 oz)	250	4	1	35	17	36	12	6	40	450	730	140	24
HORMEL														
Compleats Microwave Meals Beef Steak & Peppers w/ Noodles	1 pkg (9.9 oz)	210	5	2	50	20	22	4	2	40	580	—	—	6
Compleats Microwave Meals Chicken Breast & Dressing	1 pkg (9.9 oz)	270	7	2	45	23	29	3	2	40	800	—	—	0
Compleats Microwave Meals Chicken Breast & Gravy w/ Mashed Potatoes	1 pkg (9.9 oz)	200	3	1	35	19	24	3	2	20	950	—	—	1
Compleats Microwave Meals Homestyle Beef w/ Potatoes & Gravy	1 pkg (9.9 oz)	220	6	3	15	11	30	2	3	40	600	—	—	0

FOOD	PORTION	CALS	FAT	SAT FAT	CHOL	PROT	CARB	SUGAR	FIBER	CALCI	SOD	POTAS	FOLIC	VIT C
HORMEL (CONT.)														
Compleats Microwave Meals Meatloaf w/ Potatoes & Gravy	1 pkg (9.9 oz)	310	11	6	40	18	34	3	3	40	940	—	—	0
Compleats Microwave Meals Salisbury Steak w/ Slice Potato & Gravy	1 pkg (9.9 oz)	280	11	5	50	16	30	1	2	20	980	—	—	0
Compleats Microwave Meals Santa Fe Chicken w/ Rice & Beans	1 pkg (9.9 oz)	280	4	1	40	20	41	6	4	60	550	—	—	0
Compleats Microwave Meals Swedish Meatballs	1 pkg (9.9 oz)	350	18	8	70	15	32	4	1	60	980	—	—	0
Compleats Microwave Meals Sweet & Sour Chicken w/ Rice	1 pkg (9.9 oz)	290	2	1	35	13	54	23	2	20	960	—	—	0
Compleats Microwave Meals Teriyaki Chicken w/ Rice	1 pkg (9.9 oz)	270	2	1	20	13	50	20	2	20	930	—	—	1
Compleats Microwave Meals Tuna Casserole	1 pkg (9.9 oz)	240	7	4	35	17	26	3	2	20	880	—	—	0
Compleats Microwave Meals Turkey & Dressing w/ Gravy	1 pkg (9.9 oz)	290	9	3	45	20	31	4	2	40	960	—	—	0
Compleats Microwave Meals Turkey & Hearty Vegetables	1 pkg (9.9 oz)	180	4	1	25	14	24	3	4	20	1200	—	—	1
IAN'S														
Chicken Finger Meal Allergen Free	1 pkg (7 oz)	368	9	2	40	17	56	14	3	40	420	—	—	9
Chicken Nugget Meal	1 pkg (8 oz)	440	14	2	50	18	50	21	2	0	320	—	—	6
Fish Stick Meal	1 pkg (8.4 oz)	480	11	2	25	17	79	23	4	100	480	—	—	9
Hamburger Meal	1 pkg (7 oz)	296	9	2	25	12	45	13	3	20	260	—	—	6
Pizza Meal	1 pkg (6.7 oz)	340	7	3	25	9	60	23	4	40	290	—	—	5
Popcorn Turkey Dog Meal Allergen Free	1 pkg (7 oz)	442	17	2	21	8	67	27	1	20	460	—	—	2

FOOD	PORTION	CALS	FAT	SAT FAT	CHOL	PROT	CARB	SUGAR	FIBER	CALCI	SOD	POTAS	FOLIC	VIT C
JOY OF COOKING														
Braised Beef Tips & Egg Noodles	1 cup (7.7 oz)	220	7	3	75	17	24	3	1	—	650	—	—	—
Roasted Herb Chicken	1 cup (7.7 oz)	170	3	1	25	11	27	4	3	—	640	—	—	—
KASHI														
Black Bean Mango	1 pkg (10 oz)	340	8	1	0	8	58	11	7	40	430	430	—	60
Lemon Rosemary Chicken	1 pkg (10 oz)	330	9	2	15	17	45	1	5	40	640	360	—	60
Lime Cilantro Shrimp	1 pkg (10 oz)	250	8	2	0	12	33	8	6	60	690	300	—	5
Southwest Style Chicken	1 pkg (10 oz)	240	5	0	30	16	32	3	6	40	680	540	—	24
Sweet & Sour Chicken	1 pkg (10 oz)	320	4	1	35	18	55	25	6	60	380	600	—	42
LEAN CUISINE														
Cafe Cuisine Chicken & Vegetables	1 pkg (10.5 oz)	220	4	2	30	18	29	5	3	150	580	640	—	2
Cafe Cuisine Chicken Marsala	1 pkg (8.1 oz)	250	9	3	25	14	29	4	2	60	620	430	—	1
Cafe Cuisine Lemon Pepper Fish	1 pkg (9 oz)	290	8	2	25	15	40	4	2	60	520	490	—	18
Cafe Cuisine Orange Chicken	1 pkg (9 oz)	300	7	2	25	14	46	11	2	40	580	270	—	9
Cafe Cuisine Roasted Garlic Chicken	1 pkg (8.8 oz)	170	6	2	40	17	11	3	0	150	580	680	—	2
Cafe Cuisine Steak Tips Portabello	1 pkg (7.5 oz)	150	4	2	20	15	14	4	3	40	430	590	—	36
Casual Cuisine Flatbread Melts Steakhouse Ranch	1 pkg (6.25 oz)	350	9	4	30	22	46	7	4	350	550	450	—	6
Comfort Classics Baked Chicken	1 pkg (8.6 oz)	240	7	2	30	14	30	4	2	40	600	770	—	0
Comfort Cuisine Beef Pot Roast	1 pkg (9 oz)	210	6	2	25	14	26	3	3	40	550	830	—	12
Comfort Cuisine Meatloaf w/ Gravy & Whipped Potatoes	1 pkg (9.4 oz)	250	8	3	45	20	25	2	3	60	590	930	—	0
Comfort Cuisine Roasted Turkey Breast w/ Dressing	1 pkg (9.75 oz)	290	4	1	20	14	49	27	3	20	630	410	—	54

FOOD	PORTION	CALS	FAT	SAT FAT	CHOL	PROT	CARB	SUGAR	FIBER	CALCI	SOD	POTAS	FOLIC	VIT C
LEAN CUISINE (CONT.)														
Comfort Cuisine Salisbury Steak w/ Mac & Cheese	1 pkg (9.5 oz)	260	8	4	40	23	23	3	3	100	540	640	—	0
Dinnertime Selects Balsamic Glazed Chicken	1 pkg (12 oz)	330	7	3	40	25	41	11	4	100	660	490	—	15
Dinnertime Selects Chicken Florentine	1 pkg (13.25 oz)	410	9	4	45	28	54	13	6	350	840	700	—	0
Dinnertime Selects Chicken Portabello	1 pkg (12 oz)	390	8	1	55	32	48	2	2	40	560	600	—	12
Dinnertime Selects Salisbury Steak	1 pkg (12.5 oz)	270	9	4	45	19	27	10	5	100	650	950	—	4
Market Creations Chicken Poblano	1 pkg (10.5 oz)	300	5	2	40	24	40	7	5	200	640	690	—	15
Market Creations Shrimp Scampi	1 pkg (10.5 oz)	250	7	4	58	15	32	4	4	80	690	420	—	27
Market Creations Sweet & Spicy Ginger Chicken	1 pkg (10.5 oz)	280	3	1	30	21	43	12	4	60	680	490	—	15
Simple Favorites Quesadilla BBQ Chicken	1 pkg (5 oz)	280	6	3	20	17	37	7	2	300	580	390	—	18
Simple Favorites Stuffed Cabbage	1 pkg (9.5 oz)	210	6	2	15	10	28	6	3	80	670	740	—	1
Simple Favorites Swedish Meatballs	1 pkg (9.1 oz)	290	8	3	35	19	35	4	3	80	670	570	—	0
Spa Cuisine Chicken Mediterranean	1 pkg (10.5 oz)	240	4	1	25	16	34	7	5	80	620	880	—	12
Spa Cuisine Chicken In Peanut Sauce	1 pkg (9 oz)	280	6	1	25	21	35	5	5	80	550	640	—	9
Spa Cuisine Chicken Pecan	1 pkg (9 oz)	310	7	1	35	18	43	13	5	60	580	560	—	4
Spa Cuisine Lemon Chicken	1 pkg (9 oz)	290	9	2	25	13	40	8	5	40	550	370	—	5
Spa Cuisine Lemongrass Chicken	1 pkg (9.4 oz)	250	5	1	25	18	35	7	5	60	600	680	—	30
Spa Cuisine Rosemary Chicken	1 pkg (8.25 oz)	210	4	2	30	16	27	5	5	60	510	490	—	0
Spa Cuisine Salmon w/ Basil	1 pkg (9.5 oz)	210	5	2	20	15	25	2	5	150	590	540	—	0

FOOD	PORTION	CALS	FAT	SAT FAT	CHOL	PROT	CARB	SUGAR	FIBER	CALCI	SOD	POTAS	FOLIC	VIT C
MARIE CALLENDER'S														
Chicken Fried Beef	1 meal	540	28	11	45	19	51	11	6	100	1510	—	—	48
Chicken Teriyaki	1 meal	430	4	1	45	19	78	27	5	100	1230	—	—	4
Golden Battered Filet Dinner	1 meal	450	16	5	35	22	53	9	4	150	1170	—	—	21
Herb Roasted Chicken	1 meal	460	25	7	65	30	26	3	5	60	1030	—	—	15
Meat Loaf w/ Gravy	1 meal	480	22	9	60	31	39	6	3	80	1080	—	—	2
Old Fashioned Beef Pot Roast	1 meal	330	10	4	45	27	32	tr	9	100	970	—	—	18
Salisbury Steak	1 meal	400	16	6	50	27	38	6	7	80	820	—	—	0
Slow Roasted Beef	1 meal	370	13	5	40	25	37	6	7	80	1370	—	—	0
Sweet & Sour Chicken	1 meal	600	20	18	25	22	88	28	10	40	860	—	—	18
Turkey w/ Stuffing	1 meal	400	9	3	65	32	45	9	4	100	1230	—	—	5
MEAL MART														
Stuffed Cabbage Beef Hungarian Style	¼ pkg (2.5 oz)	210	5	1	30	11	30	12	2	40	600	—	—	18
MEALS TO LIVE														
Grilled White Chicken w/ Brown Rice & Vegetables Gluten Free	1 pkg (9 oz)	260	5	1	30	17	30	16	5	—	470	—	—	40
Grilled White Chicken w/ Red Roasted Potatoes & Green Beans	1 pkg (8 oz)	200	3	0	30	14	30	1	3	—	470	—	—	30
Shrimp Jambalaya Gluten Free	1 pkg (9 oz)	220	4	0	90	13	31	5	4	—	480	—	—	42
Sliced Turkey w/ Balsamic Sauce & Butternut Squash Gluten Free	1 pkg (7 oz)	230	5	1	40	17	28	9	4	—	450	—	—	54
Stacked Eggplant w/ Seasoned White Chicken	1 pkg (9 oz)	200	5	2	20	14	28	5	3	—	480	—	—	48
White Chicken Fajita w/ Santa Fe Rice Gluten Free	1 pkg (9 oz)	240	5	1	30	17	34	5	5	—	480	—	—	84
MON CUISINE														
Vegan Moroccan Couscous	1 pkg (10 oz)	280	4	1	0	20	46	10	10	—	440	—	—	—

FOOD	PORTION	CALS	FAT	SAT FAT	CHOL	PROT	CARB	SUGAR	FIBER	CALCI	SOD	POTAS	FOLIC	VIT C
MON CUISINE (CONT.)														
Vegan Veal Schnitzel In Sauce	1 pkg (10 oz)	300	8	1	0	24	38	2	7	—	440	—	—	—
Vegetarian Stuffed Cabbage In Tomato Sauce	1 pkg (10 oz)	220	5	0	0	13	36	8	5	—	260	—	—	—
MOOSEWOOD														
Organic Vegetarian Moroccan Stew	1 pkg (10 oz)	150	3	0	0	5	29	11	5	80	400	—	—	36
ORGANIC BISTRO														
Alaskan Salmon Cakes	1 pkg (10 oz)	410	16	3	70	28	39	7	8	100	250	690	—	24
Chicken Citron	1 pkg (13.5 oz)	490	17	2	60	31	53	15	6	80	400	630	—	9
Ginger Chicken	1 pkg (13.25 oz)	490	17	2	60	31	53	15	6	80	400	630	—	9
Jamaican Shrimp Cakes	1 pkg (12 oz)	380	8	2	130	23	55	10	7	100	140	550	—	72
Savory Turkey	1 pkg (12 oz)	430	14	2	65	35	43	5	8	100	290	730	—	15
Spiced Chicken Morocco	1 pkg (12.2 oz)	390	11	2	50	26	46	5	7	100	330	230	—	9
Wild Salmon	1 pkg (13.1 oz)	500	23	3	95	35	41	7	8	80	80	814	—	42
ORGANIC CLASSICS														
Chicken Marsala w/ Mashed Potatoes	1 pkg (9.5 oz)	330	16	8	60	14	31	3	3	60	530	—	—	9
Jamaican Style Jerk Chicken w/ Wehani Rice	1 pkg (9.5 oz)	270	7	1	40	16	37	8	4	40	620	—	—	42
Lemon Chicken w/ Wehani Rice	1 pkg (9.5 oz)	320	8	2	35	14	49	1	3	0	320	—	—	2
SEEDS OF CHANGE														
Chicken Teriyaki	1 pkg (10 oz)	300	4	1	30	19	47	11	4	60	770	—	—	15
Mushroom Wild Pilaf	1 pkg (11 oz)	350	16	9	45	13	40	5	5	160	800	—	—	9
Seven Grain Pilaf	1 pkg (11 oz)	390	14	8	20	15	52	7	10	300	500	—	—	12
SIMPLY SENSIBLE														
Beef Pot Roast & Gravy w/ Mashed Potatoes	½ pkg (8.5 oz)	220	5	2	40	23	16	1	1	40	500	—	—	12
Beef Tips & Gravy w/ Brown Rice	1 cup (7 oz)	200	4	1	30	19	21	0	1	20	260	—	—	0
Zing Chicken & Brown Rice	1 cup (7 oz)	230	2	0	35	16	38	10	3	40	530	—	—	9

FOOD	PORTION	CALS	FAT	SAT FAT	CHOL	PROT	CARB	SUGAR	FIBER	CALCI	SOD	POTAS	FOLIC	VIT C
SOUTH BEACH														
Chicken Santa Fe Style Rice & Beans	1 pkg (8.9 oz)	340	12	4	80	22	35	3	4	—	750	—	—	—
Meatloaf w/ Gravy	1 pkg (8.9 oz)	210	9	3	50	16	17	5	4	—	910	—	—	—
Roasted Turkey	1 pkg (9.4 oz)	240	9	2	50	17	27	2	4	—	920	—	—	—
STOUFFER'S														
Beef Stew	1 pkg (11 oz)	280	9	3	40	21	28	4	4	40	1000	—	—	0
Beef Stroganoff	1 pkg (9.75 oz)	380	17	5	70	22	34	4	2	80	990	—	—	0
Chicken A La King	1 pkg (11.5 oz)	360	12	4	35	18	44	7	0	100	800	—	—	0
Corner Bistro Bourbon Steak Tips	1 pkg (12 oz)	520	22	6	50	25	56	26	3	150	1000	—	—	6
Corner Bistro Sesame Chicken	1 pkg (12.63 oz)	510	15	3	75	22	72	19	5	80	1380	—	—	6
Country Fried Beef Steak	1 pkg (16 oz)	610	33	10	40	22	55	12	6	200	1330	—	—	9
Creamed Chipped Beef	½ pkg (5.5 oz)	140	7	4	35	9	9	5	0	100	590	—	—	0
Fish Filet	1 pkg (9 oz)	400	16	5	55	27	36	7	4	150	1050	—	—	0
Fried Chicken Breast	1 pkg (8.88 oz)	360	18	5	45	20	30	2	2	20	880	—	—	0
Green Pepper Steak	1 pkg (10.5 oz)	240	4	2	30	18	32	5	3	40	910	—	—	6
Grilled Chicken Teriyaki	1 pkg (9.38 oz)	300	4	1	40	21	45	12	3	60	880	—	—	4
Grilled Lemon Pepper Chicken	1 pkg (9 oz)	240	8	2	40	19	24	3	4	40	670	—	—	42
Pork Cutlet	1 pkg (10 oz)	370	21	4	25	13	31	2	3	20	1110	—	—	08
Roast Pork	1 pkg (9.5 oz)	320	11	3	50	17	39	18	4	60	960	—	—	9
Roast Turkey Breast	1 pkg (16 oz)	390	13	4	40	21	48	10	6	80	1290	—	—	4
Salisbury Steak	1 pkg (16 oz)	470	24	8	65	29	34	9	6	60	1050	—	—	6
Stuffed Pepper	1 pkg (10 oz)	220	10	4	20	11	22	9	2	60	1000	—	—	6
Swedish Meatballs	1 pkg (11.5 oz)	560	27	12	100	32	47	6	3	100	1250	—	—	2
SUKHIS														
Tikka Masala Chicken	1 serv (5 oz)	170	6	3	75	25	46	2	0	20	750	—	—	4
SWANSON														
Chicken & Dumplings	1 cup	230	10	5	35	11	24	2	2	40	990	—	—	0
Chicken A La King	1 can	270	18	4	20	14	12	2	2	0	1370	—	—	0

FOOD	PORTION	CALS	FAT	SAT FAT	CHOL	PROT	CARB	SUGAR	FIBER	CALCI	SOD	POTAS	FOLIC	VIT C
TASTE ABOVE														
Meatless Zesty BBQ w/ Veggie Beef & Rice	1 pkg (10 oz)	280	6	1	0	16	48	18	7	80	310	—	—	54
TASTYBITE														
Beans Marsala & Basmati Rice	1 pkg (12 oz)	426	8	2	0	14	75	5	13	110	600	—	—	4
Spinach Dal & Basmati Rice	1 pkg (12 oz)	372	9	1	0	12	62	4	8	140	640	—	—	5
Stir Fry Vegetables & Jasmine Rice	1 pkg (12 oz)	450	16	2	0	7	67	8	3	40	480	—	—	1
Vegetable Supreme & Basmati Rice	1 pkg (12 oz)	317	6	1	4	11	55	3	11	60	410	—	—	2
THE FILLO FACTORY														
Fillo Pie Spinach & Cheese	⅕ pie (4.8 oz)	270	14	7	30	10	26	1	2	200	400	—	—	2
WEIGHT WATCHERS														
Smart Ones Chicken w/ Broccoli & Cheese	1 pkg (11.8 oz)	340	8	4	65	31	37	6	3	250	730	—	—	48
YVES														
Meatless Santa Fe Beef	1 pkg (10.5 oz)	360	9	1	0	15	57	12	5	80	750	450	—	12
ZATARAIN'S														
Blackened Chicken w/ Yellow Rice	1 pkg (10.5 oz)	470	13	2	25	16	71	3	3	20	1310	—	—	12
Jambalaya w/ Sausage	1 pkg (12 oz)	500	14	4	25	13	79	3	3	40	1020	—	—	9
Red Beans & Rice w/ Sausage	1 pkg (12 oz)	510	20	7	30	16	68	5	5	80	1200	—	—	15
Rice Bowl Big Easy	1 pkg (10 oz)	430	12	5	45	22	56	3	5	40	870	—	—	15
Sausage & Chicken Gumbo w/ Rice	1 pkg (12 oz)	300	14	4	30	14	36	3	2	40	1330	—	—	12

DIP

FOOD	PORTION	CALS	FAT	SAT FAT	CHOL	PROT	CARB	SUGAR	FIBER	CALCI	SOD	POTAS	FOLIC	VIT C
shrimp cream cheese	¼ cup (2 oz)	152	14	6	74	5	2	1	tr	55	245	70	7	2
spinach sour cream	¼ cup	155	15	4	13	2	4	1	1	52	166	115	29	5
CABOT														
French Onion	2 tbsp	50	5	3	15	1	1	0	0	20	200	—	—	0
Ranch	2 tbsp	50	5	3	15	1	1	1	0	20	140	—	—	0

FOOD	PORTION	CALS	FAT	SAT FAT	CHOL	PROT	CARB	SUGAR	FIBER	CALCI	SOD	POTAS	FOLIC	VIT C
CEDARLANE														
Organic Five Layer Mexican	2 tbsp	60	3	2	10	3	4	2	1	60	100	—	—	2
EMERALD VALLEY														
Organic Black Bean	1 tbsp (1 oz)	45	2	1	0	2	6	0	1	20	120	—	—	0
FRITOS														
Bean	2 tbsp (1.2 oz)	35	1	0	0	2	5	0	2	0	190	—	—	0
Chili Cheese	2 tbsp (1.2 oz)	45	3	1	1	1	3	1	tr	20	290	—	—	0
GUILTLESS GOURMET														
Black Bean Mild	2 tbsp (1.1 oz)	40	0	0	0	2	7	0	2	20	125	—	—	1
HEALTH IS WEALTH														
Vegetarian Spinach & Artichoke	3 tbsp (1 oz)	30	2	1	5	1	3	2	0	20	50	—	—	1
KRAFT														
Green Onion	2 tbsp	60	5	3	0	tr	3	tr	0	0	170	—	—	0
LAY'S														
Country Ranch Mix as prep w/ sour cream	2 tbsp (1.1 oz)	70	6	4	10	1	2	0	0	20	160	—	—	0
French Onion	2 tbsp (1.2 oz)	60	5	0	<5	1	2	0	0	0	230	—	—	0
LITEHOUSE														
Avocado	2 tbsp	140	15	2	15	1	2	1	0	20	210	—	—	1
Caramel Low Fat	1 tbsp	110	0	0	0	1	27	16	0	20	140	—	—	0
Caramel Original	2 tbsp	110	2	2	0	1	25	15	1	20	125	—	—	0
Dilly	2 tbsp	150	16	2	15	1	1	1	0	20	200	—	—	0
Fruit Dip Chocolate Yogurt	2 tbsp	110	6	0	0	1	14	9	0	20	95	—	—	0
Fruit Dip Vanilla Yogurt	2 tbsp	60	2	0	0	1	10	7	0	20	50	—	—	0
Lite Ranch Veggie	2 tbsp	70	7	1	10	1	3	1	0	20	125	—	—	0
Organic Ranch	2 tbsp	130	13	2	10	1	2	2	0	20	200	—	—	0
MARIE'S														
French Onion Roasted	2 tbsp	100	10	3	15	1	2	1	0	40	220	—	—	0
Guacamole	2 tbsp	40	3	2	5	1	3	1	1	0	140	—	—	2
Honey Vanilla Cream Fruit Dip	2 tbsp	60	5	3	15	1	5	3	0	40	20	—	—	0
Spinach Parmesan	2 tbsp	90	9	3	15	2	2	1	0	40	200	—	—	0
NATURALLY FRESH														
Caramel	2 tbsp	100	4	2	5	0	15	13	0	—	130	25	—	—
Chocolate	2 tbsp	70	0	0	0	1	17	14	0	—	40	45	—	—
Cream Cheese Strawberry	2 tbsp	90	4	3	10	1	14	10	0	—	45	—	—	—

FOOD	PORTION	CALS	FAT	SAT FAT	CHOL	PROT	CARB	SUGAR	FIBER	CALCI	SOD	POTAS	FOLIC	VIT C
NATURALLY FRESH (CONT.)														
Ranch Lite	2 tbsp	80	8	2	5	1	2	1	0	—	240	30	—	—
Ranch Vegetable	2 tbsp	120	12	3	15	1	2	1	0	—	150	0	—	—
ROAD'S END ORGANICS														
Nacho Cheese Gluten Free	2 tbsp	20	0	0	0	2	3	0	tr	0	110	—	28	1
ROBERT ROTHCHILD FARM														
Artichoke	2 tbsp	60	5	1	<5	2	2	1	tr	40	65	—	—	4
SALPICA														
Chipotle Hummus Bean	2 tbsp (1 oz)	40	1	0	0	2	6	0	1	0	135	—	—	1
Cowgirl White Bean	2 tbsp (1 oz)	25	0	0	0	2	5	0	1	20	170	—	—	1
Salsa Con Queso	2 tbsp (1 oz)	20	1	0	0	1	4	4	0	10	160	—	—	5
SNYDER'S OF HANOVER														
Three Bean	2 tbsp	25	0	0	0	1	5	1	1	0	150	—	—	5
TOSTITOS														
Creamy Spinach	2 tbsp (1.1 oz)	50	4	0	<5	1	2	tr	tr	0	200	—	—	0
Dip Creations Mix Freshly Made Guacamole as prep w/ avocados	2 tbsp (1.1 oz)	50	4	1	0	1	3	0	2	0	120	—	—	2
Zesty Bean & Cheese Medium	2 tbsp (1.2 oz)	45	2	1	0	2	5	tr	2	20	230	110	—	0
UTZ														
Jalapeno Cheddar	2 tbsp	260	4	1	0	0	2	0	0	20	260	—	—	0
Sour Cream & Onion	2 tbsp	60	5	3	20	1	2	1	0	20	250	—	—	0
WALDEN FARMS														
Blue Cheese Calorie Free	2 tbsp (1 oz)	0	0	0	0	0	0	0	0	0	210	—	—	0
Ranch No Calorie	2 tbsp (1 oz)	0	0	0	0	0	0	0	0	0	230	—	—	0
WANT'EMS														
Sweet Chili Fusion	2 tbsp (1.1 oz)	50	0	0	0	0	12	11	0	0	40	—	—	5
Thai Mango Fusion	2 tbsp (1.1 oz)	40	0	0	0	0	9	8	0	0	115	—	—	9
WILD THYMES FARM														
Indian Vindaloo Curry	1 tbsp	12	1	tr	0	tr	1	tr	tr	10	51	—	—	1
Indonesian Peanut Sauce	1 tbsp	32	2	1	0	1	2	1	tr	0	74	—	—	3
DOCK														
fresh cooked	3½ oz	20	1	—	0	2	3	—	—	38	3	321	—	26
raw chopped	½ cup	15	tr	—	0	1	2	—	—	29	3	261	—	32
DOUGHNUTS														
chocolate glazed	1 med (1.5 oz)	175	8	2	24	2	24	13	1	89	143	45	19	0

FOOD	PORTION	CALS	FAT	SAT FAT	CHOL	PROT	CARB	SUGAR	FIBER	CALCI	SOD	POTAS	FOLIC	VIT C
chocolate w/ chocolate icing	1 med (2 oz)	218	12	4	4	3	26	13	1	17	243	77	35	1
creme filled	1 (3 oz)	307	21	5	20	5	26	12	1	21	263	68	60	0
custard filled	1 (2.3 oz)	235	16	4	16	4	20	9	1	16	201	52	46	0
french cruller glazed	1 med (1.4 oz)	169	8	2	5	1	24	14	1	11	141	32	17	0
jelly filled	1 (3 oz)	289	16	4	22	5	33	18	1	21	249	67	58	0
old fashioned plain	1 med (2 oz)	226	13	4	5	3	25	9	1	14	301	61	43	1
plain chocolate frosted	1 med (1.5 oz)	194	11	6	8	2	22	11	1	10	187	86	28	1
plain glazed	1 med (1.6 oz)	192	10	3	14	2	23	—	1	27	181	46	21	0
whole wheat sugared	1 med (1.6 oz)	162	9	1	9	3	19	10	1	22	160	67	9	tr
ENTENMANN'S														
Crumb	1 (1.9 oz)	230	10	4	10	2	34	20	tr	40	190	—	—	0
Glazed	1 (2 oz)	250	13	6	10	2	32	20	tr	40	190	—	—	0
Mini Rich Frosted Chocolate	1 (1.1 oz)	170	12	7	5	1	14	8	0	0	95	—	—	0
Old Fashion Plain	1 (1.7 oz)	230	14	6	15	2	23	10	tr	0	220	—	—	0
Pop'Ems Cinnamon	4 (2 oz)	250	13	6	0	3	31	16	tr	40	240	—	—	0
Pop'Ems Glazed Crullers	2 (1.6 oz)	210	12	5	10	1	25	17	0	40	140	—	—	0
Pop'Ems Holes Rich Frosted	4 (2.1 oz)	320	23	14	10	2	28	17	tr	0	180	—	—	0
Rich Frosted	1 (1.9 oz)	240	19	11	10	2	27	16	tr	0	170	—	—	0
TAKE-OUT														
andagi okinawan doughnut	1 (0.7 oz)	84	5	1	7	1	10	—	0	9	109	25	10	0
malasada portuguese ball	1 (1.1 oz)	118	5	1	22	2	16	—	0	14	49	31	25	0

DRINK MIXERS

FOOD	PORTION	CALS	FAT	SAT FAT	CHOL	PROT	CARB	SUGAR	FIBER	CALCI	SOD	POTAS	FOLIC	VIT C
whiskey sour mix not prep	1 pkg (0.6 oz)	64	0	0	0	tr	16	—	—	45	46	3	0	1
whiskey sour mix	2 oz	55	0	0	0	0	14	—	0	1	66	18	0	2
ANGOSTURA														
Bloody Mary	4 oz	20	0	0	0	0	4	1	0	20	560	—	—	9
Daiquiri	2 oz	72	0	0	0	0	18	18	0	0	5	—	—	0
Daiquiri Strawberry	8 oz	120	0	0	0	0	31	31	0	0	240	—	—	0
Grenadine	1 tsp	10	0	0	0	0	3	3	0	0	5	—	—	0
Margarita	4 oz	80	0	0	0	0	30	28	0	0	5	—	—	0
Pina Colada	4 oz	60	0	0	0	0	16	16	0	0	120	—	—	0
ARIZONA														
Pina Colada Virgin Cocktail	8 oz	90	1	0	0	0	23	20	0	0	10	—	—	60

FOOD	PORTION	CALS	FAT	SAT FAT	CHOL	PROT	CARB	SUGAR	FIBER	CALCI	SOD	POTAS	FOLIC	VIT C
DAVE'S GOURMET														
Bloody Mary Original	2 oz	25	0	0	0	1	5	3	tr	0	210	—	—	0
FEVER-TREE														
Bitter Lemon	1 bottle (6.8 oz)	75	0	0	0	tr	18	18	0	—	2	—	—	—
GO COCKTAILS!														
On-The-Go Sugar Free Appletini	1 pkg (1.9 g)	5	0	0	0	0	tr	0	0	0	15	—	—	0
On-The-Go Sugar Free Cosmo	1 pkg (2.2 g)	5	0	0	0	0	tr	0	0	0	35	—	—	0
On-The-Go Sugar Free Lemon Drop	1 pkg (2.5 g)	5	0	0	0	0	tr	0	0	0	133	—	—	0
On-The-Go Sugar Free Margarita	1 pkg (2.78 g)	5	0	0	0	0	tr	0	0	0	33	—	—	0
MARGARITAVILLE														
Margarita Mix Mango	4 oz	120	0	0	0	0	29	26	—	—	75	—	—	—
Margarita Mix Original Lime	4 oz	110	0	0	0	0	27	26	—	—	70	—	—	—
MCILHENNY														
Bloody Mary Mix as prep	1 cup	70	0	0	0	2	15	9	2	4	1930	—	—	12
MODMIX														
Mojito	2 oz	50	0	0	0	0	13	13	0	—	10	—	—	2
Organic Citrus Margarita	2 oz	70	0	0	0	0	19	18	0	—	0	—	—	9
Organic French Martini	2 oz	50	0	0	0	0	13	12	0	—	10	—	—	—
Organic Lavender Lemon Drop	2 oz	55	0	0	0	0	14	13	0	—	0	—	—	1
Organic Pomegranate Cosmopolitan	2 oz	55	0	0	0	0	14	13	0	—	10	—	—	—
Organic Wasabi Bloody Mary	2 oz	20	0	0	0	1	4	3	0	—	150	—	—	2
MONIN														
Grenadine	1 oz	90	0	0	0	0	22	22	—	—	0	—	—	—
Mojito Mix	1 oz	84	0	0	0	0	21	21	—	—	0	—	—	—
White Sangria Mix	1 oz	91	0	0	0	0	22	22	—	—	0	—	—	—
OLD ORCHARD														
Daiquiri Mixer Strawberry frzn as prep	8 oz	120	0	0	0	0	32	30	—	0	0	—	—	0
Margarita Mixer frzn as prep	8 oz	120	0	0	0	0	32	30	—	0	0	—	—	0

FOOD	PORTION	CALS	FAT	SAT FAT	CHOL	PROT	CARB	SUGAR	FIBER	CALCI	SOD	POTAS	FOLIC	VIT C
OLD ORCHARD (CONT.)														
Pina Colada Mixer frzn as prep	8 oz	120	0	0	0	0	32	30	—	0	0	—	—	0
PROMETHEUS SPRINGS														
Capsaicin Spiced Elixir Citrus Cayenne	8 oz	70	0	0	0	0	17	17	—	—	50	—	—	—
Capsaicin Spiced Elixir Lychee Wasabi	8 oz	80	0	0	0	0	20	20	—	—	50	—	—	—
Capsaicin Spiced Elixir Mango Chili	8 oz	70	0	0	0	0	17	16	—	—	50	—	—	—
Capsaicin Spiced Elixir Spicy Pear	8 oz	70	0	0	0	0	17	16	—	—	50	—	—	—
DRUM														
freshwater fillet baked	5.4 oz	236	10	2	126	35	0	0	0	118	148	543	—	—
freshwater baked	3 oz	130	5	1	70	19	0	0	0	65	82	300	—	—
DUCK														
boneless roasted	½ duck (7.8 oz)	444	25	9	197	52	0	0	0	27	144	557	22	0
boneless w/o skin roasted	3.5 oz	201	11	4	89	23	0	0	0	12	65	252	10	0
boneless w/o skin roasted diced	1 cup (4.9 oz)	281	16	6	125	33	0	0	0	17	91	353	14	0
chinese pressed	3 oz	162	8	3	28	6	16	9	1	12	188	156	12	3
chinese pressed	1 cup (4.9 oz)	267	14	4	46	10	26	14	1	20	309	256	20	6
pekin breast boneless w/ skin roasted	1 (4.2 oz)	242	13	4	163	29	0	0	0	10	101	—	—	3
pekin breast w/o skin broiled	3 oz	133	2	1	136	26	0	0	0	9	100	—	—	3
pekin leg w/ skin w/o bone roasted	1 (3.2 oz)	200	10	3	105	25	0	0	0	9	101	—	—	1
pekin leg w/o skin & bone roasted	1 (2.6 oz)	134	5	1	79	22	0	0	0	8	81	—	—	2
w/ skin & bone roasted	½ duck (13 oz)	1287	108	37	321	73	0	0	0	42	225	779	23	0
w/ skin & bone roasted	1 serv (6 oz)	583	49	17	145	33	0	0	0	19	102	353	10	0
wing roasted bone removed	1 (1.1 oz)	101	8	3	25	6	0	0	0	3	66	61	2	0
GRIMAUD FARMS														
Muscovy Duck Confit	1 serv (3 oz)	170	10	4	95	20	tr	—	—	0	140	420	—	0
Muscovy Duck Whole	1 serv (3.7 oz)	200	14	5	130	19	tr	—	—	0	125	360	—	0

FOOD	PORTION	CALS	FAT	SAT FAT	CHOL	PROT	CARB	SUGAR	FIBER	CALCI	SOD	POTAS	FOLIC	VIT C
TAKE-OUT														
breast battered & fried bone removed	½ (3.2 oz)	199	10	3	94	20	6	tr	tr	16	310	238	26	0
leg battered & fried bone removed	1 (2.5 oz)	155	8	3	73	16	5	tr	tr	13	242	186	20	0

DUMPLING

FOOD	PORTION	CALS	FAT	SAT FAT	CHOL	PROT	CARB	SUGAR	FIBER	CALCI	SOD	POTAS	FOLIC	VIT C
CRAZY CUIZINE														
Potstickers Chicken w/ Sauce	8 (5 oz)	220	6	2	25	13	31	2	1	20	790	—	—	15
Potstickers Pork w/o Sauce	8 (5 oz)	240	8	3	20	10	32	1	1	40	620	—	—	24
FUJISAN														
Chicken Shumai Dumplings	3 (3 oz)	130	2	0	20	8	18	2	0	20	440	—	—	1
HEALTH IS WEALTH														
Potstickers Vegan	2 (1.6 oz)	90	3	0	0	6	13	tr	2	20	280	—	—	4
HEALTHY CHOICE														
Sweet Asian Potstickers Entree	1 pkg (9.9 oz)	340	5	1	0	8	66	14	5	40	560	220	100	5
JOYCE CHEN														
Chinese Style Potstickers Chicken & Vegetable	6	170	2	0	15	8	30	2	2	20	125	—	—	12
Chinese Style Potstickers Pork & Vegetable	6	170	3	1	15	8	30	2	2	20	125	—	—	12
KAHIKI														
Potstickers Chicken	5 (3.3 oz)	230	11	2	10	7	24	1	1	20	520	—	—	5
Samosas Coconut Curry Chicken	4 (2.8 oz)	170	3	1	15	8	26	1	1	20	520	—	—	5
LEAN CUISINE														
Market Creations Pot Stickers Chicken	1 pkg (10 oz)	270	6	1	14	11	42	16	5	60	750	510	—	4
Simple Favorites Asian Pot Stickers	1 pkg (9 oz)	260	4	1	10	8	49	9	2	40	530	180	—	6
PANNI														
Spaetzle Authentic German not prep	2 oz	200	2	1	55	8	39	0	2	20	20	—	—	0
PEPPERIDGE FARM														
Apple	1	230	11	6	0	3	29	13	1	0	220	—	—	0
Peach	1	250	11	6	0	3	34	18	1	0	220	—	—	2

FOOD	PORTION	CALS	FAT	SAT FAT	CHOL	PROT	CARB	SUGAR	FIBER	CALCI	SOD	POTAS	FOLIC	VIT C
TRAVELING CHEF														
Potstickers Chicken + Dipping Sauce	5 pieces + 1 tbsp sauce	285	7	1	20	13	42	11	1	20	840	—	—	5
TAKE-OUT														
apple	1 (6.7 oz)	661	34	7	0	7	83	30	3	13	614	118	78	2
bread dumpling	1 lg	330	10	—	—	—	28	—	—	—	—	—	—	—
cherry	1 (2.7 oz)	238	12	2	0	3	31	13	1	8	216	58	30	1
cornmeal	1 (2.8 oz)	134	4	1	62	5	20	1	2	69	278	82	44	0
fried pork	1 (3.5 oz)	338	21	5	27	13	25	1	1	33	363	197	40	tr
fried puerto rican style	1 med (1.1 oz)	117	7	1	0	2	11	1	tr	46	182	35	16	tr
gyoza potstickers vegetable	8 (4.9 oz)	210	4	1	0	8	34	7	5	40	500	—	—	0
peach	1 (2.7 oz)	253	12	2	0	3	33	12	1	6	248	88	31	2
piroshki meat filled	1 (3.4 oz)	348	22	6	23	12	25	tr	1	11	425	114	43	0
steamed meat	1 (1.3 oz)	41	1	tr	18	4	4	tr	tr	7	161	70	7	1
DURIAN														
fresh	3.5 oz	141	2	—	0	3	29	—	—	12	1	601	—	42
EDAMAME														
(*see* SOYBEANS)														
EEL														
fresh cooked	3 oz	200	13	3	137	20	0	0	0	22	55	297	—	—
fresh cooked	1 fillet (5.6 oz)	375	24	5	257	38	0	0	0	41	104	555	—	—
raw	3 oz	156	10	2	107	16	0	0	0	17	43	232	—	—
smoked	3.5 oz	330	28	7	—	19	0	0	0	—	—	—	—	—
EGG														
(*see also* EGG DISHES, EGG SUBSTITUTES)														
CHICKEN														
fresh large	1 (1.8 oz)	72	5	2	186	6	tr	tr	0	28	71	69	24	0
fresh medium	1 (1.5 oz)	63	4	1	164	6	tr	tr	0	25	62	61	21	0
fresh small	1 (1.3 oz)	54	4	1	141	5	tr	tr	0	21	54	52	18	0
hard or soft cooked	1	77	5	2	186	6	1	1	0	25	139	63	22	0
pickled	1	72	5	2	198	6	1	1	0	24	131	59	21	0
poached	1	73	5	2	184	6	tr	tr	0	26	147	66	18	0
scrambled plain	1 (2 oz)	61	7	2	169	6	1	1	0	40	88	81	22	0
sunny side up	2	155	12	3	365	11	1	1	0	46	414	116	30	0
white raw	1 (1.1 oz)	17	tr	0	0	4	tr	tr	0	2	55	54	1	0
yolk raw	1 (0.5 oz)	55	4	2	184	3	1	tr	0	22	8	19	25	0
DAVIDSON'S														
Pasteurized Shell Eggs	1 lg	75	5	2	213	6	0	0	0	—	60	—	—	—
EGG INNOVATIONS														
100% Organic Cage Free Large	1 (1.8 oz)	70	5	2	215	6	1	0	0	20	65	—	—	0

FOOD	PORTION	CALS	FAT	SAT FAT	CHOL	PROT	CARB	SUGAR	FIBER	CALCI	SOD	POTAS	FOLIC	VIT C
EGG-LAND'S BEST														
Extra Large	1 (2 oz)	80	5	2	200	7	0	0	0	20	75	—	24	0
Hard-Cooked Peeled	1 med (1.5 oz)	60	4	1	160	5	0	0	0	20	55	—	—	0
Large	1 (1.8 oz)	70	4	1	175	6	0	0	0	—	60	—	40	0
GOOD EARTH ORGANICS														
Organic Instant Whites	1 pkg (0.5 oz)	50	0	0	0	12	1	1	0	20	0	—	—	0
HORIZON ORGANIC														
Jumbo	1 (2.2 oz)	90	5	2	270	8	1	0	0	40	80	—	—	0
JAKE & AMOS														
Pickled Red Beet Eggs	2 (5.3 oz)	200	8	3	345	10	21	21	0	40	170	—	—	0
LAND O LAKES														
Farm Fresh Brown Extra Large	1 (1.8 oz)	70	5	2	215	6	1	—	—	20	65	—	—	0
ORGANIC VALLEY														
Egg Whites Pasteurized	¼ cup	25	0	0	0	5	1	0	0	0	90	—	—	0
Large Omega-3	1	70	5	2	225	7	tr	—	—	20	85	—	—	0
PETE & GERRY'S														
Organic Large	1 (1.8 oz)	70	5	2	215	6	1	—	—	20	65	—	—	0
SAFEST CHOICE														
Pasteurized Fresh	1 lg (1.8 oz)	70	5	2	186	6	0	0	0	20	70	—	16	0
TREE OF LIFE														
White Large Natural Omega 3	1 (1.8 oz)	70	5	0	250	<6	tr	0	0	20	65	—	—	0
OTHER POULTRY														
duck 100 year old	1 (1 oz)	49	3	—	173	4	1	—	—	18	154	43	—	—
duck cooked	1 (2.5 oz)	129	10	3	616	9	1	1	0	45	210	155	42	0
duck preserved hard core	1 (1.8 oz)	80	6	2	220	6	1	0	0	0	350	—	—	0
duck preserved soft core	1 (1.8 oz)	80	6	2	220	7	1	0	0	0	350	—	—	0
duck salted	1 (1 oz)	54	4	—	184	4	2	—	—	34	769	52	—	—
goose cooked	1 (5 oz)	265	19	5	1223	20	2	1	0	86	420	301	82	0
quail canned	1 (0.3 oz)	14	1	tr	75	1	tr	tr	0	6	47	12	6	0
quail cooked	1 (0.5 oz)	24	2	1	42	2	0	0	0	11	24	23	—	0
turkey raw	1 (2.8 oz)	135	9	3	737	11	1	—	0	78	119	112	56	0
EGG DISHES														
AUNT JEMIMA														
Eggs & Sausage	1 pkg (6.2 oz)	320	21	5	310	16	17	3	2	60	900	—	—	5
Omelet Ham & Cheese	1 pkg (5.2 oz)	240	14	6	195	12	17	2	2	150	710	—	—	6
Scramble Ham & Egg	1 pkg (6.8 oz)	260	13	4	195	16	21	4	2	200	920	—	—	9

FOOD	PORTION	CALS	FAT	SAT FAT	CHOL	PROT	CARB	SUGAR	FIBER	CALCI	SOD	POTAS	FOLIC	VIT C
CEDARLANE														
Zone Omelette Cheese	1 pkg (10.4 oz)	350	14	8	40	25	31	5	2	400	720	—	—	12
JIMMY DEAN														
Breakfast Skillets Bacon as prep	1 serv (4.5 oz)	370	24	7	336	10	14	2	2	60	840	—	—	18
Breakfast Skillets Ham as prep	1 serv (4.5 oz)	270	15	4	336	8	16	1	2	40	792	—	—	18
Breakfast Skillets Smoked Sausage as prep	1 serv (4.5 oz)	380	25	7	345	8	20	1	3	60	792	—	—	12
Breakfast Bowls D-Lights Sausage	1 pkg	230	7	3	20	23	19	1	2	150	730	—	—	2
Breakfast Bowls Eggs Potato Sausage & Cheddar Cheese	1 pkg	490	34	13	370	23	20	1	3	250	1210	—	—	4
Breakfast Bowls Eggs Potato & Ham	1 pkg	390	23	9	360	24	23	1	3	250	1170	—	—	5
Omelets Ham & Cheese	1 (4.2 oz)	280	19	7	295	16	4	1	0	200	770	—	—	0
Omelets Sausage & Cheese	1 (4.3 oz)	270	22	8	295	15	5	1	0	150	570	—	—	1
MEALS TO LIVE														
Spinach Omelet w/ Turkey Sausage Gluten Free	1 pkg (7.5 oz)	190	6	2	20	17	18	5	2	—	480	—	—	6
WEIGHT WATCHERS														
Smart Ones Smart Morning Wrap Egg Sausage & Cheese	2 (4 oz)	240	8	3	30	11	32	2	7	80	560	—	—	0
TAKE-OUT														
deviled	1 half	62	5	1	121	4	tr	tr	0	15	94	37	13	0
eggs benedict	2	825	64	30	784	35	26	3	2	182	1654	441	119	4
omelet cheese	3 eggs	387	29	11	588	25	6	6	0	342	1134	356	52	0
omelet mushroom	3 eggs	251	17	5	511	18	6	4	1	125	796	293	50	0
omelet mushroom & onion	3 eggs	294	20	6	600	20	7	5	1	146	780	326	57	1
omelet plain	3 eggs	338	25	7	736	24	4	4	0	154	854	312	64	0
omelet spanish	3 eggs	496	38	9	626	23	17	11	3	175	876	767	79	45
omelet spinach	3 eggs	279	19	6	568	20	6	4	1	177	687	438	108	22
omelet western	3 eggs	355	23	7	537	24	6	4	tr	127	1007	381	48	11
salad	½ cup	353	34	6	344	10	2	1	0	46	402	110	37	0
scotch egg	1 (4.2 oz)	301	21	—	—	14	16	—	2	60	—	—	—	—

FOOD	PORTION	CALS	FAT	SAT FAT	CHOL	PROT	CARB	SUGAR	FIBER	CALCI	SOD	POTAS	FOLIC	VIT C
tortilla de amarillo omelet w/ plantain	3 eggs	536	35	7	467	16	43	21	3	64	1017	742	55	17
EGG ROLLS														
egg roll wrapper fresh	1 (1.1 oz)	93	tr	tr	3	3	19	—	1	15	183	26	28	0
BLUE HORIZON ORGANIC														
Spring Rolls Chinese Shrimp	3 (2.1 oz)	130	4	2	0	3	16	1	1	20	210	—	—	15
Spring Rolls Indian	3 (2.1 oz)	110	4	2	0	3	15	1	1	20	250	—	—	1
Spring Rolls Thai	3 (2.1 oz)	110	4	2	0	3	16	1	1	20	210	—	—	15
Spring Rolls Thai Shrimp	3 (2.1 oz)	130	4	2	0	3	15	1	1	20	250	—	—	1
HEALTH IS WEALTH														
Spinach	1 (3 oz)	170	8	1	0	8	18	1	3	100	310	—	—	9
Thai Spring Roll	2 (1.6 oz)	90	3	1	0	3	13	1	1	0	300	—	—	5
KAHIKI														
Chicken	1 (3 oz)	160	6	1	10	7	19	2	1	20	730	—	—	5
Chipotle Lime Chicken	1 (3 oz)	170	4	2	10	8	26	3	2	40	380	—	—	5
Lemongrass Chicken Stix	3 (2.6 oz)	100	2	0	20	7	13	3	tr	20	380	—	—	6
Pork & Shrimp	1 (3 oz)	140	4	1	30	8	20	2	1	20	630	—	—	6
Vegetable	1 (3 oz)	90	4	1	0	2	12	2	1	20	410	—	—	9
LEAN CUISINE														
Casual Cuisine Spring Rolls Fajita Chicken	½ pkg	200	7	2	30	15	20	3	2	20	580	300	—	1
Casual Cuisine Spring Rolls Garlic Chicken	½ pkg	200	8	2	20	10	24	4	2	40	580	320	—	1
Simple Favorites Eggroll Vegetable	1 pkg (9 oz)	320	4	1	0	8	62	12	2	0	630	110	—	6
TAKE-OUT														
chicken	1 (3 oz)	140	4	2	15	7	20	5	4	40	510	—	—	1
lobster	1 (4.8 oz)	270	7	2	0	8	43	4	6	20	460	—	—	2
lumpia vegetable & shrimp	2 (3 oz)	120	0	0	10	4	26	1	2	0	300	—	—	2
meat & shrimp	1 (4.8 oz)	320	12	3	10	10	41	3	4	20	470	—	—	5
pork & shrimp	1 (5 oz)	300	10	4	15	13	41	6	7	40	890	—	—	0
shrimp	1 (2.2 oz)	156	7	2	11	5	18	4	2	28	320	147	41	8
spicy pork	1 (3 oz)	200	9	2	5	6	23	3	3	20	410	—	—	0
spring roll deep fried	1 (0.8 oz)	70	4	2	3	1	7	—	1	8	141	23	—	0
vegetable	1 (3 oz)	170	4	1	0	5	28	4	4	20	520	—	—	0

FOOD	PORTION	CALS	FAT	SAT FAT	CHOL	PROT	CARB	SUGAR	FIBER	CALCI	SOD	POTAS	FOLIC	VIT C
EGG SUBSTITUTES														
BOB'S RED MILL														
Egg White Dried	2 tsp	15	0	0	0	3	0	0	0	—	45	—	—	—
Vegetarian Egg Replacer	1 tbsp	30	1	0	0	3	2	1	1	—	20	—	—	—
EGG BEATERS														
Original	¼ cup (2.1 oz)	30	0	0	0	6	1	tr	0	20	115	95	60	0
EGGPRO														
Powder	1 tbsp	15	0	0	0	4	tr	0	0	—	55	50	—	—
FANTASTIC														
Tofu Scrambler not prep	1 tbsp	35	0	0	0	1	7	0	1	0	260	—	—	1
HORIZON ORGANIC														
Liquid Egg	¼ cup	35	0	0	0	6	1	0	0	40	100	—	32	0
QUICK EGGS														
Fat Free Cholesterol Free	¼ cup	30	0	0	0	6	1	tr	0	20	115	—	60	0
EGGNOG														
eggnog	1 qt	1368	76	45	596	39	138	—	—	1321	553	1678	9	15
eggnog	1 cup	342	19	11	149	10	34	—	—	330	138	420	2	4
eggnog flavor mix as prep w/ milk	9 oz	260	8	5	33	8	39	—	—	291	163	369	12	2
FARMLAND														
Egg Nog	½ cup	180	8	5	50	4	23	22	0	150	150	—	—	0
HOOD														
Fat Free Sugar Free	1 cup	110	0	0	<5	8	18	12	0	300	210	—	—	0
Golden	½ cup	180	9	5	65	4	22	20	0	150	100	—	—	0
Light	½ cup	140	4	3	45	4	22	21	0	150	100	—	—	0
HORIZON ORGANIC														
Lowfat	½ cup	140	3	2	45	6	22	22	0	200	135	—	—	0
LACTAID														
Eggnog	½ cup (4 oz)	170	9	5	60	4	20	19	0	150	95	—	—	0
ORGANIC VALLEY														
Ultra Pasteurized	½ cup	180	10	6	90	5	18	17	0	150	85	—	—	0
STRAUS														
Organic	4 oz	160	10	5	70	5	13	13	0	150	55	—	—	0
TAKE-OUT														
eggnog	1 cup	306	22	14	63	5	16	—	0	49	95	93	3	tr
EGGNOG SUBSTITUTES														
SILK														
Nog	½ cup (4 oz)	90	2	0	0	3	15	12	0	20	75	150	—	0
EGGPLANT														
cubed cooked w/ oil	1 cup	133	8	1	0	2	17	6	5	12	1000	240	27	3

FOOD	PORTION	CALS	FAT	SAT FAT	CHOL	PROT	CARB	SUGAR	FIBER	CALCI	SOD	POTAS	FOLIC	VIT C
pickled	½ cup	33	tr	tr	0	1	7	3	2	17	1138	8	14	0
slices grilled	1 (2 oz)	36	2	tr	0	tr	5	2	1	3	268	64	7	1
CEDARLANE														
Eggplant Mediterranean	1 pkg (10 oz)	230	10	4	20	13	22	7	6	200	590	—	—	12
CELENTANO														
Eggplant Parmigiana	1 serv (7 oz)	330	22	5	25	9	26	9	5	100	480	—	—	27
PELOPONNESE														
Baba Ganoush	2 tbsp	40	3	0	0	1	2	0	1	0	250	63	—	0
STONEWALL KITCHEN														
Eggplant Spread	1 tbsp	25	1	—	—	0	4	4	—	—	90	—	—	1
TASTYBITE														
Punjab Eggplant	½ pkg (5 oz)	144	9	1	0	4	13	4	2	50	515	—	—	4
THE GRACIOUS GOURMET														
Tapenade Roasted Eggplant	2 tbsp (1 oz)	35	4	1	0	1	3	1	tr	0	135	—	—	2
TAKE-OUT														
baba ghannouj	¼ cup	55	4	—	0	2	5	—	—	—	95	—	—	—
caponata	2 tbsp (1 oz)	30	2	—	0	1	3	2	—	—	115	—	—	4
iman bayildi eggplant w/ onion & tomato	1 serv (15.6 oz)	345	28	4	0	3	25	6	2	43	552	773	59	29
indian eggplant raita	1 serv	180	14	4	0	2	13	1	1	30	228	527	13	15
moussaka	1 serv (9 oz)	372	24	6	54	20	18	6	5	119	415	611	46	15
papoutsaki little shoes	1 serv (15.5 oz)	245	16	7	40	12	15	1	1	144	751	669	37	12
tempura	1 serv (1.5 oz)	118	10	5	0	1	5	0	1	6	13	73	—	0
ELDERBERRIES														
fresh	1 cup	105	1	—	0	1	27	—	—	55	—	406	—	52
ELDERBERRY JUICE														
elderberry	7 oz	76	0	0	0	4	16	—	—	10	2	576	12	52
ELK														
eye of round roasted	3.5 oz	151	3	1	63	31	1	0	0	4	50	369	1	0
ground cooked	3.5 oz	143	3	1	70	29	0	0	0	5	56	379	1	0
NATURAL FRONTIER FOODS														
Filet	1 (4 oz)	140	3	1	95	26	0	0	0	0	60	—	—	0
EMU														
cooked	3 oz	130	—	—	111	—	—	—	—	6	97	270	—	tr

FOOD	PORTION	CALS	FAT	SAT FAT	CHOL	PROT	CARB	SUGAR	FIBER	CALCI	SOD	POTAS	FOLIC	VIT C
ENERGY BARS														

(*see also* CEREAL BARS, FRUIT AND NUT BARS, NUTRITION SUPPLEMENTS)

FOOD	PORTION	CALS	FAT	SAT FAT	CHOL	PROT	CARB	SUGAR	FIBER	CALCI	SOD	POTAS	FOLIC	VIT C
ACTIVEX														
Organic All Flavors	1 (1.6 oz)	200	12	3	0	8	17	8	2	20	75	—	—	0
ATTUNE														
Wellness Chocolate Crisp	1 (0.7 oz)	100	6	4	0	2	11	8	1	200	20	—	—	2
Wellness Cool Mint Chocolate	1 (0.7 oz)	100	6	4	0	2	11	8	1	200	20	—	—	2
BALANCE														
100 Calories Peanut Butter Crisp	1 (1 oz)	100	5	3	<5	6	14	4	5	200	180	45	—	60
100 Calories Vanilla Crisp	1 (1 oz)	100	4	3	<5	5	15	5	5	200	180	25	—	60
Carbwell Chocolate Fudge	1 (1.8 oz)	190	6	4	<5	14	23	1	2	100	190	95	100	60
Gold Chocolate Peanut Butter	1 (1.8 oz)	210	6	4	<5	14	23	14	tr	100	125	125	100	60
Gold S'mores Crunch	1 (1.8 oz)	210	6	4	<5	15	23	12	0	100	140	115	100	60
Organic Apricot Mango Crisp	1 (1.6 oz)	180	7	3	0	10	23	11	5	100	120	120	100	15
Organic Cranberry Pomegranate Crisp	1 (1.6 oz)	180	7	3	0	10	23	12	5	100	100	95	100	15
Original Almond Brownie	1 (1.8 oz)	200	6	2	<5	14	22	17	2	100	75	220	100	60
Original Mocha Crisp	1 (1.8 oz)	200	6	4	0	15	21	18	tr	100	95	130	100	60
Pure Banana Cashew	1 (1.6 oz)	180	6	1	0	9	23	18	2	40	80	—	—	0
Pure Cherry Pecan	1 (1.6 oz)	190	7	1	0	9	22	18	2	40	75	—	—	0
BELLY-BAR														
Baby Needs Chocolate	1	170	6	3	0	8	22	12	2	250	280	—	800	21
Berry Nutty Cravings	1	170	4	1	0	8	26	13	2	250	70	35	800	21
Mellow Oat	1	180	5	2	0	8	26	11	2	250	70	40	800	21
BOOMI BAR														
Almond Protein Plus	1	270	18	1	15	12	20	15	4	110	12	—	—	0
Cashew Almond Delicacy	1	260	17	2	0	8	23	3	1	60	55	250	16	9
Cranberry Apple	1	210	9	1	0	4	28	18	4	60	50	—	—	1
Merry Macadamia	1	220	14	2	0	3	26	21	3	80	25	—	—	2

FOOD	PORTION	CALS	FAT	SAT FAT	CHOL	PROT	CARB	SUGAR	FIBER	CALCI	SOD	POTAS	FOLIC	VIT C
BOOMI BAR (CONT.)														
Pistachio Pineapple	1	200	9	2	0	5	28	17	3	20	50	—	—	6
BORA BORA														
Organic Island Brazil Nut Almond	1 (1.4 oz)	200	12	2	0	5	18	10	2	20	5	100	—	0
Organic Peanut Peanut	1 (1.4 oz)	230	17	3	0	6	10	5	2	0	10	—	—	0
Organic Sesame Raisin	1 (1.4 oz)	170	11	2	0	5	17	12	3	10	15	—	—	0
CLIF														
Apricot	1 (2.4 oz)	230	3	1	0	10	45	21	5	250	125	310	80	60
Black Cherry Almond	1 (2.4 oz)	250	5	2	0	10	44	20	5	250	110	220	80	60
Builders Chocolate	1 (2.4 oz)	270	8	5	0	20	30	20	4	250	230	220	80	60
Builders Lemon	1 (2.4 oz)	270	8	4	0	20	31	23	1	250	240	140	80	60
Chocolate Almond Fudge	1 (2.4 oz)	250	5	2	0	10	44	20	5	250	140	300	80	60
Chocolate Chip Peanut Crunch	1 (2.4 oz)	260	6	2	0	11	42	21	5	250	200	260	80	60
Crunchy Peanut Butter	1 (2.4 oz)	250	6	1	0	11	42	20	5	250	230	270	80	60
Mojo Chocolate Peanut	1 (1.6 oz)	210	10	4	0	9	22	11	3	60	190	190	—	0
Mojo Honey Roasted Peanuts	1 (1.6 oz)	200	10	2	0	10	20	9	2	80	200	210	—	1
Mojo Mountain Mix	1 (1.6 oz)	180	8	2	0	9	21	12	2	80	220	240	—	1
Mojo Peanut Butter & Jelly	1 (1.6 oz)	220	11	4	0	9	21	12	2	80	115	190	—	0
Nectar Cherry Pomegranate	1 (1.6 oz)	150	5	1	0	3	29	20	7	20	0	370	—	0
Nectar Dark Chocolate Walnut	1 (1.6 oz)	160	6	2	0	3	27	18	6	20	0	370	—	0
Oatmeal Raisin Walnut	1 (2.4 oz)	240	5	1	0	10	43	20	5	250	130	310	80	60
Spiced Pumpkin Pie	1 (2.4 oz)	240	5	2	0	10	45	23	5	250	140	250	80	60
Vanilla Almond	1 (2.4 oz)	270	8	5	0	20	30	22	3	250	240	170	80	60
Zbar Blueberry	1 (1.3 oz)	120	3	0	0	3	23	11	3	300	90	80	80	21
Zbar Honey Graham	1 (1.3 oz)	130	3	1	0	3	26	10	3	300	95	115	80	21
Zbar Spooky S'mores	1 (1.3 oz)	130	4	2	0	2	23	11	3	300	80	85	80	21

FOOD	PORTION	CALS	FAT	SAT FAT	CHOL	PROT	CARB	SUGAR	FIBER	CALCI	SOD	POTAS	FOLIC	VIT C
GLENNY'S														
Fruit & Nut Mixed Nut	1	230	16	3	—	6	14	6	3	—	50	—	—	—
GLUCERNA														
All Flavors	1 (0.7 oz)	80	3	1	0	4	12	4	tr	100	60	50	40	9
GRANOLA GOURMET														
Chocolate Espresso	1 (1.23 oz)	150	6	1	0	4	20	10	3	80	15	—	—	0
Ultimate Berry	1 (1.2 oz)	150	6	1	0	5	19	9	3	40	20	—	—	0
Ultimate Cran-Orange	1 (1.2 oz)	140	5	1	0	5	19	11	3	40	30	—	—	1
Ultimate Fudge Brownie	1 (1.3 oz)	150	6	2	0	5	19	10	3	20	30	—	—	0
Ultimate Mocha Fudge	1 (1.2 oz)	150	6	2	0	5	19	10	3	20	35	—	—	0
GREEN SUPERFOOD														
Whole Food	1 (2.1 oz)	220	8	2	0	5	36	25	4	40	25	350	—	12
Whole Food Chocolate	1 (2.1 oz)	230	9	3	0	5	37	27	0	40	25	330	—	9
HALO														
Honey Graham	1 (1.3 oz)	150	5	1	0	4	24	8	2	20	200	—	—	0
Nutty Marshmallow	1 (1.3 oz)	150	6	1	0	4	22	9	2	20	250	—	—	0
Rocky Road	1 (1.3 oz)	160	8	2	0	5	20	9	2	20	125	—	—	0
S'Mores	1 (1.3 oz)	150	5	1	0	3	25	13	2	20	190	—	—	0
JOJOBAR														
Chocolate Cashew	1 (1.8 oz)	220	14	5	10	11	18	6	2	40	55	—	—	1
Peanut Butter & Jelly	1 (1.8 oz)	220	13	4	10	13	17	6	3	60	25	—	—	1
KASHI														
GoLean Chocolate Almond Toffee	1 (2.7 oz)	290	6	5	0	13	45	31	6	80	250	250	—	0
GoLean Cookies 'N Cream	1 (2.7 oz)	290	6	4	0	13	50	35	6	80	200	250	—	0
GoLean Crunchy Chocolate Peanut	1 (1.8 oz)	180	5	2	0	9	30	13	6	200	250	—	100	9
GoLean Malted Chocolate Chip	1 (2.7 oz)	290	6	4	0	13	49	35	6	80	200	270	—	1
GoLean Oatmeal Raisin Cookie	1 (2.7 oz)	280	5	3	0	13	49	33	6	100	140	250	—	0
GoLean Peanut Butter & Chocolate	1 (2.7 oz)	290	6	5	0	13	48	31	6	80	280	250	—	0
GoLean Roll Caramel Peanut	1 (1.9 oz)	200	5	2	0	12	29	14	6	200	210	120	100	9
GoLean Roll Fudge Sundae	1 (1.9 oz)	190	5	2	0	12	27	13	6	200	260	60	100	9

FOOD	PORTION	CALS	FAT	SAT FAT	CHOL	PROT	CARB	SUGAR	FIBER	CALCI	SOD	POTAS	FOLIC	VIT C
KASHI (CONT.)														
TLC Chewy Granola Cherry Dark Chocolate	1 (1.2 oz)	120	2	1	0	5	24	8	4	0	75	—	—	0
TLC Crunchy Granola Honey Toasted 7 Grain	1 (1.4 oz)	180	6	1	0	7	26	7	4	0	160	—	—	0
TLC Crunchy Granola Pumpkin Spice	1 (1.4 oz)	180	6	1	0	6	26	7	4	0	150	—	—	0
TLC Crunchy Granola Roasted Almond	1 (1.4 oz)	180	6	1	0	7	26	7	4	0	160	—	—	0
LARABAR														
Jocalat Chocolate	1 (1.7 oz)	190	10	2	0	5	24	18	5	40	0	270	16	0
LEAN BODY														
Gold Caramel Cookie Twist	1 (2.9 oz)	330	7	6	0	30	36	10	2	150	430	—	—	0
LIVING HARVEST														
Organic Hemp Protein Forbidden Fruit	1 (1.6 oz)	170	6	1	0	6	25	18	4	20	100	—	—	1
LUNA														
Berry Almond	1 (1.7 oz)	170	4	0	0	9	29	11	3	100	115	170	—	9
Chai Tea	1 (1.7 oz)	190	5	3	0	9	26	12	3	350	95	150	400	12
Dulce De Leche	1 (1.7 oz)	170	4	2	0	9	28	13	3	350	120	135	400	12
Mini Caramel Nut Brownie	1 (0.7 oz)	70	3	1	0	3	11	5	2	150	50	60	160	5
Mini S'mores	1 (0.7 oz)	80	2	1	0	4	11	5	1	150	60	65	160	5
Sunrise Apple Cinnamon	1 (1.7 oz)	180	5	2	0	8	27	11	5	350	100	110	200	30
Sunrise Strawberry Crunch	1 (1.7 oz)	170	5	2	0	8	26	12	5	350	105	130	200	30
Toasted Nuts 'N Cranberry	1 (1.7 oz)	170	5	1	0	9	26	11	3	350	180	180	400	12
MOMMY MUNCHIES														
Chocolate Mint	1 (1.8 oz)	180	7	2	5	12	32	13	5	500	35	400	320	48
Cinnamon Bun	1 (1.8 oz)	180	6	3	0	12	23	15	5	500	40	390	320	48
MRS. MAY'S														
Trio Blueberry	1 (1.2 oz)	170	12	2	0	5	15	6	2	20	45	—	—	0
Trio Tropical	1 (1.2 oz)	170	12	9	0	5	14	6	2	20	45	—	—	1
MUSCLE MILK														
Light Chocolate Peanut Caramel	1 (1.59 oz)	170	6	4	0	15	18	9	4	60	105	110	—	0

FOOD	PORTION	CALS	FAT	SAT FAT	CHOL	PROT	CARB	SUGAR	FIBER	CALCI	SOD	POTAS	FOLIC	VIT C
NOGII														
No Gluten High Protein Peanut Butter & Chocolate	1 (2 oz)	230	8	3	0	20	20	10	2	100	250	—	—	0
NUTIVA														
Organic Flax & Raisin	1 (1.4 oz)	200	15	2	0	7	15	8	4	80	0	—	—	0
Organic Flaxseed Flax Chocolate	1 (1.4 oz)	200	12	2	0	6	19	10	5	80	5	—	—	0
Organic Original Hempseed	1 (1.4 oz)	210	14	2	0	9	11	5	5	0	5	—	—	0
ODWALLA														
Berries GoMega	1	220	5	1	0	5	41	20	5	250	230	—	100	0
Carrot	1	220	4	2	0	4	43	21	4	250	115	—	100	0
Choco-walla	1	240	6	2	0	5	42	20	5	250	80	220	100	12
Cranberry C Monster	1	220	3	1	0	4	44	21	3	250	85	250	100	150
Super Protein	1	230	5	2	0	16	31	16	4	250	160	200	100	12
Superfood	1	230	4	2	0	4	43	20	3	250	110	300	100	12
OH MAMA!														
Chocolate Peanut Butter	1 (1.8 oz)	190	6	3	0	9	26	13	3	500	170	—	400	60
Frosted White Lemon	1 (1.8 oz)	180	5	4	0	9	28	13	3	500	160	—	400	60
Frosted White Raspberry	1 (1.8 oz)	180	5	4	0	10	26	10	3	500	180	—	400	60
PERFECT 10														
Bliss Apricot	1 (1.8 oz)	215	9	2	2	5	29	24	5	78	10	506	—	2
Bliss Cranberry	1 (1.8 oz)	215	12	3	2	4	26	20	4	72	10	256	—	2
Natural Apricot	1 (1.8 oz)	205	10	1	0	5	27	20	4	80	5	506	—	2
Natural Cranberry	1 (1.8 oz)	164	10	1	0	4	17	11	4	72	3	238	—	2
Natural Lemon	1 (1.8 oz)	210	12	1	0	5	24	18	5	80	5	340	—	2
POM														
Pomegranate Dipped In Chocolate	1 (1.8 oz)	210	8	3	0	3	31	18	4	60	5	390	—	0
POMX														
Coconut Dipped In Yogurt	1 (1.8 oz)	230	12	5	0	3	28	22	3	60	15	260	—	0
Pomegranate Dipped In Yogurt	1 (1.8 oz)	210	8	3	0	3	31	23	4	60	15	340	—	0
PREMIER														
Protein Bar Double Chocolate Crunch	1 (2.5 oz)	270	6	4	20	30	26	9	2	100	330	340	—	0

FOOD	PORTION	CALS	FAT	SAT FAT	CHOL	PROT	CARB	SUGAR	FIBER	CALCI	SOD	POTAS	FOLIC	VIT C
PREMIER (CONT.)														
Protein Bar Yogurt Peanut Crunch	1 (2.5 oz)	290	8	5	10	30	24	10	1	60	410	140	—	0
PUREFIT														
Almond Crunch	1 (2 oz)	230	6	1	0	18	25	16	3	80	190	180	—	0
Peanut Butter Crunch	1 (2 oz)	240	7	2	0	18	26	16	2	60	200	160	—	0
RISE BAR														
Energy + Cherry Almond	1 (1.6 oz)	200	11	2	0	5	23	11	3	60	55	160	—	0
Protein + Almond Honey	1 (2.1 oz)	280	16	2	0	20	20	13	4	150	25	0	—	0
Protein + Crunchy Carob Chip	1 (2.1 oz)	260	15	1	5	17	22	13	5	150	25	0	—	0
SENCHA NATURALS														
Green Tea Bar Lively Lemongrass	1 (2 oz)	220	8	2	0	9	29	12	3	60	115	250	—	0
Green Tea Bar Original	1 (2 oz)	220	9	2	0	9	29	12	3	60	120	240	—	1
SIMPLY NUTRILITE														
Sweet & Salty	1 (1.6 oz)	170	6	2	0	4	27	21	4	40	310	—	—	60
SNICKERS														
Marathon Chewy Chocolatey Peanut	1 (1.94 oz)	210	8	3	5	13	26	15	5	450	170	170	400	60
SOUTH BEACH														
Energy Mix	1 pkg (1 oz)	160	13	3	0	6	8	3	2	—	45	—	—	—
SOYJOY														
Soy & Fruit Banana	1 (1.1 oz)	130	6	3	20	4	16	12	2	20	50	240	—	0
Soy & Fruit Blueberry	1 (1.1 oz)	140	6	3	20	4	17	12	4	20	45	220	—	0
Soy & Fruit Mango Coconut	1 (1.1 oz)	140	6	4	20	4	16	11	3	20	45	230	—	4
SUNRIDGE FARMS														
Energy Nuggets	2 (1.4 oz)	200	11	2	0	6	18	11	4	60	0	—	—	0
THINK5														
Red Berry	1 (2.5 oz)	240	4	1	0	4	48	7	3	300	140	610	40	72
Red Berry Chocolate Covered	1 (2.8 oz)	290	8	4	0	4	52	16	3	300	140	630	32	72
THINKPINK														
Blueberry Dark Chocolate	1 (2.1 oz)	240	8	4	0	20	26	0	2	300	80	135	100	15
Lemon Burst	1 (2.1 oz)	230	7	4	0	20	27	0	2	250	150	27	100	15

FOOD	PORTION	CALS	FAT	SAT FAT	CHOL	PROT	CARB	SUGAR	FIBER	CALCI	SOD	POTAS	FOLIC	VIT C
THINKPINK (CONT.)														
Peanut Butter Caramel	1 (2.1 oz)	230	8	4	5	20	26	0	1	250	280	80	100	15
White Chocolate Raspberry	1 (2.1 oz)	240	8	4	0	20	28	1	3	250	100	95	100	15
TITAN														
High Protein Chocolate Peanut Butter Crunch	1 (2.8 oz)	320	13	7	10	26	32	5	1	150	160	—	—	0
High Protein Cookies And Cream	1 (2.8 oz)	330	9	7	5	26	34	5	tr	100	200	—	—	0
ZOE'S														
Chocolate Delight	1 (1.7 oz)	190	7	3	0	8	27	13	5	50	70	235	—	0
ENERGY DRINKS														
180														
Blue w/ Acai	1 can (8.2 oz)	120	0	0	0	0	31	—	—	—	—	—	—	—
Blue w/ Acai Low Calorie	1 can (8.2 oz)	15	0	0	0	0	4	—	—	—	—	—	—	—
Orange Citrus Blast	1 can (8.2 oz)	120	0	0	0	0	33	—	—	—	—	—	—	—
Orange Citrus Blast Sugar Free	1 can (8.2 oz)	5	0	0	0	0	1	—	—	—	—	—	—	—
Red w/ Gogi	1 can (8.2 oz)	130	0	0	0	0	31	—	—	—	—	—	—	—
1IN3TRINITY														
Energy Drink	1 can (8.4 oz)	10	0	0	0	0	3	3	0	0	0	—	—	60
ARIZONA														
Energy Low Carb	1 can (8 oz)	10	0	0	0	0	3	3	—	—	10	—	—	60
Rx Energy Fast Shot Natural Green Tea	1 bottle (2 oz)	10	0	0	0	0	3	3	—	—	—	—	400	—
Sports Orange	8 oz	50	0	0	0	0	14	13	0	0	110	30	—	15
B52														
Zero Sugar Citrus Berry	8 oz	10	0	0	0	0	1	0	—	—	190	20	—	—
BAI														
Antioxidant Infusion Jamaica Blueberry	8 oz	70	0	0	0	0	18	18	—	—	10	—	—	60
Antioxidant Infusion Kenya Peach	8 oz	70	0	0	0	0	17	17	—	—	10	—	—	60
Antioxidant Infusion Mango Kauai	8 oz	70	0	0	0	0	18	18	—	—	10	—	—	60

FOOD	PORTION	CALS	FAT	SAT FAT	CHOL	PROT	CARB	SUGAR	FIBER	CALCI	SOD	POTAS	FOLIC	VIT C
BAWLS														
Guarana	8 oz	90	0	0	0	0	25	25	—	—	30	—	—	—
Guaranexx Sugar Free	1 bottle (10 oz)	0	0	0	0	0	0	0	0	—	15	—	—	—
BING														
Energy Drink	1 can (12 oz)	40	0	0	0	0	10	10	—	—	20	—	—	60
BLOOM														
All Flavors	1 can (10.5 oz)	100	0	0	0	tr	24	20	—	100	115	—	—	60
BLOX														
Black Cherry	8 oz	86	0	0	0	0	25	16	—	—	38	—	—	—
Orange Rush	8 oz	103	0	0	0	0	25	24	—	79	40	—	—	24
Original	8 oz	105	0	0	0	0	26	26	—	—	40	—	—	—
BOOST														
Beauty	1 bottle (12 oz)	220	0	0	tr	2	52	40	tr	50	30	—	—	24
High Protein Vanilla	8 oz	240	6	—	10	15	33	16	0	330	170	380	140	60
Youth	1 bottle (12 oz)	200	0	0	tr	2	48	36	tr	40	30	—	—	0
BOOZER														
Hangover Remedy	1 can (8.4 oz)	110	0	0	0	0	28	28	—	—	10	—	200	252
BRAIN TONIQ														
Functional Drink	1 can (8.4 oz)	80	0	0	0	0	20	20	—	—	0	—	—	—
C1.5														
Extreme	1 can (8.4 oz)	120	0	0	0	0	30	30	—	—	50	—	—	—
CELSIUS														
Ginger Ale	1 bottle (12 oz)	10	—	—	—	—	—	—	—	50	6	—	—	60
Orange	1 bottle (12 oz)	10	—	—	—	—	—	—	—	50	6	—	—	60
CINTRON														
Citrus Mango	8 oz	110	0	0	0	tr	27	26	0	—	200	tr	—	—
Citrus Mango Sugar Free	8 oz	0	0	0	0	tr	0	0	0	—	200	tr	—	—
CLIF														
Quench Fruit Punch	8 oz	45	0	0	0	0	11	10	0	—	130	35	—	—
Quench Orange	8 oz	45	0	0	0	0	11	10	0	—	130	35	—	—
COCA-COLA														
Zero	8 oz	1	0	0	0	0	tr	0	0	—	28	31	—	—
COOLAH														
Original	8 oz	120	0	0	0	0	31	30	—	—	40	—	—	—
CYTOMAX														
Performance Drink Cool Citrus	1 pkg (1.4 oz)	140	0	0	0	0	35	19	0	10	190	95	—	96
DNA ENERGY														
Low Carb Citrus	8 oz	0	0	0	0	0	0	0	—	—	96	—	400	—

FOOD	PORTION	CALS	FAT	SAT FAT	CHOL	PROT	CARB	SUGAR	FIBER	CALCI	SOD	POTAS	FOLIC	VIT C
DR. TIM'S														
ISO-5	1 bottle (11.2 oz)	60	0	0	0	0	15	15	—	50	35	660	—	—
Jungle Juice	1 bottle (4 oz)	20	0	0	0	2	8	4	0	0	30	—	—	0
EMU														
Energy Drink	1 bottle (8.4 oz)	170	0	0	0	tr	41	41	—	—	220	—	—	—
EQ THIRST EQUALIZER														
All Flavors	8 oz	60	0	0	0	0	15	11	—	—	15	380	—	—
EX														
Aqua Vitamins Lemon Lime	1 bottle (16.9 oz)	110	0	0	0	0	27	26	—	—	5	—	—	—
Chillout	1 can (8.4 oz)	80	0	0	0	0	20	20	—	—	0	—	—	12
Pure Energy	1 can (8.4 oz)	70	0	0	0	0	17	15	—	—	5	—	165	50
Slim Energy	1 can (8.4 oz)	20	0	0	0	0	5	2	—	—	10	—	165	50
FACEDRINK														
The Social Drink	1 bottle (2.5 oz)	3	0	0	0	0	1	0	—	—	48	—	400	250
FEVER														
Stimulation Beverage All Flavors	8 oz	130	0	0	0	0	31	31	—	—	10	—	—	—
FITNESS EDGE														
Tropical Orange	1 bottle (12 oz)	170	2	1	5	20	17	15	1	150	85	—	—	60
FUNCTION														
Alternative Energy	8 oz	60	0	0	0	0	15	14	—	—	65	—	200	60
Brainiac Carambola Punch	8 oz	60	0	0	0	0	15	14	—	—	—	—	—	—
Urban Detox Citrus Prickly Pear	8 oz	60	0	0	0	0	17	17	—	40	48	—	40	24
Youth Trip Acai Grape	8 oz	60	0	0	0	0	15	14	—	100	10	—	—	60
FUZE														
Refresh Banana Coconut	8 oz	90	0	0	0	0	25	23	—	250	15	—	—	30
Refresh Peach Mango	8 oz	90	0	0	0	0	23	22	—	250	15	—	—	30
Refresh Strawberry Banana	8 oz	100	0	0	0	0	25	24	—	250	15	—	—	30
Slenderize Cranberry Raspberry	8 oz	5	0	0	0	0	2	1	—	—	5	—	—	60
Slenderize Low Carb Tropical Punch	8 oz	5	0	0	0	0	tr	0	—	—	5	—	—	60

FOOD	PORTION	CALS	FAT	SAT FAT	CHOL	PROT	CARB	SUGAR	FIBER	CALCI	SOD	POTAS	FOLIC	VIT C
FUZE (CONT.)														
Slenderize Tangerine Grapefruit	8 oz	10	0	0	0	0	2	1	—	—	10	—	—	60
Vitalize Blackberry Grape	8 oz	100	0	0	0	0	26	25	—	150	10	150	—	90
Vitalize Orange Mango	8 oz	100	0	0	0	0	25	25	—	40	10	150	—	90
GATORADE														
All Flavors	8 oz	50	0	0	0	0	14	14	—	—	110	30	—	—
GINGER BOOST														
Ginger Orange	8 oz	110	0	0	0	1	24	21	1	20	15	185	—	30
GLEUKOS														
Performance All Flavors	8 oz	70	0	0	0	0	17	17	0	—	40	50	—	—
GO GIRL														
Bliss	1 can (11.5 oz)	35	0	0	0	0	8	8	—	—	30	—	—	—
Glo	1 can (12 oz)	35	0	0	0	0	9	8	0	100	80	—	40	0
Sugar Free	1 can (12 oz)	<5	0	0	0	0	tr	0	—	—	100	—	—	—
GUAYAKI														
Organic Raspberry Revolution	8 oz	50	0	0	0	0	12	12	tr	—	11	—	—	—
Organic Unsweetened	8 oz	15	0	0	0	0	3	tr	tr	—	11	—	—	—
HEALTHY SHOT														
Double Protein Peach	1 bottle (2.5 oz)	100	0	0	0	24	1	0	0	60	80	—	100	15
High Protein All Flavors	1 bottle (2.5 oz)	110	0	0	0	12	17	16	0	20	40	—	100	15
HIRO														
Thermo	1 can (8.33 oz)	10	0	0	0	0	2	tr	—	206	83	101	—	5
Vitality	1 can (8.33 oz)	10	0	0	0	0	2	1	—	—	48	143	—	90
HONEYDROP														
Alive Blood Orange & Honey	8 oz	40	0	0	0	0	11	10	—	—	0	—	—	—
Strong Blueberries & Honey	8 oz	40	0	0	0	0	11	10	—	—	0	—	—	30
HOOAH!														
Soldier Fuel All Flavors	1 can (12 oz)	160	0	0	0	0	41	12	—	—	40	—	—	30
HYDRIVE														
All Flavors	1 bottle (11.2 oz)	25	0	0	0	0	5	5	—	—	135	55	—	—
ICHILL														
Relaxation Shot Blissful Berry	1 bottle (2 oz)	0	0	0	0	0	0	0	0	—	—	—	—	—

FOOD	PORTION	CALS	FAT	SAT FAT	CHOL	PROT	CARB	SUGAR	FIBER	CALCI	SOD	POTAS	FOLIC	VIT C
KIDSTRONG														
All Flavors	8 oz	30	0	0	0	0	7	3	1	50	90	225	80	24
KING 888														
Original	8 oz	110	0	0	0	0	28	28	—	—	25	—	—	—
Sugar Free	8 oz	0	0	0	0	0	0	0	0	—	25	—	—	—
LIV NATURALS														
All Flavors	8 oz	70	0	0	0	0	16	13	0	—	105	45	—	—
MAMMA CHIA														
All Flavors	8 oz	120	4	—	0	4	20	14	6	100	12	40	—	0
MARQUIS PLATINUM														
Vitality Drink	1 can	30	0	0	0	0	16	7	1	—	—	—	—	—
ME														
Curious Blueberry Lime	1 can	70	0	0	0	0	17	16	—	—	10	—	—	—
Vivacious Tangerine Pineapple	1 can	70	0	0	0	0	17	17	—	—	10	—	—	4
MIX1														
All Flavors	1 bottle (11 oz)	200	3	0	—	15	29	22	3	200	125	370	140	42
MR. RE														
Restorative	1 can (11 oz)	80	0	0	0	0	22	21	0	0	0	—	4	60
NAWGAN														
Berry Caffeine Free	1 can (11.5 oz)	40	0	0	0	0	10	10	—	—	0	—	—	—
Torocco Orange	1 can (11.5 oz)	45	0	0	0	0	15	11	—	—	80	—	—	—
NEURO														
Bliss	1 bottle (14.5 oz)	35	0	0	0	0	9	9	—	—	—	—	800	48
Gasm	1 bottle (14.5 oz)	35	0	0	0	0	9	9	—	—	—	—	800	120
Sleep	1 bottle (14.5 oz)	35	0	0	0	0	9	9	—	—	—	—	—	—
Sonic	1 bottle (14.5 oz)	35	0	0	0	0	9	9	—	—	—	—	800	120
Sport	1 bottle (14.5 oz)	35	0	0	0	0	9	9	—	30	72	70	—	—
Trim	1 bottle (14.5 oz)	35	0	0	0	0	9	9	1	—	—	—	—	—
NOS														
High Performance	1 bottle (11 oz)	150	0	0	0	2	38	37	—	—	160	—	140	84
OCEAN SPRAY														
Cranergy Cranberry	8 oz	35	0	0	0	0	8	8	—	—	50	—	—	60
Cranergy Pomegranate Cranberry Lift	8 oz	35	0	0	0	0	9	9	—	0	50	0	—	60

FOOD	PORTION	CALS	FAT	SAT FAT	CHOL	PROT	CARB	SUGAR	FIBER	CALCI	SOD	POTAS	FOLIC	VIT C
OCEAN SPRAY (CONT.)														
Cranergy Raspberry Cranberry Lift	8 oz	20	0	0	0	0	9	9	—	0	50	0	—	60
ODWALLA														
Berries GoMega	8 oz	160	2	0	0	3	34	24	5	20	15	—	—	15
Mo' Beta	8 oz	150	0	0	0	1	37	26	1	0	15	270	—	300
Super Protein Original	8 oz	190	1	0	0	10	35	29	1	350	180	420	—	90
Superfood	8 oz	130	1	0	0	1	30	25	0	20	10	370	—	36
Wellness	8 oz	150	1	0	0	2	33	24	1	20	35	350	—	150
OOBA														
All Flavors	8 oz	90	0	0	0	0	22	20	—	20	5	—	—	30
PALO														
Mamajuana	7 oz	50	0	0	0	0	15	13	—	—	10	—	—	—
PHASE III RECOVERY														
Chocolate	1 bottle (14.5 oz)	330	5	3	35	35	36	32	3	800	120	500	—	60
Vanilla	1 bottle (14.5 oz)	320	5	3	35	35	34	33	1	900	125	340	—	60
PICKLE JUICE														
Dill	8 oz	0	0	0	0	0	1	0	—	—	820	35	—	—
Sport	8 oz	7	0	0	0	0	2	0	—	—	1640	70	—	18
PIMPJUICE														
Energy Drink	1 can (8 oz)	140	0	0	0	0	35	34	—	—	5	—	—	60
PJ Tight	1 can (8 oz)	20	0	0	0	0	3	3	—	—	5	—	—	60
POMX														
Shot Antioxidant Supplement	1 bottle (3 oz)	100	0	0	0	—	25	21	—	—	—	—	—	—
POWER TRIP														
Xtreme	1 can (10.5 oz)	140	0	0	0	1	35	33	—	—	200	—	—	—
PREMIER														
Nitro Shot	1 (1.8 oz)	75	0	0	0	—	15	15	0	—	—	—	400	—
Rocket Shot Berry Blast	1 (1.8 oz)	30	0	0	0	0	7	7	—	—	—	—	—	—
PURITY ORGANIC														
Acerola Cherry	1 bottle	60	0	0	0	0	15	14	—	—	—	—	—	—
Pomegranate Blueberry	1 bottle	60	0	0	0	0	15	14	—	—	—	—	—	—
Pomegranate Raspberry	1 bottle	60	0	0	0	0	15	14	—	—	—	—	—	120
QUENCH AID														
Berry	1 pkg	10	0	0	0	0	2	2	—	—	76	105	—	12
Dragonfruit	1 pkg	10	0	0	0	0	2	2	—	—	90	—	—	150

FOOD	PORTION	CALS	FAT	SAT FAT	CHOL	PROT	CARB	SUGAR	FIBER	CALCI	SOD	POTAS	FOLIC	VIT C
RECHARGE														
Lemon as prep	8 oz	10	0	0	0	0	1	tr	—	20	30	50	—	6
Tropical as prep	8 oz	10	0	0	0	0	1	tr	—	20	30	50	—	6
RED BULL														
Original	1 can (8.3 oz)	110	0	0	0	0	28	27	—	—	200	—	—	—
Sugar Free	1 can (8.3 oz)	10	0	0	0	tr	3	0	—	—	200	—	—	—
REHAB														
Recovery Supplement	1 can (12 oz)	150	0	0	0	0	38	37	—	50	60	20	—	45
RESURRECT														
Daily Detox & Anti-Hangover Elixir	1 can (12 oz)	5	0	0	0	0	2	0	—	—	45	—	400	60
ROCKSTAR														
Energy Drink	8 oz	140	0	0	0	0	31	31	—	—	40	—	—	—
Juiced	8 oz	90	0	0	0	0	22	21	0	30	15	—	—	60
RONIN														
Diet	1 can (16 oz)	15	0	0	0	0	2	—	—	40	370	—	400	300
Original	1 can (16 oz)	180	0	0	0	0	46	43	—	40	370	—	400	300
SIMPLY NUTRILITE														
Berry Antioxidant	1 can (8.4 oz)	120	0	0	0	1	29	29	0	20	15	—	—	60
SOCAL														
Just Chill	1 can (8.4 oz)	50	0	0	0	0	12	12	—	—	—	—	—	60
SOL MATE														
All Flavors	1 bottle	90	0	0	0	0	22	21	—	—	0	—	—	—
SOLIXIR														
Blackberry	1 can	50	0	0	0	0	12	11	—	—	10	—	—	—
Orange	1 can	55	0	0	0	0	13	12	—	—	0	—	—	—
Pomegranate	1 can	60	0	0	0	0	14	13	—	—	0	—	—	—
SOURCE BURN														
2	8 oz	130	0	0	0	1	31	30	—	—	10	65	—	15
Energy Drink	8 oz	140	0	0	0	0	36	28	—	—	20	—	—	—
Sugar Free	8 oz	10	0	0	0	1	0	0	0	—	15	—	—	60
STEAZ														
Organic Fuel	8 oz	90	0	0	0	0	23	23	—	—	35	—	—	36
SUM POOSIE														
Energy Drink	1 bottle (12 oz)	170	0	0	0	0	44	43	—	—	45	—	—	—
SVELTE														
Protein Drink All Flavors	1 bottle (15.9 oz)	260	10	2	0	16	35	9	5	350	190	—	—	0
T-FUSION														
Energy Tea	8 oz	0	0	0	0	0	1	0	0	0	50	—	—	0
THERAFIZZ														
Energy	1 pkg	8	—	—	—	—	—	—	—	—	150	170	—	100
Vitamin C	1 pkg	5	0	0	0	0	tr	—	—	50	—	200	13	1000

FOOD	PORTION	CALS	FAT	SAT FAT	CHOL	PROT	CARB	SUGAR	FIBER	CALCI	SOD	POTAS	FOLIC	VIT C
UNDERWAY														
Appetite Suppressing All Flavors	8 oz	10	0	0	0	0	2	—	1	—	0	—	—	—
UNWIND														
All Flavors	1 can (12 oz)	40	0	0	0	0	10	10	—	—	25	—	—	—
VENGA														
Brainstorm	8 oz	130	0	0	0	0	31	29	—	96	50	—	—	—
Calorie Burn	8 oz	10	0	0	0	0	2	—	—	—	5	—	—	106
Energize	8 oz	100	0	0	0	0	24	24	—	—	—	—	—	72
Health&Zen	8 oz	80	0	0	0	0	20	20	—	—	50	—	80	—
VIB														
Chill-N	1 can (8 oz)	40	0	0	0	0	10	10	0	0	0	—	—	0
WHO'S YOUR DADDY														
Original	8 oz	110	0	0	0	0	29	29	—	—	50	—	—	60
Sugar Free	8 oz	0	0	0	0	0	0	0	0	—	50	—	—	60
XCYTO														
Sugar Free	1 can (12.5 oz)	10	0	0	0	tr	2	0	0	—	35	—	—	60
XOOD														
Endurance Drink All Flavors as prep	1 serv	135	0	0	0	3	30	10	—	60	105	95	12	50
YOUTH JUICE														
Drink	2 oz	10	0	0	0	tr	3	2	1	—	5	—	400	60
ZENERGIZE														
Chill	1 tablet	2	0	0	0	0	1	0	0	100	300	—	800	—
Energy+	1 tablet	2	0	0	0	0	1	0	0	50	220	—	400	1000
Hydrate	1 tablet	2	0	0	0	0	1	0	0	—	390	50	400	600
ENGLISH MUFFIN														
READY-TO-EAT														
crumpets	1 (1.5 oz)	80	0	0	0	3	16	1	tr	20	270	—	—	0
plain	1 (2 oz)	129	1	tr	0	5	25	2	2	93	206	62	54	1
whole wheat	1 (2.3 oz)	134	1	tr	0	6	27	5	4	175	240	139	32	0
AUNT GUSSIE'S														
Gluten Free Cinnamon Raisin	1 (3 oz)	200	3	0	0	3	41	8	4	20	400	—	—	0
Gluten Free Original	1 (3 oz)	200	3	0	0	3	41	6	4	0	440	—	—	0
FIBER ONE														
100% Whole Wheat	1 (2 oz)	100	0	0	0	5	22	3	6	60	230	—	0	0
FOODS BY GEORGE														
Gluten Free Multigrain	1 (3.6 oz)	220	5	0	0	5	39	4	2	150	280	—	80	0

FOOD	PORTION	CALS	FAT	SAT FAT	CHOL	PROT	CARB	SUGAR	FIBER	CALCI	SOD	POTAS	FOLIC	VIT C
FOODS BY GEORGE (CONT.)														
Gluten Free No-Rye Rye	1 (3.6 oz)	210	4	0	0	4	40	4	2	20	270	—	—	0
MATTHEW'S														
Golden White	1 (2.1 oz)	140	2	0	0	5	28	2	0	80	240	—	8	0
MILTON'S														
Healthy Multi-Grain	1 (2 oz)	150	1	0	0	4	33	7	3	20	180	—	—	4
PEPPERIDGE FARM														
100% Whole Wheat	1	140	2	1	0	6	26	4	3	20	190	—	24	0
Original	1	130	2	1	0	5	25	1	1	0	170	—	40	0
ROMAN MEAL														
English Muffin	1 (2.3 oz)	140	1	0	0	6	29	4	3	100	320	—	60	0
RUDI'S ORGANIC BAKERY														
MultiGrain w/ Flax	1 (2 oz)	130	1	0	0	5	25	2	2	0	220	—	8	0
Whole Grain Wheat	1 (2 oz)	120	1	0	0	5	23	2	3	0	220	—	8	0
SUN-MAID														
Raisin	1 (2.5 oz)	170	1	0	0	5	36	13	2	20	180	—	60	0
THOMAS'														
10 Grain	1 (2.1 oz)	130	1	0	0	6	29	2	6	80	200	—	32	0
100 Calories	1	100	1	0	0	4	24	tr	5	80	220	—	—	0
100% Whole Wheat	1 (2 oz)	120	1	0	0	6	23	2	3	60	220	—	—	0
Griller Multi-Grain	1 (3.2 oz)	210	2	0	0	7	41	5	3	150	250	—	—	0
Griller Onion	1 (3.2 oz)	200	1	0	0	7	40	2	2	150	320	—	—	0
Hearty Grains Honey Wheat	1	130	1	0	0	5	27	3	2	60	190	—	—	0
Light Multi-Grain	1 (2 oz)	100	1	0	0	5	25	tr	8	150	170	—	40	0
Multi-Grain	1 (2 oz)	150	3	0	0	5	27	3	2	80	160	—	—	0
Oatmeal & Honey	1	130	1	0	0	5	25	3	2	60	180	—	—	0
Original	1 (2 oz)	120	1	0	0	4	25	1	1	80	200	—	—	0
Raisin Cinnamon	1 (2.1 oz)	140	1	0	0	4	29	8	1	40	170	—	—	0
TAKE-OUT														
w/ butter	1 (2.2 oz)	189	6	2	13	5	30	—	—	103	386	69	57	1
w/ cheese & sausage	1 (4 oz)	365	22	9	46	14	27	2	1	227	721	193	55	0
w/ egg cheese & canadian bacon	1 (4.9 oz)	307	13	5	234	19	30	3	1	268	773	211	99	2
w/ egg cheese & sausage	1 (5.8 oz)	472	30	11	269	22	29	2	tr	277	776	243	94	0

FOOD	PORTION	CALS	FAT	SAT FAT	CHOL	PROT	CARB	SUGAR	FIBER	CALCI	SOD	POTAS	FOLIC	VIT C
EPAZOTE														
fresh	1 tbsp (1 g)	<1	0	—	0	0	tr	—	tr	2	tr	5	2	0
fresh sprig	1 (2 g)	1	tr	—	0	tr	tr	—	tr	6	1	13	4	tr
EPPAW														
raw	½ cup	75	1	—	0	2	16	—	—	55	6	170	—	7
FALAFEL														
FALAFEL REPUBLIC														
Traditional	3 (3 oz)	210	7	0	0	11	26	1	6	80	630	—	—	1
NEAR EAST														
Falafel Patties Vegetarian as prep	2.5	220	13	2	0	10	18	3	5	40	552	—	—	0
VEGGIE PATCH														
Falafel	4 (3 oz)	180	9	1	0	5	21	3	6	60	380	—	—	6
TAKE-OUT														
falafel	1 (1.2 oz)	57	3	tr	0	2	5	—	—	9	50	99	13	tr
FAT														
(*see also* BUTTER, BUTTER SUBSTITUTES, MARGARINE, OIL)														
bacon grease	1 tbsp	116	13	5	12	0	0	0	0	0	19	0	0	0
beef shortening	1 tbsp	115	13	6	13	0	0	0	0	0	0	0	0	0
beef suet	1 oz	242	27	15	19	tr	0	0	0	1	2	5	0	0
chicken	1 tbsp (0.4 oz)	115	13	4	11	0	0	0	0	0	0	0	0	0
duck	1 tbsp (0.4 oz)	113	13	4	13	0	0	0	0	0	0	0	0	0
goose	1 tbsp	115	13	4	13	0	0	0	0	0	0	0	0	0
goose	1 oz	257	29	2	—	0	0	0	0	—	—	—	—	—
lamb new zealand	1 oz	182	19	10	25	2	0	0	0	6	6	15	—	—
lard	1 tbsp (0.5 oz)	115	13	5	12	0	0	0	0	tr	0	0	—	—
lard	1 cup (7.2 oz)	1849	205	80	195	0	0	0	0	tr	tr	tr	—	—
meat pan drippings	½ tbsp	124	14	6	14	0	0	0	0	0	76	0	0	0
pork raw	1 oz	230	25	9	16	1	0	0	0	1	3	18	0	0
salt pork	1 cube (1 oz)	215	23	8	26	2	0	0	0	2	383	19	0	0
shortening	1 cup	1812	205	41	0	0	0	0	0	—	—	—	—	—
shortening	1 tbsp	113	13	3	0	0	0	0	0	—	—	—	—	—
turkey	1 tbsp	116	13	4	13	0	0	0	0	0	0	0	0	0
ucuhuba butter	1 tbsp	120	14	12	—	0	0	0	0	—	—	—	—	—
whale blubber	1 oz	248	28	—	0	tr	0	0	0	—	—	—	—	—
CRISCO														
Butter Flavor	1 tbsp	110	12	3	0	0	0	0	0	—	0	—	—	—
Shortening	1 tbsp	110	12	3	0	0	0	0	0	—	0	—	—	—
EARTH BALANCE														
Natural Shortening	1 tbsp	130	14	5	0	0	0	0	0	—	0	—	—	—

FOOD	PORTION	CALS	FAT	SAT FAT	CHOL	PROT	CARB	SUGAR	FIBER	CALCI	SOD	POTAS	FOLIC	VIT C
NEBRASKA LAND														
Pork Fatback	½ oz	110	11	4	5	1	0	0	0	0	280	—	—	0
FAVA BEANS														
canned	½ cup	91	tr	tr	0	7	16	—	—	33	580	310	42	2
fava fresh cooked	½ cup	94	tr	tr	0	6	17	2	5	31	4	228	88	tr
PROGRESSO														
Fava Beans	½ cup (4.6 oz)	110	1	0	0	6	20	—	5	20	250	—	—	—
FEIJOA														
fresh	1 (1.75 oz)	25	tr	—	0	1	5	—	—	8	2	78	19	7
puree	1 cup	119	2	—	0	3	26	—	—	41	7	378	93	32
FENNEL														
fresh bulb	1 (8.2 oz)	73	tr	—	0	3	17	—	7	115	122	969	63	28
fresh sliced	1 cup	27	tr	—	0	1	6	—	3	43	45	360	23	10
leaves	1 oz	7	tr	—	—	tr	1	—	1	31	25	—	29	27
seed	1 tsp	7	tr	tr	0	tr	1	—	1	24	2	34	—	tr
stir fried	1 cup	85	6	1	0	2	9	5	3	89	669	600	46	13
OCEAN MIST														
Fennel Sweet Anise Sliced Fresh	1 cup	27	1	0	0	1	6	0	3	40	45	—	—	10
FENUGREEK														
seed	1 tsp	12	tr	tr	0	1	2	—	1	6	2	28	2	tr
FIBER														
BENEFIBER														
Supplement	1 pkg (4 g)	20	0	0	0	0	4	—	3	—	20	—	—	—
FIBER SUPREME														
Fiber	1 round tbsp (0.5 oz)	36	tr	0	0	1	12	0	7	—	tr	—	—	0
ND LABS														
Apple Fiber	1 round tbsp (7 g)	15	tr	0	0	0	7	0	4	—	tr	—	—	0
Liquid Fiber Flow	1 tbsp (0.5 oz)	42	0	0	0	0	11	0	7	—	3	0	—	—
UNIFIBER														
Natural Fiber	1 pkg (4 g)	4	0	0	0	0	tr	—	3	—	—	—	—	—
WELLEMENTS														
Fiber-Psyll	1 scoop (0.5 oz)	55	0	0	0	0	14	0	12	—	0	—	—	—
FIDDLEHEAD FERNS														
fresh	3.5 oz	34	tr	—	0	5	6	—	—	32	1	370	—	27
FIG JUICE														
SMART JUICE														
Organic 100% Juice	8 oz	131	0	0	0	1	35	29	1	70	2	—	—	2
FIGS														
calimyrna	3 (5.4 oz)	120	0	0	0	1	28	11	4	60	0	—	—	4

FOOD	PORTION	CALS	FAT	SAT FAT	CHOL	PROT	CARB	SUGAR	FIBER	CALCI	SOD	POTAS	FOLIC	VIT C
canned in heavy syrup	½ cup	114	tr	tr	0	tr	30	27	3	35	1	128	3	1
canned in light syrup	½ cup	87	tr	tr	0	tr	23	20	2	34	1	129	3	1
canned water pack	½ cup	66	tr	tr	0	1	17	15	3	35	1	128	2	1
dried california	½ cup (3.5 oz)	200	1	—	0	4	58	—	17	150	11	710	24	2
dried cooked	½ cup	139	1	tr	0	2	36	30	5	91	5	381	1	6
dried small	1 (1.4 oz)	30	tr	tr	0	tr	8	7	1	14	0	93	2	1
dried whole	1 (8 g)	21	tr	tr	0	tr	5	4	1	14	1	57	1	tr
fresh large	1 (2.2 oz)	47	tr	tr	0	tr	12	10	2	22	1	148	4	1
BLUE RIBBON														
California Figs	1 pkg (1.5 oz)	120	0	0	0	1	28	21	5	60	0	—	—	0
CALIFORNIA FRESH														
Fresh	3 (5.4 oz)	120	0	0	0	1	31	25	4	80	0	—	—	1
HERMES														
Organic Adriatic Fig Spread	1 tbsp	60	0	0	0	0	15	14	0	10	0	—	—	0
JENNY														
Kalamata Crown Natural Sundried	4 (1.5 oz)	120	0	0	0	1	28	21	5	60	5	260	—	—
NUTA FIGS														
Mission	¼ cup (1.4 oz)	110	0	0	0	1	26	20	5	60	0	240	—	0
ORCHARD CHOICE														
Mission	4 5 (1.4 oz)	110	0	0	0	1	26	20	5	60	0	240	8	0
SUN-MAID														
California Mission	4 (1.5 oz)	110	0	0	0	1	26	20	5	60	0	240	—	0
Calimyrna	3 (1.5 oz)	120	0	0	0	1	28	21	5	60	0	260	—	0
FIREWEED														
leaves chopped	¼ cup (0.2 oz)	6	tr	—	0	tr	1	—	1	25	2	28	6	tr
plant	1 (0.8 oz)	23	1	—	0	1	4	—	2	94	7	109	25	1
FISH														

(*see also individual names,* FISH SUBSTITUTES, SUSHI)

FOOD	PORTION	CALS	FAT	SAT FAT	CHOL	PROT	CARB	SUGAR	FIBER	CALCI	SOD	POTAS	FOLIC	VIT C
FROZEN														
breaded fillet	1 (2 oz)	155	7	2	64	9	14	—	—	11	332	149	10	—
sticks	1 stick (1 oz)	76	3	1	31	4	7	—	—	6	163	73	5	—
DR. PRAEGER'S														
Fillets Lightly Breaded	1 (2.1 oz)	100	4	1	15	5	12	1	0	0	250	—	—	1
Fish Sticks Potato Crusted	3 (2.3 oz)	120	6	1	25	6	7	0	tr	20	220	—	—	0
Fishies Lightly Breaded	3 (1.5 oz)	90	4	1	10	4	9	1	0	0	210	—	—	0

FOOD	PORTION	CALS	FAT	SAT FAT	CHOL	PROT	CARB	SUGAR	FIBER	CALCI	SOD	POTAS	FOLIC	VIT C
GORTON'S														
Classic Crispy Battered Fillets	2	230	10	3	25	6	22	3	5	20	650	—	—	—
Classic Crunchy Golden Fillets	2	140	12	3	36	9	23	5	—	20	500	160	—	—
Fillets Beer Battered	2 (3.6 oz)	250	17	4	20	8	17	4	1	20	600	120	—	—
Fillets Breaded Lemon Herb	2 (3.6 oz)	240	13	3	25	9	21	4	—	20	720	130	—	—
Fillets Potato Crunch	2 (3.6 oz)	240	14	4	25	9	20	3	2	20	790	150	—	—
Fish Sticks Classic Breaded	6	290	18	4	25	10	19	2	1	20	340	—	—	—
Grilled Fillets Cajun Blackened	1 (3.8 oz)	100	3	1	60	17	1	0	0	20	330	360	—	—
Grilled Fillets Lemon Pepper	1 (3.8 oz)	90	3	1	60	16	0	0	0	20	310	360	—	—
Tenders Original Batter	3 pieces (3.6 oz)	230	12	3	20	8	23	3	2	20	660	130	—	—
IAN'S														
Fillets	1 (3.4 oz)	260	8	1	20	14	32	4	2	100	410	—	—	1
Fish Sticks	5 pieces	190	6	1	15	11	24	3	1	80	310	—	—	1
Fish Sticks Allergy Free	5 pieces	190	6	1	15	11	24	3	1	80	310	—	—	1
SEAPAK														
Popcorn	8 (3 oz)	190	9	2	30	9	18	1	1	0	370	—	—	0
VAN DE KAMP'S														
Battered Tenders	4 (4 oz)	210	10	4	20	9	22	5	1	20	700	—	—	0
Crisp & Healthy Breaded Fish Sticks	6 (3.6 oz)	140	1	1	25	9	24	3	1	20	380	—	—	0
Crunchy Fillets	2 (3.5 oz)	230	13	5	20	8	21	2	tr	0	440	—	—	0
Sticks	6 (4 oz)	260	13	5	30	11	26	3	1	20	410	—	—	0
TAKE-OUT														
amuk bok kum korean stir fried fish cake	1 cup (7.6 oz)	267	7	1	65	18	31	—	3	37	1959	569	22	8
fish cake	1 (4.7 oz)	166	7	2	—	18	6	—	—	179	—	—	—	5
jamaican brown fish stew	1 serv	426	22	5	84	48	9	—	2	—	419	—	—	—
kedgeree	5.6 oz	242	11	—	—	21	15	—	1	58	—	—	—	0
mousse	1 serv (3.5 oz)	185	14	—	—	13	3	tr	tr	40	540	250	—	tr
stew	1 cup (7.9 oz)	157	4	2	—	19	10	—	—	32	—	—	—	11
taramasalata	2 tbsp	124	14	—	10	1	1	—	—	6	182	16	2	0
FISH OIL														
cod liver	1 tbsp	123	14	3	78	0	0	0	0	0	0	0	0	0
herring	1 tbsp	123	14	3	104	0	0	0	0	0	0	0	0	0

FOOD	PORTION	CALS	FAT	SAT FAT	CHOL	PROT	CARB	SUGAR	FIBER	CALCI	SOD	POTAS	FOLIC	VIT C
menhaden	1 tbsp	123	14	4	71	0	0	0	0	0	0	0	0	0
salmon	1 tbsp	123	14	3	66	0	0	0	0	0	0	0	0	0
sardine	1 tbsp	123	14	4	97	0	0	0	0	0	0	0	0	0
shark	1 oz	270	29	—	—	0	0	0	0	—	—	—	—	—
whale beluga	1 oz	256	29	4	—	0	0	0	0	0	0	0	0	0
whale bowhead	1 oz	252	28	—	—	0	0	0	0	0	—	—	—	—
GENESIS TODAY														
Omega-3 Vitamin Super Chews	1	20	0	0	—	—	4	3	—	—	—	—	—	30
NORDIC NATURALS														
Nordic Omega-3 Gummies Tangerine Treats	2 pieces	20	0	0	0	0	4	3	—	—	10	—	—	—
Omega 3-6-9 Junior	2 pieces	9	1	tr	—	0	0	0	0	—	—	—	—	—
Omega-3 Effervescent as prep	1 pkg (9.7 g)	39	2	0	—	0	3	—	—	—	209	—	—	—

FISH PASTE
FOOD	PORTION	CALS	FAT	SAT FAT	CHOL	PROT	CARB	SUGAR	FIBER	CALCI	SOD	POTAS	FOLIC	VIT C
fish paste	2 tsp	15	1	—	—	1	tr	—	0	25	—	—	—	0

FLAXSEED
FOOD	PORTION	CALS	FAT	SAT FAT	CHOL	PROT	CARB	SUGAR	FIBER	CALCI	SOD	POTAS	FOLIC	VIT C
ARROWHEAD MILLS														
Organic	3 tbsp (1 oz)	140	9	1	0	6	9	0	7	—	0	150	—	—
BOB'S RED MILL														
Flaxseed Meal	2 tbsp	60	5	0	0	3	4	0	4	—	0	—	—	—
CARRINGTON FARMS														
Organic Flax Paks	1 pkg (0.4 oz)	50	5	tr	0	2	3	0	3	16	5	90	—	0
FLAX USA														
Flax Sprinkles	2 tbsp (0.5 oz)	70	5	1	0	2	4	0	3	20	0	—	—	0
NATURAL OVENS														
Flax Complete Supplement	1 tbsp (0.4 oz)	60	4	—	4	2	4	1	2	20	—	—	400	90
TREE OF LIFE														
Flax Seed	3 tbsp (1 oz)	140	10	1	0	5	11	0	6	80	0	—	—	0

FLOUNDER
FOOD	PORTION	CALS	FAT	SAT FAT	CHOL	PROT	CARB	SUGAR	FIBER	CALCI	SOD	POTAS	FOLIC	VIT C
FRESH														
cooked	1 fillet (4.5 oz)	148	2	tr	86	31	0	0	0	23	133	436	—	—
cooked	3 oz	99	1	tr	58	21	0	0	0	16	89	292	—	—
FROZEN														
MRS. PAUL'S														
Filets Lightly Breaded	1 (2.7 oz)	150	7	4	25	8	12	3	1	0	290	—	—	0
TAKE-OUT														
breaded & fried	3.2 oz	211	11	3	31	13	15	—	—	17	484	292	51	0
stuffed w/ crab	1 piece (7.6 oz)	332	11	2	160	43	14	2	1	124	903	792	59	6

FOOD	PORTION	CALS	FAT	SAT FAT	CHOL	PROT	CARB	SUGAR	FIBER	CALCI	SOD	POTAS	FOLIC	VIT C
FLOUR														
all-purpose enriched bleached	½ cup (2.2 oz)	228	1	tr	0	6	48	tr	2	9	1	97	114	0
all-purpose self-rising	½ cup (2.2 oz)	221	1	tr	0	6	46	tr	2	211	794	78	122	0
all-purpose unbleached	½ cup (2.2 oz)	228	1	tr	0	6	48	tr	2	9	1	67	114	0
arrowroot	½ cup (2.2 oz)	228	tr	tr	0	tr	56	—	2	26	1	7	4	0
bread flour	½ cup (2.4 oz)	247	1	tr	0	8	50	tr	2	10	1	68	23	0
buckwheat whole groat	½ cup (2.1 oz)	201	2	tr	0	8	42	2	6	25	7	346	32	0
cake	½ cup (2.4 oz)	248	1	tr	0	6	53	tr	1	10	1	72	127	0
carob	½ cup (1.8 oz)	114	tr	tr	0	2	46	25	21	179	18	426	15	tr
carob	1 tbsp (0.2 oz)	13	tr	tr	0	tr	5	3	2	21	2	50	2	0
chickpea besan	½ cup (1.6 oz)	178	3	tr	0	10	27	5	5	21	29	389	201	0
peanut lowfat	½ cup (1.1 oz)	128	7	1	0	10	9	—	5	39	0	407	40	0
potato	½ cup (2.8 oz)	286	tr	tr	0	6	66	3	5	52	44	801	20	3
rice brown	½ cup (2.8 oz)	287	2	tr	0	6	60	1	4	9	6	228	13	0
rice white	½ cup (2.8 oz)	289	1	tr	0	5	63	tr	2	8	0	60	3	0
rye dark	½ cup (2.2 oz)	207	2	tr	0	9	44	1	15	36	1	467	38	0
rye light	½ cup (1.8 oz)	187	1	tr	0	4	41	1	7	11	1	119	11	0
soy lowfat	½ cup (1.5 oz)	165	4	1	0	20	15	5	7	125	4	920	127	0
triticale whole grain	½ cup (2.3 oz)	220	1	tr	0	9	48	—	10	23	1	303	48	0
whole wheat	½ cup (2.1 oz)	203	1	tr	0	8	44	tr	7	20	3	243	26	0
ARROWHEAD MILLS														
Organic Barley	⅓ cup	95	1	0	0	3	19	0	4	0	0	125	—	—
Organic Brown Rice	⅓ cup	130	1	0	0	3	27	0	2	—	0	75	—	—
Organic Kamut	⅓ cup	130	1	0	0	5	25	0	4	0	0	150	—	0
Organic Oat	⅓ cup	120	3	1	0	4	21	0	3	20	0	105	—	0
Organic Rye	¼ cup	110	1	0	0	3	24	0	4	20	0	—	—	0
Organic Spelt	⅓ cup	130	1	0	0	4	25	0	4	0	0	150	—	—
Organic Unbleached White	¼ cup	120	1	0	0	3	26	0	tr	—	0	35	—	0
Organic White Rice	⅓ cup	120	0	0	0	2	28	0	tr	0	0	25	—	0
AZUKAR ORGANICS														
Coconut	3.5 oz	413	9	8	0	19	65	9	39	—	80	—	—	—
BOB'S RED MILL														
Brown Rice	¼ cup	140	1	0	0	3	31	0	1	—	5	—	—	—
Corn	¼ cup	160	1	0	0	2	22	0	4	—	2	—	—	—
Graham	¼ cup	120	1	0	0	5	21	0	3	—	1	—	—	—
Kamut Organic	¼ cup	94	1	0	0	3	21	0	3	—	0	—	—	—

FOOD	PORTION	CALS	FAT	SAT FAT	CHOL	PROT	CARB	SUGAR	FIBER	CALCI	SOD	POTAS	FOLIC	VIT C
BOB'S RED MILL (CONT.)														
Sorghum Sweet White Gluten Free	¼ cup	120	1	0	0	4	25	0	3	—	0	—	—	—
Spelt	¼ cup	120	1	0	0	4	22	0	4	—	1	—	—	—
Whole Wheat	¼ cup	110	1	0	0	4	23	1	4	—	0	—	—	—
Whole Wheat Hard White Organic	¼ cup	120	1	0	0	4	24	0	4	—	0	—	—	—
CERESOTA														
100% Whole Wheat	¼ cup (1 oz)	100	1	0	0	4	21	0	3	—	0	—	—	—
All Purpose Unbleached	¼ cup (1 oz)	100	0	0	0	3	22	tr	tr	—	0	35	40	—
DOMATA LIVING FLOUR														
Gluten Free Casein Free	¼ cup	110	0	0	0	tr	26	0	tr	0	20	—	—	0
GOLD MEDAL														
All Purpose	¼ cup (1 oz)	100	0	0	0	3	22	tr	tr	—	0	40	40	—
Self Rising	¼ cup (1 oz)	100	0	0	0	3	23	—	tr	60	400	35	40	—
Wondra	¼ cup (1 oz)	100	0	0	0	3	23	—	tr	—	0	—	40	—
HECKERS														
100% Whole Wheat	¼ cup (1 oz)	100	1	0	0	4	21	0	3	—	0	—	—	—
All Purpose Unbleached	¼ cup (1 oz)	100	0	0	0	3	22	tr	tr		0	35	40	—
KING ARTHUR														
All Purpose	¼ cup	110	0	0	0	4	22	tr	tr	0	0	—	40	0
Organic Artisan	¼ cup	110	0	0	0	3	23	tr	tr	0	0	—	—	0
Organic White Whole Wheat	¼ cup	100	1	0	0	4	18	tr	3	20	0	—	—	0
Organic Whole Wheat	½ cup	110	1	0	0	4	23	0	4	20	0	—	—	0
Self-Rising	¼ cup	120	0	0	0	2	27	0	1	80	440	—	40	0
White Whole Wheat	¼ cup	100	1	0	0	4	18	tr	3	20	0	—	—	0
Whole Wheat	¼ cup	110	1	0	0	4	21	1	4	0	0	—	—	0
LUNDBERG														
Brown Rice	¼ cup	110	2	0	0	2	26	tr	1	0	0	150	—	0
MANITOBA HARVEST														
Hemp Seed Flour	¼ cup	120	4	0	0	10	14	tr	12	40	0	—	—	0
PILLSBURY														
All Purpose	¼ cup (1.1 oz)	110	0	0	0	3	23	tr	tr	0	0	—	40	0
Bread Flour	¼ cup (1.1 oz)	110	0	0	0	4	22	0	tr	0	0	—	40	0
Self Rising	¼ cup (1.1. oz)	100	0	0	0	3	22	0	tr	100	370	—	40	0
Whole Wheat	¼ cup (1.1 oz)	110	1	0	0	4	22	tr	3	0	0	—	8	0

FOOD	PORTION	CALS	FAT	SAT FAT	CHOL	PROT	CARB	SUGAR	FIBER	CALCI	SOD	POTAS	FOLIC	VIT C
SIMPLI														
Whole Oat Gluten Free	¼ cup (1.1 oz)	110	3	0	0	4	17	0	3	20	0	—	—	0
FOOD COLORS														
blue	1 tsp	0	0	0	0	0	0	0	0	—	86	—	—	—
orange	1 tsp	0	0	0	0	0	0	0	0	—	91	—	—	—
red	1 tsp	<1	0	0	0	0	tr	0	0	—	38	tr	—	tr
yellow	1 tsp	tr	0	0	0	tr	0	0	0	—	28	tr	—	—
FRENCH BEANS														
dried cooked	1 cup	228	1	tr	0	12	43	—	17	111	11	655	132	2
FRENCH FRIES														
(see POTATO)														
FRENCH TOAST														
french toast frzn	1 slice (2 oz)	126	4	1	48	4	19	—	2	63	292	79	14	—
AUNT JEMIMA														
Cinnamon Sticks	4 (3.1 oz)	270	10	3	0	5	41	11	1	60	280	—	—	0
Homestyle	2 slices (4.1 oz)	220	5	1	75	8	37	7	1	100	350	—	60	0
Whole Grain	2 slices (4 oz)	210	5	2	75	9	34	8	3	100	330	—	8	0
FARM RICH														
Original Sticks	5 (4.2 oz)	330	15	2	0	6	42	10	2	200	490	—	32	0
IAN'S														
Sticks	5 (3.2 oz)	250	9	2	5	6	38	5	6	60	330	—	—	0
JIMMY DEAN														
French Toast Duos	1 serv (3.2 oz)	210	10	3	105	12	19	8	1	40	440	—	—	0
French Toast Griddlers Sandwich	1 (3.6 oz)	210	8	2	60	8	27	6	0	20	390	—	—	0
WEIGHT WATCHERS														
Smart Ones French Toast w/ Turkey Sausage	1 pkg (4.4 oz)	280	8	3	120	14	38	18	2	60	570	—	—	0
TAKE-OUT														
plain	1 slice	151	7	2	75	7	16	—	—	64	311	86	15	tr
sticks	5 (4.9 oz)	513	29	5	75	8	58	—	3	78	499	127	82	0
w/ butter	2 slices	356	19	8	116	10	36	—	—	73	513	177	73	tr
FROG LEGS														
frog legs	3 oz	175	—	—	1	15	—	—	—	—	—	—	—	—
TAKE-OUT														
as prep w/ seasoned flour & fried	1 (0.8)	70	5	—	12	4	15	—	—	5	—	—	tr	0
FRUCTOSE														
liquid	1 oz	84	0	0	0	0	23	23	0	0	1	0	0	0
powder	¼ cup (1.7 oz)	180	0	0	0	0	49	45	0	0	6	0	0	0
powder	1 tsp (4.2 g)	15	0	0	0	0	4	4	0	0	1	0	0	0

FOOD	PORTION	CALS	FAT	SAT FAT	CHOL	PROT	CARB	SUGAR	FIBER	CALCI	SOD	POTAS	FOLIC	VIT C
BOB'S RED MILL														
Fructose	1 tsp	15	0	0	0	0	4	4	0	—	0	—	—	—
TREE OF LIFE														
Fructose	1 tsp (4 g)	15	0	0	0	0	4	4	0	0	0	—	—	0

FRUIT AND NUT BARS

(*see also* CEREAL BARS, ENERGY BARS)

FOOD	PORTION	CALS	FAT	SAT FAT	CHOL	PROT	CARB	SUGAR	FIBER	CALCI	SOD	POTAS	FOLIC	VIT C
CAVEWOMAN BARS														
Baklava	1 (2 oz)	190	9	1	0	4	33	26	5	40	0	—	—	1
PB&J	1 (2 oz)	210	7	1	0	4	36	27	4	20	45	—	—	4
Pineapple Upside Down Cake Raw	1 (2 oz)	190	6	0	0	2	39	31	4	40	0	—	—	1
KIND														
Apple Cinnamon Nut	1 (1.4 oz)	180	10	1	0	3	22	12	5	40	20	140	—	9
Blueberry Vanilla & Cashew	1 (1.4 oz)	180	9	2	0	3	24	11	2	20	25	—	—	1
Blueberry Pecan + Fiber	1 (1.4 oz)	180	10	1	0	3	23	12	5	40	25	—	—	1
Mango Macadamia	1 (1.4 oz)	190	12	5	0	2	20	15	3	200	20	180	200	0
Mini Bar Almond & Apricot	1 (0.8 oz)	110	7	3	0	2	13	7	3	20	10	—	—	1
Mini Bar Almond & Coconut + Omega-3	1 (0.8 oz)	107	6	1	0	2	12	8	2	20	0	75	—	0
Mini Bar Cranberry Almond + Antioxidants	1 (0.8 oz)	115	8	1	0	2	12	7	2	20	10	70	—	18
Mini Bar Fruit & Nut Delight	1 (0.8 oz)	108	6	1	0	3	12	7	2	20	10	—	—	1
Pomegranate Blueberry Pistachio + Antioxidants	1 (1.4 oz)	170	8	1	0	3	24	13	4	40	25	—	8	30
ORCHARD BAR														
Blueberry Pomegranate & Almond	1 (1.6 oz)	180	6	0	0	6	26	19	2	40	70	—	—	12
Pineapple Coconut & Macadamia	1 (1.6 oz)	190	7	2	0	5	25	18	2	40	65	—	—	12
Strawberry Raspberry & Walnut	1 (1.6 oz)	190	7	1	0	5	26	18	2	40	80	—	—	12
PURE														
Organic Apple Cinnamon	1 (1.7 oz)	190	8	1	0	5	28	20	3	40	40	210	8	1

FOOD	PORTION	CALS	FAT	SAT FAT	CHOL	PROT	CARB	SUGAR	FIBER	CALCI	SOD	POTAS	FOLIC	VIT C
PURE (CONT.)														
Organic Chocolate Almond	1 (1.7 oz)	190	8	1	0	7	25	17	5	40	5	320	—	0
Organic Cranberry Orange	1 (1.7 oz)	190	8	1	0	6	27	19	3	40	5	160	8	4
Organic Peanut Raisin Crunch	1 (1.5 oz)	200	12	2	0	7	18	9	5	20	230	260	—	0
Organic Superfruit Nutty Crunch	1 (1.5 oz)	190	11	2	0	5	22	12	5	20	95	95	—	1
Organic Wild Blueberry	1 (1.7 oz)	190	8	1	0	6	26	19	3	40	5	180	8	1

FRUIT DRINKS

(see also individual names, SMOOTHIES, YOGURT DRINKS)

FROZEN
CHIQUITA

FOOD	PORTION	CALS	FAT	SAT FAT	CHOL	PROT	CARB	SUGAR	FIBER	CALCI	SOD	POTAS	FOLIC	VIT C
Banana Colada as prep	8 oz	125	2	2	0	0	25	24	1	0	35	230	—	60
Mixed Berry as prep	8 oz	120	0	0	0	0	28	27	—	20	40	—	—	60
Peach Mango as prep	8 oz	120	0	0	0	1	28	27	—	20	40	210	—	60
DOLE														
Orange Peach Mango not prep	¼ cup	120	0	0	0	tr	29	23	0	0	25	190	—	120
MIX														
AQUAFULL														
Pomegranate Orange Dietary Supplement	1 pkg (9 g)	30	0	0	0	—	8	—	4	—	—	—	—	—
BIO FRUIT														
Mix	1 scoop (8 g)	42	1	—	0	—	5	2	1	20	—	—	—	106
CRYSTAL LIGHT														
Fusion Fruit Punch as prep	8 oz	5	0	0	0	0	0	0	0	—	10	—	—	—
Immunity Cherry Pomegranate as prep	8 oz	5	0	0	0	0	1	0	—	—	10	—	—	—
SOUTH BEACH														
Tide Me Over Strawberry Banana	1 pkg	30	0	0	0	3	6	0	5	—	20	—	—	—
Tide Me Over Tropical Breeze	1 pkg	30	0	0	0	3	6	0	5	—	25	—	—	—

FOOD	PORTION	CALS	FAT	SAT FAT	CHOL	PROT	CARB	SUGAR	FIBER	CALCI	SOD	POTAS	FOLIC	VIT C
TANG														
Orange Pineapple as prep	1 serv (8 oz)	100	0	0	0	0	24	24	0	60	45	—	—	60
READY-TO-DRINK														
fruit punch	6 oz	87	tr	0	0	tr	22	—	—	14	41	47	2	55
AFTER THE FALL														
Banana Casablanca	8 oz	150	0	0	0	1	37	30	—	150	20	300	—	60
Mango Montage	8 oz	150	0	0	0	1	37	33	—	150	15	190	—	60
APPLE & EVE														
100% Cranberry Apple Juice	8 oz	100	0	0	0	1	24	20	—	100	15	—	—	60
Mango Passion 100% Juice	8 oz	120	0	0	0	0	30	26	—	—	25	—	—	60
BACK TO NATURE														
100% Juice Berry	1 pkg (6 oz)	90	0	0	0	0	21	17	—	—	20	—	—	—
BOLTHOUSE														
Bom Dia Acai Berry 100% Juice	8 oz	140	0	0	0	0	33	30	1	40	15	170	—	12
BRAZSOY														
Fruit Juice w/ Soy	8 oz	94	1	0	0	1	21	19	—	—	13	—	—	32
CAPRI SUN														
Fruit Punch	1 pkg (7 oz)	90	0	0	0	0	25	25	—	—	15	—	—	—
CERES														
100% Juice Apple Berry Cherry	8 oz	130	0	0	0	0	32	29	0	0	10	210	—	36
100% Juice Medley Of Fruits	8 oz	130	0	0	0	0	31	29	2	0	10	270	—	60
CRAYONS														
Kiwi Strawberry	1 bottle (12 oz)	130	0	0	0	0	45	28	4	150	15	—	—	90
Outrageous Orange Mango	1 bottle (12 oz)	140	0	0	0	0	45	28	4	150	15	—	—	102
Redder Than Ever Fruitpunch	1 bottle (12 oz)	130	0	0	0	0	45	28	4	150	15	—	—	90
DOLE														
Orange Peach Mango	8 oz	120	0	0	0	tr	29	23	0	0	25	290	—	60
Paradise Blend	8 oz	120	0	0	0	tr	29	24	0	20	40	300	—	60
Pina Colada	8 oz	120	0	0	0	1	29	24	0	20	10	320	—	60
Strawberry Kiwi	8 oz	120	0	0	0	0	31	26	0	0	25	250	—	60
DRENCHERS														
Super Fruit Endurance Grape Apple	8 oz	120	0	0	0	1	29	27	1	150	25	320	60	102

FOOD	PORTION	CALS	FAT	SAT FAT	CHOL	PROT	CARB	SUGAR	FIBER	CALCI	SOD	POTAS	FOLIC	VIT C
DRENCHERS (CONT.)														
Super Juice Fit 'N Lean Heart Healthy Tropical Passion	8 oz	10	0	0	0	0	2	1	0	100	5	35	40	96
Super Juice Fit 'N Lean Power Protein Orange Cream	8 oz	20	0	0	0	2	2	0	0	150	10	50	40	102
Super Juice Immunity Fruit & Veggie Berry	8 oz	110	0	0	0	1	26	22	1	150	35	410	60	102
EARTHWISE														
Orange Carrot Mango	8 oz	110	0	0	0	0	30	27	0	20	15	—	—	15
ESSN														
Sparkling Blood Orange & Cranberry	1 can (8.4 oz)	160	0	0	0	1	38	34	tr	20	15	—	—	24
FIZZ ED.														
Pomegranate Cherry	1 can (8.4 oz)	90	0	0	0	0	22	20	—	—	30	—	—	6
FIZZY LIZZY														
Raspberry Lemon	1 bottle (12 oz)	120	0	0	0	0	28	28	—	—	5	—	—	60
FRUTZZO														
Organic 100% Juice Pomegranate Passionfruit	1 bottle (12 oz)	140	0	0	0	0	34	32	0	20	10	370	—	15
Organic 100% Juice Pomegranate Acai	1 bottle (12 oz)	140	0	0	0	0	35	32	0	0	10	410	—	2
GENESIS TODAY														
Boost Pomegranate Berry 100% Juice	8 oz	130	0	0	0	0	31	27	1	40	30	300	200	60
GOODBELLY														
Blueberry Acai Probiotic Drink	1 bottle (2.7 oz)	50	0	0	0	tr	12	9	tr	100	5	40	400	60
Cranberry Watermelon Probiotic Drink	8 oz	100	0	0	0	tr	24	21	1	20	30	120	—	60
Peach Mango Probiotic Drink	1 bottle (2.7 oz)	50	0	0	0	tr	13	9	tr	100	10	40	400	60
Strawberry Rosehips Probiotic Drink	1 bottle (2.7 oz)	50	0	0	0	tr	12	9	tr	100	10	40	400	60

FOOD	PORTION	CALS	FAT	SAT FAT	CHOL	PROT	CARB	SUGAR	FIBER	CALCI	SOD	POTAS	FOLIC	VIT C
HONEST ADE														
Superfruit Punch	8 oz	48	0	0	0	0	12	12	—	—	5	—	—	—
HONEST KIDS														
Organic Tropical Tango Punch	1 pkg (6.75 oz)	40	0	0	0	0	10	10	—	—	5	—	—	60
HOOD														
Fruit Punch	1 cup	120	0	0	0	0	30	28	0	0	10	—	—	60
JUICY JUICE														
Harvest Surprise Orange Mango	8 oz	130	0	0	0	1	31	27	1	20	70	230	—	72
LAKEWOOD														
Lean Green	6 oz	90	0	0	0	1	26	24	2	30	7	325	24	7
Organic Acai Amazon Berry	6 oz	95	3	0	0	2	21	16	3	50	24	280	32	60
LAND O LAKES														
Juice Cranberry Apple	1 cup (8 oz)	120	0	0	0	0	30	26	0	0	15	—	—	60
MINUTE MAID														
Pomegranate Blueberry 100% Juice	8 oz	120	1	—	0	0	31	29	—	—	20	260	—	60
MOTO BAR														
Strawberry Kiwi	8 oz	110	0	0	0	0	28	28	0	20	10	—	—	9
MOTT'S														
Apple Blueberry	8 oz	130	0	0	0	0	15	14	—	100	35	20	—	60
Fruit Medley	1 bottle (14 oz)	230	0	0	0	1	54	54	0	40	20	550	—	60
NANTUCKET NECTARS														
100% Juice Peach Orange	8 oz	130	0	0	0	0	32	32	0	20	30	—	—	15
100% Juice Pomegranate Cherry	8 oz	120	0	0	0	0	29	27	0	0	30	—	—	0
Kiwi Berry	8 oz	120	0	0	0	0	29	28	0	0	25	—	—	60
Organic Banana Mango Carrot	8 oz	140	0	0	0	0	32	30	0	0	30	—	—	30
Pineapple Orange Guava	8 oz	120	0	0	0	0	29	29	0	0	25	—	—	60
NOBLE														
Organic 100% Juice Orange Tangerine	8 oz	120	0	0	0	1	29	25	—	20	0	440	20	60
NORTHLAND														
100% Juice Cranberry Pomegranate	8 oz	140	0	0	0	0	34	30	—	—	25	180	—	60

FOOD	PORTION	CALS	FAT	SAT FAT	CHOL	PROT	CARB	SUGAR	FIBER	CALCI	SOD	POTAS	FOLIC	VIT C
NUTRASHAKE														
Fruit Punch Plus Fiber	1 pkg (8 oz)	120	0	0	0	0	29	24	10	10	8	295	—	60
OCEAN SPRAY														
100% Juice Cranberry & Concord Grape	8 oz	150	0	0	0	0	37	37	—	0	35	90	—	60
100% Juice Fruit & Veggie Tropical Citrus	8 oz	130	0	0	0	0	32	27	—	0	70	270	—	60
100% Juice Fruit & Veggie Tropical Citrus Light	8 oz	60	0	0	0	0	15	11	—	0	35	150	—	60
Cran-Apple	8 oz	130	0	0	0	0	32	32	—	0	80	15	—	60
Cran-Apple Light	8 oz	40	0	0	0	0	10	10	—	0	70	20	—	60
Cran-Cherry	8 oz	120	0	0	0	0	30	30	—	0	35	15	—	60
Cran-Grape	8 oz	120	0	0	0	0	31	31	—	0	80	15	—	60
Cran-Grape Light	8 oz	40	0	0	0	0	10	10	—	0	75	30	—	60
Cran-Pomegranate	8 oz	120	0	0	0	0	30	30	—	0	35	40	—	60
Cran-Pomegranate Light	8 oz	40	0	0	0	0	10	10	—	0	35	30	—	60
Cran-Raspberry	8 oz	110	0	0	0	0	28	28	0	0	70	25	—	60
Cran-Raspberry Light	8 oz	40	0	0	0	0	10	10	—	0	70	50	—	60
Ruby Tangerine	8 oz	110	0	0	0	0	28	28	—	—	65	50	—	60
White Cranberry Peach	8 oz	110	0	0	0	0	27	27	—	0	50	30	—	60
ODWALLA														
Quenchers AntioxiDance	8 oz	90	0	0	0	0	23	23	0	0	10	—	—	228
Quenchers B Berrier	8 oz	120	0	0	0	0	30	27	0	0	15	—	—	0
OLD ORCHARD														
100% Juice Acai Pomegranate	8 oz	130	0	0	0	0	31	29	—	0	25	280	—	72
100% Juice Berry Blend	8 oz	130	0	0	0	0	31	29	—	0	25	280	—	72
100% Juice Cherry Pomegranate	8 oz	130	0	0	0	0	31	29	—	0	25	280	—	72
Cranberry Grape Cocktail	8 oz	31	0	0	0	0	6	6	—	0	9	62	—	60
Healthy Balance Apple Kiwi Strawberry Cocktail	8 oz	31	0	0	0	0	6	6	—	0	9	62	—	60

FOOD	PORTION	CALS	FAT	SAT FAT	CHOL	PROT	CARB	SUGAR	FIBER	CALCI	SOD	POTAS	FOLIC	VIT C
OLD ORCHARD (CONT.)														
Pomegranate Blueberry Acai Cocktail	8 oz	31	0	0	0	0	6	6	—	0	9	62	—	60
Very Cherre 100% Juice Tart Cherry Cranberry	8 oz	130	0	0	0	0	31	21	—	30	45	245	—	72
PACIFIC CHAI														
Pomegranate Blueberry	8 oz	100	0	0	0	0	27	26	0	20	10	—	—	0
R.W. KNUDSEN														
Razzleberry 100% Juice	8 oz	120	0	0	0	0	28	27	0	100	15	280	—	60
Sensible Sippers Organic Fruit Punch	1 box (4.23 oz)	30	0	0	0	0	7	7	—	—	0	80	—	2
SABOR LATINO														
Guava Mango Drink	1 box (7 oz)	110	0	0	0	0	29	28	—	—	15	—	—	—
Nectar Strawberry Banana + Calcium	8 oz	150	0	0	0	0	37	37	1	1000	10	110	—	60
Pina Colada	8 oz	130	0	0	0	0	32	31	—	—	15	—	—	60
SANTA CRUZ														
Organic Cranberry Goji	8 oz	120	0	0	0	0	30	28	0	—	15	250	—	2
SMART JUICE														
Organic 100% Juice Pomegranate Purple Carrot	8 oz	137	0	0	0	1	35	33	0	30	20	340	—	—
SNAPPLE														
100% Juice Fruit Punch	8 oz	170	0	0	0	0	42	40	—	150	15	310	—	60
Juice Drink Acai Blackberry	8 oz	110	0	0	0	0	27	27	—	—	5	—	—	—
Juice Drink Cranberry Raspberry	8 oz	100	0	0	0	0	26	26	—	—	5	—	—	—
SSIPS														
Cherry Berry	1 box (7 oz)	110	0	0	0	0	26	26	—	—	10	—	—	—
SUN SHOWER														
100% Juice Nectarine Mango	8 oz	93	0	0	0	1	21	17	2	10	15	350	—	60
SUNDIA														
Tropical Medley	½ cup	70	0	0	0	1	18	15	2	0	10	—	—	60

FOOD	PORTION	CALS	FAT	SAT FAT	CHOL	PROT	CARB	SUGAR	FIBER	CALCI	SOD	POTAS	FOLIC	VIT C
TREE RIPE														
Organic Fruit Punch	8 oz	150	0	0	0	1	36	35	0	20	15	210	8	15
TROPICAL GROVE														
Fruit Punch	8 oz	110	0	0	0	0	26	26	—	—	40	—	—	—
TROPICANA														
Fruit Punch	1 cup	130	0	0	0	0	32	32	0	0	15	—	—	60
Fruit Punch Light	8 oz	10	0	0	0	0	3	1	0	0	5	—	—	60
Orange Tangerine Juice	8 oz	110	0	0	0	2	25	22	0	20	0	450	60	72
Orchard Berry	8 oz	110	0	0	0	1	27	24	0	0	25	230	—	60
Organic Orchard Medley	8 oz	120	0	0	0	0	29	25	0	0	25	280	—	60
Twister Berry Blast	8 oz	120	0	0	0	tr	29	29	0	0	10	—	—	60
Twister Citrus Spark	8 oz	120	0	0	0	0	30	29	0	0	10	—	—	60
Twister Fruit Fury	8 oz	120	0	0	0	tr	30	28	0	0	30	—	—	60
Twister Light Strawberry Spiral	8 oz	40	0	0	0	0	10	10	0	0	70	—	—	60
V8														
Light Peach Mango	8 oz	50	0	0	0	0	13	10	0	20	40	125	8	60
Splash Diet Berry Blend	8 oz	10	0	0	0	0	3	1	0	0	35	80	—	60
Splash Mango Peach	8 oz	80	0	0	0	0	20	20	0	0	40	30	—	60
V-Fusion Acai Mixed Berry	8 oz	110	0	0	0	0	27	26	0	20	70	240	—	60
V-Fusion Cranberry Blackberry	8 oz	110	0	0	0	0	27	26	—	20	70	240	—	60
V-Fusion Light Peach Mango	8 oz	50	0	0	0	0	13	10	—	20	40	160	8	60
VRUIT														
Apple Carrot	1 box (8.45 oz)	120	0	0	0	1	29	27	—	20	50	334	—	60
Berry Veggie	1 box (8.45 oz)	110	0	0	0	1	27	20	—	20	25	370	—	60
Orange Veggie	1 box (8.45 oz)	110	1	—	0	1	26	25	—	20	20	355	—	60
Tropical Blend	1 box (8.45 oz)	110	0	0	0	1	27	19	—	20	20	380	—	60
WADDA JUICE														
All Flavors	1 bottle (4 oz)	25	0	0	0	0	7	7	—	100	4	70	—	60
WALNUT ACRES														
Organic Orange Carrot	8 oz	110	0	0	0	0	27	24	—	20	30	410	—	12
WELCH'S														
100% Black Cherry Concord Grape	8 oz	160	0	0	0	1	40	39	—	—	20	—	—	60

FOOD	PORTION	CALS	FAT	SAT FAT	CHOL	PROT	CARB	SUGAR	FIBER	CALCI	SOD	POTAS	FOLIC	VIT C
WELCH'S (CONT.)														
Light Strawberry Mango	8 oz	50	0	0	0	0	13	12	—	—	80	—	—	60

FRUIT MIXED

(see also individual names, FRUIT AND NUT BARS)

FOOD	PORTION	CALS	FAT	SAT FAT	CHOL	PROT	CARB	SUGAR	FIBER	CALCI	SOD	POTAS	FOLIC	VIT C
CANNED														
fruit cocktail in heavy syrup	½ cup	93	tr	tr	0	1	24	—	—	8	7	112	—	2
fruit cocktail juice pack	½ cup	56	tr	tr	0	1	15	—	—	10	4	118	—	3
fruit cocktail water pack	½ cup	40	tr	tr	0	1	10	—	—	6	5	115	—	3
fruit salad in heavy syrup	½ cup	94	tr	tr	0	tr	24	—	—	8	7	103	—	3
fruit salad in light syrup	½ cup	73	tr	tr	0	tr	19	—	—	8	7	104	—	3
fruit salad juice pack	½ cup	62	tr	tr	0	1	16	—	—	14	7	144	—	4
fruit salad water pack	½ cup	37	tr	tr	0	tr	10	—	—	8	4	95	—	2
mixed fruit in heavy syrup	½ cup	92	tr	tr	0	tr	24	—	—	1	5	108	—	88
tropical fruit salad in heavy syrup	½ cup	110	tr	—	0	1	29	—	—	17	3	168	—	22
BUDDY FRUITS														
100% Fruit Apple & Banana	1 pkg (3.2 oz)	50	0	0	0	0	13	12	1	—	10	—	—	—
DEL MONTE														
Carb Clever Fruit Cocktail	½ cup (4.2 oz)	40	0	0	0	0	11	10	1	0	10	—	—	48
Chunky Mixed Fruit In 100% Juice	½ cup (4.4 oz)	60	0	0	0	0	15	14	1	0	10	—	—	2
Chunky Mixed Fruit In Heavy Syrup	½ cup (4.5 oz)	100	0	0	0	0	24	23	1	0	10	—	—	2
Fruit Cocktail In 100% Juice	½ cup (4.4 oz)	60	0	0	0	0	15	14	1	0	10	—	—	2
Fruit Cocktail In Heavy Syrup	½ cup (4.5 oz)	100	0	0	0	0	24	23	1	0	10	—	—	2
Fruit Cocktail In Light Syrup	½ cup (4.5 oz)	60	0	0	0	0	21	20	1	0	10	—	—	5
Fruit Cocktail In Pear Juice	½ cup (4.4 oz)	60	0	0	0	0	15	14	1	0	10	—	—	2
Fruit Cocktail Lite	½ cup (4.4 oz)	60	0	0	0	0	15	14	1	0	10	—	—	2
Fruit Naturals Apples & Oranges	½ cup (4.4 oz)	70	0	0	0	0	18	15	<2	20	10	—	—	90

FOOD	PORTION	CALS	FAT	SAT FAT	CHOL	PROT	CARB	SUGAR	FIBER	CALCI	SOD	POTAS	FOLIC	VIT C
DEL MONTE (CONT.)														
Fruit Naturals Citrus Salad	½ cup (4.4 oz)	70	0	0	0	0	20	17	0	0	20	—	—	60
Fruit Naturals Tropical Medley	½ cup (4.4 oz)	70	0	0	0	tr	18	16	tr	0	5	—	—	60
Mixed Fruit In Light Syrup	½ cup (4.4 oz)	80	0	0	0	0	18	15	1	0	5	—	—	1
Mixed Fruit In Cherry Gel	1 pkg (4.5 oz)	90	0	0	0	0	23	20	0	20	40	—	—	18
Snack Cups Cherry Mixed Fruit	1 pkg (4 oz)	70	0	0	0	tr	18	15	tr	0	10	—	—	60
Superfruit Mixed Fruit Chunks Mango & Passion	1 pkg (6 oz)	120	0	0	0	2	29	20	3	20	25	240	—	60
Superfruit Peach Chunks Pomegranate & Orange	1 pkg (6 oz)	100	0	0	0	2	26	12	3	0	15	140	—	60
Superfruit Pear Chunks Acai & Blackberry	1 pkg (6 oz)	120	0	0	0	2	31	24	3	100	15	100	—	60
Tropical Fruit Salad	½ cup (4.3 oz)	60	0	0	0	0	16	14	1	40	15	—	—	30
DOLE														
Cherry Mixed Fruit In Fruit Juice	1 pkg (4 oz)	70	0	0	0	0	17	16	1	0	5	85	—	27
Tropical Fruit In Fruit Juice	1 pkg (4 oz)	60	0	0	0	tr	15	14	1	0	5	160	—	27
HOMEMADE HARVEY'S														
Crushed Fruit Apple Pear & Spices	1 pkg (4.5 oz)	60	0	0	0	0	17	13	2	0	0	120	—	5
Crushed Fruit Mango Pineapple Banana & Passion Fruit	1 pkg (4.5 oz)	90	0	0	0	1	22	19	2	20	5	230	—	36
Crushed Fruit Strawberries Bananas & Kiwis	1 pkg (4.5 oz)	100	1	0	0	1	23	19	2	20	10	290	—	21
MOTT'S														
Healthy Harvest Pomegranate	1 pkg (3.9 oz)	50	0	0	0	0	13	11	1	—	0	70	—	15
POLAR														
Mixed Fruit Light Syrup	½ cup (4.9 oz)	50	0	0	0	0	12	11	2	0	20	—	—	0

FOOD	PORTION	CALS	FAT	SAT FAT	CHOL	PROT	CARB	SUGAR	FIBER	CALCI	SOD	POTAS	FOLIC	VIT C
S&W														
Chunky Mixed In Sweetened Juice	½ cup (4.3 oz)	80	0	0	0	tr	19	16	3	0	20	—	—	1
Fruit Cocktail	½ cup (4.4 oz)	80	0	0	0	0	20	18	2	0	20	—	—	1
DRIED														
mixed	11 oz pkg	712	1	tr	0	7	188	—	—	110	52	2332	—	11
BROTHERS-ALL-NATURAL														
Crisps Strawberry Banana	1 pkg (0.42 oz)	45	0	0	0	1	10	6	2	10	0	—	—	25
CRUNCHIES														
Freeze Dried Mixed Fruit	¼ cup (7 g)	25	0	0	0	0	6	4	1	0	0	—	—	18
ELIZABETH'S NATURAL														
Fancy Mixed	5 pieces	80	0	0	0	1	20	7	2	0	10	—	—	1
FRUITACEUTICALS														
PomaCrans	¼ cup	100	0	0	0	0	24	18	1	0	0	—	—	0
FUN-YUMS														
Fresh Crispy Mixed Fruit	1 serv (0.9 oz)	25	5	3	—	—	18	2	1	30	54			re
MARIANI														
Berries 'N Cherries	¼ cup	140	0	0	0	tr	38	25	2	20	0	75	—	48
SUN-MAID														
Fruit Bits	¼ cup (1.4 oz)	120	0	0	0	1	29	24	2	20	20	310	—	1
Mixed	¼ cup (1.4 oz)	100	0	0	0	1	26	21	3	20	35	290	—	1
SUNSWEET														
Antioxidant Blend	¼ cup (1.4 oz)	130	0	0	0	1	31	22	1	20	5	150	—	0
Berry Blend	¼ cup (1.4 oz)	120	0	0	0	1	32	24	3	40	5	115	—	9
FRESH														
CHIQUITA														
Apple & Grape Bites	1 pkg (2.5 oz)	40	0	0	0	0	10	8	1	20	0	—	—	12
FROZEN														
mixed fruit sweetened	1 cup	245	tr	tr	0	4	61	—	—	18	8	327	—	188
FRUIT SNACKS														
fruit leather	1 bar (0.8 oz)	81	1	1	0	tr	18	—	—	7	18	32	—	16
fruit leather pieces	1 oz	97	2	tr	0	tr	22	—	—	5	114	48	—	16
fruit leather pieces	1 pkg (0.9 oz)	92	2	tr	0	tr	21	—	—	5	109	44	—	15
fruit leather rolls	1 lg (0.7 oz)	73	1	tr	0	tr	18	—	—	7	13	62	—	1
fruit leather rolls	1 sm (0.5 oz)	49	tr	tr	0	tr	12	—	—	4	8	41	—	1
ANNIE'S HOMEGROWN														
Orchard Fruit Bites Grape	1 pkg (0.6 oz)	60	0	0	0	0	15	12	1	—	5	—	—	12
Orchard Fruit Bites Strawberry	1 pkg (0.6 oz)	60	0	0	0	0	15	12	1	—	5	—	—	12

FOOD	PORTION	CALS	FAT	SAT FAT	CHOL	PROT	CARB	SUGAR	FIBER	CALCI	SOD	POTAS	FOLIC	VIT C
ANNIE'S HOMEGROWN (CONT.)														
Organic Bunny Fruit Snacks Lemonade	1 pkg (0.6 oz)	70	0	0	0	0	18	10	—	—	45	—	—	—
Organic Bunny Fruit Tropical Treat	1 pkg (0.8 oz)	70	0	0	0	0	18	10	—	—	45	—	—	60
BARE FRUIT														
Bananas & Cherries	1 pkg (0.6 oz)	55	1	0	0	2	12	6	2	10	0	—	—	2
CLIF														
Twisted Fruit Grape	1 piece (0.7 oz)	70	0	0	0	0	16	9	1	0	5	240	24	6
Twisted Fruit Pineapple	1 piece (0.7 oz)	70	0	0	0	0	16	9	1	0	5	240	24	6
Twisted Fruit Tropical Twist	1 piece (0.7 oz)	70	0	0	0	0	16	9	1	0	5	240	24	6
DOLE														
Real Fruit Bites Apple	1 pkg (0.7 oz)	80	2	2	0	5	16	11	0	0	35	10	—	9
FROOSE														
All Flavors	1 pkg (0.9 oz)	70	0	0	0	0	19	9	3	20	5	—	—	15
FRUITZIO														
Apples & Strawberries	1 pkg (0.9 oz)	100	0	0	0	1	23	19	2	20	0	—	—	35
Apricots	1 pkg (0.35 oz)	40	0	0	0	0	9	7	1	10	0	—	—	2
Peach	1 pkg (0.35 oz)	40	0	0	0	0	9	7	1	40	0	—	—	2
Strawberries	1 pkg (0.9 oz)	100	0	0	0	2	22	17	3	40	0	—	—	66
FUNKY MONKEY														
Applemon	1 pkg (0.42 oz)	40	0	0	0	0	11	9	1	0	15	0	—	0
Bananamon	1 pkg (0.42 oz)	45	0	0	0	0	11	9	1	0	1	144	—	1
Carnaval Mix	1 pkg (0.42 oz)	45	0	0	0	0	11	9	1	10	2	104	—	8
Jivealime	1 pkg (0.42 oz)	45	0	0	0	0	11	8	1	20	0	118	—	4
MangoOJ	1 pkg (0.42 oz)	35	0	0	0	0	10	8	1	0	0	0	—	9
Pink Pineapple	1 pkg (0.42 oz)	45	0	0	0	0	11	9	1	0	0	0	—	24
Purple Funk	1 pkg (0.42 oz)	50	0	0	0	0	11	8	1	0	0	144	—	1
JELLY BELLY														
Fruit Snacks	1 pkg (2.5 oz)	220	0	0	0	0	58	37	1	—	105	—	—	108
KAIA FOODS														
Fruit Leather Lime Ginger	1 (1 oz)	50	0	0	0	1	12	7	2	20	0	—	—	30
Fruit Leather Vanilla Pear	1 (1 oz)	60	0	0	0	1	15	9	3	0	0	—	—	4
KETTLE VALLEY														
100% Fruit Bar All Flavors	1 (0.7 oz)	70	0	0	0	tr	16	12	1	0	15	—	—	60

FOOD	PORTION	CALS	FAT	SAT FAT	CHOL	PROT	CARB	SUGAR	FIBER	CALCI	SOD	POTAS	FOLIC	VIT C
KETTLE VALLEY (CONT.)														
Fruit Twists All Flavors	1 (0.6 oz)	60	0	0	0	0	15	12	1	0	40	—	—	60
PEELED SNACKS														
Fruit & Nuts FigSated	⅓ cup	150	6	1	0	3	20	15	3	40	60	—	—	—
Fruit & Nuts Plu-what?	⅓ cup	150	6	1	0	3	22	13	3	—	50	—	—	1
REVOLUTION FOODS														
Organic Mashups Berry	1 pkg (3.2 oz)	40	0	0	0	0	10	8	1	0	5	—	—	6
Organic Mashups Strawberry Banana	1 pkg (3.2 oz)	60	0	0	0	1	13	9	1	0	3	135	—	4
STRETCH ISLAND														
Fruit Leather Bountiful Blueberry	1 pkg (0.5 oz)	45	0	0	0	0	12	8	1	0	0	95	—	2
Fruit Leather Harvest Grape	1 pkg (0.5 oz)	45	0	0	0	0	12	9	1	0	0	120	—	2
Fruit Leather Mango Sunrise	1 pkg (0.5 oz)	45	0	0	0	0	11	9	1	0	0	85	—	2
Fruit Leather Truly Tropical	1 pkg (0.5 oz)	45	0	0	0	0	11	8	1	0	0	100	—	1
Organic Smooshed Fruit Apple	1 piece (0.4 oz)	40	0	0	0	0	10	8	1	0	0	80	—	0
Organic Smooshed Fruit Strawberry	1 piece (0.4 oz)	40	0	0	0	0	10	8	tr	0	0	85	—	0
SUN-RYPE														
Fruit Bar Mango Strawberry	1 (1.3 oz)	120	0	0	0	tr	31	27	3	20	45	230	—	1
Fruit Bar Strawberry	1 (1.3 oz)	130	0	0	0	0	32	29	2	0	20	180	—	1
TAHITIAN NONI														
Soft Chews Raspberry	1 pkg (2 oz)	240	3	2	0	2	50	44	0	—	20	—	—	—
TASTY														
All Flavors	1 pkg (0.8 oz)	130	0	0	0	0	32	17	0	0	70	—	—	102
THAT'S IT														
Bar 1 Apple + 1 Pear	1 (1.2 oz)	100	0	0	0	1	27	24	3	20	15	—	—	2
Bar 1 Apple + 10 Cherries	1 (1.2 oz)	100	0	0	0	1	26	22	3	20	20	—	—	6
Bar 1 Apple + 3 Apricots	1 (1.2 oz)	100	0	0	0	1	27	23	3	20	15	—	—	1

FOOD	PORTION	CALS	FAT	SAT FAT	CHOL	PROT	CARB	SUGAR	FIBER	CALCI	SOD	POTAS	FOLIC	VIT C
TROPICANA														
Fruit Wise Bars All Flavors	1 bar (1.4 oz)	140	0	0	0	0	36	32	2	20	10	300	—	60
Fruit Wise Strips All Flavors	1 strip (0.7 oz)	70	0	0	0	0	17	15	1	0	0	135	—	60
WELCH'S														
Fruit'N Yogurt Strawberry	1 pkg (0.9 oz)	90	2	2	—	1	17	14	—	100	20	—	—	60
Mixed Fruit	1 pkg (0.9 oz)	80	0	0	0	1	19	15	—	—	10	10	—	60
GARLIC														
clove	1	4	tr	tr	0	tr	1	tr	tr	5	1	12	tr	1
fresh chopped	1 tbsp	18	tr	tr	0	1	4	tr	tr	22	2	48	0	4
powder	1 tsp	9	tr	tr	0	tr	2	1	tr	2	1	31	0	1
GARLIC IT!														
Caramelized	1 tbsp (0.5 oz)	80	8	1	0	0	2	0	0	0	230	—	—	1
Dijon	1 tbsp (0.5 oz)	80	8	1	0	0	2	0	0	0	125	—	—	1
Savory Basil	1 tbsp (0.5 oz)	80	8	1	0	0	2	0	0	0	230	—	—	1
Thai Peanut	1 tbsp (0.5 oz)	90	9	1	0	2	2	0	0	0	80	—	—	2
Tomato Curry	1 tbsp (0.5 oz)	50	3	tr	0	0	7	6	tr	0	350	—	—	1
JAKE & AMOS														
Sweet Pickled Garlic	1 oz	36	0	0	0	0	9	7	0	20	70	—	—	0
MCSWEET														
Pickled	8 pieces (1 oz)	40	0	0	0	0	5	tr	0	40	420	—	—	0
SPICE WORLD														
Ajo Garlic Clove	1 (3 g)	5	0	0	0	0	1	—	—	20	0	—	—	2
GEFILTE FISH														
sweet	1 piece (1.5 oz)	35	1	tr	12	4	3	—	—	10	220	38	1	—
MRS. ADLER'S														
Gefilte Fish	1 piece (1.8 oz)	50	2	1	20	5	3	1	1	20	200	—	—	—
UNGAR'S														
Gefilte Fish	2 slices (1.8 oz)	83	5	1	41	6	5	3	0	0	263	—	—	0
Lite	2 slices (2.4 oz)	80	3	0	20	7	5	3	2	0	190	—	—	1
No Sugar	2 slices (1.8 oz)	70	4	1	15	6	3	tr	0	0	180	—	—	0
GELATIN														
READY-TO-EAT														
DOLE														
Mixed Fruit In Cherry Gel Sugar Free	1 pkg (4.3 oz)	60	0	0	0	0	14	5	1	0	45	90	—	15
Mixed Fruit In Peach Gel	1 pkg (4.3 oz)	100	0	0	0	1	24	22	1	0	25	65	—	15
Pineapple In Lime Gel	1 pkg (4.3 oz)	90	0	0	0	0	23	22	1	0	50	60	—	15

FOOD	PORTION	CALS	FAT	SAT FAT	CHOL	PROT	CARB	SUGAR	FIBER	CALCI	SOD	POTAS	FOLIC	VIT C
JELL-O														
Sugar Free Lemon Lime	1 serv (3.2 oz)	10	0	0	0	1	0	0	0	—	45	—	—	—
KOZY SHACK														
Gel Treats Sugar Free Strawberry	1 pkg (3.5 oz)	10	0	0	0	0	2	0	0	17	15	90	—	0
Smart Gels Cherry	1 pkg (3.5 oz)	80	0	0	0	0	21	20	0	14	10	70	—	0
Smart Gels Orange	1 pkg (3.5 oz)	80	0	0	0	0	24	22	0	14	10	84	—	0
Smart Gels Strawberry	1 pkg (3.5 oz)	80	0	0	0	0	24	22	0	14	10	70	—	0
Smart Gels Sugar Free Orange	1 pkg (3.5 oz)	5	0	0	0	0	1	0	0	16	15	87	—	0
Tropical	1 pkg (3.5 oz)	80	0	0	0	0	21	20	0	20	10	—	—	0
Tropical Sugar Free	1 pkg (3.5 oz)	5	0	0	0	0	1	0	1	20	15	—	—	0
SNACK PACK														
Gels Cherry No Sugar Added	1 pkg (3.5 oz)	10	0	0	0	0	2	0	tr	20	65	—	—	0
Gels Strawberry	1 pkg (3.5 oz)	100	0	0	0	0	25	22	0	0	40	—	—	0
GIBLETS														
capon simmered	1 cup (5 oz)	238	8	3	629	38	0	0	0	19	80	222	601	13
chicken fried	1 cup (5 oz)	402	20	6	647	47	6	—	0	26	164	478	550	13
chicken simmered	1 cup (5 oz)	289	17	6	419	30	1	0	0	9	93	392	486	20
turkey simmered	1 cup (5 oz)	243	7	2	606	39	3	—	—	18	85	291	501	3
GINGER														
ground	1 tsp	6	tr	tr	0	tr	1	tr	tr	2	1	24	1	tr
pickled	1 tbsp (0.3 oz)	9	0	0	0	0	2	—	0	1	24	25	1	0
preserved	1.5 oz	34	0	0	0	0	8	7	1	19	8	0	—	0
root fresh	5 slices	9	tr	tr	0	tr	2	tr	tr	2	1	46	1	1
root fresh sliced	¼ cup	19	tr	tr	0	tr	4	tr	1	4	3	100	3	1
DOROT														
Crushed Cubes frzn	1 (3.5 g)	0	0	0	0	0	tr	—	—	—	10	—	—	—
FRIEDA'S														
Crystallized	9 pieces (1.1 oz)	100	0	0	0	0	26	11	0	40	10	—	—	0
TREE OF LIFE														
Crystallized Pieces	7 (1.4 oz)	150	0	0	0	0	37	33	1	40	25	—	—	2
GINKGO NUTS														
canned	1 oz	32	tr	tr	0	1	6	—	—	1	87	51	—	—
dried	1 oz	99	tr	tr	0	3	21	—	—	6	4	283	—	8
raw	1 oz	52	tr	tr	0	1	11	—	—	1	1	145	—	4

FOOD	PORTION	CALS	FAT	SAT FAT	CHOL	PROT	CARB	SUGAR	FIBER	CALCI	SOD	POTAS	FOLIC	VIT C
GINSENG														
dried	1 oz	90	tr	—	—	5	20	—	2	64	16	296	—	2
fresh	1 oz	28	tr	—	—	1	6	—	tr	32	5	92	—	4
GIZZARDS														
chicken simmered	1 cup (5 oz)	212	4	1	536	44	0	0	0	25	81	260	7	0
turkey simmered	1 (3 oz)	103	3	1	171	18	tr	0	0	6	56	279	11	5
FOSTER FARMS														
Chicken Gizzards & Hearts fresh	4 oz	150	8	—	150	19	0	0	0	—	85	—	—	4
PERDUE														
Fresh Chicken	3 oz	130	3	1	165	23	1	0	—	0	55	—	—	1
GNOCCHI														
spinach	12 (4 oz)	220	1	0	0	6	50	2	5	40	330	—	—	2
RACCONTO														
Potato Whole Wheat as prep w/o salt	1 cup (5.8 oz)	248	0	0	0	1	60	tr	8	0	450	—	—	0
SOLTERRA														
Original Potato	¼ pkg (3 oz)	100	0	0	0	2	22	1	2	20	60	—	—	18
Spinach	¼ pkg (3 oz)	100	0	0	0	2	24	1	2	0	95	—	—	18
VANTIA														
Gnocchi Whole Wheat	¾ cup	210	1	0	0	5	46	0	4	0	630	—	—	0
GOAT														
diced boiled	1 cup (4.7 oz)	190	4	1	100	36	0	0	0	23	332	540	7	0
fried boneless	3 oz	130	4	1	62	23	0	0	0	14	342	336	4	0
ribs cooked	3 (4.8 oz)	196	4	1	104	37	0	0	0	23	342	556	7	0
roasted boneless	3 oz	122	3	1	64	23	0	0	0	14	73	344	4	0
TAKE-OUT														
stew puerto rican style	1 cup (6.2 oz)	460	31	6	112	40	4	2	1	37	1267	683	12	7
GOJI BERRIES														
dried	1 oz	106	3	—	0	2	19	—	2	32	—	323	—	25
KOPALI														
Organic Dark Chocolate Covered	½ pkg (1 oz)	120	6	4	0	2	18	13	2	20	13	—	—	2
NAVITAS NATURALS														
Dried	1 oz	90	0	0	0	4	18	14	1	0	140	—	—	9
SUNFOOD														
Organic	1 oz	90	0	0	0	4	18	14	3	20	105	—	—	2
SUPERFOOD SNACKS														
Organic Chocolate Goji Treats	3 pieces (1.4 oz)	150	4	1	5	4	24	12	7	40	55	—	—	0

FOOD	PORTION	CALS	FAT	SAT FAT	CHOL	PROT	CARB	SUGAR	FIBER	CALCI	SOD	POTAS	FOLIC	VIT C
TREE OF LIFE														
Organic	1 oz	110	0	0	0	<4	25	15	<5	50	130	—	—	12
GOJI JUICE														
ARTHUR'S														
Goji Plus	1 bottle (11 oz)	210	tr	0	0	3	49	38	2	20	160	590	200	9
GOJILANIA														
Organic	8 oz	110	0	0	0	5	23	23	0	20	110	—	—	108
GOOSE														
boneless roasted	2.7 oz	231	17	5	69	19	0	0	0	10	176	249	2	0
meat only raw	6.5 oz	298	13	5	155	42	0	0	0	24	161	777	57	13
w/ skin & bone roasted	1 serv (6.6 oz)	573	41	13	171	47	0	0	0	24	132	619	4	0
wild boneless roasted diced	1 cup (4.9 oz)	426	31	10	127	35	0	0	0	18	325	459	3	0
GOOSEBERRIES														
canned in light syrup	1 cup	184	1	tr	0	2	47	—	6	40	5	194	8	25
fresh	1 cup	66	1	tr	0	1	15	—	7	38	2	297	9	42
KOPALI														
Organic Goldenberry	1 pkg (1.8 oz)	150	0	0	0	4	31	4	18	0	45	—	—	4
NAVITAS NATURALS														
Cape Gooseberry Dried	1 oz	80	0	0	0	2	17	9	3	0	25	—	—	2
GRAINS														
KASHI														
7 Whole Grain Pilaf Fiery Fiesta	1 cup (4.9 oz)	210	5	1	0	8	40	3	7	0	400	—	—	0
7 Whole Grain Pilaf Moroccan Curry	1 cup (4.9 oz)	220	5	3	0	8	42	3	7	0	400	—	—	0
7 Whole Grain Pilaf Original	1 cup (4.9 oz)	220	4	1	0	8	45	1	7	0	0	—	—	0
VILLAGE HARVEST														
Wheatberry & Barley	½ cup	260	3	1	0	7	57	0	10	20	10	—	—	0
Whole Grain Creations w/ Cranberries & Almonds	¾ cup (4.3 oz)	220	4	1	0	5	44	6	6	20	5	—	—	0
Whole Grain Medley Farro & Red Rice	1 cup (5 oz)	290	3	0	0	8	60	0	4	20	5	—	—	0
GRAPE JUICE														
bottled unsweetened	1 cup	154	tr	tr	0	1	38	38	tr	23	8	334	8	tr

FOOD	PORTION	CALS	FAT	SAT FAT	CHOL	PROT	CARB	SUGAR	FIBER	CALCI	SOD	POTAS	FOLIC	VIT C
APPLE & EVE														
Vintage Concord	8 oz	150	0	0	0	0	40	38	—	—	15	—	—	60
CASCADIAN FARM														
Organic frzn as prep	8 oz	150	0	0	0	0	38	37	—	—	5	320	—	—
FIZZY LIZZY														
Yakima Grape	1 bottle (12 oz)	120	0	0	0	0	30	30	—	—	10	—	—	60
JUICY JUICE														
Harvest Surprise	8 oz	120	0	0	0	1	28	27	0	20	80	105	—	72
KEDEM														
Organic	8 oz	140	0	0	0	0	35	33	—	—	10	—	—	—
LAKEWOOD														
Organic Concord	6 oz	105	0	0	0	1	25	23	1	20	5	360	—	0
LANGERS														
Plus 100% Juice	8 oz	160	0	0	0	0	40	36	—	100	15	—	—	60
White Grape Plus 100% Juice	8 oz	160	0	0	0	0	40	36	—	100	15	—	—	60
MOTT'S														
100% Juice Grape Medley	1 bottle (14 oz)	230	0	0	0	1	55	55	0	40	20	550	—	60
NANTUCKET NECTARS														
Grapeade	8 oz	140	0	0	0	0	33	33	0	0	25	—	—	60
Organic Concord Grape	8 oz	130	0	0	0	0	31	31	0	20	35	—	—	0
OLD ORCHARD														
100% Juice	8 oz	130	0	0	0	0	31	29	—	0	25	280	—	72
100% Juice White	8 oz	130	0	0	0	0	31	29	—	0	25	280	—	72
R.W. KNUDSEN														
100% Juice	8 oz	130	0	0	0	1	32	31	tr	100	15	300	—	60
SANTA CRUZ														
Organic Concord Grape	8 oz	160	0	0	0	tr	40	39	0	20	15	250	—	5
SNAPPLE														
100% Juice Grape	8 oz	170	0	0	0	0	43	41	—	150	15	310	—	60
Grapeade	8 oz	100	0	0	0	0	26	26	—	—	5	—	—	—
TANG														
Drink Mix as prep	1 serv (8 oz)	110	0	0	0	0	28	28	0	40	10	—	—	60
TREE RIPE														
Organic 100% Juice	6 oz	120	0	0	0	1	28	27	0	20	10	—	0	0
TROPICANA														
Grape	1 bottle (14 oz)	270	0	0	0	tr	67	62	0	0	25	—	—	72
WALNUT ACRES														
Organic	8 oz	120	0	0	0	0	31	28	0	—	0	—	—	—

FOOD	PORTION	CALS	FAT	SAT FAT	CHOL	PROT	CARB	SUGAR	FIBER	CALCI	SOD	POTAS	FOLIC	VIT C
WELCH'S														
100% Juice	8 oz	140	0	0	0	1	38	36	—	20	15	210	—	72
100% White	8 oz	160	0	0	0	0	39	38	—	—	20	—	—	72
GRAPE LEAVES														
canned	1 (4 g)	3	tr	tr	0	tr	tr	—	—	12	114	1	3	1
fresh raw	1 (3 g)	3	tr	tr	0	tr	1	tr	tr	11	0	8	2	tr
GALIL														
Stuffed	5 (4.2 oz)	200	11	1	0	2	23	2	3	30	571	—	—	1
TAKE-OUT														
dolmas w/ beef & rice	1 (0.7 oz)	50	4	1	5	2	2	1	1	21	14	47	7	2
dolmas w/ lamb & rice	1 (0.7 oz)	56	4	1	5	2	3	1	1	22	14	41	5	2
dolmas w/ rice	1 (2 oz)	92	6	1	0	1	8	2	2	50	93	86	21	3
GRAPEFRUIT														
CANNED														
sections juice pack	½ cup (4.4 oz)	46	tr	tr	0	1	11	11	1	19	9	210	11	42
sections light syrup	½ cup (4.5 oz)	76	tr	tr	0	1	20	19	1	18	3	164	11	27
sections water pack	½ cup (4.3 oz)	44	tr	tr	0	1	11	11	1	18	2	161	11	27
DEL MONTE														
Fruit Bowls Grapefruit Duo	½ cup (4.4 oz)	60	0	0	0	1	16	14	1	20	10	—	—	60
Red In Light Syrup	½ cup (4.4 oz)	90	0	0	0	1	21	17	1	20	0	—	—	60
SunFresh Red No Sugar Added	½ cup (4.2 oz)	40	0	0	0	tr	10	6	1	0	15	110	—	60
FRESH														
pink or red	½ (4.6 oz)	52	tr	tr	0	1	13	8	2	27	0	166	16	38
sections pink or red	1 cup (8.1 oz)	97	tr	tr	0	2	25	16	4	51	0	310	30	72
sections white	1 cup (8.1 oz)	76	tr	tr	0	2	19	17	3	28	0	340	23	77
white	½ (4.1 oz)	39	tr	tr	0	1	10	9	1	14	0	175	12	39
OCEAN SPRAY														
Sweet Ruby	½ med (5.4 oz)	60	0	0	0	1	16	10	6	20	0	—	—	66
GRAPEFRUIT JUICE														
canned sweetened	1 cup (8.8 oz)	115	tr	tr	0	1	28	28	tr	20	5	405	25	67
canned unsweetened	1 cup (8.7 oz)	94	tr	tr	0	1	22	22	tr	17	2	378	25	72
pink fresh	1 cup (8.7 oz)	96	tr	tr	0	1	23	—	—	22	2	400	25	94
white fresh	1 cup (8.7 oz)	96	tr	tr	0	1	23	22	tr	22	2	400	25	94
APPLE & EVE														
Ruby Red	8 oz	130	0	0	0	0	32	32	—	—	35	—	—	78
FIZZY LIZZY														
Grapefruit	1 bottle (12 oz)	100	0	0	0	0	25	25	—	—	0	—	—	60
OCEAN SPRAY														
100% Juice Pink	8 oz	100	0	0	0	1	23	23	—	—	35	220	—	60

FOOD	PORTION	CALS	FAT	SAT FAT	CHOL	PROT	CARB	SUGAR	FIBER	CALCI	SOD	POTAS	FOLIC	VIT C
OCEAN SPRAY (CONT.)														
100% Juice White	8 oz	90	0	0	0	2	21	17	—	20	35	340	—	60
Ruby Drink Light	8 oz	40	0	0	0	0	10	10	—	0	65	60	—	0
ODWALLA														
100% Juice	8 oz	90	0	0	0	2	20	16	0	20	5	—	—	78
OLD ORCHARD														
Ruby Red Cocktail	8 oz	31	0	0	0	0	6	6	—	0	9	62	—	60
SUNDIA														
Ruby	½ cup	70	0	0	0	1	18	14	1	20	0	—	—	60
TROPICANA														
Sweet	8 oz	130	0	0	0	1	31	27	0	20	20	300	40	60
GRAPES														
muscadine	10–12 (3.5 oz)	76	0	0	0	5	14	—	3	24	7	167	—	6
scuppernongs	10–12 (3.5 oz)	68	0	0	0	5	12	—	3	17	5	163	—	7
seedless red or green	20	69	tr	tr	0	1	18	15	1	10	2	191	2	11
seedless red or green	1 cup	110	tr	tr	0	1	29	24	1	16	3	306	3	17
thompson seedless in heavy syrup	½ cup	93	tr	tr	0	1	25	24	1	13	6	132	4	1
thompson seedless water pack	½ cup	49	tr	tr	0	1	13	12	1	12	7	131	4	1
with seeds red or green	20	80	tr	tr	0	1	21	18	1	12	2	222	2	13
with seeds red or green	1 cup	106	tr	tr	0	1	28	24	1	15	3	294	3	17
CHIQUITA														
Grapes	1 cup (3.2 oz)	62	0	0	0	1	16	15	1	10	2	176	—	4
CRUNCH PAK														
Sweet Seedless	⅓ pkg	40	0	0	0	1	10	9	tr	0	0	—	—	0
DOLE														
Fresh	26 (4.4 oz)	90	0	0	0	tr	23	20	1	20	0	—	—	15
EARTHBOUND FARMS														
Organic Black	1½ cups	190	1	0	0	1	24	23	1	20	0	—	—	15
REVOLUTION FOODS														
Organic Mashups Grape	1 pkg (3.2 oz)	60	0	0	0	0	14	12	0	0	5	—	—	0
GRAVY														
CANNED														
beef	1 cup	124	6	3	7	9	11	—	—	14	1305	189	—	0
beef	1 can (10 oz)	155	7	3	9	11	14	—	—	17	1630	236	—	0
chicken	1 cup	189	14	3	5	5	13	—	—	48	1375	260	—	0
mushroom	1 cup	120	6	1	0	3	13	—	—	17	1259	253	—	0
turkey	1 cup	122	5	1	5	6	12	—	—	10	—	—	—	0

FOOD	PORTION	CALS	FAT	SAT FAT	CHOL	PROT	CARB	SUGAR	FIBER	CALCI	SOD	POTAS	FOLIC	VIT C
BOSTON MARKET														
Roasted Chicken	¼ cup	25	2	1	<5	0	3	—	—	—	280	—	—	—
CAMPBELL'S														
Au Jus	¼ cup	5	0	0	0	1	0	0	0	0	230	—	—	0
Chicken	¼ cup	40	3	1	5	0	3	1	0	0	260	—	—	0
Fat Free Beef	¼ cup	15	0	0	0	1	3	0	0	0	300	—	—	0
Fat Free Turkey	¼ cup	20	0	0	0	1	4	0	0	0	290	—	—	0
Mushroom	¼ cup	20	1	0	<5	0	3	1	0	0	280	—	—	0
FRANCO-AMERICAN														
Fat Free Slow Roast Chicken	¼ cup	20	0	0	0	tr	4	0	0	0	250	—	—	0
Slow Roast Chicken	¼ cup	20	1	0	<5	1	3	0	0	0	240	—	—	0
HEINZ														
Classic Chicken Fat Free	¼ cup	15	0	0	0	0	3	0	0	0	320	—	—	0
HomeStyle Classic Chicken	¼ cup	25	1	0	0	0	4	0	0	0	340	—	—	0
HomeStyle Roasted Turkey	¼ cup (2.1 oz)	25	1	0	<5	1	3	0	0	0	290	—	—	0
Roasted Turkey Fat Free	¼ cup (2.1 oz)	20	0	0	0	1	3	0	0	0	260	—	—	0
MIX														
au jus as prep w/ water	1 cup	32	1	1	1	1	4	—	—	23	964	—	—	—
brown as prep w/ water	1 cup	75	2	1	2	2	13	—	—	66	1076	57	—	—
chicken as prep	1 cup	83	2	1	3	3	14	—	—	39	1133	—	—	—
mushroom as prep	1 cup	70	1	1	1	2	14	—	—	49	1402	—	—	—
onion as prep w/ water	1 cup	77	1	tr	tr	2	16	—	—	72	1013	—	—	—
pork as prep	1 cup	76	2	1	3	2	13	—	—	32	1235	—	—	—
turkey as prep	1 cup	87	2	1	3	3	15	—	—	50	1498	—	—	—
BOURNVITA														
Extract tsp	2 heaping	34	1	—	—	1	7	—	—	8	—	—	—	0
BOVRIL														
Extract tsp	1 heaping	9	0	—	—	2	tr	—	0	2	—	—	—	0
BUTTERBALL														
Turkey	¼ cup (2 oz)	30	0	0	—	0	6	0	0	—	510	—	—	—
KNORR														
Au Jus Instant as prep	2 oz	10	0	0	0	tr	2	—	—	—	470	—	—	—
Beef Instant as prep	2 oz	20	1	tr	0	1	3	—	—	—	330	—	—	—
Brown Instant as prep	2 oz	25	0	0	0	1	6	—	—	—	410	—	—	—

FOOD	PORTION	CALS	FAT	SAT FAT	CHOL	PROT	CARB	SUGAR	FIBER	CALCI	SOD	POTAS	FOLIC	VIT C
KNORR (CONT.)														
Brown Low Sodium Instant as prep	2 oz	25	tr	0	0	1	5	—	—	—	115	—	—	—
Chicken Instant as prep	2 oz	25	tr	0	0	tr	5	—	—	—	395	—	—	—
Chicken Low Sodium Instant as prep	2 oz	25	1	tr	5	1	4	—	—	—	120	—	—	—
LEAHEY GARDENS														
No Beef Brown Gluten Free	¼ cup	9	tr	0	0	tr	3	tr	—	—	114	—	—	—
No Chicken Golden	¼ cup	18	2	0	0	tr	3	tr	—	0	275	—	—	0
LONEY'S														
Brown as prep	¼ cup (2.1 oz)	15	0	0	0	tr	3	0	0	0	200	—	—	0
Turkey as prep	¼ cup (2.1 oz)	20	0	0	0	tr	4	0	0	0	200	—	—	0
MARMITE														
Extract	1 heaping tsp	9	0	—	—	2	tr	—	—	5	—	—	—	0
ROAD'S END ORGANICS														
Savory Herb Cholesterol Free Gluten Free	¼ cup	25	0	0	0	tr	5	0	0	0	210	—	—	0
TAKE-OUT														
au jus	1 cup	62	6	2	6	1	1	tr	tr	4	290	34	5	0
giblet gravy	¼ cup	45	3	1	23	3	3	tr	tr	7	313	73	18	1
GREAT NORTHERN BEANS														
canned	1 cup	299	1	tr	0	19	55	—	13	139	11	919	213	3
dried cooked	1 cup	209	1	tr	0	15	37	—	12	121	4	692	181	2
HAMBEENS														
Great Northerns as prep	½ cup	120	1	0	0	7	22	1	11	60	63	490	—	1
GREEN BEANS														
CANNED														
drained	1 cup	27	tr	tr	0	2	6	1	3	35	354	147	43	7
ALLENS														
No Salt	½ cup	15	0	0	0	0	3	1	2	40	10	—	—	2
DEL MONTE														
Cut No Salt Added	½ cup (4.2 oz)	20	0	0	0	1	4	2	2	20	10	—	—	2
French Style	½ cup (4.2 oz)	20	0	0	0	1	4	2	2	20	390	—	—	2
Fresh Cut Italian	½ cup	30	0	0	0	1	6	2	3	20	390	—	—	2
GERTIE'S FINEST														
Pickled	1 oz	15	0	0	0	1	3	3	1	20	160	—	—	0
GREEN GIANT														
50% Less Sodium Cut	½ cup	20	0	0	0	1	4	2	1	20	200	—	—	2

FOOD	PORTION	CALS	FAT	SAT FAT	CHOL	PROT	CARB	SUGAR	FIBER	CALCI	SOD	POTAS	FOLIC	VIT C
MCSWEET														
Dilly Beans Whole	5 (1 oz)	30	0	0	0	0	7	6	tr	0	330	—	—	1
S&W														
Cut	½ cup (4.2 oz)	20	0	0	0	1	4	2	2	20	390	—	—	2
Dilled	1 oz	20	0	0	0	0	5	3	1	0	125	—	—	0
FRESH														
cooked w/o salt	1 cup	44	tr	tr	0	2	10	2	4	55	1	183	41	12
raw	1 cup	34	tr	tr	0	2	8	2	4	41	7	230	41	18
raw whole beans	10	17	tr	tr	0	1	4	1	2	20	3	115	20	9
GREENLINE														
Fresh Trimmed	3 oz	25	0	0	0	1	5	3	2	40	0	—	—	5
READY PAC														
Fast 'N Fresh as prep	1 cup (3 oz)	30	0	0	0	2	7	1	3	40	0	—	—	9
FROZEN														
cooked	1 cup	38	tr	tr	0	2	9	2	4	66	12	170	31	6
BIRDS EYE														
Steamfresh Whole	1 cup (2.9 oz)	35	0	0	0	1	5	2	2	40	0	—	—	5
C&W														
French Cut	1 cup	30	0	0	0	1	5	2	2	40	0	—	—	4
CASCADIAN FARM														
Organic Petite Whole	1 cup	25	0	0	0	1	5	1	2	20	90	140	—	4
GREEN GIANT														
Green Bean Casserole	⅔ cup	110	8	3	0	2	8	2	1	20	460	—	—	4
TAKE-OUT														
casscrole w/ mushroom sauce	1 cup	108	6	2	2	3	11	3	3	79	525	176	21	4
pickled	½ cup	19	tr	tr	0	1	4	1	2	22	160	128	19	8

GREENS

FOOD	PORTION	CALS	FAT	SAT FAT	CHOL	PROT	CARB	SUGAR	FIBER	CALCI	SOD	POTAS	FOLIC	VIT C
ALLENS														
Seasoned Mixed	½ cup	45	1	0	0	4	6	2	1	150	830	—	—	12

GROUNDCHERRIES

FOOD	PORTION	CALS	FAT	SAT FAT	CHOL	PROT	CARB	SUGAR	FIBER	CALCI	SOD	POTAS	FOLIC	VIT C
fresh	½ cup	37	tr	—	0	1	8	—	—	6	—	—	—	8

GROUPER

FOOD	PORTION	CALS	FAT	SAT FAT	CHOL	PROT	CARB	SUGAR	FIBER	CALCI	SOD	POTAS	FOLIC	VIT C
cooked	3 oz	100	1	tr	40	21	0	0	0	18	45	403	—	—
cooked	1 fillet (7.1 oz)	238	3	1	95	50	0	0	0	42	107	959	—	—
raw	3 oz	78	1	tr	31	16	0	0	0	23	45	410	—	—

GUAR GUM

FOOD	PORTION	CALS	FAT	SAT FAT	CHOL	PROT	CARB	SUGAR	FIBER	CALCI	SOD	POTAS	FOLIC	VIT C
BOB'S RED MILL														
Guar Gum	1 tbsp	20	0	0	0	0	6	0	6	—	2	—	—	—

FOOD	PORTION	CALS	FAT	SAT FAT	CHOL	PROT	CARB	SUGAR	FIBER	CALCI	SOD	POTAS	FOLIC	VIT C
GUAVA														
fresh	1 (1.9 oz)	37	1	tr	0	1	8	5	3	10	1	229	27	126
fresh cut up	1 cup (5.8 oz)	112	2	tr	0	4	24	15	9	30	3	688	81	377
fresh strawberry	1 (6 g)	4	tr	tr	0	tr	1	—	tr	1	2	18	—	2
fresh strawberry cut up	1 cup (8.6 oz)	168	1	tr	0	1	42	—	13	51	90	712	—	90
guava paste	1 piece (1.1 oz)	90	tr	tr	0	tr	23	23	tr	1	1	22	1	14
GUAVA JUICE														
nectar canned	8 oz	143	tr	—	—	tr	37	31	3	28	18	95	8	49
APPLE & EVE														
Nectar	5 oz	130	0	0	0	0	32	25	—	—	35	—	—	60
CERES														
100% Juice	8 oz	120	0	0	0	0	30	27	2	0	10	250	—	60
OKF														
Sparkling Fresh Guava	1 bottle (8.3 oz)	20	0	0	0	0	13	1	3	0	3	—	—	0
SABOR LATINO														
Nectar + Calcium	8 oz	160	0	0	0	0	39	38	—	200	20	55	—	60
GUINEA HEN														
boneless w/o skin raw	½ hen (9.3 oz)	290	7	2	166	54	0	0	0	29	182	581	16	5
w/ skin raw	½ hen (12 oz)	545	22	6	255	81	0	0	0	38	231	666	17	5
GRIMAUD FARMS														
Guinea Fowl	1 serv (3.7 oz)	130	4	2	105	25	tr	—	—	0	40	410	—	0
HADDOCK														
fresh broiled	4 oz	127	1	tr	84	27	0	0	0	48	99	452	15	0
roe raw	1 oz	37	tr	—	103	7	tr	—	—	—	—	—	—	4
smoked	1 oz	33	tr	tr	22	7	0	0	0	14	216	118	4	0
VAN DE KAMP'S														
Battered Fillets	2 (3.6 oz)	210	11	4	20	9	21	5	2	0	580	—	—	0
TAKE-OUT														
breaded & fried	4 oz	229	10	2	88	23	10	1	1	66	528	380	24	0
HAGGIS														
scottish haggis	1 serv (6.4 oz)	473	32	15	77	16	31	3	5	—	456	—	—	—
CALEDONIAN KITCHEN														
Highland Beef	3 oz	173	10	5	4	8	12	2	2	50	460	—	—	0
Vegetarian	3 oz	190	13	2	5	7	12	0	3	40	320	—	—	0
HOUSE OF KENTON														
Vegetarian	1 serv (3.5 oz)	249	20	—	—	3	14	—	—	—	—	—	—	—
MACSWEEN														
Traditional	1 (8 oz)	260	16	7	—	12	18	0	—	—	710	—	—	—
Vegetarian	1 (8 oz)	238	12	3	—	7	22	1	—	—	450	—	—	—

FOOD	PORTION	CALS	FAT	SAT FAT	CHOL	PROT	CARB	SUGAR	FIBER	CALCI	SOD	POTAS	FOLIC	VIT C
HALIBUT														
atlantic & pacific cooked	½ fillet (5.6 oz)	223	5	1	65	42	0	0	0	95	110	916	—	—
atlantic & pacific cooked	3 oz	119	2	tr	35	23	0	0	0	51	59	490	—	—
atlantic & pacific raw	3 oz	93	2	tr	27	18	0	0	0	40	46	382	—	—
greenland baked	3 oz	203	15	2	50	16	0	0	0	3	87	292	1	—
greenland baked	5.6 oz	380	28	5	94	29	0	0	0	6	163	546	2	—
FROZEN														
VAN DE KAMP'S														
Battered Fillets	3 (4 oz)	230	11	4	25	10	22	3	0	0	630	—	—	0
HAM														
boneless extra lean roasted	3 oz	123	5	2	45	18	1	0	0	7	1023	244	3	0
boneless roasted	3 oz	151	8	3	50	19	0	0	0	7	1275	348	3	0
canned extra lean roasted	3 oz	116	4	1	26	18	tr	—	0	5	965	296	4	0
canned lean roasted	3 oz	142	7	2	35	18	tr	—	0	6	908	298	4	0
center slice lean & fat roasted	3 oz	173	11	4	46	17	tr	—	0	6	1179	287	3	0
deviled	¼ cup	188	17	6	35	7	1	0	0	3	724	121	3	1
ham salad spread	2 tbsp	65	5	2	11	3	3	0	0	2	274	45	0	0
patty grilled	1 patty (2 oz)	205	19	7	43	8	1	0	0	5	638	146	2	0
prosciutto	4 slices (1.3 oz)	72	3	1	26	10	tr	0	0	4	992	188	2	0
sliced	3 slices (2.9 oz)	137	7	2	48	14	3	0	1	20	1095	241	6	3
sliced extra lean	3 slices (2.2 oz)	69	2	1	30	11	2	0	0	6	697	221	3	0
westphalian smoked	1 oz	105	10	—	—	5	0	0	0	3	398	70	—	—
whole roasted	3 oz	207	14	5	53	18	0	0	0	6	1009	243	3	0
APPLEGATE FARMS														
Organic Uncured	2 oz	70	2	1	35	10	1	0	0	0	530	—	—	0
BOAR'S HEAD														
Black Forest Smoked	2 oz	60	1	0	30	10	2	2	0	0	580	—	—	0
Deluxe	2 oz	60	1	0	25	9	2	2	0	0	590	—	—	0
Deluxe 42% Lowered Sodium	2 oz	60	1	0	25	10	2	2	0	0	460	—	—	0
Fresh Seasoned	2 oz	90	3	2	35	14	1	1	0	0	310	—	—	0
Maple Glazed Honey	2 oz	60	1	0	20	10	3	3	0	0	570	—	—	0
Pepper	2 oz	60	1	0	20	10	2	1	0	0	610	—	—	0
Virginia Smoked	2 oz	60	1	0	25	9	2	2	0	0	590	—	—	0

FOOD	PORTION	CALS	FAT	SAT FAT	CHOL	PROT	CARB	SUGAR	FIBER	CALCI	SOD	POTAS	FOLIC	VIT C
CARL BUDDIG														
Ham Sliced	2 oz	85	5	—	—	10	1	—	—	—	—	—	—	—
Honey Ham Sliced	2 oz	90	5	—	—	10	2	—	—	—	—	—	—	—
DIETZ & WATSON														
Boneless Old Fashioned	3 oz	110	5	2	40	14	1	1	0	0	720	—	—	0
Smoked	2 oz	80	3	1	30	11	1	1	0	0	480	—	—	0
Steak Our Traditional	5 oz	100	3	1	50	18	2	2	0	0	680	—	—	0
HEALTHY ONES														
Honey 97% Fat Free	7 slices (2 oz)	90	2	1	20	9	2	2	—	—	410	—	—	—
HORMEL														
Chunk Ham canned	2 oz	90	6	2	30	9	0	0	0	0	620	—	—	0
Deli Cooked	4 slices (2 oz)	70	2	1	30	10	1	1	0	0	500	—	—	0
Deli Honey	4 slices (2 oz)	70	2	1	25	9	3	3	0	0	500	—	—	0
Deli Smoked	4 slices (2 oz)	60	2	1	25	9	1	1	0	0	500	—	—	0
Dinner	2 oz	70	2	0	30	10	2	1	0	0	550	—	—	0
JONES														
Steak Extra Lean	3 oz	100	4	1	50	14	2	—	—	—	760	—	—	21
ORGANIC PRAIRIE														
Hardwood Smoked Bone In Spiral Cut	3 oz	110	3	1	40	19	tr	tr	0	0	940	—	—	0
OSCAR MAYER														
Ham Brown Sugar Thin Sliced	⅓ pkg (2 oz)	70	2	0	25	10	4	4	—	—	830	—	—	—
Virginia Shaved	2 oz	50	1	1	25	9	1	0	0	0	570	—	—	0
SARA LEE														
Bavarian Oven Roasted Honey	2 oz	70	4	1	40	9	2	2	0	0	560	—	—	9
Brown Sugar	2 oz	70	3	0	20	10	5	4	0	0	600	—	—	0
Homestyle Baked	2 oz	60	2	1	25	10	2	2	0	0	600	—	—	12
Virginia Baked	4 slices (1.8 oz)	60	2	1	20	10	2	1	0	0	550	—	—	0
TYSON														
Glazed Ham Maple & Brown Sugar	1 serv (5 oz)	180	5	2	60	17	18	16	0	20	780	—	—	0
Honey Ham	2 slices (1.6 oz)	50	2	1	25	9	1	1	0	0	740	—	—	0
TAKE-OUT														
croquette	1 (2.2 oz)	149	9	2	18	9	8	2	tr	43	532	148	11	tr
salad	½ cup	287	23	5	237	16	5	—	tr	33	671	232	22	1
spam musubi	1 serv (6 oz)	253	6	2	14	6	42	—	1	19	283	134	7	1
thick slice fried	1 (2.2 oz)	140	9	3	33	13	tr	0	0	4	756	202	2	0

HAMBURGER

FOOD	PORTION	CALS	FAT	SAT FAT	CHOL	PROT	CARB	SUGAR	FIBER	CALCI	SOD	POTAS	FOLIC	VIT C
APPLEGATE FARMS														
Organic Beef Cooked	1 (3 oz)	195	12	5	70	21	0	0	0	0	85	—	—	0
Organic Turkey Burger	1 (4 oz)	190	11	3	75	22	0	0	0	20	70	—	—	0
FARM RICH														
Cheeseburgers Mini Bacon	2 (2.2 oz)	150	7	4	15	7	14	2	1	80	470	—	—	1
FOSTER FARMS														
Cheeseburgers Mini Chicken w/ BBQ Sauce	1 (1.3 oz)	90	4	2	18	5	9	1	0	—	200	—	—	—
HOT POCKETS														
Cheeseburger	1 (4.5 oz)	310	13	6	25	11	37	9	2	150	630	—	60	—
IAN'S														
Mini	2 (4.6 oz)	360	12	4	25	23	42	5	1	0	450	—	—	0
Mini Cheeseburger	2 (5 oz)	420	17	6	65	25	42	5	1	100	540	—	—	0
LEAN POCKETS														
Cheeseburger	1 (4.5 oz)	280	7	4	25	12	40	12	3	200	560	—	—	—
OSCAR MAYER														
Lunchables All-Star Burgers	1 pkg	420	14	9	35	14	60	38	1	200	980	—	—	0
QUAKER MAID														
Pure Beef Patties	1 (4 oz)	240	18	7	50	19	0	0	0	0	40	—	—	0
TAKE-OUT														
cheeseburger + condiments	1 reg (4.5 oz)	347	17	7	46	17	28	5	1	164	644	221	26	1
double hamburger + condiments	1 reg (5.8 oz)	384	19	7	66	23	30	7	2	98	809	339	30	3
single patty + condiments	1 reg (4 oz)	299	11	4	33	15	35	8	2	104	589	277	67	5

HAMBURGER SUBSTITUTES

(see also MEAT SUBSTITUTES)

FOOD	PORTION	CALS	FAT	SAT FAT	CHOL	PROT	CARB	SUGAR	FIBER	CALCI	SOD	POTAS	FOLIC	VIT C
AMY'S														
All American Burger	1 (2.5 oz)	120	3	0	0	10	15	2	3	40	390	—	—	4
Cheddar Veggie Burger	1 (2.5 oz)	160	5	2	5	8	20	2	3	80	430	—	—	2
Texas Burger	1 (2.5 oz)	120	3	0	0	12	14	2	3	40	350	—	—	1
ASHERAH'S GOURMET														
Organic Quinoa Vegan Burgers	1 (4 oz)	180	5	3	0	6	30	3	5	60	190	400	60	5

FOOD	PORTION	CALS	FAT	SAT FAT	CHOL	PROT	CARB	SUGAR	FIBER	CALCI	SOD	POTAS	FOLIC	VIT C
BOCA														
Cheeseburger	1 (2.5 oz)	100	5	2	5	12	5	0	3	0	360	—	—	5
Ground Burger	1 serv (2 oz)	60	1	0	0	13	6	0	3	60	270	—	—	0
DR. PRAEGER'S														
Texmex	1 (4 oz)	170	6	1	0	7	20	3	6	80	370	—	—	4
Veggie Burger Bombay	1 (4 oz)	170	6	1	0	7	20	3	6	80	370	—	—	4
Veggie Burger California	1 (4 oz)	170	6	0	0	7	21	2	5	60	310	—	—	0
Veggie Burger California Slider	1 (1.6 oz)	80	4	0	0	3	8	1	2	30	150	—	—	4
FANTASTIC														
Natures Burger Mix not prep	¼ cup	170	3	0	0	8	30	2	5	60	320	—	—	2
Tofu Burger Mix not prep	3 tbsp	80	3	0	0	3	13	0	1	40	400	—	—	0
GARDENBURGER														
Black Bean Chipotle	1 (2.5 oz)	80	3	0	0	5	13	1	5	20	250	—	—	5
Flame Grilled	1 (2.5 oz)	90	4	0	0	11	5	0	4	60	420	—	—	0
GardenVegan	1 (2.5 oz)	100	1	0	0	10	12	0	3	40	230	—	—	0
Original	1 (2.5 oz)	100	4	1	5	5	14	1	5	20	420	—	—	1
Portabella	1 (2.5 oz)	90	3	1	5	5	15	1	5	60	360	—	—	1
HARMONY VALLEY														
Vegetarian Hamburger Mix as prep	1 (3 oz)	120	5	3	0	14	8	1	4	40	360	—	—	0
LIGHTLIFE														
Light Burgers	1 (3 oz)	120	2	0	0	16	11	0	3	—	500	520	—	—
Smart Menu Burger	1	80	1	0	0	4	14	1	2	—	360	200	—	—
MORNINGSTAR FARMS														
Classic Burger	1 (2.2 oz)	150	7	1	0	14	10	2	3	0	340	350	—	0
Okara Pattie	1 (2.2 oz)	120	5	1	0	12	6	tr	3	0	300	240	—	0
Vegan Burger	1 (2.5 oz)	100	2	0	0	13	8	2	5	20	460	260	—	0
SUNSHINE														
Organic Garden Burger	1 (2.6 oz)	250	13	2	0	8	14	2	3	40	320	—	—	6
SUNSHINE BURGERS														
Original	1 (2.6 oz)	190	13	2	0	8	14	3	3	40	320	—	—	6
VEGGIE BITES														
Garlic Portabella	1 (2.5 oz)	120	6	1	0	11	8	1	4	200	320	—	—	1
WILDWOOD														
Organic Original Burgers Tofu-Veggie	1 (3.2 oz)	180	13	2	0	12	8	1	1	20	330	0	—	4

FOOD	PORTION	CALS	FAT	SAT FAT	CHOL	PROT	CARB	SUGAR	FIBER	CALCI	SOD	POTAS	FOLIC	VIT C
YVES														
Meatless Chicken Burger	1 (2.6 oz)	100	3	0	0	15	5	tr	2	80	420	240	—	5

HAZELNUTS

FOOD	PORTION	CALS	FAT	SAT FAT	CHOL	PROT	CARB	SUGAR	FIBER	CALCI	SOD	POTAS	FOLIC	VIT C
chocolate hazelnut spread	2 tbsp (1.3 oz)	200	11	11	0	2	23	20	2	40	15	151	5	0
chopped	¼ cup (1 oz)	181	17	1	0	4	5	1	3	33	0	196	32	2
ground	¼ cup (0.7 oz)	118	11	1	0	3	3	1	1	21	0	128	21	1
whole	¼ cup (1.2 oz)	212	21	2	0	5	6	1	3	38	0	230	38	2
whole nuts	21 (1 oz)	178	17	1	0	4	5	1	3	32	0	193	32	2
CHUKAR CHERRIES														
Chocolate Covered Spiced	3 tbsp (1.4 oz)	228	17	7	4	4	21	16	2	10	15	—	—	1
FISHER														
Chopped	¼ cup (1 oz)	180	17	1	0	4	5	1	3	40	0	—	—	1
FUNDELINA														
Choco-Hazelnut Spread All Flavors	2 tbsp (1.3 oz)	200	11	4	0	3	23	21	2	40	14	—	—	0
KETTLE														
Butter Creamy Unsalted	2 tbsp	180	17	1	0	4	5	1	3	40	0	—	—	1
LOVE'N BAKE														
Hazelnut Praline	2 tbsp	170	12	1	0	3	13	10	2	10	0	—	—	1

HEART

FOOD	PORTION	CALS	FAT	SAT FAT	CHOL	PROT	CARB	SUGAR	FIBER	CALCI	SOD	POTAS	FOLIC	VIT C
beef simmered	3 oz	140	4	1	180	24	tr	0	0	4	50	186	4	0
chicken cooked	1 (3 g)	5	tr	tr	6	1	0	0	0	0	11	7	0	0
chicken diced simmered	½ cup	134	6	2	175	19	tr	—	0	14	35	96	58	1
lamb braised	3 oz	157	7	3	212	21	2	—	0	12	54	160	2	6
pork braised	1 (4.5 oz)	191	7	2	285	30	1	—	0	9	45	266	5	3
turkey simmered	½ cup	94	3	1	133	16	tr	0	0	5	65	211	6	2
veal braised	3 oz	158	6	2	150	25	tr	—	0	7	49	169	2	9
RUMBA														
Beef	4 oz	130	4	2	155	19	3	0	0	20	70	—	—	6

HEARTS OF PALM

FOOD	PORTION	CALS	FAT	SAT FAT	CHOL	PROT	CARB	SUGAR	FIBER	CALCI	SOD	POTAS	FOLIC	VIT C
canned	½ cup	20	tr	tr	0	2	3	—	2	42	311	129	28	6
canned	1 (1.2 oz)	9	tr	tr	0	1	2	—	1	19	141	58	13	3
DEL MONTE														
Hearts Of Palm	2–3 pieces (4.4 oz)	20	0	0	0	2	3	0	2	40	450	—	—	9
NATIVE FOREST														
Organic	1 oz	15	0	0	0	1	2	0	1	40	125	—	—	2

FOOD	PORTION	CALS	FAT	SAT FAT	CHOL	PROT	CARB	SUGAR	FIBER	CALCI	SOD	POTAS	FOLIC	VIT C
HEMP														
LIVING HARVEST														
Organic Hemp Nuts	2 tbsp (1 oz)	170	12	1	0	10	5	1	0	20	0	—	—	1
Organic Protein Powder	2 scoops (1 oz)	110	3	0	0	14	9	8	1	60	0	—	—	1
MANITOBA HARVEST														
Hemp Seed Butter	2 tbsp	160	10	1	0	11	7	1	1	0	10	—	—	0
Organic Pro Fiber	4 tbsp (1 oz)	127	3	tr	0	11	14	0	14	40	10	—	—	1
Organic Protein Dark Chocolate	4 tbsp (1 oz)	120	3	1	0	8	17	6	9	40	10	—	—	1
Shelled Seed	2 tbsp	160	10	1	0	11	7	1	1	0	10	—	—	0
NUTIVA														
Organic Protein Powder	2 scoops (1 oz)	120	3	0	0	11	14	0	14	40	15	—	—	—
Shelled Hempseed	2 tbsp	110	8	1	0	6	2	tr	1	—	0	210	—	—
HERBAL TEA														
(*see* TEA/HERBAL TEA)														
HERBS/SPICES														
(*see also individual names*)														
cajun seasoning	1 tbsp	19	1	—	—	1	3	—	1	—	5	—	—	—
chinese five spice	1 tsp	7	tr	—	—	0	2	—	tr	4	1	23	—	—
garam masala	1 tsp	8	tr	—	0	tr	1	—	—	15	2	29	0	0
poultry seasoning	1 tsp	5	tr	tr	0	tr	1	tr	tr	15	tr	10	2	tr
pumpkin pie spice	1 tsp (1.7 g)	6	tr	tr	0	tr	1	tr	tr	12	1	11	1	tr
BRAGG														
Herb & Spice Seasoning	¼ tsp	0	0	0	0	0	0	0	0	—	0	—	—	—
CHEF PAUL PRUDHOMME'S														
Magic Blackened Redfish	¼ tsp	0	0	0	0	0	0	0	0	—	95	—	—	—
Magic Pork & Veal	¼ tsp	0	0	0	0	0	0	0	0	—	130	—	—	—
DAVE'S GOURMET														
Insanity Spice	¼ tsp (1 g)	5	0	0	0	0	0	0	0	0	0	—	—	0
LAWRY'S														
Spices & Seasonings Chimichurri Burrito Casserole	1 tbsp (7 g)	20	0	0	0	tr	5	—	—	—	460	—	—	—
Spices & Seasonings Tuscan Chicken Marsala	1 tbsp (7 g)	20	0	0	0	tr	5	—	—	—	460	—	—	—
MCCORMICK														
Grill Mates Rub Applewood	2 tsp	15	0	0	0	0	3	1	0	—	350	—	—	—

FOOD	PORTION	CALS	FAT	SAT FAT	CHOL	PROT	CARB	SUGAR	FIBER	CALCI	SOD	POTAS	FOLIC	VIT C
MCCORMICK (CONT.)														
Meat Tenderizer Seasoned	¼ tsp (1 g)	0	0	0	0	0	0	0	0	—	300	—	—	—
Perfect Pinch Salt Free Original	¼ tsp	0	0	0	0	0	0	0	0	—	0	—	—	—
MODERN DAY MASALA														
Organic Garam Masala	1 tsp (3 g)	10	0	0	0	0	2	—	1	20	0	—	—	—
MRS. DASH														
Grilling Blend Steak	¼ tsp (0.7 g)	0	0	0	0	0	0	0	0	—	0	5	—	—
Original Blend	¼ tsp (0.7 g)	0	0	0	0	0	0	0	0	—	0	10	—	—
Seasoning Blends Caribbean Citrus	¼ tsp (0.7 g)	0	0	0	0	0	0	0	0	—	0	5	—	—
Seasoning Blends Garlic & Herb	¼ tsp (0.7 g)	0	0	0	0	0	0	0	0	—	0	10	—	—
Seasoning Blends Italian Medley	¼ tsp (0.7 g)	0	0	0	0	0	0	0	0	—	0	10	—	—
Seasoning Blends Table Blend	¼ tsp (0.7 g)	0	0	0	0	0	0	0	0	—	0	10	—	—
OLD BAY														
Seasoning	¼ tsp (0.6 g)	0	0	0	0	0	0	0	0	—	160	—	—	—
Seasoning 30% Less Sodium	¼ tsp (0.6 g)	0	0	0	0	0	0	0	0	—	95	—	—	—
RIBBER CITY														
Rib-A-Dub-Rub Dry Rub Seasoning	¼ tsp (0.8 oz)	3	0	0	0	0	1	0	0	—	57	—	—	—
SPICE HUNTER														
All Purpose Blend	¼ tsp	0	0	0	0	0	0	0	0	—	0	—	—	—
Greek Seasoning Salt Free	¼ tsp	0	0	0	0	0	0	0	0	—	0	—	—	—
HERRING														
atlantic baked	4 oz	230	13	3	87	26	0	0	0	84	130	475	14	1
dried salted	1 fillet (1.4 oz)	161	9	2	61	18	0	0	0	62	680	331	9	1
pickled	1 oz	74	5	1	4	4	3	—	0	22	247	20	1	0
pickled in cream sauce	1 oz	72	5	1	5	3	2	tr	0	24	200	24	1	tr
roe	1 tbsp	39	2	tr	105	6	tr	0	0	6	25	62	21	4
smoked kippered	1 oz	62	4	1	23	7	0	0	0	24	260	127	4	tr
TAKE-OUT														
breaded fried	1 serv (4 oz)	225	14	3	67	15	9	1	1	68	432	264	17	tr
HIBISCUS														
flowers dried sweetened	⅓ cup	100	0	0	0	0	23	21	2	40	15	—	—	0

FOOD	PORTION	CALS	FAT	SAT FAT	CHOL	PROT	CARB	SUGAR	FIBER	CALCI	SOD	POTAS	FOLIC	VIT C
SANTA CRUZ														
Organic Hibiscus Cooler	8 oz	100	0	0	0	tr	24	24	0	—	40	70	—	—
HICKORY NUTS														
dried	1 oz	187	18	2	0	4	5	—	—	17	0	124	—	—
HOMINY														
white canned	1 cup	119	1	tr	0	2	24	3	4	16	246	15	2	0
yellow canned	½ cup	115	1	tr	0	2	23	—	4	16	336	14	2	0
ALLENS														
White	½ cup	100	1	0	0	2	22	1	4	0	340	—	—	0
BUSH'S														
Golden	½ cup	60	0	0	0	1	13	0	3	20	550	—	—	1
HONEY														
honey	1 tbsp (0.7 oz)	64	0	0	0	tr	17	17	—	1	1	11	0	tr
honey	¼ cup (3 oz)	258	0	0	0	tr	70	70	tr	5	3	44	2	tr
orange blossom	1 tbsp	60	0	0	0	0	17	16	0	0	0	—	—	0
wild honey	1 tbsp	60	0	0	0	0	17	16	—	—	0	—	—	—
COMFORT CARE														
Raw Clover	1 tbsp (0.7 oz)	60	0	0	0	0	17	16	—	—	0	—	—	—
DUTCH GOLD														
Clover	1 tbsp	60	0	0	0	0	17	16	0	—	0	—	—	—
MAPLE GROVE FARMS														
Honey Maple Spread	2 tbsp (1.5 oz)	160	0	0	0	0	42	37	—	40	60	—	—	—
STEEL'S														
Sugar Free	1 tbsp (0.5 oz)	24	0	0	0	0	11	0	0	0	0	—	—	0
SUEBEE														
Honey	1 tbsp (0.7 oz)	60	0	0	0	0	17	16	—	—	0	—	—	—
TASTES LIKE HONEY														
Sugar Free	1 tbsp (0.7 oz)	21	0	0	0	0	0	0	0	—	0	—	—	—
TREE OF LIFE														
Alfalfa Honey Raw Unfiltered	1 tbsp	60	0	0	0	0	17	16	—	—	0	—	—	—
Avocado Honey Raw Unfiltered	1 tbsp (0.7 oz)	60	0	0	0	0	17	16	0	0	0	—	—	0
Buckwheat Honey Raw Unfiltered	1 tbsp	60	0	0	0	0	17	16	—	—	0	—	—	—
Tupelo Honey Raw Unfiltered	1 tbsp	60	0	0	0	0	17	16	—	—	0	—	—	—
WHOLESOME SWEETENERS														
Organic Fair Trade Amber	1 tbsp	60	0	0	0	0	17	16	0	0	0	—	—	—
Organic Fair Trade Raw	1 tbsp (0.7 oz)	60	0	0	0	0	17	16	0	0	0	—	—	—

FOOD	PORTION	CALS	FAT	SAT FAT	CHOL	PROT	CARB	SUGAR	FIBER	CALCI	SOD	POTAS	FOLIC	VIT C
HONEYDEW														
balls frzn	1 cup (8 oz)	83	tr	tr	0	1	21	19	2	14	41	524	44	41
fresh cut up	1 cup	61	tr	tr	0	1	15	14	1	10	31	388	32	31
fresh wedge	⅛ melon (4.5 oz)	45	tr	tr	0	1	11	10	1	8	22	285	24	23
whole fresh	1 (35 oz)	360	1	tr	0	5	91	81	8	60	180	2280	190	180
CHIQUITA														
Fresh Cut Up	1 cup (6.2 oz)	64	0	0	0	1	16	14	1	10	32	404	—	32
DOLE														
Fresh	⅒ med (4.7 oz)	50	0	0	0	tr	12	11	1	20	25	—	—	24
HORSE														
roasted	3 oz	149	5	2	58	24	0	0	0	7	47	322	—	2
HORSERADISH														
japanese wasabi	¼ tsp	1	—	—	0	—	tr	—	0	2	0	5	tr	1
sauce	1 tbsp	7	tr	tr	0	tr	2	1	1	8	47	37	9	4
wasabi root raw	1 (5.9 oz)	184	1	—	0	8	40	—	13	216	29	960	30	71
wasabi root raw sliced	½ cup (2.3 oz)	71	tr	—	0	3	15	—	5	83	11	369	12	27
BOAR'S HEAD														
Horseradish	1 tsp (5 g)	0	0	0	0	0	0	0	0	0	30	—	—	0
Horseradish Sauce Pub Style	1 tsp	15	2	0	5	0	1	0	0	0	15	—	0	—
Horseradish & Beets	1 tsp	0	0	0	0	0	0	0	0	0	30	—	—	0
DIETZ & WATSON														
Cranberry Horseradish Sauce	1 tsp (5 g)	10	1	0	0	0	1	1	0	0	5	—	—	0
GOLD'S														
Horse Radish	1 tsp (5 g)	0	0	0	0	0	0	0	0	—	30	—	—	—
ROBERT ROTHCHILD FARM														
Sauce	1 tsp	20	2	1	<5	0	1	tr	0	0	30	—	—	0
SARA LEE														
Horseradish Sauce	1 tbsp	20	2	0	0	0	0	0	0	0	45	—	—	0
ZATARAIN'S														
Prepared	1 tbsp (0.5 oz)	15	0	0	0	0	2	0	0	0	90	—	—	0
HOT CHOCOLATE														
mix not prep	1 pkg (1 oz)	111	1	1	0	2	23	18	1	37	141	199	2	tr
mix w/ no calorie sweetener as prep w/ water	8 oz	72	1	tr	0	3	14	7	2	120	180	528	2	0
mix w/ sugar as prep w/ nonfat milk	8 oz	209	1	1	5	9	30	29	1	360	128	432	12	4

FOOD	PORTION	CALS	FAT	SAT FAT	CHOL	PROT	CARB	SUGAR	FIBER	CALCI	SOD	POTAS	FOLIC	VIT C
mix w/ sugar as prep w/ water	8 oz	138	1	1	0	2	29	23	1	52	182	245	2	0
HERSHEY'S														
Goodnight Hugs	1 pkg (1.2 oz)	140	3	2	<5	3	27	26	—	100	190	—	—	0
NESTLE														
Hot Cocoa Milk Chocolate	1 pkg (1 oz)	80	3	2	0	tr	15	13	tr	20	180	—	—	0
Hot Cocoa Rich Milk Chocolate as prep w/ water	1 pkg (0.7 oz)	80	3	2	0	tr	14	12	tr	350	180	—	—	0
Hot Cocoa Mix Fat Free as prep	1 pkg	20	0	0	0	1	4	4	tr	350	130	—	—	0
SILHOUETTE SOLUTION														
Down East not prep	1 pkg (0.88 oz)	90	2	1	0	15	5	1	1	250	300	150	—	0
STARBUCKS														
Hot Cocoa Mix	1 pkg	130	2	1	0	4	28	24	2	80	170	—	—	1
SWISS MISS														
Cocoa Caramel as prep	1 pkg	120	3	2	0	1	22	17	tr	0	160	—	—	0
Cocoa No Sugar Added as prep	1 pkg	60	1	1	0	2	10	7	1	300	170	—	—	0
Cocoa Rich Creamy as prep	1 pkg	110	2	2	<5	2	22	16	tr	150	170	—	—	0
Cocoa w/ Marshmallows as prep	1 pkg	120	2	2	0	1	24	16	1	40	150	—	—	0
Cocoa w/ Marshmallows Fat Free as prep	1 pkg	140	3	2	0	1	29	21	1	40	160	—	—	0
French Vanilla as prep	1 pkg	110	2	2	0	2	24	18	tr	60	160	—	—	0
Milk Chocolate as prep	1 pkg	120	3	2	0	1	23	17	1	40	170	—	—	0
TAKE-OUT														
chocolate caliente w/ lowfat milk	1 serv (8.4 oz)	221	9	6	12	11	27	25	1	384	158	487	10	1
chocolate caliente w/ whole milk	1 serv (8.4 oz)	276	17	10	38	10	25	23	1	353	149	458	10	2
hot chocolate	1 cup (8.7 oz)	192	6	4	20	9	30	24	3	262	110	492	12	1
mexican hot chocolate	1 cup	173	6	4	18	10	20	—	1	306	150	442	13	2
HOT DOG														
(see also HOT DOG SUBSTITUTES)														
beef	1 (1.5 oz)	149	13	5	24	5	2	2	0	6	513	70	2	0
beef & pork	1 (1.5 oz)	137	12	5	23	5	1	0	1	5	504	75	2	0

FOOD	PORTION	CALS	FAT	SAT FAT	CHOL	PROT	CARB	SUGAR	FIBER	CALCI	SOD	POTAS	FOLIC	VIT C
beef lowfat	1 (2 oz)	133	11	5	23	7	1	0	0	5	593	74	2	1
chicken	1 (1.5 oz)	116	9	2	45	6	3	0	0	43	617	38	2	0
fat free	1 (2 oz)	62	1	tr	23	7	6	0	0	31	455	125	3	14
low sodium	1 (2 oz)	180	16	7	35	7	1	0	0	11	177	95	2	0
lowfat	1 (2 oz)	88	6	2	25	6	3	0	0	6	716	86	2	0
pork and beef cheese smokie	1 (1.5 oz)	141	12	5	29	6	1	1	0	25	465	89	1	0
turkey	1 (1.5 oz)	102	8	3	48	6	1	0	0	48	642	81	4	0
ABELES&HEYMANN														
Beef Uncured Reduced Fat & Sodium	1 (1.7 oz)	120	9	4	30	8	1	0	0	20	110	—	—	6
APPLEGATE FARMS														
The Great Uncured Beef	1 (2 oz)	110	8	3	30	7	0	0	0	0	330	—	—	0
The Great Uncured Chicken	1 (1.7 oz)	70	4	1	35	8	0	0	0	0	420	—	—	0
The Great Uncured Turkey	1 (1.7 oz)	60	4	1	25	7	1	0	0	0	370	—	—	0
Uncured Big Apple	1 (2 oz)	110	9	4	30	7	1	0	0	0	360	—	—	0
Uncured Beef	1 (1.5 oz)	70	6	2	20	6	0	0	0	0	330	—	—	0
BALL PARK														
Franks	1 (2 oz)	180	16	6	40	6	3	3	0	40	560	340	—	4
Franks Beef	1 (2 oz)	180	16	7	35	6	3	2	0	0	550	360	—	4
Franks Bun Size	1 (2 oz)	180	16	6	40	6	3	3	0	40	560	340	—	4
Franks Smoked White Turkey	1 (1.8 oz)	45	0	0	10	6	5	3	0	0	420	450	—	4
Franks Fat Free	1 (1.8 oz)	40	0	0	10	5	4	2	0	0	420	430	—	4
Franks Lite	1 (1.8 oz)	100	7	3	25	6	3	1	0	20	460	340	—	4
Franks Singles Cheese	1 (1.6 oz)	150	13	5	30	5	2	2	0	60	460	280	—	2
Grillmaster Hearty Beef	1	250	23	9	50	9	3	1	0	0	780	520	—	8
Grillmaster Smokehouse	1	210	24	9	50	9	3	2	0	0	790	540	—	6
BOAR'S HEAD														
Beef	1 (2 oz)	160	14	6	30	7	1	0	0	0	440	—	—	0
Beef Cocktail	5 (2 oz)	170	15	6	30	8	0	0	0	0	430	—	—	—
Beef Lite	1 (1.6 oz)	90	6	3	25	7	0	0	0	0	270	—	—	0
Pork & Beef	1 (2 oz)	150	14	5	25	7	0	0	0	0	460	—	—	0
DIETZ & WATSON														
Beef Foot Long	1 (4 oz)	310	26	10	60	14	4	4	0	0	980	—	—	0
Black Forest Wieners	1 (2 oz)	180	16	6	30	8	0	0	0	0	480	—	—	0

FOOD	PORTION	CALS	FAT	SAT FAT	CHOL	PROT	CARB	SUGAR	FIBER	CALCI	SOD	POTAS	FOLIC	VIT C
DIETZ & WATSON (CONT.)														
Gourmet Lite	1 (2 oz)	60	2	1	15	7	5	1	0	0	390	—	—	0
Super Franks	1 (3.2 oz)	270	24	8	40	11	3	3	0	0	780	—	—	0
FOSTER FARMS														
Chicken	1 (2 oz)	140	12	—	30	7	1	tr	0	100	550	—	—	—
Corn Dog Chili Cheese	1 (2.6 oz)	190	9	3	25	7	21	4	1	80	670	—	—	—
Corn Dog Extreme Cheese	1 (2.6 oz)	200	10	4	20	6	22	4	0	80	650	—	—	—
Corn Dogs Honey Crunchy	1 (2.6 oz)	180	9	3	25	7	19	6	0	60	540	—	—	—
Corn Dogs Mini	4 (2.7 oz)	210	12	—	45	7	18	0	1	40	490	—	—	—
Turkey	1 (2 oz)	140	12	—	25	7	1	tr	0	80	560	—	—	—
HEALTHY ONES														
Beef	1 (1.8 oz)	70	3	1	20	6	7	2	0	0	430	—	—	2
Franks	1 (1.8 oz)	70	3	1	20	6	6	2	0	0	430	—	—	2
IAN'S														
Popcorn Turkey Corn Dog	5 pieces (3 oz)	237	13	2	20	6	25	5	0	0	340	—	—	0
JOHNSONVILLE														
Stadium Beef	1 (2.7 oz)	240	22	8	50	9	2	0	—	20	760	—	—	0
ORGANIC PRAIRIE														
Beef Uncured	1 (1.5 oz)	120	11	4	25	5	0	0	0	0	360	—	—	4
OSCAR MAYER														
Beef	1 (1.6 oz)	140	13	6	30	5	1	1	0	0	460	—	—	0
Beef Light	1 (1.6 oz)	90	6	6	20	5	2	1	—	—	500	—	—	—
Cheese Dogs	1 (1.6 oz)	140	13	4	35	5	1	0	0	60	540	—	—	0
Corn Dogs	1	210	12	4	25	6	21	6	1	40	590	—	—	0
Smokies	1 (1.8 oz)	150	13	5	30	6	1	1	0	0	500	—	—	0
TAKE-OUT														
corndog	1	460	19	5	79	17	56	—	—	101	972	262	60	0
w/ bun chili	1	297	13	5	51	14	31	—	—	19	480	166	50	3
w/ bun plain	1	242	15	5	44	10	18	—	—	24	671	143	30	tr

HOT DOG SUBSTITUTES

FOOD	PORTION	CALS	FAT	SAT FAT	CHOL	PROT	CARB	SUGAR	FIBER	CALCI	SOD	POTAS	FOLIC	VIT C
HEALTH IS WEALTH														
Vegetarian Cocktail Franks	3 (2.4 oz)	220	16	2	0	8	16	0	3	0	200	—	—	0
LOMA LINDA														
Big Franks	1 (1.8 oz)	110	6	1	0	11	3	0	2	0	220	50	—	0
Big Franks Low Fat Vegan	1 (1.8 oz)	80	3	1	0	12	3	0	2	0	240	50	—	0
MORNINGSTAR FARMS														
Veggie Dogs	1 (1.4 oz)	50	1	0	0	7	4	2	tr	0	430	15	—	0

FOOD	PORTION	CALS	FAT	SAT FAT	CHOL	PROT	CARB	SUGAR	FIBER	CALCI	SOD	POTAS	FOLIC	VIT C
YVES														
Meatless Hot Dog	1	50	1	0	0	10	2	tr	0	20	400	150	—	0
Tofu Dogs	1	45	1	0	0	8	2	0	0	20	300	120	—	0
HUMMUS														
ATHENOS														
Artichoke & Garlic	2 tbsp (0.9 oz)	50	3	0	0	1	4	1	1	0	210	—	—	1
Cucumber Dill	2 tbsp (0.9 oz)	50	3	0	0	1	5	1	1	0	160	—	—	1
Greek Style	2 tbsp (0.9 oz)	50	3	0	0	1	5	1	1	0	140	—	—	1
Original	2 tbsp (0.9 oz)	50	3	0	0	1	5	1	1	0	160	—	—	1
Roasted Red Pepper	2 tbsp (0.9 oz)	50	3	0	0	1	5	1	1	0	150	—	—	9
CEDAR'S														
Artichoke Spinach	2 tbsp (1 oz)	70	4	0	0	2	5	1	1	40	105	—	—	6
EMERALD VALLEY														
Organic Greek Olive & Roasted Garlic	2 tbsp (1 oz)	60	3	0	0	2	6	1	2	20	190	—	—	0
Organic Original	2 tbsp (1 oz)	50	2	0	0	2	7	1	2	20	200	—	—	0
Organic Spinach Feta	2 tbsp (1 oz)	50	2	1	0	2	6	1	2	40	190	—	—	0
FOUNTAIN OF HEALTH														
Traditional	1 oz	70	5	1	0	2	6	1	1	20	115	—	—	0
GUILTLESS GOURMET														
Original	2 tbsp (1.1 oz)	50	2	0	0	2	8	1	2	20	110	—	—	0
MARGARITAVILLE														
Cilantro Jalapeno	1 oz	70	5	1	0	2	4	1	1	20	150	—	—	0
Island Lemon	1 oz	70	6	1	0	1	4	1	1	20	105	—	—	0
NASOYA														
Super Classic Original	2 tbsp (1 oz)	50	3	0	0	4	2	1	1	20	120	—	—	0
SABRA														
Greek Olive	2 tbsp (1 oz)	70	6	1	0	2	4	0	1	0	130	—	—	0
Roasted Pine Nut	2 tbsp (1 oz)	80	7	1	0	2	4	0	1	0	125	—	—	0
Spinach & Artichoke	2 tbsp (1 oz)	70	6	1	0	1	4	0	1	0	150	—	—	0
TRIBE														
40 Spices	2 tbsp	50	4	0	0	1	3	0	1	0	140	—	—	0
French Onion	2 tbsp	50	4	0	0	1	4	0	1	0	120	—	—	1
Organic Classic	2 tbsp	50	4	0	0	2	4	0	1	0	100	—	—	1
Organic Roasted Red Peppers	2 tbsp	40	3	0	0	1	3	0	1	0	95	—	—	6
Roasted Eggplant	2 tbsp	35	3	0	0	1	3	0	1	0	150	—	—	1
Scallion	2 tbsp	50	4	0	0	1	4	0	1	0	125	—	—	1
Zesty Lemon	2 tbsp	50	3	0	0	1	4	0	1	0	130	—	—	1

FOOD	PORTION	CALS	FAT	SAT FAT	CHOL	PROT	CARB	SUGAR	FIBER	CALCI	SOD	POTAS	FOLIC	VIT C
WHOLESOME VALLEY														
Organic Classic	2 tbsp (1 oz)	60	4	0	0	2	5	tr	1	20	115	—	—	0
WILD GARDEN														
Hummus Dip	2 tbsp	35	2	0	0	2	4	tr	1	20	70	—	—	0
WILDWOOD														
Organic Low Fat	2 tbsp	50	2	0	0	2	6	2	1	20	130	0	—	1
Organic Mid-Eastern	2 tbsp	65	4	1	0	2	6	2	1	20	120	0	—	1
TAKE-OUT														
hummus	¼ cup (2.2 oz)	109	5	1	0	3	12	tr	3	30	149	106	36	5

HYACINTH BEANS

FOOD	PORTION	CALS	FAT	SAT FAT	CHOL	PROT	CARB	SUGAR	FIBER	CALCI	SOD	POTAS	FOLIC	VIT C
dried cooked	1 cup	228	1	—	0	16	40	—	—	77	13	653	—	0

ICE CREAM AND FROZEN DESSERTS

(*see also* ICES AND ICE POPS, SHERBET, YOGURT FROZEN)

FOOD	PORTION	CALS	FAT	SAT FAT	CHOL	PROT	CARB	SUGAR	FIBER	CALCI	SOD	POTAS	FOLIC	VIT C
chocolate	½ cup (4 fl oz)	143	7	4	22	3	19	13	—	72	50	164	10	1
dixie cup chocolate	1 (3.5 fl oz)	125	6	4	20	2	16	11	—	63	44	145	9	tr
dixie cup strawberry	1 (3.5 fl oz)	112	5	—	17	2	16	9	—	70	35	109	7	5
dixie cup vanilla	1 (3.5 fl oz)	116	6	4	25	2	14	9	—	74	46	115	3	tr
freeze dried ice cream chocolate strawberry & vanilla	1 pkg (0.75 oz)	158	5	2	1	2	24	10	1	20	97	—	—	0
strawberry	½ cup (4 fl oz)	127	6	—	19	2	18	10	—	79	40	124	8	5
vanilla	½ cup (4 fl oz)	132	7	4	29	2	16	10	—	85	53	131	3	tr
vanilla soft serve	½ cup	111	2	1	10	4	19	—	—	138	62	194	6	1
ARCTIC ZERO														
Chocolate	½ cup (2.6 oz)	37	0	0	0	4	7	6	2	20	15	—	—	0
Chocolate Coated Bars All Flavors	1 (2 oz)	85	5	4	5	3	7	5	1	20	100	—	—	0
Coffee	½ cup (2.6 oz)	37	0	0	0	4	6	5	2	20	80	—	—	0
Mint Chocolate Cookie	½ cup (2.6 oz)	37	0	0	0	4	6	5	2	20	80	—	—	0
Pumpkin Spice	½ cup (2.6 oz)	45	0	0	10	4	7	7	2	20	95	—	—	2
Vanilla Maple	½ cup (2.6 oz)	37	0	0	0	4	7	7	2	20	15	—	—	0
BLUE BUNNY														
Bar Candy Center Crunch	1 (3.2 oz)	370	29	22	20	3	28	21	1	—	75	170	—	—
Bar English Toffee	1 (1.4 oz)	130	9	7	15	1	12	9	0	—	40	65	—	—
Bar Homemade Vanilla	1 (2.3 oz)	190	13	10	20	3	16	16	0	—	50	130	—	—
Bar Orange Dream	1 (2.1 oz)	80	2	1	5	1	16	14	0	—	35	65	—	—
Bar Strawberry Sundae Crunch	1 (2.2 oz)	170	9	4	15	2	20	13	0	—	55	55	—	—

FOOD	PORTION	CALS	FAT	SAT FAT	CHOL	PROT	CARB	SUGAR	FIBER	CALCI	SOD	POTAS	FOLIC	VIT C
BLUE BUNNY (CONT.)														
Blendz Peanut Butter Cup	1 (4.4 oz)	270	11	6	25	5	40	35	tr	150	160	180	—	—
Caramel Sundae Bite Size	4 bars (3.1 oz)	340	23	15	25	4	30	25	1	100	75	180	—	—
Chocolate	½ cup	130	7	—	25	2	17	14	0	—	55	110	—	—
Cone Bunny Tracks	1 (4.8 oz)	420	21	12	35	7	51	36	2	—	180	190	—	—
Cone The Champ Chocolate Lovers	1 (3.5 oz)	300	15	11	40	5	38	28	1	—	130	200	—	—
Cone Vanilla Nutty Sundae	1 (3 oz)	250	11	7	10	5	34	22	1	—	120	135	—	—
Cups Vanilla & Chocolate	1 (1.7 oz)	100	5	4	20	2	13	11	0	—	50	85	—	—
Mint Chip	½ cup	140	7	5	25	2	17	14	0	—	55	130	—	—
Neapolitan	½ cup	130	6	4	25	2	16	14	0	—	50	115	—	—
Orange Dream	½ cup	130	5	4	20	2	19	15	0	—	45	85	—	—
Premium All Natural Vanilla	½ cup	160	9	6	55	3	16	16	0	100	50	150	—	—
Premium Bunny Tracks	½ cup	190	11	6	25	4	21	19	tr	80	95	130	—	—
Premium Butter Pecan	½ cup	150	9	4	25	3	15	13	0	80	70	135	—	—
Premium Cookies & Cream	½ cup	150	8	5	25	3	19	15	0	80	75	135	—	—
Premium Double Strawberry	½ cup	140	6	4	25	2	20	18	0	80	40	120	—	4
Premium Exquisite Mint	½ cup	170	8	5	25	3	22	20	0	80	65	120	—	—
Premium Rocky Road	½ cup	150	7	5	20	3	21	16	0	60	90	105	—	—
Premium Toasted Almond Fudge	½ cup	160	9	5	25	3	18	14	tr	80	55	115	—	—
Sandwich Big Vanilla	1 (3.7 oz)	260	10	6	35	4	39	23	0	—	160	160	—	—
Sandwich Chips Galore	1 (3.4 oz)	310	16	8	35	3	40	27	1	—	170	115	—	—
Strawberry	½ cup	120	6	4	25	2	17	14	0	—	50	115	—	—
BREYERS														
Butter Pecan	½ cup	150	10	5	20	2	14	14	0	80	110	—	—	0
Carb Smart Chocolate	½ cup	90	6	4	15	2	13	4	4	80	75	—	—	0
Carb Smart Fudge Bar	1 (3.5 oz)	100	7	5	20	3	9	3	1	60	50	—	—	0
Carb Smart Vanilla	½ cup	90	6	4	15	2	13	4	4	60	45	—	—	0

FOOD	PORTION	CALS	FAT	SAT FAT	CHOL	PROT	CARB	SUGAR	FIBER	CALCI	SOD	POTAS	FOLIC	VIT C
BREYERS (CONT.)														
Carb Smart Vanilla Bar Chocolate Coated	1 (3 oz)	170	15	11	15	2	9	5	2	350	45	—	—	0
Cherry Vanilla	½ cup	130	6	4	15	2	18	17	0	80	55	—	—	0
Chocolate Crackle	½ cup	160	10	7	15	2	15	15	0	80	30	—	—	0
Chocolate Extra Creamy	½ cup	140	7	5	30	2	17	15	1	80	50	—	—	0
Coffee	½ cup	130	7	4	20	2	15	15	0	80	45	—	—	0
Cookies & Cream	½ cup	150	7	5	15	2	19	16	0	60	90	—	—	0
Double Churn ½ Fat Chocolate Mocha Silk	½ cup	130	5	3	20	3	19	15	1	80	50	—	—	0
Double Churn ½ Fat Creamy Vanilla	½ cup	100	3	2	10	2	17	13	0	80	65	—	—	0
Double Churn ½ Fat Mint Chocolate Chip	½ cup	130	5	4	10	2	19	15	1	80	50	—	—	0
Double Churn ½ Fat Rocky Road	½ cup	130	5	3	10	3	22	16	1	80	45	—	—	0
Double Churn Fat Free Chocolate Fudge Brownie	½ cup	110	0	0	0	3	25	15	4	80	75	—	—	0
Double Churn Fat Free Creamy Vanilla	½ cup	90	0	0	0	3	21	12	3	100	50	—	—	0
Double Churn Fat Free French Chocolate	½ cup	90	0	0	0	3	22	13	4	100	55	—	—	0
Double Churn No Sugar Added Vanilla	½ cup	80	4	3	10	2	14	4	4	60	45	—	—	0
Dulce De Leche	½ cup	150	6	4	15	2	21	19	0	80	105	—	—	0
French Vanilla	½ cup	140	7	5	45	3	14	14	0	100	35	—	—	0
Heath English Toffee	½ cup	160	6	4	10	2	25	20	0	80	130	—	—	0
Overload Very Chocolate Cherry	½ cup	120	3	2	5	2	21	16	1	80	50	—	—	0
Overload Waffle Cone	½ cup	130	3	2	5	2	22	16	0	80	95	—	—	0
Peach	½ cup	120	5	3	15	2	17	16	0	60	30	—	—	0
Sandwich Mrs. Fields Brownie	1 (6 oz)	450	19	11	20	5	64	39	2	60	140	—	—	0
Sandwich Mrs. Fields Cookie	1 (3 oz)	190	8	5	10	2	29	17	0	40	125	—	—	0

FOOD	PORTION	CALS	FAT	SAT FAT	CHOL	PROT	CARB	SUGAR	FIBER	CALCI	SOD	POTAS	FOLIC	VIT C
BREYERS (CONT.)														
Sandwich Oréo	1 (3 oz)	170	6	3	10	2	26	13	1	60	190	—	—	0
Snicker	½ cup	170	8	5	20	3	20	16	0	80	80	—	—	0
Strawberry	½ cup	120	5	3	15	2	15	15	0	60	35	—	—	6
Strawberry Cheesecake Sara Lee	½ cup	150	6	3	10	2	20	17	0	80	75	—	—	1
Vanilla Fudge Brownie	½ cup	150	7	4	15	2	20	17	1	80	50	—	—	0
Vanilla Lactose Free	½ cup	130	7	5	20	2	14	14	0	80	20	—	—	0
CELESTIAL SEASONINGS														
Tea Dreams Cinnamon Apple Spice	½ cup	140	6	0	0	0	24	6	1	20	55	—	—	0
Tea Dreams Vanilla Ginger Spice Chai	½ cup	140	6	1	0	0	24	5	1	20	70	—	—	0
Tea Dreams Bars Chocolate Caramel Chai	1 (2.7 oz)	240	15	9	0	tr	28	17	2	0	65	—	—	0
CIAO BELLA														
Gelato Chocolate	1 pkg (3.5 oz)	210	13	7	39	4	22	18	1	90	53	—	—	0
Gelato Hazelnut	1 pkg (3.5 oz)	210	13	7	39	3	21	17	1	90	61	—	—	0
Gelato Vanilla	1 pkg (3.5 oz)	184	11	11	39	3	19	16	0	90	61	—	—	0
CLEMMY'S														
Bar Sugar Free Cherry Vanilla	1 (1.9 oz)	70	3	2	15	0	16	0	5	0	10	—	—	0
Bar Sugar Free Chocolate Fudge	1 (2.2 oz)	70	3	2	10	1	18	0	5	0	20	—	—	0
Bar Sugar Free Orange Creme	1 (2 oz)	70	3	2	15	0	16	0	5	0	10	—	—	0
Butter Pecan Sugar Free	½ cup (2.6 oz)	180	14	7	60	1	19	0	5	20	45	—	—	0
Chocolate Sugar Free	½ cup (2.6 oz)	160	11	7	65	2	20	0	5	20	30	—	—	0
Ice Cream Os Sugar Free	1 (1.75 oz)	100	7	5	10	1	12	0	2	0	25	—	—	0
Peanut Butter Chocolate Chip Sugar Free	½ cup (2.6 oz)	200	15	8	55	2	20	0	5	20	60	—	—	0
Toasted Almond Sugar Free	½ cup (2.7 oz)	180	13	7	65	1	22	0	5	20	40	—	—	0
Vanilla Bean Sugar Free	½ cup (2.5 oz)	150	11	7	65	1	19	0	5	20	25	—	—	0
DIPPIN' DOTS														
Banana Split	½ cup	170	10	7	32	3	16	14	0	100	22	—	—	0
Chocolate	½ cup	165	10	7	29	3	15	14	0	100	16	—	—	0

FOOD	PORTION	CALS	FAT	SAT FAT	CHOL	PROT	CARB	SUGAR	FIBER	CALCI	SOD	POTAS	FOLIC	VIT C
DIPPIN' DOTS (CONT.)														
Fudge Fat Free No Sugar Added	½ cup	92	0	0	2	4	18	7	0	80	95	—	—	0
Horchata	½ cup	170	10	7	32	3	16	14	0	100	22	—	—	0
Java Delight	½ cup	170	10	7	32	3	16	14	0	100	22	—	—	0
Root Beer Float	½ cup	111	3	2	13	1	20	16	0	40	34	—	—	0
Vanilla	½ cup	170	10	7	32	3	16	14	0	100	22	—	—	0
ESKIMO PIE														
Milk Chocolate	1 bar (1.8 oz)	160	11	9	20	2	12	11	0	60	35	—	—	0
FAT BOY														
Casco Nut Sundae On A Stick	1 (3 oz)	310	24	10	15	7	21	15	2	40	40	—	—	0
Casco Nut Sundae On A Stick Cherry Cordial	1 (3 oz)	300	22	15	15	3	26	20	1	80	45	—	—	0
Sandwich Chocolate	1 (3 oz)	210	9	5	20	4	31	12	1	60	150	—	—	0
Sandwich Egg Nog	1 (3 oz)	220	10	5	35	4	31	18	tr	40	160	—	—	0
Sandwich Jr. Vanilla	1 (1.6 oz)	120	5	3	15	2	17	10	0	20	25	—	—	0
Sandwich Vanilla	1 (3 oz)	220	10	5	20	4	30	17	1	40	160	—	—	0
GLACE DE VINO														
Chocolate Amaretto Cream Sherry	½ cup	180	7	4	20	2	21	7	0	60	50	—	—	1
Raspberry Merlot Cheesecake	½ cup	180	7	4	20	2	22	6	0	60	50	—	—	0
GOOD HUMOR														
Bar Chocolate Eclair	1 (3 oz)	160	8	4	5	2	21	11	1	40	35	—	—	0
Bar Cookies & Cream	1 (3 oz)	190	11	7	10	2	21	14	1	60	75	—	—	0
Bar King Heath	1 (4 oz)	310	20	12	20	3	31	26	1	80	85	—	—	0
Bar Vanilla Chocolate Coated	1 (4 oz)	260	17	12	20	3	24	20	1	80	50	—	—	0
Cone King Giant	1 (8 oz)	390	21	13	30	7	44	30	2	150	135	—	—	0
Cone King Vanilla	1 (4.6 oz)	250	13	8	15	4	30	19	1	80	100	—	—	0
Cone Sundae	1 (4.3 oz)	260	15	9	15	4	29	18	1	60	80	—	—	0
Sandwich Oreo	1 (4.5 oz)	240	10	4	10	4	36	19	2	60	310	—	—	0
Sandwich Vanilla	1 (3 oz)	130	2	1	5	2	26	12	2	80	80	—	—	0
Sandwich Giant Vanilla	1 (6 oz)	220	4	2	0	4	43	23	1	100	150	—	—	0
Swirlwind	1 (6 oz)	160	3	2	10	4	31	23	0	150	110	—	—	0

FOOD	PORTION	CALS	FAT	SAT FAT	CHOL	PROT	CARB	SUGAR	FIBER	CALCI	SOD	POTAS	FOLIC	VIT C
GOODBODY														
Chocolate Banana	1 bar (3.5 oz)	120	1	0	0	7	25	19	4	300	170	510	80	66
Chocolate Double Dutch	1 bar (3.5 oz)	130	1	0	0	7	26	21	4	300	160	430	80	60
Chocolate Peanut Butter	1 bar (3.5 oz)	180	7	1	0	10	26	18	5	300	220	460	80	60
Vanilla & Raspberry Sorbet	1 bar (3.5 oz)	120	0	0	0	7	25	20	4	300	90	180	80	60
Vanilla & Strawberry Sorbet	1 bar (3.5 oz)	120	0	0	0	7	25	20	4	300	90	180	80	60
Vanilla & Tropical Sorbet	1 bar (3.5 oz)	120	0	0	0	7	25	20	4	300	90	180	80	60
GREEN & BLACK'S														
Organic Chocolate Covered Chocolate	1 bar (3.5 oz)	214	14	9	—	4	19	19	2	—	tr	—	—	—
Organic Chocolate Covered Vanilla	1 bar (3.5 oz)	233	16	10	—	4	19	18	2	—	tr	—	—	—
HAAGEN-DAZS														
Bailey's Irish Cream	½ cup (3.6 oz)	260	17	10	100	5	21	21	0	100	50	—	—	0
Bar Chocolate & Dark Chocolate	1 (3 oz)	290	20	12	65	4	24	20	2	60	30	—	—	0
Bar Vanilla & Almonds	1 (3 oz)	310	22	13	65	5	22	20	tr	100	65	—	—	0
Bar Vanilla & Milk Chocolate	1 (3 oz)	290	21	14	75	4	22	21	0	100	55	—	—	0
Butter Pecan	½ cup (3.7 oz)	310	23	11	110	5	21	18	tr	150	110	—	—	0
Caramel Cone	½ cup (4 oz)	320	19	10	100	4	32	27	0	100	190	—	—	0
Cherry Vanilla	½ cup (3.5 oz)	240	15	9	100	4	23	22	0	100	60	—	—	1
Chocolate Chip Cookie Dough	½ cup (3.6 oz)	310	20	12	95	4	29	24	0	100	125	—	—	0
Chocolate Peanut Butter	½ cup (3.8 oz)	360	24	11	100	8	27	24	2	100	100	—	—	0
Cookies & Cream	½ cup (3.6 oz)	270	17	10	105	5	23	21	0	150	95	—	—	0
Dulce De Leche	½ cup (3.7 oz)	290	17	10	100	5	28	28	0	150	95	—	—	0
Five Coffee	½ cup (3.6 oz)	220	12	7	70	5	23	21	0	100	70	—	—	0
Five Milk Chocolate	½ cup (3.6 oz)	220	12	7	75	6	22	20	tr	100	75	—	—	0
Five Mint	½ cup (3.6 oz)	220	12	7	70	5	24	23	0	100	50	—	—	0
Five Passion Fruit	½ cup (3.6 oz)	220	11	6	70	4	25	24	0	100	45	—	—	2
Five Vanilla	½ cup (3.7 oz)	270	18	11	120	5	21	21	0	150	70	—	—	0
Green Tea	½ cup (3.6 oz)	250	17	10	105	5	20	19	0	100	50	—	—	0
Mango	½ cup (3.7 oz)	250	14	8	85	4	28	27	tr	100	50	—	—	5

FOOD	PORTION	CALS	FAT	SAT FAT	CHOL	PROT	CARB	SUGAR	FIBER	CALCI	SOD	POTAS	FOLIC	VIT C
HAAGEN-DAZS (CONT.)														
Rocky Road	½ cup (3.6 oz)	300	18	9	90	5	29	24	1	100	75	—	—	0
Strawberry	½ cup (3.7 oz)	250	16	10	95	4	23	22	tr	150	65	—	—	6
Vanilla Honey Bee	½ cup (3.6 oz)	270	17	10	110	5	23	20	1	100	50	—	—	0
HAWAIIAN PUNCH														
Cream Surfers	1 bar	90	2	1	5	1	16	9	0	40	35	—	—	15
HEALTHY CHOICE														
Bar Fudge	1 (2.2 oz)	80	2	1	5	3	13	4	4	100	65	200	—	0
Bar Low Fat Sorbet & Cream	1 (2.2 oz)	80	1	0	<5	1	18	12	tr	100	25	70	—	0
Sandwich Vanilla	1 (2.4 oz)	150	2	1	<5	4	30	14	0	100	120	115	—	0
HERSHEY'S														
Banana Split	½ cup (2.5 oz)	160	9	5	35	2	18	16	0	100	55	—	—	2
Chocolate	½ cup (2.5 oz)	140	8	5	30	3	15	13	tr	100	55	—	—	0
Cookies And Cream	½ cup (2.5 oz)	160	9	6	35	2	16	15	0	80	70	—	—	0
Fudge Royale	½ cup (2.5 oz)	180	9	5	35	2	19	18	0	80	80	—	—	0
Mint Moose Tracks	½ cup (2.5 oz)	200	14	7	35	3	21	19	tr	100	75	—	—	0
Raspberry	½ cup (2.5 oz)	170	9	5	35	2	21	18	0	80	55	—	—	0
Tally-Ho Low Fat Butter Pecan	½ cup (2.5 oz)	90	2	2	10	3	14	14	0	100	95	—	—	0
Vanilla	½ cup (2.5 oz)	150	9	5	35	3	14	14	0	100	60	—	—	0
HOOD														
Butterscotch Blast	½ cup	160	7	5	25	2	20	15	0	80	60	—	—	0
Chocolate	½ cup	140	7	5	25	2	17	12	0	80	45	—	—	0
Chocolate Eclair	1 bar (2.2 oz)	150	10	4	5	1	14	8	0	20	45	—	—	0
Cookie Dough Delight	½ cup	160	8	5	25	2	20	14	0	60	60	—	—	0
Creamy Coffee	½ cup	140	7	5	30	2	16	12	0	80	50	—	—	0
Fat Free Chocolate Passion	½ cup	100	0	0	0	3	22	14	0	80	70	—	—	0
Fat Free Very Vanilla	½ cup	100	0	0	0	2	23	14	0	80	70	—	—	0
Fudge Twister	½ cup	150	7	4	25	2	20	15	0	80	50	—	—	0
Grasshopper Pie	½ cup	160	7	4	25	2	22	14	0	80	70	—	—	0
Hoodsie Cups	1 (1.7 oz)	100	5	4	20	2	12	9	0	40	35	—	—	0
Light Butter Pecan	½ cup	140	6	2	10	3	18	11	0	80	100	—	—	0
Light Creamy Vanilla	½ cup	110	3	2	10	2	18	12	0	100	60	—	—	0
Low Fat No Sugar Added Vanilla Dream	½ cup	90	2	1	5	3	20	4	3	100	70	—	—	0
Maple Walnut	½ cup	160	9	5	25	3	17	12	0	80	45	—	—	0

FOOD	PORTION	CALS	FAT	SAT FAT	CHOL	PROT	CARB	SUGAR	FIBER	CALCI	SOD	POTAS	FOLIC	VIT C
HOOD (CONT.)														
No Sugar Added Chocolate Chip	½ cup	100	3	2	5	3	21	4	3	100	65	—	—	0
Nutty Royale	1 cone (2.5 oz)	220	12	7	15	4	26	18	tr	60	75	—	—	0
Orange Cream	1 bar (2.2 oz)	90	2	1	5	1	19	13	0	40	40	—	—	0
Sandwich Vanilla	1	180	6	4	20	3	29	14	tr	60	120	—	—	0
Sandwich Vanilla Light	1 (2.2 oz)	160	3	2	10	3	29	14	tr	60	125	—	—	0
Sandwich Vanilla Lowfat	1 (2.8 oz)	80	2	1	<5	2	15	2	2	40	70	—	—	0
Spumoni	½ cup	140	7	5	25	2	17	13	0	80	50	—	—	0
JULIE'S														
Organic Gluten Free Sandwich Vanilla	1 (2.6 oz)	220	11	7	40	3	30	20	1	60	95	—	—	0
KLONDIKE														
Bar Caramel Pretzel	1 (4 oz)	260	14	11	10	3	30	21	1	80	170	—	—	0
Bar Original Vanilla	1 (4.5 oz)	250	17	13	20	3	22	18	0	80	55	—	—	0
Bar Reese's	1 (4 oz)	260	16	10	10	4	26	21	1	80	95	—	—	0
Bar Whitehouse Cherry	1 (4.5 oz)	250	17	13	20	2	24	20	0	80	55	—	—	0
Cone Crunchy Vanilla	1 (4.3 oz)	280	16	9	15	5	30	20	1	80	85	—	—	0
Slim A Bear 100 Calorie Sandwich Vanilla	1 (3 oz)	100	2	1	0	2	21	10	2	40	65	—	—	0
Slim A Bear Bar Vanilla	1 (4 oz)	170	9	8	5	6	21	7	4	150	65	—	—	0
LACTAID														
Butter Pecan	½ cup (4 oz)	170	11	5	30	2	16	11	0	60	75	—	—	0
Chocolate	½ cup (2.5 oz)	160	8	5	30	3	19	13	0	80	35	—	—	0
Vanilla	½ cup (4 oz)	150	8	5	35	2	16	12	0	80	35	—	—	0
LAND O LAKES														
Vanilla	½ cup (2.4 oz)	150	8	5	30	2	17	16	0	80	40	—	—	tr
Vanilla Light	½ cup (2.3 oz)	100	3	2	15	3	17	13	0	100	50	—	—	0
LIFEWAY														
Frozen Kefir Tart And Tangy Mango	½ cup (2.5 oz)	90	1	0	5	4	18	16	0	150	55	—	—	1
Frozen Kefir Tart And Tangy Original	½ cup (2.5 oz)	90	1	1	5	4	18	16	0	150	60	—	—	1
Frozen Kefir Tart And Tangy Pomegranate	½ cup (2.5 oz)	90	1	0	5	4	18	16	0	150	60	—	—	1

FOOD	PORTION	CALS	FAT	SAT FAT	CHOL	PROT	CARB	SUGAR	FIBER	CALCI	SOD	POTAS	FOLIC	VIT C
LIFEWAY (CONT.)														
Frozen Kefir Tart And Tangy Strawberry	½ cup (2.5 oz)	90	1	0	5	4	18	16	0	150	55	—	—	1
MAGNUM														
Classic	1 bar (2.7 oz)	240	16	10	25	3	22	21	tr	80	45	—	—	0
Dark	1 bar (2.7 oz)	240	17	11	25	3	20	18	2	80	40	—	—	0
Double Caramel	1 bar (3.2 oz)	320	20	14	25	3	32	29	1	100	85	—	—	0
White	1 bar (2.7 oz)	250	16	14	25	3	23	23	0	100	60	—	—	0
MOLLI COOLZ														
Cup Banana Cream Pie	1	120	9	4	35	2	9	8	1	80	35	—	—	0
Cup Chocolate Fusion	1	140	10	6	25	2	10	7	1	80	55	—	—	0
Cup Chocolate Peanut Butter	1	160	12	6	45	2	12	10	0	80	55	—	—	0
Ionz Cotton Candy	1 cup	100	7	3	35	2	8	5	0	80	30	—	—	0
Ionz S'mores	1 cup	110	9	4	30	2	7	5	1	80	50	—	—	0
Rocks Cherry Blue Raz & Lemon	1 cup	80	2	1	0	tr	15	8	0	20	23	—	—	0
Rocks Lemon Lime	1 cup	80	2	1	0	tr	15	8	0	20	23	—	—	0
Shakers Chocolate	1 (10.2 oz)	250	11	5	35	3	35	17	5	120	72	—	—	0
NATURAL CHOICE														
Organic Double Chocolate	½ cup	230	14	8	35	3	25	23	0	150	65	—	—	2
Organic Strawberry	½ cup	210	13	8	35	2	22	21	0	150	65	—	—	5
Organic Vanilla	½ cup	220	14	9	35	2	22	22	0	150	70	—	—	2
POPSICLE														
Creamsicle	1 (2.5 oz)	100	2	1	5	1	20	12	0	40	35	—	—	9
PURELY DECADENT														
Dairy Free Bar Chocolate Coated Vanilla	1 (2.7 oz)	200	9	3	0	2	26	22	3	0	10	—	—	0
Dairy Free Bar Chocolate Coated Vanilla Almond	1 (2.7 oz)	210	10	3	0	2	28	22	4	0	10	—	—	0
Organic Coconut Milk Chocolate	½ cup	150	9	8	0	1	20	12	6	0	5	—	—	0
Organic Coconut Milk Vanilla Bean	½ cup	150	8	7	0	1	19	12	6	0	5	—	—	0

FOOD	PORTION	CALS	FAT	SAT FAT	CHOL	PROT	CARB	SUGAR	FIBER	CALCI	SOD	POTAS	FOLIC	VIT C
PURELY DECADENT (CONT.)														
Organic Dairy Free Belgian Chocolate	½ cup	180	7	2	0	1	30	25	4	0	15	—	—	0
Organic Dairy Free Chocolate Obsession	½ cup	210	9	3	0	2	36	20	5	0	15	—	—	0
Organic Dairy Free Gluten Free Cookie Dough	½ cup	230	8	4	0	1	36	27	5	0	75	—	—	0
Organic Dairy Free Mocha Almond Fudge	½ cup	200	9	1	0	3	32	22	6	20	45	—	—	0
Organic Dairy Free Snickerdoodle	½ cup	190	6	2	0	1	34	20	5	0	65	—	—	0
Organic Dairy Free Vanilla	½ cup	170	8	1	0	1	29	18	6	0	20	—	—	0
RICE DREAM														
Bar Vanilla Chocolate Coating	1 (3 oz)	230	15	9	0	1	24	16	tr	0	70	—	—	1
Bar Vanilla Nutty	1 (3.3 oz)	320	24	11	0	5	27	15	2	20	65	—	—	1
Carob Almond	½ cup	180	10	1	0	0	26	2	2	40	70	—	—	0
Frozen Pie Chocolate	1 (3.4 oz)	330	19	8	0	3	40	14	2	0	50	—	—	1
Mint Carob Chip	½ cup	170	8	1	0	1	25	19	0	0	85	—	—	0
Strawberry	½ cup	160	8	0	0	0	25	2	2	20	70	—	—	0
SHEER BLISS														
Bar Pomegranate	1 (3.1 oz)	260	16	10	30	3	24	22	tr	100	55	—	—	1
Blissbites	2 (1.1 oz)	100	7	5	10	1	9	8	0	20	15	—	—	0
Blisswich	1 (3.3 oz)	270	10	5	20	3	39	21	tr	80	55	—	—	1
Freedom	½ cup (4 oz)	290	16	11	65	3	32	29	0	80	60	—	—	1
Mediterranean Coffee	½ cup (4 oz)	260	18	12	65	3	25	23	0	80	65	—	—	0
Pomegranate	½ cup (4 oz)	290	16	11	55	3	32	29	0	80	60	—	—	1
Vanilla	½ cup (4 oz)	300	19	13	65	6	29	27	0	80	65	—	—	0
SKINNY COW														
Bar Dippers Vanilla & Caramel	1	80	3	2	3	2	11	7	2	60	30	—	—	—
Bar Truffle Caramel	1	100	2	2	5	3	19	12	3	80	50	—	—	—
Bar Truffle French Vanilla	1	100	2	2	20	3	18	12	3	80	45	—	—	—
Cone Chocolate w/ Fudge	1	150	3	2	5	4	29	17	3	200	95	—	—	0

FOOD	PORTION	CALS	FAT	SAT FAT	CHOL	PROT	CARB	SUGAR	FIBER	CALCI	SOD	POTAS	FOLIC	VIT C
SKINNY COW (CONT.)														
Cone Vanilla w/ Caramel	1	150	3	2	5	4	29	18	3	200	80	—	—	0
Fudge Bar	1	100	1	1	3	4	22	13	4	100	45	—	—	0
Sandwich Chocolate Peanut Butter	1	150	2	1	5	4	30	15	3	80	100	—	—	0
Sandwich Cookies 'N Cream	1	150	2	1	3	4	31	15	3	80	105	—	—	0
Sandwich Vanilla	1	140	2	1	1	4	30	15	3	80	95	—	—	0
Sandwich Vanilla No Sugar Added	1	140	2	1	15	4	30	5	5	60	115	—	—	0
SODELICIOUS														
Dairy Free Sandwich Minis Pomegranate	1 (1.4 oz)	90	2	1	0	2	18	8	1	0	75	—	—	0
Dairy Free Sandwich Mint	1 (2.2 oz)	150	3	1	0	3	28	13	2	0	125	—	—	0
Dairy Free Sandwich Vanilla	1 (2 oz)	150	3	1	0	3	28	13	2	0	105	—	—	0
Dairy Free Sugar Free Chocolate Coated Vanilla Bar	1 (2.2 oz)	150	14	8	0	2	15	0	6	100	50	—	—	0
Dairy Free Sugar Free Fudge Bar	1 (2 oz)	80	5	1	0	2	12	0	6	100	50	—	—	0
Organic Dairy Free Sandwich Neapolitan	1 (2.2 oz)	150	3	1	0	3	28	13	2	0	110	—	—	0
SOY DREAM														
Butter Pecan	½ cup	140	9	2	0	1	17	9	tr	20	130	—	—	0
Sandwich Lil' Dreamers Chocolate	1 (1.4 oz)	100	5	1	0	1	15	8	tr	0	60	—	—	0
Vanilla	½ cup	140	7	2	0	1	18	10	tr	20	140	—	—	0
STARBUCKS														
Caramel Macchiato	½ cup (3.6 oz)	240	13	8	60	3	27	21	0	80	105	—	—	0
Coffee	½ cup (3.5 oz)	210	13	8	65	3	21	19	0	100	55	—	—	0
Java Chip Frappuccino	½ cup (3.5 oz)	250	15	10	60	3	25	22	0	80	50	—	—	0
Mocha Frappuccino	½ cup (3.5 oz)	220	13	8	55	3	23	20	tr	100	65	—	—	0
Mocha Bar	1	280	19	11	50	4	26	23	1	100	60	—	—	0

FOOD	PORTION	CALS	FAT	SAT FAT	CHOL	PROT	CARB	SUGAR	FIBER	CALCI	SOD	POTAS	FOLIC	VIT C
STONYFIELD FARM														
Gotta Have Java	1 serv (4 oz)	250	16	10	60	3	22	20	0	100	45	160	—	0
Strawberry Licious	1 serv (4 oz)	220	13	8	50	3	23	21	0	100	35	150	—	0
Vanilla Chai	1 serv (4 oz)	240	16	10	60	3	21	20	0	100	45	150	—	0
STRAUS														
I'm Organic Coffee	4 oz	240	15	10	70	4	19	19	0	100	55	—	—	0
I'm Organic Raspberry	½ cup (4 oz)	230	14	9	65	4	19	19	1	100	50	—	—	4
I'm Organic Vanilla Bean	4 oz	240	15	10	70	4	19	19	0	100	55	—	—	0
Organic Brown Sugar Banana	½ cup (3.2 oz)	250	11	7	55	3	32	31	0	100	45	—	—	1
THE GREEK GODS														
Pagoto Ice Krema Baklava	½ cup (4 oz)	240	12	7	40	5	29	27	1	150	60	220	—	1
Pagoto Ice Krema Chocolate Fig	½ cup (4 oz)	240	11	7	40	4	32	30	0	150	60	240	—	1
Pagoto Ice Krema Honey Pomegranate	½ cup (4 oz)	230	11	7	40	4	31	30	0	150	60	260	—	0
TOFUTTI														
Cuties Chocolate	1 (1.3 oz)	130	1	0	0	2	16	9	0	—	110	—	—	—
Cuties Vanilla	1 (1.3 oz)	130	6	1	0	2	17	9	0	—	121	—	—	—
Flowers Chocolate Covered	1 (1.4 oz)	180	8	2	0	2	23	19	2	—	105	—	—	—
Marry Me Dessert Bars	1 bar (2.5 oz)	168	8	3	0	2	22	18	tr	—	105	—	—	—
Yours Truly Cones	1 (2.6 oz)	220	13	3	0	2	24	21	2	—	135	—	—	—
TURKEY HILL														
Banana Split	½ cup	150	7	4	25	2	19	15	1	60	40	—	—	0
Choco Mint Chip	½ cup	160	9	6	25	2	17	13	1	60	45	—	—	0
Chocolate All Natural	½ cup	150	8	5	30	3	18	17	0	100	45	—	—	0
Chocolate Marshmallow	½ cup	160	6	4	20	2	24	18	1	60	100	—	—	0
Coconut Cream Pie	½ cup	170	9	6	30	2	20	20	0	80	95	—	—	0
Cookies 'N Cream	½ cup	150	8	5	25	2	19	13	0	60	60	—	—	0
Duetto Cherry	½ cup	120	3	2	10	1	21	19	0	40	35	—	—	0
Duetto Lemon	½ cup	120	4	2	10	1	21	19	0	10	35	—	—	0
Duetto Root Beer	½ cup	120	3	2	10	0	21	19	0	40	35	—	—	0
French Vanilla	½ cup	140	7	5	50	2	16	12	0	80	45	—	—	0
Light Banana Split	½ cup	110	3	1	5	2	19	15	1	200	50	—	—	0
Light Dulce De Chocolate	½ cup	120	3	2	5	2	22	17	1	200	110	—	—	0

FOOD	PORTION	CALS	FAT	SAT FAT	CHOL	PROT	CARB	SUGAR	FIBER	CALCI	SOD	POTAS	FOLIC	VIT C
TURKEY HILL (CONT.)														
Light Moose Tracks	½ cup	140	6	3	5	3	20	15	1	200	65	—	—	0
Light Vanilla Bean	½ cup	100	2	2	5	2	17	13	1	250	55	—	—	0
No Sugar Added Cherry Fudge Ripple	½ cup	80	0	0	0	3	22	5	4	100	70	—	—	0
No Sugar Added Vanilla Bean	½ cup	70	0	0	0	3	19	6	5	100	75	—	—	0
Original Vanilla	½ cup	140	7	5	30	2	16	12	0	80	45	—	—	0
Peanut Butter Ripple	½ cup	170	11	5	25	3	16	11	1	60	90	—	—	0
Rocky Road	½ cup	170	8	5	20	3	23	17	1	80	125	—	—	0
Sandwich Chocolate Chunk	1 (3.2 oz)	320	15	7	30	3	44	29	1	60	290	—	—	0
Sandwich Vanilla Bean	1 (2.5 oz)	190	7	4	20	3	29	15	1	60	95	—	—	0
Sandwich Light Vanilla Bean	1 (2.5 oz)	160	3	2	10	3	32	15	3	200	95	—	—	0
Sundae Cone Vanilla Fudge	1 (3.3 oz)	320	18	10	20	6	35	20	2	80	120	—	—	1
Tin Roof Sundae	½ cup	150	8	5	25	2	19	15	0	60	65	—	—	0
WEIGHT WATCHERS														
Smart Ones Sundae Chocolate Fudge Brownie	1 (2.3 oz)	140	3	2	5	3	26	14	tr	80	70	—	—	0
Smart Ones Sundae Turtle	1 (2.2 oz)	130	3	1	5	3	23	10	0	80	75	—	—	0
TAKE-OUT														
cone vanilla light soft serve	1 (4.6 oz)	164	6	4	28	4	24	—	—	153	92	169	5	1
gelato chocolate hazelnut	½ cup (5.3 oz)	370	29	4	92	9	26	21	2	179	49	352	35	1
gelato vanilla	½ cup (3 oz)	211	15	8	151	3	18	18	0	67	78	77	15	tr
ice cream pie no crust	1 slice (3.4 oz)	218	14	9	56	3	21	18	1	119	74	182	5	1
mud pie	⅛ pie (8 oz)	698	32	15	53	9	96	64	3	181	560	443	18	1
sundae caramel	1 (5.4 oz)	303	9	5	25	7	49	—	—	189	195	318	12	3
sundae hot fudge	1 (5.4 oz)	284	9	5	21	6	48	—	—	207	182	395	9	2
sundae strawberry	1 (5.4 oz)	269	8	4	21	6	45	—	—	161	92	270	18	2

ICE CREAM CONES AND CUPS

FOOD	PORTION	CALS	FAT	SAT FAT	CHOL	PROT	CARB	SUGAR	FIBER	CALCI	SOD	POTAS	FOLIC	VIT C
brown sugar cone	1 (10 g)	40	tr	tr	0	1	8	3	tr	4	32	14	14	0
wafer cone	1	17	tr	tr	0	tr	3	tr	tr	1	6	4	7	0
waffle cone	1 lg	121	2	tr	0	2	23	2	1	7	41	32	50	0

FOOD	PORTION	CALS	FAT	SAT FAT	CHOL	PROT	CARB	SUGAR	FIBER	CALCI	SOD	POTAS	FOLIC	VIT C
KEEBLER														
Cone Sugar	1	50	1	0	0	1	10	4	0	—	55	—	—	—
Ice Creme Cone	1	15	0	0	0	0	4	0	0	0	20	—	—	0
Waffle Bowl	1	50	1	0	0	tr	10	4	0	—	25	—	—	—
Waffle Cone	1	50	1	0	0	tr	10	4	0	—	25	—	—	—

ICE CREAM TOPPINGS

FOOD	PORTION	CALS	FAT	SAT FAT	CHOL	PROT	CARB	SUGAR	FIBER	CALCI	SOD	POTAS	FOLIC	VIT C
butterscotch	2 tbsp (1.4 oz)	103	tr	tr	—	1	27	—	—	22	143	—	—	—
caramel	2 tbsp (1.4 oz)	103	tr	tr	—	1	27	—	—	22	143	—	—	—
marshmallow cream	1 oz	88	tr	—	0	1	23	—	—	1	13	1	0	—
marshmallow cream	1 jar (7 oz)	615	tr	—	0	3	157	—	—	6	90	9	2	—
nuts in syrup	2 tbsp	184	9	1	0	2	24	15	1	14	17	62	11	tr
pineapple	1 cup (11.5 oz)	861	—	—	0	1	226	—	—	75	214	1078	9	199
pineapple	2 tbsp (1.5 oz)	106	tr	tr	0	tr	28	9	tr	3	18	18	1	1
strawberry	2 tbsp (1.5 oz)	107	tr	—	0	tr	28	—	—	10	9	31	1	11
strawberry	1 cup (11.5 oz)	863	1	—	0	1	225	—	—	81	73	248	5	85
HERSHEY'S														
Sundae Syrup Caramel	2 tbsp (1.4 oz)	100	0	0	0	—	25	20	0	0	95	—	—	0
SANDERS														
Butterscotch Caramel	2 tbsp	90	4	2	10	0	15	11	0	20	95	—	—	—
SMUCKER'S														
Plate Scrapers Chocolate Fudge	2 tbsp (1.4 oz)	120	3	1	0	1	22	14	tr	20	60	—	—	0
STEEL'S														
Sugar Free Fudge Sauce	2 tbsp (0.9 oz)	110	6	4	10	1	13	10	1	20	5	—	—	0

ICED TEA

MIX

FOOD	PORTION	CALS	FAT	SAT FAT	CHOL	PROT	CARB	SUGAR	FIBER	CALCI	SOD	POTAS	FOLIC	VIT C
AQUAFULL														
Zesty Lemon Dietary Supplement	1 pkg (9 g)	20	0	0	0	—	8	1	4	—	15	—	—	—
CRYSTAL LIGHT														
Antioxidant Sugar Free Green Tea Raspberry as prep	8 oz	5	0	0	0	0	1	0	—	—	5	—	—	6
On The Go White Peach Tea as prep	8 oz	5	0	0	0	0	0	0	0	—	10	—	—	6
Pure Sugar Free Mixed Berry as prep	8 oz	15	0	0	0	0	4	3	0	—	10	—	—	—

FOOD	PORTION	CALS	FAT	SAT FAT	CHOL	PROT	CARB	SUGAR	FIBER	CALCI	SOD	POTAS	FOLIC	VIT C
LIPTON														
Chailatta Chocolate as prep	8 oz	120	2	0	<5	3	21	19	—	80	180	—	—	—
Chailatta Hazelnut as prep	8 oz	120	2	0	<5	3	21	19	—	60	200	—	—	—
Chailatta Original as prep	8 oz	120	2	0	<5	3	21	19	—	80	180	—	—	—
Chailatta Vanilla as prep	8 oz	120	2	0	<5	3	21	19	—	80	200	—	—	—
Decaffeinated Lemon as prep	1 serv	70	0	0	0	0	18	18	—	—	0	—	—	—
To Go Green Sugar Free Mandarin Mango	½ pkg (0.7 oz)	0	0	0	0	0	0	0	0	—	0	—	—	—
To Go w/ Honey & Lemon	1 pkg	0	0	0	0	0	0	0	0	—	0	—	—	—
To Go w/ Mandarin & Mango	1 pkg	0	0	0	0	0	tr	—	—	—	0	—	—	—
Unsweetened as prep	1 serv	0	0	0	0	0	0	0	0	—	0	—	—	—
NESTEA														
Lemon Liquid Concentrate as prep	8 oz	80	0	0	0	0	19	18	—	—	0	—	—	—
Peach Liquid Concentrate as prep	8 oz	90	0	0	0	0	21	20	—	—	0	—	—	—
Sugar Free w/ Lemon	2 tsp	5	0	0	0	0	2	0	—	—	0	—	—	—
Sweetened w/ Lemon	1⅓ tbsp	60	0	0	0	0	15	15	—	—	0	—	—	—
Unsweetened w/ Lemon	2 tsp	5	0	0	0	0	1	0	—	—	0	—	—	—
READY-TO-DRINK														
ARIZONA														
Black & White	8 oz	50	0	0	0	0	14	14	0	0	10	—	—	15
Diet Black Tea Peach	8 oz	0	0	0	0	0	tr	tr	0	0	20	—	—	15
Green Tea Lemonade	8 oz	50	0	0	0	0	14	13	0	0	25	—	—	60
Organic Green Tea	8 oz	50	0	0	0	0	14	13	0	0	10	—	—	30
BINA														
Lemon	8 oz	70	0	0	0	0	17	17	—	—	25	—	—	—
Peach	8 oz	114	0	0	0	0	29	29	—	—	0	—	—	—

FOOD	PORTION	CALS	FAT	SAT FAT	CHOL	PROT	CARB	SUGAR	FIBER	CALCI	SOD	POTAS	FOLIC	VIT C
BOLTHOUSE FARMS														
Perfectly Protein Vanilla Chai Tea w/ Soy	8 oz	160	3	1	0	10	25	21	0	300	60	530	—	108
BOMBILLA & GOURD														
Organic Eco Teas All Flavors	8 oz	40	0	0	0	0	11	10	—	—	0	—	—	—
C+SWISS														
Hemp Ice Tea	1 can (8.4 oz)	90	0	0	0	0	23	21	—	—	<10	—	—	—
CAFE SEPIA														
Matcha Latte	1 can (8.6 oz)	130	3	1	10	3	23	21	1	80	50	0	—	72
DELTA BLUES														
Tea Punch Black Tea Sumptuous Spearmint	8 oz	90	0	0	0	0	21	20	0	—	0	—	—	0
Tea Punch Green Tea Peach & Delectable Lemongrass	8 oz	90	0	0	0	0	22	21	—	—	0	—	—	0
Tea Punch Green Tea Peach Apricot Pineapple Quince	8 oz	100	0	0	0	0	24	21	—	—	0	—	—	0
FUZE														
Antioxidant Tea	8 oz	60	0	0	0	0	15	15	—	—	0	—	100	60
Green Tea	8 oz	60	0	0	0	0	16	16	—	—	0	—	100	30
White Tea	8 oz	60	0	0	0	0	15	15	—	—	0	—	100	60
GOLD PEAK TEA														
Green Tea Sweetened	1 bottle (16.9 oz)	170	0	0	0	0	45	44	—	—	45	—	—	—
HAWAIIAN														
Iced Tea	1 can (11.5 oz)	120	0	0	0	0	35	35	0	0	50	—	—	60
HONEST TEA														
Assam Black	8 oz	17	0	0	0	0	5	5	—	—	5	—	—	—
Green Dragon	8 oz	30	0	0	0	0	8	8	—	—	5	—	—	—
Green Tea Zero Calorie Passion Fruit	8 oz	0	0	0	0	0	0	0	0	—	0	—	—	—
Half & Half	8 oz	48	0	0	0	0	12	12	—	—	5	—	—	—
Heavenly Lemon Tulsi	8 oz	30	0	0	0	0	8	8	—	—	5	—	—	—
Jasmine Green Energy	8 oz	17	0	0	0	0	5	5	—	—	5	—	—	—
Just Green	8 oz	0	0	0	0	0	0	0	0	—	5	—	—	—
Pearfect White	8 oz	35	0	0	0	0	9	9	—	—	5	—	—	—
White Mango Acai	8 oz	35	0	0	0	0	9	9	—	—	5	—	—	—

FOOD	PORTION	CALS	FAT	SAT FAT	CHOL	PROT	CARB	SUGAR	FIBER	CALCI	SOD	POTAS	FOLIC	VIT C
HOOD														
Iced Tea	1 cup	100	0	0	0	0	25	24	0	0	10	—	—	72
ITO EN														
Dark Green Tea Oi Ocha	8 oz	0	0	0	0	0	0	0	0	—	20	—	—	72
Golden Oolong	8 oz	0	0	0	0	0	0	0	0	—	20	—	—	60
Green Tea Jasmine	8 oz	0	0	0	0	0	0	0	0	—	20	—	—	60
Green Tea Oi Ocha	8 oz	0	0	0	0	0	0	0	0	—	20	—	—	72
Sencho Shot Japanese Green Tea	1 can (6.4 oz)	0	0	0	0	0	0	0	0	—	20	—	—	84
KOMBUCHA														
Wonder Drink Asian Pear Ginger	1 bottle (8.5 oz)	65	0	0	0	0	16	8	—	—	0	—	—	—
Wonder Drink Rooibus Red Peach	1 bottle (8.5 oz)	60	0	0	0	0	15	13	—	—	10	—	—	—
LIPTON														
Diet Green Tea w/ Citrus	8 oz	0	0	0	0	0	0	0	0	—	25	—	—	—
Diet Green Tea w/ Watermelon	8 oz	0	0	0	0	0	0	0	—	—	25	—	—	—
Diet Sweet	8 oz	0	0	0	0	0	0	0	0	—	0	—	—	—
Extra Sweet	8 oz	100	0	0	0	0	24	24	—	—	5	—	—	—
Green Tea 100% Natural Citrus	8 oz	70	0	0	0	0	19	18	—	—	20	—	—	—
Green Tea 100% Natural Passionfruit Mango	8 oz	50	0	0	0	0	13	13	—	—	20	—	—	—
NANTUCKET NECTARS														
Half & Half	8 oz	90	0	0	0	0	22	22	0	0	25	—	—	60
Original Lemon	8 oz	80	0	0	0	0	22	21	0	0	25	—	—	60
NESTEA														
Green Tea Diet Peach	8 oz	0	0	0	0	0	0	0	0	—	30	—	—	—
Green Tea Peach	1 bottle (20 oz)	220	0	0	0	0	57	57	—	—	75	—	—	—
Lemon	1 bottle (20 oz)	210	0	0	0	0	56	55	—	—	75	—	—	—
Lemon Diet	8 oz	0	0	0	0	0	0	0	—	—	30	—	—	—
Sweetened	8 oz	60	0	0	0	0	17	17	—	—	25	—	—	—
Sweetened Diet Green Tea	8 oz	0	0	0	0	0	0	0	0	—	0	—	—	—
Sweetened Green Tea	8 oz	80	0	0	0	0	20	18	—	—	0	—	—	—

FOOD	PORTION	CALS	FAT	SAT FAT	CHOL	PROT	CARB	SUGAR	FIBER	CALCI	SOD	POTAS	FOLIC	VIT C
OLD ORCHARD														
Green Tea w/ Lemon & Honey	8 oz	45	0	0	0	0	12	12	0	0	9	—	—	0
Red Tea w/ Currant	8 oz	45	0	0	0	0	12	12	—	0	9	—	—	0
OSTEO														
Fruit Tea All Flavors	1 can (12 oz)	120	0	0	0	0	32	32	0	500	5	—	1000	60
PIXIE														
Black Tea Mate Lemon Ginger	8 oz	35	0	0	0	0	8	6	0	—	15	—	—	—
Yerba Mate Authentic	8 oz	30	0	0	0	0	7	7	0	—	5	—	—	—
POMX														
Green Tea Pomegranate Lychee	8 oz	70	0	0	0	0	18	16	—	0	5	—	—	0
Light Green Tea Pomegranate Hibiscus	8 oz	35	0	0	0	0	16	8	—	0	0	—	—	0
ROOIBEE RED TEA														
Lemon Honey	1 bottle (12.5 oz)	80	0	0	0	0	21	20	—	—	10	—	—	60
Peach	1 bottle (12.5 oz)	80	0	0	0	0	21	21	—	—	10	—	—	60
Unsweet	1 bottle (12.5 oz)	0	0	0	0	0	0	0	0	—	10	—	—	60
SANTA CRUZ														
Organic (12.5 oz)	8 oz	60	0	0	0	0	15	14	0	—	0	—	—	—
Organic Peppermint	8 oz	60	0	0	0	0	15	14	0	—	0	—	—	—
Organic TeaZer Passionfruit	1 bottle (12 oz)	90	0	0	0	0	22	21	0	—	0	0	—	—
Organic TeaZer Pear	1 bottle (12 oz)	90	0	0	0	0	21	21	0	—	0	0	—	—
SNAPPLE														
Black Tea Lemon	8 oz	80	0	0	0	0	21	21	—	—	65	—	—	—
Diet Lemon Tea	8 oz	10	0	0	0	0	0	0	—	—	5	—	—	—
Diet Lemonade Iced Tea	8 oz	10	0	0	0	0	2	2	—	—	5	—	—	—
Diet Peach	8 oz	0	0	0	0	0	0	0	—	—	5	—	—	—
Diet Plum-A-Granate	8 oz	5	0	0	0	0	0	0	0	—	5	—	—	—
Green Tea Mango Metabolism	8 oz	60	0	0	0	0	15	15	—	—	5	—	—	—
Peach	8 oz	90	0	0	0	0	23	23	—	—	5	—	—	—

FOOD	PORTION	CALS	FAT	SAT FAT	CHOL	PROT	CARB	SUGAR	FIBER	CALCI	SOD	POTAS	FOLIC	VIT C
SNAPPLE (CONT.)														
Red Tea Pomegranate Raspberry	8 oz	80	0	0	0	0	21	21	—	—	60	—	—	—
White Tea Apple Plum	8 oz	80	0	0	0	0	21	21	—	—	60	—	—	9
SOKENBICHA														
All Flavors	1 bottle	0	0	0	0	0	0	0	0	—	10	—	—	—
SOLEBURY HOME														
Organic All Flavors	8 oz	33	0	0	0	0	8	8	—	—	0	—	—	60
SPINDRIFT														
Sparkling Half & Half	8 oz	80	0	0	0	0	21	20	0	0	0	—	—	0
SSIPS														
Diet Green Tea w/ Honey & Ginseng	1 box (7 oz)	0	0	0	0	0	0	0	0	—	10	—	—	—
Green Tea w/ Honey & Ginseng	1 box (7 oz)	60	0	0	0	0	15	14	—	—	10	—	—	—
Lemon	8 oz	100	0	0	0	0	24	23	0	0	10	—	—	0
SWEET LEAF														
Diet Mint & Honey Green Tea	8 oz	0	0	0	0	tr	tr	0	0	—	0	—	—	30
Lemon & Lime Unsweet	8 oz	0	0	0	0	0	0	0	0	—	0	—	—	60
Original Sweet	8 oz	70	0	0	0	0	18	17	—	—	10	—	—	60
Pomegranate Green Tea	8 oz	60	0	0	0	tr	16	14	—	—	0	—	—	120
SWISS TEA														
Diet	8 oz	0	0	0	0	0	1	0	0	—	20	—	—	—
Diet Decafe	8 oz	0	0	0	0	0	0	0	0	—	15	—	—	—
Green Tea w/ Ginseng & Honey	8 oz	80	0	0	0	0	20	20	0	0	10	—	—	0
Sweet Tea Southern Style	8 oz	90	0	0	0	0	23	23	0	—	10	—	—	—
W/ Lemon	8 oz	100	0	0	0	0	24	23	0	—	15	—	—	—
White Tea Sweetened w/ Raspberry	8 oz	90	0	0	0	0	24	23	0	—	15	—	—	—
TEAS' TEA														
Green Hoji	8 oz	0	0	0	0	0	0	0	0	—	30	—	—	60
Lemongrass Green	8 oz	0	0	0	0	0	0	0	0	—	20	—	—	72

FOOD	PORTION	CALS	FAT	SAT FAT	CHOL	PROT	CARB	SUGAR	FIBER	CALCI	SOD	POTAS	FOLIC	VIT C
TEAS' TEA (CONT.)														
Pure Black	8 oz	0	0	0	0	0	0	0	0	—	15	—	—	57
Pure Green	8 oz	0	0	0	0	0	0	0	0	—	20	—	—	84
TRUE BREW														
Cranberry Orange	8 oz	72	0	0	0	0	18	18	0	—	—	—	—	—
Green Tea	8 oz	64	0	0	0	0	16	16	0	—	—	—	—	—
Sweet Tea	8 oz	76	0	0	0	0	19	19	0	—	—	—	—	—
TURKEY HILL														
Decaffeinated	8 oz	80	0	0	0	0	20	20	—	—	15	—	—	—
Diet Decaffeinated	8 oz	0	0	0	0	0	0	0	0	—	15	—	—	—
Nature's Accents Blueberry Oolong	8 oz	100	0	0	0	0	24	24	—	—	10	—	—	—
Nature's Accents Chai Spiced Zero Calorie	8 oz	0	0	0	0	0	1	0	—	—	10	—	—	—
Nature's Accents Green Tea	8 oz	70	0	0	0	0	17	17	—	—	20	—	—	—
Southern Brew Extra Sweet	8 oz	90	0	0	0	0	21	19	—	—	10	—	—	—
VIDATEA														
All Flavors	1 can	90	0	0	0	0	24	23	—	—	—	—	—	30
VITAZEST														
Green Tea Vitamin Enriched	8 oz	0	0	0	0	0	0	0	0	—	0	—	—	30
WEIL FOR TEA														
Gyokuro	1 can (8.6 oz)	0	0	0	0	0	0	0	0	0	30	0	—	108
Turmeric	1 can (8.6 oz)	0	0	0	0	0	0	0	0	0	15	0	—	66

ICES AND ICE POPS

FOOD	PORTION	CALS	FAT	SAT FAT	CHOL	PROT	CARB	SUGAR	FIBER	CALCI	SOD	POTAS	FOLIC	VIT C
BLUE BUNNY														
Bar Big Fudge	1 (2.7 oz)	110	2	1	5	3	21	17	0	100	75	170	—	—
Chill Cups Double Lemon	1 (4 oz)	100	0	0	0	0	26	19	0	—	20	—	—	60
FrozFruit Creamy Coconut	1 bar (3 oz)	150	10	8	25	1	14	13	tr	40	20	45	—	—
Pop Banana	1 (1.9 oz)	35	0	0	0	0	9	7	0	—	5	—	—	—
Pop Jolly Rancher	1 (4 oz)	120	0	0	0	0	24	20	0	—	30	—	—	—
Pop Root Beer	1 (1.9 oz)	40	0	0	0	0	10	8	0	—	10	—	—	—
The Original Bomb	1 (1.8 oz)	50	0	0	0	0	11	9	0	—	5	—	—	—
BREEZE FREEZE														
100% Fruit Juice	1 (8 oz)	54	0	0	0	0	13	—	0	50	24	—	—	60
Fruit Granita	1 (8 oz)	120	0	0	0	1	28	27	tr	50	15	—	—	60

FOOD	PORTION	CALS	FAT	SAT FAT	CHOL	PROT	CARB	SUGAR	FIBER	CALCI	SOD	POTAS	FOLIC	VIT C
BREYERS														
Pure Fruit Pop Lemon Lime	1 (1.75 oz)	40	0	0	0	0	10	9	—	—	0	—	—	6
Pure Fruit Pop Pomegranate Blends	1 (1.75 oz)	40	0	0	0	0	10	9	—	—	0	—	—	6
DIPPIN' DOTS														
Cherry Berry	½ cup	90	0	0	0	0	23	12	0	0	0	—	—	0
Watermelon	½ cup	90	0	0	0	0	23	12	0	0	0	—	—	0
DOLE														
Fruit Bars Strawberry	1 (2.75 oz)	90	0	0	0	0	23	22	0	0	0	—	—	18
Super Fruit Bars Acai Blueberry	1 (2.75 oz)	90	0	0	0	0	22	21	0	0	0	—	—	24
HAAGEN-DAZS														
Fat Free Sorbet Mango	½ cup (4 oz)	120	0	0	0	0	37	36	0	0	10	—	—	6
Fat Free Sorbet Raspberry	½ cup (3.7 oz)	120	0	0	0	0	30	26	2	0	0	—	—	2
Fat Free Sorbet Zesty Lemon	½ cup (4 oz)	110	0	0	0	0	29	28	tr	20	25	—	—	2
Lowfat Sorbet Chocolate	½ cup (3.7 oz)	130	1	0	0	2	28	20	2	0	70	—	—	0
HAWAIIAN PUNCH														
Arctic Surfers	1 pop	50	0	0	0	0	12	8	0	0	5	—	—	15
HENDRIE'S														
Citrus N' Berry Stix	1 (1.9 oz)	15	0	0	0	0	3	0	0	0	5	—	—	27
Fudge Stix Fat Free	1 bar (1.8 oz)	70	0	0	0	1	14	11	0	60	60	—	—	0
HOOD														
Hoodsie Pop	1 (3.3 oz)	60	0	0	0	0	16	13	0	0	5	—	—	0
LUIGI'S														
Italian Ice Cherry	1 (6 oz)	130	0	0	0	0	32	25	tr	0	15	—	—	1
Italian Ice Lemon Strawberry	1 (6 oz)	120	0	0	0	0	31	24	tr	0	10	—	—	1
Italian Ice No Sugar Added Lemon	1 (6 oz)	60	0	0	0	0	20	1	0	0	10	—	—	1
Italian Ice Pina Colada	1 (6 oz)	130	0	0	0	0	33	30	0	0	40	—	—	2
Swirl Blue Ribbon Lemonade	1 (6 oz)	150	0	0	0	0	39	32	0	0	10	—	—	0
MR. J														
All Flavors	1 bar (2.25 oz)	50	tr	—	—	tr	12	5	—	5	5	71	—	60

FOOD	PORTION	CALS	FAT	SAT FAT	CHOL	PROT	CARB	SUGAR	FIBER	CALCI	SOD	POTAS	FOLIC	VIT C
NATURAL CHOICE														
Organic Vegan Fruit Bars Coconut	1 (2.75 oz)	90	4	3	0	0	16	15	1	20	10	—	—	0
Organic Vegan Fruit Bars Pink Lemonade	1 (2.75 oz)	50	0	0	0	0	13	13	0	20	5	—	—	18
Organic Vegan Grape	1 (2.75 oz)	50	0	0	0	0	13	13	0	20	5	—	—	18
Organic Vegan Sorbet Blueberry	½ cup	110	0	0	0	0	29	27	tr	20	10	—	—	5
Organic Vegan Sorbet Lemon	½ cup	110	0	0	0	0	30	27	0	20	15	—	—	15
Organic Vegan Sorbet Mango	½ cup	110	0	0	0	0	29	27	1	20	10	—	—	12
PICKLESICKLE														
Pop	1 (2 oz)	3	0	0	0	0	1	0	0	10	245	—	—	0
POPSICLE														
Creamsicle Pop No Sugar Added	2 (1.65 oz)	45	1	0	<5	1	10	3	2	40	25	—	—	6
Creamsicle Pop Sugar Free	2 (1.65 oz)	40	2	2	0	1	10	0	6	20	5	—	—	—
Diet Soda Pops	1 (1.6 oz)	15	0	0	0	0	3	0	—	—	0	—	—	6
Firecracker	1 (1.6 oz)	35	0	0	0	0	9	6	—	—	0	—	—	6
Fudgsicle Bar	1 (2.5 oz)	100	2	1	0	2	17	14	1	150	75	—	—	0
Fudgsicle Pops No Sugar Added	1 (1.65 oz)	40	1	0	0	2	10	2	2	100	45	—	—	0
Lifesavers Pop	1 (3.5 oz)	90	0	0	0	0	22	15	—	—	10	—	—	6
Pop Ups Orange Burst	1 (2.75 oz)	90	1	1	5	1	18	10	0	20	20	—	—	1
Rainbow Pops	1 (1.65 oz)	40	0	0	0	0	10	7	—	—	5	—	—	6
Snow Cone	1 (7 oz)	30	0	0	0	0	7	5	—	—	5	—	—	—
POWER OF FRUIT														
Fruit Bar Banana Berry	1 (1.75 oz)	27	tr	0	0	tr	7	5	1	102	2	95	—	13
Fruit Bar Original	1 (1.75 oz)	28	tr	0	0	tr	7	5	1	56	1	83	—	16
Fruit Bar Tropical	1 (1.75 oz)	30	tr	0	0	tr	8	6	1	49	1	88	—	14
SODELICIOUS														
Dairy Free Creamy Orange Bar	1 (2.2 oz)	80	2	0	0	1	18	12	2	100	30	—	—	6
SWEET NOTHINGS														
Bar Mango Raspberry	1 (2.6 oz)	100	0	0	0	1	23	12	0	0	10	—	—	5

FOOD	PORTION	CALS	FAT	SAT FAT	CHOL	PROT	CARB	SUGAR	FIBER	CALCI	SOD	POTAS	FOLIC	VIT C
TURKEY HILL														
Venice Mango	½ cup	100	0	0	0	0	23	22	0	0	30	—	—	1
Venice Pomegranate Blueberry w/ Acai	½ cup	100	0	0	0	0	25	23	0	0	5	—	—	0

INDIAN FOOD

(*see* ASIAN FOOD)

JACKFRUIT

FOOD	PORTION	CALS	FAT	SAT FAT	CHOL	PROT	CARB	SUGAR	FIBER	CALCI	SOD	POTAS	FOLIC	VIT C
canned in syrup	½ cup (3.1 oz)	82	tr	—	0	tr	21	—	1	39	10	85	12	tr
fresh sliced	1 cup (5.8 oz)	157	1	tr	0	3	38	31	3	40	3	739	40	23

JALAPENO

(*see* PEPPERS)

JAM/JELLY/PRESERVES

FOOD	PORTION	CALS	FAT	SAT FAT	CHOL	PROT	CARB	SUGAR	FIBER	CALCI	SOD	POTAS	FOLIC	VIT C
apple butter	1 tbsp (0.6 oz)	31	tr	tr	0	tr	8	6	tr	3	3	16	0	tr
jam all flavors	1 pkg (0.5 oz)	39	tr	tr	0	tr	10	7	tr	3	4	11	2	1
jam all flavors	1 tbsp (0.7 oz)	56	tr	tr	0	tr	14	10	tr	4	6	15	2	2
jam apricot	1 tbsp (0.7 oz)	48	tr	tr	0	tr	13	9	tr	4	8	15	0	2
jam diet all flavors	1 tbsp (0.5 oz)	18	tr	tr	0	tr	8	5	tr	1	0	10	1	0
jelly all flavors	1 tbsp (0.7 oz)	51	0	0	0	tr	13	10	tr	1	6	10	0	tr
jelly reduced sugar all flavors	1 tbsp (0.7 oz)	34	tr	tr	0	tr	9	9	tr	1	0	13	0	0
jelly diet all flavors	1 tbsp (0.7 oz)	25	tr	tr	0	tr	10	7	1	2	0	13	2	0
orange marmalade	1 tbsp (0.7 oz)	49	0	0	0	tr	13	12	tr	8	11	7	2	1
preserves all flavors	1 tbsp (0.7 oz)	56	tr	tr	0	tr	14	10	tr	4	6	15	2	2
BETH'S FARM KITCHEN														
Apple Butter	2 tbsp (1 oz)	15	0	0	0	0	4	3	1	—	0	—	—	1
Jam Gooseberry	2 tbsp (1 oz)	45	0	0	0	0	11	10	1	0	0	—	—	5
Jam Sour Cherry	2 tbsp (1 oz)	15	0	0	0	0	4	3	1	0	0	—	—	1
Jam Strawberry Rhubarb	2 tbsp (1 oz)	40	0	0	0	0	11	10	0	20	0	—	—	9
Marmalade Bitter Orange	2 tbsp (1 oz)	40	0	0	0	0	10	10	0	0	0	—	—	2
CASCADIAN FARM														
Organic Fruit Spread Blackberry	1 tbsp	45	0	0	0	0	11	10	—	—	0	—	—	—
Organic Fruit Spread Raspberry	1 tbsp	45	0	0	0	0	11	10	—	—	0	—	—	—
Organic Sweet Orange Marmalade	1 tbsp	45	0	0	0	0	11	10	—	—	0	—	—	2
CHUKAR CHERRIES														
Preserves No Sugar Added Cherry Amaretto	1 tbsp	24	0	0	0	0	18	1	tr	10	97	—	—	1

FOOD	PORTION	CALS	FAT	SAT FAT	CHOL	PROT	CARB	SUGAR	FIBER	CALCI	SOD	POTAS	FOLIC	VIT C
CHUKAR CHERRIES (CONT.)														
Preserves Red Sour Cherry	1 tbsp	40	0	0	0	0	10	8	tr	0	0	—	—	1
Preserves Vanilla Peach	1 tbsp	28	0	0	0	0	19	6	tr	10	109	—	—	9
COLUMBIA EMPIRE FARMS														
Marionberry Seedless Preserves	1 tbsp	60	0	0	0	0	14	9	—	—	5	—	—	—
COMFORT CARE														
Country Apple Butter	1 tbsp (1 oz)	40	0	0	0	0	11	10	1	0	0	—	—	1
DELICIA														
Fruit Spread Black Cherry	1 tbsp (0.7 oz)	40	0	0	0	0	10	10	—	—	0	—	—	—
EDEN														
Organic Butter Apple Cherry	1 tbsp	25	0	0	0	0	6	5	tr	—	0	40	—	—
GEDNEY														
State Fair Preserves Strawberry Rhubarb	1 tbsp	50	0	0	0	0	12	11	0	0	0	—	—	0
HERO														
Swiss Preserves Black Cherry	1 tbsp (0.7 oz)	50	0	0	0	tr	13	10	2	—	2	—	—	—
JAKE & AMOS														
Jam Fig	1 tbsp (0.5 oz)	35	0	0	0	0	9	8	0	0	0	—	—	0
Jam Hot Pepper	1 tbsp	43	0	0	0	0	9	8	—	—	3	—	—	—
Jam Rhubarb	1 tbsp (0.7 oz)	40	0	0	0	0	12	11	0	0	0	—	—	0
JENKINS JELLIES														
Hell Fire Pepper Jelly	1 tbsp (0.7 oz)	40	0	0	0	0	11	10	1	—	3	—	—	—
POLANER														
All Fruit w/ Fiber Grape	1 tbsp (0.6 oz)	30	0	0	0	0	9	6	3	—	0	—	—	—
REVOLUTION FOODS														
Organic Jelly Grape	1 tbsp (0.7 oz)	60	0	0	0	0	14	14	0	0	5	—	—	0
Organic Preserves Strawberry	1 tbsp (0.7 oz)	60	0	0	0	0	14	13	0	0	0	—	—	0
ROBERT ROTHCHILD FARM														
Preserves Cherry Acai	1 tbsp	35	0	0	0	0	9	9	0	0	0	—	—	1

FOOD	PORTION	CALS	FAT	SAT FAT	CHOL	PROT	CARB	SUGAR	FIBER	CALCI	SOD	POTAS	FOLIC	VIT C
SARABETH'S														
Spreadable Fruit Blood Orange Marmalade	1 tbsp (0.7 oz)	35	0	0	0	0	8	5	1	—	0	—	—	1
Spreadable Fruit Chunky Apple	1 tbsp (0.7 oz)	30	0	0	0	0	7	7	—	—	0	—	—	—
Spreadable Fruit Orange Apricot Marmalade	1 tbsp (0.7 oz)	30	0	0	0	0	8	8	—	—	0	—	—	2
Spreadable Fruit Pineapple Mango	1 tbsp (0.7 oz)	35	0	0	0	0	9	9	0	—	0	—	—	2
Spreadable Fruit Strawberry Rhubarb	1 tbsp (0.7 oz)	40	0	0	0	0	10	9	tr	—	<5	—	—	—
Spreadable Fruit Strawberry Peach	1 tbsp (0.7 oz)	30	0	0	0	0	8	7	—	—	0	—	—	—
SMUCKER'S														
Jam Blackberry	1 tbsp (0.7 oz)	50	0	0	0	0	13	12	—	—	0	—	—	—
Jam Concord Grape	1 tbsp (0.7 oz)	50	0	0	0	0	13	12	—	—	0	—	—	—
Jam Red Plum	1 tbsp (0.7 oz)	50	0	0	0	0	13	12	—	—	5	—	—	—
Jam Seedless Red Raspberry	1 tbsp (0.7 oz)	50	0	0	0	0	13	12	—	—	0	—	—	—
Jelly Apple	2 tbsp (0.7 oz)	50	0	0	0	0	13	12	—	—	0	—	—	—
Jelly Concord Grape	1 tbsp (0.7 oz)	50	0	0	0	0	13	12	—	—	5	—	—	—
Jelly Strawberry	1 tbsp (0.7 oz)	50	0	0	0	0	13	12	—	—	0	—	—	—
Orange Marmalade Low Sugar	2 tbsp (0.7 oz)	25	0	0	0	0	6	5	—	—	0	—	—	—
Preserves Apricot Low Sugar	1 tbsp (0.6 oz)	25	0	0	0	0	6	5	—	—	0	—	—	—
Simply Fruit Black Cherry	1 tbsp (0.7 oz)	40	0	0	0	0	10	8	—	—	0	—	—	—
Simply Fruit Peach	1 tbsp (0.7 oz)	40	0	0	0	0	10	8	—	—	0	—	—	—
Simply Fruit Strawberry	1 tbsp (0.7 oz)	40	0	0	0	0	10	8	—	—	0	—	—	—
TRAPPIST														
Jelly Pomegranate	1 tbsp (0.7 oz)	50	0	0	0	0	14	11	—	—	5	—	—	—
TREE OF LIFE														
Organic Fruit Spread Grape	1 tbsp (0.6 oz)	30	0	0	0	8	8	7	0	0	0	—	—	9
Organic Fruit Spread Peach	1 tbsp (0.6 oz)	30	0	0	0	8	8	7	0	0	0	—	—	9
WELCH'S														
Grape Jelly	1 tbsp	50	0	0	0	0	13	13	—	—	15	—	—	—

JERKY

FOOD	PORTION	CALS	FAT	SAT FAT	CHOL	PROT	CARB	SUGAR	FIBER	CALCI	SOD	POTAS	FOLIC	VIT C
JAPANESE FOOD														
(*see* ASIAN FOOD, SUSHI)														
JELLY														
(*see* JAM/JELLY/PRESERVES)														
JELLYFISH														
pickled	½ cup (1 oz)	10	tr	tr	1	2	0	0	0	1	2810	1	0	0
JERKY														
beef	1 oz	122	8	3	14	10	3	3	1	6	664	179	40	0
pork	1 oz	122	8	3	14	10	3	3	1	6	664	179	40	0
venison	1 oz	119	7	3	39	10	4	4	0	5	888	117	2	0
APPLEGATE FARMS														
Natural Joy Stick	1 (1 oz)	100	7	3	25	9	0	tr	tr	—	700	—	—	—
DAKOTA GOURMET														
Fruit Jerky Strawberry Kiwi	1	70	0	0	0	tr	16	12	1	0	15	130	—	12
FRANK'S REDHOT														
Chile'N Lime Steak Strips	1 oz	80	4	2	30	10	2	1	0	0	370	—	—	0
Original Beef	1 oz	80	1	0	20	11	5	4	0	20	750	—	—	1
GARY WEST														
Beef Strips Hickory Smoked	1 oz	70	1	1	30	12	5	5	0	<20	780	—	—	0
Buffalo Strips	½ pkg (1 oz)	60	0	0	0	11	3	2	0	0	460	—	—	0
Elk Strips	½ pkg (1 oz)	70	1	0	10	13	4	2	0	0	640	—	—	0
JERKY FOR LIFE														
Beef Steak Black Pepper & Garlic	¼ pkg (1 oz)	50	2	1	5	9	0	0	0	—	350	—	—	—
Beef Steak Jalapeno	¼ pkg (1 oz)	50	2	1	5	9	tr	0	—	—	370	—	—	—
KING KALIBUR														
Black Angus Beef Sticks	1 (1.2 oz)	93	5	3	14	8	4	4	0	20	240	0	—	0
MATADOR														
Beef Original	1 pkg (1.4 oz)	110	2	1	40	15	8	7	0	0	850	—	—	0
Snack Stick Original	1 (1 oz)	150	13	5	30	6	2	0	0	20	420	—	—	0
OSTRIM														
Stick Beef & Ostrich	1 (1.5 oz)	80	2	1	25	14	3	2	—	20	430	650	—	—
OUTPOST														
Beef	1 oz	70	1	0	30	13	4	3	0	0	790	—	—	0
Beef Steak	1 pkg (0.9 oz)	60	3	1	20	8	2	tr	0	0	550	—	—	0
Beef Stick	1 (0.4 oz)	60	5	2	10	2	2	1	0	0	190	—	—	0

FOOD	PORTION	CALS	FAT	SAT FAT	CHOL	PROT	CARB	SUGAR	FIBER	CALCI	SOD	POTAS	FOLIC	VIT C
PERKY JERKY														
Beef	1 pkg (1 oz)	90	2	1	25	11	6	5	0	20	530	—	—	0
Turkey	1 pkg (1 oz)	50	0	0	0	9	2	2	0	0	110	—	—	0
PRIMAL														
Meatless Vegan Hickory Smoke	1 pkg (1 oz)	99	3	1	0	10	8	3	1	40	344	—	—	0
Meatless Vegan Mesquite Lime	1 pkg (1 oz)	74	2	0	0	10	7	4	0	30	347	—	—	0
Meatless Vegan Texas BBQ	1 pkg (1 oz)	81	1	1	0	10	11	5	1	40	383	—	—	0
Meatless Vegan Thai Peanut	1 pkg (1 oz)	74	2	1	0	10	8	4	1	20	353	—	—	0
SLIM JIM														
Beef	7 pieces	130	8	4	35	11	3	tr	0	0	770	—	—	0
Beef Jerky Hickory Smoked	1 oz	80	2	1	30	12	4	3	0	0	470	—	—	0
Classic Handipack	1 box	210	19	7	50	8	3	tr	tr	40	610	—	—	—
Giant Caddy Pepperoni	1 pkg	150	13	5	35	6	3	tr	0	20	450	—	—	—
Twin Pack Cheese & Pepperoni	1 pkg	150	12	7	40	9	2	0	1	150	620	—	—	—
SUNRICH NATURALS														
Fruit Bar Sour Apple	1 (0.7 oz)	70	0	0	0	tr	16	12	1	0	15	130	—	—
Fruit Bar Strawberry Kiwi	1 (0.7 oz)	70	0	0	0	tr	16	12	1	0	15	130	—	12
TANKA														
Natural Buffalo Cranberry Bar	1 (1 oz)	70	2	1	17	7	7	6	1	10	360	—	—	2
Natural Buffalo Cranberry Bite	1 (0.5 oz)	35	1	0	9	4	3	3	0	0	180	—	—	1
TOFURKY														
Jurky Original	4 pieces (1 oz)	100	2	—	—	12	9	3	1	—	260	—	—	—
TONY'S SMOKEHOUSE														
Salmon	1 pkg (0.5 oz)	40	1	0	12	7	2	1	1	tr	247	—	—	tr
UMPQUA INDIAN FOODS														
Brew Pub Steak Jerky Beef Flavored	¼ pkg (1 oz)	90	3	1	15	10	6	5	—	—	360	—	—	—
Steak Jerky Original	¼ pkg (1 oz)	60	2	1	15	9	0	0	0	—	340	—	—	—
JICAMA														
fresh	1 sm (12.8 oz)	139	tr	tr	0	3	32	7	18	44	15	548	44	74
raw sliced	1 cup	46	tr	tr	0	1	11	2	6	14	5	180	14	24
JUJUBE														
dried	1 oz	82	tr	—	0	1	21	—	—	23	3	151	—	4

FOOD	PORTION	CALS	FAT	SAT FAT	CHOL	PROT	CARB	SUGAR	FIBER	CALCI	SOD	POTAS	FOLIC	VIT C
JUTE														
cooked	1 cup	32	tr	tr	0	3	6	1	2	184	10	479	90	29
KALE														
chopped cooked w/o salt	1 cup	36	1	tr	0	2	7	2	3	94	30	296	17	53
fresh cooked w/ fat	1 cup	69	4	1	0	2	7	2	2	93	339	297	18	53
scotch chopped cooked w/o salt	1 cup	36	1	tr	0	2	7	—	2	172	58	356	17	69
ALLENS														
Seasoned	½ cup	35	1	0	0	3	5	1	1	150	830	—	—	6
GLORY														
Fresh Greens	1 serv (2.8 oz)	40	1	0	0	3	8	2	2	100	35	—	—	96
Seasoned canned	½ cup	35	1	0	0	2	5	2	1	40	490	—	—	24
KANGAROO														
kangaroo	3 oz	120	2	—	56	24	—	—	—	—	—	—	—	—
KEFIR														
kefir	8 oz	98	2	1	10	8	12	12	0	284	257	370	12	2
EVOLVE														
Plain	8 oz	120	3	2	10	11	15	10	5	400	190	—	—	0
Strawberry	8 oz	180	2	2	10	10	31	27	5	400	180	—	—	0
GREEN VALLEY														
Organic Lactose Free Blueberry Pom Acai	1 pkg (6 oz)	150	3	2	10	7	25	19	0	250	70	—	—	1
Organic Lactose Free Plain	8 oz	90	3	2	10	8	10	4	0	300	75	—	—	0
HELIOS														
Organic Blueberry	8 oz	160	2	2	10	11	25	21	3	300	125	—	—	2
Organic Nonfat Plain w/ Omega 3s	8 oz	80	0	0	18	9	10	10	0	310	90	—	—	0
Organic Plain	8 oz	120	4	3	15	8	12	10	2	300	85	—	—	0
Organic Raspberry	8 oz	160	4	3	15	8	26	23	2	300	85	—	—	0
LIFEWAY														
BioKefir Shot Digestion Vanilla	1 bottle (3.5 oz)	60	0	0	0	5	10	9	2	300	50	125	—	2
BioKefir Shot Heart Health Black Cherry	1 bottle (3.5 oz)	60	0	0	0	5	10	10	—	300	50	125	—	2
BioKefir Shot Heart Health Blackberry	1 bottle (3.5 oz)	60	0	0	0	5	10	10	—	300	50	125	—	2
Greek Style	8 oz	210	14	9	55	8	12	12	—	300	120	—	—	2
Lowfat Blueberry	8 oz	140	2	2	10	11	20	20	—	300	125	—	—	2
Lowfat Cappuccino	8 oz	140	2	2	10	11	20	20	—	300	125	—	—	2

FOOD	PORTION	CALS	FAT	SAT FAT	CHOL	PROT	CARB	SUGAR	FIBER	CALCI	SOD	POTAS	FOLIC	VIT C
LIFEWAY (CONT.)														
Lowfat Pomegranate	8 oz	140	2	2	10	11	20	20	—	300	125	—	—	2
Nonfat Peach	8 oz	180	0	0	5	11	33	30	3	300	125	—	—	2
Nonfat Plain	8 oz	90	0	0	5	11	12	12	—	300	120	—	—	2
Nonfat Raspberry	8 oz	150	0	0	0	11	27	27	—	300	125	—	—	2
Organic Lowfat Plain	8 oz	110	2	2	10	11	12	12	—	300	125	—	—	2
Organic Lowfat Wildberry	8 oz	160	2	2	10	11	25	21	3	300	125	—	—	2
Original	8 oz	150	8	5	30	8	12	12	0	300	125	—	—	—
Plain Lowfat	8 oz	110	2	2	10	11	12	12	—	300	125	—	—	2
Plain Whole Milk	8 oz	160	8	5	30	10	12	12	—	300	125	—	—	2
Probugs Goo-Berry Pie	1 bottle (5 oz)	130	5	3	19	9	15	13	2	300	78	—	—	2
Slim6 Mixed Berry	8 oz	110	2	2	10	14	8	6	2	300	125	—	—	2
Slim6 Plain	8 oz	110	2	2	10	14	8	6	2	300	125	—	—	2
NANCY'S														
Organic Lowfat Blackberry	1 cup	180	3	2	15	7	34	32	2	250	80	—	—	6
Organic Lowfat Plain	1 cup	110	3	3	15	8	14	13	1	300	105	—	—	0
Organic Lowfat Raspberry	1 cup	180	3	2	15	7	35	32	3	250	80	—	—	9
YAKULT														
Drink	1 bottle (2.7 oz)	50	0	0	—	1	12	11	0	20	20	—	—	—
KETCHUP														
banana	1 tsp	10	0	0	0	0	2	2	0	—	75	—	—	—
ketchup	1 pkg (0.2 oz)	6	tr	tr	0	tr	2	—	tr	1	71	29	1	1
ketchup	1 tbsp	15	tr	tr	0	tr	4	3	0	3	167	57	2	2
low sodium	1 tbsp	15	tr	tr	0	tr	4	3	0	3	3	57	2	2
ANNIE'S HOMEGROWN														
Organic	1 tbsp (0.6 oz)	15	0	0	0	0	5	4	—	—	170	—	—	—
FISCHER & WIESER														
Chipotle Chili	1 tbsp (0.7 oz)	15	0	0	0	0	3	2	—	—	120	—	—	—
HEINZ														
Ketchup	1 tbsp	15	0	0	0	0	4	4	0	0	190	—	—	0
No Salt Added	1 tbsp (0.6 oz)	20	0	0	0	0	5	4	0	0	0	190	—	0
Reduced Sugar	1 tbsp (0.6 oz)	5	0	0	0	0	1	1	0	0	170	—	—	0
HUNT'S														
Ketchup No Salt Added	1 tbsp (0.6 oz)	25	0	0	0	0	6	4	0	0	0	—	—	0
Squeeze	1 tbsp (0.6 oz)	20	0	0	0	0	5	4	0	0	190	—	—	0
MUIR GLEN														
Organic	1 tbsp	20	0	0	0	0	4	3	0	0	230	—	—	1

FOOD	PORTION	CALS	FAT	SAT FAT	CHOL	PROT	CARB	SUGAR	FIBER	CALCI	SOD	POTAS	FOLIC	VIT C
NATURE'S HOLLOW														
Sugar Free	1 tbsp (0.7 oz)	0	0	0	0	0	2	0	0	—	130	—	—	—
ORGANICVILLE														
No Added Sugar	1 tbsp (0.6 oz)	20	0	0	0	0	4	3	0	0	125	—	—	4
TEXAS SASSY														
Tequila Ketchup	1 tbsp (0.5 oz)	20	0	0	0	0	5	5	—	—	5	—	—	—
TREE OF LIFE														
Organic	1 tbsp (0.6 oz)	20	0	0	0	0	4	4	0	0	210	—	—	0
WALDEN FARMS														
Calorie Free	1 tbsp (0.5 oz)	0	0	0	0	0	0	0	0	0	170	—	—	0
WHOLEMATO														
Organic Agave	1 tbsp	15	0	0	0	0	3	3	0	0	230	—	—	1
KIDNEY														
beef simmered	3 oz	134	4	1	609	23	0	0	0	16	80	115	71	0
lamb braised	3 oz	116	3	1	480	20	1	—	0	15	128	151	69	10
pork braised	3 oz	128	4	1	408	22	0	0	0	11	68	122	35	9
veal braised	3 oz	139	5	1	672	22	0	0	0	25	94	135	18	7
RUMBA														
Beef	4 oz	120	4	1	320	19	2	0	0	0	200	—	—	9
KIDNEY BEANS														
canned	½ cup	108	1	tr	0	7	19	2	6	44	379	303	46	2
dried cooked w/o salt	½ cup	112	tr	tr	0	8	20	tr	6	31	1	358	115	1
B&M														
Red Kidney Baked Beans	½ cup (4.6 oz)	200	3	1	<5	8	36	10	6	60	460	—	—	0
EDEN														
Chili Beans	½ cup	130	0	0	0	9	21	1	7	60	250	400	—	—
Organic	½ cup	100	0	0	0	8	18	tr	10	60	15	440	—	—
Organic Refried	½ cup	80	1	0	—	7	15	—	6	40	180	410	—	—
PROGRESSO														
Cannellini	½ cup (4.6 oz)	110	0	0	0	8	20	2	6	60	340	—	—	—
VAN CAMP'S														
New Orleans	½ cup	90	0	0	0	6	19	1	6	60	450	—	—	0
KIWI														
fresh	1 lg (3.2 oz)	56	tr	tr	0	1	13	8	3	31	3	284	23	84
fresh	1 med (2.6 oz)	46	tr	tr	0	·1	11	7	2	26	2	237	19	71
CHIQUITA														
Fresh	1 (2.7 oz)	46	0	0	0	1	11	7	2	30	2	237	—	70
FRUITZIO														
Kiwi	1 pkg (0.88 oz)	40	0	0	0	0	8	3	1	0	0	—	—	48
KIWI JUICE														
AUNA														
Kiwifruit Juice	1 bottle (12 oz)	120	0	0	0	0	33	25	4	20	25	—	8	336

FOOD	PORTION	CALS	FAT	SAT FAT	CHOL	PROT	CARB	SUGAR	FIBER	CALCI	SOD	POTAS	FOLIC	VIT C
KNISH														
GABILA'S														
Potato	1 (4.5 oz)	180	3	0	0	4	36	tr	2	20	428	—	—	6
TAKE-OUT														
cheese	1 (2.1 oz)	205	12	3	56	6	19	tr	1	22	268	60	36	0
meat	1 (1.8 oz)	174	11	3	53	7	13	tr	1	13	202	84	26	tr
potato	1 lg (7 oz)	332	12	3	72	8	49	5	1	54	470	358	35	8
potato	1 (2.1 oz)	212	12	3	59	5	21	tr	1	13	210	94	35	1
KOHLRABI														
raw sliced	1 cup	36	tr	tr	0	2	8	4	4	32	27	472	22	84
sliced cooked w/o salt	1 cup	48	tr	tr	0	3	11	5	2	41	35	561	20	89
TAKE-OUT														
creamed	1 cup	150	9	2	6	5	14	6	1	122	555	485	19	58
KRILL														
fresh	1 oz	22	1	—	—	3	tr	—	0	114	119	81	—	1
KUMQUATS														
canned in syrup	1	13	tr	tr	0	tr	3	3	1	5	1	15	1	3
fresh	1	13	tr	tr	0	tr	3	2	1	12	2	35	3	8
KUZU														
EDEN														
Root Starch	1 tbsp	30	0	0	0	0	8	0	—	—	0	0	—	—
LAMB														
cubed lean & fat braised	4 oz	253	10	4	122	38	0	0	0	17	79	295	24	0
cubed lean broiled	4 oz	211	8	3	102	32	0	0	0	15	86	380	26	0
ground broiled	4 oz	321	22	9	110	28	0	0	0	25	92	384	22	0
leg roasted	4 oz	213	15	6	74	19	0	0	0	13	182	225	16	0
loin chop lean & fat broiled	1 chop (4 oz)	222	16	7	72	17	0	0	0	15	278	201	10	0
rib chop lean & fat broiled	1 chop (1.6 oz)	165	14	6	46	10	0	0	0	9	109	124	6	0
rib roast baked	4 oz	386	31	13	109	25	0	0	0	25	84	314	18	0
shank lean & fat braised	4 oz	360	20	8	157	42	0	0	0	30	107	380	25	0
shoulder chop lean & fat cooked	1 chop (5.5 oz)	274	20	8	91	22	0	0	0	20	388	249	21	0
shoulder w/ bone braised	4 oz	231	17	7	77	19	0	0	0	17	192	210	18	0
LAMB DISHES														
TAKE-OUT														
keema w/ coconut milk	1 serv (8 oz)	380	28	18	88	13	18	9	6	57	392	194	—	—
moroccan pilaf w/ bulgur	1 serv	327	13	2	54	—	—	—	—	—	303	—	—	—

FOOD	PORTION	CALS	FAT	SAT FAT	CHOL	PROT	CARB	SUGAR	FIBER	CALCI	SOD	POTAS	FOLIC	VIT C
moussaka	4 in sq (16 oz)	659	43	11	96	35	32	10	8	210	737	1089	82	27
shepherd's pie	1 (21.3 oz)	742	31	8	103	42	76	9	9	103	2092	1806	67	43
stew w/ potatoes & vegetables	1 cup	260	6	2	58	22	29	3	4	33	728	592	30	9

LAMBSQUARTERS

chopped cooked w/ salt	1 cup	58	1	tr	0	6	9	—	4	464	477	518	25	67

LECITHIN

lecithin	1 tbsp	104	14	2	0	0	0	0	0	—	—	—	—	—
BOB'S RED MILL														
Lecithin Granules	1 tbsp	60	4	1	0	0	1	0	0	—	0	—	—	—
TREE OF LIFE														
Granules	1 tbsp (0.3 oz)	55	4	0	0	0	1	0	0	100	2	—	—	0

LEEKS

chopped cooked w/o salt	¼ cup	8	tr	tr	0	tr	2	—	tr	8	3	23	6	1
cooked	1 (4.4 oz)	38	tr	tr	0	1	9	—	1	37	12	108	30	5
freeze dried	1 tbsp	1	0	0	0	tr	tr	—	0	1	0	5	1	tr

LEMON

fresh	1 med (4 oz)	22	tr	tr	0	1	12	—	5	66	3	157	—	83
peel	1 tbsp	3	tr	tr	0	tr	1	tr	1	8	0	10	1	8
peel	1 tsp	1	0	0	0	tr	tr	tr	tr	3	0	3	0	3
wedge	1 (7 g)	2	tr	tr	0	tr	1	tr	tr	2	0	10	1	4
TRUE LEMON														
Crystallized Lemon	1 pkg (1 g)	0	0	0	0	0	tr	—	—	—	0	—	—	15

LEMON CURD

lemon curd made w/ egg	2 tsp	29	1	—	—	tr	4	—	0	2	—	—	—	1
ROBERT ROTHCHILD FARM														
Lemon Curd & Tart Filling	1 tbsp	50	2	1	10	0	8	7	0	0	5	—	—	2

LEMON JUICE

bottled	1 oz	6	tr	tr	0	1	2	1	tr	3	6	31	3	8
bottled	1 tbsp	3	tr	tr	0	tr	1	tr	tr	2	3	15	2	4
fresh	1 oz	8	0	0	0	tr	3	1	tr	2	0	38	4	14
from 1 lemon	1.6 oz	12	0	0	0	tr	4	1	tr	3	0	58	6	22
from wedge	6 g	1	0	0	0	tr	1	tr	0	0	0	7	1	3
CANARINO														
Italian Hot Lemon Beverage as prep	1 cup	0	0	0	0	0	0	0	0	—	0	—	—	—
ESSN														
Sparkling Meyer Lemon Juice	1 can (8.4 oz)	170	0	0	0	1	41	36	—	20	20	—	—	12

FOOD	PORTION	CALS	FAT	SAT FAT	CHOL	PROT	CARB	SUGAR	FIBER	CALCI	SOD	POTAS	FOLIC	VIT C
ITALIAN VOLCANO														
Organic	2 tbsp (1 oz)	9	0	0	0	0	2	1	0	0	0	—	—	5
IZZE														
Esque Sparkling Limon	1 bottle (12 oz)	50	0	0	0	0	12	11	—	—	10	—	—	—
NATALIE'S ORCHID ISLAND JUICE														
100% Juice	1 tsp	1	0	0	0	0	0	0	0	0	0	6	0	2
SANTA CRUZ														
Organic 100% Juice	1 tsp	0	0	0	0	0	0	0	0	—	0	5	—	—
VOLCANO														
Organic Lemon Burst	2 tbsp (1 oz)	0	0	0	0	0	1	0	0	0	0	—	—	5

LEMONADE

MIX

CRYSTAL LIGHT

FOOD	PORTION	CALS	FAT	SAT FAT	CHOL	PROT	CARB	SUGAR	FIBER	CALCI	SOD	POTAS	FOLIC	VIT C
Sugar Free as prep	8 oz	5	0	0	0	0	0	0	0	—	35	—	—	—
HANSEN'S														
Fruit Stix Strawberry Lemonade	½ pkg (2 g)	5	0	0	0	0	1	—	—	—	20	15	—	60

READY-TO-DRINK

APPLE & EVE

FOOD	PORTION	CALS	FAT	SAT FAT	CHOL	PROT	CARB	SUGAR	FIBER	CALCI	SOD	POTAS	FOLIC	VIT C
Organic	8 oz	130	0	0	0	0	32	27	—	—	5	—	—	—
EARTHWISE														
Harvest Lemonade	8 oz	100	0	0	0	0	26	25	0	0	5	—	—	0
HONEST ADE														
Classic Zero Calorie	8 oz	0	0	0	0	0	0	0	0	—	5	—	—	30
HOOD														
Lemonade	1 cup	110	0	0	0	0	28	28	0	0	5	—	—	72
MIKE'S														
Hard Lemonade	1 bottle (12 oz)	220	0	0	0	—	32	—	—	—	—	—	—	—
MINUTE MAID														
Lemonade	1 can (12 oz)	150	0	0	0	0	42	40	—	—	50	—	—	—
NANTUCKET NECTARS														
Lemonade	8 oz	110	0	0	0	0	28	28	0	0	20	—	—	60
NATALIE'S ORCHID ISLAND JUICE														
Lemonade	8 oz	130	0	0	0	0	33	33	0	—	0	0	24	9
NESBITT'S														
Honey	1 bottle (12 oz)	180	0	0	0	0	44	44	—	—	120	—	—	—
ODWALLA														
PomaGrand	8 oz	110	0	0	0	0	28	27	0	0	10	—	—	0
Pure Squeezed	8 oz	120	0	0	0	0	30	28	0	0	10	—	—	12

FOOD	PORTION	CALS	FAT	SAT FAT	CHOL	PROT	CARB	SUGAR	FIBER	CALCI	SOD	POTAS	FOLIC	VIT C
RAAW														
Carrot Lemonade	8 oz	110	0	0	0	1	27	26	1	—	60	—	—	—
SANTA CRUZ														
Organic Sparkling	8 oz	110	0	0	0	0	27	27	0	—	0	215	—	4
SIMPLY														
Lemonade	8 oz	120	0	0	0	0	30	28	—	—	15	—	—	—
SPINDRIFT														
Sparkling	8 oz	80	0	0	0	0	21	19	0	0	0	—	—	6
SSIPS														
Lemonade	8 oz	110	0	0	0	0	27	24	0	0	5	—	—	60
SWEET LEAF														
Half & Half Lemonade Tea	8 oz	85	0	0	0	0	20	19	—	—	10	—	—	60
Original	8 oz	90	0	0	0	tr	24	22	—	—	0	—	—	60
TROPICANA														
Light	1 cup	10	0	0	0	0	2	1	0	0	5	—	—	60
Orchard Style	8 oz	120	0	0	0	0	31	29	0	0	20	—	—	60
Trop50 Raspberry	8 oz	50	0	0	0	0	12	12	—	—	15	—	—	60
Twister Light	8 oz	50	0	0	0	0	12	12	0	0	10	—	—	60
TURKEY HILL														
Lemonade	8 oz	120	0	0	0	0	29	29	—	—	10	—	—	—
UNCLE MATT'S														
Organic	8 oz	120	0	0	0	tr	30	27	0	0	10	310	—	0
LEMONGRASS														
fresh	1 tbsp	5	tr	tr	0	tr	1	—	—	3	0	35	4	tr
LENTILS														
dried cooked	1 cup	230	1	tr	0	18	40	4	16	38	4	731	358	3
EDEN														
Organic Green w/ Onion & Bay Leaf	½ cup	90	0	0	0	8	13	0	4	40	210	230	—	—
NEAR EAST														
Lentil Pilaf as prep	1 cup	200	3	2	9	11	36	3	8	20	672	—	—	1
TASTYBITE														
Jodhpur Lentils	½ pkg (5 oz)	106	4	2	0	6	12	3	7	30	664	—	—	3
Madras Lentils	½ pkg (5 oz)	120	5	3	3	6	14	3	5	40	450	—	—	2
TRUROOTS														
Organic Sprouted Green not prep	¼ cup (1.4 oz)	140	1	0	0	10	25	1	7	40	10	—	—	5
TAKE-OUT														
lentil loaf	1 slice (1.6 oz)	83	4	tr	0	4	10	1	3	17	40	155	63	1
middle eastern lentil salad	1 serv (4.5 oz)	158	3	tr	0	—	—	—	—	—	382	—	—	—

FOOD	PORTION	CALS	FAT	SAT FAT	CHOL	PROT	CARB	SUGAR	FIBER	CALCI	SOD	POTAS	FOLIC	VIT C
yemiser selatta ethiopian lentil salad	1 serv (3 oz)	115	7	1	0	4	11	1	2	19	536	234	73	56

LETTUCE

(see also SALAD)

FOOD	PORTION	CALS	FAT	SAT FAT	CHOL	PROT	CARB	SUGAR	FIBER	CALCI	SOD	POTAS	FOLIC	VIT C
arugula	6 leaves (0.4 oz)	3	tr	tr	0	tr	tr	tr	tr	19	3	44	12	2
arugula shredded	1 cup	5	tr	tr	0	1	1	tr	tr	32	5	74	19	3
boston	1 head (5.7 oz)	21	tr	tr	0	2	4	2	2	57	8	388	119	6
boston chopped	6 leaves	7	tr	tr	0	1	1	1	1	19	3	131	40	2
cornsalad field salad	1 cup (1.9 oz)	7	tr	—	0	1	1	—	1	19	2	232	80	19
iceberg	6 med leaves	7	tr	tr	0	tr	1	1	1	9	5	68	14	1
iceberg	1 lg head (26.5 oz)	106	1	tr	0	7	22	15	9	136	76	1065	219	21
iceberg shredded	1 cup	10	tr	tr	0	1	2	1	1	13	7	102	21	2
looseleaf outer leaves	6 (5 oz)	22	tr	tr	0	2	4	1	2	52	40	279	55	26
looseleaf shredded	1 cup	5	tr	tr	0	tr	1	tr	1	13	10	70	14	7
red leaf	6 leaves (3.6 oz)	16	tr	tr	0	1	2	tr	1	34	26	191	37	4
red leaf shredded	1 cup	4	tr	tr	0	tr	1	tr	tr	9	7	52	10	1
romaine	3 leaves (3 oz)	14	tr	tr	0	1	3	1	2	28	7	207	114	20
romaine heart	6 leaves (1.3 oz)	6	tr	tr	0	tr	1	tr	1	12	3	89	49	9
romaine shredded	1 cup	8	tr	tr	0	1	2	1	1	16	4	116	64	11
ANDY BOY														
Romaine Hearts	6 leaves (3 oz)	20	1	0	0	1	3	2	1	40	0	140	—	2
DOLE														
Just Lettuce	1½ cups (3 oz)	15	0	0	0	1	3	1	1	20	10	—	60	9
Romaine Chopped	1½ cups (3 oz)	15	0	0	0	1	3	2	1	40	5	—	120	21
EARTHBOUND FARMS														
Organic Baby Romaine Salad	2 cups	15	0	0	0	1	2	0	1	40	50	—	—	54
FRESH EXPRESS														
5 Lettuce Mix	3 cups	15	0	0	0	1	1	1	1	20	20	—	—	12
Lettuce Trio	2½ cups	15	0	0	0	1	3	1	1	20	10	—	0	12
Organic Baby Arugula	3 cups	20	1	0	0	2	3	2	1	150	25	—	—	12
Organic Hearts Of Romaine	1½ cups	15	0	0	0	1	2	0	1	40	5	—	—	21
Premium Romaine	2 cups	15	0	0	0	1	3	1	2	40	10	—	—	21
Shreds Iceberg	1½ cups	15	0	0	0	1	3	2	1	20	10	—	0	5
Sweet Butter	2½ cups	10	0	0	0	1	2	1	1	20	0	—	—	5
MANN'S														
Green Leaf Singles	6 leaves (3 oz)	15	0	0	0	2	3	2	2	40	30	—	—	4

FOOD	PORTION	CALS	FAT	SAT FAT	CHOL	PROT	CARB	SUGAR	FIBER	CALCI	SOD	POTAS	FOLIC	VIT C
OCEAN MIST														
Butter Leaf Shredded	1 cup (2 oz)	7	0	0	0	1	1	1	1	20	3	—	—	2
Green Or Green Leaf Shredded	1 cup (1.3 oz)	5	0	0	0	0	1	0	0	10	10	—	—	7
Iceberg	⅙ head (3 oz)	15	0	0	0	1	3	2	1	20	10	—	—	4
READY PAC														
Baby Arugula	4 cups (3 oz)	20	0	0	0	2	3	2	1	150	25	—	—	12
Shredded Iceberg	1 cup (3 oz)	10	0	0	0	1	3	1	1	20	10	—	—	2
Simply Lettuce	2½ cups (3 oz)	15	0	0	0	1	3	1	1	20	10	—	—	9
LILY ROOT														
dried	1 oz	89	1	—	—	2	21	—	tr	9	25	195	—	5
fresh	1 oz	32	tr	—	—	1	8	—	tr	1	3	—	—	6
LIMA BEANS														
CANNED														
lima beans	½ cup	95	tr	tr	0	6	18	—	6	25	405	265	60	0
ALLENS														
Baby Butter Beans	½ cup	120	1	0	0	7	22	2	6	20	460	—	—	0
Medium Green	½ cup	140	1	0	0	9	26	0	7	20	270	230	—	0
EAST TEXAS FAIR														
Green	½ cup	120	0	0	0	7	23	0	8	40	370	—	—	0
HANOVER														
Butter Beans In Sauce	½ cup	100	0	0	0	7	18	0	5	0	390	—	—	0
DRIED														
cooked	½ cup	150	tr	tr	0	6	20	1	5	27	14	484	22	9
FROZEN														
C&W														
Baby	½ cup	110	0	0	0	6	20	2	5	40	240	—	—	9
GREEN GIANT														
Baby & Butter Sauce as prep	⅔ cup	100	2	1	<5	5	18	1	5	20	420	—	—	9
LIME														
fresh	1 (2.4 oz)	20	tr	tr	0	tr	7	1	1	22	1	68	5	20
wedge	1 (8 g)	2	tr	tr	0	tr	1	tr	tr	3	0	8	1	2
TRUE LIME														
Crystallized Lime	1 pkg	0	0	0	0	0	0	0	0	—	0	—	—	15
LIME JUICE														
bottled	1 oz	6	tr	tr	0	tr	2	tr	tr	4	5	23	2	2
fresh	1 oz	8	tr	tr	0	tr	3	1	tr	4	1	36	3	9
from 1 lime	1.1 oz	11	tr	tr	0	tr	4	1	tr	6	1	51	4	13
ANGOSTURA														
Lime Mixer	1 tsp	5	0	0	0	0	2	2	0	0	0	—	—	0

FOOD	PORTION	CALS	FAT	SAT FAT	CHOL	PROT	CARB	SUGAR	FIBER	CALCI	SOD	POTAS	FOLIC	VIT C
HONEST ADE														
Limeade	8 oz	48	0	0	0	0	12	12	—	—	5	—	—	—
NATALIE'S ORCHID ISLAND JUICE														
100% Juice	1 tsp	0	0	0	0	0	0	0	0	0	0	6	0	1
SABOR LATINO														
Limeade	8 oz	160	0	0	0	0	39	38	—	—	5	0	—	60
SANTA CRUZ														
Organic 100% Juice	1 tsp	0	0	0	0	0	0	0	0	—	0	0	—	—
SIMPLY														
Limeade	8 oz	120	0	0	0	0	31	28	—	—	15	—	—	—
SWEET LEAF														
Limeade Cherry	8 oz	90	0	0	0	tr	24	22	—	—	0	—	—	60
TURKEY HILL														
Limonade	8 oz	120	0	0	0	0	29	27	—	—	10	—	—	2
VOLCANO														
Organic Lime Burst	2 tbsp (1 oz)	0	0	0	0	0	1	0	0	0	0	—	—	2
LING														
blue raw	3.5 oz	83	1	—	—	17	0	0	0	—	—	—	—	—
fresh baked	3 oz	95	1	—	—	21	0	0	0	37	147	413	—	—
fresh fillet baked	5.3 oz	168	1	—	—	37	0	0	0	66	261	734	—	—
LINGCOD														
baked	3 oz	93	1	tr	57	19	0	0	0	15	64	476	—	—
fillet baked	5.3 oz	164	2	tr	101	34	0	0	0	27	114	846	—	—
LIQUOR														
(see ALCOHOL DRINKS, BEER AND ALE, CHAMPAGNE, MALT, WINE)														
LITCHI JUICE														
CERES														
100% Juice	8 oz	120	0	0	0	0	30	26	1	0	10	190	—	60
LIVER														
(see also PATE)														
beef braised	1 slice (2.4 oz)	130	4	1	269	20	3	0	0	4	54	239	172	1
beef pan-fried	1 slice (2.8 oz)	142	4	1	309	21	4	0	0	5	62	284	211	1
chicken fried	3 oz	146	5	2	479	22	1	0	0	8	78	268	476	2
chicken simmered	3 oz	142	6	2	479	21	1	0	0	9	65	224	491	24
duck raw	1 (1.5 oz)	60	2	1	227	8	2	—	0	5	62	101	325	2
goose raw	1 (3.3 oz)	125	4	1	484	15	6	—	0	40	132	216	694	4
lamb braised	3 oz	187	7	3	426	26	2	—	0	7	48	188	62	3
lamb fried	3 oz	202	11	4	419	22	3	—	0	8	105	299	340	11
moose braised	3 oz	132	4	—	331	21	3	—	—	6	60	200	—	19
pork braised	3 oz	140	4	1	302	22	3	—	0	8	42	128	139	20
turkey simmered	1 liver (2.9 oz)	227	17	6	322	17	1	0	0	4	46	175	574	19

FOOD	PORTION	CALS	FAT	SAT FAT	CHOL	PROT	CARB	SUGAR	FIBER	CALCI	SOD	POTAS	FOLIC	VIT C
veal braised	1 slice (2.8 oz)	154	5	2	409	23	3	0	0	5	62	263	265	1
veal pan fried	1 slice (2.4 oz)	129	4	1	325	18	3	0	0	5	57	237	234	1
ORGANIC PRAIRIE														
Beef	2 oz	80	2	1	155	11	2	0	0	0	40	—	—	1
PERDUE														
Chicken Fresh	4 oz	130	6	2	395	19	0	0	0	0	80	—	—	21
RUMBA														
Beef	4 oz	160	5	2	365	22	7	0	0	0	80	—	—	24
TAKE-OUT														
calves liver w/ onions	1 serv (5 oz)	177	4	1	335	24	10	2	1	17	390	399	236	3
LLAMA														
llama	3 oz	120	3	—	60	22	—	—	—	—	—	—	—	—
LOBSTER														
northern cooked	1 cup	142	1	tr	104	30	2	—	—	88	551	510	16	—
northern cooked	3 oz	83	1	tr	61	17	1	—	—	52	323	299	9	—
northern raw	3 oz	77	1	—	81	77	tr	—	—	—	—	—	—	—
northern raw	1 lobster (5.3 oz)	136	1	—	143	28	1	—	—	—	—	—	—	—
spiny steamed	1 (5.7 oz)	233	3	tr	146	43	5	—	—	102	370	—	—	—
spiny steamed	3 oz	122	2	tr	76	22	3	—	—	53	193	—	—	—
TAKE-OUT														
newburg	1 cup	485	27	—	455	46	13	—	—	218	127	271	—	—
LOGANBERRIES														
fresh	½ cup (2.5 oz)	40	tr	tr	0	1	9	6	4	19	1	104	19	11
frzn thawed	½ cup (2.6 oz)	40	tr	tr	0	1	10	6	4	19	1	107	19	11
LONGANS														
fresh	1	2	0	0	0	tr	tr	—	—	0	0	9	—	3
LOQUATS														
fresh	1 sm (0.5 oz)	6	tr	tr	0	tr	2	—	tr	2	0	36	2	tr
fresh	1 lg (0.7 oz)	9	tr	tr	0	tr	2	—	tr	3	0	53	35	tr
fresh cubed	½ cup (2.6 oz)	35	tr	tr	0	tr	9	—	1	12	1	198	10	1
LOTUS														
root raw sliced	10 slices	45	tr	tr	0	2	14	—	—	36	33	450	—	36
root sliced cooked	10 slices	59	tr	tr	0	1	14	—	—	23	40	323	—	24
seeds dried	1 oz	94	1	tr	0	4	18	—	—	46	1	389	—	0
LOX														
(*see* SALMON)														
LUPINES														
dried cooked	1 cup	197	5	1	0	26	16	—	—	85	7	407	—	—
LYCHEES														
canned in syrup	½ cup (4.4 oz)	114	tr	tr	0	1	29	28	1	5	1	126	6	41
canned in syrup	1 (0.7 oz)	19	tr	tr	0	tr	5	5	tr	1	0	21	1	7

FOOD	PORTION	CALS	FAT	SAT FAT	CHOL	PROT	CARB	SUGAR	FIBER	CALCI	SOD	POTAS	FOLIC	VIT C
dried	1 (2.5 g)	7	tr	tr	0	tr	2	2	tr	1	0	28	0	5
fresh	1 (0.3 oz)	6	tr	tr	0	tr	2	1	tr	0	0	16	1	7
fresh cut up	½ cup (3.3 oz)	63	tr	tr	0	1	16	14	1	5	1	162	13	68
POLAR														
Lychee	1	110	0	0	0	tr	27	26	1	0	45	—	—	12

MACA ROOT

NAVITAS NATURALS

FOOD	PORTION	CALS	FAT	SAT FAT	CHOL	PROT	CARB	SUGAR	FIBER	CALCI	SOD	POTAS	FOLIC	VIT C
Powder Gelatinized	1 tsp (5 g)	20	0	0	0	1	3	1	1	20	0	—	—	1
Raw Powder	1 tsp (5 g)	20	0	0	0	1	4	1	1	20	0	—	—	1

MACADAMIA NUTS

FOOD	PORTION	CALS	FAT	SAT FAT	CHOL	PROT	CARB	SUGAR	FIBER	CALCI	SOD	POTAS	FOLIC	VIT C
dry roasted w/ salt	11 nuts (1 oz)	200	22	4	0	2	4	2	1	20	80	100	—	—
oil roasted	1 oz	204	22	3	0	2	4	—	—	13	3	94	—	0
CHUKAR CHERRIES														
Extra Dark Chocolate Covered	3 tbsp (1.4 oz)	216	20	7	0	2	14	9	3	10	4	—	—	0
EMILY'S														
Milk Chocolate Covered	4 (1.5 oz)	260	19	9	<5	3	21	18	2	40	20	—	—	—
FISHER														
Macadamia Nuts	¼ cup (1 oz)	200	21	3	0	2	4	1	3	20	110	—	—	0
HAWAIIAN HOST														
White Choco	3 pieces (1.4 oz)	230	15	9	0	1	22	21	0	40	40	—	—	0
MAUNA LOA														
Dry Roasted Salted	¼ cup (1 oz)	230	24	4	0	2	4	1	2	20	105	—	—	0
Dry Roasted Unsalted	¼ cup (1 oz)	230	24	4	0	2	4	1	2	20	0	—	—	0
Honey Roasted	¼ cup (1 oz)	200	19	3	0	2	9	6	2	0	85	—	—	0
Kona Coffee	¼ cup (1 oz)	180	15	3	<5	1	12	8	1	0	75	—	—	0
Maui Onion & Garlic	1 pkg (1.2 oz)	230	23	4	0	2	5	1	3	20	190	—	—	—

MACE

FOOD	PORTION	CALS	FAT	SAT FAT	CHOL	PROT	CARB	SUGAR	FIBER	CALCI	SOD	POTAS	FOLIC	VIT C
ground	1 tsp	8	1	tr	0	tr	1	—	tr	4	1	8	1	tr

MACKEREL

CANNED

FOOD	PORTION	CALS	FAT	SAT FAT	CHOL	PROT	CARB	SUGAR	FIBER	CALCI	SOD	POTAS	FOLIC	VIT C
jack	1 can (12.7 oz)	563	23	7	285	84	0	0	0	870	1368	700	19	3
jack	1 cup	296	12	4	150	44	0	0	0	458	720	369	10	2
CHICKEN OF THE SEA														
Jack In Water	⅓ cup	90	4	2	55	13	0	0	0	250	280	—	—	0
POLAR														
Jack	⅓ cup	90	4	2	55	13	0	0	0	250	280	—	—	0

FOOD	PORTION	CALS	FAT	SAT FAT	CHOL	PROT	CARB	SUGAR	FIBER	CALCI	SOD	POTAS	FOLIC	VIT C
FRESH														
atlantic cooked	3 oz	223	15	4	64	20	0	0	0	13	71	341	—	tr
atlantic raw	3 oz	174	12	3	60	16	0	0	0	10	76	267	—	tr
jack baked	3 oz	171	9	2	51	22	0	0	0	25	94	442	2	—
jack fillet baked	6.2 oz	354	18	5	106	45	0	0	0	52	194	916	4	—
king baked	3 oz	114	2	tr	58	22	0	0	0	34	172	474	7	—
king fillet baked	5.4 oz	207	4	1	105	40	0	0	0	61	312	859	14	—
pacific baked	3 oz	171	9	2	51	22	0	0	0	25	94	442	2	—
pacific fillet baked	6.2 oz	354	18	5	106	45	0	0	0	52	194	916	4	—
spanish cooked	3 oz	134	5	2	62	20	0	0	0	11	56	471	—	—
spanish fillet cooked	1 (5.1 oz)	230	9	3	107	34	0	0	0	19	96	808	—	—
spanish raw	3 oz	118	5	2	65	16	0	0	0	10	50	379	—	—
SMOKED														
atlantic	3.5 oz	296	24	5	93	19	0	0	0	20	384	310	1	0
MAHI MAHI														
fresh baked	4 oz	192	13	4	49	18	1	tr	0	22	464	377	14	2
MALANGA														
dasheen mashed	1 cup	226	tr	tr	0	3	53	1	8	84	743	1075	29	6
dasheen pieces boiled	1 cup	212	tr	tr	0	3	50	1	8	78	694	1004	27	6
pieces fried	1 cup	304	11	2	0	1	52	1	8	27	442	721	21	6
root raw	1 (10.7 oz)	299	1	tr	0	5	72	—	5	27	64	1824	52	16
MALT														
malt liquor	1 bottle (12 oz)	148	0	0	0	1	13	tr	tr	18	14	90	22	0
nonalcoholic	1 bottle (12 oz)	133	tr	tr	0	1	29	29	0	25	47	29	50	2
MALTED MILK														
chocolate as prep w/ milk	1 cup	179	5	3	16	8	27	15	1	266	136	437	21	1
chocolate flavor powder	3 heaping tsp (0.7 oz)	79	1	tr	0	1	18	5	1	13	53	130	11	tr
natural flavor as prep w/ milk	1 cup	186	6	3	21	9	24	22	tr	308	181	463	19	1
natural flavor powder	3 heaping tsp (0.7 oz)	87	2	1	7	2	16	12	tr	63	104	159	10	1
MAMMY APPLE														
fresh	1	431	4	—	0	4	106	—	—	93	127	398	—	118
MANGO														
dried	1 slice (5 g)	16	tr	tr	0	tr	4	4	tr	1	0	23	1	1
dried	½ cup (1.8 oz)	74	tr	tr	0	1	41	38	3	15	3	229	10	8
fresh	1 (7.3 oz)	135	1	tr	0	1	35	31	4	21	4	323	29	57
fresh sliced	½ cup (3 oz)	54	tr	tr	0	tr	14	12	2	8	2	129	12	23
pickled	1 slice (1 oz)	38	tr	tr	0	tr	10	9	tr	2	1	34	3	5

FOOD	PORTION	CALS	FAT	SAT FAT	CHOL	PROT	CARB	SUGAR	FIBER	CALCI	SOD	POTAS	FOLIC	VIT C
C&W														
Chunks	¾ cup	90	0	0	0	tr	24	21	3	0	0	—	—	36
CRISPY GREEN														
Crispy Mangoes	1 pkg (0.35 oz)	40	0	0	0	1	8	7	1	10	0	—	—	11
CRUNCHIES														
Freeze Dried	¼ cup (6 g)	20	0	0	0	0	5	3	1	0	0	—	—	36
CRUNCHY N'YUMMY														
Organic Freeze Dried	1 pkg (1 oz)	100	0	0	0	1	20	0	tr	11	7	277	—	80
DEL MONTE														
SunFresh In Extra Light Syrup	½ cup (4.4 oz)	70	0	0	0	0	19	17	tr	0	15	190	—	60
DOLE														
Chunks frzn	¾ cup (4.9 oz)	90	0	0	0	0	24	21	2	20	0	—	—	36
Fresh	½ (3.6 oz)	70	0	0	0	tr	18	15	2	20	0	—	—	30
KOPALI														
Organic Dried	1 pkg (1.8 oz)	140	0	0	0	0	38	34	4	100	0	—	—	1
PEELED SNACKS														
Fruit Picks Go-Mango-Man-Go	1 pkg (1.4 oz)	120	0	0	0	2	28	20	2	20	0	—	—	12
PHILLIPPINE BRAND														
Dried	6 pieces (1.5 oz)	160	0	0	0	tr	19	15	1	0	26	—	—	8
Dried Green	1 pkg (0.7 oz)	75	0	0	0	0	19	4	1	0	5	—	—	6
POLAR														
Sliced	3 pieces (5 oz)	100	0	0	0	0	24	21	2	40	20	—	—	9
SUNSWEET														
Philippine dried	6 pieces (1.4 oz)	130	0	0	0	1	32	27	1	0	85	170	—	24
MANGO JUICE														
nectar canned	1 cup (8.8 oz)	128	tr	tr	0	tr	33	31	1	43	13	60	18	38
CERES														
100% Juice	8 oz	120	0	0	0	0	30	26	1	0	10	190	—	60
GOODBELLY														
Mango Probiotic Drink	8 oz	100	0	0	0	tr	25	21	1	20	15	130	—	60
OLD ORCHARD														
Nectar Cocktail	8 oz	75	0	0	0	0	17	17	—	0	12	62	—	60
SNAPPLE														
Juice Drinks Mango Madness	8 oz	100	0	0	0	0	26	25	—	—	10	—	—	—
ULTRA LO-GLY														
Mango Mojito	1 bottle (10 oz)	35	0	0	0	0	8	7	0	20	10	—	—	0
MANGOSTEEN														
canned in syrup	½ cup (3.4 oz)	72	1	—	0	tr	18	—	2	12	7	47	30	3

FOOD	PORTION	CALS	FAT	SAT FAT	CHOL	PROT	CARB	SUGAR	FIBER	CALCI	SOD	POTAS	FOLIC	VIT C
XANGO														
Single Supplement	1 pkg (1 oz)	13	0	0	0	0	3	3	—	—	—	—	—	—
MARGARINE														
margarine butter blend	1 tbsp (0.5 oz)	101	11	2	2	tr	tr	0	0	1	89	3	0	0
squeeze	1 pkg (0.2 oz)	36	4	1	0	tr	0	0	0	3	39	5	0	0
squeeze liquid	1 tbsp (0.5 oz)	102	11	2	0	tr	0	0	0	9	111	13	0	tr
stick	1 stick (4 oz)	810	91	17	0	tr	1	0	0	3	1066	20	1	tr
stick	1 tbsp (0.5 oz)	100	11	2	0	tr	tr	0	0	0	132	3	0	0
tub diet	1 tbsp (0.5 oz)	26	3	tr	0	0	tr	0	0	0	110	4	0	0
tub fat free	1 tbsp (0.5 oz)	27	tr	tr	0	tr	1	0	0	1	85	5	0	0
tub light	1 tbsp (0.5 oz)	59	7	1	0	tr	tr	—	0	1	90	5	0	0
tub salted	1 tbsp (0.5 oz)	101	11	2	0	tr	tr	0	0	0	93	2	0	0
whipped salted	1 tbsp (0.3 oz)	67	8	1	0	tr	tr	0	0	0	62	2	0	0
BENECOL														
Spread Light	1 tbsp	50	5	1	0	0	0	0	0	—	110	—	—	—
Spread Regular	1 tbsp	70	8	1	0	0	0	0	0	—	110	—	—	—
BRUMMEL & BROWN														
Creamy Fruit Spread Strawberry	1 tbsp	50	4	1	0	0	3	3	—	—	45	—	—	—
Spread w/ Natural Yogurt	1 tbsp (0.5 oz)	45	5	1	0	0	0	0	0	—	90	—	—	—
COUNTRY CROCK														
Light	1 tbsp (0.5 oz)	50	5	2	0	0	0	0	0	—	85	—	—	—
Regular	1 tbsp (0.5 oz)	90	7	2	0	0	0	0	0	—	110	—	—	—
Spread w/ Calcium + Vitamin D	1 tbsp (0.5 oz)	50	5	1	0	0	0	0	0	100	95	—	—	—
EARTH BALANCE														
Butter Blend Salted	1 tbsp	100	11	5	15	0	0	0	0	—	100	—	—	—
Buttery Spread Original	1 tbsp	100	11	4	0	0	0	0	0	—	120	—	—	—
Buttery Spread Soy Garden	1 tbsp	100	11	4	0	0	0	0	0	—	120	—	—	—
Buttery Sticks Vegan	1 tbsp	100	11	5	0	0	0	0	0	—	120	—	—	0
I CAN'T BELIEVE IT'S NOT BUTTER														
Original	1 tbsp (0.5 oz)	70	8	2	0	0	0	0	0	—	90	—	—	—
Original Soft	1 tbsp (0.5 oz)	70	8	2	0	0	0	0	0	—	90	—	—	—
Original Squeeze	1 tbsp ((0.4 oz)	60	7	1	—	0	0	0	0	—	80	—	—	—
Spray	2 sprays (1 g)	0	0	0	0	0	0	0	0	—	24	—	—	—
LAND O LAKES														
Soft	1 tbsp (0.5 oz)	100	11	3	0	0	0	0	0	0	125	—	—	0
Stick	1 tbsp (0.5 oz)	100	11	2	0	0	0	0	0	0	105	—	—	0

FOOD	PORTION	CALS	FAT	SAT FAT	CHOL	PROT	CARB	SUGAR	FIBER	CALCI	SOD	POTAS	FOLIC	VIT C
MOVE OVER BUTTER														
Spread	1 tbsp	50	6	1	0	0	0	0	0	—	75	—	—	—
PARKAY														
Original Spread	1 tbsp (0.4 oz)	70	7	2	0	0	0	0	0	—	80	—	—	—
Spray	5 sprays (1 g)	0	0	0	0	0	0	0	0	—	15	—	—	—
Squeeze	1 tbsp (0.5 oz)	70	8	2	0	0	0	0	0	—	110	—	—	—
Stick	1 tbsp (0.5 oz)	80	9	2	0	0	0	0	0	—	130	—	—	—
PROMISE														
Buttery Spread	1 tbsp (0.5 oz)	80	8	2	0	0	0	0	0	—	85	—	—	—
Buttery Spread Activ	1 tbsp	70	8	1	<5	0	0	0	0	—	85	—	—	—
Fat Free	1 tbsp	5	0	0	0	0	0	0	0	—	90	—	—	—
Light	1 tbsp	45	5	1	0	0	0	0	0	—	85	—	—	—
Light Activ	1 tbsp	45	5	1	<5	0	0	0	0	—	85	—	—	—
SMART BALANCE														
Butter Blend Stick	1 tbsp (0.5 g)	100	11	5	15	0	0	0	0	—	100	—	—	—
Buttery Spread 37% Light	1 tbsp (0.5 oz)	45	5	2	0	0	0	0	0	—	85	—	—	—
Buttery Spread 67%	1 tbsp (0.5 oz)	80	9	3	0	0	0	0	0	—	90	—	—	—
Buttery Spread Low Sodium	1 tbsp (0.4 oz)	65	7	2	0	0	0	0	0	—	30	—	—	—
Buttery Spread Omega Plus	1 tbsp (0.5 oz)	80	9	3	0	0	0	0	0	—	90	—	—	—
Buttery Spread Omega-3 w/ Extra Virgin Olive Oil	1 tbsp (0.4 oz)	60	7	2	0	0	0	0	0	—	70	—	—	—
Buttery Spread w/ Flax Oil	1 tbsp (0.5 oz)	80	9	3	0	0	0	0	0	—	85	—	—	—
Spray Buttery Burst w/ Organic Soy	5 sprays (1 g)	0	0	0	0	0	0	0	0	—	24	—	—	—

MARINADE

(*see* SAUCE)

MARJORAM

FOOD	PORTION	CALS	FAT	SAT FAT	CHOL	PROT	CARB	SUGAR	FIBER	CALCI	SOD	POTAS	FOLIC	VIT C
dried	1 tsp	2	tr	tr	0	tr	tr	tr	tr	12	0	9	2	tr

MARLIN

FOOD	PORTION	CALS	FAT	SAT FAT	CHOL	PROT	CARB	SUGAR	FIBER	CALCI	SOD	POTAS	FOLIC	VIT C
raw	3 oz	110	3	—	—	20	0	0	0	8	—	—	—	1

MARSHMALLOW

FOOD	PORTION	CALS	FAT	SAT FAT	CHOL	PROT	CARB	SUGAR	FIBER	CALCI	SOD	POTAS	FOLIC	VIT C
chocolate coated	1 (0.4 oz)	41	1	1	0	tr	8	6	tr	1	7	10	0	0
coconut coated	1 (0.4 oz)	33	1	tr	0	tr	7	5	tr	0	11	6	0	0
marshmallow regular	1 (0.3 oz)	23	tr	tr	0	tr	6	4	0	0	6	0	0	0
miniatures	10 (0.3 oz)	22	tr	tr	0	tr	6	4	0	0	6	0	0	0
miniatures	1 cup (1.8 oz)	159	tr	tr	0	1	41	29	tr	2	40	2	0	0

MATZO

FOOD	PORTION	CALS	FAT	SAT FAT	CHOL	PROT	CARB	SUGAR	FIBER	CALCI	SOD	POTAS	FOLIC	VIT C
brie	1 piece (1.8 oz)	54	3	1	21	1	5	3	tr	4	47	10	2	0
egg	1 (1 oz)	109	1	tr	23	3	22	—	1	11	6	42	7	0
matzo ball	1 med (1.2 oz)	48	2	tr	36	2	6	tr	tr	6	12	20	4	0
plain	1 (1 oz)	111	tr	tr	0	3	23	—	1	4	1	31	5	0
whole wheat	1 (1 oz)	98	tr	tr	0	4	22	—	3	6	1	88	10	0
HOLIDAY CANDIES														
Dark Chocolate Coated	1 oz	130	5	3	0	2	20	9	1	0	0	—	—	0
MANISCHEWITZ														
Egg & Onion	1 (1 oz)	100	1	0	10	3	23	2	2	10	200	50	60	0
Matzo Ball Mix	2 tbsp	50	0	0	0	1	11	0	1	40	700	—	—	0
Thin Unsalted	1 (0.8 oz)	90	0	0	0	2	20	1	0	0	0	35	64	0
YEHUDA														
Organic	1 (1 oz)	110	1	0	0	4	23	0	3	0	5	—	—	0

MAYONNAISE

FOOD	PORTION	CALS	FAT	SAT FAT	CHOL	PROT	CARB	SUGAR	FIBER	CALCI	SOD	POTAS	FOLIC	VIT C
diet	1 tbsp	36	3	1	4	tr	3	1	0	0	78	2	0	0
imitation	1 tbsp	35	3	tr	4	tr	2	1	0	0	75	2	0	0
mayonnaise	1 tbsp	99	11	2	5	tr	1	tr	0	2	78	5	1	0
BACONNAISE														
Lite	1 tbsp (0.5 oz)	30	3	0	5	0	2	0	0	0	105	—	—	0
Regular	1 tbsp (0.5 oz)	80	9	2	10	0	1	0	0	0	85	—	—	0
CAINS														
All Natural	1 tbsp	100	11	2	5	0	0	0	0	0	75	—	—	0
Light	1 tbsp	50	5	0	5	0	2	1	0	0	130	—	—	0
DIETZ & WATSON														
Mixed Pepper Mayo	1 tbsp (0.5 oz)	100	11	2	5	0	1	0	0	0	85	—	—	0
HELLMAN'S														
Light	1 tbsp (0.5 oz)	35	4	1	<5	0	tr	—	—	—	125	—	—	—
Real	1 tbsp	90	10	2	5	0	0	0	0	—	90	—	—	—
Real Canola No Cholesterol	1 tbsp	90	10	1	5	0	0	0	0	0	90	—	—	0
Reduced Fat	1 tbsp	20	2	0	0	0	2	tr	—	—	125	—	—	—
W/ Extra Virgin Olive Oil	1 tbsp	50	5	1	5	0	tr	—	—	—	120	—	—	—
HOLLYWOOD														
Canola	1 tbsp	100	11	1	5	0	0	0	0	—	100	—	—	—
Safflower	1 tbsp	100	11	2	5	0	0	0	0	—	100	—	—	—
KRAFT														
Mayo	1 tbsp	90	10	2	<5	0	0	0	0	0	70	—	—	0
Mayo w/ Olive Oil	1 tbsp	45	4	0	<5	0	2	tr	0	0	95	—	—	0
MIRACLE WHIP														
Free	1 tbsp	15	0	0	0	0	3	2	—	—	125	—	—	—

FOOD	PORTION	CALS	FAT	SAT FAT	CHOL	PROT	CARB	SUGAR	FIBER	CALCI	SOD	POTAS	FOLIC	VIT C
MIRACLE WHIP (CONT.)														
Light	1 tbsp	25	2	0	0	0	3	2	0	0	140	—	—	0
Original	1 pkg (0.4 oz)	35	3	0	<5	0	2	1	—	—	85	—	—	—
NASOYA														
Nayonaise Original	1 tbsp (0.5 oz)	35	4	0	1	tr	1	0	0	0	115	—	—	0
NATURENAISE														
Organic Spread	1 tbsp (0.5 oz)	40	3	1	0	1	2	—	—	—	105	—	—	—
SMART BALANCE														
Omega Plus Light	1 tbsp (0.5 oz)	50	5	0	5	0	2	—	—	—	115	—	—	—
VEGENAISE														
Grapeseed Oil	1 tbsp (0.5 oz)	90	9	1	0	0	0	0	0	0	85	—	—	0
Organic	1 tbsp (0.5 oz)	90	9	2	0	0	0	0	0	0	85	—	—	0
Original	1 tbsp (0.5 oz)	90	9	1	0	0	0	0	0	0	85	—	—	0

MEAT SUBSTITUTES

(*see also* BACON SUBSTITUTES, CANADIAN BACON SUBSTITUTES, CHICKEN SUBSTITUTES, HAMBURGER SUBSTITUTES, MEATBALL SUBSTITUTES, SAUSAGE SUBSTITUTES, TURKEY SUBSTITUTES)

FOOD	PORTION	CALS	FAT	SAT FAT	CHOL	PROT	CARB	SUGAR	FIBER	CALCI	SOD	POTAS	FOLIC	VIT C
AMY'S														
Veggie Loaf w/ Mashed Potatoes & Vegetables	1 pkg (10 oz)	290	8	1	0	9	47	6	7	40	690	—	—	30
FANTASTIC														
Sloppy Joe Mix not prep	¼ cup	70	1	0	0	10	11	3	3	60	450	—	—	9
Taco Filling not prep	¼ cup	80	1	0	0	11	10	1	4	80	430	—	—	2
GARDEIN														
BBQ Pulled Shreds	1 serv (4.5 oz)	160	2	0	0	19	16	10	1	100	480	—	—	2
Beefless Tips	1 serv (3.5 oz)	120	3	0	0	18	7	0	3	100	440	—	—	1
Seasoned Bites	1 serv (4.4 oz)	130	3	0	0	20	8	0	2	80	410	—	—	5
GARDENBURGER														
BBQ Riblets w/ Sauce	1 serv (5 oz)	240	5	0	0	17	33	27	5	150	580	—	—	27
HELEN'S KITCHEN														
GardenSteak Tofu Steak	1 (3 oz)	150	2	0	0	12	14	1	3	300	190	—	—	0
LIGHTLIFE														
Smart Deli Pastrami Style	4 slices (2 oz)	60	0	0	0	13	1	0	0	—	400	330	—	—
Smart Ground Original	⅓ cup (1.9 oz)	80	1	0	0	11	7	1	3	—	280	330	—	—
Smart Ground Taco Burrito	⅓ cup (2 oz)	70	0	0	0	10	5	1	4	—	210	310	—	—
Smart Menu Crumbles	⅓ cup	80	1	0	0	11	7	1	3	—	330	280	—	—
Smart Tex Mex	¼ cup	50	0	0	0	6	6	2	2	—	170	250	—	—

FOOD	PORTION	CALS	FAT	SAT FAT	CHOL	PROT	CARB	SUGAR	FIBER	CALCI	SOD	POTAS	FOLIC	VIT C
LOMA LINDA														
Dinner Cuts	2 slices (3.2 oz)	90	1	0	0	18	4	0	2	0	500	20	—	0
Swiss Stake	1 piece (3.2 oz)	130	6	1	0	9	9	tr	3	0	430	200	—	0
MORNINGSTAR FARMS														
Meal Starters Steak Strips	12 pieces (3 oz)	140	3	1	0	23	5	1	1	40	720	460	—	0
VEAT														
Gourmet Bites	1 serv (2.5 oz)	90	3	0	0	8	8	2	1	60	420	—	—	0
Vegetarian Fillet	1 (1.8 oz)	170	5	1	0	15	19	1	1	30	90	—	—	0
VIANA														
Cowgirl Veggie Steaks	1 (3.7 oz)	260	14	3	0	29	6	5	4	60	890	—	—	0
Veggie Cevapcici	4 pieces (2.8 oz)	240	14	2	0	23	5	3	3	40	680	—	—	0
Veggie Doner Kebab	½ cup (3 oz)	210	14	3	0	18	3	2	2	—	810	—	—	—
Veggie Gyros	24 strips (3 oz)	220	11	2	0	26	5	2	2	40	1050	—	—	0
Veggie Kebab	½ cup	210	14	3	0	18	3	2	2	10	810	—	—	0
WORTHINGTON														
Bolono	3 slices (2 oz)	80	3	1	0	11	3	1	2	20	660	100	—	0
Choplets	2 slices (3.2 oz)	90	1	0	0	18	4	0	2	0	500	40	—	0
Corned Beef Vegetarian	3 slices (2 oz)	140	9	1	0	10	5	1	0	0	460	130	—	0
Dinner Roast	1 slice (3 oz)	180	11	2	0	14	6	1	3	20	580	120	—	0
Multigrain Cutlets	2 slices (3.2 oz)	100	1	1	0	17	5	0	3	0	290	30	—	0
Prime Stakes	1 piece (3.2 oz)	120	6	1	0	9	7	0	1	0	440	90	—	0
Vegetable Skallops	½ cup (3 oz)	90	1	0	0	17	4	0	3	0	390	10	—	0
Wham	2 slices (2 oz)	110	7	1	0	10	3	2	0	60	400	110	—	0
YVES														
Meatless Beef Skewers	1 (2.8 oz)	100	1	0	0	14	10	5	3	80	400	290	—	0
Meatless Bologna	4 slices	60	3	0	0	14	2	tr	0	20	460	200	—	0
Meatless Pepperoni	6 slices	90	1	0	0	14	4	tr	0	40	390	150	—	0
Meatless Ground Round Original	⅓ cup	60	1	0	0	10	5	1	2	40	270	250	—	0

MEATBALL SUBSTITUTES

FOOD	PORTION	CALS	FAT	SAT FAT	CHOL	PROT	CARB	SUGAR	FIBER	CALCI	SOD	POTAS	FOLIC	VIT C
meatless	2 (1.3 oz)	71	3	1	0	8	3	tr	2	9	198	65	28	0
FRANKLIN FARMS														
Portabella Veggiballs Gluten Free	3 (3 oz)	140	1	0	0	16	18	3	4	60	470	—	—	60
GARDENBURGER														
Mama Mia Meatballs	6 (3 oz)	110	5	1	0	12	7	0	4	60	400	—	—	0

FOOD	PORTION	CALS	FAT	SAT FAT	CHOL	PROT	CARB	SUGAR	FIBER	CALCI	SOD	POTAS	FOLIC	VIT C
LIGHTLIFE														
Smart Menu Meatless Meatballs	5	160	7	1	0	19	6	1	2	—	630	150	—	—
LOMA LINDA														
Tender Rounds	6 (2.8 oz)	120	5	1	0	13	6	1	1	20	340	80	—	0
MORNINGSTAR FARMS														
Meal Starters Veggie Meatballs	5 (2.8 oz)	130	5	1	0	15	7	tr	3	60	390	180	—	0
VEGGIE PATCH														
Meatless	4 (3 oz)	120	5	1	0	16	7	1	4	250	480	—	—	1

MEATBALLS

FOOD	PORTION	CALS	FAT	SAT FAT	CHOL	PROT	CARB	SUGAR	FIBER	CALCI	SOD	POTAS	FOLIC	VIT C
beef cocktail	1 (0.2 oz)	18	1	tr	6	2	0	0	0	2	28	21	1	0
beef lg	1 (1.5 oz)	111	7	3	37	11	0	0	0	10	167	126	4	0
beef med	1 (1 oz)	74	5	2	25	7	0	0	0	7	111	84	3	0
chicken cocktail	1 (0.2 oz)	12	tr	tr	6	1	1	tr	0	4	32	15	1	tr
chicken lg	1 (1.5 oz)	71	3	1	36	8	3	1	tr	21	192	91	8	1
chicken med	1 (1 oz)	47	2	tr	24	6	2	1	tr	14	128	61	6	1
turkey med	1 (1 oz)	47	2	tr	24	6	2	1	tr	14	128	61	6	1
venison	1 (1.5 oz)	69	3	1	37	8	3	1	tr	18	168	129	5	tr
BUTTERBALL														
Seasoned Italian frzn	6 (3 oz)	170	6	2	50	21	6	1	1	60	560	—	—	—
COLEMAN														
Chicken Buffalo Style	4	160	12	4	60	12	1	0	0	40	390	—	—	2
Chicken Chipotle Cheddar	4 (2.6 oz)	180	14	4	55	12	1	0	0	60	450	—	—	2
Chicken Italian w/ Parmesan	7 (2.6 oz)	150	10	3	60	14	1	0	1	100	550	—	—	1
Chicken Pesto Parmesan	4 (2.6 oz)	170	12	4	60	13	1	0	0	80	350	—	—	2
Chicken Spinach Fontina Cheese & Roasted Garlic	4 (2.6 oz)	130	9	3	55	13	0	0	0	40	470	—	—	2
Chicken Sun-Dried Tomato Basil & Provolone	4 (2.6 oz)	150	9	3	65	13	2	0	0	60	500	—	—	1
DELGROSSO														
Italian Style	3 (3 oz)	180	12	5	65	13	5	0	0	40	960	—	—	2
FARM RICH														
Original	6 (3 oz)	240	20	8	45	14	3	1	2	80	410	—	—	1
Turkey	5 (3.1 oz)	150	9	4	55	12	4	1	2	150	440	—	—	5
FOSTER FARMS														
Turkey	3 (2.9 oz)	150	7	—	40	15	8	tr	0	60	460	—	—	—

FOOD	PORTION	CALS	FAT	SAT FAT	CHOL	PROT	CARB	SUGAR	FIBER	CALCI	SOD	POTAS	FOLIC	VIT C
HANS ALL NATURAL														
Chicken Buffalo Style	4	160	12	4	60	21	1	0	0	40	390	—	—	2
Chicken Sweet Basil Parmesan	4	170	12	4	60	13	1	0	0	80	350	—	—	2
HONEYSUCKLE WHITE														
Turkey Italian Style frzn	3 (3 oz)	190	10	3	65	17	6	1	1	—	600	—	—	—
IAN'S														
Italian	3 (2.2 oz)	145	4	1	70	16	10	1	1	20	250	—	—	1
MAMA LUCIA														
Homestyle	4	207	20	8	50	14	8	2	1	40	610	—	—	0
Italian Style	4	280	23	10	50	11	8	1	0	40	640	—	—	0
Sausage Beef	8	220	17	7	50	14	3	0	1	40	690	—	—	0
MOM MADE														
Bite-Size Turkey	9 (3 oz)	140	4	2	65	17	9	1	0	20	135	—	—	0
ORGANIC CLASSICS														
Italian Beef	3 (3 oz)	180	11	5	50	17	5	1	1	80	430	—	—	0
PERDUE														
Turkey Italian Style	4 (3 oz)	180	10	4	45	15	5	0	—	40	520	—	—	0
SHADY BROOK														
Turkey Meatballs Appetizer Size + Sweet & Sour Sauce	6 + 2 tbsp sauce	235	10	3	65	17	17	11	tr	60	770	—	—	2
TYSON														
Italian Style Chicken	6 (3 oz)	180	11	3	45	13	6	1	2	0	610	—	—	0
TAKE-OUT														
albondigas w/ sauce	3 + sauce (5.3 oz)	372	27	8	102	21	11	3	1	38	1194	480	22	4
porcupine + tomato sauce	3 + sauce	160	7	3	34	11	14	3	1	19	591	213	21	5
swedish w/ cream sauce	3 + sauce (4.7 oz)	215	12	5	86	17	9	2	tr	73	678	317	16	2
sweet & sour	3 + sauce (4.5 oz)	188	11	3	67	15	8	1	1	46	609	268	14	tr

MELON
sprite	1 (10.6 oz)	110	0	0	0	1	29	27	1	0	190	—	—	90

MEXICAN FOOD

(*see* SALSA, SPANISH FOOD, TORTILLA)

MILK
CANNED														
condensed sweetened	1 cup (10.7 oz)	982	27	17	104	24	166	166	0	869	389	1135	34	8

FOOD	PORTION	CALS	FAT	SAT FAT	CHOL	PROT	CARB	SUGAR	FIBER	CALCI	SOD	POTAS	FOLIC	VIT C
condensed sweetened	1 tbsp (0.7 oz)	61	2	1	6	2	10	10	0	54	24	71	2	1
evaporated nonfat	1 cup (9 oz)	200	1	tr	10	19	29	29	0	742	294	850	23	3
evaporated nonfat	1 tbsp (0.5 oz)	12	tr	tr	1	1	2	2	1	46	18	53	1	tr
BORDEN														
Sweetened Condensed	2 tbsp (1.4 oz)	130	3	2	10	3	22	22	0	100	40	—	—	0
Sweetened Condensed Low Fat	2 tbsp	120	2	1	5	3	23	23	0	100	40	—	—	0
CARNATION														
Evaporated	2 tbsp (1 oz)	40	2	2	10	2	3	3	—	80	30	90	—	—
Evaporated Fat Free	2 tbsp (1 oz)	25	0	0	0	2	4	4	—	80	30	110	—	—
Evaporated Lowfat 2%	2 tbsp (1 oz)	25	1	0	5	2	3	3	—	80	35	100	—	—
MEYENBERG														
Goat Evaporated	4 oz	145	8	5	27	8	10	10	—	298	112	—	80	—
DRIED														
buttermilk	¼ cup (1 oz)	111	2	1	20	10	14	14	0	341	149	458	14	2
buttermilk	1 tbsp (0.2 oz)	25	tr	tr	4	2	3	3	0	77	34	103	3	tr
nonfat instant	1 tbsp (0.6 oz)	61	tr	tr	3	6	9	9	0	209	93	290	8	1
nonfat instant	1 pkg (3.2 oz)	326	1	tr	16	32	47	47	0	1120	500	1552	46	5
whole milk	¼ cup (1.1 oz)	159	9	5	31	8	12	12	0	292	119	426	12	3
ALBA														
Instant Non-Fat as prep	1 cup	80	0	0	0	8	11	11	0	250	120	—	—	1
BOB'S RED MILL														
Buttermilk Sweet Cream as prep	8 oz	60	1	1	10	5	7	0	0	—	85	—	—	—
Non Fat as prep	8 oz	80	0	0	0	7	11	11	0	—	110	—	—	—
CARNATION														
Instant Nonfat as prep	1 cup	80	0	0	<5	8	12	12	0	300	125	390	—	1
MEYENBERG														
Goat Powdered	1 scoop (1 oz)	90	0	0	10	8	11	11	0	300	95	—	80	0
ORGANIC VALLEY														
Buttermilk	3 tbsp	110	1	0	0	10	16	12	0	100	45	—	—	0
Nonfat	3 tbsp	90	0	0	0	9	13	12	0	300	130	—	—	1
SANALAC														
Powder	¼ cup (0.8 oz)	80	0	0	5	8	13	12	0	300	105	—	—	2
REFRIGERATED														
1%	1 cup (8.6 oz)	102	3	2	12	8	12	13	0	290	107	366	12	0
2%	1 cup (8.6 oz)	122	5	3	20	8	11	12	0	287	100	368	12	1
buffalo	7 oz	224	16	—	—	8	10	—	—	390	80	200	—	6
buttermilk lowfat	1 cup (8.6 oz)	98	2	1	10	8	12	12	0	284	257	370	12	3

FOOD	PORTION	CALS	FAT	SAT FAT	CHOL	PROT	CARB	SUGAR	FIBER	CALCI	SOD	POTAS	FOLIC	VIT C
camel	7 oz	160	8	—	—	10	10	—	—	264	60	188	—	—
donkey	7 oz	86	2	—	—	4	12	—	—	220	—	—	—	4
fat free	1 cup (8.6 oz)	83	tr	tr	5	8	12	12	0	306	103	382	12	0
goat	1 cup (8.6 oz)	168	10	7	27	9	11	11	0	327	122	498	2	3
human	1 cup (8.6 oz)	172	11	5	34	3	17	07	0	79	42	125	12	12
indian buffalo	1 cup (8.6 oz)	237	17	11	46	9	13	—	0	412	127	434	15	6
mare	7 oz	98	4	—	—	4	12	—	—	220	—	128	—	30
sheep	1 cup (8.6 oz)	265	17	11	66	15	13	—	0	473	108	336	17	10
whole	1 cup (8.6 oz)	146	8	5	24	8	11	14	0	276	98	349	12	0
ACTIVE LIFESTYLE														
Fat Free w/ Plant Sterols	8 oz	90	0	0	<0	8	13	12	0	300	125	—	—	2
DAIRY EASE														
Fat Free Lactose Free	1 cup (8 oz)	90	0	0	5	8	12	12	0	300	125	460	—	0
Reduced Fat 2% Lactose Free	1 cup (8 oz)	130	5	3	15	9	12	12	0	300	130	440	—	0
Whole Lactose Free	1 cup (8 oz)	160	9	5	20	8	11	11	0	300	125	430	—	0
FARMLAND														
Buttermilk	8 oz	160	4	3	20	12	19	18	0	450	190	—	—	4
Fat Free	8 oz	80	0	0	5	8	12	12	0	300	130	—	—	1
Special Request 1% Plus Omega-3	8 oz	130	3	2	10	11	17	16	0	400	170	—	—	1
Special Request Skim Plus	8 oz	110	0	0	5	11	17	16	0	400	170	—	—	1
Special Request Skim Plus 100% Lactose Free	8 oz	110	0	0	5	11	17	16	0	400	170	—	—	1
Whole	8 oz	160	4	3	20	12	19	18	0	450	190	—	—	4
FRIENDSHIP														
Buttermilk Lowfat	1 cup	120	4	3	15	9	12	12	0	300	125	—	—	2
HOOD														
1%	1 cup	110	3	2	15	8	13	12	0	300	125	—	—	6
2%	1 cup	130	5	3	20	8	13	12	0	300	125	—	—	6
Buttermilk Fat Free	1 cup	90	0	0	<5	9	13	12	0	300	220	—	—	2
Fat Free	1 cup	80	0	0	<5	8	13	12	0	300	125	—	—	6
Simply Smart 0% Fat	1 cup	90	0	0	<5	10	13	12	0	350	130	—	—	0
Simply Smart 1% Fat	1 cup	120	3	2	15	10	13	12	0	350	130	—	—	0
Whole	1 cup	150	8	5	35	8	12	12	0	300	125	—	—	6
HORIZON														
Fat Free	8 oz	90	0	0	<5	9	12	12	0	300	130	—	—	1
Lowfat 1%	8 oz	100	3	2	10	8	12	12	0	300	125	0	—	1

FOOD	PORTION	CALS	FAT	SAT FAT	CHOL	PROT	CARB	SUGAR	FIBER	CALCI	SOD	POTAS	FOLIC	VIT C
HORIZON (CONT.)														
Reduced Fat 2%	8 oz	120	5	3	20	8	12	12	0	300	125	—	—	1
Whole	8 oz	150	8	5	35	8	12	12	0	300	125	—	—	1
LACTAID														
Fit & Creamy Lowfat	8 oz	120	3	2	15	10	12	12	0	350	120	420	—	0
Whole	8 oz	160	8	5	35	8	12	12	0	300	125	350	—	0
LAND O LAKES														
1%	1 cup (8 oz)	100	3	2	15	8	13	13	0	300	125	410	—	2
2%	1 cup (8 oz)	120	5	3	20	8	12	12	0	300	125	400	—	2
Skim	1 cup (8 oz)	90	0	0	<5	8	13	13	0	300	125	410	—	2
Whole	1 cup (8 oz)	150	8	5	35	8	12	12	0	300	125	400	—	2
MEYENBERG														
Goat Low Fat	8 oz	89	2	2	8	7	9	9	—	268	100	—	—	—
Goat Whole	8 oz	142	7	4	25	8	11	11	—	307	115	—	—	—
ORGANIC VALLEY														
Buttermilk Lowfat 1%	1 cup	100	3	2	15	8	12	12	0	300	250	—	—	2
Fat Free	1 cup	90	0	0	5	8	13	12	0	300	125	390	—	1
Lactose Free Fat Free	1 cup	90	0	0	0	8	14	13	0	300	130	390	—	0
Whole Nonhomogenized	1 cup	150	8	5	35	8	12	12	0	300	125	—	—	1
OVER THE MOON														
Fat Free	8 oz	100	0	0	5	10	15	14	0	350	150	470	—	0
Low Fat	8 oz	120	3	2	15	10	14	13	0	350	150	470	—	0
SMART BALANCE														
1% Lowfat w/ HeartRight	1 cup (8 oz)	120	3	3	5	10	14	14	—	350	150	—	—	—
1% Lowfat w/ Omega-3s & Vitamin E	1 cup (8 oz)	140	3	2	5	11	15	15	—	300	170	—	—	—
Fat Free w/ Omega-3s & Vitamin E	1 cup (8 oz)	120	0	0	5	10	15	15	—	350	160	—	—	—
STRAUS														
Organic Cream Top Whole	8 oz	150	8	5	35	8	11	11	0	300	120	—	—	2
Organic Fat Free	8 oz	90	0	0	5	9	12	12	0	320	130	—	—	2
Organic Whole Milk	8 oz	170	7	5	35	12	14	7	0	350	125	—	—	0
SUNMILK														
Heart Healthy 1% Sunflower Oil	8 oz	120	2	0	<5	11	15	15	0	400	160	460	—	2
Heart Healthy 2% Sunflower Oil	8 oz	120	3	0	<5	10	15	15	0	350	150	460	—	2

FOOD	PORTION	CALS	FAT	SAT FAT	CHOL	PROT	CARB	SUGAR	FIBER	CALCI	SOD	POTAS	FOLIC	VIT C
TURKEY HILL														
Cool Moos Whole Milk	8 oz	160	3	2	10	8	27	26	0	300	140	—	—	2
VALIO														
100% Lactose Free 0% Fat	8 oz	80	0	0	<5	11	7	7	0	300	125	—	—	0
100% Lactose Free 2% Fat	8 oz	120	5	3	20	11	7	7	0	300	125	—	—	0
WELSH FARMS														
Fat Free	8 oz	80	0	0	5	8	12	12	0	300	130	—	—	1
SHELF-STABLE														
PARMALAT														
2% Reduced Fat	8 oz	130	5	3	20	8	12	12	0	300	130	—	—	1
Fat Free	8 oz	80	0	0	5	8	12	12	0	300	130	—	—	1
Lactose Free 2% Reduced Fat	8 oz	130	5	3	20	8	12	12	0	300	130	—	—	1

MILK DRINKS

FOOD	PORTION	CALS	FAT	SAT FAT	CHOL	PROT	CARB	SUGAR	FIBER	CALCI	SOD	POTAS	FOLIC	VIT C
chocolate milk	1 cup (8.8 oz)	208	8	5	30	8	26	24	2	280	150	418	12	2
chocolate milk lowfat	1 cup (8.8 oz)	158	3	2	8	8	26	25	1	288	152	425	12	2
BRAVO!														
Blenders Creamy Double Chocolate	1 bottle (11 oz)	180	4	3	20	17	19	16	2	500	350	800	100	30
Blenders Creamy French Vanilla	1 bottle (11 oz)	160	4	3	20	17	20	16	2	500	260	970	100	30
COCIO														
Chocolate Milk	8 oz	140	4	3	15	6	20	17	0	250	80	—	—	2
DOVE														
Bravo! Dark Chocolate	1 bottle	310	16	—	60	8	37	34	2	250	140	550	—	1
Bravo! Milk Chocolate	1 bottle	310	16	—	60	8	36	34	1	—	105	530	—	1
DRSEARS														
Cool Fuel Chocolate	1 pkg (8 oz)	190	6	1	0	8	25	9	4	200	75	980	100	54
Cool Fuel Chocolate Banana	1 pkg (8 oz)	190	6	1	0	8	28	9	4	200	75	890	100	54
Cool Fuel Vanilla	1 pkg (8 oz)	190	6	1	0	8	28	9	4	200	75	840	100	54
FARMLAND														
Really Really Good! Chocolate Milk	8 oz	160	3	2	10	8	25	24	0	300	150	—	—	2
HOOD														
Chocolate Lowfat	1 cup	170	3	2	15	9	28	26	tr	500	170	—	—	0
Chocolate Milk	1 cup	230	9	5	35	9	31	29	tr	500	170	—	—	0

FOOD	PORTION	CALS	FAT	SAT FAT	CHOL	PROT	CARB	SUGAR	FIBER	CALCI	SOD	POTAS	FOLIC	VIT C
HORIZON ORGANIC														
Lowfat Chocolate Milk	8 oz	170	3	2	15	8	27	27	tr	200	140	—	—	18
Strawberry	8 oz	200	5	3	20	8	31	31	0	250	130	—	—	0
LACTAID														
Chocolate Milk 1% Fat	8 oz	150	3	2	15	8	24	23	tr	300	230	440	—	0
LAND O LAKES														
2% Swiss Chocolate	1 cup (8.4 oz)	190	5	3	20	8	26	26	tr	300	220	—	—	4
Chocolate Skim	1 cup (8 oz)	160	0	0	<5	8	31	28	tr	300	220	—	—	2
Strawberry	1 cup (8 oz)	190	8	5	30	7	22	22	0	300	220	—	—	4
MOJOMILK														
Chocolate Mix not prep	1 pkg (4.5 g)	20	1	0	0	0	4	2	0	2	40	40	—	0
Probiotic Chocolate Milk not prep	1 pkg (4.5 g)	20	1	0	0	0	4	2	0	20	40	40	—	0
NESQUIK														
Chocolate Powder No Sugar Added as prep w/ lowfat milk	1 cup (8 oz)	160	5	3	21	1	18	3	1	400	168	—	—	9
Chocolate Powder as prep w/ lowfat milk	1 cup (8 oz)	180	5	3	21	tr	27	13	tr	400	120	—	—	9
Ready-To-Drink Banana	1 cup (8 oz)	200	5	3	20	7	30	29	0	400	120	—	—	0
Ready-To-Drink Chocolate	1 cup (8 oz)	200	5	3	15	8	32	30	tr	400	150	—	—	1
Ready-To-Drink Strawberry	1 cup (8 oz)	200	5	3	15	8	33	31	0	400	120	—	—	1
Ready-To-Drink Vanilla	1 cup (8 oz)	200	5	3	15	8	30	29	0	400	120	—	—	1
Strawberry Powder as prep w/ lowfat milk	1 cup (8 oz)	190	4	3	21	0	27	15	0	400	96	—	—	9
Strawberry Powder not prep	2 tbsp (0.6 oz)	60	0	0	0	0	15	15	0	100	0	—	—	6
OVER THE MOON														
Chocolate Milk Fat Free	8 oz	150	0	0	5	11	27	25	tr	400	250	530	—	0
PARMALAT														
Chocolate Milk 2% Reduced Fat	1 cup	190	5	3	20	8	28	27	1	300	130	—	—	1
SIPAHH														
Straw Banana	1 straw	15	0	0	0	0	3	2	—	—	0	—	—	—

FOOD	PORTION	CALS	FAT	SAT FAT	CHOL	PROT	CARB	SUGAR	FIBER	CALCI	SOD	POTAS	FOLIC	VIT C
SIPAHH (CONT.)														
Straw Cookies and Cream	1 straw	15	0	0	0	0	3	2	—	—	0	—	—	—
TRUMOO														
Chocolate Milk Fat Free	8 oz	130	0	0	5	8	24	22	0	300	200	440	8	1
Chocolate Milk Lowfat	8 oz	150	3	2	10	8	24	22	0	300	180	430	8	1
Strawberry Milk Fat Free	8 oz	130	0	0	5	8	23	22	0	300	125	400	8	1
TURKEY HILL														
Cool Moos 2% Reduced Fat	8 oz	120	5	3	20	8	12	12	0	300	125	—	—	2
Cool Moos Chocolate	8 oz	180	3	2	10	8	32	30	0	300	210	—	—	1

MILK SUBSTITUTES

FOOD	PORTION	CALS	FAT	SAT FAT	CHOL	PROT	CARB	SUGAR	FIBER	CALCI	SOD	POTAS	FOLIC	VIT C
soy milk	1 cup	79	5	1	0	7	4	—	—	10	30	338	4	0
BRAZSOY														
Condensed Soy Milk	1 serv (0.7 oz)	54	1	0	0	1	10	9	0	—	11	—	—	—
Soy Cream	1 tbsp (0.5 oz)	27	3	tr	0	0	0	0	0	—	15	—	—	—
DARIFREE														
Fat Free as prep	8 oz	70	0	0	0	0	20	2	0	300	120	50	—	6
Fat Free Chocolate as prep	8 oz	110	0	0	5	0	27	11	tr	300	125	360	—	9
EDENSOY														
Organic Chocolate	8 oz	180	4	1	0	8	28	14	tr	100	105	410	40	—
Organic Original	8 oz	140	5	1	0	11	14	7	tr	100	105	440	40	—
Organic Original Unsweetened	8 oz	120	6	1	0	12	5	2	tr	40	5	460	60	
Organic Vanilla	8 oz	150	3	1	0	7	24	16	tr	80	85	320	40	—
LIVING HARVEST														
Hempmilk Original	1 cup	130	3	1	0	4	20	15	1	460	120	113	25	0
Hempmilk Vanilla	1 cup	130	3	1	0	4	20	18	1	460	120	113	25	0
LUNDBERG														
Organic Drink Rice Original	8 oz	120	3	0	0	1	22	13	tr	300	85	85	—	0
MANITOBA HARVEST														
Hemp Bliss Chocolate	8 oz	160	7	1	0	5	17	16	1	40	120	—	—	0
Hemp Bliss Original	1 cup	110	7	1	0	5	7	6	1	20	95	—	—	0
Hemp Bliss Vanilla	8 oz	150	7	1	0	5	14	13	1	20	120	—	—	0
ODWALLA														
Soy Smart Chai	8 oz	150	4	1	—	6	22	20	—	300	30	410	—	—

FOOD	PORTION	CALS	FAT	SAT FAT	CHOL	PROT	CARB	SUGAR	FIBER	CALCI	SOD	POTAS	FOLIC	VIT C
ODWALLA (CONT.)														
Soy Smart Vanilla	8 oz	120	4	1	—	6	15	14	—	300	55	290	—	—
Soymilk Plain	8 oz	110	4	1	0	7	12	—	3	300	65	380	60	0
Soymilk Vanilla Being	8 oz	100	3	0	0	4	13	10	3	300	65	310	40	0
ORGANIC VALLEY														
Soy Original	1 cup	100	3	1	0	7	11	6	3	300	95	280	24	1
Soy Unsweetened	1 cup	80	4	1	0	7	3	1	1	300	110	280	24	0
PACIFIC FOODS														
7 Grain Original Organic	1 cup (8 oz)	140	2	0	0	3	27	16	1	350	75	130	80	0
Almond Original Unsweetened Organic	8 oz	35	3	0	0	1	2	0	0	0	180	0	—	0
Hazelnut Original	8 oz	110	4	0	0	2	18	14	1	300	120	60	—	0
Hemp Original	8 oz	140	5	1	0	3	20	14	1	500	130	170	—	0
Oat Original Organic	1 cup (8 oz)	130	3	0	0	4	24	19	2	350	110	120	—	0
Rice All Natural Plain	1 cup (8 oz)	130	2	0	0	1	27	14	0	300	60	—	—	0
Soy Original Unsweetened Organic	1 cup (8 oz)	90	5	1	0	9	4	2	2	20	15	410	—	0
Soy Ultra Plain	1 cup (8 oz)	120	4	1	0	10	11	8	1	500	150	380	—	0
PEARL														
Organic Soymilk Coffee	8 oz	150	4	1	0	6	24	22	0	300	190	210	60	0
Organic Soymilk Green Tea	8 oz	110	4	1	0	7	13	10	1	300	95	280	100	0
Organic Soymilk Original	8 oz	110	4	1	0	7	12	9	1	300	110	300	80	0
RICE DREAM														
Carob	8 oz	150	3	0	0	1	30	26	tr	0	80	—	—	0
Heartwise Vanilla	8 oz	140	2	0	0	1	30	10	3	300	80	30	—	0
Horchata	8 oz	130	4	1	0	7	16	9	2	40	150	140	—	0
Original	8 oz	120	3	0	0	1	24	11	0	20	100	—	—	0
Original Enriched	8 oz	120	3	0	0	1	23	10	0	300	100	—	—	0
Vanilla Enriched	8 oz	130	3	0	0	1	26	12	0	300	105	—	—	0
SILK														
Chocolate	1 cup (8 oz)	140	4	1	0	5	23	19	2	300	100	350	24	0
Plain	8 oz	100	4	1	0	7	8	6	1	300	120	300	24	0
Soy Heart Health	1 cup	80	2	0	0	6	10	7	1	300	95	300	24	0
Soy Plain Light	1 cup	70	2	0	0	6	8	6	1	300	120	300	24	0
Soy Plus DHA Omega-3	1 cup	110	5	1	0	7	8	6	1	350	120	350	80	21

FOOD	PORTION	CALS	FAT	SAT FAT	CHOL	PROT	CARB	SUGAR	FIBER	CALCI	SOD	POTAS	FOLIC	VIT C
SILK (CONT.)														
Soy Pumpkin Spice	1 cup	170	4	1	0	6	28	24	0	40	150	300	—	0
Soy Unsweetened	1 cup	80	4	1	0	7	4	1	1	300	85	300	24	0
Vanilla	1 cup (8 oz)	100	4	1	0	6	10	7	1	300	95	300	24	0
SIMPLI														
Naked Oat Vanilla	8 oz	100	3	0	0	2	18	10	2	300	75	—	—	0
SNO*E														
Tofu as prep	8 oz	80	5	2	0	2	20	2	0	300	130	95	—	6
Tofu Low Fat as prep	8 oz	70	3	0	0	2	10	1	0	300	135	86	—	6
SOL														
Sunflower Original	8 oz	70	4	1	0	1	9	7	1	300	115	410	80	0
Sunflower Unsweetened	8 oz	45	4	1	0	1	2	0	1	300	115	410	80	0
Sunflower Vanilla	8 oz	90	4	1	0	1	14	12	1	300	115	410	80	0
SOY DREAM														
Classic Vanilla	8 oz	140	4	1	0	7	18	10	2	40	135	140	—	0
Original Enriched	8 oz	100	4	1	0	7	8	4	2	350	135	250	—	0
SUNRICH NATURALS														
Soymilk Original Plain	8 oz	110	5	1	0	8	11	9	1	300	125	360	24	0
Soymilk Vanilla	8 oz	130	5	1	0	8	14	11	1	300	125	360	24	0
VITASOY														
Organic Lite Plus Original	8 oz	60	2	tr	0	4	6	5	0	300	130	190	—	0
Organic Lite Plus Vanilla	8 oz	80	2	tr	0	4	12	11	0	300	120	190	—	0
Organic Mint Chocolate	8 oz	160	4	1	0	5	27	24	1	20	125	320	—	0
Organic Original	8 oz	90	4	1	0	7	9	7	1	300	160	410	—	0
Organic Vanilla	8 oz	110	4	1	0	7	14	12	1	300	125	340	—	0
WILDWOOD														
Organic Probiotic Soymilk Blueberry	8 oz	190	3	0	0	7	33	19	4	300	60	0	0	0
Organic Probiotic Soymilk Pomegranate	8 oz	180	3	0	0	7	31	17	4	300	55	0	0	0
Organic Soymilk Plain	8 oz	100	4	1	0	7	8	6	1	300	80	290	32	0
Organic Soymilk Unsweetened	8 oz	72	4	1	0	7	3	2	1	300	70	300	32	0
ZENSOY														
Soy Milk Cappuccino	8 oz	150	4	1	0	7	22	17	1	300	160	—	—	0

FOOD	PORTION	CALS	FAT	SAT FAT	CHOL	PROT	CARB	SUGAR	FIBER	CALCI	SOD	POTAS	FOLIC	VIT C
ZENSOY (CONT.)														
Soy Milk Chocolate	8 oz	170	4	1	0	7	27	23	2	300	160	—	—	0
Soy Milk Plain	8 oz	90	4	1	0	7	9	6	1	300	80	—	—	0
Soy Milk Vanilla	8 oz	110	4	1	0	7	14	12	1	300	80	—	—	0
Soy On The Go Vanilla w/ Omega 3	1 pkg (8.25 oz)	110	4	1	0	7	14	12	1	300	80	—	—	0
MILKFISH (AWA)														
baked	4 oz	215	10	—	76	30	0	0	0	73	104	423	20	0
MILKSHAKE														
chocolate	1 serv (10.6 oz)	357	8	5	33	9	63	63	1	396	333	672	15	0
malted milk shake	1 serv (10 oz)	402	14	8	51	9	62	58	1	311	201	487	20	1
vanilla	1 (11 oz)	351	9	6	38	12	56	56	0	457	297	573	22	0
BUFFY'S COOL COW														
Chocolate	1 pkg (8 oz)	150	3	2	5	9	23	17	tr	450	135	—	—	4
Vanilla	1 pkg (8 oz)	150	3	2	5	9	24	18	0	450	135	—	—	4
LEAN BODY														
Hi-Protein Chocolate Ice Cream	1 (17 oz)	260	9	1	25	40	9	0	5	400	600	600	100	15
MOLLI COOLZ														
Shakers Vanilla as prep w/ skim milk	1 (10.2 oz)	240	10	6	35	3	30	17	5	120	96	—	—	0
NESQUIK														
Ready-To-Drink Chocolate	1 cup (8 oz)	170	5	3	15	8	26	23	tr	400	180	—	—	1
SILHOUETTE SOLUTION														
Colossal Chocolate not prep	1 pkg (1.05 oz)	110	3	1	35	15	8	4	2	100	230	380	—	15
Vanilla Creme not prep	1 pkg (1.02 oz)	100	2	1	40	15	8	5	2	100	230	320	80	15
MILLET														
cooked	1 cup (6.1 oz)	207	2	tr	0	6	41	—	2	5	3	108	33	0
ARROWHEAD MILLS														
Organic Hulled not prep	¼ cup	150	2	0	0	4	33	0	1	20	0	110	—	0
MINERAL WATER														
(*see* WATER)														
MISO														
dried	1 oz	86	3	—	—	7	10	—	1	51	2130	219	—	0
miso	½ cup	284	8	1	0	16	39	—	7	92	5036	226	46	0

FOOD	PORTION	CALS	FAT	SAT FAT	CHOL	PROT	CARB	SUGAR	FIBER	CALCI	SOD	POTAS	FOLIC	VIT C
EDEN														
Hacho	1 tbsp	40	2	tr	0	3	4	0	tr	20	680	180	—	2
Organic Mugi	1 tbsp	25	1	0	0	2	4	1	tr	0	640	60	—	0
Organic Shiro	1 tbsp	30	1	0	0	1	6	4	tr	0	330	15	—	0
MOLASSES														
blackstrap	1 tbsp (0.7 oz)	47	0	0	0	0	12	—	—	172	11	498	0	—
molasses	1 tbsp (0.7 oz)	58	tr	tr	0	0	15	11	0	41	7	293	0	0
molasses	¼ cup (3 oz)	244	tr	tr	0	0	63	47	0	173	31	1233	0	0
TREE OF LIFE														
Blackstrap Unsulphured	1 tbsp	45	0	0	0	0	11	8	—	140	15	—	—	—
MONKFISH														
baked	3 oz	82	2	—	27	16	0	0	0	8	20	436	7	1
MOOSE														
roasted	4 oz	142	1	tr	83	31	0	0	0	6	73	355	4	5
MOTH BEANS														
dried cooked	1 cup	207	1	tr	0	14	37	—	—	6	17	538	—	2
MOUSSE														
TAKE-OUT														
chocolate	½ cup	454	32	18	283	8	32	30	1	194	77	289	30	tr
fish timbale	1 cup	329	25	15	210	22	3	1	0	75	394	422	19	2
MUFFIN														
MIX														
BETTY CROCKER														
Banana Nut as prep	1	120	3	1	0	2	22	10	0	—	240	35	16	—
Blueberry as prep	1	120	3	1	0	2	23	11	—	—	230	25	16	—
Cornbread Muffin as prep	1	160	6	3	48	2	24	5	tr	20	210	25	32	—
Fiber One Banana Nut as prep	1	170	7	1	36	2	27	12	5	—	230	70	8	—
Fiber One Blueberry as prep	1	160	6	2	36	2	30	13	5	—	240	45	8	—
Lemon Poppyseed as prep	1	200	8	1	36	2	29	17	—	40	210	30	24	—
DUNCAN HINES														
Blueberry Streusel as prep	1	210	8	2	35	3	32	19	3	0	230	—	—	—
Cinnamon Swirl 100% Whole Grain as prep	1	220	8	2	35	3	34	21	3	0	230	—	—	0
Triple Chocolate Chunk 100% Whole Grain as prep	1	240	11	4	35	4	35	23	3	40	290	—	—	—

FOOD	PORTION	CALS	FAT	SAT FAT	CHOL	PROT	CARB	SUGAR	FIBER	CALCI	SOD	POTAS	FOLIC	VIT C
GLORY														
Golden Sweet Corn as prep	1	170	5	1	36	2	27	7	1	40	360	—	—	0
KING ARTHUR														
Cranberry Orange Whole Grain not prep	¼ cup	180	1	0	0	4	41	20	3	100	130	—	—	2
MARTHA WHITE														
Whole Grain Apple Cinnamon not prep	¼ cup (1.2 oz)	140	4	2	5	2	24	13	1	100	150	—	32	0
Whole Grain Blueberry not prep	¼ cup (1.2 oz)	140	4	2	5	2	24	13	1	100	150	—	24	0
Yellow Corn not prep	¼ cup (1.2 oz)	140	3	1	0	2	26	6	1	60	230	—	0	0
MIRACLE MUFFINS														
Banana w/ Splenda as prep	1	86	3	0	0	9	12	0	7	—	130	—	—	—
VITAMUFFIN														
Deep Chocolate as prep	1 (2 oz)	100	2	1	0	4	26	11	9	100	140	—	200	30
Golden Corn as prep	1 (2 oz)	100	0	0	0	3	24	7	5	100	125	—	200	30
READY-TO-EAT														
DO GOODIE														
Gluten Free Banana Nut	1	180	9	3	45	2	24	20	1	20	220	—	—	2
FOODS BY GEORGE														
Gluten Free Blueberry	1 (2.8 oz)	220	8	1	25	3	33	11	1	40	450	—	—	0
HOSTESS														
100 Calorie Pack Mini Banana Streusel	1 pkg (1.2 oz)	100	4	1	10	2	19	7	4	0	120	—	—	0
100 Calorie Pack Mini Blueberry Streusel	1 pkg (1.2 oz)	100	3	1	10	2	20	7	4	0	120	—	—	0
UDI'S														
Gluten Free Double Chocolate	1 (4 oz)	350	15	6	80	4	52	32	3	80	250	—	—	0
UNCLE WALLY'S														
Apple Cinnamon Rich & Moist	1 (4 oz)	380	18	4	70	4	51	29	1	20	320	—	—	0
Blueberry Rich & Moist	1 (4 oz)	370	18	3	60	4	49	27	1	20	330	—	—	0

FOOD	PORTION	CALS	FAT	SAT FAT	CHOL	PROT	CARB	SUGAR	FIBER	CALCI	SOD	POTAS	FOLIC	VIT C
UNCLE WALLY'S (CONT.)														
Cheesecake Rich & Moist	1 (4 oz)	390	19	5	70	5	50	27	0	20	360	—	—	0
Chocolate Passion Fat Free	½ (2 oz)	120	0	0	0	3	28	16	0	20	260	—	—	0
Corn Rich & Moist	1 (4 oz)	400	18	3	70	5	55	27	1	20	330	—	—	0
Cranberry Apple Smart Portion	1 (1.1 oz)	80	1	0	0	2	17	9	2	20	130	—	—	0
Cranberry Orange Supreme Fat Free	½ (2 oz)	140	0	0	0	2	32	19	1	20	210	—	—	0
Fiber One Banana Chocolate Chip	1 (2.3 oz)	180	5	2	30	3	36	19	7	20	190	—	—	0
Fiber One Wild Blueberry & Oats	1 (2.3 oz)	170	4	1	30	3	33	16	7	20	200	—	—	0
Honey Raisin Bran Fat Free	½ (2 oz)	140	0	0	0	2	32	19	1	20	210	—	—	0
My Sweet Multi Bran Sugar Free	1 (2 oz)	120	3	1	10	3	28	1	1	20	280	—	—	0
Pineapple Coconut Rich & Moist	1 (4 oz)	390	19	5	70	4	51	19	1	20	340	—	—	0
Sweet Chocolate Dreams Sugar Free	1 (2 oz)	130	3	1	15	3	29	1	1	20	290	—	—	0
Wild Blueberry Bliss Fat Free	½ (2 oz)	110	0	0	0	2	25	14	1	20	210	—	—	0
VITAMUFFIN														
Banana Nut	1 (2 oz)	100	2	0	0	5	19	3	5	20	120	50	200	30
Banana Nut Sugar Free	1 (2 oz)	90	3	0	0	5	21	0	5	20	125	65	200	30
VITATOP														
Apple Crumb	1 (2 oz)	100	1	0	0	3	25	7	8	20	105	20	200	30
BlueBran	1 (2 oz)	100	1	0	0	4	20	9	5	20	140	60	200	30
CranBran	1 (2 oz)	100	1	0	0	4	22	11	5	20	140	60	200	30
Deep Chocolate	1 (2 oz)	100	2	1	0	4	26	11	9	200	140	10	200	30
Golden Corn	1 (2 oz)	100	1	0	0	3	27	9	10	20	120	15	200	30
Raisin Bran	1 (2 oz)	100	1	0	0	4	22	11	5	20	140	80	200	30
TAKE-OUT														
blueberry	1 (5 oz)	546	27	5	56	7	69	38	2	49	485	133	67	1
corn	1 lg (5 oz)	424	12	2	36	8	71	10	5	103	890	96	111	0
oat bran	1 lg (5 oz)	375	10	2	0	10	67	11	6	88	546	705	124	0
pumpkin w/ raisins & nuts	1 med (4 oz)	351	8	1	81	5	67	43	2	59	297	168	42	1

FOOD	PORTION	CALS	FAT	SAT FAT	CHOL	PROT	CARB	SUGAR	FIBER	CALCI	SOD	POTAS	FOLIC	VIT C
MULBERRIES														
fresh	20 (1 oz)	13	tr	tr	0	tr	3	2	1	12	3	58	2	11
fresh	½ cup (2.5 oz)	30	tr	tr	0	1	7	6	1	27	7	136	4	26
KOPALI														
Organic Dark Chocolate Covered	½ pkg (1 oz)	140	6	4	0	2	20	15	2	20	8	—	—	21
Organic Dried	1 pkg (1.7 oz)	240	1	0	0	5	38	22	6	120	36	—	—	138
NAVITAS NATURALS														
Dried	1 oz	91	0	0	0	3	21	12	3	70	25	—	—	81
MULLET														
striped cooked	3 oz	127	4	1	54	21	0	0	0	26	61	389	—	—
striped raw	3 oz	99	3	1	42	16	0	0	0	34	55	304	7	—
MUNG BEANS														
dried cooked	1 cup	213	1	tr	0	14	39	—	—	55	4	536	321	2
TRUROOTS														
Organic Sprouted not prep	¼ cup (1.4 oz)	140	1	0	0	10	30	1	7	40	10	—	—	6
MUNGO BEANS														
dried cooked	1 cup	190	1	tr	1	14	33	—	—	95	13	416	170	2
MUSHROOMS														
CANNED														
caps	8 (1.6 oz)	12	tr	tr	0	1	2	1	1	5	200	61	6	0
caps pickled	6 (0.8 oz)	5	tr	tr	0	1	1	tr	tr	1	53	59	2	tr
chanterelle	3.5 oz	12	1	—	0	1	tr	—	6.	5	165	155	—	3
pickled	1 cup	33	tr	tr	0	4	5	2	1	5	351	395	14	2
pieces	½ cup	20	tr	tr	0	1	2	1	1	9	332	101	9	0
straw	1 cup	58	1	tr	0	7	8	—	5	18	699	142	69	0
GREEN GIANT														
Pieces & Stems	½ cup	25	0	0	0	2	4	1	1	0	440	—	—	0
JAKE & AMOS														
Pickled Dill Mushrooms	1 serv (1 oz)	5	0	0	0	0	1	0	tr	—	244	—	—	—
POLAR														
Straw	½ cup	20	0	0	0	3	4	0	2	10	460	—	—	2
Whole Button	½ cup	30	0	0	0	3	4	1	2	0	320	—	—	0
Whole Shiitake	½ cup	30	1	0	0	1	4	0	tr	0	620	—	—	1
SUNNY DELL														
Portabella Sliced	½ cup	20	0	0	0	1	4	0	2	0	460	—	—	2
DRIED														
chanterelle	1 oz	25	tr	—	0	5	tr	—	17	24	9	1	—	tr
shiitake	1 (3.6 g)	11	tr	tr	0	tr	3	tr	tr	0	0	55	6	tr
tree ear	½ cup (0.4 oz)	36	tr	—	0	1	10	—	—	14	8	85	19	0
wood ear mok yee	½ cup (0.4 oz)	25	tr	—	—	2	8	—	4	30	6	91	—	—

FOOD	PORTION	CALS	FAT	SAT FAT	CHOL	PROT	CARB	SUGAR	FIBER	CALCI	SOD	POTAS	FOLIC	VIT C
EDEN														
Maitake Sliced	10 pieces (0.3 oz)	35	0	0	0	2	7	0	4	0	0	230	—	0
Shiitake Sliced	3 pieces (0.3 oz)	35	0	0	0	2	7	2	5	0	0	200	—	0
OCEAN SPRING														
Fresh Crispy Mixed Mushrooms	1 serv (0.9 oz)	113	4	2	—	—	18	2	1	33	46	—	—	tr
FRESH														
brown italian or crimini sliced	1 cup	19	tr	tr	0	2	3	1	tr	13	4	323	10	0
brown italian or crimini whole	1 (0.7 oz)	5	tr	tr	0	1	1	tr	tr	4	1	90	3	0
chanterelle	3.5 oz	11	tr	—	0	2	tr	—	6	8	3	507	—	6
enoki raw	1 lg (5 g)	2	tr	tr	0	tr	tr	tr	tr	0	0	18	3	0
enoki sliced	1 cup	29	tr	tr	0	2	5	tr	2	1	2	239	34	0
enoki whole	1 cup	28	tr	tr	0	2	5	tr	2	1	2	236	33	0
maitake diced	1 cup	26	tr	tr	0	1	5	1	2	1	1	143	20	0
maitake whole	1 (6.6 g)	2	tr	tr	0	tr	tr	tr	tr	0	0	13	2	0
morel	3.5 oz	9	tr	—	0	2	0	—	7	11	2	390	—	5
oyster	1 sm (0.5 oz)	5	tr	tr	0	1	1	tr	tr	0	3	63	4	0
oyster sliced	1 cup	30	tr	tr	0	3	6	1	2	3	15	361	23	0
portabella raw	1 cap (3 oz)	22	tr	tr	0	2	4	2	1	7	5	407	18	0
portabella sliced grilled	1 cup (4.2 oz)	42	1	tr	0	5	6	0	3	5	12	630	23	0
shiitake cooked	4 (2.5 oz)	40	tr	tr	0	1	10	3	2	2	3	84	15	tr
shiitake pieces cooked	1 cup	81	tr	tr	0	2	21	5	3	4	6	170	30	tr
white	1 (0.6 oz)	4	tr	tr	0	1	1	tr	tr	1	1	57	3	tr
white sliced cooked	1 cup	28	tr	tr	0	4	4	0	2	4	13	428	22	0
white sliced raw	½ cup	8	tr	tr	0	1	1	1	tr	1	2	111	6	1
DOLE														
Raw	½ cup (1.2 oz)	9	0	0	0	1	1	0	0	0	0	130	—	0
GIORGIO														
Mushrooms	3 oz	20	0	0	0	2	3	1	1	0	10	—	—	0
GOLDEN GOURMET														
Beech Brown	4 oz	20	1	—	0	3	7	—	—	—	1	417	—	—
Beech White	4 oz	13	1	—	0	3	6	—	—	—	1	440	—	—
King Trumpet	4 oz	20	0	0	0	3	7	—	—	—	2	316	—	—
Maitake	4 oz	20	1	—	0	3	8	—	—	—	1	317	—	—

FOOD	PORTION	CALS	FAT	SAT FAT	CHOL	PROT	CARB	SUGAR	FIBER	CALCI	SOD	POTAS	FOLIC	VIT C
HOKTO														
Organic Bunashimeji Beech Mushrooms	1 pkg (3.5 oz)	30	1	—	0	3	3	—	3	—	0	270	—	—
Organic Maitake Hen Of The Wood	1 pkg (3.5 oz)	30	1	—	0	2	4	—	3	—	0	280	—	—
FROZEN														
FARM RICH														
Breaded	5 (3 oz)	120	2	0	0	3	23	0	1	0	430	—	—	0
TAKE-OUT														
battered fried	1 lg (0.6 oz)	39	3	tr	1	1	3	1	tr	4	29	37	5	tr
creamed	1 cup	171	11	3	7	6	15	7	3	128	853	306	22	1
stuffed	1 (0.8 oz)	67	4	1	3	3	6	1	1	39	142	90	8	1
MUSKRAT														
roasted	3 oz	199	10	—	—	26	0	0	0	31	81	272	—	6
MUSSELS														
blue raw	1 cup	129	3	1	42	18	6	—	—	39	429	479	—	—
blue raw	3 oz	73	2	tr	24	10	3	—	—	22	243	272	—	—
fresh blue cooked	3 oz	147	4	1	48	20	6	—	—	28	313	228	—	—
POLAR														
Mussels	2 oz	60	3	0	15	10	tr	0	0	20	90	—	—	0
MUSTARD														
dry mustard	1 tsp	15	1	tr	0	1	1	—	—	17	tr	23	—	—
hot chinese	1 tsp	3	tr	tr	0	tr	tr	tr	tr	4	56	8	0	tr
organic yellow	1 tsp	5	0	0	0	0	0	0	0	—	70	—	—	—
seed	1 tsp	15	1	tr	0	1	1	tr	1	17	0	23	3	tr
yellow prepared	1 tbsp	3	tr	tr	0	tr	tr	tr	tr	3	57	7	0	tr
ANNIE'S HOMEGROWN														
Organic Dijon	1 tsp (5 g)	5	0	0	0	0	1	—	—	—	120	—	—	—
BOAR'S HEAD														
Delicatessen Style	1 tsp (5 g)	0	0	0	0	0	0	0	0	0	40	—	—	0
Honey	1 tsp (5 g)	10	0	0	0	0	2	1	0	0	25	—	—	0
BONE SUCKIN'														
Fat Free Gluten Free	1 tbsp	25	0	0	0	0	5	4	0	0	95	—	—	0
DAVE'S GOURMET														
Insanity	1 tsp (5 g)	5	0	0	0	0	1	—	—	0	55	—	—	0
DIETZ & WATSON														
Champagne Dill	1 tsp (5 g)	5	0	0	0	0	0	0	0	0	120	—	—	0
Yellow	1 tsp (5 g)	0	0	0	0	0	0	0	0	0	80	—	—	0
D'ONI														
Bold As Love Honey Habanero	1 tsp	5	0	0	0	0	2	1	—	—	45	—	—	—

FOOD	PORTION	CALS	FAT	SAT FAT	CHOL	PROT	CARB	SUGAR	FIBER	CALCI	SOD	POTAS	FOLIC	VIT C
EDEN														
Yellow	1 tsp	0	0	0	0	0	0	0	0	—	80	—	—	—
FRENCH'S														
Classic Yellow	1 tsp	0	0	0	0	0	0	0	0	—	55	—	—	—
Honey	1 tsp	10	0	0	0	0	1	tr	—	—	30	—	—	—
Honey Dijon	1 tsp	10	0	0	0	0	1	—	—	—	40	—	—	—
Horseradish	1 tsp	5	0	0	0	0	0	0	0	—	80	—	—	—
Spicy Brown	1 tsp	5	0	0	0	0	0	0	0	—	80	—	—	—
GULDEN'S														
Spicy Brown	1 tsp	5	0	0	0	0	0	0	0	—	50	—	—	—
HELLMAN'S														
Deli	1 tsp	5	0	0	0	0	tr	—	0	0	55	—	—	0
Dijonnaise	1 tsp	5	0	0	0	0	1	—	0	0	70	—	—	0
Honey Mustard	1 tsp	10	0	0	0	0	2	—	0	0	25	—	—	0
JACK & AMOS														
Sweet Dipping	1 tbsp (0.5 oz)	30	1	0	10	1	5	4	0	0	10	—	—	0
ROBERT ROTHCHILD FARM														
Champagne Garlic	1 tsp	6	0	0	0	0	1	1	0	0	120	—	—	2
SARA LEE														
Country Honey	1 tbsp	10	0	0	0	0	2	2	0	0	25	—	—	0
Cranberry Honey	1 tbsp	10	0	0	0	0	2	2	0	0	25	—	—	0
SCHOOL HOUSE KITCHEN														
Sweet Smooth Hot	1 tsp	15	1	0	0	0	1	1	0	0	10	—	—	0
TEXAS SASSY														
Mustard Sauce	2 tbsp (1 oz)	15	0	0	0	0	3	3	—	—	260	—	—	—
VIVI'S														
Classic	1 tbsp (0.5 oz)	15	0	0	0	0	4	3	0	0	190	—	—	1
Sizzlin' Chipotle	1 tbsp (0.5 oz)	15	0	0	0	0	4	3	0	0	200	—	—	1
ZATARAIN'S														
Creole	1 tsp (7 g)	10	1	0	0	0	tr	0	0	0	150	—	—	0
MUSTARD GREENS														
canned	1 cup	23	tr	tr	0	3	3	tr	3	113	428	308	112	38
fresh as prep w/ fat	1 cup	50	3	1	0	3	3	tr	3	112	459	302	108	38
fresh chopped boiled w/o salt	1 cup	21	tr	tr	0	3	3	tr	3	104	22	283	102	35
fresh raw chopped	1 cup	15	tr	tr	0	2	3	1	2	58	14	198	105	39
frozen chopped boiled w/o salt	1 cup	28	tr	tr	0	3	5	tr	4	152	38	208	105	21
ALLENS														
Seasoned	½ cup	45	1	0	0	4	6	2	1	150	830	—	—	12
GLORY														
Seasoned	½ cup	35	0	0	0	2	3	1	1	40	490	—	—	15
SYLVIA'S														
Specially Seasoned	½ cup	30	0	0	0	2	5	2	2	60	220	95	—	6

FOOD	PORTION	CALS	FAT	SAT FAT	CHOL	PROT	CARB	SUGAR	FIBER	CALCI	SOD	POTAS	FOLIC	VIT C
NATTO														
HOUSE														
Natto	2 oz	120	6	1	0	10	5	0	0	60	25	—	—	0
NAVY BEANS														
canned	1 cup	296	1	tr	0	20	54	—	—	123	1173	755	163	2
dried cooked	1 cup	259	1	tr	0	16	48	—	—	128	2	669	255	2
EDEN														
Organic	½ cup	110	0	0	0	7	20	—	7	80	15	300	—	—
NECTARINE														
fresh	1 lg (5.5 oz)	69	1	tr	0	2	16	12	3	9	0	314	8	8
fresh	1 sm (4.5 oz)	57	tr	tr	0	1	14	10	2	8	0	259	6	7
fresh sliced	1 cup (5 oz)	63	tr	tr	0	2	15	11	2	9	0	287	7	8
CHIQUITA														
Fresh	1 (5 oz)	63	0	0	0	2	15	11	2	10	0	287	—	8
DOLE														
Fresh	1 med (5 oz)	60	0	0	0	1	15	11	2	0	0	—	—	15
NECTARINE JUICE														
SUN SHOWER														
100% Juice	8 oz	93	0	0	0	1	21	17	2	10	15	350	—	60
NEUFCHATEL														
neufchatel	1 oz	72	6	4	21	3	1	1	0	33	95	43	4	0
neufchatel	1 pkg (3 oz)	215	19	11	63	8	3	3	0	99	284	129	12	0
ORGANIC VALLEY														
Soft	2 tbsp	70	6	4	20	2	2	2	0	20	140	—	—	0
NONI JUICE														
LAKEWOOD														
Noni Pure Juice	2 oz	8	0	0	0	0	2	2	0	10	5	17	—	—
SNAPPLE														
Juice Drink Low Calorie Metabolism Noni Berry	8 oz	15	0	0	0	0	2	1	—	—	5	—	—	—
TREE OF LIFE														
100% Juice Concentrate	2 tbsp	15	0	0	0	0	4	3	0	0	10	—	—	6
NOODLES														
cellophane	1 cup	492	tr	tr	0	tr	121	—	—	35	14	14	—	0
chow mein	1 cup (1.6 oz)	237	14	2	0	4	25	—	2	9	189	52	39	0
egg	1 cup (38 g)	145	2	tr	36	5	27	—	—	12	8	89	11	0
egg cooked	1 cup (5.6 oz)	213	2	tr	53	8	40	—	2	19	11	45	102	0
japanese soba cooked	1 cup (4 oz)	113	tr	tr	0	6	24	—	—	5	68	40	8	0
japanese somen cooked	1 cup (6.2 oz)	231	tr	tr	0	7	48	—	—	14	283	51	4	0

FOOD	PORTION	CALS	FAT	SAT FAT	CHOL	PROT	CARB	SUGAR	FIBER	CALCI	SOD	POTAS	FOLIC	VIT C
korean acorn noodles not prep	2 oz	195	tr	—	—	7	41	—	tr	—	—	—	—	0
rice cooked	1 cup (6.2 oz)	192	tr	tr	0	2	44	—	2	7	33	7	5	0
spinach/egg cooked	1 cup (5.6 oz)	211	3	1	53	8	39	—	4	30	19	59	102	0
ANNIE CHUN'S														
Noodle Express Chinese Chow Mein	½ pkg	160	4	1	0	5	27	3	1	0	510	—	—	0
Noodle Express Singapore Curry	½ pkg	160	3	0	0	4	28	3	2	20	550	—	—	0
Noodle Express Spicy Szechuan	½ pkg	170	3	0	0	4	29	4	1	0	470	—	—	2
GLUTEN FREE CAFE														
Asian Noodles	1 pkg (9.2 oz)	340	10	3	0	8	53	11	5	350	720	—	120	15
HOUSE														
Shirataki Tofu Noodles	2 oz	20	1	0	0	1	3	0	2	100	15	—	—	1
Shirataki Yam Noodles	2 oz	5	0	0	0	0	1	0	0	0	0	—	—	0
KRASDALE														
Egg Wide not prep	1 cup (2 oz)	210	2	0	0	8	41	2	2	0	0	—	120	0
LA CHOY														
Chow Mein Noodles	½ cup (1 oz)	130	5	2	0	3	19	0	tr	0	230	—	—	0
Rice	½ cup	130	4	1	0	2	21	1	tr	0	350	—	—	0
LIGHT 'N FLUFFY														
Egg Extra Wide not prep	⅙ pkg (2 oz)	210	3	1	70	8	40	2	2	—	15	—	100	—
NO YOLKS														
Dumplings	2 oz	210	1	0	0	8	41	3	3	0	30	—	120	0
NOOODLE														
All Natural	1 serv (1.6 oz)	0	0	0	0	0	1	tr	0	0	0	—	—	0
PENNSYLVANIA DUTCH														
Fine Egg not prep	1 cup (2 oz)	220	3	1	65	8	40	2	2	20	15	—	—	0
RONZONI														
Healthy Harvest Whole Grain Extra Wide not prep	2 oz	180	1	0	0	8	41	0	6	0	15	—	—	0
STREIT'S														
Egg Wide not prep	1¾ cups (2 oz)	210	3	1	60	8	39	2	2	20	20	—	120	0
NUTMEG														
ground	1 tsp	12	1	1	0	tr	1	1	1	4	0	8	2	tr
nutmeg butter	1 tbsp	120	14	12	0	0	0	0	0	0	0	0	0	0

FOOD	PORTION	CALS	FAT	SAT FAT	CHOL	PROT	CARB	SUGAR	FIBER	CALCI	SOD	POTAS	FOLIC	VIT C
NUTRITION SUPPLEMENTS														
(*see also* CEREAL BARS, ENERGY BARS, ENERGY DRINKS)														
BE HAPPY														
Health Guard	1 bottle (2 oz)	40	0	0	0	0	10	9	0	—	25	—	—	—
BOOST														
Breeze	8 oz	160	0	0	0	8	31	31	—	150	50	230	80	60
CIRKU														
Beverage Mix Summer Citrus	1 pkg (0.23 oz)	15	0	0	0	0	3	—	—	—	—	—	—	60
CLIF														
Shot Bloks Black Cherry	3 (1 oz)	100	0	0	0	0	24	12	0	0	70	20	—	0
Shot Bloks Cola	3 (1 oz)	100	0	0	0	0	24	12	0	0	70	20	—	0
Shot Bloks Margarita	3 (1 oz)	90	0	0	0	0	24	12	0	0	210	20	—	0
Shot Bloks Orange	3 (1 oz)	100	0	0	0	0	24	12	0	0	70	20	—	0
ENSURE														
Shake Creamy Milk Chocolate	1 bottle (8 oz)	250	6	1	5	9	40	22	1	300	190	390	100	30
Shake Strawberries & Cream	1 bottle (8 oz)	250	6	1	5	9	40	23	0	300	200	370	100	30
GLOWELLE														
Beauty Drink All Flavors	1 bottle	100	0	0	0	0	24	13	—	—	25	—	—	250
GLUCERNA														
Shake Creamy Chocolate Delight	1 bottle (8 oz)	200	7	1	<5	10	27	6	5	250	210	400	100	60
Shake Homemade Vanilla	1 bottle (8 oz)	200	7	1	<5	10	26	6	5	250	210	380	100	60
JELLY BELLY														
Sport Beans Lemon Lime	1 pkg (1 oz)	100	0	0	0	0	25	19	—	—	80	40	—	6
JOINT JUICE														
Cranberry Pomegranate	1 bottle (8 oz)	20	0	0	0	0	5	2	—	—	120	50	—	60
Easy Shot Glucosamine Chondrotin	2.5 tbsp (1.25 oz)	15	0	0	0	0	3	2	—	—	20	—	—	60
Easy Shot Hyal-Joint	2.5 tbsp (1.25 oz)	15	0	0	0	0	3	2	—	—	3	—	—	60
On The Go Blueberry Acai	1 pkg (6 g)	20	0	0	0	tr	4	—	—	100	30	10	—	60
LUNA														
Electrolyte Splash	1 pkg	80	0	0	0	0	20	20	—	100	200	50	—	60

FOOD	PORTION	CALS	FAT	SAT FAT	CHOL	PROT	CARB	SUGAR	FIBER	CALCI	SOD	POTAS	FOLIC	VIT C
LUNA (CONT.)														
Moons Energy Chews Watermelon	6 (1 oz)	100	0	0	0	0	24	12	0	0	70	20	—	0
Recovery Smoothie	1 pkg	120	0	0	0	0	21	14	1	150	150	130	200	60
ORGAIN														
Organic Meal Replacement All Flavors	1 pkg (11 oz)	255	7	0	20	16	32	12	2	250	260	320	100	15
OXYLENT														
Oxygenating Multivitamin Drink	1 pkg	10	0	0	0	0	2	2	—	128	35	225	400	1000
PREMIER														
Protein Shake Chocolate	1 (11 oz)	160	3	1	25	30	5	1	3	500	340	500	100	15
Protein Shake Strawberry	1 (11 oz)	160	3	1	25	30	3	1	2	500	330	390	100	15
Protein Shake Vanilla	1 (11 oz)	160	3	1	25	30	3	1	2	500	330	390	100	15
S/7														
Prenatal Vitamin Drink Berry	1 pkg (0.5 oz)	45	1	—	—	0	9	8	—	125	55	110	400	60
SLIM-FAST														
Optima Ready-To-Drink Creamy Milk Chocolate	1 can (11 oz)	190	6	3	5	10	25	18	5	500	200	605	120	60
TO GO														
Extreme Berries	½ pkg (3.15 g)	12	tr	—	—	tr	3	1	tr	—	1	2	—	30
NUTS MIXED														
(*see also individual names*)														
dry roasted w/ peanuts salted	¼ cup	203	18	2	0	6	9	—	3	24	229	204	17	tr
dry roasted w/ peanuts w/o salt	¼ cup	203	18	2	0	6	9	—	3	24	4	204	17	tr
mixed nuts chocolate covered	¼ cup (1.5 oz)	240	17	7	5	4	20	17	2	80	25	—	—	0
oil roasted w/o peanuts salted	¼ cup	221	20	3	0	6	8	2	2	38	110	196	20	tr
oil roasted w/o peanuts w/o salt	¼ cup	221	20	3	0	6	8	—	2	38	4	196	20	tr
BACK TO NATURE														
Tuscan Herb Roast	1 oz	170	15	2	0	5	7	2	2	40	100	—	—	0

FOOD	PORTION	CALS	FAT	SAT FAT	CHOL	PROT	CARB	SUGAR	FIBER	CALCI	SOD	POTAS	FOLIC	VIT C
DAVE'S GOURMET														
Burning Nuts	1 oz	200	17	8	—	9	7	1	3	40	135	—	—	0
EMILY'S														
Roasted Mixed Nuts	¼ cup (1.3 oz)	230	20	3	0	6	8	2	2	40	80	—	—	—
FRITO LAY														
Deluxe Mixed	¼ cup	170	16	3	0	4	6	1	2	20	115	—	—	0
MAUNA LOA														
Mixed Nuts	¼ cup (1 oz)	180	16	2	0	5	6	1	2	20	85	—	—	0
NUTTZO														
Multi-Nut Butter Organic	2 tbsp (1.1 oz)	180	16	2	—	7	7	1	3	20	70	—	—	—
ORGANIC TRAILS														
Tamari Roasted Nuts & Seeds	¼ cup	190	15	2	0	7	10	1	5	40	130	—	—	0
PEANUT BETTER														
Mixed Nut Butter Creamy & Crunchy	2 tbsp	190	17	2	0	8	5	1	3	60	135	—	—	0
PLANTERS														
Bar Big Triple Nut	1 (1.6 oz)	220	12	2	0	8	22	12	3	20	220	—	—	0
Lightly Salted	1 oz	170	15	2	0	6	5	1	2	40	55	—	—	0
Mixed	1 oz	170	15	2	0	6	5	1	2	40	110	—	—	0
Unsalted	1 oz	170	15	2	0	6	5	1	2	40	0	—	—	0
TRUE NORTH														
Clusters Pecan Almond Peanut	8 (1 oz)	170	13	2	0	5	13	5	2	20	75	—	—	0

OCTOPUS

FOOD	PORTION	CALS	FAT	SAT FAT	CHOL	PROT	CARB	SUGAR	FIBER	CALCI	SOD	POTAS	FOLIC	VIT C
dried boiled	3 oz	144	2	tr	84	26	4	0	0	107	695	703	31	10
fresh steamed	3 oz	139	2	tr	81	25	4	0	0	26	111	169	7	2
smoked	1 oz	40	1	tr	23	7	1	0	0	26	111	169	7	2
MATIZ														
Pulpo In Olive Oil	½ pkg (2 oz)	107	5	1	36	12	3	0	0	80	264	—	—	0
TAKE-OUT														
ensalada de pulpo	1 cup	299	21	3	52	17	10	4	2	79	232	535	32	15

OHELOBERRIES

FOOD	PORTION	CALS	FAT	SAT FAT	CHOL	PROT	CARB	SUGAR	FIBER	CALCI	SOD	POTAS	FOLIC	VIT C
fresh	1 cup	39	tr	—	0	1	10	—	—	10	2	54	—	8

OIL

FOOD	PORTION	CALS	FAT	SAT FAT	CHOL	PROT	CARB	SUGAR	FIBER	CALCI	SOD	POTAS	FOLIC	VIT C
almond	1 cup	1927	218	1	0	0	0	0	0	—	—	—	—	—
almond	1 tbsp	120	14	1	0	0	0	0	0	—	—	—	—	—
apricot kernel	1 tbsp	120	14	1	0	0	0	0	0	—	—	—	—	—
apricot kernel	1 cup	1927	218	14	0	0	0	0	0	—	—	—	—	—
avocado	1 tbsp	124	14	2	0	0	0	0	0	—	—	—	—	—
avocado	1 cup	1927	218	25	0	0	0	0	0	—	—	—	—	—
babassu palm	1 tbsp	120	14	11	0	0	0	0	0	—	—	—	—	—
butter oil	1 tbsp	112	13	8	33	tr	0	0	0	—	—	—	—	—

FOOD	PORTION	CALS	FAT	SAT FAT	CHOL	PROT	CARB	SUGAR	FIBER	CALCI	SOD	POTAS	FOLIC	VIT C
butter oil	1 cup	1795	204	127	524	1	0	0	0	—	—	—	—	—
canola	1 tbsp	124	14	2	0	0	0	0	0	—	—	—	—	—
canola	1 cup	1927	218	15	0	0	0	0	0	—	—	—	—	—
coconut	1 tbsp	117	14	12	0	0	0	0	0	0	0	0	0	0
corn	1 cup	1927	218	28	0	0	0	0	0	—	—	—	—	—
corn	1 tbsp	120	14	2	0	0	0	0	0	—	—	—	—	—
cottonseed	1 cup	1927	218	56	0	0	0	0	0	—	—	—	—	—
cottonseed	1 tbsp	120	14	4	0	0	0	0	0	—	—	—	—	—
cupu assu	1 tbsp	120	14	7	0	0	0	0	0	—	—	—	—	—
garlic oil	1 tbsp	150	17	1	0	0	0	0	0	—	0	—	—	—
grapeseed	1 tbsp	120	14	1	0	0	0	0	0	0	0	0	0	0
hazelnut	1 tbsp	120	14	1	0	0	0	0	0	—	—	—	—	—
hazelnut	1 cup	1927	218	1	0	0	0	0	0	—	—	—	—	—
mustard	1 cup	1927	218	25	0	0	0	0	0	—	—	—	—	—
mustard	1 tbsp	124	14	2	0	0	0	0	0	—	—	—	—	—
oat	1 tbsp	120	14	3	0	0	0	0	0	—	—	—	—	—
olive	1 tbsp	119	14	2	0	0	0	0	0	tr	0	—	—	—
olive	1 cup	1909	216	26	0	0	0	0	0	tr	tr	—	—	—
palm	1 cup	1927	218	107	0	0	0	0	0	—	—	—	—	—
palm	1 tbsp	120	14	7	0	0	0	0	0	—	—	—	—	—
palm kernel	1 tbsp	117	14	11	0	0	0	0	0	—	—	—	—	—
palm kernel	1 cup	1879	218	178	0	0	0	0	0	—	—	—	—	—
peanut	1 cup	1909	216	36	0	0	0	0	0	tr	tr	tr	—	—
pcanut	1 tbsp	119	14	2	0	0	0	0	0	tr	tr	0	—	—
peppermint	1 tsp	42	4	—	0	—	0	0	0	—	—	—	—	—
poppyseed	1 tbsp	120	14	2	0	0	0	0	0	—	—	—	—	—
pumpkin seed	1 oz	217	29	—	—	0	0	0	0	—	—	—	—	—
rice bran	1 tbsp	120	14	3	0	0	0	0	0	—	—	—	—	—
safflower	1 cup	1927	218	20	0	0	0	0	0	—	—	—	—	—
safflower	1 tbsp	120	14	1	0	0	0	0	0	—	—	—	—	—
sesame	1 tbsp	120	14	2	0	0	0	0	0	—	—	—	—	—
sheanut	1 tbsp	120	14	6	0	0	0	0	0	—	—	—	—	—
soybean	1 cup	1927	218	31	0	0	0	0	0	tr	tr	—	—	—
soybean	1 tbsp	120	14	2	0	0	0	0	0	tr	0	—	—	—
sunflower	1 cup	1927	218	23	0	0	0	0	0	—	—	—	—	—
sunflower	1 tbsp	120	14	1	0	0	0	0	0	—	—	—	—	—
teaseed	1 tbsp	120	14	3	0	0	0	0	0	—	—	—	—	—
tomatoseed	1 tbsp	120	14	3	0	0	0	0	0	—	—	—	—	—
vegetable	1 cup	1927	218	2	0	0	0	0	0	—	—	—	—	—
vegetable	1 tbsp	120	14	2	0	0	0	0	0	—	—	—	—	—
walnut	1 tbsp	120	14	1	0	0	0	0	0	—	—	—	—	—
walnut	1 cup	1927	218	20	0	0	0	0	0	—	—	—	—	—
wheat germ	1 tbsp	120	14	3	0	0	0	0	0	—	—	—	—	—

FOOD	PORTION	CALS	FAT	SAT FAT	CHOL	PROT	CARB	SUGAR	FIBER	CALCI	SOD	POTAS	FOLIC	VIT C
ANNIE'S HOMEGROWN														
Basil Oil	1 tbsp (0.5 oz)	120	14	2	—	0	0	0	0	—	0	—	—	—
Dipping Oil	1 tbsp (0.5 oz)	100	11	2	—	0	0	0	0	—	0	—	—	—
AZUKAR ORGANICS														
Virgin Coconut	1 tbsp (0.5 oz)	125	14	13	0	0	0	0	0	—	0	—	—	—
BELL PLANTATION														
Extra Virgin Roasted Peanut	1 tbsp	120	14	3	0	0	0	0	0	0	0	—	—	0
BELLA SUN LUCI														
Olive Extra Virgin Cold Pressed	1 tbsp (0.5 oz)	120	14	2	0	0	0	0	0	—	0	—	—	—
BRAGG														
Olive Extra Virgin	1 tbsp	120	14	2	0	0	2	2	0	—	0	—	—	—
CARAPELLI														
Grapeseed	1 tbsp	120	14	1	0	0	0	0	0	0	0	—	—	0
Olive Extra Virgin	1 tbsp	120	14	2	0	0	0	0	0	0	0	—	—	0
CAROTINO														
Palm Fruit Oil	1 tbsp (0.5 oz)	121	14	6	0	0	0	0	0	—	0	—	—	—
Red Palm & Canola	1 tbsp	120	14	2	0	0	0	0	0	—	0	—	—	—
COLAVITA														
Olive Extra Virgin	1 tbsp (0.5 oz)	120	14	2	0	0	0	0	0	—	0	—	—	—
CRISCO														
Cooking Spray Original	⅓ sec spray	0	0	0	0	0	0	0	0	—	0	—	—	—
Frying Oil Blend	1 tbsp	130	14	3	0	0	0	0	0	—	0	—	—	—
Light Olive	1 tbsp	120	14	2	0	0	0	0	0	—	0	—	—	—
Peanut	1 tbsp	120	14	3	0	0	0	0	0	—	0	—	—	—
Pure Vegetable	1 tbsp	120	14	2	0	0	0	0	0	—	0	—	—	—
EDEN														
Organic Soybean	1 tbsp	120	14	2	0	0	0	0	0	—	0	—	—	—
Toasted Sesame	1 tbsp	120	14	2	0	0	0	0	0	—	0	—	—	—
GAEA														
Olive Carbon Neutral	1 tbsp (0.5 oz)	130	14	2	0	0	0	0	0	—	0	—	—	—
GOURME MIST														
Extra Virgin Olive Cold Pressed	1 sec spray	4	tr	tr	0	0	0	0	0	—	0	—	—	—
HOLLYWOOD														
Canola Enriched	1 tbsp	120	14	1	0	0	0	0	0	—	0	—	—	—
Peanut Enriched Gold	1 tbsp	120	14	2	0	0	0	0	0	—	0	—	—	—
Safflower Expeller Pressed	1 tbsp	120	14	1	0	0	0	0	0	—	0	—	—	—

FOOD	PORTION	CALS	FAT	SAT FAT	CHOL	PROT	CARB	SUGAR	FIBER	CALCI	SOD	POTAS	FOLIC	VIT C
HOUSE OF TSANG														
Mongolian Fire	1 tsp	45	5	1	0	0	0	0	0	0	0	0	—	0
Wok Oil	1 tbsp	130	14	3	0	0	0	0	0	0	0	0	—	0
KINLOCH PLANTATION														
100% Virgin Pecan	1 tbsp	130	14	2	0	0	0	0	0	0	0	—	—	0
LIVING HARVEST														
Organic Hemp Oil	2 tbsp	250	28	3	0	0	0	0	0	0	0	—	—	0
LOUANA														
Canola	1 tbsp (0.5 oz)	120	14	1	0	0	0	0	0	—	0	—	—	—
LUCINI														
Extra Virgin Premium Select	1 tbsp (0.5 oz)	120	14	2	0	0	0	0	0	—	0	—	—	—
MANITOBA HARVEST														
Hemp Seed Oil	1 tbsp	126	14	2	0	0	0	0	0	0	0	—	—	0
MARTINIS														
Kalamata Olive Extra Virgin Cold Pressed	1 tbsp (0.5 oz)	120	15	2	0	0	0	0	0	—	0	—	—	—
MAZOLA														
Corn	1 tbsp	120	14	2	0	0	0	0	0	—	0	—	—	—
MONINI														
Grapeseed	1 tbsp (0.5 oz)	120	14	2	0	0	0	0	0	—	0	—	—	—
NAVITAS NATURALS														
Organic Virgin Coconut	1 tbsp (0.5 oz)	120	14	13	0	0	0	0	0	0	0	—	—	0
NUTIVA														
Organic Coconut Extra Virgin	1 tbsp	120	14	13	0	0	0	0	0	—	0	—	—	—
Organic Hemp Cold Pressed	1 tbsp	120	14	1	0	0	0	0	0	—	0	—	—	—
OLIVO														
Spray Olive Oil 100% Extra Virgin	⅓ sec spray	0	0	0	0	0	0	0	0	—	0	—	—	—
PAM														
All Varieties	¼ sec spray	0	0	0	0	0	0	0	0	—	0	—	—	—
PENNY'S POPSURPRISE														
Organic Extra Virgin Olive Spicy	1 tbsp (0.5 oz)	130	14	2	0	0	0	0	0	—	0	—	—	—
PILLSBURY														
Baking Spray w/ Flour	⅙ sec spray	0	0	0	0	0	0	0	0	—	0	—	—	—
PLANTERS														
100% Pure Peanut	1 tbsp (0.5 oz)	120	14	3	0	0	0	0	0	—	0	—	—	—

FOOD	PORTION	CALS	FAT	SAT FAT	CHOL	PROT	CARB	SUGAR	FIBER	CALCI	SOD	POTAS	FOLIC	VIT C
POMPEIAN														
Olive	1 tbsp	130	14	—	0	—	—	—	—	0	—	—	—	—
ROBERT ROTHCHILD FARM														
Basil Infused	1 tbsp	120	14	2	0	0	0	0	0	0	0	—	—	0
SMART BALANCE														
Omega Oil	1 tbsp (0.5 oz)	120	14	1	0	0	0	0	0	—	90	—	—	—
TREE OF LIFE														
Almond Expeller Pressed	1 tbsp (0.5 oz)	120	14	2	0	0	0	0	0	0	0	—	—	0
Avocado Expeller Pressed	1 tbsp (0.5 oz)	120	14	2	0	0	0	0	0	0	0	—	—	0
Macadamia Nut Expeller Pressed	1 tbsp (0.5 oz)	120	14	2	0	0	0	0	0	0	0	—	—	0
Organic Coconut Expeller Pressed	1 tbsp	120	14	12	0	0	0	0	0	—	0	—	—	—
Walnut Expeller Pressed	1 tbsp (0.5 oz)	120	14	2	0	0	0	0	0	0	0	—	—	0
WESSON														
Canola	1 tbsp	120	14	1	0	0	0	0	0	—	0	—	—	—
OKRA														
CANNED														
pickled	6 pods (2.3 oz)	18	tr	tr	0	1	4	1	2	44	150	161	32	9
ALLENS														
Cut	½ cup	30	0	0	0	1	6	1	3	60	400	—	—	12
MCILHENNY														
Spicy Pickled	1 oz	10	0	0	0	0	2	1	1	40	270	—	—	0
TRAPPEY'S														
Creole Gumbo	½ cup	35	0	0	0	2	6	1	3	60	290	—	—	9
FRESH														
cooked w/ salt	8 pods	19	tr	tr	0	2	4	2	2	65	205	115	39	14
luffa chinese okra cooked	1 cup	39	tr	tr	0	3	8	4	4	137	422	239	82	29
sliced cooked w/ salt	½ cup	18	tr	tr	0	2	4	2	2	62	193	108	37	13
FROZEN														
MCKENZIE'S														
Cut	1 serv (3 oz)	25	0	0	0	1	5	1	3	—	35	—	—	—
TAKE-OUT														
batter dipped fried	10 pieces (2.6 oz)	142	10	1	2	2	12	3	2	50	100	155	36	8
OLIVES														
black	2 med (0.3 oz)	8	1	tr	0	tr	tr	0	tr	7	70	1	50	9
greek	1 (0.5 oz)	16	1	tr	0	tr	1	0	tr	14	132	1	0	tr
green	2 lg (0.3 oz)	11	1	tr	0	tr	tr	tr	tr	4	121	3	0	0
green	1 sm (0.2 oz)	8	1	tr	0	tr	tr	tr	tr	3	90	2	0	tr

FOOD	PORTION	CALS	FAT	SAT FAT	CHOL	PROT	CARB	SUGAR	FIBER	CALCI	SOD	POTAS	FOLIC	VIT C
green	2 med (0.2 oz)	10	1	tr	0	tr	tr	tr	tr	4	106	3	0	0
green	2 extra lg (0.5 oz)	19	2	tr	0	tr	1	tr	tr	7	205	6	0	0
green chopped	¼ cup (1.2 oz)	48	5	1	0	tr	1	tr	1	17	517	14	1	0
green olive tapenade	1 tbsp	25	3	0	0	0	1	1	0	20	210	—	—	2
green stuffed	2 lg (0.3 oz)	12	1	tr	0	tr	tr	tr	tr	4	123	5	0	1
green stuffed	¼ cup (1.3 oz)	47	5	1	0	tr	1	tr	1	17	493	21	1	4
green stuffed	2 med (0.3 oz)	10	1	tr	0	tr	tr	tr	tr	4	107	5	0	tr
green stuffed	2 sm (0.2 oz)	9	1	tr	0	tr	tr	tr	tr	3	91	4	0	1
ripe	2 extra lg (0.4 oz)	12	1	tr	0	tr	1	0	tr	10	97	1	0	tr
ripe	2 lg (0.3 oz)	10	1	tr	0	tr	1	0	tr	8	81	1	0	tr
ripe	2 sm (0.2 oz)	7	1	tr	0	tr	tr	0	tr	6	60	1	0	tr
ripe sliced	¼ cup (1.2 oz)	35	3	tr	0	tr	2	0	1	30	297	3	0	tr
spanish stuffed	5 (0.5 oz)	15	1	0	0	0	1	0	0	20	320	—	—	0
DAVE'S GOURMET														
Olives In Pain	⅛ jar (0.5 oz)	15	2	—	—	0	0	0	0	0	270	—	—	0
MARTINIS														
Kalamata Pitted	4 (0.5 oz)	40	4	1	0	tr	tr	0	tr	10	148	—	—	0
MATIZ														
Olivada Spread Sweet	2 tbsp	87	6	1	0	tr	9	9	1	40	288	—	—	tr
Olivada Spread Traditional & Hot	2 tbsp	114	12	3	0	tr	3	tr	2	40	288	—	—	tr
PELOPONNESE														
Amfissa	3	45	5	0	0	0	1	0	0	0	200	—	—	0
Ionian Green	3	25	3	0	0	0	1	0	0	0	250	—	—	0
Kalamata Pitted	5	45	5	0	0	0	1	0	0	0	210	—	—	0
Kalamata Spread	1 tsp	15	2	0	0	0	0	0	0	0	160	—	—	0
PRIORAT NATUR														
Natural Olives	10	30	3	0	0	0	1	tr	1	0	120	—	—	0
PROGRESSO														
Tapenade	1 tbsp (0.5 oz)	20	2	0	0	0	1	0	0	0	180	—	—	0
STONEWALL KITCHEN														
Mixed Olive Spread	1 tbsp	35	2	0	—	0	5	3	—	—	150	—	—	1
ZATARAIN'S														
Cocktail	7 (0.5 oz)	25	3	1	0	0	0	0	0	0	350	—	—	0
Stuffed	6 (0.5 oz)	25	3	1	0	0	0	0	0	0	280	—	—	0
ONION														
CANNED														
cocktail	½ cup	41	tr	tr	0	2	9	4	2	20	257	153	14	5

FOOD	PORTION	CALS	FAT	SAT FAT	CHOL	PROT	CARB	SUGAR	FIBER	CALCI	SOD	POTAS	FOLIC	VIT C
BOAR'S HEAD														
Sweet Vidalia In Sauce	1 tbsp	10	0	0	0	0	2	2	0	0	15	—	—	0
DIETZ & WATSON														
Sweet Vidalia In Sauce	1 tbsp (0.5 oz)	12	0	0	0	0	3	0	0	0	0	—	—	0
FRENCH'S														
Original French Fried	2 tbsp	45	4	2	0	0	3	0	0	—	60	—	—	—
MCSWEET														
Pickled Onions	4 (1 oz)	10	0	0	0	0	2	tr	0	0	1060	—	—	0
THE GRACIOUS GOURMET														
Balsamic Four Onion Spread	1 tbsp (0.5 oz)	20	0	0	0	0	6	4	0	0	45	—	—	1
DRIED														
flakes	1 tbsp	17	tr	tr	0	tr	4	2	1	13	1	81	8	4
powder	1 tsp	7	tr	tr	0	tr	2	1	tr	9	1	23	4	tr
shallots	1 tbsp	3	0	0	0	tr	1	—	—	2	1	15	1	tr
BOB'S RED MILL														
Minced	1 tbsp	40	1	0	0	1	8	0	1	—	4	—	—	—
SENECA														
Crisp Onions	1 tbsp (7 g)	40	3	0	0	0	4	1	0	0	35	—	—	0
FRESH														
cooked w/o salt	1 lg (4.5 oz)	56	tr	tr	0	2	13	6	2	28	4	212	19	7
cooked w/o salt	1 sm (2 oz)	26	tr	tr	0	1	6	3	1	13	2	100	9	3
cooked w/o salt	1 med (3.3 oz)	41	tr	tr	0	1	10	4	1	21	3	156	14	5
cooked w/o salt chopped	1 tbsp	7	tr	tr	0	tr	2	1	tr	3	0	25	2	1
raw chopped	½ cup	32	tr	tr	0	1	7	3	1	18	3	117	15	6
raw chopped	1 tbsp	4	tr	tr	0	tr	1	tr	tr	2	0	15	2	1
raw slice	1 (0.5 oz)	6	tr	tr	0	tr	1	1	tr	3	1	20	3	1
raw sliced	½ cup	23	tr	0	0	1	5	2	1	13	2	84	11	4
scallions raw	1 med (0.5 oz)	5	tr	tr	0	tr	1	tr	tr	11	2	41	10	3
scallions raw chopped	¼ cup	8	tr	tr	0	tr	2	1	1	18	4	69	16	5
shallots raw chopped	¼ cup	29	tr	tr	0	1	7	—	—	15	5	134	14	3
sweet whole raw	1 (11.6 oz)	106	tr	tr	0	3	25	17	3	66	26	394	76	16
whole raw	1 med (4 oz)	44	tr	tr	0	1	10	5	2	25	4	161	21	8
whole raw	1 lg (5.3 oz)	60	tr	tr	0	2	14	6	3	34	6	219	28	11
whole raw	1 sm (2.5 oz)	28	tr	tr	0	1	7	3	1	16	3	102	13	5
BLAND FARMS														
Vidalia Sweet	1 (5 oz)	60	0	0	0	1	14	5	3	40	10	—	—	12
BLUE RIBBON														
Yellow	1 med (5.2 oz)	60	0	0	0	2	14	9	3	40	5	—	—	12

FOOD	PORTION	CALS	FAT	SAT FAT	CHOL	PROT	CARB	SUGAR	FIBER	CALCI	SOD	POTAS	FOLIC	VIT C
EARTHBOUND FARMS														
Organic Green Onions	¼ cup	10	0	0	0	0	2	1	1	0	5	—	—	5
Organic Red	1 med (5.2 oz)	60	0	0	0	2	14	9	3	40	5	—	—	12
OCEAN MIST														
Green Onions Chopped	¼ cup	10	0	0	0	0	2	1	1	0	5	—	—	5
OSOSWEET														
Onion	1 med (5 oz)	60	0	0	0	2	14	9	3	40	5	—	—	12
REALSWEET														
Vidalia	1 (5.2 oz)	45	0	0	0	1	11	9	3	40	5	50	—	12
FROZEN														
C&W														
Petite Whole	⅔ cup (3 oz)	30	0	0	0	0	6	3	tr	0	10	—	—	0
FARM RICH														
Petals Breaded + Sauce	10 (3 oz)	200	12	2	5	2	22	3	1	20	700	—	—	4
IAN'S														
Rings & Strings	5–9 pieces (2.5 oz)	152	7	1	0	2	16	1	1	20	180	—	—	0
TAKE-OUT														
creamed	1 cup	187	9	2	7	5	22	10	2	132	306	369	27	8
fried	½ cup	57	5	—	0	tr	3	tr	1	9	5	58	—	1
rings breaded & fried	8 to 9 (3 oz)	276	16	7	14	4	31	—	—	73	430	129	55	1
OPOSSUM														
roasted	3 oz	188	9	—	—	26	0	0	0	—	—	—	—	—
ORANGE														
CANNED														
DEL MONTE														
Mandarin In Lite Orange Gel	1 pkg (4.5 oz)	60	0	0	0	0	14	12	0	20	40	—	—	18
SunFresh Mandarin In Light Syrup	½ cup (4.5 oz)	70	0	0	0	tr	17	15	0	0	10	95	—	60
DOLE														
Mandarin In Fruit Juice	1 pkg (4 oz)	80	0	0	0	tr	19	18	1	40	10	75	—	27
FRESH														
california valencia	1 (4.2 oz)	59	tr	tr	0	1	14	—	3	48	0	217	47	59
california valencia sections	½ cup (3.2 oz)	44	tr	tr	0	1	11	—	2	36	0	161	35	44
florida	1 (5.3 oz)	69	tr	tr	0	1	17	14	4	65	0	255	26	65
florida sections	½ cup (3.2 oz)	43	tr	tr	0	1	11	8	2	40	0	156	16	42
fresh	1 lg (6.5 oz)	86	tr	tr	0	2	22	17	4	74	0	333	55	98
fresh	1 sm (3.4 oz)	45	tr	tr	0	1	11	9	2	38	0	174	29	51

FOOD	PORTION	CALS	FAT	SAT FAT	CHOL	PROT	CARB	SUGAR	FIBER	CALCI	SOD	POTAS	FOLIC	VIT C
fresh	1 med (4.6 oz)	62	tr	tr	0	1	15	12	3	52	0	237	39	70
navel	1 (4.9 oz)	69	tr	tr	0	1	18	12	3	60	1	232	48	83
navel sections	1 cup (5.8 oz)	81	tr	tr	0	2	21	14	4	71	2	274	56	98
peel	1 tbsp (0.2 oz)	3	tr	tr	0	tr	1	tr	1	8	0	10	1	8
DARLING														
Mandarine	1 med (3.8 oz)	50	0	0	0	1	13	9	3	40	0	160	24	27
DOLE														
Orange	1 med (4.2 oz)	60	0	0	0	1	14	13	3	40	0	—	40	60
SUNKIST														
Cara Cara	1 med (5.4 oz)	80	0	0	0	1	19	14	3	20	0	250	60	90

ORANGE JUICE

FOOD	PORTION	CALS	FAT	SAT FAT	CHOL	PROT	CARB	SUGAR	FIBER	CALCI	SOD	POTAS	FOLIC	VIT C
chilled bottled	1 cup (8.7 oz)	112	1	tr	0	2	26	21	1	27	2	496	74	124
fresh	1 cup (8.7 oz)	112	1	tr	0	2	26	21	1	27	2	496	74	124
mandarin orange	7 oz	94	tr	—	—	2	20	—	—	38	—	—	—	64
AFTER THE FALL														
24 Karrot Orange	8 oz	120	0	0	0	1	28	25	—	150	55	390	—	90
DOLE														
100% Juice w/ Calcium	8 oz	120	0	0	0	tr	27	—	0	300	10	450	—	72
FLORIDA'S NATURAL														
Calcium & Vitamin D	8 oz	110	0	0	0	2	26	22	0	350	0	450	60	72
GENESIS TODAY														
Omega Orange 100% Juice	8 oz	90	0	0	0	1	23	13	3	20	0	310	200	120
HOOD														
100% Juice	1 cup	120	0	0	0	0	30	30	0	0	20	—	—	72
ITALIAN VOLCANO														
Organic Blood Orange	8 oz	101	0	0	0	1	25	23	—	—	0	430	—	48
IZZE														
Esque Sparkling Mandarin	1 bottle (12 oz)	50	0	0	0	0	12	11	—	—	10	—	—	—
LAND O LAKES														
Juice	1 cup (8 oz)	110	0	0	0	1	25	23	0	20	45	—	—	60
Juice w/ Calcium	1 cup (8 oz)	120	0	0	0	1	29	28	0	350	0	—	—	60
MOTT'S														
100% Juice Sunkist Orange Sensation	1 bottle (14 oz)	210	0	0	0	0	50	49	0	40	15	610	—	60
MR. J														
100% Juice Calcium Fortified	1 pkg (4 oz)	60	0	0	0	0	19	14	—	151	—	—	4	30

FOOD	PORTION	CALS	FAT	SAT FAT	CHOL	PROT	CARB	SUGAR	FIBER	CALCI	SOD	POTAS	FOLIC	VIT C
NUTRABALANCE														
Fortified	1 pkg (4 oz)	60	0	0	0	1	17	—	4	250	25	250	—	60
OCEAN SPRAY														
Juice	8 oz	100	0	0	0	0	31	31	—	2	35	400	—	60
ODWALLA														
100% Juice	8 oz	110	0	0	0	1	25	24	0	20	15	450	—	144
OLD ORCHARD														
100% Juice	8 oz	130	0	0	0	0	31	29	—	0	25	280	—	72
ORGANIC VALLEY														
W/ Calcium	1 cup	110	0	0	0	2	26	26	0	300	0	450	80	72
SIMPLY														
Orange Calcium Fortified	8 oz	110	0	0	0	2	26	22	—	350	0	450	60	84
Orange Original	8 oz	110	0	0	0	2	26	22	—	20	0	450	60	84
SNAPPLE														
Orangeade	8 oz	100	0	0	0	0	26	26	—	—	5	—	—	—
SSIPS														
Orangeade	8 oz	120	0	0	0	0	31	29	—	—	10	40	—	60
TREE RIPE														
100% Juice + Calcium & Vitamins	8 oz	120	0	0	0	1	29	28	0	350	0	480	40	120
TROPICANA														
Antioxidant Vitamins	8 oz	110	0	0	0	2	26	22	0	20	0	450	60	144
Calcium + Vitamin D	8 oz	110	0	0	0	2	26	22	0	350	0	450	60	72
Fiber	8 oz	120	0	0	0	2	29	22	3	20	0	450	60	72
Healthy Heart	8 oz	120	0	0	0	2	26	22	0	20	0	450	60	60
Healthy Kids	8 oz	110	0	0	0	2	26	22	0	350	0	450	60	72
Light'n Healthy w/ Calcium	8 oz	50	0	0	0	tr	13	10	0	200	10	450	24	72
No Pulp	8 oz	110	0	0	0	2	26	22	0	20	0	450	60	72
Orangeade	8 oz	111	0	0	0	0	33	30	0	0	0	—	—	60
Organic	8 oz	120	0	0	0	1	28	22	0	20	25	450	60	72
Trop50 Orange Juice Beverage	8 oz	50	0	0	0	tr	13	10	0	0	10	450	28	72
UNCLE MATT'S														
Organic 100% Juice Pulp Free	8 oz	110	0	0	0	2	26	22	0	0	10	450	60	72
Organic 100% Juice w/ Pulp	8 oz	110	0	0	0	2	26	22	0	0	10	450	60	72
WELSH FARMS														
Juice	8 oz	110	0	0	0	0	27	23	—	—	—	—	—	78
TAKE-OUT														
orange julius	1 cup (9.2 oz)	212	tr	tr	0	14	39	35	tr	472	196	938	84	61

FOOD	PORTION	CALS	FAT	SAT FAT	CHOL	PROT	CARB	SUGAR	FIBER	CALCI	SOD	POTAS	FOLIC	VIT C
OREGANO														
crumbled	1 tsp	3	tr	tr	0	tr	1	tr	tr	16	0	17	3	1
ground	1 tsp	6	tr	tr	0	tr	1	tr	1	28	0	30	5	1
ORGAN MEATS														
(*see* BRAINS, GIBLETS, GIZZARDS, HEART, KIDNEY, LIVER, SWEETBREAD)														
OSTRICH														
cooked	4 oz	195	8	2	92	29	0	0	0	9	450	358	16	0
cooked diced	1 cup (4.7 oz)	215	9	2	111	35	0	0	0	11	543	432	19	0
NATURAL FRONTIER FOODS														
Filets	1 (4 oz)	130	3	1	50	28	0	0	0	0	75	—	—	0
Ground Lean	4 oz	130	3	1	50	28	0	0	0	0	75	—	—	0
OYSTERS														
canned eastern	1 cup	112	4	1	89	11	6	0	0	73	181	371	15	8
eastern baked	6 med	47	1	tr	22	4	4	—	0	33	96	90	14	4
eastern raw	6 med	50	1	tr	21	4	5	—	0	37	150	104	15	4
eastern sauteed	6 med	76	5	1	36	5	3	0	0	30	342	106	6	2
smoked	6	33	1	tr	26	3	2	0	0	22	259	75	5	2
CHICKEN OF THE SEA														
Smoked In Oil	1 can (3.75 oz)	170	8	2	45	10	8	0	0	20	280	—	—	0
Whole	¼ can (2 oz)	80	3	1	35	7	6	0	0	20	220	—	—	0
POLAR														
Whole	¼ cup	70	3	2	3	7	4	0	0	0	150	—	—	0
Whole Smoked	⅓ cup	95	5	2	10	8	4	0	0	20	160	—	—	0
TAKE-OUT														
breaded & fried	6	368	18	5	108	13	40	—	—	28	677	182	31	4
fritter	1 (1.4 oz)	121	6	1	36	4	12	tr	tr	62	276	58	21	1
oysters rockefeller	1 cup	302	17	8	90	18	22	2	4	226	1113	627	143	27
stew	1 cup	208	13	8	78	11	11	9	0	235	892	380	15	3
PANCAKE/WAFFLE SYRUP														
light	¼ cup	98	0	0	0	0	27	20	0	1	120	2	0	0
pancake syrup	¼ cup	209	tr	tr	0	0	55	50	0	4	48	5	0	0
pancake syrup	1 pkg (2 oz)	156	tr	tr	0	0	41	38	0	4	36	4	0	0
AUNT JEMIMA														
Butter Lite	¼ cup (2.1 oz)	100	0	0	0	0	26	25	1	—	210	—	—	—
LOG CABIN														
Lite	¼ cup (2 oz)	100	0	0	0	0	25	22	—	—	160	—	—	—
NATURALLY FRESH														
Maple Mountain Sugar Free	2 tbsp	0	0	0	0	0	0	0	0	—	70	5	—	—
SMUCKER'S														
Breakfast Syrup Sugar Free	¼ cup (2.1 oz)	20	0	0	0	0	8	0	—	—	150	—	—	—
WHOLESOME SWEETENERS														
Organic	¼ cup	240	0	0	0	0	60	60	0	0	90	—	—	—

PANCAKES

FOOD	PORTION	CALS	FAT	SAT FAT	CHOL	PROT	CARB	SUGAR	FIBER	CALCI	SOD	POTAS	FOLIC	VIT C
FROZEN														
AUNT JEMIMA														
Blueberry	3 (3.7 oz)	260	6	1	25	7	44	13	1	60	460	—	—	0
Buttermilk	3 (3.7 oz)	250	6	1	30	6	41	9	1	60	460	—	—	0
Buttermilk Lowfat	3 (3.6 oz)	200	2	0	25	7	41	8	1	60	440	—	—	0
Oatmeal	3 (3.7 oz)	230	4	2	25	8	42	11	4	80	380	—	—	0
Whole Grain	3 (3.6 oz)	240	6	1	20	6	42	9	3	40	440	—	—	0
DR. PRAEGER'S														
Broccoli	1 (2 oz)	80	4	0	0	2	9	1	2	0	170	—	—	9
Potato	1 (2.2 oz)	100	4	0	15	2	13	1	3	0	190	—	—	12
Sweet Potato Bites	1 (2 oz)	80	2	0	0	2	12	6	3	20	140	—	—	2
GOLDEN														
Potato Latkes	1 (1.3 oz)	70	3	0	<5	2	10	2	1	0	190	—	—	0
Zucchini	1 (1.3 oz)	70	3	1	0	2	8	tr	1	0	170	—	—	1
IAN'S														
Blueberry	1 (1.3 oz)	100	2	0	<5	3	19	7	1	60	150	—	—	0
Pancake	1 (1.3 oz)	100	2	0	<5	3	19	7	1	60	150	—	—	0
JIMMY DEAN														
Breakfast Bowls Pancake & Sausage Links	1 pkg	710	31	11	45	13	93	34	3	20	890	—	—	0
Griddle Cake Sandwich Sausage Egg & Cheese	1 (4 oz)	370	23	8	40	8	32	13	1	60	640	—	—	0
Griddle Sticks	1 (2.5 oz)	160	6	2	25	7	21	8	0	20	410	—	—	0
PILLSBURY														
Blueberry	3 (4 oz)	230	4	1	10	5	46	14	2	100	430	—	40	0
Buttermilk	3 (4 oz)	240	4	1	10	6	47	13	2	100	470	—	40	0
Original	3 (4 oz)	250	4	1	10	6	49	14	2	100	450	—	40	0
RATNER'S														
Potato Latkes	1 (1.5 oz)	80	2	0	25	2	15	tr	tr	—	380	—	—	—
MIX														
ARROWHEAD MILLS														
Gluten Free Pancake & Waffle as prep	2 (5 in)	240	6	1	57	11	42	1	0	150	312	105	—	0
BATTER BLASTER														
Organic Original Pancake & Waffle Batter not prep	¼ cup (2 oz)	112	1	0	10	3	23	7	2	0	95	—	—	0
BISQUICK														
Shake 'N Pour Buttermilk as prep	3	220	3	1	0	6	42	7	1	250	800	—	60	—

FOOD	PORTION	CALS	FAT	SAT FAT	CHOL	PROT	CARB	SUGAR	FIBER	CALCI	SOD	POTAS	FOLIC	VIT C
KING ARTHUR														
Multi-Grain Buttermilk not prep	6 tbsp	160	2	0	5	7	31	2	5	150	180	—	—	0
MAPLE GROVE FARMS														
Buttermilk & Honey as prep	1	220	7	1	69	4	32	36	tr	60	576	—	—	0
Mix Gluten Free as prep	1	200	8	2	60	4	30	4	2	200	360	—	—	0
TAKE-OUT														
bu chu jun korean w/ vegetables	1 (4 oz)	83	4	1	21	2	11	—	1	14	230	53	29	3
buckwheat	1 (7 in)	142	5	1	45	5	19	4	2	175	366	160	14	0
norwegian lefse	1 (9 in) (2.7 oz)	163	5	2	8	3	27	2	2	13	134	199	31	4
pindaettok korean mung bean	1 (3.9 oz)	204	11	2	3	6	20	—	6	28	33	231	120	3
plain	1 (7 in)	183	3	1	7	4	35	10	1	50	407	58	33	tr
potato	1 (1.3 oz)	70	4	1	26	2	8	tr	1	9	151	165	9	6
w/ butter & syrup	2 (8.1 oz)	520	14	6	58	8	91	—	—	128	1104	251	30	4
whole wheat	1 (7 in)	183	8	2	47	6	23	5	3	155	489	188	14	0

PANCREAS

(*see* SWEETBREAD)

PANINI

(*see* SANDWICHES)

PAPAYA

FOOD	PORTION	CALS	FAT	SAT FAT	CHOL	PROT	CARB	SUGAR	FIBER	CALCI	SOD	POTAS	FOLIC	VIT C
canned in syrup	½ cup (2.3 oz)	50	tr	tr	0	tr	13	11	1	11	2	102	9	14
dried	1 strip (0.8 oz)	59	tr	tr	0	1	15	9	3	37	5	391	29	19
fresh	1 lg (13.3 oz)	148	1	tr	0	2	37	22	7	91	11	977	144	235
fresh	1 sm (5.3 oz)	59	tr	tr	0	1	15	9	3	36	5	391	58	94
fresh cubed	1 cup (4.9 oz)	55	tr	tr	0	1	14	8	3	34	4	360	53	87
green cooked	½ cup (2.3 oz)	18	tr	tr	0	tr	5	3	1	11	2	107	9	20
CRUNCHY N'YUMMY														
Organic Papaya	1 pkg (1 oz)	55	0	0	0	1	13	0	2	33	4	630	—	64
DOLE														
Fresh	½ (4.9 oz)	60	0	0	0	tr	15	9	3	40	5	390	60	96

PAPAYA JUICE

FOOD	PORTION	CALS	FAT	SAT FAT	CHOL	PROT	CARB	SUGAR	FIBER	CALCI	SOD	POTAS	FOLIC	VIT C
nectar	1 cup (8.8 oz)	142	tr	tr	0	tr	36	35	2	25	12	78	5	8
CERES														
100% Juice	8 oz	120	0	0	0	0	31	25	0	0	15	220	—	60
LAKEWOOD														
Red	8 oz	80	0	0	0	1	20	16	2	30	6	315	48	60
Yellow	8 oz	105	0	0	0	2	26	22	2	50	5	390	160	90
OLD ORCHARD														
Nectar Cocktail	8 oz	75	0	0	0	0	17	17	—	0	12	62	—	60

FOOD	PORTION	CALS	FAT	SAT FAT	CHOL	PROT	CARB	SUGAR	FIBER	CALCI	SOD	POTAS	FOLIC	VIT C
PAPRIKA														
dried	1 tsp	1	tr	tr	0	tr	tr	re	tr	7	2	19	1	1
BOB'S RED MILL														
Hungarian	½ tsp	11	0	0	0	0	2	0	1	—	0	—	—	—
PARSLEY														
dried	1 tbsp	4	tr	tr	0	tr	1	tr	1	23	7	61	3	2
freeze dried	1 tbsp	1	tr	—	0	tr	tr	—	tr	1	2	25	1	1
fresh chopped	1 tbsp	1	tr	tr	0	tr	tr	tr	tr	5	2	21	6	5
fresh chopped	¼ cup	5	tr	tr	0	tr	1	tr	1	21	8	83	23	20
fresh sprigs	5 (1.8 oz)	18	tr	tr	0	1	3	tr	2	69	28	277	76	67
DOROT														
Chopped Cubes frzn	1 cube (4 g)	5	tr	tr	0	tr	tr	—	tr	—	17	—	—	—
PARSNIPS														
fresh sliced cooked w/o salt	½ cup (2.7 oz)	55	tr	tr	0	1	13	4	3	29	8	286	45	10
whole cooked	1 (5.6 oz)	114	tr	tr	0	2	27	8	6	59	16	587	93	21
TAKE-OUT														
creamed	1 cup (8 oz)	237	11	3	7	6	31	10	5	166	652	620	82	17
PASSION FRUIT														
fresh	1 (0.6 oz)	17	tr	tr	0	tr	4	2	2	2	5	63	3	5
fresh cut up	½ cup (4.1 oz)	114	1	tr	0	3	28	13	12	14	33	411	17	35
PASSION FRUIT JUICE														
nectar	1 cup (8.8 oz)	168	tr	tr	0	tr	44	43	tr	8	10	280	8	30
yellow lilikoi	1 cup (8.7 oz)	138	tr	tr	0	1	35	34	1	10	15	687	20	59
CERES														
100% Juice	8 oz	130	0	0	0	0	32	27	0	0	15	220	—	36
EARTHWISE														
Passionfruit Aloe	8 oz	110	0	0	0	0	28	26	0	20	30	—	—	2
SANTA CRUZ														
Organic 100% Juice Nectar	8 oz	150	0	0	0	1	40	36	0	20	15	125	—	—
PASTA														
(*see also* NOODLES, PASTA DINNERS, PASTA SALAD)														
DRY														
corn cooked	1 cup (4.9 oz)	176	1	tr	0	4	39	—	7	1	0	43	8	0
elbows not prep	1 cup	389	2	tr	0	13	78	—	—	19	8	170	19	0
elbows cooked	1 cup (4.9 oz)	197	1	tr	0	7	40	—	2	10	1	43	98	0
shells small cooked	1 cup (4 oz)	162	1	tr	0	5	33	—	2	8	1	36	81	0
spaghetti cooked	1 cup (4.9 oz)	197	1	tr	0	7	40	—	2	10	1	43	98	0
spinach spaghetti cooked	1 cup (4.9 oz)	182	1	tr	0	6	37	—	—	42	20	81	17	0
spirals cooked	1 cup (4.7 oz)	189	tr	tr	0	6	38	—	2	9	1	42	94	0
vegetable cooked	1 cup (4.7 oz)	172	tr	tr	0	6	36	—	6	15	8	42	87	0

FOOD	PORTION	CALS	FAT	SAT FAT	CHOL	PROT	CARB	SUGAR	FIBER	CALCI	SOD	POTAS	FOLIC	VIT C
whole wheat all shapes cooked	1 cup	174	tr	tr	0	7	37	—	4	21	4	62	7	0
AMISH NATURAL														
Fettuccine Fiber Rich not prep	2 oz	200	1	0	0	6	42	3	11	0	50	—	—	0
Fettuccine not prep	2 oz	201	1	0	0	8	41	5	2	0	5	—	—	0
Fettuccine Whole Wheat not prep	2 oz	210	2	0	0	8	41	2	7	20	5	—	—	0
ANNIE CHUN'S														
Soba Noodles not prep	2 oz	200	1	0	0	8	39	1	3	0	390	—	—	0
BARILLA														
Lasagne not prep	2 pieces (1.8 oz)	180	0	0	0	7	37	1	2	0	0	—	120	0
Piccolini Mini Penne not prep	2 oz	210	1	0	0	7	43	2	6	0	0	—	120	0
Plus Spaghetti not prep	2 oz	210	2	0	0	10	38	2	4	20	25	—	160	0
Rotini Whole Grain not prep	2 oz	200	2	0	0	7	41	2	6	—	0	—	—	—
Spaghetti Whole Grain not prep	½ box (2 oz)	200	2	0	0	7	41	2	6	—	0	—	—	—
Tortellini Three Cheese not prep	⅔ cup (2 oz)	230	8	3	35	8	32	2	3	80	500	—	—	0
DEBOLES														
Angel Hair Rice Pasta not prep	¼ pkg (2 oz)	210	1	0	0	4	46	0	tr	40	15	80	—	0
Elbow Corn Pasta Wheat Free not prep	⅙ pkg (2 oz)	200	2	0	0	4	43	0	5	0	15	170	—	0
Fettuccine not prep	¼ pkg (2 oz)	210	1	0	0	7	41	2	1	0	0	—	—	0
Organic Angel Hair Whole Wheat not prep	¼ pkg (2 oz)	210	2	0	0	7	42	2	5	20	10	220	—	0
Organic Eggless Ribbon not prep	1 cup (2 oz)	210	1	0	0	7	43	2	1	0	5	130	—	0
Organic Fettucini Spinach not prep	¼ pkg (2 oz)	210	1	0	0	7	43	1	3	60	20	180	—	0
Organic Lasagna not prep	¼ pkg (2.5 oz)	260	1	0	0	9	54	2	1	20	5	170	—	0
Organic Rigatoni Whole Wheat not prep	1 cup (2 oz)	210	2	0	0	7	42	2	5	20	10	220	—	0
Rigatoni not prep	¼ pkg (2 oz)	210	1	0	0	7	41	2	1	0	0	—	—	0

FOOD	PORTION	CALS	FAT	SAT FAT	CHOL	PROT	CARB	SUGAR	FIBER	CALCI	SOD	POTAS	FOLIC	VIT C
DREAMFIELDS														
Lasagna not prep	2 pieces (2 oz)	190	1	0	0	7	42	1	5	0	15	—	160	0
Rotini not prep	⅔ cup (2 oz)	190	1	0	0	7	42	1	5	0	15	—	120	0
EDEN														
Bifun Pasta not prep	2 oz	200	1	0	5	5	44	0	0	0	5	10	—	0
Harusame Pasta not prep	2 oz	190	0	0	0	0	47	0	0	0	5	10	—	0
Organic Rigatoni Kamut & Buckwheat not prep	½ cup (2 oz)	200	2	tr	0	9	39	3	5	20	10	220	16	—
Organic Spaghetti 100% Whole Wheat not prep	2 oz	210	2	0	0	10	40	2	6	20	0	260	—	0
Organic Spirals Flax Rice not prep	½ cup (2 oz)	200	2	0	0	9	40	0	4	20	10	240	24	—
Organic Vegetable Shells not prep	½ cup (2 oz)	210	2	0	0	9	40	1	4	0	20	280	24	0
Organic Ziti Rigati Spelt not prep	½ cup (2 oz)	210	2	0	0	7	41	1	5	0	10	260	24	0
GILLIAN'S														
Penne Brown Rice Pasta Wheat Gluten Egg Free not prep	2 oz	200	2	0	0	4	43	0	2	0	0	—	—	0
HEARTLAND														
Gluten Free not prep	2 oz	200	1	0	0	3	45	0	1	0	0	—	—	—
Naturals Penne not prep	¾ cup (2 oz)	210	1	0	0	7	41	2	2	0	0	—	—	0
Perfect Balance Elbow Macaroni not prep	½ cup (2 oz)	200	1	0	0	7	41	2	3	20	0	—	100	0
Whole Wheat Rotini not prep	¾ cup (2 oz)	210	2	0	0	7	41	2	5	20	0	—	—	0
JOVIAL														
Organic Einkorn All Shapes	2 oz	200	2	0	0	9	35	1	4	20	0	260	—	0
Organic Einkorn White All Shapes	2 oz	200	2	0	0	8	40	1	2	20	0	125	—	0
Organic Gluten Free Brown Rice All Shapes	2 oz	210	2	0	0	5	43	0	2	0	0	—	—	0

FOOD	PORTION	CALS	FAT	SAT FAT	CHOL	PROT	CARB	SUGAR	FIBER	CALCI	SOD	POTAS	FOLIC	VIT C
LUNDBERG														
Organic Spaghetti Brown Rice not prep	2 oz	210	2	1	0	4	44	3	3	0	5	190	—	0
MADDY'S														
Gluten Free not prep	4 oz	310	2	2	0	5	66	4	2	0	120	—	—	0
MAGNOODLES														
Organic Smart not prep	2 oz	204	1	—	—	7	41	—	5	18	11	164	1	3
MARA'S PASTA														
100% Whole Wheat not prep	2 oz	190	1	0	0	8	40	0	7	0	0	—	—	0
MUELLER'S														
Elbow Macaroni not prep	½ cup	210	1	0	0	7	41	2	2	0	0	—	100	0
RACCONTO														
Essentials Heart Health not prep	2 oz	190	1	0	0	8	41	0	7	0	0	—	—	0
Essentials Heart Health Rigatoni not prep	⅙ pkg (2 oz)	190	1	0	0	8	41	0	7	0	0	—	—	0
RICE SELECT														
Orzo Original not prep	⅓ cup	210	1	—	0	7	42	—	—	—	0	—	—	—
RONZONI														
Alphabets not prep	⅓ cup (2 oz)	210	1	0	0	7	42	2	2	—	0	—	100	—
Bow Ties not prep	1 cup (2 oz)	210	1	0	0	7	42	2	2	—	0	—	100	—
Elbows not prep	½ cup (2 oz)	210	1	0	0	7	42	2	2	—	0	—	100	—
Garden Delight Radiatore not prep	2 oz	190	1	0	0	7	40	2	4	20	15	—	140	2
Garden Delight Spaghetti not prep	2 oz	190	1	0	0	7	40	2	4	20	15	—	140	2
Quick Cook Penne Rigate not prep	¾ cup (2 oz)	210	1	0	0	7	42	2	2	—	0	—	100	—
Smart Taste Angel Hair not prep	½ pkg (2 oz)	170	1	0	0	6	40	1	5	300	0	—	120	—
Smart Taste Rotini not prep	2 oz	180	1	0	0	6	43	1	7	300	5	—	140	0
THAI KITCHEN														
Stir-Fry Rice Linguini not prep	2 oz	210	1	0	0	4	46	0	0	0	20	—	—	0

FOOD	PORTION	CALS	FAT	SAT FAT	CHOL	PROT	CARB	SUGAR	FIBER	CALCI	SOD	POTAS	FOLIC	VIT C
WACKY MAC														
Veggie Bows not prep	⅙ pkg (2 oz)	200	1	0	0	8	41	0	1	0	15	—	120	0
FRESH														
cooked	2 oz	75	1	tr	33	3	14	—	—	3	3	14	36	0
spinach cooked	2 oz	74	1	tr	19	3	14	—	—	10	3	21	36	0
BUITONI														
Angel Hair	⅓ pkg (2.8 oz)	230	2	0	40	9	44	1	2	20	170	—	—	0
Ravioli Four Cheese	1 serv (3.7 oz)	340	12	4	55	15	42	2	3	150	630	—	—	0
Reserva Quattro Formaggi Agnolotti	1 serv (4.4 oz)	360	17	9	90	17	35	2	2	300	698	—	—	0
Tortellini Spinach Cheese	1 serv (3.7 oz)	320	7	4	55	15	49	4	3	200	510	—	—	0
Tortelloni Whole Wheat Cheese	1 serv (3.7 oz)	330	10	3	60	16	45	3	6	150	500	—	—	0
MONTEREY GOURMET														
Whole Wheat Ravioli Vegetable & Cheese	1 cup (3.5 oz)	240	6	2	25	12	35	1	4	100	340	—	—	5
Whole Wheat Tortellini Italian Cheese	1 cup (3.5 oz)	290	6	3	35	13	48	1	5	150	290	—	—	0
NASOYA														
Pasta Zero Plus Silken	⅔ cup (4 oz)	20	0	0	0	1	4	0	3	100	0	—	40	0
PASTA PRIMA														
Ravioli Butternut Squash	½ pkg (4 oz)	250	6	4	45	12	36	2	2	200	410	—	—	4
Ravioli Gluten Free Butternut Squash	1 cup (3.5 oz)	180	4	3	30	6	30	2	2	100	340	—	—	4
Ravioli Gluten Free Five Cheese	1 cup (3.5 oz)	230	10	6	55	11	24	1	2	25	410	—	—	0
Ravioli Italian Sausage	½ pkg (4 oz)	290	13	6	60	16	25	1	2	300	570	—	—	1
Ravioli Lobster	½ pkg (4 oz)	250	7	4	55	14	31	2	2	200	650	—	—	2
Ravioli Spinach & Cheese	1 cup (3.5 oz)	210	7	3	35	9	29	1	2	80	430	—	—	1
FROZEN														
PASTA PRIMA														
Ravioli Spinach & Mozzarella	1 cup (4 oz)	200	5	2	27	9	29	0	4	150	390	—	—	6
SOLTERRA														
Fettuccine Gluten Free	⅓ pkg (4 oz)	330	6	2	150	12	54	1	3	40	490	—	—	0

FOOD	PORTION	CALS	FAT	SAT FAT	CHOL	PROT	CARB	SUGAR	FIBER	CALCI	SOD	POTAS	FOLIC	VIT C
TOFUTTI														
Ravioli Dairy Free	4 (3.2 oz)	210	10	3	0	2	28	1	1	—	300	—	—	—

PASTA DINNERS

(*see also* PASTA SALAD)

CANNED

ANNIE'S HOMEGROWN

FOOD	PORTION	CALS	FAT	SAT FAT	CHOL	PROT	CARB	SUGAR	FIBER	CALCI	SOD	POTAS	FOLIC	VIT C
Organic Cheesy Ravioli	1 cup (8.5 oz)	180	4	2	5	6	31	9	3	80	730	—	—	2
Organic P'sghetti Loops	1 cup (8.4 oz)	190	4	1	0	9	29	9	2	60	650	—	—	4
CHEF BOYARDEE														
99% Fat Free Beef Ravioli	1 cup	170	2	1	10	7	33	6	2	20	880	—	—	0
Beef Ravioli	1 cup (8.6 oz)	230	8	3	15	8	31	5	3	20	750	450	40	0
Beefaroni	1 cup (8.7 oz)	240	10	4	15	9	30	5	3	20	720	470	80	0
Mini Ravioli	1 cup (8.8 oz)	250	9	4	15	8	35	5	3	20	950	—	—	0
Mini-Bites Spaghetti & Meatballs	1 cup (8.8 oz)	240	10	4	15	10	28	6	3	20	750	840	—	0
Spaghetti & Meat Balls	1 cup (9 oz)	260	11	4	15	10	30	7	4	20	750	570	—	0
HORMEL														
Kid's Kitchen Microwave Meals Cheezy Mac 'N Beef	1 pkg (7.5 oz)	250	6	4	20	14	34	8	1	100	840	—	—	0
Kid's Kitchen Microwave Meals Cheezy Mac 'N Cheese	1 pkg (7.5 oz)	270	14	9	40	11	24	3	1	150	750	—	—	0
Kid's Kitchen Microwave Meals Mini Beef Ravioli	1 pkg (7.5 oz)	240	6	3	20	8	38	6	1	40	950	—	—	1
Kid's Kitchen Microwave Meals Spaghetti Rings & Franks	1 pkg (7.5 oz)	240	8	4	25	9	32	11	1	80	840	—	—	0
Lasagna w/ Meat Sauce	1 pkg (7.5 oz)	210	5	2	10	9	31	14	3	60	840	—	—	1
Spaghetti w/ Meat Sauce	1 pkg (7.5 oz)	210	5	3	15	10	31	14	3	60	750	—	—	2
SPAGHETTIOS														
A to Z's w/ Meatballs	1 cup	260	9	4	20	11	33	12	3	150	990	—	100	6
A to Z's w/ Sliced Franks	1 cup	230	6	3	20	9	32	9	2	150	990	—	100	6

FOOD	PORTION	CALS	FAT	SAT FAT	CHOL	PROT	CARB	SUGAR	FIBER	CALCI	SOD	POTAS	FOLIC	VIT C
SPAGHETTIOS (CONT.)														
Mini Beef Ravioli In Meat Sauce	1 cup	260	5	2	10	11	43	14	5	40	1060	—	60	1
Pasta	1 cup	180	1	0	5	6	37	13	3	20	630	—	100	0
Plus Calcium	1 cup	170	1	1	5	6	35	13	3	300	620	—	80	6
Sliced Franks	1 cup (8.8 oz)	220	6	2	20	9	32	9	4	150	600	840	100	6
FROZEN														
4REAL														
Mac+Cheese	1 pkg (8 oz)	230	5	3	5	8	33	1	2	60	410	—	—	0
Meat Sauce w/ Beef Ravioli	1 pkg (8 oz)	190	4	1	30	8	32	5	2	40	410	—	—	6
Spaghetti Rings	1 pkg (8 oz)	180	1	0	0	6	37	5	2	20	310	—	—	6
AMY'S														
Bowls Baked Ziti	1 pkg	390	12	2	0	9	62	8	6	100	590	—	—	24
Bowls Stuffed Pasta Shells	1 pkg	310	13	7	30	19	30	7	5	400	740	—	—	24
Lasagna Cheese	1 pkg (10.2 oz)	380	14	8	45	20	44	8	4	450	680	—	—	12
Lasagna Tofu Vegetable	1 pkg (9.4 oz)	310	11	2	0	13	41	6	6	100	680	—	—	21
Macaroni & Cheese	1 pkg (8.9 oz)	410	16	10	40	16	47	6	3	300	590	—	—	1
Macaroni & Cheese Light In Sodium	1 pkg (8.9 oz)	400	16	10	40	16	47	6	3	300	290	—	—	1
Macaroni & Soy Cheese	1 pkg (8.9 oz)	370	15	2	0	16	42	2	4	150	500	—	—	1
Rice Mac & Cheese	1 pkg (9 oz)	400	16	10	50	16	47	6	1	300	590	—	—	1
BANQUET														
Lasagna Family Entree	1 cup	510	16	5	15	25	63	7	3	100	730	—	—	1
Macaroni & Cheese	1 cup	200	6	3	10	7	30	7	3	80	750	—	—	0
Noodles & Beef	1 cup	160	4	2	30	8	20	0	2	0	900	—	—	0
BIRDS EYE														
Steamfresh Meals For Two Shrimp Alfredo	½ pkg (11.9 oz)	420	12	7	100	21	55	7	4	150	900	—	—	18
Steamfresh Meals For Two Shrimp Pasta Primavera	½ pkg (11.9 oz)	450	24	14	130	15	39	6	3	60	770	—	—	42
BLUE HORIZON ORGANIC														
Penne Alfredo w/ Shrimp	½ pkg (9.9 oz)	430	22	8	115	17	39	0	2	100	380	—	—	1
Penne Alla Vodka w/ Shrimp	½ pkg (9.9 oz)	270	6	3	75	17	38	0	3	60	280	—	—	12

FOOD	PORTION	CALS	FAT	SAT FAT	CHOL	PROT	CARB	SUGAR	FIBER	CALCI	SOD	POTAS	FOLIC	VIT C
BLUE HORIZON ORGANIC (CONT.)														
Pesto Farfalle w/ Shrimp	½ pkg (9.9 oz)	280	6	2	70	17	38	0	3	150	430	—	—	9
Scampi Rotini w/ Shrimp	½ pkg (9.9 oz)	410	19	6	85	18	44	0	4	60	640	—	—	15
BUITONI														
Braised Beef & Sausage Ravioli w/ Creamy Marinara Sauce	½ pkg (11.9 oz)	590	19	9	120	33	72	9	5	250	1200	—	—	1
Chicken & Mushroom Ravioli w/ Marsala Wine Sauce	½ pkg (10.9 oz)	530	20	11	110	29	59	7	5	250	1140	—	—	0
Four Cheese & Spinach Ravioli w/ Tomato Basil Sauce	½ pkg (12.9 oz)	550	21	12	100	24	55	12	7	350	1270	—	—	15
Grilled Chicken w/ Spinach Cannelloni w/ Alfredo Sauce	½ pkg (10.9 oz)	560	26	15	145	35	46	7	3	450	1070	—	—	5
CAESAR'S														
Gluten Free Lasagna Cheese In Marinara Sauce	1 pkg (11.5 oz)	520	14	7	50	14	84	8	4	300	570	—	—	9
Gluten Free Lasagna Vegetable In Marinara Sauce	1 pkg (11.5 oz)	510	13	6	45	13	84	8	5	250	510	—	—	12
Gluten Free Manicotti w/ Cheese In Marinara Sauce	1 pkg (11 oz)	380	18	9	105	16	42	10	3	300	640	—	—	12
Gluten Free Stuffed Shells w/ Cheese In Marinara Sauce	1 pkg (11 oz)	370	18	9	65	16	37	10	3	350	660	—	—	9
CANDLE CAFE														
Macaroni & Vegan Cheese	1 pkg (9 oz)	300	12	5	0	8	41	tr	5	60	880	—	—	0
Tofu Spinach Ravioli	1 pkg (9 oz)	320	10	3	0	11	48	4	4	150	750	—	—	1
CEDARLANE														
Zone Chicken & Vegetables Pasta & Ginger	1 pkg (10 oz)	340	12	5	140	24	35	2	3	150	650	—	—	15

FOOD	PORTION	CALS	FAT	SAT FAT	CHOL	PROT	CARB	SUGAR	FIBER	CALCI	SOD	POTAS	FOLIC	VIT C
CEDARLANE (CONT.)														
Zone Lasagna Vegetable	1 pkg (10.9 oz)	310	12	5	15	24	33	12	5	250	910	—	—	18
CELENTANO														
Cheese Ravioli	4 (4.3 oz)	220	5	3	30	11	34	1	2	100	280	—	—	0
CONTESSA														
Ravioli Portabello	6 (6.7 oz)	360	17	8	65	14	39	4	2	100	640	—	—	0
GLORY														
Macaroni & Cheese	1 pkg	480	23	6	90	21	47	10	1	450	1300	—	—	0
GLUTEN FREE CAFE														
Fettuccini Alfredo	1 pkg (9.2 oz)	400	16	7	45	4	55	tr	2	450	390	—	120	0
Pasta Primavera	1 pkg (9.2 oz)	270	9	5	25	4	42	4	4	350	260	—	135	24
GLUTINO														
Gluten Free Duo Mushroom Penne	1 pgk (10.5 oz)	380	6	2	5	8	73	1	5	60	720	—	—	1
Gluten Free Macaroni & Cheese	1 pkg (8.8 oz)	430	20	9	45	19	44	5	2	500	1430	—	—	0
Gluten Free Penne Alfredo	1 pkg (9.1 oz)	340	8	4	50	15	48	2	3	300	830	—	—	1
GREEN GIANT														
Skillet Meal Chicken & Cheesy Pasta as prep	1¼ cups	270	6	3	33	15	42	7	4	100	740	—	—	5
HEALTHY CHOICE														
Chicken Fettuccini Alfredo	1 pkg (11.4 oz)	300	7	3	45	20	39	16	7	100	580	670	60	6
Hearty Beef Stroganoff	1 pkg (10.9 oz)	280	7	3	40	20	33	17	6	40	600	700	100	4
Lobster Cheese Ravioli	1 pkg (8.9 oz)	270	6	3	15	11	41	9	4	200	600	590	60	6
Roasted Red Pepper Marinara	1 pkg (8.5 oz)	270	6	2	5	9	43	6	5	150	560	420	60	6
Tortellini Primavera Parmesan	1 pkg (8.9 oz)	240	5	2	20	10	37	7	6	250	490	530	60	12
HELEN'S KITCHEN														
Farfalle & Basil Pasta w/ Tofu Steaks	1 pkg (9 oz)	320	11	4	30	20	70	5	5	450	370	—	—	6
JOY OF COOKING														
Al Dente Cavatappi Bolognese	1 cup (7.7 oz)	280	12	4	55	14	29	5	2	—	700	—	—	—

FOOD	PORTION	CALS	FAT	SAT FAT	CHOL	PROT	CARB	SUGAR	FIBER	CALCI	SOD	POTAS	FOLIC	VIT C
JOY OF COOKING (CONT.)														
Best Loved Macaroni & Cheese	1 cup (5.4 oz)	280	18	6	25	10	36	4	1	—	520	—	—	—
Cheese Ravioli Pomodoro	1 cup (7.7 oz)	250	7	4	30	13	34	5	3	—	710	—	—	—
Creamy Fettuccine Carbonara	1 cup (7.5 oz)	330	16	9	100	15	31	3	3	—	620	—	—	—
KASHI														
Chicken Pasta Pomodoro	1 pkg (10 oz)	280	6	2	25	19	38	5	6	100	470	510	—	18
LEAN CUISINE														
Cafe Cuisine Three Cheese Stuffed Rigatoni	1 pkg (9 oz)	230	6	4	20	13	32	6	4	200	370	420	—	9
Dinnertime Selects Chicken Fettuccini	1 pkg (12 oz)	330	6	3	40	26	42	3	4	150	770	430	—	18
Market Creations Tortelloni Mushroom	1 pkg (10 oz)	280	7	3	30	15	43	7	5	200	690	580	—	9
Simple Favorites Alfredo Pasta w/ Chicken & Broccoli	1 pkg (10 oz)	300	6	3	30	16	45	5	3	150	660	370	—	12
Simple Favorites Angel Hair Pomodoro	1 pkg (10 oz)	250	5	2	5	8	42	10	4	150	620	470	—	4
Simple Favorites Cheese Ravioli	1 pkg (8.5 oz)	220	5	3	35	11	33	8	3	200	620	530	—	9
Simple Favorites Chicken Fettuccini	1 pkg (9.25 oz)	270	6	3	40	22	32	6	0	200	690	520	—	0
Simple Favorites Fettuccini Alfredo	1 pkg (9.25 oz)	330	7	3	15	12	54	6	3	150	600	270	—	0
Simple Favorites Lasagna Chicken Florentine	1 pkg (10 oz)	280	6	2	30	20	36	6	3	200	650	540	—	2
Simple Favorites Lasagna Classic Five Cheese	1 pkg (11.5 oz)	350	7	3	20	20	51	11	4	300	620	650	—	6
Simple Favorites Lasagna w/ Meat Sauce	1 pkg (10.5 oz)	320	8	4	30	17	45	8	4	150	630	710	—	6
Simple Favorites Macaroni & Cheese	1 pkg (10 oz)	290	7	4	20	15	41	7	1	300	630	560	—	0

FOOD	PORTION	CALS	FAT	SAT FAT	CHOL	PROT	CARB	SUGAR	FIBER	CALCI	SOD	POTAS	FOLIC	VIT C
LEAN CUISINE (CONT.)														
Simple Favorites Spaghetti w/ Meat Sauce	1 pkg (11.5 oz)	300	4	1	15	15	49	9	4	80	690	480	—	9
Simple Favorites Spaghetti w/ Meatballs	1 pkg (9.5 oz)	270	6	2	25	16	38	6	3	40	580	510	—	6
Spa Cuisine Ravioli Butternut Squash	1 pkg (9.9 oz)	260	7	2	20	11	40	11	5	150	550	420	—	6
MARIE CALLENDER'S														
Fettucine Chicken & Broccoli	1 meal	630	37	15	90	30	43	5	6	200	900	—	—	18
Meat Lasagna	1 cup	240	9	5	45	14	24	9	2	150	950	—	—	0
MEALS TO LIVE														
Turkey Meatballs w/ Marinara Sauce & Whole Wheat Spaghetti	1 pkg (11 oz)	300	5	2	40	21	44	7	9	—	480	—	—	18
MILTON'S														
Lasagna Vegetable w/ Multi-Grain Pasta	1 cup (8 oz)	340	16	9	60	17	30	7	5	250	950	—	—	9
MOM MADE														
Cheesy Mac	1 pkg (7 oz)	200	3	2	10	10	36	4	4	60	340	—	—	12
Spaghetti w/ Turkey Meatballs & Sauce	1 pkg (7 oz)	180	4	1	35	10	26	3	3	40	320	—	—	6
MON CUISINE														
Vegetarian Spaghetti & Meatballs	1 pkg (10 oz)	360	4	0	0	29	54	8	9	—	440	—	—	—
MOOSEWOOD														
Organic Vegetarian Broccoli & Pasta Parmesan	1 pkg (10 oz)	380	13	6	30	14	52	7	4	250	380	—	—	27
Organic Vegetarian Farfalle & Spinach Pesto Sauce	1 pkg (10 oz)	370	11	5	20	14	56	6	4	150	370	—	—	9
Organic Vegetarian Spicy Penne Puttanesca	1 pkg (10 oz)	300	10	2	0	8	45	5	2	60	300	—	—	24
NEW YORK RAVIOLI														
Jolie Kid Shapes Ravioli Cheese	1 cup	330	9	5	35	15	47	5	4	250	270	—	—	0

FOOD	PORTION	CALS	FAT	SAT FAT	CHOL	PROT	CARB	SUGAR	FIBER	CALCI	SOD	POTAS	FOLIC	VIT C
NEW YORK RAVIOLI (CONT.)														
Jolie Kid Shapes Ravioli Cheese & Broccoli	1 cup	340	8	4	105	15	53	2	2	80	210	—	—	1
Ravioli Four Cheese	1 cup	360	6	4	80	17	58	2	2	100	250	—	—	15
Ravioli Tomato Basil & Mozzarella	1 cup	340	5	3	55	12	64	3	2	60	210	—	—	9
ORGANIC BISTRO														
Pasta Puttanesca	1 pkg (12.15 oz)	330	6	1	0	12	57	6	9	80	370	700	—	36
ORGANIC CLASSICS														
Cajun Chicken Tetrazzine w/ Penne Pasta	1 pkg (10 oz)	370	10	5	55	25	43	4	3	150	490	—	—	27
Chicken Cacciatore w/ Penne Pasta	1 pkg (10 oz)	270	4	1	40	20	37	5	3	40	390	—	—	30
Macaroni & Meat Sauce	1 pkg (10 oz)	340	9	3	20	16	49	9	3	40	580	—	—	6
PLUM ORGANICS														
Bowtie Pasta	1 pkg (6.9 oz)	230	6	3	15	7	37	2	3	40	15	—	—	15
Cheese Filled Spinach Tortellini	1 pkg (6.9 oz)	190	2	1	10	8	37	6	3	40	270	—	—	15
PUTNEY PASTA														
Ravioli Butternut Squash & Vermont Maple Syrup	1 cup	200	4	—	30	8	35	—	1	—	270	—	—	—
Ravioli Portabello & Grilled Onion	7 (5.2 oz)	240	5	—	40	11	39	—	3	—	260	—	—	—
Ravioli Whole Wheat Spinach & Cheese	9 (5 oz)	300	9	—	55	13	42	—	2	—	340	—	—	—
Skillet Meal Chicken Piccata	1 serv (9 oz)	300	11	—	30	14	35	—	2	—	350	—	—	—
Skillet Meal Shrimp Pesto	1 serv (9 oz)	540	38	—	100	18	32	—	3	—	410	—	—	—
Tortellini Spinach Mozzarella & Walnuts	1 cup	360	8	—	60	20	51	—	2	—	410	—	—	—
Tortellini Tri-Color Three Cheese	1 cup	340	8	—	55	16	51	—	1	—	500	—	—	—
SEEDS OF CHANGE														
Chicken Fettuccine Alfredo	1 pkg (10 oz)	340	10	5	50	23	40	5	3	200	670	—	—	15

FOOD	PORTION	CALS	FAT	SAT FAT	CHOL	PROT	CARB	SUGAR	FIBER	CALCI	SOD	POTAS	FOLIC	VIT C
SEEDS OF CHANGE (CONT.)														
Lasagna Vegetable	1 pkg (11 oz)	310	9	4	20	16	41	9	5	400	1020	—	—	15
Lasagna Creamy Spinach	1 pkg (11 oz)	370	16	11	35	19	36	4	7	300	750	—	—	0
Penne Marinara	1 pkg (11 oz)	290	7	3	10	13	44	11	5	250	680	—	—	12
STOUFFER'S														
Cheesy Spaghetti Bake	1 pkg (12 oz)	460	24	9	120	21	39	6	4	250	950	—	—	0
Chicken Parmigiana	1 pkg (13.13 oz)	460	18	4	35	18	56	9	4	150	1060	—	—	9
Homestyle Chicken & Noodles	1 pkg (12 oz)	340	12	3	65	25	33	10	3	150	950	—	—	4
Italian Sausage Stuffed Rigatoni	1 pkg (9.13 oz)	380	14	8	60	18	46	8	2	300	880	—	—	1
Lasagna Vegetable	1 pkg (10.5 oz)	390	18	7	25	17	40	9	4	350	730	—	—	1
Lasagna Bake w/ Meat Sauce	1 pkg (11.5 oz)	380	13	6	40	18	47	10	5	200	1080	—	—	2
Macaroni & Beef	1 pkg (11.5 oz)	330	11	5	40	19	38	12	4	100	920	—	—	6
Macaroni & Cheese	1 cup (6 oz)	350	17	7	25	15	34	2	2	300	920	—	—	0
Manicotti Cheese	1 pkg (9 oz)	360	14	6	70	18	41	8	2	250	920		—	6
Shrimp Scampi	1 pkg (14 oz)	410	11	5	80	21	57	5	6	80	990	—	—	4
Tuna Noodle Casserole	1 pkg (10 oz)	350	15	5	40	18	35	8	2	150	930	—	—	0
Turkey Tettrazini	1 pkg (10 oz)	380	20	8	60	19	32	6	1	100	970	—	—	0
TABATCHNICK														
Macaroni & Cheese	1 serv (7.5 oz)	250	8	4	20	9	34	4	tr	150	770	100	—	0
TASTE ABOVE														
Meatless Thai Peanut Coconut Sauce w/ Veggie Chicken & Vermicelli	1 pkg (10 oz)	320	19	2	0	26	22	3	8	150	300	—	—	24
Meatless Tuscan Marinara Sauce w/ Veggie Chicken & Penne Pasta	1 pkg (10 oz)	320	19	2	0	26	22	3	8	150	300	—	—	24
WEIGHT WATCHERS														
Chicken & Broccoli Alfredo	1 pkg (11.8 oz)	300	4	2	50	28	39	3	4	200	660	—	—	36
Smart Ones Sesame Chicken	1 pkg (11.8 oz)	360	7	1	30	25	49	10	6	40	490	—	—	12

FOOD	PORTION	CALS	FAT	SAT FAT	CHOL	PROT	CARB	SUGAR	FIBER	CALCI	SOD	POTAS	FOLIC	VIT C
WEIGHT WATCHERS (CONT.)														
Smart Ones Ziti w/ Meatballs & Cheese	1 pkg (11.7 oz)	390	9	4	50	25	52	8	6	300	490	—	—	9
YVES														
Meatless Lasagna	1 pkg (10.5 oz)	300	3	1	0	17	51	9	4	150	650	330	—	4
MIX														
ANNIE'S HOMEGROWN														
Gluten Free Rice Pasta & Cheddar as prep	1 cup	280	4	3	10	6	54	4	1	150	408	—	—	0
Mac & Cheese Lower Sodium as prep	1 cup	280	4	3	10	7	47	5	2	150	430	—	40	0
Organic 5-Grain Elbows & White Cheddar as prep	1 cup	270	4	2	10	7	48	5	3	150	570	—	—	0
Organic Classic Mac & Cheese as prep	1 cup	280	4	2	10	7	48	5	2	150	530	—	40	0
Organic Peace Pasta & Parmesan as prep	1 cup	270	4	2	10	11	47	4	2	150	610	—	—	0
Organic Shells & Real Aged Wisconsin Cheddar as prep	1 cup	270	4	3	10	7	47	5	2	150	570	—	40	0
Organic Skillet Meals Beef Stroganoff as prep	1 cup	360	18	8	60	7	33	3	1	150	690	—	—	2
Organic Skillet Meals Cheesy Lasagna as prep	1 cup	440	18	9	81	6	32	6	1	60	750	—	—	4
Organic Skillet Meals Tuna Spirals as prep	1 cup	320	8	5	36	8	39	4	2	150	620	—	—	1
Shells & White Cheddar as prep	1 cup	270	5	2	10	7	47	5	2	150	570	—	40	0
BACK TO NATURE														
Crazy Bugs Macaroni & Cheese as prep	1 cup	370	10	6	24	12	60	8	2	150	864	—	—	0
Harvest Wheat Elbows & Cheddar as prep	½ pkg	380	12	7	30	12	60	10	2	200	768	—	—	0
Organic Shells & Cheese as prep	½ pkg	380	12	7	30	12	60	10	2	200	750	—	—	0

FOOD	PORTION	CALS	FAT	SAT FAT	CHOL	PROT	CARB	SUGAR	FIBER	CALCI	SOD	POTAS	FOLIC	VIT C
CARAPELLI														
Penne Alfredo as prep	1 cup	240	1	1	5	9	47	6	4	60	960	—	—	0
Spirals Creamy Tomato as prep	1 cup	240	1	0	0	9	49	8	4	40	900	—	—	1
DEBOLES														
Organic Macaroni & Cheese Whole Wheat as prep	1 cup	410	14	8	42	11	60	6	9	200	384	245	—	0
Pasta & Cheese as prep	1 cup	420	15	9	51	10	60	5	6	150	384	220	—	0
Rice Shells & Cheddar as prep	½ cup	260	8	5	24	3	57	0	1	150	216	68	—	0
HAMBURGER HELPER														
Cheesy Jambalaya as prep	1 cup	330	13	5	60	4	30	2	1	100	840	455	60	—
KNORR														
Pasta & Sauce Jalapeno Jack as prep	1 cup	230	3	1	3	8	45	4	2	20	504	0	120	2
Pasta Sides w/ Whole Grains Alfredo as prep	⅔ cup	300	11	5	15	10	42	2	4	150	864	0	120	0
KRAFT														
Macaroni & Cheese White Cheddar as prep	⅓ pkg	380	15	4	10	10	48	7	0	100	744	—	—	0
LA BELLA VITA														
Chicken & Lemon Borsellini as prep	1 cup	270	6	3	70	14	39	1	2	150	430	—	—	1
NEAR EAST														
Basil & Herb as prep	1 cup	240	5	1	0	8	42	1	3	20	430	—	—	9
Spicy Tomato as prep	1 cup	230	5	1	0	7	38	2	3	20	600	—	—	12
PASTA RONI														
Angel Hair w/ Herbs as prep	1 cup	310	13	4	5	9	41	6	2	100	820	—	60	0
Chicken as prep	1 cup	300	12	4	5	9	39	4	2	60	1060	—	60	0
Chicken Quesadilla as prep	1 cup	310	13	3	5	10	40	6	2	80	860	—	80	0
Fettuccine Alfredo as prep	1 cup	450	25	7	5	11	47	6	2	100	1140	—	80	0
NATURE'S WAY														
Mushrooms In Cream Sauce as prep	1 cup	280	10	3	5	9	39	8	2	100	710	—	—	0

FOOD	PORTION	CALS	FAT	SAT FAT	CHOL	PROT	CARB	SUGAR	FIBER	CALCI	SOD	POTAS	FOLIC	VIT C
PASTA RONI (CONT.)														
Sour Cream & Chives as prep	1 cup	310	15	5	5	8	38	4	2	100	880	—	60	1
Stroganoff as prep	1 cup	350	14	5	10	12	47	7	2	150	970	—	80	0
ROAD'S END ORGANICS														
Mac & Cheese Dairy Free Gluten Free as prep	1 cup	310	1	0	0	8	63	0	5	20	310	—	60	—
Shells & Cheese as prep	1 cup	330	1	0	0	14	66	5	7	—	408	—	60	—
SIMPLY SHARI'S														
Mac & Cheese Gluten Free as prep	¼ pkg (4 oz)	280	6	3	15	18	17	1	2	180	330	0	—	0
THAI KITCHEN														
Stir-Fry Rice Noodles Thai Peanut as prep	½ pkg	310	6	1	0	9	54	13	1	20	330	—	—	0
REFRIGERATED														
COUNTRY CROCK														
Elbow Macaroni & Cheese	1 cup (8 oz)	370	17	8	40	14	40	6	1	250	940	—	—	1
Four Cheese Pasta	1 cup (8 oz)	380	17	8	40	15	41	7	2	210	1060	—	—	0
NOOODLE														
Mamma Mia! Marinara	1 pkg (10 oz)	70	3	0	0	2	13	3	4	40	480	—	—	12
Say Cheese Pleeeze!	1 pkg (10 oz)	100	10	5	25	4	6	2	4	100	190	—	—	0
Terri-Yaki Chicken	1 pkg (10 oz)	80	2	0	25	11	10	5	4	20	650	—	—	2
Ultra-Lite Primavera	1 pkg (10 oz)	30	0	0	0	2	8	3	4	20	360	—	—	24
ROZZANO														
Organic Ravioli Grilled Vegetable	1 cup (3.5 oz)	200	6	3	35	10	26	2	2	150	420	—	—	12
SIMPLY SENSIBLE														
Lasagna w/ Meat Sauce	½ pkg (8 oz)	200	5	2	20	13	28	8	2	200	440	—	—	21
Mediterranean Style Chicken	1½ cups (7.2 oz)	250	6	1	20	14	36	3	2	20	400	—	—	36
SHELF-STABLE														
ALLERGAROO														
Gluten Free Spaghetti	1 pkg (8 oz)	220	3	0	0	3	49	9	3	40	510	—	—	9
Gluten Free Spyglass Noodles	1 pkg (8 oz)	230	3	0	0	4	49	9	3	40	510	—	—	9

FOOD	PORTION	CALS	FAT	SAT FAT	CHOL	PROT	CARB	SUGAR	FIBER	CALCI	SOD	POTAS	FOLIC	VIT C
BETTY CROCKER														
Bowl Appetit! Cheddar Broccoli Pasta	1 bowl (2.8 oz)	330	11	4	10	11	49	7	2	100	1000	385	100	—
Bowl Appetit! Garlic Parmesan Pasta	1 bowl (2.8 oz)	320	9	3	10	11	50	5	1	100	1010	230	100	—
HEALTHY CHOICE														
Balsamic Vegetable Medley	1 pkg (6.9 oz)	290	3	1	0	10	56	6	7	100	510	400	—	0
Fresh Mixers Rotini & Zesty Marinara Sauce	1 pkg (9.9 oz)	300	4	1	0	10	56	11	7	40	600	930	—	0
Fresh Mixers Ziti & Meat Sauce	1 pkg (6.9 oz)	340	6	2	20	15	56	10	8	40	600	990	—	0
Pasta Margherita	1 pkg (6.9 oz)	270	4	1	0	8	52	7	4	80	600	430	—	0
HORMEL														
Compleats Microwave Meals Chicken & Noodles	1 pkg (9.9 oz)	240	8	4	60	15	27	3	2	60	990	—	—	1
TASTYBITE														
Peanut Sauce w/ Noodles	1 pkg (10 oz)	530	19	6	0	17	104	40	12	30	595	—	—	0
TAKE-OUT														
lasagna meatless	1 piece (9 oz)	356	11	7	38	19	46	8	3	335	896	425	79	10
lasagna w/ meat	1 piece (8 oz)	362	14	7	56	22	37	6	3	278	838	427	67	8
lasagna w/ vegetables	1 serv (9 oz)	315	10	6	33	17	41	8	4	302	776	512	95	20
macaroni & cheese w/ ham	1 cup	542	33	13	61	21	41	7	3	311	1375	343	66	0
manicotti cheese w/ marinara sauce	1 (5 oz)	229	10	6	83	13	22	3	1	214	615	233	40	3
manicotti cheese w/ meat sauce	1 (5 oz)	239	11	6	86	14	20	1	3	203	612	246	39	3
pasta w/ pesto sauce	1 cup	370	25	4	10	10	27	1	2	179	178	189	78	2
ravioli cheese & spinach w/ cream sauce	1 cup	362	17	6	160	15	38	5	2	238	962	356	115	3
ravioli cheese w/ tomato sauce	1 cup	335	14	6	158	14	38	4	2	162	1570	375	72	5
ravioli meat w/ marinara sauce	1 cup	372	16	5	168	22	36	5	3	72	1488	535	70	7
rigatoni w/ sausage sauce	¾ cup	260	12	4	59	10	28	—	3	44	106	286	8	16

FOOD	PORTION	CALS	FAT	SAT FAT	CHOL	PROT	CARB	SUGAR	FIBER	CALCI	SOD	POTAS	FOLIC	VIT C
spaghetti w/ red clam sauce	1 cup	285	8	1	17	13	41	3	3	64	280	379	109	14
spaghetti w/ sauce & meatballs	2 cups	670	26	8	114	34	80	15	12	188	1820	1052	60	21
spaghetti w/ white clam sauce	1 cup	456	20	3	50	25	43	1	3	82	461	513	37	16
tortellini cheese w/ tomato sauce	1 cup	332	14	6	158	14	38	4	2	150	1560	375	72	5
tortellini meat w/ marinara sauce	1 cup	281	10	3	90	14	33	3	2	92	1294	258	82	3
tortellini spinach w/ marinara sauce	1 cup	238	8	2	72	10	32	3	2	110	1190	278	104	5

PASTA SALAD

MIX

SUDDENLY SALAD

FOOD	PORTION	CALS	FAT	SAT FAT	CHOL	PROT	CARB	SUGAR	FIBER	CALCI	SOD	POTAS	FOLIC	VIT C
Caesar as prep	1 cup (1.8 oz)	310	14	2	0	6	38	3	1	—	640	—	80	—
Classic as prep	¾ cup	250	8	1	0	6	39	4	1	—	840	—	80	—
Creamy Italian as prep	¾ cup	350	20	2	15	7	36	4	2	20	410	—	80	—
Creamy Parmesan as prep	¾ cup	370	22	3	18	5	33	2	1	20	300	—	80	—

TAKE-OUT

FOOD	PORTION	CALS	FAT	SAT FAT	CHOL	PROT	CARB	SUGAR	FIBER	CALCI	SOD	POTAS	FOLIC	VIT C
pasta salad w crab vegetables mayonnaise	1 cup	317	16	2	32	10	33	2	2	46	866	179	92	2
pasta salad w/ shrimp vegetables & mayonnaise	1 cup (6.2 oz)	335	17	3	65	10	35	6	2	51	982	127	80	2
tortellini salad cheese filled w/ vinaigrette dressing	1 cup	333	18	7	144	12	30	1	1	137	1070	122	61	tr

PATE

FOOD	PORTION	CALS	FAT	SAT FAT	CHOL	PROT	CARB	SUGAR	FIBER	CALCI	SOD	POTAS	FOLIC	VIT C
chicken liver canned	1 tbsp	26	2	1	51	2	1	0	0	1	50	12	42	1
duck pate	1 oz	96	8	—	—	4	1	tr	—	—	—	—	—	—
fish pate	1 oz	76	7	—	—	3	1	—	—	52	286	45	—	—
liver w/ truffle	1 serv (2 oz)	183	16	6	59	6	4	—	—	39	452	77	34	1
mushroom pate	1 can (2.25 oz)	130	11	2	5	2	7	1	1	20	400	—	—	1
pate de foie gras smoked canned	1 tbsp	60	6	2	20	1	1	—	0	9	91	18	8	tr
pork pate	1 oz	107	10	4	51	3	1	1	0	11	189	27	29	tr
pork pate en croute	1 oz	91	7	3	32	3	3	tr	tr	—	214	—	—	—
rabbit pate	1 oz	66	5	3	21	5	1	—	—	3	97	89	—	tr
shrimp pate	1 can (2.25 oz)	140	10	2	25	6	7	1	0	20	450	—	—	1

FOOD	PORTION	CALS	FAT	SAT FAT	CHOL	PROT	CARB	SUGAR	FIBER	CALCI	SOD	POTAS	FOLIC	VIT C
PATCHWORK														
All Flavors	2 oz	270	27	9	90	5	5	0	0	40	410	—	—	0

PEACH

FOOD	PORTION	CALS	FAT	SAT FAT	CHOL	PROT	CARB	SUGAR	FIBER	CALCI	SOD	POTAS	FOLIC	VIT C
CANNED														
halves in heavy syrup	½ cup (2.6 oz)	85	tr	tr	0	1	22	20	2	3	7	104	3	3
halves in light syrup	1 half (3.4 oz)	53	tr	tr	0	tr	14	13	1	3	5	95	3	2
halves juice pack	1 half (3.4 oz)	43	tr	tr	0	1	11	10	1	6	4	125	3	4
peach sauce	½ cup	120	0	0	0	tr	32	31	1	0	0	—	—	6
pickled	½ cup (4.2 oz)	143	tr	tr	0	1	35	34	1	7	1	173	4	5
pickled whole	1 (3.1 oz)	104	tr	tr	0	1	26	25	1	5	1	126	3	4
slices juice pack	½ cup (4.4 oz)	55	tr	tr	0	1	14	13	2	7	5	159	4	5
slices light syrup	½ cup (4.4 oz)	68	tr	tr	0	1	18	17	2	4	6	122	4	3
slices water pack	½ cup (4.3 oz)	29	tr	tr	0	1	7	6	2	2	4	121	4	4
spiced in heavy syrup	½ cup (4.2 oz)	91	tr	tr	0	1	24	23	2	7	5	103	4	6
DEL MONTE														
Carb Clever Sliced	½ cup (4.2 oz)	30	0	0	0	1	7	6	1	0	10	—	—	54
Chunks Raspberry Flavor	½ cup (4.4 oz)	80	0	0	0	tr	20	19	tr	0	10	—	—	4
Clingstone Sliced In Light Syrup	½ cup (4.4 oz)	70	0	0	0	0	17	16	1	0	10	—	—	1
Fruit Bowls	½ cup (4.4 oz)	70	0	0	0	0	17	15	2	—	20	<100	—	60
Fruit Cup Diced In Water No Sugar Added	1 pkg (3.75 oz)	25	0	0	0	0	6	5	—	—	10	120	—	60
Fruit Naturals Chunks No Sugar Added	½ cup (4.2 oz)	40	0	0	0	1	12	7	2	0	0	—	—	60
Orchard Select Cinnamon Spiced	½ cup (4.4 oz)	80	0	0	0	tr	20	19	tr	0	10	120	—	60
Orchard Select Sliced Cling No Sugar Added	½ cup (4.2 oz)	40	0	0	0	1	11	8	2	0	10	120	—	60
Peaches In Peach Gel	1 pkg (4.5 oz)	90	0	0	0	0	22	21	0	20	40	—	—	18
POLAR														
White	½ cup	70	0	0	0	1	17	16	1	0	10	—	—	1
S&W														
Slices Natural Style	½ cup (4.4 oz)	80	0	0	0	1	19	18	1	0	20	—	—	1
DRIED														
halves	1 (0.5 oz)	31	tr	tr	0	tr	8	5	1	4	1	129	0	1
halves	½ cup (2.8 oz)	191	1	tr	0	3	49	33	7	22	6	797	0	4

FOOD	PORTION	CALS	FAT	SAT FAT	CHOL	PROT	CARB	SUGAR	FIBER	CALCI	SOD	POTAS	FOLIC	VIT C
halves cooked w/o sugar	½ cup (4.5 oz)	99	tr	tr	0	2	25	22	4	12	3	413	0	5
MRS. MAY'S														
Fruit Chips	1 pkg	35	0	0	0	0	8	7	1	0	0	—	—	8
STONERIDGE ORCHARDS														
Whole	⅓ cup (1.4 oz)	140	0	0	0	0	31	29	1	60	75	—	—	222
FRESH														
peach	1 med (5.3 oz)	58	tr	tr	0	1	14	13	2	9	0	285	6	10
peach	1 lg (6.1 oz)	68	tr	tr	0	2	17	15	3	10	0	332	7	12
sliced	½ cup (2.7 oz)	30	tr	tr	0	1	8	6	1	5	0	146	3	5
DOLE														
Peach	1 lg (5.2 oz)	60	0	0	0	1	14	12	2	0	0	—	—	9
FROZEN														
C&W														
Ultimate Sliced	¾ cup	50	0	0	0	1	13	9	2	0	0	—	—	168
DOLE														
Sliced	¾ cup (4.9 oz)	50	0	0	0	1	13	10	1	0	0	—	—	138
REFRIGERATED														
DOLE														
Fruit Crisp Peach	1 pkg (4 oz)	150	4	0	0	2	28	20	2	0	25	90	—	24
Parfait Peaches & Creme	1 pkg (4.3 oz)	120	2	2	0	1	23	21	1	0	10	—	—	27
PEACH JUICE														
nectar	1 cup (8.7 oz)	134	tr	tr	0	1	35	33	2	12	17	100	2	13
AFTER THE FALL														
Georgia Peach	8 oz	130	0	0	0	1	31	28	—	150	15	250	—	60
CERES														
100% Juice	8 oz	120	0	0	0	0	30	28	0	0	5	240	—	60
FROOSE														
Playful Peach	1 box (4.2 oz)	80	0	0	0	1	19	7	3	0	10	105	—	15
OKF														
Sparkling Fresh Peach	1 bottle (8.3 oz)	50	0	0	0	0	12	9	3	0	36	—	—	23
SANTA CRUZ														
Organic Nectar	8 oz	120	0	0	0	0	31	29	0	—	10	40	—	—
PEANUT BUTTER														
chunky	2 tbsp (1.1 oz)	188	16	3	0	8	7	3	3	14	156	238	29	0
no sugar added	2 tbsp (1.1 oz)	208	18	3	0	8	5	1	3	23	143	262	46	0
reduced sodium	2 tbsp (1.1 oz)	202	16	2	0	8	7	3	2	13	65	239	29	0
smooth	2 tbsp (1.1 oz)	188	16	3	0	8	7	3	2	14	147	208	24	0
ARROWHEAD MILLS														
Organic Creamy	2 tbsp	190	17	3	0	8	6	1	2	20	0	—	—	0
Organic Honey Sweetened Creamy	2 tbsp	190	16	3	0	7	7	2	2	20	100	—	—	0

FOOD	PORTION	CALS	FAT	SAT FAT	CHOL	PROT	CARB	SUGAR	FIBER	CALCI	SOD	POTAS	FOLIC	VIT C
ARROWHEAD MILLS (CONT.)														
Organic Natural Crunchy	2 tbsp	190	17	3	0	8	6	1	2	20	0	—	—	0
BETTER'N PEANUT BUTTER														
Creamy	2 tbsp (1.1 oz)	100	2	—	—	4	13	2	2	40	190	—	—	5
Low Sodium	2 tbsp (1.1 oz)	100	2	—	—	4	13	2	2	40	95	—	—	5
CHET'S														
Chocolate	2 tbsp	180	14	2	0	7	10	4	2	—	135	—	—	—
Roasted Nut	2 tbsp	180	14	3	0	7	9	4	2	—	130	—	—	—
EARTH BALANCE														
Creamy or Chunky	1 tbsp	190	17	3	0	7	7	2	3	0	110	—	—	0
JAKE & AMOS														
Schmier	1 tbsp (0.6 oz)	60	3	1	0	2	8	8	0	0	35	—	—	0
JIF														
Simply	2 tbsp (1.1 oz)	190	16	3	0	8	6	2	2	—	65	—	—	—
JUSTIN'S														
Organic Cinnamon	2 tbsp (1.1 oz)	180	15	2	0	7	8	2	3	40	65	—	—	0
Organic Classic	2 tbsp (1.1 oz)	150	17	3	0	7	7	1	2	20	0	—	—	0
KETTLE														
Organic Unsalted	2 tbsp	170	14	3	0	7	5	2	2	20	0	—	—	0
MAPLE GROVE FARMS														
Crunchy No Salt Added	2 tbsp (1.1 oz)	190	15	2	—	8	6	2	2	0	15	—	—	0
NATURALLY MORE														
Natural	2 tbsp	169	11	2	0	10	8	2	4	0	130	—	232	0
Organic	2 tbsp	170	11	2	0	10	8	2	4	0	65	—	232	0
PB2														
Powdered Chocolate	2 tbsp	52	13	tr	tr	4	6	4	1	112	60	—	—	tr
Powdered Chocolate Chip	2 tbsp	53	2	tr	0	6	3	2	tr	10	78	—	—	0
PEANUT BETTER														
Hickory Smoked	2 tbsp	190	16	3	0	9	5	1	3	0	135	—	—	0
Onion Parsley	2 tbsp	180	15	3	0	8	6	1	3	20	115	—	—	0
Peanut Praline	2 tbsp	180	15	3	0	8	8	4	3	0	0	—	—	0
Rosemary Garlic	2 tbsp	180	15	3	0	8	7	2	3	20	85	—	—	0
Spicy Southwestern	2 tbsp	190	17	3	0	8	5	1	3	0	100	—	—	0
Sweet Molasses	2 tbsp	180	14	2	0	8	8	4	2	40	0	—	—	0
Thai Ginger & Red Pepper	2 tbsp	180	15	3	0	8	7	2	3	0	110	—	—	0
PEANUT BUTTER & CO.														
Cinnamon Raisin Swirl	2 tbsp (1.1 oz)	160	11	2	0	6	13	9	2	20	35	—	—	0

FOOD	PORTION	CALS	FAT	SAT FAT	CHOL	PROT	CARB	SUGAR	FIBER	CALCI	SOD	POTAS	FOLIC	VIT C
PEANUT BUTTER & CO. (CONT.)														
Dark Chocolate Dreams	2 tbsp (1.1 oz)	170	13	3	0	6	12	7	2	20	35	—	—	0
Old Fashioned Crunchy	2 tbsp (1.1 oz)	190	16	2	0	8	6	1	2	20	40	—	—	0
The Bee's Knees	2 tbsp (1.1 oz)	180	14	3	0	6	12	8	1	20	60	—	—	0
REESE'S														
Creamy	2 tbsp (1.1 oz)	190	16	3	—	8	7	3	3	20	140	—	—	0
Peanut Butter Chips	1 tbsp (0.5 oz)	80	5	4	—	2	8	6	tr	0	35	—	—	0
REVOLUTION FOODS														
Organic Creamy & Crunchy	1 tbsp (1.1 oz)	200	16	3	0	10	5	2	2	20	120	—	—	0
SANTA CRUZ														
Organic Creamy	2 tbsp (1.1 oz)	210	16	3	0	8	6	1	2	—	50	—	—	0
SKIPPY														
Creamy	2 tbsp (1.3 oz)	190	16	3	0	7	7	3	2	0	150	—	—	0
Extra Chunky Super Chunk	2 tbsp (1.1. oz)	190	16	3	0	7	7	3	2	0	120	—	—	0
Reduced Fat Creamy	2 tbsp (1.3 oz)	180	12	2	0	7	15	4	2	0	170	—	32	0
Roasted Honey Nut Creamy	2 tbsp (1.1 oz)	190	16	3	0	7	7	3	2	0	125	—	—	0
SMART BALANCE														
Omega Creamy & Chunky	2 tbsp (1.1 oz)	200	17	3	0	7	6	1	2	0	110	190	40	0
SMUCKER'S														
Chunky	2 tbsp (1.1 oz)	200	16	3	0	7	6	1	2	0	90	—	—	0
Creamy No Salt Addded	2 tbsp (1.1 oz)	210	16	3	0	7	6	1	2	0	0	—	—	0
Creamy Reduced Fat	2 tbsp (1.2 oz)	190	12	2	0	8	12	2	2	0	115	—	24	0
Creamy Honey	2 tbsp (1.2 oz)	200	16	3	0	7	9	4	2	0	30	—	—	0
Goober Grape	3 tbsp (1.9 oz)	240	13	3	0	7	24	21	2	20	140	—	—	0
Goober Peanut Butter & Chocolate Spread	3 tbsp (2 oz)	230	11	2	0	6	27	23	2	40	135	—	—	0
WONDER														
Peanut Spread	2 tbsp	100	3	0	0	4	13	2	0	40	190	—	—	5
Peanut Spread Low Sodium	2 tbsp	100	3	0	0	4	13	2	0	40	95	—	—	5

PEANUT BUTTER SUBSTITUTES

FOOD	PORTION	CALS	FAT	SAT FAT	CHOL	PROT	CARB	SUGAR	FIBER	CALCI	SOD	POTAS	FOLIC	VIT C
NONUTS														
Golden Peabutter	1 tbsp	93	7	1	0	2	6	—	1	—	1	91	—	—

PEANUTS

FOOD	PORTION	CALS	FAT	SAT FAT	CHOL	PROT	CARB	SUGAR	FIBER	CALCI	SOD	POTAS	FOLIC	VIT C
chocolate coated	1	21	1	1	0	1	2	2	tr	4	2	20	0	0

FOOD	PORTION	CALS	FAT	SAT FAT	CHOL	PROT	CARB	SUGAR	FIBER	CALCI	SOD	POTAS	FOLIC	VIT C
chocolate coated	¼ cup	193	12	5	3	5	18	14	2	39	15	187	3	0
cooked w/ salt	½ cup	286	20	3	0	12	19	2	8	50	676	162	68	0
dry roasted w/ salt	28 (1 oz)	164	14	2	0	7	6	2	1	15	230	187	41	0
dry roasted w/o salt	28 (1 oz)	164	14	2	0	7	6	1	2	15	2	184	41	0
dry roasted w/o salt	¼ cup	214	18	3	0	9	8	2	3	20	2	240	53	0
honey roasted	¼ cup	191	16	3	0	8	8	5	3	18	95	218	36	tr
sugar coated	¼ cup	203	13	2	0	6	18	16	2	30	61	158	29	0
yogurt coated	¼ cup	230	16	7	0	6	18	15	2	65	24	203	48	tr
FISHER														
Butter Toffee	¼ cup (1 oz)	140	6	1	0	3	18	15	1	20	110	—	—	0
Honey Roasted	¼ cup (1 oz)	170	13	2	0	5	9	5	2	20	125	—	—	0
FRITO LAY														
Salted In Shells	1 oz	160	14	2	0	7	6	1	2	0	170	—	—	0
LANCE														
Salted	1 pkg (1.1 oz)	200	15	3	0	9	6	0	4	0	150	—	—	0
NUTS ARE GOOD														
Buffalo	1 oz	120	6	1	0	3	16	12	2	0	180	—	—	1
Pina Colada	1 oz	130	7	1	0	3	16	14	1	0	0	—	—	0
Raspberry	1 oz	130	7	1	0	3	16	14	1	0	0	—	—	0
Vanilla Rum	1 oz	130	7	1	0	3	17	14	1	0	0	—	—	0
PLANTERS														
Bar Big Double	1 (1.6 oz)	220	13	3	0	8	21	12	3	20	170	—	—	0
Dry Roasted	1 oz	160	14	2	0	7	5	2	2	20	190	—	—	0
Dry Roasted Lightly Salted	1 oz	160	14	2	0	7	5	1	2	20	95	—	—	0
Dry Roasted Unsalted	1 oz	170	14	2	0	8	5	1	2	20	0	—	—	0
Five Alarm Chili Dry Roasted	39 (1 oz)	160	14	2	0	8	5	2	1	20	160	200	—	0
Honey & Dry Roasted	1 oz	160	13	2	0	6	7	4	2	20	110	—	—	0
Roasted In Milk Chocolate	¼ cup (1.4 oz)	210	15	5	5	5	18	15	2	40	80	—	—	0
SUNFOOD														
Organic Wild Jungle	1 oz	174	14	2	0	7	5	1	2	30	5	—	—	0
SUNRIDGE FARMS														
Chocolate Toffee	6 (1.4 oz)	200	11	5	5	3	24	22	1	40	45	—	—	0
Yogurt Clusters	4 (1.4 oz)	220	15	6	0	6	17	14	1	10	15	—	—	0
TRUE NORTH														
Clusters	6 (1 oz)	170	13	3	0	6	9	5	2	0	75	—	—	0
VIRGINIA COCKTAIL PEANUTS														
Jalapeno	⅕ can (1 oz)	170	13	2	0	7	7	tr	5	—	85	—	—	—
Sea Salt	⅕ can (1 oz)	170	13	2	0	7	7	tr	5	—	85	—	—	—

FOOD	PORTION	CALS	FAT	SAT FAT	CHOL	PROT	CARB	SUGAR	FIBER	CALCI	SOD	POTAS	FOLIC	VIT C
VIRGINIA COCKTAIL PEANUTS (CONT.)														
Toffee	⅓ can (1 oz)	210	7	1	0	4	16	14	2	—	20	—	—	—
Unsalted	⅓ can (1 oz)	170	13	2	0	7	7	tr	5	—	0	—	—	—
PEAR														
CANNED														
halves in heavy syrup	1 (1.7 oz)	36	tr	tr	0	tr	9	8	1	3	2	32	0	1
halves in heavy syrup	½ cup (3.5 oz)	74	tr	tr	0	tr	19	17	3	6	5	66	1	1
halves in light syrup	1 (2.7 oz)	43	tr	tr	0	tr	12	9	1	4	4	50	1	1
halves juice pack	½ cup (4.4 oz)	62	tr	tr	0	tr	16	12	2	11	5	119	1	2
halves juice pack	1 (2.7 oz)	38	tr	tr	0	tr	10	7	1	7	3	73	1	1
halves light syrup	½ cup (4.4 oz)	72	tr	tr	0	tr	19	15	2	6	6	83	1	1
halves water pack	1 (2.7 oz)	22	tr	tr	0	tr	6	5	1	3	2	40	1	1
DEL MONTE														
Halves In 100% Juice	½ cup (4.4 oz)	60	0	0	0	0	15	14	1	0	10	—	—	2
Halves In Heavy Syrup	½ cup (4.6 oz)	100	0	0	0	0	24	23	1	0	10	—	—	2
Halves In Light Syrup	½ cup (4.4 oz)	80	0	0	0	0	15	14	1	0	10	—	—	2
Orchard Select Sliced Bartlett	½ cup (4.4 oz)	70	0	0	0	0	17	16	1	0	10	50	—	60
DOLE														
Diced In Fruit Juice	1 pkg (4 oz)	90	0	0	0	tr	21	18	2	0	10	20	—	27
LIBERTY GOLD														
Bartlett In Heavy Syrup	½ cup (4.5 oz)	90	0	0	0	0	23	22	2	0	10	85	—	0
S&W														
Halves Light Syrup	½ cup (4.4 oz)	80	0	0	0	0	19	17	2	0	10	—	—	1
DRIED														
halves	5 (3 oz)	229	1	tr	0	2	61	54	7	30	5	466	0	6
halves	½ cup (3.2 oz)	236	1	tr	0	2	63	56	7	31	50	480	0	6
halves	1 (0.6 oz)	47	tr	tr	0	tr	13	11	1	6	1	96	0	1
halves cooked w/o sugar	½ cup (4.5 oz)	162	tr	tr	0	1	43	35	8	20	4	329	0	5
BARE FRUIT														
Organic	1 pkg (0.6 oz)	46	0	0	0	1	12	9	2	10	0	—	—	1
BROTHERS-ALL-NATURAL														
Crisps Asian Pear	1 pkg (0.35 oz)	40	0	0	0	0	9	7	1	0	0	—	—	1
CRISPY GREEN														
Crispy Asian Pears	1 pkg (0.35 oz)	40	0	0	0	0	8	7	1	0	0	—	—	1

FOOD	PORTION	CALS	FAT	SAT FAT	CHOL	PROT	CARB	SUGAR	FIBER	CALCI	SOD	POTAS	FOLIC	VIT C
CRUNCHIES														
Freeze Dried	¼ cup (6 g)	20	0	0	0	0	5	3	1	0	0	—	—	36
FRESH														
asian	1 lg (9.6 oz)	116	1	tr	0	1	30	19	10	11	0	333	22	10
asian	1 med (9.6 oz)	51	tr	tr	0	1	13	9	4	5	0	148	10	5
pear	1 sm (5.2 oz)	86	tr	tr	0	1	23	15	5	13	1	176	10	6
pear	1 lg (8.1 oz)	133	tr	tr	0	1	36	23	7	21	2	274	16	10
pear	1 med (6.2 oz)	103	tr	tr	0	1	28	17	6	16	2	212	12	8
sliced w/ skin	1 cup (4.9 oz)	81	tr	tr	0	1	22	14	4	13	1	167	10	6
CHIQUITA														
Pear	1 (6.2 oz)	103	0	0	0	1	28	17	6	20	2	404	—	7
DOLE														
Pear	1 med (5.8 oz)	100	0	0	0	tr	26	16	5	20	0	—	—	6
PEAR JUICE														
nectar canned	1 cup (8.8 oz)	150	tr	tr	0	tr	39	38	2	12	10	32	2	3
CERES														
100% Juice	8 oz	120	0	0	0	0	31	25	2	0	10	200	—	60
FROOSE														
Perfect Pear	1 box (4.2 oz)	80	0	0	0	0	18	5	3	0	15	55	—	15
SANTA CRUZ														
Organic Nectar	8 oz	120	0	0	0	0	30	25	0	40	30	135	—	2
SMART JUICE														
Organic 100% Juice	8 oz	110	0	0	0	0	31	25	2	0	10	200	—	60
PEAS														
CANNED														
green	½ cup (4.4 oz)	66	tr	tr	0	4	12	4	4	22	310	124	36	12
green low sodium	½ cup (4.4 oz)	66	tr	tr	0	4	12	4	4	22	11	124	36	12
DEL MONTE														
Sweet No Salt Added	½ cup	60	0	0	0	3	11	6	4	20	10	—	—	9
GREEN GIANT														
50% Less Sodium Young Tender Sweet	½ cup	60	0	0	0	4	11	4	3	20	200	—	—	6
Young Tender Sweet	½ cup	60	0	0	0	4	12	5	3	20	400	—	—	6
LE SUEUR														
Very Young Small	½ cup (4.2 oz)	60	0	0	0	4	12	4	3	20	380	—	—	6
S&W														
Petit Pois	½ cup (4.4 oz)	60	0	0	0	3	10	5	4	0	360	—	—	9
DRIED														
split cooked w/o salt	1 cup (6.9 oz)	231	1	tr	0	16	41	6	16	27	4	710	127	1

FOOD	PORTION	CALS	FAT	SAT FAT	CHOL	PROT	CARB	SUGAR	FIBER	CALCI	SOD	POTAS	FOLIC	VIT C
ARROWHEAD MILLS														
Organic Green Split not prep	¼ cup	160	1	0	0	12	24	1	4	20	10	300	—	1
CRUNCHIES														
Freeze Dried Organic	¼ cup (0.5 oz)	50	1	0	0	3	9	8	3	20	3	—	—	24
GOYA														
Green Split Peas not prep	¼ cup (1.6 oz)	110	0	0	0	11	27	1	11	0	25	—	—	0
HAMPEAS														
Green Split Peas as prep	½ cup	120	1	0	0	8	21	1	4	20	63	340	—	0
JACK RABBIT														
Green Split	¼ cup (1.6 oz)	110	0	0	0	11	27	1	11	0	25	—	—	0
SNAPEA CRISPS														
Baked Original	22 (1 oz)	70	8	1	0	5	14	tr	2	60	125	—	—	4
SUNRIDGE FARMS														
Wasabi Roasted	¼ cup (1 oz)	120	1	1	0	7	20	2	2	20	75	—	—	0
TREE OF LIFE														
Wasabi Peas	¼ cup (1.1 oz)	120	4	1	0	5	17	5	2	20	130	—	—	tr
FRESH														
green cooked w/o salt	½ cup (2.8 oz)	67	tr	tr	0	4	13	5	4	22	2	217	50	11
green raw	½ cup (2.5 oz)	59	tr	tr	0	4	10	4	4	18	4	177	47	29
snap peas cooked w/o salt	1 cup (5.6 oz)	67	tr	tr	0	5	11	6	5	67	6	384	46	77
snap peas raw	10 (1.2 oz)	14	tr	tr	0	1	3	1	1	15	1	68	14	20
snap peas raw	1 cup (2.2 oz)	26	tr	tr	0	2	5	3	2	27	3	126	26	38
DOLE														
Sugar Snap Peas	1 cup (3 oz)	35	0	0	0	2	6	3	2	40	0	—	—	48
MANN'S														
Snow Peas	1 serv (3 oz)	35	0	0	0	2	6	3	2	40	0	170	32	54
FROZEN														
creamed	1 cup (4.3 oz)	132	6	2	4	6	15	6	4	79	239	159	45	7
green cooked w/o salt	½ cup (2.8 oz)	62	tr	tr	0	4	11	4	4	19	58	88	47	8
BIRDS EYE														
Baby Sweet Peas	⅔ cup (3 oz)	70	0	0	0	4	12	4	4	0	0	—	—	6
Steamfresh Garlic Baby Peas & Mushrooms	¾ cup	80	2	0	0	4	12	4	3	20	340	—	—	6
C&W														
Alfredo	½ cup	110	5	3	15	6	11	5	4	40	380	—	—	9

FOOD	PORTION	CALS	FAT	SAT FAT	CHOL	PROT	CARB	SUGAR	FIBER	CALCI	SOD	POTAS	FOLIC	VIT C
C&W (CONT.)														
Early Harvest Petite No Salt Added	⅔ cup	70	0	0	0	4	12	4	4	0	0	—	—	6
Sugar Snap	⅔ cup	40	0	0	0	2	7	3	2	40	0	—	—	9
GREEN GIANT														
Early June No Sauce	⅔ cup	50	1	0	0	5	11	3	4	20	95	—	—	12
SHELF-STABLE														
TASTYBITE														
Agra Peas & Greens	½ pkg (5 oz)	138	10	2	3	4	9	2	4	50	417	—	—	2
PECANS														
candied	1 oz	190	17	3	0	tr	10	4	5	0	75	—	—	0
dry roasted	1 oz	187	18	1	0	2	6	—	—	10	0	105	12	—
dry roasted salted	1 oz	187	18	1	0	2	6	—	—	10	260	105	12	—
halves dry roasted w/ salt	20 (1 oz)	200	21	2	0	3	4	1	3	20	110	120	8	—
halves dried	1 cup	721	73	6	0	8	20	—	7	39	1	423	42	2
oil roasted	1 oz	195	20	2	0	2	5	—	—	10	0	102	—	—
oil roasted salted	1 oz	195	20	2	0	2	5	—	—	10	252	102	—	—
EMILY'S														
Roasted & Salted	¼ cup (1 oz)	210	22	2	0	3	4	1	3	20	118	—	—	—
FISHER														
Roasted & Salted	¼ cup (1 oz)	200	21	2	0	3	4	1	3	20	110	—	—	0
PLANTERS														
Halves	1 oz	200	20	2	0	3	4	1	3	20	0	—	—	0
PECTIN														
liquid	1 oz	3	0	0	0	0	1	0	1	0	0	0	0	0
powder	1 pkg (1.75 oz)	162	tr	tr	0	0	45	—	4	4	100	4	0	0
SURE JELL														
Fruit Pectin	1 pkg (1.75 oz)	0	0	0	0	0	0	0	0	0	0	0	—	0
PEPEAO														
dried	¼ cup	18	tr	—	0	tr	5	—	—	7	4	42	10	tr
raw sliced	1 cup	25	tr	—	0	tr	7	—	—	16	9	43	19	1
PEPPER														
black	1 tsp	5	tr	tr	0	tr	1	tr	1	9	1	26	0	tr
cayenne	1 tsp	6	tr	tr	0	tr	1	tr	1	3	1	36	2	1
white	1 tsp	7	tr	tr	0	tr	2	—	1	6	0	2	0	1
MCCORMICK														
Lemon Pepper w/ Garlic & Onion California Style	¼ tsp (0.6 g)	0	0	0	0	0	0	0	0	—	30	—	—	—
PEPPERMINT														
fresh chopped	2 tbsp	2	tr	tr	0	tr	tr	—	tr	8	1	18	4	1

FOOD	PORTION	CALS	FAT	SAT FAT	CHOL	PROT	CARB	SUGAR	FIBER	CALCI	SOD	POTAS	FOLIC	VIT C
PEPPERS														
CANNED														
chili green	1 cup (5.5 oz)	29	tr	tr	0	1	6	—	2	50	552	157	75	0
chili green hot chopped	½ cup	17	tr	tr	0	1	4	—	—	5	—	—	—	46
chili pepper paste	1 tbsp	6	1	—	—	tr	1	—	1	21	1445	40	—	—
chili red hot	1 (2.6 oz)	18	tr	tr	0	1	4	—	—	5	—	—	—	50
chili red hot chopped	½ cup	17	tr	tr	0	1	4	—	—	5	—	—	—	46
green halves	½ cup	13	tr	tr	0	1	3	—	—	28	958	102	—	33
jalapeno chopped	½ cup	17	tr	tr	0	1	3	—	—	18	995	92	—	9
red halves	½ cup	13	tr	tr	0	1	3	—	—	28	958	102	—	33
B&G														
Cherry Sweet	1 (1 oz)	10	0	0	0	0	2	0	—	—	310	—	—	—
Hot Pepper Rings	7 pieces (1 oz)	0	0	0	0	0	1	0	—	—	310	—	—	—
COSTA PERUANA														
Organic Aji Paste All Flavors	1 tbsp (0.5 oz)	10	0	0	0	0	2	0	0	0	0	—	—	2
DIETZ & WATSON														
Sweet Roasted	1 oz	5	0	0	0	0	1	0	0	0	55	—	—	15
GEDNEY														
Hot & Sweet Jalapeno Peppers	¼ cup	30	0	0	0	0	5	5	0	0	260	—	—	0
Hot Banana Pepper Rings	¼ cup	10	0	0	0	0	1	0	0	0	400	—	—	0
GERTIE'S FINEST														
Piquillo	1 oz	10	0	0	0	1	2	1	tr	10	134	—	—	25
JAKE & AMOS														
Mild Sweet Stuffed	2 tbsp	15	0	0	0	0	7	0	0	0	265	—	—	0
MATIZ														
Organic Piquillo Peppers	2	20	0	0	0	1	4	3	tr	0	115	—	—	60
Piparras	½ jar (1 oz)	5	0	0	0	0	1	0	0	10	126	—	—	1
PACE														
Green Chiles Diced	2 tbsp	10	0	0	0	0	2	tr	tr	0	100	—	—	4
DRIED														
ancho	1 (0.6 oz)	48	1	tr	0	2	9	—	4	10	7	410	12	0
ancho	1 tsp	3	tr	—	0	tr	1	—	tr	1	0	24	1	0
casabel	1 tsp	3	tr	—	0	tr	1	—	tr	1	—	—	—	1
chipotle smoked	1 tsp	3	tr	—	0	tr	1	—	tr	3	—	—	—	0
green	1 tbsp	1	tr	tr	0	tr	tr	—	—	1	1	13	1	8
guajillo	1 tsp	3	tr	—	0	tr	1	—	tr	1	—	—	—	1
mulato	1 tsp	3	tr	—	0	tr	1	—	tr	1	—	—	—	1

FOOD	PORTION	CALS	FAT	SAT FAT	CHOL	PROT	CARB	SUGAR	FIBER	CALCI	SOD	POTAS	FOLIC	VIT C
pasilla	1 (7 g)	24	1	—	0	1	4	—	2	7	6	156	12	0
pasilla	1 tsp	3	tr	—	0	tr	1	—	tr	1	1	22	2	0
red	1 tbsp	1	tr	tr	0	tr	tr	—	—	1	1	13	1	8
FRESH														
banana	1 (4 in) (1.2 oz)	9	tr	tr	0	1	2	—	1	5	4	84	10	27
banana	1 cup (4.4 oz)	33	1	tr	0	2	7	—	4	17	16	317	36	27
chili green hot	1	18	tr	tr	0	1	4	—	—	8	3	153	11	109
chili green hot chopped	½ cup	30	tr	tr	0	2	7	—	—	13	5	255	18	182
chili red chopped	½ cup	30	tr	tr	0	2	7	—	—	13	5	255	18	182
chili red hot	1 (1.6 oz)	18	tr	tr	0	1	4	—	—	8	3	153	11	109
green	1 (2.6 oz)	20	tr	tr	0	1	5	—	1	7	1	131	16	95
green chopped	½ cup	13	tr	tr	0	tr	3	—	1	5	1	89	11	45
green chopped cooked	½ cup	19	tr	tr	0	1	5	—	—	6	1	113	11	51
green cooked	1 (2.6 oz)	20	tr	tr	0	1	5	—	—	7	1	121	11	54
habanero	1 tsp	9	tr	—	0	1	2	—	1	5	2	99	7	27
hungarian	1 (0.9 oz)	8	tr	tr	0	tr	2	—	0	3	tr	55	14	0
jalapeno	1 (0.5 oz)	4	tr	tr	0	tr	1	—	tr	1	tr	30	7	6
jalapeno sliced	1 cup (3.2 oz)	27	1	tr	0	1	5	—	3	9	1	197	42	6
red	1 (2.6 oz)	20	tr	tr	0	1	5	—	1	7	1	131	16	141
red chopped	½ cup	13	tr	tr	0	tr	3	—	1	5	1	69	11	95
red chopped cooked	½ cup	19	tr	tr	0	1	5	—	—	6	1	113	11	125
red cooked	1 (2.6 oz)	20	tr	tr	0	1	5	—	—	7	1	121	11	125
serrano	1 (6 g)	2	tr	0	0	tr	tr	—	tr	1	1	19	1	3
serrano chopped	1 cup (3.7 oz)	34	tr	tr	0	2	7	4	4	12	11	320	24	3
yellow	1 (6.5 oz)	50	tr	—	0	2	12	—	—	20	3	393	48	341
yellow	10 strips	14	tr	—	0	1	3	—	—	6	1	110	14	95
FROZEN														
green chopped	1 oz	6	tr	tr	0	tr	1	—	—	3	1	26	4	16
red chopped	1 oz	6	tr	tr	0	tr	1	—	—	3	1	26	4	16
C&W														
Strips	¾ cup	25	0	0	0	1	4	3	1	0	10	—	—	21
FARM RICH														
Stuffed Jalapeno	2 (1.7 oz)	120	8	3	10	2	10	1	0	20	410	—	—	18
PERCH														
FRESH														
cooked	1 fillet (1.6 oz)	54	1	tr	53	11	0	0	0	47	36	158	—	—
cooked	3 oz	99	1	tr	98	21	0	0	0	87	67	293	—	—
ocean perch atlantic cooked	1 fillet (1.8 oz)	60	1	tr	27	12	0	0	0	69	48	175	—	—
ocean perch atlantic cooked	3 oz	103	2	tr	46	20	0	0	0	117	82	298	—	—

FOOD	PORTION	CALS	FAT	SAT FAT	CHOL	PROT	CARB	SUGAR	FIBER	CALCI	SOD	POTAS	FOLIC	VIT C
ocean perch atlantic raw	3 oz	80	1	tr	36	16	0	0	0	91	64	232	—	—
raw	3 oz	77	1	tr	76	16	0	0	0	68	52	228	—	—
red raw	3.5 oz	114	4	—	—	18	0	0	0	22	80	308	—	1
FROZEN														
BELL														
Cajun Nuggets	12 (4.5 oz)	170	3	0	75	21	16	0	1	40	300	—	—	1
Fillets Breaded	1 piece (4.5 oz)	170	3	0	75	21	16	0	tr	60	510	—	—	0
Fillets Unbreaded	1 piece (3.5 oz)	80	1	0	75	18	0	0	0	40	20	—	—	0

PERSIMMONS

FOOD	PORTION	CALS	FAT	SAT FAT	CHOL	PROT	CARB	SUGAR	FIBER	CALCI	SOD	POTAS	FOLIC	VIT C
dried japanese	1 (1.2 oz)	93	tr	—	0	tr	25	—	5	8	1	273	—	0
fresh	1 (6 oz)	118	tr	tr	0	1	31	21	6	13	2	271	13	13
FRIEDA'S														
Dried Fuyu	⅓ cup (1.4 oz)	140	0	0	0	1	35	27	3	20	10	—	—	72

PHEASANT

FOOD	PORTION	CALS	FAT	SAT FAT	CHOL	PROT	CARB	SUGAR	FIBER	CALCI	SOD	POTAS	FOLIC	VIT C
breast boneless cooked	½ (4.4 oz)	312	15	4	113	41	0	0	0	20	260	343	6	3
cooked diced	1 cup	332	16	5	120	44	0	0	0	22	277	364	7	3
drumstick & thigh cooked	1 (2.6 oz)	184	9	3	67	24	0	0	0	12	154	202	4	2

PHYLLO

FOOD	PORTION	CALS	FAT	SAT FAT	CHOL	PROT	CARB	SUGAR	FIBER	CALCI	SOD	POTAS	FOLIC	VIT C
sheet	1 (0.7 oz)	57	1	tr	0	1	10	tr	tr	2	92	14	17	0
ATHENS														
Fillo Dough Sheets	5 (2 oz)	160	1	0	0	5	31	1	1	40	180	—	—	0
Kataifi Shredded Fillo Dough	⅛ pkg (2 oz)	120	2	0	0	3	22	0	tr	20	115	—	—	0
Mini Fillo Shells	2 (7 g)	25	1	0	0	1	4	0	0	0	15	—	—	0
Spanakopita Spinach & Cheese Spinach & Cheese	2 (2 oz)	160	8	2	20	4	17	1	1	60	240	—	—	5
Tyropita Three Cheese Appetizers	2 (2 oz)	180	11	5	25	6	14	1	0	80	310	—	—	0
EKIZIAN														
Sheets	2 (4 oz)	433	9	4	62	12	76	2	3	24	287	117	31	0
THE FILLO FACTORY														
Kataifi Shredded Fillo	1 (2 oz)	180	2	0	0	5	35	1	4	20	140	—	—	0
Organic	2 sheets (1.5 oz)	130	1	0	0	4	27	0	1	20	160	—	—	0
Organic Whole Wheat	2 sheets (1.8 oz)	140	1	0	0	4	30	0	2	20	200	—	—	0
Shells Large	1 (0.7 oz)	80	2	0	0	2	13	0	0	0	55	—	—	0

PICKLES

PICANTE
(see SALSA)

PICKLES

FOOD	PORTION	CALS	FAT	SAT FAT	CHOL	PROT	CARB	SUGAR	FIBER	CALCI	SOD	POTAS	FOLIC	VIT C
bread & butter	6 slices	39	tr	tr	0	tr	9	4	1	15	323	96	2	4
dill	1 lg (4.7 oz)	24	tr	tr	0	1	6	5	2	12	1731	157	1	3
dill low sodium	1 med (2.3 oz)	12	tr	tr	0	tr	3	—	1	6	12	75	1	1
dill sliced	6 slices	7	tr	tr	0	tr	2	1	1	3	497	45	0	1
sweet gherkin	1 (1.2 oz)	41	tr	tr	0	tr	11	5	tr	1	329	11	0	tr
tsukemono japanese pickles sliced	¼ cup	10	tr	tr	0	tr	2	1	1	13	180	200	9	tr
CLAUSSEN														
Bread 'N Butter Chips	1 oz	20	0	0	0	0	4	3	—	—	180	—	—	—
Kosher Dills Halves	1 (1 oz)	5	0	0	0	0	1	0	0	—	330	—	—	—
Sandwich Slices Hearty Garlic	2 (1.2 oz)	5	0	0	0	0	1	tr	—	20	320	—	—	—
Sweet Gerkins	1 (0.9 oz)	30	0	0	0	0	7	6	—	—	210	—	—	1
DIETZ & WATSON														
New Half Sours	2 pieces (1 oz)	0	0	0	0	0	0	0	0	20	360	—	—	0
GEDNEY														
Baby Dills	3 (1 oz)	5	0	0	0	0	1	0	0	0	290	—	—	0
Organic Baby Dills	2 (1 oz)	5	0	0	0	0	1	0	0	0	260	—	—	0
JAKE & AMOS														
Bread & Butter Chips	2 tbsp	20	0	0	0	0	5	2	0	—	288	—	—	—
MT. OLIVE														
Bread & Butter Spears	¾ spear (1 oz)	20	0	0	0	0	6	4	—	—	130	—	—	—
TEXAS SASSY														
Pickle Chips	1 tbsp (0.5 oz)	30	0	0	0	0	7	7	—	—	115	—	—	—
TREE OF LIFE														
Organic Sweet Bread & Butter Chips	4 (1 oz)	30	0	0	0	0	8	7	0	0	180	—	—	0
VLASIC														
Kosher Dill Spears Reduced Sodium	⅔ spear (1 oz)	0	0	0	0	0	tr	0	0	—	150	—	—	—
Stackers Kosher Dill	1 (1 oz)	0	0	0	0	0	tr	0	—	—	210	—	—	—
Stackers Kosher Dill Reduced Sodium	1 (1 oz)	0	0	0	0	0	tr	0	0	—	150	—	—	—

FOOD	PORTION	CALS	FAT	SAT FAT	CHOL	PROT	CARB	SUGAR	FIBER	CALCI	SOD	POTAS	FOLIC	VIT C
PIE														
(*see also* PIE CRUST, PIE FILLING)														
FROZEN														
EDWARDS														
Pie Slices Key Lime	1 slice (3.25 oz)	330	16	11	35	4	42	33	tr	100	240	—	—	0
MOM MADE														
Munchie Apple	1 (2.5 oz)	220	10	5	0	3	30	8	1	0	130	—	—	1
MRS. SMITH'S														
Bake & Serve No Sugar Added Apple	1 slice (4.6 oz)	310	16	7	0	3	40	7	4	—	430	—	—	—
Blueberry Crumb	1 slice (4.2 oz)	320	14	6	0	3	48	23	2	—	280	—	—	—
Cherry	1 slice (4.6 oz)	330	16	7	0	3	44	17	1	—	280	—	—	—
Cinnabon Apple Crumb	1 slice (4.6 oz)	350	16	7	0	3	49	23	2	—	340	—	—	—
Classic Cream Key Lime	1 slice (4.2 oz)	410	19	13	15	5	56	44	1	—	200	—	—	—
Coconut Custard	1 slice (4.4 oz)	300	17	9	65	6	31	15	1	—	260	—	—	—
Deep Dish Berry Burst	1 slice (4.2 oz)	340	15	7	0	3	51	28	3	—	240	—	—	—
Dutch Apple Crumb	1 slice (4.6 oz)	370	17	7	0	3	52	22	2	—	250	—	—	—
Pumpkin Custard	1 slice (4.6 oz)	300	15	7	40	5	38	18	2	—	280	—	—	—
Soda Shoppe Boston Cream	1 slice (2.7 oz)	220	9	3	30	2	32	21	0	—	160	—	—	—
Soda Shoppe Chocolate Cream	1 slice (4.6 oz)	350	17	8	15	4	47	27	1	—	270	—	—	—
Soda Shoppe Lemon Meringue	1 slice (4.2 oz)	300	10	2	40	3	51	31	0	—	190	—	—	—
READY-TO-EAT														
FOODS BY GEORGE														
Gluten Free Pecan Tarts	1 (4 oz)	470	26	7	95	6	51	26	3	40	160	—	—	0
LANCE														
Pecan	1 (3 oz)	350	17	4	25	4	46	35	3	0	200	—	—	0
LIFESTREAM														
Pie Oh-My Apple	1 (3.5 oz)	280	11	5	0	3	43	16	2	20	240	—	—	1
Pie Oh-My Pineapple	1 (3.5 oz)	280	11	5	0	3	45	16	2	20	400	—	—	9
TAKE-OUT														
apple one crust	1 slice (5.3 oz)	363	14	3	0	3	59	36	2	9	298	84	28	2
apple tart	1 (4.2 oz)	370	19	5	0	4	48	20	1	8	382	68	43	1
apple two crust	1 slice (5.3 oz)	356	17	6	0	3	51	23	2	16	399	98	40	5
apricot tart	1 (4.2 oz)	356	17	4	0	4	48	20	2	12	362	166	44	4

FOOD	PORTION	CALS	FAT	SAT FAT	CHOL	PROT	CARB	SUGAR	FIBER	CALCI	SOD	POTAS	FOLIC	VIT C
apricot two crust	1 slice (5.3 oz)	417	19	5	0	5	59	28	3	15	332	218	50	6
banana cream	1 slice (5.1 oz)	387	20	5	73	6	47	17	1	108	346	238	38	2
blackberry one crust	1 slice (4.4 oz)	341	17	4	0	4	44	18	4	20	346	113	46	10
blackberry two crust	1 slice (5.3 oz)	394	19	4	0	4	54	24	5	26	318	142	51	13
blueberry one crust	1 slice (4.8 oz)	292	12	3	0	3	45	23	3	10	211	67	30	1
blueberry tart	1 (4.2 oz)	346	17	4	0	3	47	21	2	8	341	72	38	5
blueberry two crust	1 slice (5.3 oz)	348	15	3	0	3	52	15	2	12	488	75	40	4
cherry one crust	1 slice (4.8 oz)	312	12	3	0	3	50	30	2	14	258	105	30	2
cherry two crust	1 slice (5.3 oz)	390	17	4	0	3	60	21	1	18	369	122	10	1
chess	1 slice (3 oz)	365	18	8	128	5	48	37	1	22	205	55	30	0
chocolate cream	1 slice (5 oz)	380	18	7	73	7	50	29	2	114	320	226	45	0
coconut cream	1 slice (5 oz)	429	24	10	0	3	54	52	2	42	367	94	10	0
custard	1 slice (4.8 oz)	286	16	3	45	7	28	16	2	109	326	144	27	1
grasshopper	1 slice (3.5 oz)	341	19	8	96	4	33	23	1	32	260	88	22	tr
key lime	1 slice (5 oz)	420	14	6	25	4	71	28	tr	60	210	—	—	0
lemon meringue	1 slice (4.8 oz)	367	12	2	62	2	65	33	2	77	200	122	33	4
lemon meringue tart	1 (4.1 oz)	298	14	3	68	4	41	22	1	14	276	53	33	3
mince two crust	1 slice (5.3 oz)	434	16	4	0	4	72	42	4	33	381	304	34	9
peach two crust	1 slice (5.3 oz)	334	15	2	0	3	49	9	1	12	405	188	44	1
pear two crust	1 slice (5.3 oz)	400	18	4	0	4	57	27	3	12	354	106	45	2
pecan	1 slice (4 oz)	456	21	4	36	5	65	32	4	19	483	84	39	1
pineapple two crust	1 slice (5.3 oz)	394	18	4	0	4	55	23	2	15	328	94	46	4
plum two crust	1 slice (5.3 oz)	441	21	5	0	4	61	29	2	12	46	134	50	2
prune one crust	1 slice (5.3 oz)	450	14	4	0	6	77	55	2	15	357	189	36	3
pumpkin	1 slice (5.4 oz)	323	15	3	31	6	42	21	4	92	434	237	37	2
raisin tart	1 (4.2 oz)	348	16	4	0	4	49	21	2	16	265	157	41	1
raisin two crust	1 slice (5.3 oz)	376	16	4	0	4	55	26	2	18	334	190	40	1
raspberry one crust	1 slice (4.8 oz)	330	13	3	5	3	52	29	6	22	212	129	34	17
raspberry two crust	1 slice (5.3 oz)	422	20	5	0	4	58	25	5	22	340	130	51	15
rhubarb two crust	1 slice (5.3 oz)	444	23	6	0	5	55	16	2	118	412	106	58	2
shoo-fly	1 slice (4 oz)	404	13	3	36	4	69	39	1	90	239	492	44	0
strawberry rhubarb two crust	1 slice (5.3 oz)	422	21	5	20	5	53	18	2	64	382	129	60	21
strawberry two crust	1 slice (6 oz)	386	16	4	0	4	58	29	3	22	284	181	54	51
sweet potato	1 piece (5.4 oz)	276	14	4	57	6	32	13	2	97	205	253	31	7

PIE CRUST

FOOD	PORTION	CALS	FAT	SAT FAT	CHOL	PROT	CARB	SUGAR	FIBER	CALCI	SOD	POTAS	FOLIC	VIT C
baked	⅙ crust (1 oz)	147	9	3	0	1	14	1	tr	6	185	31	16	0

FOOD	PORTION	CALS	FAT	SAT FAT	CHOL	PROT	CARB	SUGAR	FIBER	CALCI	SOD	POTAS	FOLIC	VIT C
chocolate wafer	⅛ crust (1.2 oz)	177	11	2	0	2	19	8	1	10	235	59	18	0
chocolate wafer tart shell	1 (0.8 oz)	111	7	1	0	1	12	5	tr	7	148	37	12	0
deep dish frzn	⅛ crust (1.8 oz)	266	16	5	0	3	27	—	1	12	200	53	48	—
graham cracker	⅙ crust (1.2 oz)	172	9	2	0	1	23	13	1	7	199	31	8	0
graham cracker tart shell	1 (0.8 oz)	109	5	1	0	1	14	8	tr	5	126	19	5	0
puff pastry shell	1 (1.4 oz)	223	15	2	0	3	18	tr	1	4	101	25	22	0
tart shell	1 (1 oz)	149	10	3	0	1	14	1	tr	6	188	32	16	0
HONEY MAID														
Graham Cracker Crumbs as prep	⅛ pie	160	9	2	0	1	18	4	0	0	192	—	—	0
KEEBLER														
Graham Reduced Fat	⅛ pie (0.7 oz)	100	4	1	0	1	15	6	tr	—	100	—	—	0
Ready Crust Chocolate	⅛ pie (0.7 oz)	100	5	1	0	1	14	6	tr	—	110	—	—	0
Ready Crust Graham	¹⁄₁₀ pie (0.9 oz)	130	6	2	0	1	18	7	tr	—	140	—	—	0
Ready Crust Shortbread	⅛ pie (0.7 oz)	110	5	2	0	1	14	6	0	—	110	—	—	0
MRS. SMITH'S														
Deep Dish Shell frzn	1 slice (1 oz)	130	7	4	0	2	14	2	0	—	110	—	—	—
NILLA WAFERS														
Pie Crust	⅙ (1 oz)	140	8	2	5	1	18	10	0	—	85	—	—	—
PEPPERIDGE FARM														
Puff Pastry Sheets frzn	⅙ sheet	160	10	5	0	3	16	1	1	0	140	—	—	0
Puff Pastry Shell frzn	1	180	11	6	0	3	18	1	2	0	160	—	—	0
PILLSBURY														
Crusts Just Unroll	⅛ (1 oz)	110	7	3	<5	tr	12	0	0	0	140	—	—	0
Deep Dish frzn	⅛ (0.7 oz)	90	5	2	<5	1	11	1	0	0	85	—	—	0
Pet Ritz Deep Dish frzn	⅛ (0.6 oz)	90	5	2	<5	1	11	1	0	0	85	—	—	0
PIE FILLING														
apple	1 cup	155	tr	tr	0	tr	41	34	2	8	6	124	2	4
blueberry	1 cup	474	1	tr	0	1	116	99	7	71	31	301	3	2
cherry	1 cup	317	2	tr	0	2	76	66	2	24	143	201	16	4
lemon	1 cup	923	18	4	348	13	185	166	1	59	226	207	59	28
pumpkin pie mix canned	1 cup (9.5 oz)	281	tr	tr	0	3	71	—	22	100	562	373	94	9
CHUKAR CHERRIES														
Triple Cherry	½ cup	190	1	0	0	tr	47	39	2	0	0	—	—	6

FOOD	PORTION	CALS	FAT	SAT FAT	CHOL	PROT	CARB	SUGAR	FIBER	CALCI	SOD	POTAS	FOLIC	VIT C
COMSTOCK														
Blueberry	⅓ cup	100	0	0	0	0	24	17	1	0	10	—	—	0
Country Cherry Original	⅓ cup (3.1 oz)	90	0	0	0	0	23	19	1	0	25	—	—	0
FARMER'S MARKET														
Organic Pumpkin Pie Mix	½ cup	100	0	0	0	0	25	20	2	20	0	—	—	0
PIEROGI														
potato	1 (1.3 oz)	70	2	1	22	3	11	tr	1	22	95	60	18	1
MRS. T'S														
Mini Potato & Cheddar	7 (3 oz)	130	2	1	5	4	25	1	1	20	360	—	—	5
Potato & Cheddar	4 (4 oz)	170	3	1	5	6	32	1	1	40	510	—	—	6
Potato & Onion	3 (4 oz)	160	2	0	5	5	32	1	1	20	390	—	—	6
Potato Broccoli & Cheddar	3 (4 oz)	190	5	1	5	6	31	2	2	40	530	—	—	9
Sauerkraut	3 (4 oz)	140	2	0	5	4	28	1	3	—	670	—	—	—
Sour Cream & Chive	3 (4 oz)	190	5	2	10	5	32	1	1	—	480	—	—	—
PIGEON PEAS														
dried cooked	1 cup	204	1	tr	0	11	39	—	—	72	9	644	186	0
dried cooked w/ salt	½ cup (2.9 oz)	102	tr	tr	0	6	20	—	6	36	202	323	93	0
PIGNOLIA														
(*see* PINE NUTS)														
PIG'S FEET														
cooked	1	201	14	4	93	19	0	0	0	0	204	29	2	0
pickled	1	177	14	5	70	12	tr	tr	0	28	803	204	3	0
HORMEL														
Pigs Feet	2 oz	80	6	2	45	7	0	0	0	20	590	—	—	0
PIKE														
northern cooked	½ fillet (5.4 oz)	176	1	tr	78	38	0	0	0	113	76	514	—	6
northern cooked	3 oz	96	1	tr	43	21	0	0	0	62	42	282	3	—
northern raw	3 oz	75	1	tr	33	16	0	0	0	48	33	220	—	3
roe raw	1 oz	37	tr	—	103	7	tr	—	—	—	—	—	—	4
walleye baked	3 oz	101	1	tr	94	21	0	0	0	120	56	424	—	—
walleye fillet baked	4.4 oz	147	2	tr	137	30	0	0	0	175	81	618	—	—
PILLNUTS														
canarytree dried	1 oz	204	23	9	0	3	1	—	—	41	1	144	—	—
PIMIENTOS														
canned	1 tbsp	3	tr	tr	0	tr	1	—	—	1	2	19	1	10
canned	1 slice	0	0	0	0	tr	tr	—	—	0	0	2	0	1
PINE NUTS														
pine nuts dried	¼ cup (1.2 oz)	277	23	2	0	5	4	1	1	5	1	201	11	tr

FOOD	PORTION	CALS	FAT	SAT FAT	CHOL	PROT	CARB	SUGAR	FIBER	CALCI	SOD	POTAS	FOLIC	VIT C
pinyon dried	20 (2 g)	13	1	tr	0	tr	tr	—	tr	0	1	13	1	0
pinyon dried	1 oz	178	17	3	0	3	5	—	3	2	20	178	16	1
FISHER														
Pine Nuts	¼ cup (1 oz)	190	19	2	0	4	4	1	1	0	0	—	—	0
PINEAPPLE														
CANNED														
in heavy syrup crushed sliced or chunks	1 cup (8.9 oz)	198	tr	tr	0	1	51	50	2	36	3	264	13	19
in heavy syrup slice	1 (1.7 oz)	38	tr	tr	0	tr	10	8	tr	7	0	51	2	4
in juice crushed sliced or chunks	1 cup (8.7 oz)	149	tr	tr	0	1	39	36	2	35	2	304	12	24
in light syrup crushed sliced or chunks	1 cup (8.8 oz)	131	tr	tr	0	1	34	32	2	35	3	265	13	19
in light syrup slice	1 (1.7 oz)	25	tr	tr	0	tr	6	6	tr	7	0	50	2	4
in water crushed sliced or chunks	1 cup (8.6 oz)	79	tr	tr	0	1	20	18	2	37	2	312	12	19
juice pack slice	1 (1.6 oz)	28	tr	tr	0	tr	7	7	tr	7	0	57	2	5
water pack slice	1 (1.6 oz)	15	tr	tr	0	tr	4	4	tr	7	0	60	2	4
DEL MONTE														
Chunks In Heavy Syrup	½ cup (4.3 oz)	90	0	0	0	0	24	22	1	0	10	—	—	12
Chunks In Its Own Juice	½ cup (4.3 oz)	70	0	0	0	0	17	15	1	0	10	—	—	12
Crushed In Heavy Syrup	½ cup (4.3 oz)	90	0	0	0	0	24	22	1	0	10	—	—	12
Crushed In Its Own Juice	½ cup (4.3 oz)	70	0	0	0	0	17	15	1	0	10	—	—	12
Fruit Naturals Chunks	½ cup (4.4 oz)	70	0	0	0	tr	18	15	tr	0	5	—	—	60
Slices In Heavy Syrup	2 (4 oz)	60	0	0	0	0	16	14	1	0	10	—	—	12
DOLE														
Crushed In Heavy Syrup	½ cups (4.3 oz)	90	0	0	0	0	24	22	1	0	10	—	—	12
Crushed Juice Pack	½ cup (4.3 oz)	70	0	0	0	1	18	16	1	0	0	150	—	12
Slices In Heavy Syrup	2 (4.1 oz)	90	0	0	0	0	24	22	1	0	10	—	—	12
Slices Juice Pack	2 (4 oz)	60	0	0	0	0	15	13	1	0	10	—	—	15
GEFEN														
Chunks In Juice	½ cup (4.9 oz)	80	0	0	0	0	19	17	1	20	0	—	—	6

FOOD	PORTION	CALS	FAT	SAT FAT	CHOL	PROT	CARB	SUGAR	FIBER	CALCI	SOD	POTAS	FOLIC	VIT C
LIBERTY GOLD														
Chunks Natural Juice	½ cup (4.7 oz)	80	0	0	0	tr	21	19	2	20	10	—	—	12
Slices Natural Juice	½ cup	80	0	0	0	tr	21	19	1	20	10	—	—	12
DRIED														
dried	1 piece (1 oz)	71	tr	tr	0	1	19	14	2	18	1	156	13	14
BROTHERS-ALL-NATURAL														
Crisps	1 pkg (0.53 oz)	60	0	0	0	0	14	11	1	0	0	—	—	9
CRISPY GREEN														
Crispy Pineapple	1 pkg (0.35)	35	0	0	0	0	9	7	1	0	0	—	—	11
CRUNCHIES														
Freeze Dried	1 pkg (9 g)	35	0	0	0	0	8	6	tr	0	0	—	—	24
CRUNCHY N'YUMMY														
Organic Freeze Dried	1 pkg (1 oz)	100	0	0	0	0	23	0	2	56	1	165	—	21
KOPALI														
Organic	1 pkg (1.7 oz)	170	0	0	0	0	43	36	2	20	24	—	—	0
MRS. MAY'S														
Fruit Chips	1 pkg	35	0	0	0	0	8	7	1	0	0	—	—	8
SUNSWEET														
Philippine	⅓ cup (1.4 oz)	130	0	0	0	0	33	30	2	40	95	60	—	5
FRESH														
chunks	1 cup (5.8 oz)	82	tr	tr	0	1	22	16	2	21	2	180	30	79
slice	1 slice (3 oz)	42	tr	tr	0	tr	11	8	1	11	1	92	15	40
whole	1 (2 lbs)	452	1	tr	0	5	119	89	13	118	9	986	163	433
CHIQUITA														
Bites	1 piece (2.8 oz)	40	0	0	0	1	9	7	tr	0	15	—	—	48
Cut Up	1 cup (5.8 oz)	82	0	0	0	1	22	16	2	20	2	180	—	79
DOLE														
Pineapple	2 slices (3.9 oz)	60	0	0	0	tr	15	12	2	20	0	—	—	66
FROZEN														
chunks sweetened	1 cup (8.6 oz)	211	tr	tr	0	1	54	52	3	22	5	245	27	10
DOLE														
Chunks	¾ cup (4.9 oz)	70	0	0	0	1	18	3	2	0	0	—	—	48
Tropical Gold	1 pkg (3 oz)	45	0	0	0	0	11	8	1	0	0	—	—	42
PINEAPPLE JUICE														
canned unsweetened w/ vitamin C	1 cup (8.8 oz)	132	tr	tr	0	1	32	25	1	32	5	325	45	110
frzn unsweetened as prep w/ water	1 cup (8.8 oz)	130	tr	tr	0	1	32	31	1	28	2	340	28	30
CERES														
100% Juice	8 oz	120	0	0	0	0	29	25	2	40	5	300	—	60

FOOD	PORTION	CALS	FAT	SAT FAT	CHOL	PROT	CARB	SUGAR	FIBER	CALCI	SOD	POTAS	FOLIC	VIT C
DOLE														
100% Juice	1 can (6 oz)	90	0	0	0	1	22	21	1	40	10	330	—	72
FIZZY LIZZY														
Pineapple	1 bottle (12 oz)	100	0	0	0	0	25	25	—	—	0	—	—	60
SUNDIA														
Purely	½ cup	60	0	0	0	1	15	19	1	20	0	—	—	60
WALNUT ACRES														
Organic	8 oz	130	0	0	0	0	32	31	—	40	5	330	—	1
PINK BEANS														
dried cooked	1 cup	252	1	tr	0	15	47	—	—	88	3	858	284	0
PINTO BEANS														
dried cooked	1 cup	245	1	tr	0	15	45	1	15	79	2	746	294	1
ARROWHEAD MILLS														
Organic Dried not prep	¼ cup	150	0	0	0	9	27	2	10	60	0	570	—	4
EDEN														
Organic Spicy Refried	½ cup	90	1	0	—	6	19	1	7	40	180	420	—	—
HAMBEENS														
Dried as prep	½ cup	120	1	0	0	7	22	1	6	40	63	460	—	2
TREE OF LIFE														
Organic	½ cup (4.6 oz)	120	0	0	0	8	23	2	<9	40	120	—	—	2
TAKE-OUT														
stewed w/ viandas	1 cup	222	8	2	8	11	27	2	6	51	668	546	97	8
PISTACHIOS														
dry roasted w/ salt	49 nuts (1 oz)	161	13	2	0	6	8	2	3	31	115	295	14	1
dry roasted w/o salt	49 nuts (1 oz)	162	13	2	0	6	8	2	3	31	3	295	14	1
in shells	½ cup	165	13	2	0	6	8	2	3	32	89	302	14	1
FISHER														
Shelled	¼ cup (1 oz)	160	13	2	0	6	8	2	3	10	110	—	—	1
LOVE'N BAKE														
Pistachio Paste	2 tbsp	160	11	1	0	4	14	10	2	20	0	—	—	1
PLANTERS														
Dry Roasted	1 oz	170	14	2	0	5	8	1	3	20	150	—	—	1
TRUE NORTH														
Sea Salted In Shells	½ cup	170	14	2	0	6	7	2	4	20	270	—	8	0
WONDERFUL														
Roasted & Salted In Shells	½ cup	160	14	2	0	6	8	2	3	40	160	310	—	0
PITANGA														
fresh	1 cup	57	1	—	0	1	13	—	—	16	5	178	—	46
fresh	1	2	tr	—	0	tr	1	—	—	1	0	7	—	2

PIZZA

(see also PIZZA CRUST*)*

FOOD	PORTION	CALS	FAT	SAT FAT	CHOL	PROT	CARB	SUGAR	FIBER	CALCI	SOD	POTAS	FOLIC	VIT C
4REAL														
Cheese	1 (4.2 oz)	220	4	2	5	11	38	2	5	150	350	—	—	1
Cheesy Pizza Quesadilla	1 (2.5 oz)	160	5	2	5	11	15	1	1	250	350	—	—	1
Turkey Pepperoni	1 (4.2 oz)	220	4	2	5	11	38	2	5	150	350	—	—	1
A.C.LAROCCO														
Thin Crust Whole Grain Cheese & Garlic	⅓ pie (4.8 oz)	250	8	3	15	12	40	3	9	200	340	—	—	21
Thin Crust Whole Grain Greek Sesame	⅓ pie (4.4 oz)	250	8	3	17	12	40	3	9	200	350	—	—	18
Thin Crust Whole Grain Tomato & Feta	⅓ pie (4.8 oz)	250	8	3	15	12	40	3	9	1000	340	—	—	21
Ultra Thin Sprouted Grain Bruschetta	½ pie (3.5 oz)	170	8	4	16	11	17	0	1	300	290	—	—	11
Ultra Thin Sprouted Grain Old World Veggie	½ pie (3.6 oz)	170	7	3	15	11	19	0	2	250	260	—	—	58
AMY'S														
Cheese & Pesto Whole Wheat Crust	⅓ pie (4.6 oz)	360	18	4	15	13	37	4	1	200	680	—	—	4
Margherita	1 pie (6.2 oz)	360	17	5	10	16	47	4	3	80	720	—	—	4
Non Dairy Cheese Rice Crust	1 pie (6 oz)	460	28	3	0	10	46	7	4	40	680	—	—	6
Pocket Sandwich Spinach Feta	1 (4.5 oz)	260	9	5	20	11	34	4	3	250	590	—	—	6
Roasted Vegetable No Cheese	⅓ pie (4 oz)	270	9	2	0	6	42	5	2	20	490	—	—	12
Single Serve Spinach Light In Sodium	1 (7.2 oz)	440	18	6	20	19	54	5	3	300	390	—	—	6
Soy Cheese	⅓ pie (4.3 oz)	290	11	1	0	12	37	3	2	20	590	—	—	2
Toaster Pops Cheese Pizza	5–6 pieces (1.9 oz)	160	6	1	5	5	21	2	1	60	220	—	—	1
BELLATORIA														
Fire Grilled Flatbread Buffalo Chicken	⅓ pie (5.8 oz)	340	17	7	45	20	34	4	5	300	1050	—	—	0

FOOD	PORTION	CALS	FAT	SAT FAT	CHOL	PROT	CARB	SUGAR	FIBER	CALCI	SOD	POTAS	FOLIC	VIT C
BELLATORIA (CONT.)														
Fire Grilled Flatbread Chicken Ranch w/ Uncured Bacon	¼ pie (4.5 oz)	270	13	5	45	19	25	3	3	250	750	—	—	0
Ultra Thin Crust Margherita	⅓ pie (4.9 oz)	280	16	6	30	14	23	2	1	350	500	—	—	6
Ultra Thin Crust Ultimate Pepperoni	¼ pie (4.3 oz)	300	18	8	45	16	21	3	1	300	790	—	—	2
BOLD ORGANICS														
Deluxe	½ pie (6.7 oz)	460	24	5	10	8	56	12	5	60	790	—	—	27
Meat Lovers	½ pie	450	24	5	10	7	54	11	5	60	790	—	—	12
Vegan Cheese	½ pie (5.5 oz)	380	18	3	0	4	54	11	5	60	580	—	—	12
Veggie Lovers	½ pie (6.2 oz)	390	18	3	10	5	55	12	5	60	580	—	—	27
CEDARLANE														
Zone Cheese	1 (6.5 oz)	380	14	5	30	27	39	4	6	350	700	—	—	4
DAYEINU														
Passover Pizza	1 slice (4 oz)	325	8	5	18	15	49	16	5	100	480	—	—	0
DIGIORNO														
Crispy Flatbread Tuscan Chicken	⅓ pie (4.6 oz)	280	14	6	35	14	25	2	2	250	680	—	—	0
For One Thin Crust Grilled Chicken & Vegetable	1 (8.4 oz)	520	17	8	45	28	64	7	4	250	850	—	—	6
For One Traditional Crust Supreme	1 (9.9 oz)	790	36	14	50	31	85	11	6	300	1460	—	—	6
Four Cheese	⅙ pie (4.7 oz)	310	11	5	25	15	40	6	2	200	850	—	—	2
Garlic Bread Pepperoni	⅙ pie (5 oz)	380	17	6	25	17	40	7	3	200	690	—	—	0
Rising Crust Four Cheese	⅓ pie (4 oz)	270	9	5	20	13	34	6	2	200	710	—	—	0
Rising Crust Italian Sausage	⅙ pie (5 oz)	350	14	6	30	15	40	6	2	200	960	—	—	2
Rising Crust Spinach Mushroom Garlic	⅙ pie (5 oz)	290	9	4	15	15	42	6	2	150	790	—	—	2
Rising Crust Three Meat	⅙ pie (5 oz)	350	15	6	30	16	41	6	2	150	1010	—	—	2
Stuffed Crust Pepperoni	⅕ pie (5.3 oz)	380	16	8	40	19	40	7	3	250	1040	—	—	0
Thin Crispy Crust Pepperoni	⅕ pie (4.4 oz)	320	15	7	35	16	31	5	2	250	790	—	—	0

FOOD	PORTION	CALS	FAT	SAT FAT	CHOL	PROT	CARB	SUGAR	FIBER	CALCI	SOD	POTAS	FOLIC	VIT C
DIGIORNO (CONT.)														
Thin Crispy Crust Spinach Mushroom Garlic	⅕ pie (4.6 oz)	250	9	5	20	12	32	4	3	200	540	—	—	0
Ultimate Topping Four Meat	⅕ pie (5 oz)	380	19	8	50	19	34	5	2	200	1140	—	—	2
Ultimate Topping Supreme	⅕ pie (5.3 oz)	360	18	7	45	16	35	5	2	1000	1010	—	—	6
FARM RICH														
Pizza Slices Pepperoni	2 (3.5 oz)	280	14	7	30	14	22	6	1	250	720	—	—	9
FOODS BY GEORGE														
Gluten Free Cheese	1 pie (6.5 oz)	400	15	8	30	20	44	5	2	450	860	—	—	4
GLUTINO														
Gluten Free Duo Cheese	1 (6.1 oz)	420	12	5	25	10	68	0	2	250	560	—	—	0
Gluten Free Spinach & Feta	1 (6.1 oz)	430	16	5	25	10	62	0	4	250	1000	—	—	0
HEALTH IS WEALTH														
Vegetarian Mini Pizza Bagels	4 (3.1 oz)	150	0	0	0	8	28	4	3	—	490	—	—	4
HOT POCKETS														
Croissant Five Cheese	1 (4.5 oz)	350	17	9	20	14	35	10	2	350	750	—	60	—
Croissant Pepperoni	1 (4.5 oz)	380	22	9	25	11	32	7	2	150	810	—	60	—
Sausage	1 (4.5 oz)	330	16	6	20	10	36	6	2	150	630	—	60	—
IAN'S														
Cheese	1 slice (1.5 oz)	100	3	2	10	4	14	2	1	20	200	—	—	1
JENO'S														
Crisp 'N Tasty Cheese	1 pie (6.8 oz)	440	21	5	15	16	47	5	2	300	1060	—	—	—
Crisp 'N Tasty Pepperoni	1 (6.7 oz)	490	26	6	20	16	50	5	2	150	1170	—	—	—
Crisp 'N Tasty Supreme	1 (7.2 oz)	490	25	6	20	17	49	5	2	150	1150	—	—	—
KRAFT														
Rising Crust Three Meat	⅓ pie (4.4 oz)	320	14	5	30	15	25	7	2	150	880	—	—	0
LEAN CUISINE														
Casual Cuisine Deep Dish Roasted Vegetable	1 pkg (6 oz)	320	5	2	5	16	52	6	3	200	480	320	—	12

FOOD	PORTION	CALS	FAT	SAT FAT	CHOL	PROT	CARB	SUGAR	FIBER	CALCI	SOD	POTAS	FOLIC	VIT C
LEAN CUISINE (CONT.)														
Casual Cuisine Deep Dish Spinach & Mushroom	1 pkg (6 oz)	340	7	4	10	18	52	5	2	250	430	150	—	1
Casual Cuisine Deep Dish Three Meat	1 pkg (6.4 oz)	390	9	3	25	22	55	7	3	200	610	350	—	6
Casual Cuisine Flatbread Melts Chicken Philly	1 pkg (6.5 oz)	350	9	4	35	22	46	5	5	350	620	300	—	9
Casual Cuisine Traditional Deluxe	1 pkg (6 oz)	340	8	3	20	17	49	6	4	150	510	320	—	9
Casual Cuisine Traditional Four Cheese	1 pkg (6 oz)	350	6	2	10	20	55	6	3	300	600	280	—	2
Casual Cuisine Traditional Mushroom	1 pkg (6 oz)	300	5	2	5	16	50	5	4	200	470	240	—	2
Casual Cuisine Traditional Pepperoni	1 pkg (6 oz)	380	9	3	20	20	55	6	3	200	610	320	—	6
Casual Cuisine Wood Fire Bacon Alfredo	1 pkg (6 oz)	320	9	3	15	17	42	4	2	200	670	170	—	2
Casual Cuisine Wood Fire Margherita	1 pkg (6 oz)	310	7	3	15	16	46	7	3	250	460	320	—	6
Simple Favorites French Bread Cheese	1 pkg (6 oz)	340	7	3	15	17	53	7	5	350	680	310	—	5
LEAN POCKETS														
Pepperoni	1 (4.5 oz)	260	7	3	20	15	35	9	3	250	900	—	—	—
Sausage & Pepperoni	1 (4.5 oz)	280	7	4	25	12	39	10	2	250	630	—	—	—
LUNCHABLES														
Extra Cheesy	1 pkg	280	9	5	25	17	31	6	3	350	630	—	—	1
Pizza w/ Pepperoni	1 pkg	310	13	6	30	16	31	6	3	250	760	—	—	12
MOM MADE														
Munchie Cheese Pizza	1 (2.5 oz)	160	9	4	0	5	13	2	1	20	220	—	—	4
PACIFIC FOODS														
BBQ Chicken	⅓ pie (4.5 oz)	270	9	5	25	16	30	3	1	250	520	—	—	2
Herb Garlic Chicken	⅓ pie (4.5 oz)	270	9	5	25	16	30	3	1	250	520	—	—	2
Supreme	⅓ pie (4.8 oz)	270	11	5	25	15	31	4	2	250	650	—	—	5

FOOD	PORTION	CALS	FAT	SAT FAT	CHOL	PROT	CARB	SUGAR	FIBER	CALCI	SOD	POTAS	FOLIC	VIT C
RED BARON														
Classic Crust 4 Cheese	1 pie (8.6 oz)	740	39	19	65	33	62	6	3	700	1480	—	—	0
SIMPLY SHARI'S														
Gluten Free Cheese	½ pie (5 oz)	290	11	5	65	15	35	3	2	350	780	0	—	1
Gluten Free Pepperoni	½ pie (5 oz)	320	13	6	75	17	35	3	2	350	1000	0	—	1
Gluten Free Pesto Margherita	½ pie (5 oz)	340	15	5	60	14	36	3	3	350	840	0	—	5
Gluten Free Spinach Feta	¼ pkg (5 oz)	280	10	5	65	13	35	4	2	300	890	0	—	2
Gluten Free Vegetable Margherita	¼ pie (5 oz)	220	5	2	40	5	38	4	3	100	700	0	—	9
SOLTERRA														
Cheese Margherita	½ pie (4.1 oz)	200	9	4	15	8	22	2	2	40	580	—	—	2
Vegan	½ pie (4.1 oz)	210	10	3	0	3	27	2	3	40	610	—	—	2
STOUFFER'S														
Corner Bistro Flatbread Marghcrita	1 pkg (9.13 oz)	540	22	9	40	22	65	7	4	300	800	—	—	4
Corner Bistro Flatbread Shrimp & Roasted Garlic	1 pkg (9.33 oz)	600	19	10	115	33	75	5	5	450	610	—	—	6
French Bread Grilled Vegetable	1 pkg (11.63 oz)	340	12	5	15	13	44	5	4	150	570	—	—	12
French Bread Sausage	1 pkg (4.2 oz)	420	21	7	25	15	43	5	4	150	730	—	—	4
French Bread Sausage & Pepperoni	1 pkg (4.2 oz)	460	24	8	30	17	42	5	4	150	880	—	—	2
French Bread White Pizza	1 pkg (10.13 oz)	470	23	7	40	22	44	3	4	450	900	—	—	0
TANDOOR CHEF														
Naan Pizza Margherita	½ pie (4 oz)	220	3	1	4	10	38	6	2	40	467	—	—	1
Naan Pizza Roasted Eggplant	½ pie (4.6 oz)	320	6	1	17	13	53	8	4	90	538	—	—	1
Naan Pizza Spinach & Paneer Cheese	½ pie (4.2 oz)	290	5	1	13	11	50	6	4	30	415	—	—	1
TOFUTTI														
Pan Crust Pizzaz Dairy Free	1 slice (2.7 oz)	180	7	2	0	3	24	6	1	—	320	—	—	—

FOOD	PORTION	CALS	FAT	SAT FAT	CHOL	PROT	CARB	SUGAR	FIBER	CALCI	SOD	POTAS	FOLIC	VIT C
TONY'S														
Pizza For One Cheese	1 (6.5 oz)	500	22	12	20	18	58	5	3	250	830	—	—	0
TOTINO'S														
Crisp Crust Canadian Bacon	½ pie (5.1 oz)	320	15	3	10	13	34	4	1	150	910	—	—	—
Crisp Crust Combination	½ pie (5.3 oz)	380	21	5	15	14	34	3	1	150	940	—	—	—
Crisp Crust Pepperoni Trio	½ pie (5 oz)	370	21	5	15	13	33	4	1	150	980	—	—	0
Crisp Crust Three Meat	½ pie (5.2 oz)	350	18	4	15	13	34	3	1	150	870	—	—	—
Pizza Rolls Combination	6 (3 oz)	220	11	3	10	8	24	2	1	40	470	—	—	0
Pizza Rolls Supreme	6 (3 oz)	210	9	2	10	7	25	3	2	40	390	—	—	1
Pizza Rolls Mega Ultimate Combination	3 (3.3 oz)	200	8	2	10	8	25	3	1	40	480	—	—	0
TAKE-OUT														
cheese	16 in pie	3384	144	61	294	151	372	44	23	2575	6584	1974	1067	4
cheese	⅛ of 16 in pie	423	18	8	37	19	46	5	3	322	823	247	133	1
cheese deep dish individual	1 (5.5 oz)	460	24	9	20	15	47	4	2	250	750	—	—	1
cheese & vegetables	⅛ of 16 in pie	428	16	6	19	17	55	5	3	292	967	361	97	18
ground beef	16 in pie	3753	172	68	299	151	392	25	20	2145	8642	2569	698	41
ham & pineapple	⅛ of 16 in pie	439	16	6	29	19	55	7	3	269	1110	374	92	19
no cheese	⅛ of 16 in pie	262	7	2	0	6	43	3	2	22	356	218	78	5
pepperoni	⅛ of 16 in pie	469	22	9	37	19	49	3	3	268	1080	321	87	5
white pizza	⅛ of 16 in pie	484	17	9	38	20	61	1	2	366	903	133	114	tr
PIZZA CRUST														
crust	1 slice (1.7 oz)	130	2	0	0	4	25	1	1	0	230	—	40	0
whole wheat	⅛ crust (2 oz)	120	2	0	0	4	24	0	4	20	250	—	—	2
BOBOLI														
100% Whole Wheat	⅕ crust (2 oz)	150	3	2	0	6	27	2	5	60	280	—	—	0
Original	⅛ crust (1.8 oz)	140	3	1	0	5	24	1	1	60	270	—	—	0
Original Mini	½ crust (2.5 oz)	190	3	1	0	6	35	1	1	60	380	—	—	0
Thin Crust	⅕ crust (2 oz)	170	4	2	0	6	28	1	1	80	330	—	—	0
FRENCH MEADOW BAKERY														
Gluten Free	¼ pie (1.9 oz)	160	4	1	0	2	29	2	1	0	310	—	—	2
MARTHA WHITE														
Mix not prep	¼ pkg	160	1	0	0	5	32	2	1	40	250	—	60	0
PILLSBURY														
Classic	⅙ crust (2.3 oz)	160	2	1	0	5	31	4	tr	0	470	—	—	0

FOOD	PORTION	CALS	FAT	SAT FAT	CHOL	PROT	CARB	SUGAR	FIBER	CALCI	SOD	POTAS	FOLIC	VIT C
UDI'S														
Gluten Free	½ crust (4.2 oz)	300	9	1	0	7	47	5	2	20	580	—	—	0
PLANTAINS														
cooked mashed	1 cup	232	tr	tr	0	2	62	28	5	4	10	930	52	22
sliced cooked	1 cup	179	tr	tr	0	1	48	22	4	3	8	716	40	17
DOLE														
Fresh cooked	½ med (3.2 oz)	100	0	0	0	tr	28	13	2	0	0	420	—	9
GRAB EM SNACKS														
Chips Black Pepper	1 oz	150	8	1	0	tr	19	tr	2	0	180	200	—	9
ISLENO														
Chips	1 oz	150	9	1	0	tr	17	0	2	0	35	—	—	5
TAKE-OUT														
mofongo	1 serv	320	3	1	7	9	71	31	5	21	1019	1303	63	25
ripe fried	1 serv (2.8 oz)	214	7	—	—	1	38	—	4	5	—	—	—	10
sweet baked w/ ice cream	1 serv	285	8	5	0	2	57	35	3	37	65	678	35	14
PLUM JUICE														
NANTUCKET NECTARS														
Red Plum	8 oz	120	0	0	0	0	30	30	0	0	25	—	—	0
SUNSWEET														
PlumSmart Light	8 oz	60	0	0	0	0	15	11	3	20	20	135	—	72
PlumSmart w/ Extra Fiber	8 oz	160	0	0	0	0	36	26	3	40	55	360	—	72
PLUMS														
canned purple in heavy syrup	1 cup	163	tr	tr	0	1	42	39	3	18	35	170	5	1
canned purple juice pack	1 cup	146	tr	tr	0	1	38	35	2	25	3	388	8	7
canned purple water pack	1 cup	102	tr	tr	0	1	27	25	2	17	2	314	7	7
dried japanese	1	9	tr	tr	0	tr	2	1	tr	2	96	28	0	0
fresh	1	30	tr	tr	0	tr	8	7	1	4	0	104	3	6
pickled	1	34	tr	tr	0	tr	9	9	tr	1	0	35	1	2
CHIQUITA														
Fresh	1 (2.3 oz)	30	0	0	0	0	8	7	1	0	0	104	—	6
DOLE														
Fresh	2 (5.3 oz)	70	0	0	0	1	17	15	2	0	0	—	—	15
OREGON														
Whole In Heavy Syrup	½ cup (4.6 oz)	100	0	0	0	1	25	19	2	0	25	190	—	0
SUNSWEET														
Plumsweets Dried	14 pieces (1 oz)	120	6	3	0	1	19	13	2	20	5	—	—	0
POI														
poi	1 cup	240	0	0	0	1	65	—	1	38	29	439	50	10

FOOD	PORTION	CALS	FAT	SAT FAT	CHOL	PROT	CARB	SUGAR	FIBER	CALCI	SOD	POTAS	FOLIC	VIT C
POKEBERRY SHOOTS														
cooked	½ cup	16	tr	—	0	2	3	—	—	43	—	—	—	67
fresh	½ cup	18	tr	—	0	2	3	—	—	42	—	—	—	109
POLENTA														
BOB'S RED MILL														
Corn Grits Polenta not prep	¼ cup	130	1	0	0	3	27	0	2	—	0	—	—	—
POLLACK														
atlantic baked	3 oz	100	1	tr	77	21	0	0	0	65	94	388	—	—
atlantic fillet baked	5.3 oz	178	2	tr	137	38	0	0	0	116	166	689	—	—
POMEGRANATE														
fresh	1 (5.4 oz)	105	tr	tr	0	1	26	26	1	5	5	399	9	9
NAVITAS NATURALS														
Pomegranate Powder	1 tbsp (0.5 oz)	50	0	0	0	0	13	3	0	0	35	—	—	2
POMEGRANATE JUICE														
APPLE & EVE														
Organic	8 oz	130	0	0	0	0	33	30	—	—	25	260	—	60
ARTHUR'S														
Pom Plus	1 bottle (11 oz)	220	0	0	0	1	54	33	1	60	25	790	40	27
FRUTZZO														
Organic 100% Juice	1 bottle (12 oz)	130	0	0	0	0	32	29	0	0	25	320	—	6
LANGERS														
100% Juice	8 oz	150	0	0	0	0	37	34	—	—	15	590	—	27
ODWALLA														
PomaGrand 100% Juice	8 oz	160	0	0	0	0	40	31	0	60	30	540	—	0
POM														
100% Juice	8 oz	160	0	0	0	0	40	34	0	0	10	430	—	0
Pomegranate Blueberry	8 oz	160	0	0	0	0	39	33	0	10	20	340	—	0
Pomegranate Mango	8 oz	140	0	0	0	0	36	28	0	0	10	470	—	0
SMART JUICE														
Organic 100% Juice	8 oz	149	0	0	0	1	37	33	1	40	25	360	—	12
TART IS SMART														
Concentrate	0.5 oz	37	0	0	0	0	9	9	0	—	2	137	—	—
ULTRA LO-GLY														
Pomegranate	1 bottle (10 oz)	45	0	0	0	0	10	9	0	0	10	—	—	0
Pomegranate Mojita	1 bottle (10 oz)	40	0	0	0	0	9	7	0	20	15	—	—	0
POMPANO														
smoked	2 oz	109	6	2	33	12	0	0	0	15	215	252	9	0

FOOD	PORTION	CALS	FAT	SAT FAT	CHOL	PROT	CARB	SUGAR	FIBER	CALCI	SOD	POTAS	FOLIC	VIT C
steamed or poached	4 oz	156	9	3	47	18	0	0	0	21	55	308	11	0
TAKE-OUT														
battered & fried	4 oz	304	21	6	67	20	8	tr	tr	46	132	398	26	0
breaded & fried	4 oz	242	15	4	63	16	10	1	1	46	438	319	21	0

POPCORN

(*see also* POPCORN CAKES)

FOOD	PORTION	CALS	FAT	SAT FAT	CHOL	PROT	CARB	SUGAR	FIBER	CALCI	SOD	POTAS	FOLIC	VIT C
air popped	1 cup (0.3 oz)	31	tr	tr	0	1	6	—	2	1	0	24	2	0
caramel coated	1 cup (1.2 oz)	152	5	1	—	1	28	14	2	15	72	38	—	0
caramel coated w/ peanuts	⅔ cup (1 oz)	114	2	tr	0	2	23	11	1	19	84	101	—	0
cheese	1 cup (0.4 oz)	58	4	1	1	1	6	—	1	12	98	29	—	tr
oil popped	1 cup (0.4 oz)	55	3	1	0	1	6	tr	1	1	97	25	2	0
BACHMAN														
Regular	2¾ cups (1 oz)	160	10	1	0	2	14	0	6	0	225	—	—	0
CHIP'INS														
Chips Hot Buffalo Wing	18 (1 oz)	130	5	0	0	2	21	0	1	0	230	—	—	0
Chips Jalapeno Ranch	18 (1 oz)	130	4	0	0	2	21	0	1	0	230	—	—	4
Chips Sea Salt	18 (1 oz)	120	3	0	0	2	22	0	1	0	230	—	—	0
Chips White Cheddar	18 (1 oz)	130	4	0	0	2	21	1	1	20	240	—	—	0
CRACKER JACK														
The Original	½ cup (1 oz)	120	2	0	0	2	23	15	1	0	70	—	—	0
DALE & THOMAS														
Hall Of Fame Kettlecorn	½ cup	34	1	0	0	0	6	6	1	0	22	—	—	0
North Country Cheddar	½ cup	73	5	1	1	1	7	1	1	0	68	—	—	0
Peanut Butter & White Chocolate Drizzlecorn	½ cup	115	6	3	0	1	15	12	1	0	83	—	—	0
Purepopped Natural	½ cup	26	2	0	0	1	3	0	1	0	20	—	—	0
Sweet Georgia Pecan	½ cup	96	3	1	3	1	18	10	1	0	123	—	—	0
Toffee Crunch Drizzlecorn	½ cup	107	5	2	1	3	15	11	1	0	88	—	—	0
DEEP RIVER SNACKS														
Sharp White Cheddar	1 oz	150	10	2	5	3	13	3	2	60	200	—	—	0
DIVVIES														
Caramel Corn Vegan	½ cup	80	3	1	0	tr	14	10	tr	0	35	—	—	0

FOOD	PORTION	CALS	FAT	SAT FAT	CHOL	PROT	CARB	SUGAR	FIBER	CALCI	SOD	POTAS	FOLIC	VIT C
G.H.CRETORS														
Chicago Mix	1¼ cup (1 oz)	140	8	2	10	2	17	10	1	20	220	—	—	0
Just The Cheese	2 cups (1 oz)	170	13	3	5	3	10	0	2	40	340	—	—	0
Kettle Corn	2 cups (1 oz)	130	7	1	0	2	18	6	2	0	210	—	—	0
I.M. HEALTHY														
Roasted Sweet Corn Original Lightly Salted	1 oz	120	5	1	0	3	20	1	2	0	46	—	—	0
JAY'S														
Caramel	¾ cup	110	0	0	0	tr	26	17	1	0	80	—	—	0
Ok-Ke-Doke Cheese	1 oz	160	11	3	10	2	13	1	2	20	270	—	—	0
LANCE														
White Cheddar	1 pkg (0.7 oz)	100	11	3	0	1	8	1	2	0	250	—	—	4
MRS. FIELDS														
Clusters Butter Toffee Crunch	⅔ cup	170	5	2	<5	2	31	20	3	0	180	—	—	0
NEWMAN'S OWN														
Microwave Low Sodium Butter	3½ cups	130	5	2	0	2	18	0	3	0	100	—	—	0
ORVILLE REDENBACHER'S														
Microwave Smart Pop 94% Fat Free as prep	1 cup	15	0	0	0	4	3	—	1	—	24	35	—	—
POPCORN INDIANA														
Kettlecorn Cinnamon Sugar	2½ cups (1 oz)	130	5	0	0	1	21	7	2	0	115	—	—	0
Kettlecorn Sweet & Tangy BBQ	2½ cups (1 oz)	130	5	0	0	1	21	7	2	0	160	—	—	0
Original Movie Theater	2 cups (1 oz)	160	12	2	5	2	13	0	3	0	190	—	—	0
Sea Salt	3 cups (1 oz)	130	6	0	0	3	18	0	3	0	190	—	—	0
POPCORNERS														
Butter	1 oz	120	4	0	0	2	21	1	tr	0	280	—	40	0
Jalapeno	1 oz	130	5	0	0	2	19	1	tr	20	115	—	40	0
Kettle	1 oz	120	4	0	0	2	21	2	tr	0	105	—	40	0
SeaSalt	1 oz	130	3	0	0	2	22	0	0	0	170	—	—	0
White Cheddar	1 oz	130	5	0	0	2	19	1	tr	20	115	—	40	0
POPPYCOCK														
Cashew Lovers	½ cup (1.1 oz)	148	6	0	5	2	21	12	tr	0	90	—	—	0
Original	½ cup (1.1 oz)	160	8	2	10	2	20	13	1	0	90	—	—	0
Pecan Delight	½ cup (1.1 oz)	150	8	2	10	1	20	13	0	0	90	—	—	0
SMART BALANCE														
Movie Style as prep	1 cup	35	2	1	0	—	3	0	1	0	24	—	—	0

FOOD	PORTION	CALS	FAT	SAT FAT	CHOL	PROT	CARB	SUGAR	FIBER	CALCI	SOD	POTAS	FOLIC	VIT C
SMART BALANCE (CONT.)														
Smart 'N Healthy as prep	1 cup	20	0	0	0	4	6	0	1	0	0	—	—	0
SMARTFOOD														
Kettle Corn	1¼ cups (1 oz)	140	6	1	0	tr	20	11	2	40	110	—	—	0
Reduced Fat White Cheddar	3 cups (1 oz)	130	6	1	0	3	18	0	3	20	250	60	—	0
White Cheddar	1¾ cups (1 oz)	160	10	2	<5	3	14	2	2	60	290	100	—	0
SNYDER'S OF HANOVER														
Butter	0.6 oz	100	8	1	0	1	6	0	1	0	150	—	—	0
THE WHOLE EARTH														
Organic Kettle Corn Salty & Sweet	2 cups (1 oz)	120	5	0	0	2	20	9	2	0	130	—	—	0
TREE OF LIFE														
Organic Lightly Salted	4 cups	100	2	0	0	3	21	0	5	0	350	—	—	0
UTZ														
Butter	2 cups	170	12	3	0	2	13	tr	2	0	250	—	—	0
Cheese	2 cups	160	11	2	5	2	14	1	3	0	300	—	—	0
Puff'n Corn Original Hulless	2 cups	150	17	3	0	1	11	0	0	20	150	—	—	0
WISE														
Butter	1 pkg (0.5 oz)	80	5	1	0	1	7	0	1	0	140	—	—	0
POPCORN CAKES														
(see also RICE CAKES)														
ORVILLE REDENBACHER'S														
Chocolate	1	45	0	0	0	tr	10	4	tr	0	20	—	—	0
POPOVER														
home recipe as prep w/ 2% milk	1 (1.4 oz)	87	3	1	46	4	11	—	—	38	82	65	7	tr
home recipe as prep w/ whole milk	1 (1.4 oz)	90	3	1	47	4	11	—	—	37	82	64	7	tr
mix as prep	1 (1.2 oz)	67	2	tr	—	3	10	—	—	9	143	25	—	—
POPPY SEEDS														
poppy seeds	1 tbsp	47	4	tr	0	2	2	1	1	127	2	62	5	tr
BOB'S RED MILL														
Poppy Seeds	3 tbsp	170	14	2	0	6	6	0	3	—	0	—	—	—
LOVE'N BAKE														
Poppy Seed Filling	2 tbsp	120	5	0	0	2	18	16	tr	150	15	—	—	0
PORGY														
fresh	3 oz	77	tr	—	—	18	0	0	0	41	52	415	—	—

FOOD	PORTION	CALS	FAT	SAT FAT	CHOL	PROT	CARB	SUGAR	FIBER	CALCI	SOD	POTAS	FOLIC	VIT C
PORK														
(see also HAM, JERKY, PORK DISHES*)*														
FRESH														
boneless loin lean & fat roasted	3.5 oz	195	9	3	80	26	0	0	0	7	46	348	—	0
center loin chop bone in broiled	1 (3 oz)	178	9	3	71	22	0	0	0	20	46	293	—	0
center rib chop lean & fat bone in broiled	1 (3 oz)	189	11	4	57	21	0	0	0	24	46	279	—	0
country style ribs bone in lean & fat braised	3.5 oz	288	19	7	110	28	0	0	0	36	61	299	—	0
dehydrated oriental style	1 cup (0.8 oz)	135	14	5	15	3	tr	0	0	2	151	31	0	0
fresh ham rump half lean & fat roasted	4 oz	278	16	6	106	32	0	0	0	13	69	413	3	tr
fresh ham shank half lean & fat roasted	4 oz	319	22	8	102	28	0	0	0	17	65	373	6	tr
fresh ham whole lean & fat roasted	4 oz	302	19	7	104	30	0	0	0	15	66	389	11	tr
ground cooked	4 oz	328	23	9	104	28	0	0	0	24	81	400	7	1
ham hock cooked	1	167	12	4	56	14	0	0	0	9	128	187	2	tr
shoulder chop bone in braised	1 (3 oz)	229	15	6	84	23	0	0	0	22	49	259	—	0
sirloin roast lean & fat bone in roasted	4 oz	231	13	4	89	27	0	0	0	15	57	340	—	0
spareribs bone in roasted	3 oz	304	26	8	89	18	0	0	0	16	77	225	—	0
tail simmered	3 oz	336	30	11	110	15	0	0	0	11	21	—	3	0
tenderloin roast boneless lean & fat roasted	4 oz	145	4	1	73	26	0	0	0	6	49	419	—	0
top loin chop boneless lean & fat broiled	1 (3.5 oz)	195	9	3	73	27	0	0	0	7	44	358	—	0
BOAR'S HEAD														
Smoked Shoulder Butt Roast	3 oz	170	13	5	55	13	tr	tr	—	—	760	—	—	—
DIETZ & WATSON														
Chops Boneless Smoked	3 oz	110	3	1	40	15	3	3	0	0	750	—	—	0
Shoulder Butt	3 oz	150	9	3	50	15	1	1	0	0	740	—	—	0

FOOD	PORTION	CALS	FAT	SAT FAT	CHOL	PROT	CARB	SUGAR	FIBER	CALCI	SOD	POTAS	FOLIC	VIT C
DIETZ & WATSON (CONT.)														
Spare Ribs Canadian Center Cut	1 serv (5 oz)	300	20	8	76	16	15	1	0	0	500	—	—	0
HATFIELD														
Chop Center Cut Boneless	1 (4 oz)	130	4	2	45	19	2	0	0	0	620	—	—	1
HORMEL														
Always Tender Loin Filet Honey Mustard	1 serv (4 oz)	140	5	2	45	20	4	4	0	0	510	—	—	0
Always Tender Tenderloin	1 serv (4 oz)	140	4	2	50	19	5	4	0	0	500	—	—	0
Apple Bourbon Pork Roast Au Jus	1 serv (2 oz)	90	3	1	25	8	10	10	0	0	510	—	—	0
ORGANIC PRAIRIE														
Chop Bone In	1 (3.3 oz)	220	13	5	80	26	0	0	0	20	55	—	—	0
SMITHFIELD														
Boneless Smoked Pork Chop	3 oz	110	4	1	45	15	4	3	0	20	820	—	—	1
Smoked Pork Chop	3 oz	100	3	1	30	14	2	2	0	20	1070	—	—	0
TYSON														
Baby Back Ribs Buffalo	4 oz	300	24	9	80	16	4	1	0	40	1080	—	—	1
Ground Reduced Fat	4 oz	260	20	7	65	18	0	0	0	0	320	—	—	0
Half Loin Boneless	4 oz	190	12	5	45	20	0	0	0	0	270	—	—	0
Loin Chops Bone-In Center Cut	4 oz	190	13	5	45	20	0	0	0	0	330	—	—	0
Spareribs	4 oz	290	24	9	80	16	0	0	0	40	330	—	—	0
Stew Meat	4 oz	130	5	2	65	21	0	0	0	0	300	—	—	0
FROZEN														
ORGANIC PRAIRIE														
Ribs Boneless Country Style	1 (4 oz)	160	7	3	75	23	0	0	0	20	55	—	—	1
Tenderloin	4 oz	150	6	2	75	23	0	0	0	0	55	—	—	1
TAKE-OUT														
char siu chinese style	1 piece (0.4 oz)	28	2	1	7	2	2	—	0	4	72	32	tr	0
chicharrones pork cracklings fried	1 cup	492	38	13	100	34	1	0	0	10	2102	514	2	0
chop breaded & fried	1 lg (5 oz)	441	26	8	126	30	19	2	1	76	835	453	28	tr
chop breaded & fried	1 med (3.4 oz)	304	18	5	87	20	13	1	1	53	577	313	19	tr
chop stewed	1 lg (4.6 oz)	315	18	7	106	36	0	0	0	28	63	494	4	1

FOOD	PORTION	CALS	FAT	SAT FAT	CHOL	PROT	CARB	SUGAR	FIBER	CALCI	SOD	POTAS	FOLIC	VIT C
PORK DISHES														
A LA CARTE GOURMET														
Pork Loin w/ Cream Spinach Feta Stuffing	1 serv (5 oz)	200	9	5	85	20	8	3	tr	80	600	—	—	—
TYSON														
Roast Pork w/ Vegetables	1 serv (4 oz)	190	4	2	60	21	18	0	2	40	190	—	—	12
VENTERA														
Pork Carnitas	1 serv (5 oz)	190	8	2	70	23	6	1	1	40	390	—	—	1
TAKE-OUT														
kalua pork	1 cup (7 oz)	497	34	13	157	43	1	—	0	55	3498	629	11	1
pork satay w/ peanut sauce	5 sticks (3.5 oz)	214	13	4	74	12	14	—	3	21	318	—	—	—
pulled pork w/ barbecue sauce	1 serv (5 oz)	240	14	5	55	14	15	12	1	40	680	—	—	18
spareribs barbecue w/ sauce	2 med (2.8 oz)	248	18	6	70	17	3	1	tr	32	267	230	3	2
tourtiere	1 piece (4.9 oz)	451	34	10	—	15	21	—	—	18	—	—	—	—
PORK RINDS														
(see SNACKS*)*														
POT PIE														
AMY'S														
Broccoli	1 (7.5 oz)	430	22	10	45	11	46	3	4	150	630	—	—	27
Shepherd's	1 (8 oz)	160	4	0	0	5	27	5	5	100	590	—	—	18
Shepherd's Pie Light In Sodium	1 (8 oz)	160	4	0	0	5	27	5	5	100	290	—	—	18
Vegetable	1 (7.5 oz)	360	13	2	0	10	50	3	4	60	640	—	—	3
BANQUET														
Beef	1	450	27	11	30	14	36	7	2	0	730	—	—	2
Chicken	1	370	21	9	35	10	34	5	2	20	850	—	—	0
Chicken w/ Broccoli	1	350	20	9	30	10	32	4	2	20	800	—	—	0
Turkey	1	390	21	9	35	10	36	3	2	20	840	—	—	0
BELL & EVANS														
Chicken	1 cup (7.9 oz)	520	29	13	80	16	48	3	2	40	630	—	—	5
HOT POCKETS														
Pot Pie Express Chicken	1 (4.5 oz)	330	18	6	15	8	34	8	2	100	760	—	—	—
IAN'S														
Chicken	1 pkg (9.4 oz)	510	23	10	65	26	50	2	2	40	600	—	—	1
MARIE CALLENDER'S														
Beef	½ pie	540	32	12	25	16	46	4	3	0	700	—	—	0
Cheesy Chicken	½ pie	600	37	15	30	17	46	5	3	100	850	—	—	0

FOOD	PORTION	CALS	FAT	SAT FAT	CHOL	PROT	CARB	SUGAR	FIBER	CALCI	SOD	POTAS	FOLIC	VIT C
MARIE CALLENDER'S (CONT.)														
Chicken	1	670	41	14	35	19	55	4	3	40	1000	—	—	0
Creamy Mushroom & Chicken	½ pie	560	35	13	30	15	45	4	3	60	700	—	—	0
Turkey	1	670	41	16	25	19	56	6	4	40	1000	—	—	0
MON CUISINE														
Vegan	1 pkg (9 oz)	650	39	6	0	21	60	6	8	—	850	—	—	—
PACIFIC FOODS														
Organic Beef	1 cup (8 oz)	410	21	12	80	17	40	0	6	20	660	—	—	1
Organic Turkey	1 cup (8 oz)	400	19	11	70	15	46	1	7	40	850	—	—	1
PEPPERIDGE FARM														
Chili Beans & Cornbread	1 cup	360	17	5	20	11	40	11	3	40	890	—	—	9
Reduced Fat Roasted White Meat Chicken	1 cup	470	21	7	25	14	56	9	0	40	900	—	—	5
Roasted White Meat Chicken	1 cup	510	32	9	30	13	43	7	3	60	870	—	—	4
STOUFFER'S														
Chicken White Meat	1 pkg (10 oz)	660	37	14	50	19	62	14	2	150	1060	—	—	0
TAKE-OUT														
beef	1 (14.6 oz)	938	57	13	67	34	72	4	5	42	1660	709	129	14
chicken	1 (14.6 oz)	897	52	16	113	37	69	5	6	108	1080	646	133	17
ham	1 serv (11 oz)	752	45	10	38	28	58	3	4	38	1937	588	104	12
oyster	1 serv (11.5 oz)	817	53	15	89	19	67	6	3	220	1056	515	115	4
puerto rican pastelon de carne	1 piece (5 oz)	666	48	18	93	22	35	1	2	170	1476	359	63	5
st. stephen's day pie	1 serv (16.7 oz)	549	29	16	198	35	38	5	6	90	474	—	—	41
tuna	1 (27 oz)	1715	102	30	92	71	126	10	10	192	1953	1138	231	16
vegetarian w/ meat substitute	1 (8 oz)	511	32	9	20	17	39	3	5	68	543	247	102	9

POTATO

(see also CHIPS, KNISH, PANCAKES)

FOOD	PORTION	CALS	FAT	SAT FAT	CHOL	PROT	CARB	SUGAR	FIBER	CALCI	SOD	POTAS	FOLIC	VIT C
CANNED														
potatoes	½ cup	54	tr	tr	0	1	12	—	—	5	—	206	6	5
BUTTERFIELD														
Whole White	3.5 pieces (5.8 oz)	90	0	0	0	2	20	0	2	60	330	—	—	15
DEL MONTE														
Savory Sides Au Gratin	½ cup	80	3	1	0	2	13	1	1	40	470	—	—	6
S&W														
New Whole	2 (5.5 oz)	60	0	0	0	1	13	0	2	20	360	—	—	9

FOOD	PORTION	CALS	FAT	SAT FAT	CHOL	PROT	CARB	SUGAR	FIBER	CALCI	SOD	POTAS	FOLIC	VIT C
SUNSHINE														
Whole White	3 pieces (5.9 oz)	90	0	0	0	2	20	0	2	60	330	—	—	15
FRESH														
baked skin only	1 skin (2 oz)	115	tr	tr	0	2	27	—	2	20	12	332	—	8
baked w/ skin	1 (6.5 oz)	220	tr	tr	0	5	51	—	—	20	16	844	22	26
baked w/o skin	1 (5 oz)	145	tr	tr	0	3	34	—	2	8	8	610	14	20
baked w/o skin	½ cup	57	tr	tr	0	1	13	—	1	3	3	238	6	8
boiled	½ cup	68	tr	tr	0	1	16	—	1	4	3	295	8	10
microwaved	1 (7 oz)	212	tr	tr	0	5	49	—	—	22	16	903	24	31
microwaved w/o skin	½ cup	78	tr	tr	0	2	18	—	—	4	5	321	10	12
raw w/o skin	1 (3.9 oz)	88	tr	tr	0	2	20	—	—	8	7	608	14	22
DOLE														
Idaho	1 (5.3 oz)	110	0	0	0	3	26	1	2	20	0	620	—	27
GREEN GIANT														
Klondike Gourmet	5 sm (5.3 oz)	110	0	0	0	3	26	1	2	20	0	620	—	27
Red Potatoes	1 med (5 oz)	100	0	0	0	4	26	3	3	20	0	720	—	27
MASSER'S														
Roasted Russet Triple Washed	1 (5.3 oz)	110	0	0	0	3	26	1	2	20	0	620	24	27
MELISSA'S														
Dutch Yellow Baby diced	¾ cup (3.9 oz)	80	0	0	0	2	20	tr	2	80	35	—	—	4
FROZEN														
french fries	10 strips	111	4	2	0	2	17	—	2	4	15	229	8	6
french fries thick cut	10 strips	109	4	2	0	2	17	—	—	5	23	240	9	5
hash browns	½ cup	170	9	4	—	2	22	—	—	12	27	340	—	5
potato puffs	½ cup	138	7	3	0	2	19	—	—	19	462	236	10	4
potato puffs	1	16	1	tr	0	tr	2	—	—	2	52	27	1	1
ALEXIA														
Sweet Potato Puffs	⅔ cup (3 oz)	130	4	0	0	1	23	8	2	20	230	170	—	4
BIRDS EYE														
Steamfresh Roasted Red Potatoes w/ Garlic Butter Sauce	1¼ cups (5.1 oz)	190	7	5	20	3	30	0	3	20	390	—	—	15
CASCADIAN FARM														
Organic Country Style	¾ cup	50	0	0	0	1	12	0	1	0	10	220	—	5
Organic Hash Browns	1 cup	60	0	0	0	2	14	0	1	0	10	240	—	5
FUNSTER														
BBQ Lite	14 pieces (3 oz)	140	3	0	0	2	25	tr	<2	20	500	—	—	2

FOOD	PORTION	CALS	FAT	SAT FAT	CHOL	PROT	CARB	SUGAR	FIBER	CALCI	SOD	POTAS	FOLIC	VIT C
FUNSTER (CONT.)														
Cheddar	14 pieces (3 oz)	135	3	0	0	2	25	tr	<2	30	385	—	—	2
Original	14 pieces (3 oz)	135	3	0	0	2	25	tr	2	20	230	—	—	2
GREEN GIANT														
Roasted Potatoes w/ Garlic & Herb Sauce as prep	½ cup	90	2	1	0	2	15	1	1	60	420	—	—	—
HEALTH IS WEALTH														
Twice Baked Cheddar Cheese	1 (5 oz)	200	10	3	10	4	25	2	2	60	340	—	—	15
Vegetarian Potato Skins	2 (2.7 oz)	110	7	4	15	5	8	0	1	150	440	—	—	12
IAN'S														
Alphatots	1 serv (3.5 oz)	156	7	5	0	2	23	1	1	—	160	—	—	5
JOY OF COOKING														
Elegant Scalloped	1 cup (8 oz)	300	17	11	50	9	21	2	2	—	710	—	—	—
Red Skin Mashed	1 cup (4.2 oz)	160	9	5	25	3	17	2	2	—	720	—	—	—
LARRY'S														
Mashed Broccoli & Cheddar Cheese	1 serv (5 oz)	180	8	2	0	3	22	7	2	80	390	—	—	4
Mashed Cheddar Cheese	1 serv (5 oz)	190	8	2	5	4	25	8	2	100	460	—	—	2
Mashed Old Fashioned Butter	1 serv (5 oz)	190	9	3	10	3	25	9	2	80	370	—	—	2
Mashed Sour Cream & Chives	1 serv (5 oz)	180	8	2	5	3	25	8	2	80	440	—	—	2
Mashed Sweet Potatoes	1 serv (4 oz)	140	4	2	10	2	27	11	2	200	530	—	—	4
LEAN CUISINE														
Simple Favorites Cheddar Potato w/ Broccoli	1 pkg (10.25 oz)	210	4	2	15	10	34	6	4	200	600	820	—	36
MCCAIN														
5 Minute Fries	1 serv (3 oz)	120	5	1	0	1	16	tr	1	0	290	270	—	6
Farmer's Kitchen Oven Baked Crinkles	12 pieces (2 oz)	50	1	0	0	1	11	0	1	0	130	180	—	4
Purely Potatoes Whole Baby Skin On	1 serv (3 oz)	100	0	0	0	2	16	0	tr	0	25	170	—	6
MIX														
au gratin as prep	½ cup	160	9	6	29	6	14	—	—	146	528	483	10	12
instant mashed flakes as prep w/ whole milk & butter	½ cup	118	6	4	15	2	16	—	—	52	349	245	8	10

FOOD	PORTION	CALS	FAT	SAT FAT	CHOL	PROT	CARB	SUGAR	FIBER	CALCI	SOD	POTAS	FOLIC	VIT C
instant mashed flakes not prep	½ cup	78	tr	tr	0	2	18	—	—	5	24	239	9	18
instant mashed granules as prep w/ whole milk & butter	½ cup	114	5	3	15	2	15	—	—	37	270	152	8	6
instant mashed granules not prep	½ cup	372	1	tr	0	8	86	—	—	41	67	703	40	37
scalloped	½ cup	105	5	3	14	4	13	—	—	70	409	461	10	13
BETTY CROCKER														
Au Gratin as prep	⅔ cup	150	5	1	0	2	24	0	1	40	624	—	—	2
Cheddar & Bacon as prep	⅔ cup	120	3	1	0	2	21	1	1	40	696	240	—	—
Cheesy Scalloped as prep	½ cup	120	3	1	0	2	21	1	1	40	600	270	—	—
Julienne as prep	⅔ cup	140	5	1	0	2	20	1	1	40	624	—	—	—
Mashed Creamy Butter as prep	⅔ cup	80	1	1	<5	2	17	1	3	—	460	—	—	2
Mashed Four Cheese as prep	½ cup	170	7	2	6	2	21	1	1	100	480	455	—	—
Mashed Sour Cream & Chives as prep	½ cup	170	7	2	6	2	21	1	1	100	456	420	—	—
Scalloped as prep	½ cup	130	4	1	0	2	20	1	1	40	624	280	—	1
Seasoned Skillets Hash Browns as prep	½ cup	120	4	1	0	2	19	0	2	—	456	250	—	—
IDAHOAN														
Mashed Buttery Homestyle as prep	½ cup	110	3	1	0	2	20	2	1	20	450	—	—	4
Mashed Buttery Yukon as prep	½ cup	110	3	1	0	2	21	2	2	20	400	—	—	0
Mashed Original as prep	½ cup	170	7	1	0	2	24	0	2	60	456	—	—	4
Mashed Roasted Garlic & Parmesan as prep	½ cup	110	2	1	0	3	21	1	2	20	560	—	—	4
REFRIGERATED														
BOB EVANS														
Mashed Potatoes Original	½ cup (4.4 oz)	150	7	4	15	3	20	1	2	20	410	—	—	0
COUNTRY CROCK														
Garlic Mashed	⅔ cup (5 oz)	160	7	3	10	2	22	1	2	20	430	—	—	9
Homestyle Mashed	⅔ cup (5 oz)	160	9	4	15	2	18	1	1	20	510	—	—	0
Loaded Mashed	⅔ cup (5 oz)	200	11	5	25	4	22	2	2	60	410	—	—	6

FOOD	PORTION	CALS	FAT	SAT FAT	CHOL	PROT	CARB	SUGAR	FIBER	CALCI	SOD	POTAS	FOLIC	VIT C
DINER'S CHOICE														
Mashed	⅔ cup	110	5	3	10	2	15	3	3	40	500	—	—	0
RESER'S														
Potato Express Red Skinned Mashed	½ cup	140	5	3	15	3	22	1	2	20	310	—	—	2
SIMPLY POTATOES														
Traditional Mashed	½ cup (4.4 oz)	120	6	4	20	2	15	1	2	30	420	—	—	0
SHELF-STABLE														
TASTYBITE														
Bombay Potatoes	½ pkg (5 oz)	105	4	tr	0	5	13	2	3	50	412	—	—	3
TAKE-OUT														
au gratin w/ cheese	½ cup	178	10	4	18	7	17	—	—	156	548	375	—	12
baked topped w/ cheese sauce	1	475	29	11	19	15	47	—	—	310	381	1167	28	26
baked topped w/ cheese sauce & bacon	1	451	26	10	30	18	44	—	—	309	973	1179	28	29
baked topped w/ cheese sauce & broccoli	1 (12 oz)	403	21	9	20	14	47	—	—	336	485	1441	61	49
baked topped w/ cheese sauce & chili	1	481	22	13	31	23	56	—	—	409	701	1570	50	32
baked topped w/ sour cream & chives	1	394	22	10	23	7	50	—	—	105	182	1383	32	34
cheese fries w/ ranch dressing	1 serv	3010	—	—	—	—	—	—	—	—	—	—	—	—
french fries	1 reg	235	12	4	0	3	29	—	—	12	124	541	25	4
hash browns	½ cup (2.5 oz)	151	9	4	9	2	16	—	—	7	290	267	8	6
indian yogurt potatoes	1 serv	315	9	4	18	7	52	—	0	—	216	—	—	—
mashed	½ cup	111	4	1	2	2	18	—	—	27	309	303	0	6
o'brien	1 cup	157	3	2	7	5	30	—	—	70	421	516	16	32
potato pancakes	1 (1.3 oz)	101	7	1	35	2	11	—	—	9	188	291	9	8
potato salad	½ cup	179	10	2	85	3	14	—	2	24	661	318	9	13
red new boiled	5 sm (5 oz)	120	0	0	0	3	27	3	2	20	5	680	—	24
scalloped	½ cup	127	5	—	7	4	18	—	—	66	435	401	—	13
twice baked w/ cheese	1 half (10 oz)	392	18	10	54	8	48	—	4	400	810	—	—	29
POTATO STARCH														
potato starch	1 oz	96	tr	—	0	tr	24	—	—	10	1	4	—	0
BOB'S RED MILL														
Potato Starch	1 tbsp	40	0	0	0	0	10	0	0	—	0	—	—	—

FOOD	PORTION	CALS	FAT	SAT FAT	CHOL	PROT	CARB	SUGAR	FIBER	CALCI	SOD	POTAS	FOLIC	VIT C
POUT														
ocean baked	3 oz	87	1	tr	57	18	0	0	0	11	66	436	7	0
ocean fillet baked	1 (4.8 oz)	140	2	1	92	29	0	0	0	18	107	703	11	0
PRETZELS														
chocolate covered	1 (0.4 oz)	47	1	tr	1	1	8	2	tr	7	110	23	15	0
soft	1 lg (5 oz)	483	4	1	4	12	99	tr	2	33	2008	126	34	0
twists salted	10 (2.1 oz)	229	2	tr	0	6	48	—	2	22	1029	88	50	0
twists w/o salt	10 (2.1 oz)	229	2	tr	0	5	48	1	2	22	173	88	103	0
whole wheat	2 sm (1 oz)	103	1	tr	0	3	23	—	2	8	58	122	15	tr
yogurt covered	1 cup (3 oz)	391	13	11	1	7	61	30	1	101	588	191	79	tr
yogurt covered	1 (4 g)	19	1	1	0	tr	3	1	tr	5	29	9	4	0
ANNIE'S HOMEGROWN														
Organic Bunnies	32 (1 oz)	100	1	0	0	3	19	1	1	0	360	—	—	0
BACHMAN														
Honey Wheat Splits	9 (1 oz)	110	1	0	0	3	23	3	1	0	190	—	—	0
Mini Low Sodium	17 (1 oz)	110	0	0	0	3	25	—	1	0	50	—	—	0
Original Twist	5 (1 oz)	100	1	0	0	3	22	1	1	0	440	—	—	0
Rolled Rods	2 (1 oz)	110	0	0	0	3	23	1	1	0	240	—	—	0
Thin N Rights	12 (1 oz)	120	1	0	0	3	23	1	1	100	125	—	—	0
BETTER BALANCE														
Cinnamon Toast Gluten Free	1 oz	120	5	2	0	10	9	0	3	40	150	—	—	0
Golden Butter Twists Gluten Free	1 oz	110	5	2	0	10	12	1	2	40	220	—	—	—
Jalapeno Mustard Gluten Free	1 oz	120	5	2	0	10	9	2	3	10	150	—	—	0
BRAIDS														
Honey Wheat	7 (1 oz)	110	2	0	0	3	23	4	1	0	280	—	—	0
Mini Knots	17 (1 oz)	110	1	0	0	3	23	tr	tr	0	340	—	—	0
FARM RICH														
Stuffed Bites frzn	3 (1.7 oz)	110	3	2	5	4	18	2	1	40	410	—	—	1
GLENNY'S														
Organic Original Salted	8 (1 oz)	110	0	0	0	3	23	1	1	—	480	—	—	—
Organic Sourdough	6 (1 oz)	110	0	0	0	3	23	1	1	—	480	—	—	—
GLUTINO														
Gluten Free All Shapes	44 (1.4 oz)	190	8	4	0	1	28	tr	0	0	540	—	—	0
HEALTHY HANDFULS														
Python Pretzels	1 box (1.5 oz)	170	1	0	0	5	36	0	1	0	360	—	—	0

FOOD	PORTION	CALS	FAT	SAT FAT	CHOL	PROT	CARB	SUGAR	FIBER	CALCI	SOD	POTAS	FOLIC	VIT C
NEW YORK STYLE														
Pretzel Flatz Original Salt	12	110	1	0	0	3	23	0	1	0	250	—	—	0
NEWMAN'S OWN														
Organic Salted Rounds	8	110	1	0	0	2	24	1	tr	—	400	—	—	—
ROLD GOLD														
Braided Twists Honey Wheat	8 (1 oz)	110	1	0	0	3	24	3	1	0	200	—	—	0
Rods	3 (1 oz)	110	1	0	0	3	22	1	1	0	450	90	—	0
Sourdough	1 (0.8 oz)	90	1	0	0	2	19	tr	2	0	500	—	—	0
Sticks	53 (1 oz)	100	0	0	0	2	23	1	1	0	490	70	—	0
Tiny Twists Fat Free	18 (1 oz)	110	0	0	0	3	23	tr	tr	0	450	—	—	0
SALBA SMART														
Omega-3 Enriched	1 oz	110	2	0	0	2	21	1	1	20	330	—	—	0
SNYDER'S OF HANOVER														
100 Calorie Pack Snaps	1 pkg (0.9 oz)	100	1	0	0	3	22	tr	tr	0	340	—	—	0
Dips Milk Chocolate	1 oz	140	6	4	<5	2	19	11	tr	40	100	—	—	0
Dips Special Dark Chocolate	1 oz	140	5	3	<5	2	22	8	2	0	130	—	—	0
Gluten Free Sticks	30 (1 oz)	110	2	1	0	0	25	0	tr	20	260	—	—	0
Mini Unsalted	1 oz	110	0	0	0	3	25	tr	tr	0	75	—	—	0
MultiGrain Sticks Lightly Salted	1 oz	120	2	0	0	3	23	2	3	0	160	—	—	0
MultiGrain Twists	1 oz	120	2	0	0	3	22	2	2	0	170	—	—	0
Nibblers Sourdough	1 oz	120	0	0	0	3	25	tr	tr	0	200	—	—	0
Old Tyme	1 oz	120	1	0	0	3	24	tr	1	0	120	—	—	0
Organic Honey Wheat	1 oz	130	2	0	0	3	24	4	1	0	210	—	—	0
Organic Oat Bran	1 oz	120	0	0	0	3	25	3	2	0	320	—	—	0
Pieces Garlic Bread	1 oz	140	7	3	0	3	18	0	1	0	160	—	—	0
Pieces Honey Mustard & Onions	1 oz	140	7	3	0	2	18	3	tr	0	240	—	—	0
Pieces Hot Buffalo Wing	1 oz	140	7	3	0	2	17	0	tr	0	380	—	—	0
Pretzel Sandwich Peanut Butter	1 oz	140	7	2	0	4	16	2	tr	0	140	—	—	0
Rods	1 oz	120	1	0	0	3	24	tr	1	0	290	—	—	0
Snaps	1 oz	120	1	0	0	3	25	tr	1	0	270	—	—	9

FOOD	PORTION	CALS	FAT	SAT FAT	CHOL	PROT	CARB	SUGAR	FIBER	CALCI	SOD	POTAS	FOLIC	VIT C
SNYDER'S OF HANOVER (CONT.)														
Sourdough Unsalted	1 oz	100	0	0	0	3	22	0	1	0	90	—	—	0
Sticks 12 Multi Grain	1 oz	130	2	0	0	3	22	3	3	20	180	—	—	1
SUPERPRETZEL														
Mozzarella	2 (1.8 oz)	130	4	2	5	6	20	0	1	80	420	—	—	0
Pretzelfils Pizza	2 (1.8 oz)	130	2	1	5	5	22	1	1	60	180	—	—	0
Soft	1 (2.25 oz)	160	1	0	0	5	34	1	1	0	130	—	—	0
Soft Bites	5 (1.9 oz)	150	1	0	0	3	32	1	1	0	912	—	—	0
Softstix	2 (1.8 oz)	130	3	2	1	4	22	1	1	40	260	—	—	0
TOM STURGIS														
Little Cheesers	17 (1 oz)	120	2	1	0	3	22	tr	2	0	380	—	—	0
Little Ones	17 (1 oz)	110	2	0	0	2	22	tr	tr	0	550	—	—	0
UTZ														
Braided Twists Baked Honey Wheat	1 oz	110	2	0	0	3	23	4	1	0	280	—	—	0
Chocolate Covered	6 (1.1 oz)	140	5	5	0	2	22	11	tr	0	220	—	—	0
Hard	1	90	0	0	0	2	18	tr	tr	0	470	—	—	0
Special	1 oz	110	1	0	0	3	21	tr	1	0	470	—	—	0
Special Multigrain	1 oz	110	1	0	0	3	21	1	2	0	340	—	—	0
Sticks Organic Whole Grain	1 oz	120	2	0	0	3	22	1	3	20	200	—	—	0
PRUNE JUICE														
jarred	1 cup	182	tr	tr	0	2	45	42	3	31	10	707	0	11
LAKEWOOD														
Organic	8 oz	165	0	0	0	1	40	16	3	30	5	550	—	11
LANGERS														
Plus 100% Juice	8 oz	180	0	0	0	0	41	23	1	100	10	480	—	60
SUNSWEET														
100% Juice	8 oz	180	0	0	0	2	43	19	3	20	30	530	—	0
TREE OF LIFE														
Organic 100% Juice	8 oz	180	0	0	0	1	43	23	2	20	480	—	—	—
PRUNES														
cooked w/o sugar	½ cup	133	tr	tr	0	1	35	31	4	24	1	398	0	4
dried	1	20	tr	tr	0	tr	5	3	1	4	0	61	0	tr
DEL MONTE														
Dried Pitted	5 (1.5 oz)	100	0	0	0	1	24	12	3	20	5	290	—	0
EARTHBOUND FARMS														
Organic Dried Plums	5	110	0	0	0	1	25	18	3	20	0	—	—	1

FOOD	PORTION	CALS	FAT	SAT FAT	CHOL	PROT	CARB	SUGAR	FIBER	CALCI	SOD	POTAS	FOLIC	VIT C
LOVE'N BAKE														
Prune Lekvar	2 tbsp	90	0	0	0	0	21	17	1	0	120	—	—	1
NEWMAN'S OWN														
Organic	½ cup	110	0	0	0	1	26	13	2	—	5	—	—	—
SUNSWEET														
Ones	4 (1.4 oz)	100	0	0	0	1	24	12	3	20	5	290	—	0
Pitted	5 (1.4 oz)	100	0	0	0	1	24	12	3	20	5	290	—	0
Pitted 60 Calorie Pack	1 pkg (0.9 oz)	60	0	0	0	1	16	8	2	20	0	190	—	0

PUDDING

READY-TO-EAT

JELL-O

FOOD	PORTION	CALS	FAT	SAT FAT	CHOL	PROT	CARB	SUGAR	FIBER	CALCI	SOD	POTAS	FOLIC	VIT C
100 Calorie Pack Fat Free Chocolate Vanilla Swirl	1 pkg (4 oz)	100	0	0	0	2	23	17	tr	100	190	—	—	0
100 Calorie Pack Fat Free Tapioca	1 pkg (4 oz)	100	0	0	0	1	23	17	0	100	210	—	—	0
Boston Cream Pie Sugar Free	1 pkg (4 oz)	60	1	1	0	1	13	0	0	100	170	—	—	0
Dulce De Leche Sugar Free	1 pkg (3.7 oz)	60	1	1	0	1	13	0	0	100	178	—	—	0
Vanilla	1 serv (4 oz)	110	2	2	0	1	23	18	0	100	190	—	—	0
KOZY SHACK														
Banana	1 pkg (4 oz)	130	5	3	15	3	19	15	0	115	120	146	—	0
Bread Pudding Apple Cinnamon	1 pkg (3.5 oz)	150	3	2	40	4	26	19	0	80	110	—	—	1
Chocolate Lactose Free	1 pkg (4 oz)	130	4	2	15	4	22	17	1	100	140	—	—	0
Chocolate No Sugar Added	1 pkg (4 oz)	60	1	1	10	3	10	4	4	89	130	215	—	tr
Old Fashioned Tapioca	1 pkg (4 oz)	130	3	2	10	3	23	17	0	114	130	145	—	1
Real Chocolate	1 pkg (4 oz)	140	4	2	10	4	24	19	1	110	135	240	—	tr
Rice Lactose Free	1 pkg (4 oz)	120	3	2	15	4	20	13	0	100	130	—	—	0
Rice No Sugar Added	1 pkg (4 oz)	70	1	0	10	4	11	5	3	109	120	139	—	0
Rice Original	1 pkg (4 oz)	130	3	2	15	4	21	14	0	106	120	140	—	0
Soy Chocolate	1 pkg (4.4 oz)	120	2	1	0	4	23	12	2	33	80	215	—	0
Soy Vanilla	1 pkg (4.4 oz)	110	2	0	0	4	21	12	1	28	80	75	—	0
Tapioca Lactose Free	1 pkg (4 oz)	120	3	2	15	3	20	15	0	100	135	—	—	1
Tapioca No Sugar Added	1 pkg (4 oz)	70	1	0	5	4	11	5	4	114	135	145	—	0
Vanilla	1 pkg (4 oz)	130	3	2	15	3	21	18	0	110	135	140	—	0
Vanilla No Sugar Added	1 pkg (4 oz)	90	3	2	10	3	10	5	4	106	115	135	—	0

FOOD	PORTION	CALS	FAT	SAT FAT	CHOL	PROT	CARB	SUGAR	FIBER	CALCI	SOD	POTAS	FOLIC	VIT C
SNACK PACK														
Banana Cream Pie	1 pkg (3.5 oz)	110	4	2	0	1	18	13	0	100	150	—	—	0
Butterscotch	1 pkg (3.5 oz)	110	3	2	0	1	21	16	0	100	150	—	—	0
Caramel Cream	1 pkg (3.5 oz)	120	3	2	0	1	21	17	0	40	160	—	—	0
Chocolate	1 pkg (3.5 oz)	130	3	2	0	1	23	16	tr	100	140	—	—	0
Chocolate Daredevil Triples	1 pkg (3.5 oz)	130	4	2	0	1	23	18	tr	100	125	—	—	0
Chocolate Fat Free	1 pkg (3.5 oz)	80	0	0	0	2	20	15	tr	100	140	—	—	0
Chocolate No Sugar Added	1 pkg (3.5 oz)	70	4	2	0	tr	15	0	1	100	110	—	—	0
Lemon	1 pkg (3.5 oz)	130	3	2	0	0	25	20	0	0	65	—	—	0
Tapioca	1 pkg (3.5 oz)	120	4	2	0	2	20	15	0	100	135	—	—	0
Tapioca Fat Free	1 serv (3.5 oz)	80	0	0	0	1	18	13	0	100	160	—	—	0
Vanilla	1 pkg (3.5 oz)	120	4	2	0	tr	21	14	1	100	135	—	—	0
SOYUMMI														
Dark Chocolate	1 pkg (3.5 oz)	110	3	0	0	4	17	11	4	20	80	—	—	—
Key Lime	1 pkg (3.5 oz)	115	4	0	0	4	17	11	2	20	70	—	—	—
SWISS MISS														
Chocolate	1 pkg	150	4	3	0	3	27	22	0	60	190	—	—	0
Chocolate Low Fat	1 pkg	130	2	2	0	3	26	19	0	200	180	—	—	0
Pie Lover's Banana Cream	1 pkg	130	4	4	<5	2	23	17	0	80	170	—	—	0
Pie Lover's Lemon Meringue	1 pkg	140	3	3	0	0	28	21	0	—	600	—	—	—
Swirl Chocolate Vanilla	1 pkg	140	4	3	0	2	27	20	0	60	160	—	—	0
ZENSOY														
Banana	1 pkg (4 oz)	100	1	0	0	2	21	15	1	150	75	—	—	0
Chocolate	1 pkg (4 oz)	130	1	0	0	3	29	21	2	—	75	—	—	—
Vanilla	1 pkg (4 oz)	110	1	0	0	2	23	15	1	150	75	—	—	0
TAKE-OUT														
blancmange	1 serv (4.7 oz)	154	5	—	—	4	25	—	tr	149	—	—	—	tr
bread w/ raisins	1 cup	306	9	3	124	11	47	29	2	238	472	432	40	1
coconut	1 cup	291	9	7	15	8	45	38	2	258	451	370	13	tr
corn	1 cup	328	13	6	185	11	43	17	4	100	703	440	83	9
guinataan coconut milk pudding	1 cup (9 oz)	331	11	9	0	2	59	—	3	26	20	444	20	8
indian pudding	½ cup	156	4	2	40	5	25	16	1	146	220	345	23	0
noodle pudding kugel	1 cup	297	10	2	144	9	44	15	2	39	94	194	56	2
plum pudding	1 slice (1.5 oz)	125	5	3	22	2	20	12	1	43	83	197	6	tr
pumpkin	½ cup (4.6 oz)	139	4	1	4	3	24	19	tr	86	204	183	7	2
queen of puddings	1 serv (4.4 oz)	266	10	—	—	6	41	—	tr	99	—	—	—	1
rice pudding	1 cup	302	4	2	14	8	60	37	1	225	133	403	9	tr
sweet potato	½ cup	107	3	1	1	2	19	7	3	51	310	259	7	13

FOOD	PORTION	CALS	FAT	SAT FAT	CHOL	PROT	CARB	SUGAR	FIBER	CALCI	SOD	POTAS	FOLIC	VIT C
tapioca	1 cup	236	7	3	156	10	35	31	0	211	312	291	18	0
yorkshire	1 serv (3 oz)	177	8	—	57	6	22	—	tr	37	168	45	3	0

PUFFERFISH
raw	3 oz	72	0	0	—	17	0	0	0	12	120	246	—	0

PUMMELO
fresh white	1 (21.4 oz)	231	tr	—	0	5	59	—	6	24	6	1315	—	372
sections white	1 cup (6.7 oz)	72	tr	—	0	1	18	—	2	8	2	410	—	116

PUMPKIN
butter	1 tbsp	32	0	0	0	0	8	8	—	—	0	—	—	—
canned w/o salt	1 cup (8.6 oz)	83	1	tr	0	3	20	8	7	64	12	505	29	10
cooked mashed w/o salt	1 cup (8.6 oz)	49	tr	tr	0	2	12	3	3	37	2	564	22	12
flowers cooked w/o salt	1 cup (4.7 oz)	20	tr	tr	0	1	4	3	1	50	8	142	55	7
leaves cooked w/o salt	1 cup (2.5 oz)	15	tr	tr	0	2	2	tr	2	31	6	311	18	1
FARMER'S MARKET														
Organic Puree	½ cup (4.3 oz)	50	0	0	0	1	10	4	4	40	6	—	—	5
JAKE & AMOS														
Pumpkin Butter	1 tbsp (0.5 oz)	5	0	0	0	0	1	1	0	0	0	—	—	1
LIBBY'S														
Pumpkin	½ cup (4.3 oz)	40	1	0	0	2	9	4	5	20	5	—	—	1
TREE OF LIFE														
Organic Puree	½ cup (4.3 oz)	50	0	0	0	1	10	4	4	40	5	—	—	5
TAKE-OUT														
indian sago	1 serv (2.3 oz)	75	5	2	0	2	6	3	3	49	222	213	—	1
pumpkin fritters	1 (1.2 oz)	84	3	1	3	1	14	8	tr	7	94	99	9	2

PUMPKIN SEEDS
kernels dried	¼ cup (1.1 oz)	180	16	3	0	10	3	tr	2	15	2	261	19	1
kernels roasted w/o salt	¼ cup (1 oz)	169	14	3	0	9	4	tr	2	15	5	232	17	1
whole roasted w/o salt	¼ cup (0.5 oz)	71	3	1	0	3	9	—	3	9	3	147	1	0
DAVID														
Kernels	1 pkg (2.5 oz)	280	22	4	0	15	6	tr	2	—	20	—	40	—
EDEN														
Dry Roasted & Salted	¼ cup	200	16	3	0	10	5	—	5	0	100	270	—	—
MRS. MAY'S														
Pumpkin Crunch	1 oz	164	11	2	0	9	8	4	1	20	41	—	—	0
SPITZ														
Seasoned Hulled	¼ cup (1 oz)	180	15	3	0	8	4	0	4	0	920	—	—	0
SUNRICH NATURALS														
Pepitas Lightly Salted	1 pkg (1 oz)	160	14	3	0	8	4	0	2	20	75	—	—	0

FOOD	PORTION	CALS	FAT	SAT FAT	CHOL	PROT	CARB	SUGAR	FIBER	CALCI	SOD	POTAS	FOLIC	VIT C
TREE OF LIFE														
Seeds Roasted & Salted	¼ cup (2 oz)	300	24	5	0	13	8	1	4	20	330	—	—	1
PURSLANE														
cooked	1 cup	21	tr	—	0	2	4	—	—	90	51	561	—	12
fresh	1 cup	7	tr	—	0	1	1	—	—	28	20	213	—	9
QUAIL														
cooked bone removed	1 (2.7 oz)	177	11	3	65	19	0	0	0	11	163	163	5	2
QUICHE														
LA TERRA FINA														
Cheddar & Broccoli	⅕ pie (4.6 oz)	300	18	8	25	10	24	3	2	150	460	—	—	6
Lorraine	⅕ pie (4.6 oz)	320	19	8	30	15	22	2	1	80	550	—	—	1
Spinach & Artichoke	⅕ pie (4.6 oz)	290	17	7	20	11	23	2	2	80	510	—	—	2
MRS. SMITH'S														
Pour-A-Quiche Bacon & Onion	1 serv (4.3 oz)	230	16	8	195	14	6	4	0	—	700	—	—	—
TAKE-OUT														
cheese	⅛ (9 in) pie	566	44	21	240	17	27	1	1	317	459	232	52	1
lorraine	⅛ (9 in) pie	568	44	20	242	17	27	1	1	230	695	267	52	1
mushroom	1 slice (3 oz)	256	18	—	—	9	17	—	1	180	—	—	—	tr
spinach	⅛ (9 in) pie	342	26	12	157	11	17	1	1	223	326	275	80	5
QUINCE														
fresh	1	53	tr	tr	0	tr	14	—	—	10	4	181	—	14
MATIZ														
Quince Pasta	2 tbsp	83	0	0	0	tr	20	13	1	0	0	—	—	0
QUINCE JUICE														
SMART JUICE														
Organic 100% Juice	8 oz	110	0	0	0	1	31	21	0	20	7	0	—	4
QUINOA														
cooked	1 cup (6.5 oz)	222	4	—	0	8	39	—	5	31	13	318	78	0
quinoa not prep	¼ cup (1.5 oz)	156	3	tr	0	6	27	—	3	20	2	239	78	—
ALTI PLANO GOLD														
Natural	1 pkg	170	3	0	0	6	30	9	5	—	120	—	—	—
ANCIENT HARVEST QUINOA														
Flakes not prep	¼ cup	159	2	1	0	5	28	1	3	20	8	—	—	0
Organic Inca Red not prep	¼ cup	163	3	0	0	6	29	5	4	—	5	—	—	—
Organic Traditional not prep	¼ cup	172	3	0	0	6	31	3	3	—	1	—	—	—

FOOD	PORTION	CALS	FAT	SAT FAT	CHOL	PROT	CARB	SUGAR	FIBER	CALCI	SOD	POTAS	FOLIC	VIT C
EDEN														
Quinoa not prep	¼ cup	180	4	0	0	7	29	2	11	20	10	260	32	0
SEEDS OF CHANGE														
French Herb Quinoa Blend as prep	1 cup	290	4	1	0	8	56	7	3	40	860	—	16	0
SIMPLY SHARI'S														
Quinoa + Marinara Gluten Free as prep	¼ pkg (4 oz)	175	2	0	5	10	35	4	5	50	225	0	—	33
TRUROOTS														
Organic not prep	¼ cup (1.6 oz)	172	3	0	0	5	31	3	3	0	1	—	—	0
VILLAGE HARVEST														
Whole Grain Medley Golden Quinoa	¾ cup (5 oz)	220	3	0	0	6	43	0	4	20	20	—	—	0
Whole Grain Medley Red Quinoa & Brown Rice	1 cup (5 oz)	300	4	1	0	7	58	0	3	20	10	—	—	0
RABBIT														
domestic w/o bone roasted	3 oz	167	7	2	70	25	0	0	0	16	40	325	9	0
wild w/o bone stewed	3 oz	147	3	1	104	28	0	0	0	15	38	292	—	—
RACCOON														
roasted	3 oz	217	12	—	—	25	0	0	0	—	—	—	—	—
RADICCHIO														
raw shredded	½ cup	5	tr	—	0	tr	1	—	—	4	4	60	12	2
RADISHES														
chinese dried	½ cup	157	tr	tr	0	5	37	—	—	165	161	2027	—	0
chinese raw	1 (12 oz)	62	tr	tr	0	2	14	—	—	91	71	767	—	74
chinese raw sliced	½ cup	8	tr	tr	0	tr	2	—	—	12	9	100	—	10
chinese sliced cooked	½ cup	13	tr	tr	0	tr	3	—	—	12	10	211	—	11
daikon dried	½ cup	157	tr	tr	0	5	37	—	—	365	161	2027	—	0
daikon raw	1 (12 oz)	62	tr	tr	0	2	14	—	—	91	71	767	—	74
daikon raw sliced	½ cup	8	tr	tr	0	tr	2	—	—	12	9	100	—	10
daikon sliced cooked	½ cup	13	tr	tr	0	tr	3	—	—	12	10	211	—	11
red raw	10	7	tr	tr	0	tr	2	—	—	9	11	104	12	10
red sliced	½ cup	10	tr	tr	0	tr	2	—	—	12	14	134	16	13
white icicle raw	1 (0.5 oz)	2	tr	tr	0	tr	tr	—	—	5	3	48	2	5
white icicle raw sliced	½ cup	7	tr	tr	0	1	1	—	—	14	8	140	7	15

FOOD	PORTION	CALS	FAT	SAT FAT	CHOL	PROT	CARB	SUGAR	FIBER	CALCI	SOD	POTAS	FOLIC	VIT C
CADIS														
Fresh	6 (2.6 oz)	12	tr	—	0	1	2	—	—	—	18	179	—	16
TAKE-OUT														
korean kimchee	½ cup	31	1	—	—	2	6	—	—	3	—	—	—	7
moo namul saengche korean salad	1 serv (3.7 oz)	34	tr	tr	0	1	8	6	2	19	547	247	15	13

RAISINS

FOOD	PORTION	CALS	FAT	SAT FAT	CHOL	PROT	CARB	SUGAR	FIBER	CALCI	SOD	POTAS	FOLIC	VIT C
cinnamon coated	¼ cup	108	tr	tr	0	1	29	21	1	18	4	271	2	1
cooked	¼ cup	162	tr	tr	0	1	42	35	1	18	5	232	1	1
golden seedless	¼ cup	109	tr	tr	0	1	29	21	1	19	4	270	1	1
jumbo golden	¼ cup	130	0	0	0	1	31	29	2	20	10	—	—	0
milk chocolate coated	28 (1 oz)	109	4	2	1	1	19	17	1	24	10	144	2	tr
milk chocolate coated	¼ cup	176	7	4	1	2	31	28	2	39	16	231	3	tr
seedless	55 (1 oz)	86	tr	tr	0	1	23	17	1	14	3	214	1	1
sultanas	1 oz	88	0	—	—	1	23	—	2	18	—	—	—	0
AMAZIN' RAISIN														
All Flavors	1 pkg (1 oz)	84	0	0	0	1	22	20	2	20	4	—	—	0
BOB'S RED MILL														
Unsulfured	⅓ cup	130	0	0	0	1	31	26	3	—	5	—	—	—
DOLE														
Golden Seedless	¼ cup (1.4 oz)	120	0	0	0	1	32	24	1	20	0	300	—	1
EARTHBOUND FARMS														
Organic Jumbo Flame Seedless	¼ cup	120	0	0	0	1	32	30	2	20	0	—	—	1
EMILY'S														
Milk Chocolate Covered	29 (1.4 oz)	180	8	5	<5	2	26	24	2	40	15	—	—	—
FOOL														
Cinnamon Raisin Spread	1 tbsp	20	0	0	0	0	5	4	1	—	0	—	—	—
GODIVA														
Milk Chocolate Covered	1 pkg (1.2 oz)	150	7	4	<5	2	21	20	1	60	20	—	—	0
NEWMAN'S OWN														
Organic	¼ cup	130	0	0	0	1	26	13	2	—	10	310	—	—
REVOLUTION FOODS														
Organic	1 pkg (1.2 oz)	100	0	0	0	1	28	21	1	20	0	260	—	1
SUN-MAID														
Chocolate Covered	30 (1.4 oz)	170	6	4	5	2	26	25	1	40	20	—	—	—
Golden	¼ cup (1.4 oz)	130	0	0	0	1	31	29	2	20	10	310	—	0
Jumbo	¼ cup (1.4 oz)	130	0	0	0	1	31	29	2	20	10	310	—	0

FOOD	PORTION	CALS	FAT	SAT FAT	CHOL	PROT	CARB	SUGAR	FIBER	CALCI	SOD	POTAS	FOLIC	VIT C
SUN-MAID (CONT.)														
Seedless	¼ cup (1.4 oz)	130	0	0	0	1	31	29	2	20	10	310	—	0
Snack Box	1 (1 oz)	90	0	0	0	1	22	20	2	—	5	220	—	—
RAMBUTAN														
canned in syrup	1 cup (4.3 oz)	123	tr	—	0	1	31	—	1	33	16	63	12	7
canned in syrup	1 (0.3 oz)	7	tr	—	—	tr	2	—	tr	2	1	4	1	tr
puerto rican fresh	5 (1.6 oz)	34	tr	—	—	tr	8	8	tr	4	9	38	—	27
POLAR														
In Syrup	½ cup	68	0	0	0	0	17	14	tr	20	10	—	—	1
RASPBERRIES														
black fresh	1 cup	70	1	tr	0	2	16	6	9	34	1	202	28	35
canned in heavy syrup	½ cup	116	tr	tr	0	1	30	26	4	14	4	120	14	11
canned water pack	1 cup	43	1	tr	0	1	10	4	5	21	2	111	9	15
fresh	1 pt	162	2	tr	0	4	37	14	20	78	3	471	66	82
fresh	1 cup	64	1	tr	0	1	15	5	8	31	1	186	26	32
frzn sweetened	1 cup	129	tr	tr	0	1	33	27	6	19	1	142	32	21
frzn unsweetened	1 cup	65	1	tr	0	2	15	6	8	30	1	170	25	23
C&W														
Ultimate Red	¾ cup	70	0	0	0	2	15	9	7	20	0	—	—	24
CASCADIAN FARM														
Organic frzn	1¼ cup	60	0	0	0	1	17	6	6	20	0	160	—	21
DOLE														
Fresh	1 cup (4.3 oz)	60	1	0	0	1	15	5	8	40	0	—	—	30
Raspberries frzn	1 cup (4.9 oz)	70	1	0	0	2	17	7	9	40	0	—	—	36
FRIEDA'S														
Dried	⅓ cup (1.4 oz)	145	1	0	0	0	36	25	6	30	0	—	—	5
OREGON														
In Heavy Syrup	½ cup	120	0	0	0	tr	30	22	5	20	10	140	—	6
STONERIDGE ORCHARDS														
Dried Whole	⅓ cup (1.4 oz)	130	1	—	0	1	32	29	3	100	0	—	—	12
RASPBERRY JUICE														
IZZE														
Esque Sparkling Black Raspberry	1 bottle (12 oz)	50	0	0	0	0	12	11	—	—	10	—	—	—
OLD ORCHARD														
100% Juice	8 oz	130	0	0	0	0	31	29	—	0	25	280	—	72
RED BEANS														
ALLENS														
Red Beans	½ cup	100	1	0	0	6	19	1	9	40	310	—	—	0
RELISH														
hamburger	1 tbsp	19	tr	tr	0	tr	5	—	—	1	164	11	—	tr
hamburger	½ cup	158	1	tr	0	1	42	—	—	5	1338	93	—	3
hot dog	½ cup	111	1	tr	0	2	28	—	—	7	1332	95	—	1

FOOD	PORTION	CALS	FAT	SAT FAT	CHOL	PROT	CARB	SUGAR	FIBER	CALCI	SOD	POTAS	FOLIC	VIT C
hot dog	1 tbsp	14	tr	tr	0	tr	4	—	—	1	164	12	—	tr
piccalilli	1.4 oz	13	tr	—	—	tr	2	—	1	10	—	—	—	0
sweet	½ cup	159	1	tr	0	tr	43	—	—	4	990	30	—	1
sweet	1 tbsp	19	tr	tr	0	tr	5	—	—	0	122	4	—	tr
tomato	¼ cup (2.8 oz)	119	tr	tr	0	1	28	26	1	36	1894	260	13	39
CASCADIAN FARM														
Organic Sweet Relish	1 tbsp (0.5 oz)	15	0	0	0	1	4	4	0	0	65	—	—	0
CLAUSSEN														
Sweet Pickle	1 tbsp (0.5 oz)	15	0	0	0	0	3	2	0	—	85	—	—	—
GEDNEY														
Hot Dog	1 tbsp	18	0	0	0	0	4	3	0	0	100	—	—	0
Organic Sweet	1 tbsp	15	0	0	0	0	4	3	0	0	120	—	—	0
JAKE & AMOS														
Chow Chow Sweet & Sour	1 serv (4 oz)	140	0	0	0	4	31	19	5	40	110	—	—	12
Corn	2 tbsp	40	0	0	0	1	8	6	0	—	55	—	—	—
Green Tomato	1 serv (1 oz)	25	0	0	0	0	7	6	—	—	90	—	—	—
PATAK'S														
Brinjal Eggplant Sweet Spicy	1 tbsp	70	4	1	0	0	8	6	1	0	250	—	—	0
Garlic	1 tbsp	45	3	0	0	0	4	3	0	0	300	—	—	0
Lime Mild	1 tbsp	30	3	0	0	0	0	0	0	0	530	—	—	4
Mango Mild	1 tbsp	40	4	0	0	0	1	1	0	0	660	—	—	2
PELOPONNESE														
Sun Dried Tomato	1 tbsp	25	2	0	0	0	2	1	0	0	200	—	—	0
TEXAS SASSY														
Pickle Relish	1 tbsp (0.5 oz)	30	0	0	0	0	7	7	—	—	115	—	—	—
TREE OF LIFE														
Organic Sweet Pickle	1 tbsp (0.5)	15	0	0	0	0	4	3	0	0	120	—	—	0

RENNIN

tablet	1 (0.9 g)	1	0	—	—	0	tr	—	—	34	234	3	—	0

RHUBARB

fresh	½ cup	13	tr	—	0	1	3	—	—	52	2	175	4	5
frozen	½ cup	60	tr	—	0	tr	3	—	—	132	1	73	6	3
frzn as prep w/ sugar	½ cup	139	tr	—	0	tr	37	—	—	174	2	115	6	4

RICE

(*see also* RICE CAKES, WILD RICE)

arborio	½ cup	100	0	—	0	2	22	—	—	—	5	—	—	—
brown long grain cooked	1 cup (6.8 oz)	216	2	tr	0	5	45	—	4	20	10	84	8	0
brown medium grain cooked	1 cup (6.8 oz)	218	2	tr	0	5	46	—	4	20	2	154	8	0

FOOD	PORTION	CALS	FAT	SAT FAT	CHOL	PROT	CARB	SUGAR	FIBER	CALCI	SOD	POTAS	FOLIC	VIT C
glutinous cooked	1 cup (6.1 oz)	169	tr	tr	0	4	37	—	2	3	9	17	2	0
starch	1 oz	98	0	0	0	tr	24	—	—	6	17	2	—	—
white long grain cooked	1 cup (5.5 oz)	205	tr	tr	0	4	45	—	1	16	2	55	92	0
white long grain instant cooked	1 cup (5.8 oz)	162	tr	tr	0	3	35	—	1	13	5	7	68	0
white medium grain cooked	1 cup (6.5 oz)	242	tr	tr	0	4	53	—	1	6	0	54	108	0
white short grain cooked	1 cup (6.5 oz)	242	tr	tr	0	4	53	—	—	2	0	48	110	0
AMY'S														
Bowls Brown Rice Black-Eyed Peas & Veggies	1 pkg (8.9 oz)	290	11	2	0	11	38	5	8	60	580	—	—	12
Bowls Brown Rice & Vegetables	1 pkg (9.9 oz)	260	9	1	0	9	36	7	5	80	270	—	—	21
ARROWHEAD MILLS														
Organic Brown Basmati not prep	¼ cup	140	2	0	0	3	31	1	2	0	0	—	—	0
Organic Long Grain Brown not prep	¼ cup	160	1	0	0	3	32	0	1	—	0	—	—	—
BETTY CROCKER														
Bowl Appetit! Teriyaki Rice	1 bowl (2.5 oz)	260	3	1	0	7	54	6	2	20	1160	190	60	—
BIRDS EYE														
Steamfresh Whole Grain Brown Rice as prep	1 cup (4.8 oz)	150	1	0	0	4	31	0	2	20	5	—	—	0
CAROLINA														
White Medium Grain as prep	1 cup	160	0	0	0	3	35	0	1	0	0	—	80	0
COUNTRY CROCK														
Cheddar Broccoli Rice	1 cup (7 oz)	270	11	5	20	8	35	3	1	150	790	—	—	12
FANTASTIC														
Arborio not prep	¼ cup	160	4	0	0	3	36	0	tr	0	0	—	—	0
Basmati not prep	¼ cup	160	0	0	0	3	36	0	tr	0	0	—	—	0
Jasmine not prep	¼ cup	160	0	0	0	3	36	0	tr	0	0	—	—	0
GOURMET HOUSE														
Indian Basmati as prep	¾ cup	160	0	0	0	3	35	0	0	0	0	—	80	0
Italian Arborio as prep	¾ cup	160	0	0	0	3	37	0	tr	0	0	—	80	0
Organic Brown as prep	¾ pkg	150	1	0	0	3	32	0	1	0	0	100	—	0

FOOD	PORTION	CALS	FAT	SAT FAT	CHOL	PROT	CARB	SUGAR	FIBER	CALCI	SOD	POTAS	FOLIC	VIT C
GOURMET HOUSE (CONT.)														
Organic White as prep	¾ cup	150	0	0	0	3	35	0	0	0	0	—	—	0
GOYA														
Yellow Rice not prep	¼ cup (1.6 oz)	160	0	0	0	4	35	0	tr	20	250	—	—	1
GREEN GIANT														
Rice Pilaf	1 pkg (9.9 oz)	200	3	2	5	5	40	3	3	40	1080	—	—	4
White & Wild & Green Beans	1 pkg (9.9 oz)	260	5	1	0	6	48	3	3	60	1260	—	—	4
KNORR														
Asian Side Dish Chicken Fried Rice as prep	1 cup	240	1	0	0	7	48	2	1	0	864	0	120	2
Rice Sides Rice Medley as prep	1 cup	250	5	1	<5	6	45	3	1	20	780	—	120	2
Rice Sides Sesame Chicken w/ Whole Grains as prep	⅔ cup	300	9	2	0	7	51	6	3	40	864	0	60	6
LUNDBERG														
Eco-Farmed Black Japonica not prep	¼ cup	170	2	0	0	5	38	1	3	0	0	—	—	0
Eco-Farmed California Brown Basmati not prep	¼ cup	160	2	0	0	4	34	1	2	0	0	—	—	0
Eco-Farmed White California Arborio not prep	¼ cup	160	0	0	0	6	43	0	1	0	3	—	—	0
Organic Brown Golden Rose not prep	¼ cup	160	1	0	0	3	34	0	1	20	0	—	—	0
Organic Rice Sensations Ginger Miso not prep	½ cup	116	1	0	0	3	24	1	1	0	150	59	—	0
Organic Risotto Porcini Mushroom not prep	½ cup	143	1	1	0	4	35	1	1	0	535	—	—	0
Organic White Sushi Rice not prep	¼ cup	150	0	0	0	4	36	0	1	0	0	—	—	0
Organic Wild Blend not prep	¼ cup	150	2	0	0	4	35	0	3	0	0	—	—	0
RiceXpress Chicken Herb	½ pkg (4.4 oz)	250	5	1	0	4	47	2	6	0	670	76	—	1

FOOD	PORTION	CALS	FAT	SAT FAT	CHOL	PROT	CARB	SUGAR	FIBER	CALCI	SOD	POTAS	FOLIC	VIT C
LUNDBERG (CONT.)														
RiceXpress Santa Fe Grill	½ pkg (4.4 oz)	260	5	1	0	5	50	2	3	20	472	110	—	2
Risotto Butternut Squash not prep	½ cup	143	1	1	0	4	31	2	1	20	496	35	—	1
MAHATMA														
Jasmine as prep	¾ cup	160	0	0	0	3	36	0	0	0	0	—	80	0
White as prep	¾ cup	150	0	0	0	3	35	0	0	0	0	—	80	0
Whole Grain Brown as prep	¾ cup	150	1	0	0	3	32	0	1	0	0	100	—	0
MARRAKESH EXPRESS														
Pilaf Tomato & Basil as prep	1 cup	190	0	0	0	6	41	3	0	40	570	—	—	0
Risotto Parmesan as prep	1 cup	200	1	0	0	5	42	2	1	20	870	—	—	0
MINUTE														
Brown as prep	⅔ cup	150	2	0	0	3	34	0	2	—	10	40	—	—
Ready To Serve Brown & Wild Rice	1 pkg (4.4 oz)	230	5	1	0	5	42	0	5	—	135	140	8	—
Ready To Serve Pilaf	1 pkg (4.4 oz)	220	4	0	0	5	41	3	2	40	1350	—	24	—
Ready To Serve Spanish Rice	1 pkg (4.4 oz)	230	5	1	0	6	41	1	2	—	420	140	100	—
Ready To Serve Whole Grain Brown	1 pkg (4.4 oz)	230	4	0	0	5	40	0	2	—	175	140	8	—
Steamers Broccoli & Cheese	1 cup (6.4 oz)	200	4	2	5	6	37	2	1	100	720	—	—	9
Steamers Fried Rice	1 cup (6.5 oz)	280	6	1	5	5	50	0	2	40	770	—	—	4
White as prep	1 cup	200	0	0	0	5	45	0	0	—	5	—	80	—
NEAR EAST														
Long Grain & Wild Original as prep	1 cup	220	4	2	9	5	43	0	2	20	840	—	—	2
Pilaf Curry as prep	1 cup	220	4	2	9	4	44	0	2	20	696	—	—	4
Pilaf Original as prep	1 cup	220	4	2	9	4	43	0	1	0	816	—	—	0
Pilaf Sesame Ginger as prep	1 cup	270	4	2	6	5	55	6	1	20	528	—	—	6
Pilaf Spanish Rice as prep	1 cup	310	7	5	21	5	54	2	2	20	1104	—	—	21
Whole Grains Brown Rice as prep	1 cup	210	4	2	9	5	41	1	3	20	696	—	—	0
PATAK'S														
Basmati	1 pkg	430	5	2	0	9	87	1	2	20	440	0	—	0

FOOD	PORTION	CALS	FAT	SAT FAT	CHOL	PROT	CARB	SUGAR	FIBER	CALCI	SOD	POTAS	FOLIC	VIT C
PATAK'S (CONT.)														
Coconut	1 pkg	500	12	9	0	10	87	5	4	40	880	0	—	0
Yellow	1 pkg	440	5	2	0	10	89	6	2	40	1140	0	—	0
RICE A RONI														
Beef as prep	1 cup	310	9	2	0	7	51	3	2	20	1110	—	100	0
Chicken as prep	1 cup	310	9	2	0	7	51	2	2	20	1160	—	100	0
Express Asian Fried	1 cup	280	6	1	0	6	51	2	2	20	710	—	80	4
Fried Rice as prep	1 cup	320	11	2	0	7	49	4	2	20	1490	—	100	1
Garden Vegetable as prep	1 cup	270	10	3	0	6	41	3	2	40	910	—	80	12
Long Grain & Wild as prep	1 cup	250	7	1	0	5	43	1	1	0	760	—	—	0
Lower Sodium Chicken as prep	1 cup	270	5	1	0	7	51	1	2	20	730	—	100	0
Parmesan Chicken as prep	1 cup	370	15	5	5	8	51	5	3	200	1360	—	80	2
Red Beans & Rice as prep	1 cup	290	7	2	0	8	51	3	5	60	1170	—	140	15
Savory Whole Grain Blends Spanish as prep	1 cup	250	8	1	0	5	42	4	3	20	760	—	—	30
Spanish as prep	1 cup	260	7	2	0	6	44	6	2	40	1340	—	100	2
RICE SELECT														
Jasmati	1 serv	150	0	0	0	3	34	—	—	—	0	—	—	—
Kasmati	1 serv	150	1	—	—	3	34	—	—	—	0	—	—	—
Risotto	1 serv	150	0	0	0	3	37	—	—	—	0	—	—	—
Royal Blend	1 serv	160	1	—	—	4	34	—	—	—	0	—	—	—
Royal Blend w/ Lentils	1 serv	130	1	0	0	3	28	—	1	—	5	—	—	—
Royal Blend w/ Red Beans	1 serv	130	1	0	0	4	27	—	2	—	10	—	—	—
Sushi Rice not prep	¼ cup	190	0	0	0	3	45	—	—	—	0	—	—	—
Teriyaki Fried Rice not prep	¼ cup	160	1	0	—	4	34	—	—	—	330	—	—	—
Texmati Brown	1 serv	170	1	—	—	4	35	—	2	—	0	—	—	—
Texmati Light Brown	1 serv	170	1	—	—	4	33	—	1	—	0	—	—	—
Texmati White	1 serv	150	1	—	—	3	34	—	—	—	0	—	—	—
Texmati Royal Blend Brown & Wild	1 serv	160	2	0	0	5	34	—	—	—	5	—	—	—
RIVER RICE														
Brown as prep	¾ cup	150	0	0	0	3	32	0	1	0	0	100	—	0

FOOD	PORTION	CALS	FAT	SAT FAT	CHOL	PROT	CARB	SUGAR	FIBER	CALCI	SOD	POTAS	FOLIC	VIT C
SEEDS OF CHANGE														
Moroccan Lentil Rice Pilaf as prep	1 cup	180	1	0	0	5	38	3	3	20	750	—	16	1
Tuscan Rice & Beans as prep	1 cup	180	1	0	0	4	40	3	2	20	670	—	16	0
STAHLBUSH ISLAND FARMS														
Organic Brown Rice & Black Beans frzn	1 cup (6.2 oz)	200	2	0	0	8	39	0	7	150	10	—	—	0
SUCCESS														
Boil-In-Bag Jasmine as prep	¾ cup	150	0	0	0	3	36	0	0	—	0	—	60	—
Boil-In-Bag White as prep	1 cup	190	0	0	0	4	43	0	0	20	0	—	80	—
Ready To Serve Brown	1 cup	170	5	1	0	3	28	0	2	20	5	—	8	0
TASTYBITE														
Pilaf Multigrain	½ pkg (5 oz)	200	5	1	0	9	33	3	4	0	440	—	—	1
Pilaf Tandoori	½ pkg (5 oz)	183	3	0	0	3	37	3	1	20	458	—	—	0
THAI KITCHEN														
Jasmine not prep	2 tbsp (1.5 oz)	160	0	0	0	3	36	0	tr	0	0	—	—	0
UNCLE BEN'S														
Boil-In-Bag Whole Grain Brown Rice	1 cup	170	2	0	0	4	36	0	2	0	0	—	—	0
Long Grain & Roasted Chicken as prep	1 cup	190	1	0	0	5	39	1	3	40	640	—	—	5
Long Grain & Wild Sun-Dried Tomato Florentine as prep	1 cup	180	1	0	0	6	39	1	3	4	580	—	—	9
Ready Rice Spanish	1 cup (5 oz)	200	3	0	0	4	40	3	2	80	620	240	100	1
Ready Rice Teriyaki as prep	1 cup	190	4	0	0	5	51	2	1	40	730	—	—	0
Ready Rice Whole Grain Medley	1 cup (5 oz)	210	4	0	0	5	41	1	4	40	730	220	32	0
Ready Rice Whole Grain Medley Roasted Garlic	1 cup (4.9 oz)	200	3	0	0	5	38	0	3	20	560	150	60	1
Whole Grain White Broccoli Cheddar as prep	1 cup	200	2	1	0	5	41	1	4	40	560	5	120	6

FOOD	PORTION	CALS	FAT	SAT FAT	CHOL	PROT	CARB	SUGAR	FIBER	CALCI	SOD	POTAS	FOLIC	VIT C
UNCLE BEN'S (CONT.)														
Whole Grain White Creamy Chicken as prep	1 cup	200	2	0	0	5	44	1	5	20	590	360	120	1
Whole Grain White Garden Vegetable as prep	1 cup	180	1	0	0	4	40	2	4	20	470	7	120	1
Whole Grain White Long Grain as prep	1 cup	170	1	0	0	4	38	1	4	0	5	80	100	0
Whole Grain White Sweet Tomato as prep	1 cup	210	2	1	0	5	46	4	5	20	480	6	120	1
Whole Grain White Taco as prep	1 cup	160	2	0	0	4	35	1	4	20	570	130	100	0
VILLAGE HARVEST														
Whole Grain Creations w/ Corn & Black Beans	¾ cup (4.3 oz)	140	2	0	0	4	27	4	4	0	0	—	—	4
Whole Grain Medley Brown Red & Wild Rice frzn	1 cup (5 oz)	250	3	1	0	5	52	0	3	20	20	—	—	0
WATER MAID														
Medium Grain as prep	¾ cup	160	0	0	0	3	36	0	1	0	0	—	80	0
ZATARAIN'S														
Black Eyed Peas & Rice as prep	1 cup	220	1	0	0	9	46	0	4	40	1330	—	—	6
Caribbean Rice Mix as prep	1 cup	160	2	1	0	3	34	0	tr	20	820	—	—	9
Cheddar Broccoli as prep	1 cup	220	2	1	<5	5	45	3	tr	80	820	—	—	2
Yellow as prep	1 cup	190	0	0	0	4	43	tr	tr	40	930	—	—	5
TAKE-OUT														
coconut rice	1 serv	500	42	—	—	6	30	—	2	—	27	—	—	—
congee	½ cup (4.1 oz)	44	—	—	—	1	10	—	—	4	—	13	—	—
dirty rice w/ chicken giblets	1 cup (6.9 oz)	291	10	5	107	11	38	tr	1	24	457	202	129	2
nasi goring indonesian rice & vegetables	1 cup (4.9 oz)	130	0	0	0	4	28	1	1	20	530	—	—	5
pea palau rice & peas fried in ghee	1 serv	144	5	3	21	4	21	1	2	19	145	57	—	0
pilaf	½ cup	84	3	1	22	4	11	—	3	21	362	206	24	15
rice & black beans	1 cup (5.1 oz)	220	6	1	—	7	36	1	5	54	613	327	—	—

FOOD	PORTION	CALS	FAT	SAT FAT	CHOL	PROT	CARB	SUGAR	FIBER	CALCI	SOD	POTAS	FOLIC	VIT C
risotto	1 serv (6.6 oz)	426	18	—	—	6	65	—	3	46	—	—	—	tr
spanish	¾ cup	363	27	10	35	11	19	—	—	22	1339	369	14	26

RICE CAKES

(*see also* POPCORN CAKES)

HAIN

| Mini Munchies Apple Cinnamon | 9 (0.5 oz) | 60 | 1 | 0 | 0 | 1 | 14 | 2 | tr | 100 | <5 | — | — | 0 |

LUNDBERG

Eco-Farmed Apple Cinnamon	1 (0.7 oz)	80	1	0	0	2	18	2	tr	0	0	75	—	0
Eco-Farmed Brown Rice Salt Free	1 (0.7 oz)	70	0	0	0	1	14	0	tr	0	0	63	—	0
Eco-Farmed Toasted Sesame	1 (0.7 oz)	70	0	0	0	2	15	0	1	20	65	65	—	0
Organic Caramel Corn	1 (0.7 oz)	80	1	0	0	1	18	2	1	0	40	40	—	1
Organic Green Tea w/ Lemon	1 (0.7 oz)	80	0	0	0	1	17	2	1	0	0	—	—	0
Organic Mochi Sweet	1 (0.7 oz)	70	0	0	0	1	15	0	tr	0	55	65	—	0

MOTHER'S

Caramel	1 (0.5 oz)	45	0	0	0	1	10	3	—	—	30	—	—	—
Plain Salted	1 (0.3 oz)	35	0	0	0	1	7	—	—	—	15	—	—	—
Plain Unsalted	1 (0.3 oz)	35	0	0	0	1	7	—	—	—	0	—	—	—
Salted Butter	1 (0.3 oz)	35	0	0	0	1	8	—	—	—	45	—	—	—

QUAKER

| Mini Delights Chocolatey Drizzle | 1 pkg (0.7 oz) | 90 | 4 | 4 | 0 | 1 | 14 | 6 | 1 | 0 | 85 | — | — | — |

RICEWORKS

| Sweet Chili | 10 (1 oz) | 140 | 6 | 1 | 0 | 2 | 19 | tr | 1 | 0 | 170 | — | — | 0 |
| Wasabi | 10 (1 oz) | 140 | 6 | 1 | 0 | 2 | 19 | tr | 1 | 0 | 140 | — | — | 0 |

ROCKFISH

pacific cooked	3 oz	103	2	tr	38	20	0	0	0	10	65	442	—	—
pacific cooked	1 fillet (5.2 oz)	180	3	1	66	36	0	0	0	18	114	774	—	—
pacific raw	3 oz	80	1	tr	29	16	0	0	0	8	51	344	—	—

ROE

(*see also individual fish names*)

| fresh baked | 1 oz | 58 | 2 | 1 | 136 | 8 | 1 | — | 0 | 8 | 33 | 80 | 26 | 5 |

ROLL

FROZEN

JOY OF COOKING

| Ciabatta Olive Oil Rosemary | 1 (1.7 oz) | 120 | 2 | 0 | 0 | 4 | 21 | 0 | 1 | — | 240 | — | — | — |

FOOD	PORTION	CALS	FAT	SAT FAT	CHOL	PROT	CARB	SUGAR	FIBER	CALCI	SOD	POTAS	FOLIC	VIT C
JOY OF COOKING (CONT.)														
French Baguettes Mini	1 (1.6 oz)	100	0	0	0	3	20	0	1	—	220	—	—	—
PILLSBURY														
Dinner Rolls Crusty Sourdough	1 (1.2 oz)	90	1	0	0	4	17	0	tr	0	200	—	—	0
Dinner Rolls Crusty French	1 (1.2 oz)	90	1	0	0	3	15	1	tr	0	190	—	—	0
Dinner Rolls Whole Wheat	1 (1.2 oz)	90	1	0	0	4	17	2	3	—	170	—	—	—
READY-TO-EAT														
bialy	1 (2.2 oz)	138	0	0	0	14	32	—	1	—	167	—	—	—
brioche sweet roll	1 (3.5 oz)	410	23	14	190	10	41	5	3	43	495	201	—	tr
cheese	1 (2.3 oz)	238	12	4	50	5	29	—	1	78	236	90	28	tr
cinnamon raisin	1 (2.1 oz)	223	10	2	40	4	31	19	1	43	230	67	43	1
dinner	1 (1 oz)	78	1	tr	0	3	14	2	1	39	134	26	31	0
egg	1 (1.2 oz)	107	2	1	16	3	18	2	1	21	191	36	64	0
french	1 (1.3 oz)	105	2	tr	0	3	19	tr	1	35	231	43	43	0
garlic	1 (1.5 oz)	133	3	1	2	5	22	2	1	77	229	60	43	tr
hamburger or hot dog	1 (1.5 oz)	120	2	tr	0	4	21	3	1	59	206	40	48	0
hamburger or hot dog multi grain	1 (1.5 oz)	113	3	1	0	4	19	3	2	41	197	69	48	0
hamburger or hot dog reduced calorie	1 (1.5 oz)	84	1	tr	0	4	18	2	3	25	190	34	48	tr
hamburger or hot dog whole wheat	1 (1.5 oz)	114	2	tr	0	4	22	4	3	46	206	117	13	0
hard	1 (2 oz)	167	2	tr	0	6	30	1	1	54	310	62	54	0
hoagie or submarine roll whole wheat	1 (4.7 oz)	359	6	1	0	12	69	11	10	143	645	367	40	0
hot cross bun	1	202	4	—	—	5	38	—	1	72	—	—	—	0
mexican bolillo	1 (4.1 oz)	305	2	tr	1	10	60	tr	2	15	358	98	168	0
oat bran	1 (1.2 oz)	78	2	tr	0	3	13	2	1	28	136	40	31	0
oatmeal	1 (1.3 oz)	103	2	1	7	3	17	2	1	15	145	52	28	0
pumpernickel	1 (1.3 oz)	100	1	tr	0	4	19	tr	2	24	205	75	31	0
rye	1 med (1.3 oz)	103	1	tr	0	4	19	tr	2	11	321	65	36	0
sourdough	1 (1.6 oz)	130	1	tr	0	5	25	1	1	20	292	58	67	tr
wheat	1 (1 oz)	76	2	tr	0	2	13	tr	1	49	95	32	17	0
whole wheat	1 med (1.3 oz)	96	2	tr	0	3	18	3	3	38	172	98	11	0
ARNOLD														
Whole Grains Sandwich 100% Whole Wheat	1 (2.2 oz)	160	2	1	0	8	26	4	4	80	310	—	24	0

FOOD	PORTION	CALS	FAT	SAT FAT	CHOL	PROT	CARB	SUGAR	FIBER	CALCI	SOD	POTAS	FOLIC	VIT C
CALISE														
Kaiser 100% Whole Wheat	1 (2.5 oz)	190	3	1	0	8	33	5	3	100	370	—	—	5
ECCE PANIS														
Focaccia	1 (3.2 oz)	260	5	0	0	8	49	tr	2	40	480	—	—	0
FRENCH MEADOW BAKERY														
Gluten Free Italian	1 (4.4 oz)	340	9	1	0	3	63	7	8	40	470	—	—	4
J.J. CASSONE														
Sandwich	1 (2.5 oz)	190	2	0	0	7	38	2	2	40	400	—	80	0
MRS BAIRD'S														
Home Bake	1 (1 oz)	80	2	0	0	2	13	2	tr	200	110	—	24	0
NATURAL OVENS														
Better Wheat Buns	1 (2.2 oz)	170	3	0	0	7	30	5	4	0	140	—	40	0
NATURE'S OWN														
100% Whole Grain Sugar Free	1 (1.9 oz)	110	2	1	0	6	23	0	4	40	240	—	16	0
Butter Buns	1 (1.7 oz)	120	2	2	5	5	23	2	1	40	115	—	40	0
PEPPERIDGE FARM														
Deli Flats Soft 100% Whole Wheat	1	100	2	0	0	6	19	3	5	40	170	—	16	0
Deli Flats Soft Honey Wheat	1	100	1	0	0	5	21	3	5	60	170	—	16	0
Dinner Classic	1	90	2	0	0	3	17	3	1	20	120	—	24	0
Hamburger 100% Whole Wheat	1	110	2	0	0	9	17	2	2	60	160	—	8	0
Hot Dog Top Sliced	1	150	3	1	0	7	24	4	<2	60	180	—	40	0
Sandwich Mini	1	100	2	0	0	4	18	3	1	40	130	—	32	0
Soft Hoagie	1	210	6	2	0	7	35	3	2	60	250	—	40	0
Stone Baked Artisan Ciabatta Sourdough	1	140	1	0	0	5	27	1	3	0	270	—	—	0
Stone Baked Artisan French Dinner	1	120	0	0	0	4	25	tr	1	0	300	—	60	0
Stone Baked Artisan Multi-Grain Dinner	1	120	1	0	0	6	25	5	3	0	290	—	32	0
RUDI'S ORGANIC BAKERY														
100% Whole Wheat	1 (2.3 oz)	160	2	0	0	7	29	3	5	20	240	—	16	0
Hot Dog Spelt	1 (2 oz)	140	2	0	0	5	28	3	2	0	260	—	0	1
Hot Dog Wheat	1 (2 oz)	150	2	0	0	5	28	4	2	0	260	—	8	1
Hot Dog White	1 (2 oz)	150	2	0	0	5	28	4	tr	0	280	—	8	1

FOOD	PORTION	CALS	FAT	SAT FAT	CHOL	PROT	CARB	SUGAR	FIBER	CALCI	SOD	POTAS	FOLIC	VIT C
S. ROSEN'S														
Brat & Sausage Rolls	1 (2.1 oz)	160	3	1	0	6	28	2	1	60	340	—	60	0
Klassic Kaiser	1 (2.6 oz)	230	3	1	0	6	46	7	1	60	420	—	80	0
STROEHMANN														
Hot Dog Wheat	1 (1.8 oz)	140	3	1	0	5	25	5	2	60	240	—	32	0
UDI'S														
Gluten Free Cinnamon	1 (3 oz)	260	7	3	0	3	48	25	2	40	270	—	—	0
WEIGHT WATCHERS														
Sandwich Wheat	1 (2 oz)	140	2	1	0	6	28	2	5	60	300	—	40	0
REFRIGERATED														
crescent	1 (1 oz)	78	1	tr	0	3	14	2	1	39	134	26	31	0
PILLSBURY														
Crescent Big & Buttery	1 (1.7 oz)	170	10	3	0	3	20	4	tr	0	370	—	—	0
Crescent Butter Flake	1 (1 oz)	110	6	2	0	2	11	2	0	0	220	—	—	0
Crescent Original	1 (1 oz)	110	6	2	0	2	11	2	0	0	220	—	—	0
Crescent Reduced Fat	1 (1 oz)	90	5	2	0	2	12	2	0	0	220	—	—	0
ROSE APPLE														
fresh	3.5 oz	32	tr	—	0	1	7	—	—	20	—	—	—	22
ROSE HIP														
fresh	1 oz	26	0	0	0	1	5	—	—	73	42	83	—	tr
ROSELLE														
fresh	1 cup	28	tr	—	0	1	6	—	—	123	3	118	—	7
ROSEMARY														
dried	1 tsp	4	tr	tr	0	tr	1	—	1	15	1	11	4	1
fresh	1 tbsp	1	tr	tr	0	tr	tr	—	tr	2	0	5	1	tr
ROUGHY														
orange baked	3 oz	75	1	tr	22	16	0	0	0	—	69	—	—	—
RUBS														
(se HERBS/SPICES)														
RUTABAGA														
cooked mashed	1 cup	94	1	tr	0	3	21	14	4	115	602	778	36	45
cubed cooked	1 cup	66	tr	tr	0	2	14	10	3	82	427	551	26	32
GLORY														
Cut Fresh	1 cup	50	0	0	0	2	11	8	4	60	30	—	—	36
SUNSHINE														
Diced	½ cup	30	0	0	0	tr	7	2	1	40	220	—	—	1
SABLEFISH														
baked	3 oz	213	17	3	53	15	0	0	0	—	61	390	—	—
fillet baked	5.3 oz	378	30	6	95	26	0	0	0	—	108	693	—	—

FOOD	PORTION	CALS	FAT	SAT FAT	CHOL	PROT	CARB	SUGAR	FIBER	CALCI	SOD	POTAS	FOLIC	VIT C
smoked	3 oz	218	17	4	55	15	0	0	0	—	626	401	—	—
smoked	1 oz	72	6	1	18	5	0	0	0	—	206	132	—	—

SAFFLOWER

FOOD	PORTION	CALS	FAT	SAT FAT	CHOL	PROT	CARB	SUGAR	FIBER	CALCI	SOD	POTAS	FOLIC	VIT C
seeds dried	1 oz	147	11	1	0	5	10	—	—	22	—	—	—	—

SAFFRON

FOOD	PORTION	CALS	FAT	SAT FAT	CHOL	PROT	CARB	SUGAR	FIBER	CALCI	SOD	POTAS	FOLIC	VIT C
dried	1 tsp	2	tr	tr	0	tr	tr	—	tr	1	1	12	1	1

SAGE

FOOD	PORTION	CALS	FAT	SAT FAT	CHOL	PROT	CARB	SUGAR	FIBER	CALCI	SOD	POTAS	FOLIC	VIT C
ground	1 tsp	2	tr	tr	0	tr	tr	tr	tr	12	0	7	2	tr

SALAD

(*see also* SALAD TOPPINGS)

DOLE

FOOD	PORTION	CALS	FAT	SAT FAT	CHOL	PROT	CARB	SUGAR	FIBER	CALCI	SOD	POTAS	FOLIC	VIT C
American Blend	1½ cups (3 oz)	15	0	0	0	1	3	1	2	20	10	0	100	21
Butter Bliss	1½ cups (3 oz)	15	0	0	0	1	2	1	1	20	15	—	—	6
European Blend	1½ cups (3 oz)	15	0	0	0	1	3	1	1	20	10	—	60	9
Field Greens	1½ cups (3 oz)	20	0	0	0	1	4	1	2	40	20	—	100	12
Italian Blend	1½ cups (3 oz)	15	0	0	0	1	3	2	1	20	10	—	100	18
Kit Asian Island Crunch as prep	1½ cups (3.5 oz)	130	7	1	5	2	15	9	3	40	230	—	—	18
Seven Lettuces	1½ cups (3 oz)	20	0	0	0	1	4	1	1	20	10	—	—	15
Spring Mix	1½ cups (3 oz)	20	0	0	0	2	3	2	2	40	95	—	—	4
Very Veggie Blend	1½ cups (3 oz)	20	0	0	0	1	4	2	2	20	20	—	60	18

EARTHBOUND FARMS

FOOD	PORTION	CALS	FAT	SAT FAT	CHOL	PROT	CARB	SUGAR	FIBER	CALCI	SOD	POTAS	FOLIC	VIT C
Organic Baby Arugula Salad	2 cups	20	0	0	0	2	3	2	1	150	25	—	—	12
Organic Baby Lettuce Salad	2 cups	15	0	0	0	1	3	0	1	60	60	—	—	18
Organic Baby Spinach Salad	2 cups	10	0	0	0	2	7	0	7	60	100	—	—	21
Organic Fresh Herb Salad	2 cups	15	0	0	0	2	4	0	2	80	70	—	—	36
Organic Mixed Baby Greens	2 cups	15	0	0	0	2	4	0	2	60	70	—	—	30

FRESH EXPRESS

FOOD	PORTION	CALS	FAT	SAT FAT	CHOL	PROT	CARB	SUGAR	FIBER	CALCI	SOD	POTAS	FOLIC	VIT C
50/50 Mix	3 cups	10	0	0	0	2	5	2	4	60	65	—	—	18
Asian Supreme w/ Dressing as prep	2½ cups	170	10	2	0	3	17	8	2	20	380	—	—	15
Caesar Lite w/ Dressing as prep	2½ cups	100	7	1	10	2	8	2	2	20	360	—	—	18
Caesar w/ Dressing as prep	2½ cups	150	13	2	10	2	8	2	2	60	370	—	—	18
Fancy Field Greens	3 cups	20	0	0	0	1	3	1	2	20	15	—	0	12

FOOD	PORTION	CALS	FAT	SAT FAT	CHOL	PROT	CARB	SUGAR	FIBER	CALCI	SOD	POTAS	FOLIC	VIT C
FRESH EXPRESS (CONT.)														
Gourmet Cafe Caribbean Chicken as prep	1 pkg (3.5 oz)	120	6	1	10	4	14	8	1	20	190	—	—	12
Gourmet Cafe Chicken Caesar w/ Crostini as prep	1 pkg (3.5 oz)	150	11	3	25	8	5	1	1	80	390	—	—	15
Gourmet Cafe Chopped Turkey Chef as prep	1 pkg (3.5 oz)	120	9	2	15	5	7	4	tr	40	300	—	—	9
Gourmet Cafe Orchard Harvest as prep	1 pkg (3.5 oz)	230	18	3	10	5	13	9	2	100	270	—	—	12
Gourmet Cafe Tuscan Pesto Chicken as prep	1 pkg (3.5 oz)	130	8	2	15	7	6	3	1	60	280	—	—	15
Gourmet Cafe Waldorf Chicken as prep	1 pkg (3.5 oz)	190	10	2	20	7	19	14	2	40	350	—	—	9
More Carrots American	1½ cups	15	0	0	0	1	3	2	1	20	10	—	—	12
Organic Italian	2½ cups	15	0	0	0	1	3	2	1	40	5	—	—	21
Original Iceberg Garden With Zip	1½ cups	15	0	0	0	1	3	2	4	20	0	—	—	6
Pacifica! Veggie Supreme w/ Dressing as prep	3 cups	220	15	2	10	4	18	14	2	40	340	—	—	12
Spring Mix	3 cups	15	0	0	0	1	3	1	2	40	40	—	—	15
Sweet Baby Greens	3 cups	10	0	0	0	1	2	1	1	20	10	—	—	9
Veggie Lover's	2 cups	20	0	0	0	1	4	2	1	20	15	—	0	15
LIFESTYLE FOODS														
Asian w/ Chicken	1 pkg (8.9 oz)	340	16	3	30	13	36	21	3	60	710	—	—	36
Casear	1 pkg (5 oz)	210	11	3	25	5	22	6	2	100	570	—	—	18
Garden	1 pkg (6.6 oz)	180	12	2	10	4	14	4	2	100	670	—	—	27
Greek	1 pkg (6 oz)	130	11	3	10	3	6	2	2	40	1040	—	—	24
MANN'S														
Rainbow	1 serv (3 oz)	25	0	0	0	2	5	2	2	40	25	260	48	54
READY PAC														
All American	2 cups (3 oz)	15	0	0	0	1	3	2	1	20	15	—	—	6
American Blue Cheese Mix as prep	1¾ cups (3.5 oz)	110	8	2	10	2	8	2	1	40	250	—	—	9
Baby Romaine Blend	4½ cups (3 oz)	20	0	0	0	2	3	0	2	40	90	—	—	2
Baby Spinach Mix as prep	2 cups (3.5 oz)	140	3	0	0	4	24	12	2	40	270	—	—	12
Chef	1 pkg (7.7 oz)	270	20	7	55	15	10	5	2	250	890	—	—	15

FOOD	PORTION	CALS	FAT	SAT FAT	CHOL	PROT	CARB	SUGAR	FIBER	CALCI	SOD	POTAS	FOLIC	VIT C
READY PAC (CONT.)														
Cobb	1 pkg (7.2 oz)	300	23	6	140	13	7	4	2	80	950	—	—	18
Garden	2 cups (3 oz)	15	0	0	0	1	3	2	1	20	10	—	—	5
Grand Asian Mix as prep	1¼ cups (3.5 oz)	130	6	1	0	3	19	11	2	40	260	—	—	27
Spinach Bacon	1 pkg (4.7 oz)	240	12	4	130	12	19	8	3	150	750	—	—	6
Spring Mix	4½ cups	20	0	0	0	2	4	0	2	20	25	—	—	4
Spring Mix Spinach	5 cups (3 oz)	20	0	0	0	2	4	1	2	40	45	—	80	9
Veggie Medley	2 cups (3 oz)	15	0	0	0	1	4	2	1	20	15	—	—	12
TAKE-OUT														
7-layer salad	2 cups	557	51	11	119	11	15	8	3	150	612	324	81	18
caesar	4 cups	734	61	11	173	22	28	6	7	372	1119	873	415	73
chef salad w/o dressing	3 cups	535	32	16	280	52	9	—	—	469	1487	802	202	33
cobb w/ dressing	4 cups	645	49	13	294	32	23	9	11	243	1512	1383	258	44
greek w/ dressing	4 cups	424	29	14	475	28	14	8	4	491	1638	714	160	20
mixed salad greens shredded	1 cup	9	tr	tr	0	1	2	tr	1	26	16	160	59	9
somen w/ lettuce egg fish pork	2 cups	550	17	5	429	40	57	4	4	109	1229	669	93	7
spinach w/o dressing	4 cups	429	19	6	308	20	45	5	6	181	909	926	275	26
tossed w/ avocado w/o dressing	2 cups	90	6	1	0	2	9	4	5	31	35	473	64	13
tossed w/ chicken w/o dressing	3 cups	194	4	1	86	33	5	3	2	49	108	535	51	16
tossed w/ egg w/o dressing	2 cups	93	5	1	183	7	6	4	2	49	92	347	51	10
tossed w/ shrimp w/o dressing	1½ cups (8.3 oz)	106	2	1	179	15	7	—	—	59	489	404	87	9
tossed w/ shrimp & egg w/o dressing	3 cups	185	5	1	430	30	5	3	2	219	1006	351	57	11
tossed w/o dressing	2 cups	22	tr	tr	0	1	5	3	2	31	30	240	36	5
waldorf	1 cup	242	21	3	7	2	15	10	3	26	119	196	21	5
wilted lettuce w/ bacon dressing	1 cup	99	8	3	11	3	3	1	1	38	159	236	36	16

SALAD DRESSING

(*see also* SALAD TOPPINGS)

MIX

GOOD SEASONS

FOOD	PORTION	CALS	FAT	SAT FAT	CHOL	PROT	CARB	SUGAR	FIBER	CALCI	SOD	POTAS	FOLIC	VIT C
Italian as prep	2 tbsp	130	13	2	0	0	3	tr	—	—	336	—	—	—
Italian not prep	⅛ pkg (3 g)	5	0	0	0	0	1	tr	—	—	320	—	—	—
J&D'S														
Bacon Ranch as prep	2 tbsp	120	12	2	12	0	3	—	—	20	240	—	—	0

FOOD	PORTION	CALS	FAT	SAT FAT	CHOL	PROT	CARB	SUGAR	FIBER	CALCI	SOD	POTAS	FOLIC	VIT C
READY-TO-EAT														
blue cheese	1 tbsp	77	8	2	—	1	1	—	—	12	—	—	—	tr
french	1 tbsp	67	6	2	—	tr	3	—	—	2	214	12	—	—
french reduced calorie	1 tbsp	22	1	tr	1	0	4	—	—	2	128	13	—	—
italian	1 tbsp	69	7	1	—	tr	2	—	—	1	116	2	—	—
italian reduced calorie	1 tbsp	16	2	tr	1	tr	1	—	—	0	118	2	—	—
japanese ginger salad dressing	2 tbsp	90	—	—	—	—	—	—	—	—	—	—	—	—
russian	1 tbsp	76	8	1	—	tr	2	—	—	3	133	24	—	1
russian reduced calorie	1 tbsp	23	1	tr	1	tr	5	—	—	3	141	26	—	—
sesame seed	1 tbsp	68	7	1	0	1	1	—	—	—	153	—	—	—
thousand island	1 tbsp	59	6	1	—	tr	2	—	—	2	109	18	—	—
thousand island reduced calorie	1 tbsp	24	2	tr	2	tr	3	—	—	2	153	17	—	—
ANNIE'S HOMEGROWN														
Cowgirl Ranch	2 tbsp (1 oz)	90	11	1	10	1	3	2	—	20	240	—	—	—
Tuscany Italian	2 tbsp (1 oz)	100	9	1	—	0	3	2	—	—	250	—	—	—
Vinaigrette Lite Gingerly	2 tbsp (1.1 oz)	40	3	—	—	0	3	2	—	—	280	—	—	—
Vinaigrette Lite Honey Mustard	1 tbsp (1.1 oz)	40	3	—	—	0	4	3	—	—	125	—	—	—
Vinaigrette Mango Fat Free	2 tbsp (1.1 oz)	20	0	0	0	0	5	5	—	—	5	—	—	2
Vinaigrette Roasted Red Pepper	2 tbsp (1.1 oz)	60	6	—	—	0	3	2	—	—	240	—	—	9
BERNSTEIN'S														
Chunky Blue Cheese	2 tbsp	120	13	2	5	1	2	1	0	20	180	—	—	0
Creamy Caesar	2 tbsp	120	13	1	15	0	1	0	0	20	200	—	—	0
Italian Restaurant Recipe	2 tbsp	120	12	1	5	1	1	0	0	20	360	—	—	0
Light Fantastic Roasted Garlic Balsamic	2 tbsp	45	4	0	0	0	3	2	0	0	320	—	—	0
Red Wine & Garlic Italian	2 tbsp	110	1	0	0	0	2	1	0	0	250	—	—	0
BRAGG														
Ginger & Sesame	2 tbsp	150	12	2	0	0	2	2	0	—	230	—	—	—
Organic Vinaigrette	2 tbsp	150	15	2	0	0	3	2	0	0	120	—	—	1
CAINS														
Caesar Creamy	2 tbsp	170	19	3	5	0	1	0	0	20	170	—	—	1
Caesar Fat Free	2 tbsp	30	0	0	0	0	6	2	0	20	600	—	—	1

FOOD	PORTION	CALS	FAT	SAT FAT	CHOL	PROT	CARB	SUGAR	FIBER	CALCI	SOD	POTAS	FOLIC	VIT C
CAINS (CONT.)														
Caesar Light	2 tbsp	70	6	1	5	2	5	2	0	20	490	—	—	0
Chianti Vinaigrette	2 tbsp	130	12	2	0	0	5	3	0	0	220	—	—	0
Creamy Dill Cucumber Fat Free	2 tbsp	35	0	0	0	0	8	3	0	20	370	—	—	0
French	2 tbsp	120	11	2	0	0	6	4	0	0	170	—	—	0
French Light	2 tbsp	80	5	1	0	0	10	6	0	0	170	—	—	0
Greek	2 tbsp	160	17	3	5	0	2	2	0	0	190	—	—	0
Italian Fat Free	2 tbsp	15	0	0	0	0	4	2	0	0	490	—	—	0
Ranch	2 tbsp	180	19	3	5	0	1	1	0	0	270	—	—	0
Ranch Light	2 tbsp	80	6	1	5	0	6	2	0	20	310	—	—	0
DAVID BURKE														
Flavor Spray Ranch	2 sprays	0	0	0	0	0	0	0	0	—	10	—	—	—
DAVID'S UNFORGETTABLES														
Balsamic Vinaigrette Low Fat	1 tbsp (0.5 oz)	40	3	0	0	0	3	3	0	0	190	—	—	0
Balsamic Vinaigrette Original	1 tbsp (0.5 oz)	70	7	0	0	0	3	3	0	0	190	—	—	0
FOLLOW YOUR HEART														
Lemon Herb	2 tbsp (1 oz)	100	11	1	0	0	1	0	0	—	220	—	—	2
Sesame Miso	2 tbsp (1 oz)	64	6	1	0	1	3	2	0	—	151	—	—	—
Thousand Island	2 tbsp (1 oz)	80	8	1	0	0	3	0	tr	—	230	—	—	—
GIRARD'S														
White Balsamic Vinaigrette	2 tbsp	140	13	2	0	0	5	4	—	—	190	—	—	—
GOTTA LUV IT														
Chipotle Lime	2 tbsp	110	11	1	0	0	3	2	0	0	100	—	—	1
Raspberry Balsamic Vinaigrette	2 tbsp	150	14	1	0	0	6	5	0	20	0	—	—	0
Sweet & Tangy Italian	2 tbsp	140	15	1	0	0	2	2	0	0	0	—	—	0
JAKE & AMOS														
Bacon	2 tbsp (1 oz)	90	5	1	25	1	10	10	1	0	35	—	—	0
KEN'S														
Bacon Ranch	2 tbsp	140	15	2	0	1	2	2	0	0	270	—	—	0
Caesar	2 tbsp	170	18	3	0	0	1	1	0	0	430	—	—	0
Country French w/ Vermont Honey	2 tbsp	150	12	2	0	0	10	9	0	0	220	—	—	0
Fat Free Italian	2 tbsp	25	0	0	0	0	5	4	0	0	380	—	—	0

FOOD	PORTION	CALS	FAT	SAT FAT	CHOL	PROT	CARB	SUGAR	FIBER	CALCI	SOD	POTAS	FOLIC	VIT C
KEN'S (CONT.)														
Fat Free Raspberry Pecan	2 tbsp	50	0	0	0	0	12	10	0	0	280	—	—	0
Honey Mustard	2 tbsp	130	11	2	15	0	7	6	0	0	210	—	—	0
Italian w/ Aged Romano	2 tbsp	110	12	2	0	0	11	1	0	0	300	—	—	0
Light Vinaigrette Balsamic	2 tbsp (1 oz)	60	5	1	0	0	4	4	0	0	210	—	—	0
Lite Ranch	2 tbsp	80	6	1	10	0	6	2	0	20	310	—	—	0
Lite Red Wine Vinegar & Olive Oil	2 tbsp	50	5	1	0	0	2	2	0	0	280	—	—	2
Red Wine Vinegar & Olive Oil	2 tbsp	120	12	2	0	0	2	2	0	0	360	—	—	2
Russian	2 tbsp	140	14	2	15	0	52	3	0	0	280	—	—	0
Thousand Island	2 tbsp	140	13	2	15	0	4	3	0	0	300	—	—	0
KRAFT														
Honey Dijon	2 tbsp	100	9	2	0	0	6	5	0	0	250	—	—	0
Italian Creamy	2 tbsp	100	11	2	0	0	2	2	0	0	250	—	—	0
Light Done Right Caesar	2 tbsp	60	5	1	10	1	3	1	0	0	320	—	—	0
Light Done Right Red Wine Vinaigrette	2 tbsp	45	4	0	0	0	3	2	0	0	310	—	—	0
Ranch Garlic	2 tbsp	120	12	2	0	0	3	2	0	0	360	—	—	0
Special Collection Classic Italian Vinaigrette	2 tbsp	60	4	0	0	0	5	2	0	0	430	—	—	0
Special Collection Parmesan Romano	2 tbsp	140	14	3	10	1	2	1	0	0	360	—	—	0
Special Collection Tangy Tomato Bacon	2 tbsp	100	6	1	0	0	10	9	0	0	350	—	—	0
Thousand Island w/ Bacon	2 tbsp	100	8	1	0	0	7	6	0	0	220	—	—	0
LITEHOUSE														
Bleu Cheese Bacon	2 tbsp	150	16	2	15	1	1	1	0	20	240	—	—	0
Organic Vinaigrette Raspberry Lime	2 tbsp	40	2	0	0	0	5	5	0	0	55	—	—	0
Ranch Homestyle	2 tbsp	120	12	1	10	0	2	1	0	20	240	—	—	1
Ranch Lite	2 tbsp	70	6	0	5	0	2	2	0	20	220	—	—	0
Sesame Ginger	2 tbsp	35	0	0	0	0	8	7	0	0	230	—	—	0
Spinach Salad	2 tbsp	50	0	0	0	1	11	7	0	0	260	—	—	0
Vinaigrette Huckleberry	2 tbsp	20	0	0	0	0	4	4	0	0	90	—	—	0

FOOD	PORTION	CALS	FAT	SAT FAT	CHOL	PROT	CARB	SUGAR	FIBER	CALCI	SOD	POTAS	FOLIC	VIT C
LITEHOUSE (CONT.)														
Vinaigrette Lite Honey Dijon	2 tbsp	130	13	1	10	0	3	2	0	0	250	—	—	1
LUCINI														
Delicate Cucumber & Shallots	2 tbsp (1 oz)	120	12	1	—	0	2	1	—	—	170	—	—	—
Fig & Walnut Savory Balsamic	2 tbsp (1 oz)	110	10	1	—	0	4	3	—	—	180	—	—	—
Roasted Hazelnut & Extra Virgin Olive Oil	2 tbsp (1 oz)	120	11	1	—	1	3	2	—	—	190	—	—	—
MAPLE GROVE FARMS														
Asiago & Garlic	2 tbsp (1 oz)	40	4	—	—	0	2	1	—	—	260	—	—	—
Caesar Lite	2 tbsp (1 oz)	50	5	—	—	0	4	3	—	—	260	—	—	—
Cranberry Balsamic Fat Free	2 tbsp (1 oz)	30	0	0	0	0	7	6	—	—	180	—	—	—
Creamy Ranch Sugar Free	2 tbsp (1 oz)	100	12	1	—	0	tr	—	—	—	110	—	—	—
Honey Dijon Fat Free	2 tbsp (1 oz)	35	0	0	0	0	9	8	tr	—	200	—	—	—
Poppyseed Fat Free	2 tbsp (1 oz)	35	0	0	0	0	7	7	—	—	160	—	—	—
Sesame Ginger	2 tbsp (1 oz)	45	2	—	—	tr	6	5	—	—	260	—	—	—
Strawberry Balsamic	1 tbsp (1 oz)	30	0	0	0	0	6	6	—	—	160	—	—	—
Sweet'n Sour	2 tbsp (1 oz)	90	6	—	—	0	10	9	—	—	150	—	—	—
Vidalia Onion Fat Free	2 tbsp (1 oz)	20	0	0	0	0	5	4	—	—	140	—	—	—
Vinaigrette Balsamic Sugar Free	2 tbsp (1 oz)	5	0	0	0	0	1	—	—	—	90	—	—	2
Vinaigrette Champagne	2 tbsp (1 oz)	100	11	1	—	0	2	1	—	—	130	—	—	—
MARIE'S														
Blue Cheese Lite Chunky	2 tbsp	80	6	2	5	1	7	1	4	40	280	—	—	0
Blue Cheese Vinaigrette	2 tbsp	120	11	3	5	2	4	4	0	40	200	—	—	0
Caesar	2 tbsp	170	19	4	15	1	1	0	0	0	170	—	—	0
Coleslaw	2 tbsp	120	13	2	10	0	8	7	0	0	170	—	—	0
Creamy Ranch	2 tbsp	170	19	3	15	1	1	1	0	0	150	—	—	0
Red Wine Vinaigrette	2 tbsp	60	5	1	0	0	6	5	0	0	210	—	—	0
Sesame Ginger	2 tbsp	70	8	2	0	0	7	6	0	0	250	—	—	0

FOOD	PORTION	CALS	FAT	SAT FAT	CHOL	PROT	CARB	SUGAR	FIBER	CALCI	SOD	POTAS	FOLIC	VIT C
NATURALLY FRESH														
Balsamic Vinaigrette	2 tbsp	10	0	0	0	0	2	1	0	—	250	—	—	—
Bleu Cheese	2 tbsp	170	18	4	15	1	1	0	0	—	120	5	—	—
Bleu Cheese Bacon	2 tbsp	170	18	4	15	1	1	0	0	—	150	10	—	—
Bleu Cheese Lite	2 tbsp	100	10	3	10	1	1	1	0	—	130	45	—	—
Buffalo Ranch	2 tbsp	110	10	2	10	0	4	3	0	—	350	15	—	—
Classic Oriental	2 tbsp	100	11	2	0	0	9	8	0	—	140	15	—	—
Ginger	2 tbsp	70	7	1	0	1	1	0	0	—	370	20	—	—
Greek Feta	2 tbsp	100	12	2	5	0	1	0	0	—	270	—	—	—
Honey French	2 tbsp	100	11	2	0	0	5	5	0	—	310	0	—	—
Honey Mustard	2 tbsp	140	13	2	10	1	5	4	0	—	180	—	—	—
Orange Miso	2 tbsp	100	9	2	5	0	4	3	0	—	135	—	—	—
Ranch Classic	2 tbsp	150	16	3	10	1	1	1	0	—	240	20	—	—
Ranch Lite	2 tbsp	80	8	2	5	1	2	1	0	—	240	30	—	—
Slaw	2 tbsp	90	10	2	10	0	6	6	0	—	150	5	—	—
NEWMAN'S OWN														
Balsamic Vinaigrette	2 tbsp	90	9	1	0	0	3	1	0	—	350	—	—	—
Caesar	2 tbsp	150	16	2	0	1	1	1	0	20	420	—	—	0
Lighten Up Light Balsamic Vinaigrette	2 tbsp (1 oz)	45	4	1	0	0	2	2	0	0	390	—	—	0
ORGANICVILLE														
Herbs De Provence	2 tbsp (1 oz)	100	11	2	0	0	tr	0	0	0	190	—	—	0
Miso Ginger	2 tbsp (1 oz)	100	10	2	0	0	1	tr	0	0	250	—	—	0
Orange Cranberry	2 tbsp (1 oz)	100	10	2	0	0	3	3	0	0	190	—	—	2
Pomegranate	2 tbsp (1 oz)	100	10	2	0	0	2	2	0	0	55	—	—	0
Ranch Non Dairy	2 tbsp (1 oz)	90	9	2	0	tr	1	1	0	0	240	—	—	0
Sesame Goddess	2 tbsp (1 oz)	130	13	2	0	1	2	tr	0	0	290	—	—	0
PETRINI'S														
Italian Original	2 tbsp (1 oz)	106	12	2	0	tr	tr	0	tr	240	210	—	—	0
Italian Ranch	2 tbsp (1 oz)	140	14	2	5	0	1	—	—	—	190	—	—	—
SCHOOLHOUSE KITCHEN														
Balsamic Vinaigrette Basico	2 tbsp	160	17	1	0	0	3	2	0	0	260	—	—	0
SEEDS OF CHANGE														
Vinaigrette Balsamic	2 tbsp	60	4	0	0	0	6	3	0	0	105	—	—	0
Vinaigrette Greek Feta	2 tbsp	60	5	1	0	1	5	2	0	0	270	—	—	0
Vinaigrette Roasted Garlic	2 tbsp	60	4	0	0	0	6	3	0	0	125	—	—	0

FOOD	PORTION	CALS	FAT	SAT FAT	CHOL	PROT	CARB	SUGAR	FIBER	CALCI	SOD	POTAS	FOLIC	VIT C
SEEDS OF CHANGE (CONT.)														
Vinaigrette Sweet Basil	2 tbsp	60	5	0	0	0	6	2	0	0	160	—	—	0
SONOMA														
Creamy Tomato Bacon	2 tbsp	150	15	3	5	0	3	2	0	0	310	—	—	0
SOY VAY														
Toasted Sesame	3 tbsp	190	15	3	0	2	11	9	0	40	250	—	—	0
TEXAS SASSY														
Vinaigrette	2 tbsp (1 oz)	80	8	2	—	0	4	4	—	—	10	—	—	—
THREE ACRE KITCHEN														
Balsamic Vinaigrette	2 tbsp (1.1 oz)	130	14	2	—	0	3	2	—	—	75	—	—	—
VINO DE MILO														
Gorgonzola Pear Riesling	2 tbsp	80	7	1	0	0	2	1	0	0	75	—	—	0
Pomegranate Port	2 tbsp	90	7	1	0	0	5	5	0	0	0	—	—	4
WALDEN FARMS														
Sesame Ginger Calorie Free	2 tbsp (1 oz)	0	0	0	0	0	0	0	0	0	260	—	—	0
WILD THYMES FARM														
Salad Refreshers Black Currant	1 tbsp	36	3	tr	0	tr	3	3	tr	0	4	—	—	1
Salad Refreshers Meyer Lemon	1 tbsp	35	3	tr	0	0	3	3	tr	0	4	—	—	3
Salad Refreshers Morello Cherry	1 tbsp	34	3	tr	0	tr	3	2	tr	0	6	—	—	1
Salad Refreshers Pomegranate	1 tbsp	33	3	tr	0	0	3	2	0	0	4	—	—	0
Vinaigrette Mandarin Orange Basil	1 tbsp	43	4	tr	0	0	2	1	tr	0	6	—	—	1
Vinaigrette Raspberry Pear	1 tbsp	43	4	tr	0	0	1	1	tr	0	7	—	—	1
Vinaigrette Roasted Apple Shallot	1 tbsp	42	4	tr	0	0	2	1	tr	0	6	—	—	0
Vinaigrette Toasted Sesame Wasabi	1 tbsp	42	4	tr	0	tr	1	1	tr	0	55	—	—	0
WISHBONE														
Bountifuls Berry Delight	2 tbsp	35	0	0	0	0	8	6	—	—	210	—	—	—
Bountifuls Tuscan Romano Basil	2 tbsp	25	1	—	0	0	4	3	—	—	340	—	—	2
Caesar w/ Aged Romano	2 tbsp	80	8	1	0	0	3	2	0	0	530	—	—	2

FOOD	PORTION	CALS	FAT	SAT FAT	CHOL	PROT	CARB	SUGAR	FIBER	CALCI	SOD	POTAS	FOLIC	VIT C
WISHBONE (CONT.)														
Creamy Caesar	2 tbsp	170	18	3	10	tr	1	tr	0	0	300	—	—	0
Five Cheese Italian	2 tbsp	120	10	2	0	tr	6	2	0	0	410	—	—	1
Just 2 Good Blue Cheese	2 tbsp	45	2	1	0	tr	6	2	0	0	310	—	—	0
Just 2 Good Creamy Caesar	2 tbsp	50	2	1	10	tr	7	2	0	0	300	—	—	0
Just 2 Good Thousand Island	2 tbsp	50	2	0	5	0	9	5	0	0	290	—	—	0
Western	2 tbsp (1 oz)	160	12	2	0	0	11	11	0	0	230	—	—	0
Western Fat Free	2 tbsp (1 oz)	50	0	0	0	0	12	11	0	0	280	—	—	0
Western Light Just 2 Good	2 tbsp (1 oz)	70	2	0	0	0	13	12	0	0	270	—	—	0
TAKE-OUT														
vinegar & oil	1 tbsp	72	8	2	0	0	tr	—	—	—	tr	1	—	—

SALAD TOPPINGS

FOOD	PORTION	CALS	FAT	SAT FAT	CHOL	PROT	CARB	SUGAR	FIBER	CALCI	SOD	POTAS	FOLIC	VIT C
FRESH GOURMET														
Crispy Onions Garlic Pepper	1½ tbsp	35	2	0	0	—	4	—	—	0	50	—	—	0
Tortilla Strips Lightly Salted	2 tbsp	35	2	0	0	—	5	0	0	0	25	—	—	0
Wonton Strips Wasabi Ranch	2 tbsp	35	2	0	0	1	4	0	0	0	45	—	—	0
MCCORMICK														
Salad Toppins	1.3 tbsp (7 g)	35	2	—	0	2	3	tr	0	—	70	—	—	—
Salad Toppins Garden Vegetable	1.3 tbsp (7 g)	35	2	—	0	2	3	tr	0	—	50	—	—	—
NATURALLY FRESH														
Fruit & Nut Mix	½ tbsp	45	4	0	0	1	2	1	1	—	20	—	—	—
Glazed Almond & Pecan Pieces	½ tbsp	40	3	0	0	1	3	2	1	—	0	—	—	—

SALBA

FOOD	PORTION	CALS	FAT	SAT FAT	CHOL	PROT	CARB	SUGAR	FIBER	CALCI	SOD	POTAS	FOLIC	VIT C
SALBA SMART														
Ground	2 tbsp	65	4	tr	0	3	5	—	4	92	2	79	tr	1
Whole Grain	1 tbsp	65	4	tr	0	3	5	—	4	92	2	79	tr	1

SALMON

FOOD	PORTION	CALS	FAT	SAT FAT	CHOL	PROT	CARB	SUGAR	FIBER	CALCI	SOD	POTAS	FOLIC	VIT C
CANNED														
w/ bone	½ cup	106	5	1	39	15	0	0	0	165	410	251	10	0
CHICKEN OF THE SEA														
Pink	¼ cup (2.2 oz)	90	5	1	40	12	0	0	0	100	270	—	—	0
Pink Skinless & Boneless	⅓ pkg (2 oz)	60	2	1	20	10	0	0	0	0	280	—	—	0
Pink Smoked Pacific	1 pkg (3 oz)	120	4	1	45	21	1	1	0	20	490	—	—	1
Red	¼ cup	110	7	2	40	13	0	0	0	100	270	—	—	0

FOOD	PORTION	CALS	FAT	SAT FAT	CHOL	PROT	CARB	SUGAR	FIBER	CALCI	SOD	POTAS	FOLIC	VIT C
POLAR														
Pink	¼ cup	90	5	1	40	12	0	0	0	100	270	—	—	0
Sockeye Red	¼ cup	110	7	2	40	13	0	0	0	100	270	—	—	0
TONNINO														
Wild Sockeye In Olive Oil	2 oz	220	17	5	—	16	tr	0	tr	0	450	—	—	0
WILD PLANET														
Salmon Wild Alaskan Pink	2 oz	65	2	0	25	12	0	0	0	0	220	—	—	0
Salmon Wild Alaskan Sockeye	2 oz	85	4	1	24	12	0	0	0	0	196	—	—	2
FRESH														
atlantic farmed baked	4 oz	233	14	3	71	25	0	0	0	17	69	435	39	4
coho wild poached	4 oz	209	9	2	65	31	0	0	0	52	30	516	10	1
pink baked	4 oz	169	5	1	76	29	0	0	0	19	97	469	6	0
roe raw	1 oz	59	3	—	—	7	tr	—	—	—	—	—	—	5
sockeye baked	4 oz	245	12	2	99	31	0	0	0	8	75	425	6	0
FROZEN														
GORTON'S														
Classic Grilled Fillets	1 (3 oz)	100	3	1	35	15	2	1	—	20	270	260	—	—
SEAPAK														
Burgers	1 (3.2 oz)	110	3	1	60	18	1	0	0	0	380	—	—	0
Herb Butter Fillet	1 (5 oz)	350	26	11	105	23	3	tr	0	20	280	—	—	6
SMOKED														
lox	1 oz	33	1	tr	7	5	0	0	0	3	567	50	1	0
KASILOF FISH CO.														
Wild Alaska Fillet	1 pkg (2 oz)	90	4	1	62	11	4	0	0	20	336	—	—	0
TAKE-OUT														
guisado salmon stew	1 serv (7.4 oz)	320	16	3	66	26	18	3	3	276	1130	825	34	15
roulette w/ spinach stuffing	1 serv (4 oz)	160	6	2	45	13	10	0	tr	40	400	—	—	6
salmon cake	1 (4.2 oz)	264	16	4	56	16	14	1	1	179	671	385	24	4
salmon loaf	1 slice (3.7 oz)	206	11	3	120	16	9	2	tr	192	819	287	29	2
SALSA														
black bean & corn	2 tbsp	15	0	0	0	1	3	1	tr	20	45	—	—	5
citrus	2 tbsp (1 oz)	10	0	0	0	0	2	2	0	0	7	—	—	1
peach	2 tbsp	15	0	0	0	0	4	4	0	0	90	—	—	5
tomatoless corn & chile	2 tbsp	45	0	0	0	1	10	6	tr	0	95	—	—	2
AMY'S														
Organic Black Bean & Corn	2 tbsp (1 oz)	15	0	0	0	1	3	1	tr	0	170	—	—	2
Organic Medium	2 tbsp (1 oz)	10	0	0	0	0	2	1	0	20	190	—	—	2

FOOD	PORTION	CALS	FAT	SAT FAT	CHOL	PROT	CARB	SUGAR	FIBER	CALCI	SOD	POTAS	FOLIC	VIT C
BONE SUCKIN'														
Fat Free Gluten Free	2 tbsp	40	0	0	0	0	10	8	0	0	110	—	—	0
CHI-CHI'S														
Fiesta Mild	2 tbsp	10	0	0	0	0	2	2	0	0	150	—	—	1
CHUKAR CHERRIES														
Peach Cherry	1 tbsp	13	0	0	0	0	3	2	tr	0	65	—	—	9
CLINT'S														
Texas Medium	2 tbsp (1 oz)	5	0	0	0	0	1	1	—	—	70	—	—	0
DAVE'S GOURMET														
Insanity	2 tbsp (1 oz)	15	0	0	0	tr	2	2	—	20	170	—	—	12
DEI FRATELLI														
Casera Mild	2 tbsp (1.1 oz)	5	0	0	0	0	2	1	0	0	230	—	—	4
DELGROSSO														
Chunky Hot	2 tbsp (1.1 oz)	10	0	0	0	0	3	2	tr	0	250	—	—	5
Chunky Mild	2 tbsp (1.1 oz)	10	0	0	0	0	3	2	tr	0	110	—	—	5
EMERALD VALLEY														
Organic Fiesta	1 tbsp (1 oz)	20	0	0	0	tr	4	tr	tr	0	125	—	—	6
Organic Green	2 tbsp (1 oz)	10	0	0	0	0	2	tr	tr	0	110	—	—	2
FRONTERA														
Chipotle Hot	2 tbsp (1 oz)	10	0	0	0	0	2	2	0	0	140	—	—	9
Corn & Poblano Medium	2 tbsp (1 oz)	10	0	0	0	0	2	tr	0	0	135	—	—	6
Guajillo Medium	2 tbsp (1 oz)	10	1	0	0	0	2	1	1	0	170	—	—	4
Spanish Olive Mild	2 tbsp (1 oz)	10	1	0	0	0	1	tr	0	0	170	—	—	2
JAKE & AMOS														
Black Bean	2 tbsp (1 oz)	15	0	0	0	0	3	3	0	0	60	—	—	0
Peach	2 tbsp (1 oz)	20	0	0	0	0	6	5	0	0	40	—	—	0
JALA-FRESCA														
Green Stuff Medium	2 tbsp	10	0	0	0	0	2	1	0	0	240	—	—	6
MARGARITAVILLE														
Medium	2 tbsp	10	0	0	0	0	2	2	tr	20	0	—	—	0
Peppadew Chipotle Garlic	1 oz	10	0	0	0	0	2	2	0	20	100	—	—	5
Peppadew Mild	1 oz	10	0	0	0	0	2	2	0	20	105	—	—	6
MUIR GLEN														
Organic Medium	2 tbsp	10	0	0	0	0	3	1	0	0	130	—	—	5
NEWMAN'S OWN														
Bandito Pineapple	2 tbsp	15	0	0	0	0	3	3	1	—	90	—	—	—
Bandito Roasted Garlic	2 tbsp	10	0	0	0	1	2	1	1	—	150	—	—	—

FOOD	PORTION	CALS	FAT	SAT FAT	CHOL	PROT	CARB	SUGAR	FIBER	CALCI	SOD	POTAS	FOLIC	VIT C
NUMBER 9														
Black Bean & Corn	2 tbsp (1.1 oz)	20	0	0	0	1	4	1	1	0	90	—	—	6
Hot	2 tbsp (1.1 oz)	15	0	0	0	1	2	1	1	0	85	—	—	9
Mild	2 tbsp (1.1 oz)	15	0	0	0	1	2	1	1	0	90	—	—	9
ORGANICVILLE														
Mild	2 tbsp (1 oz)	15	0	0	0	0	3	1	0	0	135	—	—	6
Pineapple	2 tbsp (1 oz)	15	0	0	0	0	4	3	0	0	130	—	—	5
PACE														
Black Bean & Corn	2 tbsp	25	0	0	0	1	5	2	1	0	150	—	—	1
Organic Picante	2 tbsp	10	0	0	0	0	2	2	tr	0	220	—	—	0
Thick & Chunky	2 tbsp	10	0	0	0	0	2	2	tr	0	230	—	—	0
READY PAC														
Pico De Gallo	2 tbsp (1 oz)	5	0	0	0	0	2	1	0	0	15	—	—	4
ROBERT ROTHCHILD FARM														
Tomatillo & Pepper	2 tbsp	20	0	0	0	0	5	2	tr	0	95	—	—	6
SALBA SMART														
Organic Omega-3 Enriched	2 tbsp	12	0	0	0	0	2	0	1	20	126	—	—	5
SEEDS OF CHANGE														
Black Bean & Tomato Mild	2 tbsp	15	0	0	0	1	3	1	tr	0	170	—	—	0
Garlic & Cilantro Mild	2 tbsp	15	0	0	0	0	2	1	tr	0	170	—	—	0
SNYDER'S OF HANOVER														
Sweet	2 tbsp	20	0	0	0	0	5	4	0	20	95	—	—	4
TOSTITOS														
All Natural Chunky Mild	2 tbsp (1.2 oz)	10	0	0	0	0	2	2	tr	0	250	—	—	6
Con Queso	2 tbsp	40	3	1	<5	tr	5	tr	tr	40	280	—	—	0
UTZ														
Sweet	2 tbsp	10	0	0	0	0	2	1	tr	0	160	—	—	4
WALNUT ACRES														
Organic Fiesta Cilantro	2 tbsp	10	0	0	0	0	2	2	0	20	135	—	—	6
Organic Sweet Southwestern Peach	2 tbsp	20	0	0	0	0	5	4	0	0	85	—	—	6
SALSIFY														
fresh sliced cooked	½ cup	46	tr	—	0	2	10	—	—	32	11	192	—	3
SALT SUBSTITUTES														
gomasio sesame salt	2 tsp	34	3	—	—	1	2	—	1	60	388	29	—	—

FOOD	PORTION	CALS	FAT	SAT FAT	CHOL	PROT	CARB	SUGAR	FIBER	CALCI	SOD	POTAS	FOLIC	VIT C
ALSOSALT														
Butter Flavored	¼ tsp	1	0	0	0	0	0	0	0	—	0	320	—	—
Garlic Flavored	¼ tsp	1	0	0	0	0	0	0	0	—	0	300	—	—
Original	¼ tsp	1	0	0	0	0	0	0	0	—	0	356	—	—
CHEF PAUL PRUDHOMME'S														
Magic Salt Free Seasoning	¼ tsp	0	0	0	0	0	0	0	0	—	0	—	—	—
FRENCH'S														
No Salt	¼ cup	0	0	0	0	0	0	0	0	—	0	650	—	—
NU-SALT														
Salt Substitute	1 pkg (1 g)	0	0	0	0	0	0	0	0	—	0	530	—	—
SALT/SEASONED SALT														
kosher	¼ tsp	0	0	0	0	0	0	0	0	—	730	—	—	—
salt	1 dash (0.4 g)	0	0	0	0	0	0	0	0	0	155	0	0	0
salt	1 tbsp (0.6 oz)	0	0	0	0	0	0	0	0	4	6976	1	0	0
salt	1 tsp (6 g)	0	0	0	0	0	0	0	0	1	2325	0	0	0
sea salt coarse	1 tsp	0	0	0	0	0	0	0	0	—	1320	—	—	—
sea salt fine	¼ tsp	0	0	0	0	0	0	0	0	—	440	—	—	—
BACONSALT														
Original	¼ tsp (1 g)	0	0	0	<5	0	0	0	0	0	135	—	—	0
Peppered	¼ tsp (1 g)	0	0	0	<5	0	0	0	0	0	130	—	—	0
BOB'S RED MILL														
Garlic Salt Blend	¼ tsp	0	0	0	0	0	0	0	0	—	335	—	—	—
Sea Salt	¼ tsp	0	0	0	0	0	0	0	0	—	390	—	—	—
DAVID'S														
Kosher Salt	¼ tsp (1.5 g)	0	0	0	0	0	0	0	0	—	590	—	—	—
FALKSALT														
Flake Salt All Flavors	¼ tsp (1.5 g)	0	0	0	0	0	0	0	0	0	580	—	—	0
LAWRY'S														
Original Seasoned Salt	¼ tsp	0	0	0	0	0	0	0	0	—	380	—	—	—
MAINE COAST														
Sea Salt w/ Sea Veg	¼ tsp	0	0	0	0	0	0	0	0	3	396	19	—	—
MCCORMICK														
Grinder Garlic Sea Salt	¼ tsp	0	0	0	0	0	0	0	0	—	125	—	—	—
Grinder Sea Salt	¼ tsp	0	0	0	0	0	0	0	0	—	400	—	—	—
MORTON														
Iodized	¼ tsp	0	0	0	0	0	0	0	0	—	590	—	—	—
NUTRASALT														
African Medley	1 serv (1g)	0	0	0	0	0	0	0	0	0	55	158	—	2
Sea Salt	1 serv (1g)	0	0	0	0	0	0	0	0	0	118	331	—	0
Seasoned Salt	1 serv (1g)	0	0	0	0	0	0	0	0	0	85	243	—	0

FOOD	PORTION	CALS	FAT	SAT FAT	CHOL	PROT	CARB	SUGAR	FIBER	CALCI	SOD	POTAS	FOLIC	VIT C
OCEAN'S FLAVOR														
Natural Sea Salt	¼ tsp	0	0	0	0	0	0	0	0	—	211	86	—	—
SPICE HUNTER														
Celery Salt	¼ tsp	0	0	0	0	0	0	0	0	—	270	—	—	—
Garlic Salt	¼ tsp	0	0	0	0	0	0	0	0	—	290	—	—	—

SANDWICHES

FOOD	PORTION	CALS	FAT	SAT FAT	CHOL	PROT	CARB	SUGAR	FIBER	CALCI	SOD	POTAS	FOLIC	VIT C
ALEXIA														
Panini Tuscan Four Cheese w/ Roasted Tomato & Basil	1 pkg (6 oz)	380	15	7	25	18	42	5	6	400	900	—	—	2
Panini Tuscan Grilled Chicken w/ Mozzarella	1 pkg (6 oz)	400	18	6	35	23	37	2	5	200	650	—	—	0
Panini Tuscan Grilled Steak w/ Mushrooms & Onions	1 pkg (6 oz)	370	12	6	40	22	43	9	5	200	350	—	—	0
Panini Tuscan Smoked Chicken w/ Fire Roasted Vegetables & Parmesan	1 pkg (6 oz)	410	19	7	35	22	37	3	5	250	700	—	—	9
AMY'S														
Pocket Sandwich Tofu Scramble	1 (4 oz)	180	6	0	0	11	23	2	tr	0	520	—	—	12
Pocket Sandwich Vegetable Pie	1 (5 oz)	300	9	2	0	8	45	5	3	20	490	—	—	5
Wrap Indian Somosa	1 (5 oz)	250	9	1	0	8	35	2	4	60	680	—	—	12
AUNT JEMIMA														
Biscuit Sausage Egg & Cheese	1 (4 oz)	340	21	7	110	12	27	2	tr	100	830	—	—	0
Griddlecake Sausage Egg & Cheese	1 (4.4 oz)	350	20	7	150	13	30	11	tr	200	900	—	—	0
Sausage Egg & Cheese On French Toast	1 (4.7 oz)	310	18	7	205	15	23	6	tr	150	690	—	—	0
AUNT TRUDY'S														
Fillo Pocket Cheese & Tomato	1 (5 oz)	320	15	5	20	11	36	1	2	200	490	—	—	9
Fillo Pocket Classic Samosa	1 (5 oz)	280	10	1	0	6	43	1	3	20	350	—	—	15
Fillo Pocket Mediterranean Olive & Veggies	1 (5 oz)	270	10	1	0	6	41	1	2	40	550	—	—	9

FOOD	PORTION	CALS	FAT	SAT FAT	CHOL	PROT	CARB	SUGAR	FIBER	CALCI	SOD	POTAS	FOLIC	VIT C
AUNT TRUDY'S (CONT.)														
Organic Fillo Pocket Roasted Sweet Potato	1 (5 oz)	310	12	2	0	5	45	0	4	40	270	—	—	9
CEDARLANE														
Wrap Low Fat Couscous & Vegetable Veggie	1 (6 oz)	220	3	0	0	14	36	2	3	100	580	—	—	36
DIGIORNO														
Flatbread Melts Chicken Parmesan	1 (6 oz)	380	14	7	35	19	45	4	2	200	750	—	—	2
FARM RICH														
Philly Cheese Steak	2 (3 oz)	220	11	5	35	11	18	3	1	200	710	—	—	1
Sandwich Melts	2 (4.2 oz)	290	14	5	35	18	22	1	1	250	910	—	—	1
GARDENBURGER														
Wrap Black Bean Chipotle	1 (4.7 oz)	240	8	2	10	13	32	2	6	250	600	—	—	0
Wrap Pizza 100% Meatless Margherita	1 (4.7 oz)	240	8	3	10	12	34	3	5	250	590	—	—	9
GUILTLESS GOURMET														
Wrap Black Bean Chipotle	1 (5.7 oz)	270	3	1	0	9	51	6	7	100	570	—	—	0
Wrap California Veggie	1 (5.7 oz)	300	5	0	0	10	53	2	6	80	260	—	—	0
Wrap Mediterranean Spinach	1 (5.7 oz)	270	5	1	<5	10	45	4	4	150	270	—	—	0
HOT POCKETS														
Bacon Egg & Cheese	1 (2.2 oz)	160	8	4	40	6	17	4	1	60	240	—	—	—
Barbecue Beef	1 (4.5 oz)	310	10	5	25	11	42	11	1	100	800	—	60	—
Biscuit Sausage Egg & Cheese	1 (4.5 oz)	270	11	5	80	10	32	7	2	150	750	—	—	—
Calzone Four Meat & Four Cheese	½ (4.2 oz)	300	13	5	25	11	35	13	2	250	750	—	—	—
Calzone Pepperoni & Three Cheese	½ (4.2 oz)	330	15	6	25	11	39	14	2	250	780	—	—	—
Chicken Melt	1 (4.5 oz)	300	11	5	30	12	36	8	1	150	610	—	60	—
Croissant Chicken Parmesan	1 (4.5 oz)	340	15	6	10	9	41	10	3	150	810	—	60	—
Croissant Turkey Bacon Club	1 (4.5 oz)	320	15	7	25	12	34	10	1	150	640	—	60	—
Ham & Cheese	1 (4.5 oz)	290	11	5	30	11	36	9	1	150	660	—	60	—

FOOD	PORTION	CALS	FAT	SAT FAT	CHOL	PROT	CARB	SUGAR	FIBER	CALCI	SOD	POTAS	FOLIC	VIT C
HOT POCKETS (CONT.)														
Meatballs & Mozzarella	1 (4.5 oz)	300	12	5	25	11	36	7	2	200	760	—	80	—
Philly Steak & Cheese	1 (4.5 oz)	270	9	3	25	12	34	6	2	150	870	—	—	—
Steak Fajita	1 (4.5 oz)	280	12	6	25	10	33	8	2	150	750	—	40	—
Turkey & Ham w/ Cheese	1 (4.5 oz)	280	10	4	30	12	35	8	1	150	660	—	60	—
IAN'S														
Mini Chicken Patty	2 (5.3 oz)	368	10	2	34	20	54	6	1	0	608	—	—	4
JIMMY DEAN														
Bagel Sausage Egg & Cheese	1 (4.8 oz)	380	21	8	115	13	34	3	1	100	770	—	—	0
Biscuit Sausage Egg & Cheese	1 (4.5 oz)	440	31	11	120	13	27	5	1	150	850	—	—	1
Croissant Sausage Egg & Cheese	1 (4.5 oz)	430	29	9	115	13	30	6	1	150	740	—	—	1
D-Lights Croissants Turkey Sausage Egg White & Cheese	1 (4.8 oz)	300	12	5	35	17	31	4	4	100	910	—	—	1
D-Lights Honey Wheat Muffin Canadian Bacon Egg White & Cheese	1 (4.5 oz)	230	6	3	15	15	30	3	2	200	790	—	—	0
Muffin Sausage Egg & Cheese	1 (4.6 oz)	350	21	8	110	13	28	3	1	250	720	—	—	1
LEAN CUISINE														
Casual Cuisine Panini Chicken Club	1 pkg (6 oz)	360	9	4	40	24	45	6	4	300	675	510	—	1
Casual Cuisine Panini Spinach Artichoke Chicken	1 pkg (6 oz)	320	9	4	25	18	40	5	5	300	700	270	—	2
Casual Cuisine Panini Steak Cheddar & Mushroom	1 pkg (6 oz)	340	9	4	30	20	43	5	5	300	660	370	—	1
LEAN POCKETS														
Bacon Egg & Cheese	1 (2.2 oz)	150	5	2	40	6	18	3	1	80	230	—	—	—
Barbecue Beef	1 (4.5 oz)	290	7	4	25	11	46	11	2	100	700	—	—	—
Chicken Cheddar & Broccoli	1 (4.5 oz)	260	7	3	20	11	40	11	2	200	490	—	—	—
Chicken Fajita	1 (4.5 oz)	240	7	3	20	10	35	6	3	150	660	—	—	—

FOOD	PORTION	CALS	FAT	SAT FAT	CHOL	PROT	CARB	SUGAR	FIBER	CALCI	SOD	POTAS	FOLIC	VIT C
LEAN POCKETS (CONT.)														
Chicken Parmesan	1 (4.5 oz)	290	7	3	25	11	45	5	3	200	500	—	—	—
Ham & Cheese	1 (4.5 oz)	270	7	4	25	12	39	11	2	200	560	—	—	—
Meatballs & Mozzarella	1 (4.5 oz)	260	7	2	20	14	35	9	4	200	880	—	—	—
Philly Steak & Cheese	1 (4.5 oz)	270	7	4	25	11	38	8	1	150	600	—	—	—
Sausage Egg & Cheese	1 (2.2 oz)	140	5	2	30	6	18	6	1	80	220	—	—	—
Steak Fajita	1 (4.5 oz)	250	7	4	20	10	36	8	4	150	670	—	—	—
Three Cheese & Chicken Quesadilla	1 (4.5 oz)	260	7	4	20	13	34	6	3	300	690	—	—	—
Turkey & Ham w/ Cheddar	1 (4.5 oz)	280	7	4	25	12	40	9	2	150	640	—	—	—
Turkey Broccoli & Cheese	1 (4.5 oz)	270	7	4	25	10	39	12	2	150	450	—	—	—
LUNCHABLES														
Cracker Stackers Bologna & American	1 pkg	390	22	9	60	14	33	11	2	250	900	—	—	6
Cracker Stackers Ham & Cheddar	1 pkg	410	21	9	50	16	39	14	1	200	970	—	—	9
Sub Sandwich Ham + American	1 pkg	240	7	3	20	11	33	7	1	150	610	—	—	0
Sub Sandwich Turkey & Cheddar	1 pkg	230	6	2	15	11	34	8	1	150	580	—	—	6
MOM MADE														
Munchies Turkey Sausage	1 (2.5 oz)	220	11	5	5	5	24	1	1	60	290	—	—	4
Munchies Chicken	1 (2.5 oz)	220	11	5	10	6	24	1	2	40	280	—	—	1
OSCAR MAYER														
Deli Creations Honey Ham & Swiss	1 pkg (6.8 oz)	440	14	5	55	28	51	15	4	300	1490	—	—	0
Deli Creations Steakhouse Cheddar	1 pkg (7.1 oz)	450	15	6	60	29	50	14	3	200	1420	—	—	1
Deli Creations Turkey & Cheddar Dijon	1 pkg (6.7 oz)	430	15	5	50	26	48	12	5	250	1410	—	—	0
PBJAMMERZ														
Peanut Butter & Jelly All Flavors	1 (2 oz)	220	13	3	0	8	22	10	3	0	150	—	—	12

FOOD	PORTION	CALS	FAT	SAT FAT	CHOL	PROT	CARB	SUGAR	FIBER	CALCI	SOD	POTAS	FOLIC	VIT C
PILLSBURY														
Toaster Scrambles Cheese Egg & Bacon	1 (1.6 oz)	180	12	3	25	4	15	1	0	0	330	—	—	0
Toaster Scrambles Cheese Egg & Sausage	1 (1.6 oz)	180	12	3	25	4	15	1	0	0	320	—	—	0
SMUCKER'S														
Uncrustables Peanut Butter & Grape Jelly On Whole Wheat	1 (2 oz)	210	9	2	0	7	26	9	3	20	230	—	—	0
Uncrustables Peanut Butter & Strawberry Jam	1 (2 oz)	210	9	2	0	6	28	9	2	20	240	—	—	0
Uncrustables Peanut Butter on Wheat Bread	1 (2 oz)	210	9	2	0	9	26	9	3	20	230	—	—	0
STOUFFER'S														
Corner Bistro Panini Philly Style Steak & Cheese	1 pkg (6 oz)	340	16	6	40	20	33	3	3	200	680	—	—	2
Corner Bistro Panini Southwestern Chicken	1 pkg (6 oz)	360	16	7	45	20	31	2	3	250	920	—	—	2
THE FILLO FACTORY														
Organic Fillo Pocket Asian Vegetable	1 (5 oz)	240	10	2	0	5	34	2	3	40	390	—	—	18
VAN'S														
Breakfast In A Pocket Sandwich Ham Egg & Cheese	1 (4.5 oz)	370	22	12	80	11	30	3	tr	80	550	—	—	0
Breakfast In A Pocket Sandwich Veggie Egg & Cheese	1 (4.5 oz)	340	19	11	80	10	31	3	1	80	510	—	—	1
Breakfast Panini Huevos Rancheros	1 (4.5 oz)	270	11	4	125	11	33	2	5	150	330	—	—	27
Breakfast Panini Sausage Egg & Cheese	1 (4.5 oz)	290	13	5	105	14	28	1	3	150	730	—	—	0
TAKE-OUT														
bacon & egg	1 (6.2 oz)	388	21	6	421	21	28	4	1	158	938	276	90	tr

FOOD	PORTION	CALS	FAT	SAT FAT	CHOL	PROT	CARB	SUGAR	FIBER	CALCI	SOD	POTAS	FOLIC	VIT C
bacon lettuce & tomato w/ mayo	1 (5.8 oz)	344	17	4	21	12	35	5	3	80	945	348	74	10
beef barbecue w/ bun	1 (6.7 oz)	417	12	4	69	32	42	6	2	123	647	468	94	2
calzone beef & cheese	1 (14 oz)	1476	76	27	187	62	131	1	6	772	1726	683	382	0
calzone cheese	1 (15 oz)	1632	93	44	254	80	117	2	5	1802	2519	560	305	0
chicken fillet	1 (6.4 oz)	515	29	9	60	24	39	—	—	60	957	353	100	9
chicken fillet w/ cheese	1 (8 oz)	632	39	12	78	29	42	—	—	258	1238	333	109	3
chicken salad	1 (5 oz)	333	16	3	49	19	28	3	2	97	565	210	70	1
crab cake w/ bun	1	308	8	2	97	21	36	4	2	174	578	311	105	4
crispy chicken fillet w/ lettuce tomato & mayo	1 (7.7 oz)	537	26	5	64	27	49	tr	3	171	1424	449	64	1
croque monsieur	1 (12.4 oz)	765	46	26	152	41	43	9	2	1089	1018	437	41	9
egg salad	1 (5.6 oz)	485	35	7	329	14	28	3	1	121	706	157	94	0
french dip w/ roll	1 (6.8 oz)	357	13	5	54	26	34	4	1	104	562	347	81	0
fried egg	1 (3.4 oz)	226	9	2	206	10	26	3	1	104	439	117	80	0
grilled cheese	1 (2.9 oz)	290	16	6	22	9	28	4	1	235	764	129	38	0
gyro	1 (13.7 oz)	593	12	4	82	44	74	8	4	179	874	800	164	12
ham & egg	1 (4.4 oz)	272	11	3	222	15	27	3	2	110	802	197	82	1
ham w/ cheese lettuce & mayo	1 (5.4 oz)	369	18	7	57	19	32	4	2	260	1525	313	68	3
hot turkey w/ gravy	1	389	10	3	88	40	32	2	2	111	1349	517	68	0
peanut butter	1 (3.3 oz)	342	17	4	0	12	38	5	3	109	568	254	92	0
peanut butter & banana	1	617	14	3	0	10	43	11	4	89	451	406	85	5
peanut butter & jelly	1 (3.3 oz)	327	14	3	0	10	42	12	3	93	483	222	78	tr
reuben w/ sauerkraut & cheese	1 (6.4 oz)	463	29	10	81	21	30	7	4	257	1377	250	63	4
roast beef w/ gravy	1 (7.8 oz)	386	16	6	69	30	30	2	2	91	1083	425	64	0
sloppy joe pork on bun	1 (6.5 oz)	318	9	3	50	23	34	6	2	93	908	404	58	6
tuna melt	1 (5.3 oz)	350	16	5	34	20	30	6	1	165	832	258	45	1
tuna salad w/ lettuce	1 (5.9 oz)	289	7	1	22	19	37	6	2	94	785	242	68	1
turkey w/ mayo	1 (5 oz)	329	11	3	67	29	26	2	1	100	565	305	64	0

SAPODILLA

FOOD	PORTION	CALS	FAT	SAT FAT	CHOL	PROT	CARB	SUGAR	FIBER	CALCI	SOD	POTAS	FOLIC	VIT C
fresh	1	140	2	—	0	1	34	—	—	36	20	328	—	25
fresh cut up	1 cup	199	3	—	0	1	48	—	—	51	29	465	—	35

SAPOTES

FOOD	PORTION	CALS	FAT	SAT FAT	CHOL	PROT	CARB	SUGAR	FIBER	CALCI	SOD	POTAS	FOLIC	VIT C
fresh	1	301	1	—	0	5	76	—	—	88	21	773	—	45

FOOD	PORTION	CALS	FAT	SAT FAT	CHOL	PROT	CARB	SUGAR	FIBER	CALCI	SOD	POTAS	FOLIC	VIT C
SARDINES														
CANNED														
atlantic in oil w/ bone	1 can (3.2 oz)	192	11	1	131	23	0	0	0	351	465	365	11	—
atlantic in oil w/ bone	2	50	3	tr	34	6	0	0	0	92	121	95	3	—
pacific in tomato sauce w/ bone	1 can (13 oz)	658	44	11	225	61	0	0	0	887	1532	1262	89	4
pacific in tomato sauce w/ bone	1 (1.3 oz)	68	5	1	23	6	0	0	0	91	157	130	9	tr
CHICKEN OF THE SEA														
In Hot Sauce	1 can (3.75 oz)	120	3	1	70	19	3	0	1	400	430	—	—	0
In Oil Lightly Smoked	1 can (3.75 oz)	150	10	2	75	16	0	0	0	400	370	—	—	0
In Tomato Sauce	1 can (3.75 oz)	90	2	1	60	14	4	2	1	300	430	—	—	0
In Water	1 can (3.75 oz)	90	2	1	70	17	0	0	0	500	370	—	—	0
KING OSCAR														
In Extra Virgin Olive Oil	1 can (3.75 oz)	150	11	3	120	14	0	0	0	200	340	—	—	0
Skinless Boneless In Soya Oil	3 pieces (1.9 oz)	120	7	2	20	13	0	0	0	80	350	—	—	1
MATIZ														
In Olive Oil	½ pkg (2 oz)	120	7	1	0	13	0	0	0	180	236	—	—	0
POLAR														
In Mustard	1 can (4.5 oz)	170	7	2	75	17	10	1	0	350	610	—	—	0
In Tomato Sauce	1 can (4.5 oz)	120	4	1	70	17	5	tr	0	350	600	—	—	2
In Water	1 can (3 oz)	100	3	0	50	20	tr	tr	0	350	140	—	—	0
WILD PLANET														
Sardines Wild In Extra Virgin Olive Oil	2 oz	110	8	2	25	10	0	0	0	200	260	—	—	0
Sardines Wild In Marinara Sauce	2 oz	60	2	1	25	11	0	0	0	150	220	—	—	0
Sardines Wild In Oil w/ Lemon	2 oz	110	8	2	25	10	0	0	0	200	250	—	—	0
Sardines Wild In Spring Water	2 oz	73	2	1	48	13	0	0	0	300	194	—	—	0
FRESH														
raw	3.5 oz	135	5	—	—	19	0	0	0	85	100	—	—	—
SAUCE														
(*see also* BARBECUE SAUCE, CURRY, GRAVY, SPAGHETTI SAUCE)														
adobo fresco	2 tbsp	81	8	1	0	1	7	tr	1	44	6175	67	3	2
bearnaise	1 oz	177	19	12	21	1	1	—	tr	49	257	63	1	tr
cheese mix as prep w/ milk	1 cup	307	17	9	53	16	23	—	—	570	1566	554	—	2

FOOD	PORTION	CALS	FAT	SAT FAT	CHOL	PROT	CARB	SUGAR	FIBER	CALCI	SOD	POTAS	FOLIC	VIT C
enchilada sauce green	¼ cup	46	4	2	11	1	3	2	1	19	113	134	0	7
enchilada sauce red	¼ cup	79	8	4	22	1	2	1	1	16	86	86	4	4
fish sauce chinese	1 tbsp	9	0	0	—	2	tr	—	0	2	1224	52	—	0
fish sauce vietnamese nuoc mam	1 tbsp	6	0	0	0	1	1	—	0	8	1390	52	9	0
hoisin	1 tbsp	35	1	—	0	1	7	—	tr	5	258	19	4	0
moroccan tagine	½ cup (4 oz)	70	3	0	0	2	10	10	1	20	1140	—	—	30
mushroom mix as prep w/ milk	1 cup	228	10	5	34	11	24	—	—	—	1533	—	—	—
oyster	1 tbsp	8	0	0	0	tr	2	—	0	5	437	9	2	0
plum sauce	0.5 oz	42	0	0	—	0	10	10	0	6	281	7	—	0
satay peanut sauce	1 oz	77	6	2	0	2	3	3	1	8	138	55	—	0
sour cream mix as prep w/ milk	1 cup	509	30	16	91	19	45	—	—	546	1007	733	—	—
stroganoff mix as prep	1 cup	271	11	7	38	12	34	—	—	521	1829	672	—	—
sweet & sour mix as prep	1 cup	294	tr	tr	0	1	73	—	—	41	779	66	—	—
teriyaki	1 tbsp	15	0	0	0	1	3	—	—	4	690	41	4	0
teriyaki mix as prep	1 cup	131	1	tr	0	4	28	—	—	112	4791	216	—	—
white sauce mix as prep w/ milk	1 cup	241	13	6	34	10	21	—	—	424	796	443	—	—
AHH!GOURMET														
Perky Savory Coffee Sauce	4 tbsp	71	0	0	0	tr	17	15	tr	5	57	—	—	0
Ritzy Kumquat Plum Sauce	4 tbsp	98	0	0	0	tr	24	21	1	10	507	—	—	0
Spicy Garlicky Sweet Sauce Paste	4 tbsp	101	4	tr	0	2	16	13	2	10	503	—	—	1
Spicy Ginger Soy Sauce Paste	4 tbsp	137	8	1	0	2	15	13	2	32	612	—	—	0
ANNIE'S HOMEGROWN														
Organic Worcestershire	1 tsp (5 g)	5	0	0	0	0	1	1	—	—	75	—	—	—
ASIAN CREATIONS														
Marvelous Mango	¼ cup	20	0	0	0	0	6	5	0	0	20	—	—	6
Pad Thai Pizzazz	2 oz	110	6	1	0	2	14	9	tr	20	310	—	—	6
Peanut Passion	¼ cup	130	9	4	0	4	12	7	1	20	420	—	—	2
BEAR-MAN														
Sap-Happy Golden Bear	2 tbsp	60	0	0	0	0	20	17	0	20	350	—	—	2

FOOD	PORTION	CALS	FAT	SAT FAT	CHOL	PROT	CARB	SUGAR	FIBER	CALCI	SOD	POTAS	FOLIC	VIT C
BOAR'S HEAD														
Ham Glaze Sugar & Spice	2 tbsp	120	0	0	0	0	30	29	0	40	95	—	—	0
BONE SUCKIN'														
Hiccuppin' Hot	1 tsp	10	0	0	0	0	2	2	0	0	25	—	—	0
Yaki Stir Fry	1 tbsp	30	0	0	0	0	7	6	0	0	260	—	—	0
BOURBON CHICKEN														
Marinade Original	1 tbsp (0.6 oz)	5	0	0	0	0	1	0	—	—	410	—	—	—
CAINS														
Tartar	2 tbsp	160	16	3	15	0	2	1	0	0	160	—	—	0
CHEF HYMIE GRANDE														
New Mexico Sweet Basting Sauce	2 tbsp (1.2 oz)	35	0	0	0	0	8	6	—	—	15	—	—	6
CHINA PRIDE														
Duck Sauce Sweet & Pungent	2 tbsp	80	0	0	0	0	19	11	1	0	260	—	—	0
DAVE'S GOURMET														
Hot Sauce Roasted Garlic	1 tsp (5 g)	0	0	0	0	0	0	0	0	0	90	—	—	1
Insanity Sauce	1 tsp (5 g)	10	1	—	—	0	0	0	0	0	0	—	—	5
Jammin' Jerk	1 tsp (5 g)	5	0	0	0	0	1	—	—	0	15	—	—	1
Steak Sauce	1 tbsp (0.6 oz)	20	0	0	0	0	5	4	—	0	220	—	—	0
DEI FRATELLI														
Sloppy Joe Sauce	¼ cup (2.2 oz)	35	0	0	0	1	9	5	1	20	360	—	—	6
DELGROSSO														
Sloppy Joe Sauce	¼ cup (2.2 oz)	60	1	0	0	1	13	10	1	0	260	—	—	9
D'ONI														
Happy Together Orange Chili Garlic	2 tbsp	50	0	0	0	0	12	11	—	—	80	—	—	—
Moondance Marinade	1 tbsp	10	0	0	0	—	0	0	—	—	150	—	—	—
EMERIL'S														
Kick It Up Red Pepper Sauce	1 tsp	0	0	0	0	0	0	0	0	—	140	—	—	—
ETHNIC GOURMET														
Punjab Saag Spinach	4 oz	60	3	1	5	2	6	3	1	40	500	—	—	15
Simmer Sauce Calcutta Masala	4 oz	90	5	2	5	2	10	8	1	40	500	—	—	15
Simmer Sauce Delhi Korma	4 oz	100	7	3	10	2	9	1	2	60	500	—	—	12
FISCHER & WIESER														
Bourbon Charred Pineapple	1 tbsp (0.7 oz)	35	0	0	0	0	8	8	0	0	0	—	—	0

FOOD	PORTION	CALS	FAT	SAT FAT	CHOL	PROT	CARB	SUGAR	FIBER	CALCI	SOD	POTAS	FOLIC	VIT C
FISCHER & WIESER (CONT.)														
Chipotle Original Roasted Raspberry	1 tbsp (0.7 oz)	40	0	0	0	0	10	9	1	0	60	—	—	2
Grilling Chipotle Plum	1 tbsp (0.7 oz)	40	0	0	0	0	10	10	—	—	15	—	—	—
Grilling Spicy Garlic Steak	1 tbsp (0.7 oz)	20	1	0	0	1	2	2	0	0	270	—	—	1
Habanero Mango Ginger	1 tbsp (0.7 oz)	40	0	0	0	0	11	9	—	—	0	—	—	2
Marinade All Purpose Vegetable & Meat	1 tbsp (0.7 oz)	35	3	0	0	0	3	2	0	0	290	—	—	1
Onion Glaze Sweet & Savory	1 tbsp (0.7 oz)	45	0	0	0	0	11	11	—	—	5	—	—	—
Roasted Blackberry Chipotle	1 tbsp (0.7 oz)	35	0	0	0	0	9	9	—	—	70	—	—	—
Soppin' Big Bold Red	1 tbsp (0.7 oz)	35	0	0	0	1	7	6	—	—	380	—	—	—
FORTUN'S														
Asian Style Pepper	¼ cup (2 oz)	40	1	0	0	1	5	2	0	0	500	—	—	12
Lemon Dill Caper w/ White Wine	¼ cup (2 oz)	20	1	0	0	0	3	1	0	0	370	—	—	2
Marsala & Mushroom	¼ cup (2 oz)	40	1	0	0	1	5	2	0	0	340	—	—	1
Spicy Mustard w/ Brandy	¼ cup (2 oz)	35	2	1	5	0	2	1	0	0	450	—	—	0
Stroganoff	¼ cup (2 oz)	45	3	1	5	1	3	1	0	20	580	—	—	1
FRANK'S														
RedHot Chile & Lime Sauce	1 tsp	0	0	0	0	0	0	0	0	—	200	—	—	—
RedHot Original Cayenne Pepper Sauce	1 tsp	0	0	0	0	0	0	0	0	—	200	—	—	—
RedHot X-tra Hot	1 tsp	0	0	0	0	0	0	0	0	—	210	—	—	—
FRENCH'S														
Worcestershire	1 tsp	0	0	0	0	0	1	0	0	0	50	—	—	0
FRONTERA														
Hot Sauce Habanero	1 tsp	5	0	0	0	0	1	0	0	0	35	—	—	0
GOOD CLEAN FOOD														
Simmer Sauce Balsamic Mushroom	⅜ cup (3 oz)	100	6	1	5	2	9	4	tr	—	250	—	—	2
Simmer Sauce Cacciatore	⅜ cup (3 oz)	70	4	1	—	2	7	4	2	200	350	—	—	24
Simmer Sauce Creole	⅜ cup (3 oz)	45	2	1	5	2	7	4	1	80	330	—	—	15

FOOD	PORTION	CALS	FAT	SAT FAT	CHOL	PROT	CARB	SUGAR	FIBER	CALCI	SOD	POTAS	FOLIC	VIT C
GOOD CLEAN FOOD (CONT.)														
Simmer Sauce Dill	⅜ cup (3 oz)	60	4	1	5	2	5	1	—	—	250	—	—	2
Simmer Sauce French Tarragon	⅜ cup (3 oz)	90	6	1	5	2	8	2	tr	20	290	—	—	2
Simmer Sauce Mediterranean	⅜ cup (3 oz)	50	3	—	—	1	6	2	1	80	180	—	—	12
HOT SQUEEZE														
Original	2 tbsp (1 oz)	110	0	0	0	1	27	25	—	—	310	—	—	2
HOUSE OF TSANG														
General Tsao	1 tsp	45	1	0	0	0	10	7	0	0	230	—	—	0
Hoisin	1 tsp	15	0	0	0	0	4	3	0	0	120	14	—	0
Kobe Steak Grill	1 tbsp	50	4	1	0	0	2	2	0	0	560	125	—	0
Korean Teriyaki Stir Fry	1 tbsp	35	2	0	0	0	5	4	0	0	460	28	—	0
Peanut Sauce Bangkok Padang	1 tbsp	45	3	1	0	1	4	3	0	0	250	41	—	0
Spicy Brown Bean	1 tbsp	15	0	0	0	0	3	2	0	0	130	17	—	0
Sweet & Sour	1 tbsp	35	0	0	0	0	8	7	0	0	50	20	—	0
Sweet Ginger Sesame	1 tbsp	40	1	0	0	0	8	7	0	0	401	47	—	0
Thai Peanut	1 tbsp	50	3	1	0	1	4	4	0	0	280	43	—	0
KEN'S														
Marinade Herb & Garlic	1 tbsp	20	1	0	0	0	3	2	0	0	370	—	—	1
Marinade Lemon & Pepper	1 tbsp	10	0	0	0	0	2	1	0	0	350	—	—	1
Marinade Teriyaki	1 tbsp	20	0	0	0	0	4	3	0	0	260	—	—	0
KIKKOMAN														
Black Bean w/ Garlic	1 tbsp (1.2 oz)	50	1	0	0	3	6	4	2	20	1120	—	—	0
Hoisan	2 tbsp (1.2 oz)	80	2	1	0	1	17	16	0	0	460	—	—	0
Katsu	1 tbsp (0.6 oz)	20	1	0	0	0	5	4	—	—	290	—	—	—
Marinade Quick & Easy Honey & Mustard	1 tbsp (0.6 oz)	30	0	0	0	1	6	5	—	—	420	—	—	—
Oyster	1 tbsp (0.6 oz)	25	0	0	0	0	5	4	0	0	860	—	—	0
Peanut Sauce Thai Style	2 tbsp (1.2 oz)	80	4	1	0	2	10	8	tr	0	650	—	—	0
Plum	2 tbsp (1.2 oz)	80	1	0	0	0	18	17	0	0	280	—	—	0
Stir-Fry	1 tbsp (0.6 oz)	20	0	0	0	tr	4	3	—	—	520	—	—	—
Sweet & Sour	2 tbsp (1.2 oz)	35	0	0	0	0	9	7	—	—	190	—	—	—
Teriyaki Less Sodium	1 tbsp (0.5 oz)	15	0	0	0	tr	3	3	—	—	320	—	—	—
Teriyaki Sauce & Marinade	1 tbsp (0.5 oz)	15	0	0	0	1	2	2	—	—	610	—	—	—
Teriyaki Takumi Original	1 tbsp (0.6 oz)	30	0	0	0	1	6	6	—	—	450	—	—	—

FOOD	PORTION	CALS	FAT	SAT FAT	CHOL	PROT	CARB	SUGAR	FIBER	CALCI	SOD	POTAS	FOLIC	VIT C
KNORR														
Alfredo Mix as prep	2 oz	60	3	2	5	2	5	—	—	—	390	—	—	—
Bearnaise Mix as prep	2 oz	35	1	tr	5	2	5	—	—	—	190	—	—	—
Demi-Glace Mix as prep	2 oz	30	1	tr	0	1	4	—	—	—	500	—	—	—
Green Peppercorn Mix as prep	2 oz	35	1	tr	5	1	5	—	—	—	390	—	—	—
Hollandaise Mix as prep	2 oz	35	1	tr	5	2	5	—	—	—	170	—	—	—
Mango Habanero	1 oz	20	0	0	0	tr	6	—	—	—	95	—	—	—
Sweet Red Chili	1 oz	80	0	0	0	1	19	—	—	—	300	—	—	—
White Mix as prep	2 oz	20	1	tr	0	tr	3	—	—	—	290	—	—	—
LA CHOY														
Sweet & Sour	2 tbsp (1.2 oz)	60	0	0	0	0	14	11	0	0	110	—	—	0
Teriyaki	1 tbsp (0.6 oz)	40	0	0	0	tr	10	8	0	0	570	—	—	0
LATINO CHEF														
Chimichurri Sun Dried Tomato	2 tbsp	120	10	1	0	2	8	5	2	20	210	—	—	5
Sofrito	2 tbsp	20	1	—	0	0	3	—	—	—	160	—	—	5
LAWRY'S														
Marinade Szechuan Sweet & Sour BBQ	1 tbsp (0.5 oz)	35	0	0	0	0	8	7	—	—	460	—	—	—
Marinade Tuscan Sun-Dried Tomato	1 tbsp (0.5 oz)	15	0	0	0	0	2	1	—	—	350	—	—	1
LEA & PERRINS														
Worcestershire	1 tsp (0.2 oz)	5	0	0	0	0	1	1	—	—	65	—	—	—
LONEY'S														
Bar-B-Q Chicken as prep	¼ cup (2.1 oz)	15	0	0	0	tr	3	0	0	0	200	—	—	0
MANWICH														
Sloppy Joe Original	¼ cup (2.2 oz)	40	0	0	0	tr	9	6	2	0	410	190	—	0
MARGARITAVILLE														
ConQueso In Paradise	1 oz	45	3	2	10	2	2	1	0	80	210	—	—	0
MATIZ														
Paella Sofrito	¼ cup	137	12	2	tr	tr	6	5	1	<10	230	—	—	1
MCCORMICK														
Cocktail For Seafood Original	¼ cup (2.1 oz)	90	1	—	0	1	19	16	1	—	970	—	—	—
Seafood Sauce Asian	2 tbsp (1.2 oz)	50	2	—	0	tr	7	4	0	—	470	—	—	—

FOOD	PORTION	CALS	FAT	SAT FAT	CHOL	PROT	CARB	SUGAR	FIBER	CALCI	SOD	POTAS	FOLIC	VIT C
MCCORMICK (CONT.)														
Seafood Sauce Cajun Style	1 tbsp (1.1 oz)	15	0	0	0	0	3	3	0	—	370	—	—	—
Seafood Sauce Scampi	1 tbsp (1 oz)	160	17	—	0	0	2	1	0	—	220	—	—	—
Tartar Fat Free	2 tbsp (1.1 oz)	30	0	0	0	0	7	5	1	—	250	—	—	—
Tartar Original	2 tbsp (1 oz)	140	14	—	20	0	3	3	0	—	190	—	—	—
MRS. DASH														
10 Minute Marinade Lemon Herb Peppercorn	1 tbsp (0.5 oz)	25	2	—	—	0	2	1	—	—	0	18	—	1
10 Minute Marinade Mesquite Grille	1 tbsp (0.5 oz)	25	2	—	—	0	2	1	—	—	0	30	—	1
10 Minute Marinade Spicy Teriyaki	1 tbsp (0.5 oz)	25	1	—	—	0	5	3	—	—	0	35	—	1
10 Minute Marinade Zesty Garlic Herb	1 tbsp (0.5 oz)	25	2	—	—	0	3	1	—	—	0	27	—	2
NATURALLY FRESH														
Seafood Cocktail	2 tbsp	25	0	0	0	0	5	5	0	—	210	0	—	—
Tartar Sauce	2 tbsp	130	14	2	10	0	2	2	0	—	85	20	—	—
NEWMAN'S OWN														
Fra Diavolo	½ cup	70	3	0	0	0	10	4	3	—	510	—	—	—
OLD BAY														
Tartar Sauce	2 tbsp (1.1 oz)	130	12	—	15	0	3	—	0	—	210	—	—	—
OLD EL PASO														
Enchilada Mild	¼ cup	25	1	0	0	0	4	1	0	0	250	—	—	0
ORGANICVILLE														
Island Teriyaki	1 tbsp (0.5 oz)	25	1	0	0	tr	4	3	0	0	240	—	—	0
PACE														
Taco Sauce Green	1 tbsp	5	0	0	0	0	1	1	0	0	100	—	—	0
Taco Sauce Red	2 tbsp	10	0	0	0	0	2	1	0	0	130	—	—	0
PATAK'S														
Jalfrezi Sweet Peppers & Coconut	½ cup	140	8	3	0	2	15	10	1	20	620	—	—	4
Korma Rich Creamy Coconut	½ cup	240	20	12	15	2	13	9	1	0	750	—	—	0
Rogan Josh Spicy Tomato & Cardamon	½ cup	90	4	0	0	2	12	6	2	20	750	—	—	1
Tikka Masala Tangy Lemon & Cilantro	½ cup	120	8	1	0	1	12	6	1	0	900	—	—	2

FOOD	PORTION	CALS	FAT	SAT FAT	CHOL	PROT	CARB	SUGAR	FIBER	CALCI	SOD	POTAS	FOLIC	VIT C
PROGRESSO														
Bruschetta	2 tbsp (1 oz)	10	1	0	0	0	1	1	0	—	100	—	—	4
ROAD'S END ORGANICS														
Alfredo Style Dairy Free Gluten Free	⅓ pkg	35	0	0	0	3	5	0	1	0	240	—	40	0
Cheddar Style Dairy Free	⅓ pkg	35	0	0	0	2	6	0	1	0	260	—	40	0
ROBERT ROTHCHILD FARM														
Anne Mae's Smoky Sweet Chipotle	2 tbsp	35	0	0	0	tr	9	8	0	60	80	—	—	9
SAUCY SUSAN														
Peach Apricot	2 tbsp (1.3 oz)	80	0	0	0	0	19	11	2	0	260	—	—	0
SIMPLY BOULDER														
Coconut Peanut	2 tbsp (1 oz)	90	7	2	0	2	6	5	0	0	140	—	—	0
Lemon Pesto	2 tbsp (1 oz)	50	5	1	0	0	3	2	0	0	200	—	—	1
Zesty Pineapple	2 tbsp (1 oz)	45	3	0	0	0	7	5	0	0	85	—	—	2
SOY VAY														
Hoisin Garlic Asian Glaze & Marinade	1 tbsp	40	1	0	0	1	7	7	0	0	400	—	—	0
Veri Veri Teriyaki	1 tbsp	35	1	0	0	0	6	5	0	0	490	—	—	0
STEEL'S														
Cocktail w/ Dill & Lemon Sugar Free Gluten Free	¼ cup (2.4 oz)	35	0	0	0	2	9	6	2	0	85	—	—	12
Hoisin No Sugar Added Gluten Free	2 tbsp (1 oz)	30	0	0	0	1	6	4	1	0	330	—	—	0
TABASCO														
Pepper Sauce	1 tsp	0	0	0	0	0	0	0	0	0	40	—	—	0
TEXAS SASSY														
Marinade Salsa	1 tbsp (0.5 oz)	15	0	0	0	0	3	3	—	—	45	—	—	—
Pickle Sauce	1 tbsp (0.5 oz)	30	0	0	0	0	7	7	—	—	115	—	—	—
THAI KITCHEN														
Pineapple & Chili	2 tbsp (1 oz)	25	0	0	0	0	7	6	0	0	160	—	—	66
Premium Fish Sauce	1 tbsp (0.5 oz)	10	0	0	0	2	0	0	0	0	1360	—	—	0
Sweet Red Chili	2 tbsp (1 oz)	70	0	0	0	0	18	14	0	0	410	—	—	0
Thai Chili & Ginger	2 tbsp (1 oz)	40	0	0	0	0	10	8	0	0	260	—	—	1
THE GRACIOUS GOURMET														
Pesto Lemon Artichoke	2 tbsp (1 oz)	50	5	1	0	1	2	0	1	20	180	—	—	4

FOOD	PORTION	CALS	FAT	SAT FAT	CHOL	PROT	CARB	SUGAR	FIBER	CALCI	SOD	POTAS	FOLIC	VIT C
THE WIZARD'S														
Organic Worcestershire Vegetarian Wheat Free	1 tsp	0	0	0	0	0	1	tr	0	0	115	—	—	0
THREE ACRE KITCHEN														
Marinade Balsamic w/ Juniper & Rosemary	1 tbsp (0.5 oz)	50	5	1	—	0	2	1	—	—	85	—	—	—
WALDEN FARMS														
Calorie Free Scampi Sauce	2 tbsp (1 oz)	0	0	0	0	0	0	0	0	0	130	—	—	0
WILD THYMES FARM														
Marinade Hawaiian Teryaki	1 tbsp	19	1	tr	0	1	3	2	tr	10	280	—	—	1
Marinade Korean Ginger Scallion	1 tbsp	20	1	tr	0	tr	3	2	tr	0	300	—	—	1
Marinade New Orleans Creole	1 tbsp	11	0	0	0	tr	3	1	tr	0	61	—	—	2
WILDWOOD														
Aioli	1 tbsp	80	9	1	0	0	0	0	0	0	80	0	—	0
Pesto Basil & Pine Nuts	¼ cup	230	23	4	8	5	2	0	1	150	360	0	—	9
WINGERS														
Hotter Than Hot	1 tsp	0	0	0	0	0	0	0	0	—	120	—	—	—
WORLD HARBORS														
Buccaneer Blends Pirate's Original	1 tbsp (0.6 oz)	20	0	0	0	0	4	10	0	0	115	—	—	2
Chimichurri	2 tbsp (1.2 oz)	40	0	0	0	0	9	8	0	0	180	—	—	1
Fajita	2 tbsp (1.1 oz)	45	0	0	0	0	10	8	0	0	290	—	—	1
Jerk	2 tbsp (1 oz)	70	0	0	0	0	18	16	0	20	200	—	—	0
Lemon Pepper & Garlic	2 tbsp (1 oz)	35	0	0	0	0	8	7	0	0	140	—	—	1
Thai	2 tbsp (1 oz)	40	0	0	0	0	8	7	0	0	350	—	—	1
TAKE-OUT														
cucumber yogurt sauce	1½ tbsp	20	0	0	2	2	3	—	0	60	20	—	—	4

SAUERKRAUT

FOOD	PORTION	CALS	FAT	SAT FAT	CHOL	PROT	CARB	SUGAR	FIBER	CALCI	SOD	POTAS	FOLIC	VIT C
canned	½ cup	22	tr	tr	0	1	5	—	—	36	780	201	—	17
BA-TAMPTE														
Kosher	2 tbsp (1 oz)	5	0	0	0	0	1	0	1	0	180	—	—	2
BOAR'S HEAD														
Sauerkraut	2 tbsp (1 oz)	5	0	0	0	0	1	0	tr	0	180	—	—	2
DEI FRATELLI														
Sauerkraut	2 tbsp (1 oz)	5	0	0	0	0	1	0	tr	20	190	—	—	4

FOOD	PORTION	CALS	FAT	SAT FAT	CHOL	PROT	CARB	SUGAR	FIBER	CALCI	SOD	POTAS	FOLIC	VIT C
GEDNEY														
Sauerkraut	½ cup	15	0	0	0	0	3	0	0	0	1020	—	—	0
TREE OF LIFE														
Organic	½ cup (3.6 oz)	15	0	0	0	0	3	0	<3	0	1000	160	—	0

SAUSAGE

FOOD	PORTION	CALS	FAT	SAT FAT	CHOL	PROT	CARB	SUGAR	FIBER	CALCI	SOD	POTAS	FOLIC	VIT C
beef & pork	1 link (2.3 oz)	196	17	4	51	8	1	0	0	5	560	187	3	0
beef & pork w/ cheddar cheese	1 link (2.7 oz)	228	20	7	49	10	2	tr	0	44	653	159	2	0
bierschinken	3.5 oz	174	11	—	—	18	tr	—	—	15	753	261	—	—
bierwurst	3.5 oz	258	21	—	—	16	0	0	0	—	—	—	—	—
blutwurst uncooked	3.5 oz	424	39	—	—	13	0	0	0	7	680	38	—	—
bockwurst	3.5 oz	276	25	—	—	12	0	0	0	—	700	—	—	—
bratwurst chicken cooked	1 (3 oz)	148	9	—	60	16	0	0	0	9	60	177	5	2
bratwurst pork cooked	1 link (2.5 oz)	226	19	7	44	10	2	2	0	34	778	197	4	0
brotwurst pork & beef	1 link (2.5 oz)	226	19	7	44	10	2	2	0	34	778	197	4	0
chipolata	3.5 oz	342	32	12	66	14	1	1	0	16	747	160	3	1
chorizo	1 link (2.1 oz)	273	23	8	53	14	1	0	0	5	741	239	1	0
fleischwurst	3.5 oz	305	29	—	—	12	0	0	0	14	829	199	—	—
free range chicken breakfast	2 links (2.7 oz)	110	6	1	45	14	1	1	0	0	570	—	—	0
gelbwurst uncooked	3.5 oz	363	33	—	—	12	0	0	0	—	640	285	—	—
italian pork cooked	1 (2.4 oz)	230	18	6	38	13	3	1	1	14	809	204	3	tr
italian turkey smoked	1 (2 oz)	88	5	—	30	8	3	2	1	12	520	110	4	17
jagdwurst	3.5 oz	211	16	—	—	16	0	0	0	14	818	260	—	—
knockwurst pork & beef	1 (2.5 oz)	221	20	7	43	8	2	0	0	8	670	143	1	0
mettwurst uncooked	3.5 oz	483	45	—	—	13	0	0	0	13	1090	213	—	—
plockwurst uncooked	3.5 oz	312	45	—	—	19	0	0	0	—	—	—	—	—
polish kielbasa	2 oz	127	10	3	39	7	2	0	0	—	672	—	—	8
pork cooked	2 links (1.7 oz)	163	14	4	40	9	0	0	0	8	360	141	1	tr
regensburger uncooked	3.5 oz	354	31	—	—	13	0	0	0	—	—	—	—	—
smoked beef cooked	1 (1.4 oz)	134	12	—	29	—	—	—	<7	4	—	—	—	—
venison patty	1 (1 oz)	84	8	3	15	3	1	0	0	8	292	46	2	4
vienna canned	1 can (4 oz)	260	22	8	98	12	3	0	0	11	1095	114	5	0
vienna canned	1 link (0.5 oz)	37	3	1	14	2	tr	0	0	2	155	16	1	0
weisswurst uncooked	3.5 oz	305	27	—	—	11	0	0	0	25	620	122	—	—

FOOD	PORTION	CALS	FAT	SAT FAT	CHOL	PROT	CARB	SUGAR	FIBER	CALCI	SOD	POTAS	FOLIC	VIT C
zungenwurst (tongue)	3.5 oz	285	24	—	—	17	0	0	0	—	—	—	—	—
AL FRESCO														
Buffalo Style	1 (3 oz)	160	8	3	50	19	4	0	—	20	630	—	—	1
Spicy Jalapeno	1 (3 oz)	120	7	2	65	19	1	1	—	—	550	—	—	—
Sundried Tomato & Basil	1 (3 oz)	180	8	2	70	19	3	2	—	20	440	—	—	1
Sweet Apple	1 (3 oz)	160	8	3	65	19	9	3	—	—	580	—	—	2
APPLEGATE FARMS														
Organic Andouille	1 (3 oz)	120	6	2	60	13	3	1	1	20	620	—	—	1
ARMOUR														
Sizzle & Serve Turkey	3 (1.8 oz)	130	9	3	35	9	2	1	0	40	380	—	—	0
BANQUET														
Brown'N Serve Lite Maple	3 (2 oz)	130	9	3	35	9	4	2	0	40	450	—	—	0
Brown'N Serve Lite Original	3 (2.1 oz)	120	9	3	25	9	2	1	0	40	430	—	—	0
Brown'N Serve Turkey	3 (2.1 oz)	110	7	2	40	9	2	1	0	60	390	—	—	0
BOAR'S HEAD														
Bratwurst	1 (4 oz)	300	25	11	75	19	0	0	0	20	650	—	—	0
Hot Smoked	1 (3.2 oz)	250	22	9	55	12	1	0	0	0	740	—	—	0
Kielbasa	2 oz	120	10	4	50	9	0	0	0	0	440	—	—	0
Knockwurst Beef	1 (4 oz)	310	27	11	70	15	1	0	0	20	950	—	—	0
BUTTERBALL														
Bratwurst Turkey	1 (3.2 oz)	140	8	2	60	17	1	—	—	—	460	—	—	—
Breakfast Turkey	3 (3 oz)	130	7	2	55	15	0	0	0	20	530	—	—	—
Polska Kielbasa Turkey	2 oz	100	6	2	30	8	4	1	0	20	610	—	—	1
Sweet Italian Turkey	1 (3.2 oz)	140	8	2	60	16	1	—	—	—	360	—	—	—
COLEMAN														
Bratwurst	1 (3 oz)	240	21	8	55	11	tr	0	0	0	650	—	—	0
Chicken Spicy Chorizo	1 (3 oz)	150	8	3	65	15	1	0	0	20	490	—	—	2
DIETZ & WATSON														
Italian	1 (2 oz)	160	14	5	30	8	1	0	0	0	480	—	—	0
Italian Chicken	1 (3.4 oz)	130	8	3	50	15	0	0	0	0	680	—	—	0
Jerk Chicken	1 (3.4 oz)	130	8	3	50	15	0	0	0	0	680	—	—	0
Polska Kielbasa	1 (2 oz)	150	13	5	30	4	1	0	0	0	550	—	—	0
Scrapple Philadelphia	2 oz	120	8	3	40	6	7	0	1	0	320	—	—	0
FOSTER FARMS														
Turkey Breakfast Links	2 (2 oz)	120	10	—	45	9	0	0	0	—	400	—	—	—

FOOD	PORTION	CALS	FAT	SAT FAT	CHOL	PROT	CARB	SUGAR	FIBER	CALCI	SOD	POTAS	FOLIC	VIT C
HANS ALL NATURAL														
Breakfast Links Skinless Chicken	2 (1.7 oz)	60	4	2	40	8	0	0	0	20	370	—	—	1
HANS ALL NATURAL (CONT.)														
Chicken Spinach & Feta	1 (2.7 oz)	130	8	2	45	13	1	0	0	40	350	—	—	4
HEALTHY ONES														
Smoked	2 oz	80	3	1	25	7	6	2	0	20	480	—	—	2
HIGH PLAINS BISON														
Bratwurst Beer & Cheddar	1 (3.2 oz)	280	21	8	55	14	3	1	0	250	820	—	—	1
Cocktail	1 (2 oz)	180	15	7	40	9	1	0	0	0	410	—	—	1
Wild Rice & Asiago	1 (3.2 oz)	260	21	10	60	13	6	0	0	100	610	—	—	0
HONEYSUCKLE WHITE														
Turkey Roll Mild Italian	2.5 oz	100	5	2	40	13	1	0	0	—	460	—	—	—
JIMMY DEAN														
Fully Cooked Original Links	3 (2.4 oz)	240	22	8	45	9	1	1	0	20	450	—	—	0
Fully Cooked Original Patties	2 (2.4 oz)	240	23	8	50	9	1	2	0	20	610	—	—	0
Fully Cooked Turkey Links	3 (2.4 oz)	120	7	2	55	13	1	1	0	20	490	—	—	0
Fully Cooked Turkey Patties	2 (2.4 oz)	120	7	2	55	13	1	1	0	40	490	—	—	1
Original Links	3 (2 oz)	170	14	5	35	7	1	1	0	20	350	—	—	0
Original Patties cooked	2 (2.4 oz)	240	23	8	50	9	1	0	0	20	610	—	—	0
Pork All Natural cooked	2 oz	190	15	5	55	12	1	1	0	20	520	—	—	0
Pork Light cooked	2 oz	140	11	4	35	9	1	0	0	0	350	—	—	0
JOHNSONVILLE														
Bratwurst Original	1 (3 oz)	270	22	8	60	15	2	1	—	—	810	—	—	—
Breakfast Patty Original	2 (2 oz)	180	15	5	40	10	1	0	—	—	450	—	—	—
Grilling Chorizo	1 (3 oz)	280	22	8	55	16	3	1	—	20	840	—	—	0
Italian Mild	1 (3 oz)	270	22	9	60	15	3	2	—	—	710	—	—	—
Original Summer	1 (2 oz)	170	15	6	45	9	1	0	0	0	680	—	—	0
Polish	1 (2.7 oz)	240	21	9	60	9	2	0	—	0	640	—	—	0
Pork	2 oz	180	15	5	40	10	1	0	—	—	440	—	—	—
Smoked Turkey	1 (3 oz)	110	6	2	45	10	4	2	0	20	710	—	—	0
JONES														
All Natural Light	3 (2.1 oz)	130	9	4	35	9	3	—	—	—	350	—	—	—
LIBBY'S														
Vienna Sausage BBQ	3	140	12	5	40	5	4	2	1	20	430	—	—	0

FOOD	PORTION	CALS	FAT	SAT FAT	CHOL	PROT	CARB	SUGAR	FIBER	CALCI	SOD	POTAS	FOLIC	VIT C
MURRAY'S														
Chicken Spinach & Garlic	3 oz	130	7	2	85	16	1	—	—	20	670	—	—	0
PERDUE														
Turkey Breakfast	2 oz	80	5	2	30	9	0	0	0	20	350	—	—	0
Turkey Sweet Italian cooked	1 link (2.8 oz)	150	8	2	70	15	4	1	—	60	440	—	—	1
WAMPLER														
Bratwurst as prep	1 (2.5 oz)	230	20	6	50	12	0	0	0	—	610	—	—	—
Breakfast Links as prep	2 (1.2 oz)	130	11	4	30	7	0	0	0	—	250	—	—	—
Breakfast Patties as prep	1 (1.1 oz)	120	11	4	25	5	0	0	0	—	135	—	—	—
Italian as prep	1 (2.5 oz)	230	20	6	50	12	0	0	0	—	610	—	—	—
SAUSAGE DISHES														
TAKE-OUT														
italian sausage w/ peppers & onions	1 cup	210	11	—	70	17	14	—	—	—	1120	—	—	—
sausage roll	1 (2.3 oz)	311	24	—	—	5	22	—	1	46	—	—	—	0
SAUSAGE SUBSTITUTES														
meatless	1 link (0.9 oz)	64	5	1	0	5	2	0	1	16	222	58	7	0
meatless	1 patty (1.3 oz)	98	7	1	0	7	4	0	1	24	337	88	10	0
GARDENBURGER														
Veggie Breakfast	1 patty (1.5 oz)	45	3	0	0	5	3	0	2	40	270	—	—	0
HARMONY VALLEY														
Vegetarian Breakfast Sausage Mix as prep	1 (2 oz)	90	4	2	0	11	6	1	3	40	430	—	—	0
LIGHTLIFE														
Gimme Lean	2 oz	50	0	0	0	8	4	1	2	—	330	—	—	—
Smart Brats	1 (2 oz)	120	5	0	0	13	5	0	1	—	580	150	—	—
Smart Menu Breakfast Patty	1	45	2	0	0	5	3	0	1	—	280	150	—	—
MORNINGSTAR FARMS														
Breakfast Patties	1 (1.3 oz)	80	3	1	0	8	4	tr	1	0	250	160	—	0
WORTHINGTON														
Saucettes Breakfast Links	1 (1.3 oz)	90	6	1	0	6	1	0	1	0	200	25	—	0
YVES														
Veggie Brats Classic	1 (3.3 oz)	160	5	0	0	19	5	2	1	40	640	260	—	0
SAVORY														
ground	1 tsp	4	tr	tr	0	tr	1	—	tr	30	0	15	—	1
SCALLOP														
raw	3 oz	75	1	tr	28	14	2	—	—	21	137	274	—	—

FOOD	PORTION	CALS	FAT	SAT FAT	CHOL	PROT	CARB	SUGAR	FIBER	CALCI	SOD	POTAS	FOLIC	VIT C
MRS. PAUL'S														
Fried	13 (3.7 oz)	260	11	4	25	12	28	3	tr	40	700	—	—	0
TAKE-OUT														
breaded & fried	2 lg	67	3	1	19	6	3	—	—	13	144	103	—	—
SCONE														
KING ARTHUR														
English Cream Tea Scone not prep	⅓ cup	180	1	0	0	5	38	10	tr	100	130	—	—	0
TAKE-OUT														
apricot	1	232	7	—	34	5	39	—	—	—	201	—	—	—
blueberry	1 (3 oz)	270	9	4	10	7	41	7	2	40	600	—	—	0
cheese	1 (3.5 oz)	364	18	—	—	10	44	—	2	250	—	—	—	tr
orange poppy	1 (3 oz)	260	6	4	30	6	47	12	2	80	400	—	—	0
plain	1 (3.5 oz)	362	14	—	—	8	54	—	2	180	—	—	—	tr
raisin	1 (3 oz)	270	8	3	10	6	43	12	2	40	490	—	—	0
SCUP														
fresh baked	3 oz	115	3	—	—	21	0	0	0	44	46	313	—	—
SEA BASS														
(*see* BASS)														
SEA CUCUMBER														
dried	1 oz	74	1	—	17	14	1	—	0	87	1411	101	—	0
fresh	1 oz	20	tr	—	14	5	tr	—	0	81	143	12	—	0
SEA URCHIN														
canned	1 oz	39	1	—	—	4	3	—	0	—	—	—	—	0
fresh	1 oz	36	1	—	—	4	3	—	tr	2	32	51	—	3
roe paste	1 tbsp	19	tr	—	—	2	3	—	0	6	658	31	—	0
SEATROUT														
(*see* TROUT)														
SEAWEED														
agar dried	1 oz	87	tr	tr	0	2	23	—	—	78	29	321	—	0
agar fresh	1 oz	<1	tr	tr	0	tr	2	—	—	15	3	64	—	0
furikake	1 tbsp (5 g)	15	1	0	1	1	2	—	0	14	239	57	5	1
hijiki rehydrated	1 tbsp (3 g)	1	0	0	0	0	0	0	0	7	7	22	tr	0
hijiki dried	1 tbsp	9	0	0	0	1	2	—	1	70	—	—	—	0
irishmoss fresh	1 oz	14	tr	tr	0	tr	4	—	—	21	19	18	—	—
kelp fresh	1 oz	12	tr	tr	0	tr	3	—	—	48	66	25	51	—
konbu dried	1 piece (5 g)	11	0	0	0	0	2	—	1	22	150	260	0	1
konbu fresh	1 oz	12	tr	tr	0	tr	3	—	—	48	66	25	51	—
laver fresh	1 oz	10	tr	tr	0	2	1	—	—	20	14	101	—	11
nori fresh	1 oz	10	tr	tr	0	2	1	—	—	20	14	101	—	11
nori sheet dried	1 (8 x 8 in)	5	0	0	0	1	1	—	1	7	18	45	—	0
ogo fresh	1 cup (2.8 oz)	24	0	0	0	1	5	—	0	472	60	34	2	0
seahair dried	1 tbsp	13	0	0	0	1	3	—	tr	38	—	—	—	—

FOOD	PORTION	CALS	FAT	SAT FAT	CHOL	PROT	CARB	SUGAR	FIBER	CALCI	SOD	POTAS	FOLIC	VIT C
spirulina dried	1 oz	83	2	1	0	16	7	—	—	—	309	388	—	13
spirulina fresh	1 oz	7	tr	tr	0	2	1	—	—	—	28	36	—	tr
tangle fresh	1 oz	12	tr	tr	0	tr	3	—	—	48	66	25	51	—
wakame rehydrated	1 tbsp (3 g)	1	0	0	0	0	0	0	0	4	26	2	6	0
ANNIE CHUN'S														
Roasted Snacks Sesame	1 pkg (1.5 g)	5	0	0	0	0	0	0	0	—	45	—	—	1
Roasted Snacks Wasabi	1 pkg (1.5 g)	10	tr	—	—	0	0	0	0	—	20	—	—	1
EDEN														
Agar Agar Bars	1 bar (7 g)	25	0	0	0	0	5	0	5	—	0	—	—	—
Agar Agar Flakes	1 tbsp	0	0	0	0	0	1	0	1	20	10	10	—	0
Arame Wild	½ cup	30	0	0	0	1	7	0	7	100	120	180	—	0
Hiziki Wild	½ cup	30	0	0	0	0	6	0	6	100	160	480	—	0
Kombu Wild	½ piece (3.3 g)	5	0	0	0	0	1	0	1	20	90	170	—	0
Nori Sheets	1 (2.5 g)	10	0	0	0	1	0	0	0	0	5	90	—	6
Organic Dulse Flakes	1 tsp	3	0	0	0	0	0	0	0	0	15	80	—	0
MAINE COAST														
Organic Alaria Whole Leaf	⅓ cup	18	tr	—	—	1	3	—	3	77	297	522	—	tr
Organic Dulse Whole Leaf	½ cup	19	tr	—	—	2	3	—	2	15	122	547	—	tr
Organic Dulse Granules	1 tsp	6	0	0	0	0	2	—	—	4	22	156	—	—
Organic Kelp Whole Leaf	⅓ cup	17	tr	—	—	1	3	—	2	66	312	784	—	tr
Organic Kelp Granules	½ tsp	5	0	0	0	0	2	—	—	30	45	167	—	—
Organic Laver Whole Leaf	⅓ cup	22	tr	—	—	2	3	—	2	13	113	188	—	1
SEA'S GIFT														
Roasted	1 pkg (5 g)	30	2	0	0	1	1	0	1	20	50	—	—	12
Roasted Snack Organic	1 pkg (5 g)	30	2	0	0	1	1	0	1	0	50	—	—	12
Roasted Snack Wasabi	1 pkg (5 g)	30	2	0	0	1	1	0	1	0	60	—	—	12
Sweet Snack	1 pkg (6 g)	35	3	0	0	1	2	tr	1	20	70	—	—	12
SEEDS														
SAVISEED														
Cocoa Kissed	⅓ pkg (1 oz)	170	13	4	0	5	10	5	4	40	80	—	—	0
Karmalized	⅓ pkg (1 oz)	160	11	1	0	6	11	8	3	30	120	—	—	0
Oh Natural	⅓ pkg (1 oz)	190	15	1	0	8	5	0	5	40	170	—	—	0

SEITAN

(*see* WHEAT)

FOOD	PORTION	CALS	FAT	SAT FAT	CHOL	PROT	CARB	SUGAR	FIBER	CALCI	SOD	POTAS	FOLIC	VIT C
SEMOLINA														
dry	1 cup (5.9 oz)	601	2	tr	0	21	122	—	7	28	2	311	129	0
SESAME														
seeds	1 tsp	16	2	—	0	1	tr	—	—	4	1	11	—	—
sesame butter	1 tbsp	95	8	1	0	3	4	—	1	154	2	93	—	0
sesame crunch candy	20 pieces (1.2 oz)	181	12	2	0	4	18	—	—	—	—	—	—	—
sesame crunch candy	1 oz	146	9	1	0	3	14	—	—	—	—	—	—	—
tahini from roasted & toasted kernels	1 tbsp	89	8	1	0	3	3	—	—	64	17	62	—	0
tahini from stone ground kernels	1 tbsp	86	7	1	0	3	4	—	—	63	11	62	—	0
tahini from unroasted kernels	1 tbsp	85	8	1	0	3	3	—	—	20	0	64	—	—
ARROWHEAD MILLS														
Organic Seeds	¼ cup	210	19	3	0	9	3	0	1	100	15	140	—	0
Organic Tahini	2 tbsp	190	18	3	0	8	3	1	tr	—	10	—	—	0
MRS. MAY'S														
Black Sesame Crunch	1 oz	165	11	2	0	4	14	5	4	300	43	—	—	0
PELOPONNESE														
Tahini	1 tbsp	100	9	1	0	4	2	0	1	20	50	—	—	0
TREE OF LIFE														
Organic Sesame Tahini	2 tbsp	108	15	2	—	5	8	—	5	40	10	—	—	—
Seeds	¼ cup (1.3 oz)	210	18	3	0	6	8	0	3	350	10	—	—	0
SESBANIA														
flower	1 (3 g)	1	0	0	0	tr	tr	—	—	1	0	6	3	2
flowers	1 cup (0.7 oz)	5	tr	—	0	tr	1	—	—	4	3	37	20	15
flowers cooked	1 cup	23	tr	—	0	1	5	—	—	23	11	111	—	39
SHAD														
american baked	3 oz	214	15	—	—	18	0	0	0	51	56	418	—	—
cooked	1 oz	55	3	1	121	7	1	tr	0	7	149	74	22	5
roe baked w/ butter & lemon	1 oz	36	1	—	—	6	tr	—	—	4	21	38	—	—
SHALLOTS														
(*see* ONION)														
SHARK														
fin dried	1 oz	32	tr	—	—	7	—	—	—	48	5	16	—	0
raw	3 oz	111	4	1	43	18	0	0	0	29	67	136	—	—
TAKE-OUT														
batter-dipped & fried	3 oz	194	12	3	50	16	5	—	—	52	103	132	—	—

FOOD	PORTION	CALS	FAT	SAT FAT	CHOL	PROT	CARB	SUGAR	FIBER	CALCI	SOD	POTAS	FOLIC	VIT C
SHEEPSHEAD FISH														
cooked	1 fillet (6.5 oz)	234	3	1	—	48	0	0	0	70	136	952	—	—
cooked	3 oz	107	1	tr	—	22	0	0	0	32	62	435	—	—
raw	3 oz	92	2	1	—	17	0	0	0	18	61	344	—	—
SHELLFISH														
(*see individual names*, SHELLFISH SUBSTITUTES)														
SHELLFISH SUBSTITUTES														
crab imitation	1 cup (4.4 oz)	144	1	tr	60	17	16	0	tr	53	1065	304	3	0
scallop imitation	3 oz	84	tr	—	18	11	9	—	—	7	676	88	—	—
shrimp imitation	3 oz	86	1	tr	31	11	8	—	0	16	599	76	2	0
surimi	3 oz	84	1	—	25	13	6	—	—	7	122	95	—	—
LOUIS KEMP														
Crab Delights Flake Style	½ cup (3 oz)	90	0	0	5	6	15	3	0	0	340	—	—	1
Crab Delights Leg Style	½ cup (3 oz)	90	0	0	5	6	15	3	0	0	340	—	—	1
Crab Delights Snack Delights	1 stick (1.5 oz)	35	0	0	<5	4	5	2	0	0	230	—	—	0
Lobster Delights Chunk Style	½ cup (3 oz)	90	0	0	5	6	15	3	0	0	340	—	—	1
TAKE-OUT														
crab salad	1 cup	395	26	4	77	18	21	1	1	77	1739	426	19	1
SHELLIE BEANS														
canned	½ cup	37	tr	tr	0	2	8	—	—	36	408	133	—	4
SHERBET														
orange	½ gal	2158	31	19	113	17	469	—	—	827	706	1585	111	31
orange	½ cup (4 fl oz)	132	2	1	5	1	29	—	—	52	44	92	4	4
orange	1 bar (2.75 fl oz)	91	1	1	3	1	20	—	—	36	30	63	3	3
BLUE BUNNY														
Cool Tubes Orange Sherbet	1 (3 oz)	110	1	1	5	0	24	20	0	—	30	45	—	—
Lime	½ cup	110	0	0	0	0	25	20	0	20	30	45	—	—
Raspberry	½ cup	110	0	0	0	0	26	20	0	20	30	50	—	—
CIAO BELLA														
Lemon	1 pkg (3.5 oz)	120	0	0	0	0	31	29	—	—	0	—	—	12
Mango	1 pkg (3.5 oz)	100	0	0	0	0	25	24	1	—	0	—	—	18
Raspberry	1 pkg (3.5 oz)	110	0	0	0	1	28	25	2	—	0	—	—	4
DIPPIN' DOTS														
Lemon Lime	½ cup	97	1	1	3	1	22	19	0	40	16	—	—	0
HERSHEY'S														
Lemon	½ cup (3.4 oz)	100	1	1	<5	tr	23	22	tr	40	40	—	—	0
Orange	½ cup (3.4 oz)	100	1	1	<5	tr	23	22	0	40	40	—	—	0
Strawberry	½ cup (3.4 oz)	110	1	1	<5	tr	25	24	tr	40	40	—	—	2

FOOD	PORTION	CALS	FAT	SAT FAT	CHOL	PROT	CARB	SUGAR	FIBER	CALCI	SOD	POTAS	FOLIC	VIT C
HOLA FRUTA														
Bar Pomegranate & Blueberry	1 (2.5 oz)	100	1	1	0	1	22	14	0	—	20	—	—	—
Mango	½ cup	130	0	1	<5	1	31	20	0	—	20	—	—	—
Margarita	½ cup	140	1	1	0	1	30	21	0	—	20	—	—	—
Peach	½ cup	130	1	1	0	8	30	19	0	—	35	—	—	—
Pomegranate	½ cup	140	1	1	0	1	32	21	0	—	20	—	—	—
HOOD														
Orange Burst	½ cup	120	1	1	<5	1	27	20	0	40	40	—	—	0
LAND O LAKES														
Orange	½ cup (3.2 oz)	130	2	1	5	2	28	27	1	40	35	—	—	tr
TURKEY HILL														
Fruit Rainbow	½ cup	120	1	1	5	0	26	17	0	40	15	—	—	12
Orange Grove	½ cup	120	1	1	5	1	26	18	0	40	20	—	—	12

SHRIMP

(*see also* ASIAN FOOD, EGG ROLLS)

FOOD	PORTION	CALS	FAT	SAT FAT	CHOL	PROT	CARB	SUGAR	FIBER	CALCI	SOD	POTAS	FOLIC	VIT C
CANNED														
canned drained	1 can (6 oz)	113	2	tr	285	23	0	0	0	164	878	90	10	5
canned drained	10 (1.1 oz)	32	tr	tr	81	7	0	0	0	46	249	26	3	1
canned drained	1 cup (4.5 oz)	128	2	tr	323	26	0	0	0	186	995	102	12	5
chinese shrimp paste	1 tbsp	46	0	0	9	1	10	8	tr	26	273	30	—	0
CHICKEN OF THE SEA														
Medium	½ can (2 oz)	45	1	0	145	10	1	1	0	40	400	—	—	0
Small	½ can (2 oz)	45	1	0	145	10	1	1	0	40	400	—	—	0
Tiny	½ can (2 oz)	45	1	0	145	10	1	1	0	40	400	—	—	0
POLAR														
Tiny Peeled	¼ cup (2 oz)	44	0	0	113	10	1	1	0	50	650	—	—	0
WILD PLANET														
Shrimp Wild Pink	2 oz	50	1	0	125	11	0	0	0	20	330	—	—	2
DRIED														
dried	1 oz	72	1	tr	181	15	0	0	0	104	559	58	7	3
dried	10 (5 g)	13	tr	tr	32	3	0	0	0	18	98	10	1	1
FRESH														
broiled jumbo	3 (1 oz)	44	1	tr	55	7	tr	0	0	19	155	67	1	1
broiled small	3 (0.4 oz)	18	1	tr	22	3	tr	0	0	8	62	27	0	tr
broiled tiny popcorn	3 (3 g)	4	tr	tr	5	1	tr	0	0	2	16	7	0	3
prawn broiled	3 (0.6 oz)	27	1	tr	33	4	tr	0	0	12	93	40	1	tr
steamed jumbo	3 (1 oz)	41	1	tr	59	8	tr	0	0	20	177	51	1	1
steamed large	3 (0.6 oz)	25	tr	tr	36	5	tr	0	0	12	106	30	1	tr
steamed medium	3 (0.5 oz)	21	tr	tr	30	4	tr	0	0	10	88	25	0	9
CHICKEN OF THE SEA														
Ring w/ Cocktail Sauce	⅓ pkg (3 oz)	100	1	0	130	16	6	3	0	40	580	—	—	0

FOOD	PORTION	CALS	FAT	SAT FAT	CHOL	PROT	CARB	SUGAR	FIBER	CALCI	SOD	POTAS	FOLIC	VIT C
FROZEN														
BLUE HORIZON ORGANIC														
Garlic Shrimp	1 serv (3.5 oz)	160	2	0	80	15	21	0	1	20	360	—	—	1
Panko Shrimp	1 serv (3.5 oz)	160	2	0	80	15	22	0	1	20	360	—	—	1
Popcorn Shrimp	1 serv (3.5 oz)	160	2	0	80	15	21	0	1	20	360	—	—	1
Tempura Shrimp	1 serv (3.5 oz)	160	2	0	85	15	21	0	1	20	290	—	—	1
CHICKEN OF THE SEA														
Tempura w/ Soy Dipping Sauce	3	200	13	3	50	9	14	1	0	50	245	—	—	0
CONTESSA														
Orange Shrimp	11 to 13 (6 oz)	250	8	2	95	14	33	12	5	60	1150	—	—	2
Ragin' Cajun	8 to 10 (4 oz)	170	10	3	100	11	9	0	3	40	910	—	—	0
Shrimp Scampi	8 to 10 (4 oz)	290	27	7	85	9	4	1	2	150	810	—	—	0
GORTON'S														
Popcorn Crunchy Golden	20 (3.2 oz)	240	12	4	55	8	24	2	0	20	630	95	—	0
Temptations Breaded Butterfly	5 (3.5 oz)	250	11	3	55	11	27	4	4	100	430	140	—	–
Temptations Scampi Sauced	1 serv (4 oz)	120	6	1	65	10	8	—	tr	20	630	150	—	—
MARGARITAVILLE														
Island Lime	6 (4 oz)	240	11	3	115	12	5	2	0	80	330	—	—	0
Jammin' Jerk	7 (4 oz)	210	10	6	120	12	4	—	1	40	1040	—	—	1
Plum Crazy + Sauce	7 + 2 oz sauce	270	12	2	55	8	33	13	1	100	770	—	—	1
MRS. PAUL'S														
Butterfly	7 (4 oz)	250	11	4	65	12	27	3	1	40	540	—	—	0
SEAPAK														
Butterfly	7 (3 oz)	210	10	2	60	10	20	2	tr	20	480	—	—	1
Coconut + Sauce	4 (3.7 oz)	310	14	4	65	12	36	19	1	40	140	—	—	2
Popcorn	15 (3 oz)	210	10	2	60	10	20	2	1	20	480	—	—	1
Scampi	8 (4 oz)	350	29	10	155	15	2	0	0	60	460	—	—	1
Tempura + Sauce	4 (4.1 oz)	240	8	2	35	9	35	13	7	0	570	—	—	1
SHRIMP BURGERS														
Cajun	1 (4 oz)	160	3	1	185	23	8	0	0	80	650	—	—	0
Original	1 (4 oz)	160	3	1	180	23	8	0	0	60	570	—	—	5
Teriyaki	1 (4 oz)	150	3	1	175	22	8	2	0	60	500	—	—	4
VAN DE KAMP'S														
Battered	6 (4 oz)	200	6	2	90	14	22	tr	1	40	750	—	—	2
Breaded Popcorn	20 (4 oz)	260	11	5	80	11	30	3	2	40	780	—	—	0
TAKE-OUT														
battered jumbo	3 (3 oz)	268	17	3	95	13	16	1	1	50	778	129	22	1
battered large	3 (1.8 oz)	152	9	2	54	7	9	tr	1	29	441	73	13	1
battered medium	3 (1.2 oz)	98	5	1	35	5	6	tr	tr	18	285	47	8	tr
battered small	3 (0.6 oz)	54	3	1	19	3	3	tr	tr	10	156	26	4	tr

FOOD	PORTION	CALS	FAT	SAT FAT	CHOL	PROT	CARB	SUGAR	FIBER	CALCI	SOD	POTAS	FOLIC	VIT C
battered tiny popcorn	3 (6 g)	18	1	tr	6	1	1	tr	tr	3	52	9	2	tr
breaded & fried	1 lg (0.6 oz)	44	3	0	30	3	2	—	0	7	81	26	5	0
cocktail w/ cocktail sauce	4 shrimp (3.2 oz)	78	1	tr	114	10	7	3	2	75	727	170	11	11
creole w/o rice	1 cup (8.6 oz)	335	13	3	293	40	11	3	2	138	1134	480	22	18
gingered	4	80	tr	tr	140	—	—	—	—	—	920	—	—	—
jambalaya w/ rice	1 cup (8.5 oz)	294	9	2	262	25	28	2	2	192	1001	292	87	15
scampi	1 cup	310	22	13	246	26	1	tr	0	72	330	239	3	3
shish kabob w/ vegetables	1 (7.1 oz)	184	5	1	184	26	9	5	2	85	1040	537	20	28
shrimp cake	1 (4.2 oz)	238	13	3	194	16	14	1	1	113	695	244	18	6
shrimp egg patty torta de cameron seco	2 (1.3 oz)	152	11	2	171	9	3	1	tr	33	289	87	17	tr
shrimp in garlic sauce	1 cup (7.4 oz)	649	54	9	267	36	6	1	tr	108	1124	413	17	29
shrimp newburg	1 cup (8.6 oz)	605	50	30	417	30	11	tr	tr	246	886	534	49	3
shrimp salad	1 cup (6.4 oz)	258	16	2	291	24	4	2	1	186	1043	209	25	6
shrimp w/ crab stuffing	3 (1.7 oz)	94	5	1	76	10	3	tr	tr	40	240	123	19	1
tempura	1 (0.9 oz)	65	4	1	43	4	3	—	0	11	119	38	7	0
toast fried	3 pieces (2.5 oz)	219	14	2	35	8	16	2	2	59	678	120	33	2

SMELT

FOOD	PORTION	CALS	FAT	SAT FAT	CHOL	PROT	CARB	SUGAR	FIBER	CALCI	SOD	POTAS	FOLIC	VIT C
rainbow cooked	3 oz	106	3	tr	76	19	0	0	0	65	65	316	—	—
rainbow raw	3 oz	83	2	tr	60	15	0	0	0	51	51	247	—	—

SMOOTHIES

(*see also* FRUIT DRINKS, YOGURT DRINKS)

ARIZONA

FOOD	PORTION	CALS	FAT	SAT FAT	CHOL	PROT	CARB	SUGAR	FIBER	CALCI	SOD	POTAS	FOLIC	VIT C
Smoothie Mix Orchard Peach as prep	8 oz	150	0	0	0	0	39	38	0	0	10	—	—	15

ARTHUR'S

FOOD	PORTION	CALS	FAT	SAT FAT	CHOL	PROT	CARB	SUGAR	FIBER	CALCI	SOD	POTAS	FOLIC	VIT C
Carrot Energizer	1 bottle (11 oz)	200	1	0	0	2	47	37	3	0	60	910	280	90
Green Energy	1 bottle (11 oz)	230	1	tr	0	2	53	39	3	20	15	780	320	15

BOLTHOUSE FARMS

FOOD	PORTION	CALS	FAT	SAT FAT	CHOL	PROT	CARB	SUGAR	FIBER	CALCI	SOD	POTAS	FOLIC	VIT C
Green Goodness	8 oz	140	0	0	0	2	33	27	1	20	25	470	—	63
Mango Lemonade	8 oz	120	0	0	0	tr	30	30	tr	20	0	35	—	9
Passion Fruit Apple Carrot Juice	8 oz	120	0	0	0	2	29	28	2	20	95	270	—	21

C&W

FOOD	PORTION	CALS	FAT	SAT FAT	CHOL	PROT	CARB	SUGAR	FIBER	CALCI	SOD	POTAS	FOLIC	VIT C
Berry Blend	½ cup	90	2	1	10	2	15	11	2	150	65	—	—	21
Peach	½ cup	80	2	1	10	2	15	12	1	150	65	—	—	5

FOOD	PORTION	CALS	FAT	SAT FAT	CHOL	PROT	CARB	SUGAR	FIBER	CALCI	SOD	POTAS	FOLIC	VIT C
DEL MONTE														
Ready-To-Blend Mango Pineapple	1 (6 oz)	115	0	0	0	0	29	26	3	0	15	210	—	60
Ready-To-Blend Strawberry Peach	1 (6 oz)	120	0	0	0	0	30	21	4	0	25	290	—	60
Ready-To-Blend Strawberry Peach Lite	1 (6 oz)	80	0	0	0	0	20	15	4	0	20	220	—	60
DOLE														
Shakers Mixed Berry not prep	1 pkg (4 oz)	100	2	1	10	5	17	13	3	100	40	—	—	30
E4B														
100% Fruit Puree Blueberry Raspberry	4 oz	70	0	0	0	0	18	14	3	20	10	—	—	9
100% Fruit Puree Kiwi	4 oz	70	0	0	0	0	16	13	1	40	15	—	—	15
100% Fruit Puree Mango	4 oz	70	0	0	0	0	18	16	1	20	10	—	—	12
100% Fruit Puree Pear Caramel	4 oz	70	0	0	0	0	18	16	1	40	15	—	—	4
100% Fruit Puree Strawberry Banana	4 oz	70	0	0	0	0	18	16	1	40	10	—	—	15
HORIZON ORGANIC														
Tropical Punch	1 bottle (6.2 oz)	120	0	0	0	4	25	23	1	150	75	—	—	60
JAMBA JUICE														
Mango-A-Go-Go not prep	½ pkg (4 oz)	70	0	0	0	1	17	15	1	40	15	—	—	60
Razzmatazz not prep	½ pkg (4 oz)	60	0	0	0	2	14	10	2	40	15	—	—	60
Strawberries Wild not prep	½ pkg (4 oz)	60	0	0	0	2	15	11	1	40	20	—	—	60
KIDZ DREAM														
Orange Cream	1 box	120	2	0	0	4	21	17	tr	350	30	240	—	6
MAIN ST CAFE														
Protein Smoothie Mixed Berry	1 bottle (11 oz)	270	2	2	15	10	33	42	1	300	300	330	—	1
Protein Smoothie Peach	1 bottle (11 oz)	260	2	2	15	10	54	43	1	300	300	350	—	5
Protein Smoothie Strawberry	1 bottle (11 oz)	280	2	2	15	10	58	48	1	300	300	330	—	1
NUTIVA														
Organic HempShake Amazon Acai not prep	4 tbsp	100	3	0	0	9	15	3	8	20	5	—	—	0

FOOD	PORTION	CALS	FAT	SAT FAT	CHOL	PROT	CARB	SUGAR	FIBER	CALCI	SOD	POTAS	FOLIC	VIT C
NUTIVA (CONT.)														
Organic HempShake Chocolate not prep	4 tbsp	80	2	tr	0	7	19	7	12	20	5	—	—	0
ODWALLA														
Bluberry B Monster	8 oz	140	0	0	0	0	33	27	0	—	10	—	16	15
Citrus C Monster	8 oz	150	0	0	0	2	36	27	0	20	15	640	—	600
Mango Tango	8 oz	150	1	1	0	1	34	30	0	20	10	—	—	18
SAMBAZON														
Acai Amazon Cherry	8 oz	156	0	0	0	5	16	15	1	20	5	—	—	900
Acai Mango Banana	8 oz	190	5	1	0	2	38	29	3	40	90	—	—	72
Acai Mango Uprising	8 oz	190	5	1	0	2	38	29	3	40	90	—	—	72
Acai Protein Warrior Vanilla	8 oz	215	6	1	0	8	33	27	3	50	142	—	—	4
Acai Shaman's Immunity	8 oz	90	0	0	0	1	24	22	1	10	28	—	—	1050
Acai Soy Energy	8 oz	210	6	1	0	6	25	19	4	200	142	—	—	102
Acai Strawberry Sensation	8 oz	210	4	1	0	1	42	37	2	40	10	123	—	5
Acai Supergreens Revolution	8 oz	200	4	1	0	2	40	29	3	40	12	—	—	10
Organic Acai	1 bottle	155	3	1	0	1	31	22	2	40	16	—	—	5
SIMPLI														
OatShake Tropical Fruits	1 (8.4 oz)	160	2	1	0	2	30	23	8	300	15	—	—	78
SMOOZE														
Mango + Coconut	1 box (8.5 oz)	250	10	10	0	2	33	33	0	0	—	—	—	60
Passion Fruit + Coconut	1 box (8.5 oz)	225	8	8	0	2	33	28	3	0	38	—	—	77
Pineapple + Coconut	1 box (8.5 oz)	200	8	8	0	2	33	23	0	0	25	—	—	68
SOY FUSION														
Berry	1 box (8.45 oz)	120	1	—	—	2	24	21	—	150	20	150	40	60
Matcha Green Tea	1 box (8.45 oz)	110	2	—	—	3	19	16	—	200	120	150	100	60
TROPICANA														
Fruit Smoothie Mixed Berry	1 bottle (11 oz)	220	0	0	0	1	54	44	2	20	30	630	—	120
Fruit Smoothie Tropical Fruit	1 bottle (11 oz)	220	0	0	0	1	53	42	1	20	15	790	—	120
V8														
Splash Tropical Colada	8 oz	100	0	0	0	3	21	18	1	100	50	60	—	60

FOOD	PORTION	CALS	FAT	SAT FAT	CHOL	PROT	CARB	SUGAR	FIBER	CALCI	SOD	POTAS	FOLIC	VIT C
SNACKS														
cheese puffs	1 oz	122	3	1	0	2	21	2	3	101	364	81	27	6
oriental mix	1 oz	155	12	—	0	6	9	—	—	22	235	147	25	tr
pork skins	1 oz	154	9	3	27	17	0	0	0	8	521	36	—	tr
pork skins barbecue	1 oz	152	9	3	33	16	1	—	—	12	756	51	—	tr
ANNIE'S HOMEGROWN														
Organic Cheddar Snack Mix	40 pieces (1 oz)	140	5	1	0	3	20	1	0	20	300	—	—	0
Organic Pizza Snack Mix	½ cup (1 oz)	140	5	1	0	3	18	1	0	0	240	—	—	0
BACHMAN														
Baked Cheese Curls	23 (1 oz)	140	7	1	0	2	17	2	0	40	300	—	—	0
Onion Rings	½ pkg (1 oz)	130	6	1	0	2	19	1	1	0	290	—	—	0
BAKEN-ETS														
Pork Skins Hot 'N Spicy	9 (0.5 oz)	80	5	2	20	7	0	0	0	0	470	—	—	0
Pork Skins Traditional	9 (0.5 oz)	80	5	3	20	7	0	0	0	0	310	—	—	0
BARBARA'S BAKERY														
Cheese Puffs Bakes Original	¾ cup	160	11	2	0	2	13	1	—	40	190	—	—	2
Cheese Puffs Original	¾ cup (1 oz)	150	10	2	0	2	16	0	—	20	130	—	—	2
BETTER BALANCE														
Kruncheeze White Cheddar Gluten Free	1 oz	130	6	1	0	9	10	0	2	40	200	—	—	0
CAROLE'S														
Soycrunch Cinnamon & Raisins	½ cup	110	1	0	0	6	19	12	2	40	0	—	—	0
Soycrunch Original	½ cup	120	2	0	0	5	16	10	2	40	0	—	—	0
Soycrunch Toffee	½ cup	110	2	0	0	7	15	13	2	40	15	—	—	0
CHEETOS														
Baked Crunchy	34 (1 oz)	130	5	1	0	2	20	tr	tr	100	150	—	—	0
Corn BBQ	29 (1 oz)	150	10	2	0	2	16	tr	1	40	280	—	—	0
Natural White Cheddar	1 oz	150	9	2	0	2	16	1	tr	20	290	—	—	0
Puffs	13 (1 oz)	160	10	2	0	2	13	1	0	20	350	—	—	0
CHEEZ-IT														
Right Bites Party Mix	1 pkg (0.74 oz)	100	4	1	0	2	15	tr	tr	0	200	—	—	0

FOOD	PORTION	CALS	FAT	SAT FAT	CHOL	PROT	CARB	SUGAR	FIBER	CALCI	SOD	POTAS	FOLIC	VIT C
CHESTER'S														
Puffcorn Butter	1 oz	160	11	2	0	1	14	0	tr	0	300	—	—	0
Snack Mix Crazy Cheddar	1¼ cups (1 oz)	140	7	1	0	2	17	tr	1	0	250	—	—	0
DRSEARS														
Popumz BBQ	1 pkg (0.74 oz)	70	2	0	0	3	11	1	2	0	105	—	—	2
Popumz Caramel Drizzle	1 pkg (0.75 oz)	90	3	2	0	3	13	5	2	20	100	—	—	2
Popumz Cheddar	1 pkg (0.74 oz)	80	3	1	5	4	11	1	2	40	190	—	—	2
Popumz Cool Ranch	1 pkg (0.74 oz)	80	2	0	0	4	12	2	2	20	200	—	—	2
Popumz Vanilla Drizzle	1 pkg (0.74 oz)	90	3	2	0	3	13	5	2	20	95	—	—	2
FULLBITES														
Bold Cheddar	1 pkg (1.3 oz)	150	6	1	<5	8	21	2	5	20	270	—	—	0
Savory BBQ	1 pkg (1.3 oz)	150	5	1	0	8	22	2	5	0	220	—	—	0
FUNYUNS														
Onion Rings	13 (1 oz)	140	7	1	0	2	18	tr	tr	0	240	—	—	0
KAY'S NATURALS														
Snack Mix Sweet BBQ Gluten Free	1 oz	120	5	1	0	10	11	5	2	20	230	—	—	0
LANCE														
Cheese Puffs	9 (1 oz)	170	12	3	0	2	13	1	0	20	380	—	—	0
Gold-N-Chees	1 oz	150	8	1	0	2	17	0	tr	20	240	35	—	0
LIFESTYLE FOODS														
Awake	1 pkg (5 oz)	170	0	0	2	3	55	38	5	40	65	—	—	66
Essential	1 pkg (5.6 oz)	200	10	4	2	9	21	13	3	60	230	—	—	72
Miami	1 pkg (7.5 oz)	180	0	0	0	5	36	29	3	100	70	—	—	78
Power Up	1 pkg (6.7 oz)	170	33	4	0	18	77	17	9	0	430	—	—	78
MEDORA SNACKS														
Corners Sea Salt	1 oz	130	3	0	0	2	22	0	0	0	170	—	—	0
Pucci Garlic	1 oz	120	4	2	5	4	17	2	1	20	420	—	—	0
Pucci Tomato Basil	1 oz	120	4	2	5	4	17	2	1	20	440	—	—	0
Sotos Cheese Olive Oil & Lemon	1 oz	120	4	1	0	2	19	3	2	0	420	—	—	0
MICHAEL SEASON'S														
Cheese Puffs & Curls	1½ cups	180	13	3	5	3	13	3	2	40	270	—	—	0
MUNCHIES														
Snack Mix Totally Ranch	¾ cup (1 oz)	140	7	1	0	2	18	1	2	20	180	75	—	0
ROBERT'S AMERICAN GOURMET														
Booty Barbeque	1 oz	130	5	1	0	2	20	1	1	—	90	—	—	—
Booty Pirate's	1 oz	130	5	1	0	2	18	0	1	0	150	—	—	2

FOOD	PORTION	CALS	FAT	SAT FAT	CHOL	PROT	CARB	SUGAR	FIBER	CALCI	SOD	POTAS	FOLIC	VIT C
ROBERT'S AMERICAN GOURMET (CONT.)														
Booty Veggie	1 oz	130	6	1	0	1	17	1	1	20	150	—	—	6
Smart Puffs	1 oz	130	6	1	0	2	17	1	0	20	150	—	—	0
Tings	1 oz	160	8	1	0	1	17	0	0	0	85	—	—	0
SABRITONES														
Puffed Wheat Chili & Lime	23 pieces (1 oz)	150	10	3	0	2	13	0	1	20	690	—	—	0
SILHOUETTE SOLUTION														
Puffs BBQ	1 pkg (1.06 oz)	120	4	0	0	15	8	3	0	300	420	110	—	0
SNIKIDDY														
Puffs Grilled Cheese	1 pkg (0.6 oz)	80	3	1	0	2	10	0	1	20	160	—	—	0
Puffs Rockin' Ranch	1 pkg (0.6 oz)	83	0	0	0	1	11	0	1	0	160	—	—	0
SNYDER'S OF HANOVER														
CheddAirs	1 oz	130	5	1	0	3	20	0	tr	20	140	—	—	0
MultiGrain Cheese Puffs	1 oz	130	6	1	0	2	19	2	2	0	200	—	—	0
SUNRIDGE FARMS														
Mocha Marble Crunch	¼ pkg (1.4 oz)	220	16	5	0	5	17	12	3	60	25	—	—	0
SWEET EMOTIONS														
Chocolate Passion	1 pkg (0.5 oz)	60	3	1	0	1	10	2	2	100	200	—	—	0
Cinnamon Joy	1 pkg (0.5 oz)	60	3	1	0	1	10	2	2	100	200	—	—	0
T.G.I. FRIDAY'S														
Mozzarella Sticks	20 (1 oz)	150	9	2	0	2	14	1	1	20	250	—	—	0
UTZ														
Cheese Balls	50 (1 oz)	150	9	3	0	2	16	tr	tr	0	260	—	—	0
Cheese Curls	18 (1 oz)	150	9	3	0	2	16	tr	tr	0	260	—	—	0
Onion Rings	41 (1 oz)	130	5	1	0	1	20	2	0	0	500	—	—	0
Party Mix	1 oz	150	7	1	0	2	19	tr	1	20	250	—	—	0
Pork Cracklins	0.5 oz	90	7	3	15	6	0	0	0	—	300	—	—	—
Pork Rinds Original	0.5 oz	80	5	2	15	9	0	0	0	—	210	—	—	—
WISE														
Cheez Doodles Crunchy	1 pkg (1 oz)	150	9	3	0	1	17	1	0	150	220	—	—	0
SNAIL														
cooked	3 oz	233	1	tr	110	41	13	—	—	96	350	590	10	—
raw	3 oz	117	tr	tr	55	20	7	—	—	48	175	295	5	—
TAKE-OUT														
escargot cooked	5	25	0	0	15	4	1	—	0	5	25	95	0	0
SNAKE														
fresh	3 oz	78	tr	—	—	17	3	—	0	15	57	303	—	3

FOOD	PORTION	CALS	FAT	SAT FAT	CHOL	PROT	CARB	SUGAR	FIBER	CALCI	SOD	POTAS	FOLIC	VIT C
SNAPPER														
cooked	3 oz	109	1	tr	40	22	0	0	0	34	48	444	—	—
cooked	1 fillet (6 oz)	217	3	1	80	45	0	0	0	69	96	887	—	—
raw	3 oz	85	1	tr	31	17	0	0	0	27	54	355	—	—
SODA														
club	12 oz	0	0	0	0	0	0	0	0	17	75	6	0	0
cola	12 oz	151	tr	—	0	tr	39	—	—	9	14	4	0	0
cream	12 oz	191	0	0	0	0	49	—	—	19	43	4	0	0
diet cola	12 oz	2	0	0	0	tr	tr	—	—	12	21	0	0	0
ginger ale	12 oz	124	0	—	0	tr	32	—	—	12	25	5	0	0
grape	12 oz	161	0	0	0	0	42	—	—	12	57	3	0	0
lemon lime	12 oz	149	0	0	0	0	38	—	—	9	41	4	0	0
orange	12 oz	177	0	0	0	0	46	—	—	19	49	9	0	0
pepper type	12 oz	151	tr	—	0	0	38	—	—	12	38	2	0	0
quinine	12 oz	125	0	0	0	0	32	—	—	5	15	1	0	0
root beer	12 oz	152	0	0	0	tr	39	—	—	19	49	3	0	0
shirley temple	1 serv	159	0	0	0	0	41	—	0	11	34	23	—	—
tonic water	12 oz	125	0	0	0	0	32	—	—	5	15	1	0	0
ALE 8 ONE														
Soft Drink	1 bottle (12 oz)	120	0	0	0	0	30	30	—	—	15	—	—	—
BARQ'S														
Diet French Vanilla Creme	8 oz	1	0	0	0	0	tr	tr	0	—	44	tr	—	—
Diet Red Creme	8 oz	4	0	0	0	0	0	0	0	—	43	0	—	—
Diet Root Beer	8 oz	1	0	0	0	0	tr	tr	0	—	48	9	—	—
Floatz	8 oz	127	0	0	0	0	34	34	0	—	44	2	—	—
French Vanilla Creme	8 oz	112	0	0	0	0	30	30	0	—	44	0	—	—
Red Creme	8 oz	115	0	0	0	0	31	31	0	—	43	0	—	—
Root Beer	8 oz	111	0	0	0	0	30	30	0	—	48	tr	—	—
CAPE COD DRY														
Cranberry	8 oz	120	0	0	0	0	29	29	—	—	0	—	—	—
Diet Cranberry	8 oz	10	0	0	0	0	2	2	—	—	0	—	—	—
CARVER'S														
Ginger Ale	8 oz	94	0	0	0	0	24	24	0	—	22	15	—	—
CELSIUS														
Cola	1 bottle (12 oz)	5	—	—	—	—	—	—	—	50	6	—	—	60
COCA-COLA														
C2	8 oz	45	0	0	0	0	12	12	—	—	30	28	—	—
Classic	8 oz	97	0	0	0	0	27	27	0	—	33	0	—	—
W/ Lime	8 oz	98	0	0	0	0	27	27	0	—	25	34	—	—
COKE														
Cherry	8 oz	104	0	0	0	0	28	28	0	—	28	0	—	—
Diet	8 oz	1	0	0	0	0	tr	0	0	—	28	12	—	—

FOOD	PORTION	CALS	FAT	SAT FAT	CHOL	PROT	CARB	SUGAR	FIBER	CALCI	SOD	POTAS	FOLIC	VIT C
COKE (CONT.)														
Diet Cherry	8 oz	1	0	0	0	0	tr	tr	0	—	28	19	—	—
Diet Plus	8 oz	0	0	0	0	0	0	0	0	—	30	—	—	—
Diet Vanilla	8 oz	1	0	0	0	0	tr	tr	0	—	28	19	—	—
Diet w/ Lime	8 oz	2	0	0	0	0	tr	tr	0	—	28	19	—	—
Vanilla	8 oz	100	0	0	0	0	28	28	0	—	25	0	—	—
DRY														
Vanilla Bean	1 bottle (12 oz)	60	0	0	0	0	16	16	—	—	0	—	—	—
FANTA														
Apple	8 oz	121	0	0	0	0	33	33	0	—	39	0	—	—
Citrus	8 oz	91	0	0	0	0	25	25	0	—	16	1	—	—
Orange	8 oz	111	0	0	0	0	35	35	0	—	35	0	—	—
FRESCA														
Soda	8 oz	2	0	0	0	0	tr	tr	0	—	24	59	—	—
FRESH GINGER														
Ginger Ale Jasmine Green Tea	1 bottle (12 oz)	160	0	0	0	0	40	37	0	0	5	—	—	4
Ginger Ale Original	1 bottle (12 oz)	160	0	0	0	0	40	37	0	0	0	—	—	4
Ginger Ale Pomegranate w/ Hibiscus	1 bottle (12 oz)	160	0	0	0	0	41	37	0	20	10	—	—	4
GOYA														
Ginger Beer	1 bottle (12 oz)	190	0	0	0	0	43	27	0	—	30	—	—	—
GUS														
Dry Cola	1 bottle (12 oz)	95	0	0	0	0	24	24	—	—	10	—	—	—
Dry Crimson Grape	1 bottle (12 oz)	90	0	0	0	0	22	22	—	—	10	—	—	—
Dry Valencia Orange	1 bottle (12 oz)	95	0	0	0	0	24	24	—	—	10	—	—	60
Star Ruby Grapefruit	1 bottle (12 oz)	90	0	0	0	0	22	22	—	—	10	—	—	—
HANSEN'S														
Blackberry	1 bottle	150	0	0	0	tr	37	—	—	40	55	—	—	9
HEALTH COLA														
Soda	1 bottle (12 oz)	140	0	0	0	0	35	35	—	—	0	—	—	90
HOTLIPS														
Apple	1 bottle	136	0	0	0	0	34	—	—	20	50	—	—	2
Boysenberry	1 bottle	152	0	0	0	1	37	—	—	10	1	—	—	5
Pear	1 bottle	142	1	—	0	tr	34	—	—	20	35	—	—	4
INCA KOLA														
Diet	8 oz	1	0	0	0	0	tr	tr	0	—	34	7	—	—
Soda	8 oz	96	0	0	0	0	26	26	0	—	31	0	—	—

FOOD	PORTION	CALS	FAT	SAT FAT	CHOL	PROT	CARB	SUGAR	FIBER	CALCI	SOD	POTAS	FOLIC	VIT C
JOIA														
Grapefruit Chamomile & Cardamom	1 bottle (12 oz)	110	0	0	0	0	31	28	—	—	0	—	—	—
Lime Hibiscus & Clove	1 bottle (12 oz)	120	0	0	0	0	35	28	—	—	0	—	—	—
Pineapple Coconut & Nutmeg	1 bottle (12 oz)	110	0	0	0	0	38	26	—	—	0	—	—	—
JONES SODA														
Blue Bubble Gum	1 bottle (12 oz)	190	0	0	0	0	48	48	0	—	25	—	—	—
Cream	1 bottle (12 oz)	190	0	0	0	0	48	48	0	—	25	—	—	—
Crushed Melon	1 bottle (12 oz)	190	0	0	0	0	48	48	0	—	25	—	—	—
FuFu Berry	1 bottle (12 oz)	190	0	0	0	0	46	46	0	—	70	—	—	—
Green Apple	1 bottle (12 oz)	180	0	0	0	0	46	46	0	—	25	—	—	—
Orange Cream	1 bottle (12 oz)	180	0	0	0	0	46	46	0	—	25	—	—	—
LUCOZADE														
Soda	7 oz	136	0	0	0	0	36	—	0	10	—	—	—	0
MANZANA MIA														
Soda	8 oz	99	0	0	0	0	27	27	0	—	47	3	—	—
MELLO YELLOW														
Diet	8 oz	3	0	0	0	0	tr	tr	0	—	25	51	—	—
Soda	8 oz	118	0	0	0	0	32	32	0	—	33	20	—	—
MR. PIBB														
Diet	8 oz	1	0	0	0	0	tr	tr	0	—	26	20	—	—
NORTHERN NECK														
Diet Ginger Ale	8 oz	4	0	0	0	0	0	0	0	—	24	13	—	—
Ginger Ale	8 oz	94	0	0	0	0	24	24	0	—	22	15	—	—
NUTRISODA														
Calm Sparkling Wild Berry & Citron	1 can (8.7 oz)	0	0	0	0	0	1	0	—	—	0	20	200	4
Flex Sparkling Black Cherry & Apple	1 can (8.7 oz)	5	0	0	0	0	1	0	—	—	0	20	—	—
Immune Sparkling Tangerine & Lime	1 can (8.7 oz)	15	0	0	0	2	1	0	—	—	0	20	200	4
Slender Sparkling Guava & Grapefruit	1 can (8.7 oz)	10	0	0	0	0	1	0	—	300	15	110	200	18
OOGAVE NATURAL														
All Flavors	8 oz	68	0	0	0	0	17	17	0	—	0	—	—	—
ORANGINA														
Sparkling Citrus	8 oz	100	0	0	0	0	26	26	—	—	40	—	—	—

FOOD	PORTION	CALS	FAT	SAT FAT	CHOL	PROT	CARB	SUGAR	FIBER	CALCI	SOD	POTAS	FOLIC	VIT C
PEPSI														
Cola	8 oz	100	0	0	0	0	28	28	—	—	20	5	—	—
Diet	8 oz	0	0	0	0	0	0	0	0	—	25	20	—	—
Diet Vanilla	8 oz	0	0	0	0	0	0	0	0	—	25	30	—	—
One	8 oz	1	0	0	0	0	0	0	—	—	25	35	—	—
Wild Cherry	8 oz	100	0	0	0	0	28	28	—	—	20	10	—	—
PIBB														
Zero	8 oz	2	0	0	0	0	tr	tr	0	—	31	22	—	—
POLAR														
Birch Beer	8 oz	110	0	0	0	0	28	28	—	—	0	—	—	—
Bitter Lemon Mixer	8 oz	120	0	0	0	0	29	29	—	—	0	—	—	—
Collins Mixer	8 oz	90	0	0	0	0	22	22	—	—	0	—	—	—
Cream	8 oz	120	0	0	0	0	30	30	—	—	0	—	—	—
Diet Pomegranate Dry	8 oz	10	0	0	0	0	2	2	—	—	0	—	—	—
Orange	8 oz	130	0	0	0	0	32	32	—	—	0	—	—	—
Pomegranate Dry	8 oz	120	0	0	0	0	30	30	—	—	0	—	—	—
Seltzer All Flavors	8 oz	0	0	0	0	0	0	0	0	—	0	—	—	—
Strawberry	8 oz	120	0	0	0	0	30	30	—	—	0	—	—	—
Tonic Water	8 oz	90	0	0	0	0	23	23	—	—	0	—	—	—
Vichy Water	8 oz	0	0	0	0	0	0	0	0	—	300	—	—	—
RED FLASH														
Soda	8 oz	105	0	0	0	0	28	28	0	—	21	12	—	—
REED'S														
Ginger Brew Original	1 bottle (12 oz)	145	0	0	0	0	37	37	0	—	5	—	—	—
SANTA CRUZ														
Organic Cherry	1 can (12 oz)	140	0	0	0	0	34	32	0	—	20	75	—	1
Organic Ginger Ale	1 can (12 oz)	150	0	0	0	0	37	35	0	0	10	15	—	4
Organic Root Beer	1 can (12 oz)	150	0	0	0	0	36	36	0	—	10	25	—	0
Organic Vanilla Creme	1 can (12 oz)	160	0	0	0	0	38	38	0	40	10	0	—	60
SPINDRIFT														
Sparkling Cranberry Raspberry	8 oz	60	0	0	0	0	16	16	0	0	0	—	—	6
Sparkling Grapefruit	8 oz	80	0	0	0	0	21	21	0	0	0	—	—	6
Sparkling Mango Orange	8 oz	80	0	0	0	0	21	21	0	0	0	—	—	24
Sprakling Blackberry	8 oz	70	0	0	0	0	18	17	0	0	0	—	—	0
SPRITE														
Diet Zero	8 oz	0	0	0	0	0	0	0	0	—	25	—	—	—

FOOD	PORTION	CALS	FAT	SAT FAT	CHOL	PROT	CARB	SUGAR	FIBER	CALCI	SOD	POTAS	FOLIC	VIT C
SPRITE (CONT.)														
ReMix Aruba Jam	8 oz	97	0	0	0	0	26	26	—	—	44	0	—	—
Soda	8 oz	96	0	0	0	0	26	26	0	—	47	0	—	—
STEAZ														
Organic Green Tea Soda Cola	8 oz	90	0	0	0	0	23	23	—	—	35	—	—	36
Organic Green Tea Soda Diet Black Cherry	8 oz	20	0	0	0	0	5	5	—	—	20	—	—	42
Organic Green Tea Soda Ginger Ale	8 oz	90	0	0	0	0	23	23	—	—	35	—	—	42
Organic Green Tea Soda Lemon	8 oz	90	0	0	0	0	23	23	—	—	35	—	—	36
STEWART'S														
Birch Beer	1 bottle (12 oz)	170	0	0	0	0	42	42	—	—	40	—	—	—
STIRRINGS														
Ginger Ale	8 oz	120	0	0	0	0	31	30	0	0	0	—	—	0
TAB														
Soda	8 oz	1	0	0	0	0	tr	tr	—	—	28	12	—	—
TAVA														
Sparkling Brazilian Samba	8 oz	0	0	0	0	0	0	0	0	—	35	—	—	—
Sparkling Mediterranean Fiesta	8 oz	0	0	0	0	0	0	0	0	—	40	—	—	—
TAYLOR'S TONICS														
Chai Cola	1 bottle (12 oz)	135	0	0	0	0	32	32	—	—	45	—	—	—
Cola Azteca	1 bottle (12 oz)	95	0	0	0	0	28	28	—	—	30	—	—	—
Mate Mojito Mint & Lime Shoppe	1 bottle (12 oz)	98	0	0	0	0	28	28	—	—	20	—	—	—
THE POP														
Cola	1 bottle (12 oz)	180	0	0	0	0	46	45	—	—	20	—	—	—
Cream	1 bottle (12 oz)	190	0	0	0	0	47	46	—	—	20	—	—	—
Lime Ricky	1 bottle (12 oz)	150	0	0	0	07	38	37	—	—	20	—	—	—
Pineapple	1 bottle (12 oz)	240	0	0	0	0	60	58	—	—	20	—	—	—
THOMAS KEMPER														
Black Cherry	1 bottle (12 oz)	170	0	0	0	0	40	40	—	—	40	—	—	—
Ginger Ale	1 bottle (12 oz)	150	0	0	0	0	36	35	—	—	45	—	—	—
Orange Cream	1 bottle (12 oz)	170	0	0	0	0	42	40	—	—	50	—	—	—
Root Beer	1 bottle (12 oz)	160	0	0	0	0	41	40	—	—	45	—	—	—
Root Beer Low Calorie	1 bottle (12 oz)	20	0	0	0	0	5	1	—	—	70	—	—	—
Vanilla Cream	1 bottle (12 oz)	150	0	0	0	0	38	34	—	—	55	—	—	—
TROPICANA														
Twister Orange	1 can (12 oz)	180	0	0	0	0	52	52	—	—	35	—	—	—

FOOD	PORTION	CALS	FAT	SAT FAT	CHOL	PROT	CARB	SUGAR	FIBER	CALCI	SOD	POTAS	FOLIC	VIT C
VIGNETTE														
Wine Country Soda Chardonnay	1 bottle (12 oz)	130	0	0	0	0	33	31	—	—	20	—	—	—
Wine Country Soda Pinot Noir	1 bottle (12 oz)	130	0	0	0	0	31	31	—	—	15	—	—	—
VIRGIL'S														
Micro Brewed Root Beer	1 bottle (12 oz)	160	0	0	0	0	42	42	—	—	0	—	—	—
ZEVIA														
Dr. Zevia	1 can (12 oz)	0	0	0	0	0	7	0	0	—	20	—	—	—
SOLE														
cooked	1 fillet (4.5 oz)	148	2	tr	86	31	0	0	0	23	133	436	—	—
cooked	3 oz	99	1	tr	58	21	0	0	0	16	89	292	—	—
lemon raw	3.5 oz	85	1	—	—	17	0	0	0	—	80	298	—	—
TAKE-OUT														
breaded & fried	3.2 oz	211	11	3	31	13	15	—	—	17	484	292	51	0
SORGHUM														
sorghum	1 cup (6.7 oz)	651	6	1	0	22	143	—	—	54	12	672	—	0
SOUFFLE														
GARDEN LITES														
Roasted Vegetable	1 pkg (7 oz)	140	2	0	0	8	24	8	3	60	350	—	—	54
HEAVENLY SOUFFLE														
Chocolate	1 (2.6 oz)	262	16	9	103	3	29	26	0	10	128	—	—	1
TAKE-OUT														
cheese	1 cup	194	15	6	134	9	6	3	tr	178	307	124	19	0
chicken	1 cup (5.6 oz)	278	18	5	218	20	9	4	tr	110	560	262	29	0
corn	1 cup	257	11	3	152	10	34	11	3	92	666	417	54	6
lime chilled	1 cup	388	18	3	306	11	48	45	2	53	102	184	30	6
seafood	1 cup	245	15	4	231	17	9	4	tr	137	668	251	33	1
spinach	1 cup	124	8	2	97	6	7	3	1	98	170	171	47	1
SOUP														
CANNED														
ALLENS														
Chicken Broth	1 cup	10	0	0	0	1	1	1	0	0	620	—	—	0
AMY'S														
Organic Butternut Squash Light In Sodium	1 cup (8.6 oz)	100	3	0	0	2	20	4	2	40	290	—	—	6
Organic Chunky Tomato Bisque	1 cup (8.4 oz)	120	4	2	10	2	21	14	2	80	680	—	—	24
Organic Chunky Tomato Bisque Light In Sodium	1 cup (8.6 oz)	120	4	2	10	2	21	14	2	80	340	—	—	24

FOOD	PORTION	CALS	FAT	SAT FAT	CHOL	PROT	CARB	SUGAR	FIBER	CALCI	SOD	POTAS	FOLIC	VIT C
AMY'S (CONT.)														
Organic Cream Of Mushroom	¾ cup (6.5 oz)	150	9	2	10	3	13	3	2	20	590	—	—	5
Organic Lentil Light In Sodium	1 cup (8.6 oz)	180	5	1	0	8	25	3	6	20	290	—	—	6
Organic No Chicken Noodle Soup	1 cup (8.6 oz)	100	3	0	0	5	13	3	2	20	540	—	—	6
Organic Pasta & 3 Bean	1 cup (8.6 oz)	150	4	1	0	5	22	5	4	60	680	—	—	5
Organic Southwestern Vegetable	1 cup (8.7 oz)	140	4	1	0	4	21	4	4	40	680	—	—	15
Organic Split Pea	1 cup (8.6 oz)	100	0	0	0	7	19	4	3	20	670	—	—	4
Split Pea Light In Sodium	1 cup (8.6 oz)	100	0	0	0	7	19	4	4	20	280	—	—	4
Tom Kha Phak Thai Coconut	1 cup (7 oz)	140	10	8	0	4	9	4	2	40	580	—	—	4
BUTTERBALL														
Chicken Broth 99% Fat Free	1 cup	10	0	0	0	tr	2	0	0	—	840	—	—	—
CAMPBELL'S														
25% Less Sodium Chicken Noodle as prep	1 cup	60	2	1	15	3	8	1	1	0	660	—	—	0
25% Less Sodium Cream Of Mushroom as prep	1 cup	110	8	1	5	2	8	1	2	0	650	—	—	0
98% Fat Free Cream Of Celery as prep	1 cup	60	3	1	5	1	8	1	1	0	580	—	—	0
98% Fat Free Cream Of Chicken as prep	1 cup	70	3	1	10	2	10	1	1	0	590	—	—	0
100% Natural Caramelized French Onion	1 cup (8.4 oz)	80	3	1	5	3	12	4	1	60	480	—	—	1
100% Natural Chicken Tuscany	1 cup	90	2	1	10	7	12	4	4	40	480	—	—	1
100% Natural Chicken w/ Egg Noodles	1 cup	100	3	1	25	8	11	2	1	20	480	—	—	0
100% Natural Chicken w/ Whole Grain Pasta	1 cup (8.4 oz)	100	2	1	20	7	14	1	1	20	410	700	—	0

FOOD	PORTION	CALS	FAT	SAT FAT	CHOL	PROT	CARB	SUGAR	FIBER	CALCI	SOD	POTAS	FOLIC	VIT C
CAMPBELL'S (CONT.)														
100% Natural Creole Chicken w/ Red Beans & Rice	1 cup (8.4 oz)	130	3	2	30	7	18	4	2	60	650	—	—	0
100% Natural Harvest Tomato w/ Basil	1 cup (8.4 oz)	100	0	0	0	3	22	15	2	20	410	630	—	6
100% Natural Light Minestrone w/Whole Grain Pasta	1 cup	80	1	0	0	4	14	4	4	40	480	—	—	1
100% Natural Light Savory Chicken w/ Vegetables	1 cup	80	1	1	10	5	15	3	4	20	480	—	—	0
100% Natural Light Southwestern Style Vegetable	1 cup	50	0	0	0	2	13	4	3	40	480	—	—	2
100% Natural Light Vegetable & Pasta	1 cup (8.4 oz)	60	0	0	0	3	13	3	4	60	480	—	—	1
100% Natural Light Vegetable Beef & Barley	1 cup (8.4 oz)	80	2	1	5	5	14	4	4	20	480	—	—	6
100% Natural Southwest White Chicken Chili	1 cup (8.4 oz)	140	2	1	10	10	21	3	5	60	650	—	—	1
Cheddar Cheese as prep	1 cup	110	5	2	5	2	12	2	1	40	890	—	—	0
Chicken & Stars as prep	1 cup	70	2	1	5	3	11	1	1	0	480	—	—	0
Chicken Alphabet as prep	1 cup	70	2	1	5	3	12	1	1	0	480	—	—	1
Chicken Noodle O's as prep	1 cup	90	3	1	20	3	15	2	1	0	480	—	—	0
Chunky Creamy Chicken & Dumplings	1 cup (8.4 oz)	170	8	2	30	7	17	3	3	20	880	180	—	1
Chunky Healthy Request Chicken Noodle	1 cup (8.4 oz)	120	3	1	10	8	17	3	2	20	410	700	—	1
Chunky Italian Wedding	1 cup (8.4 oz)	130	3	1	15	6	21	6	3	60	410	900	—	1
Chunky Roadhouse Beef & Bean Chili	1 cup	230	8	4	30	15	25	11	8	40	870	—	—	1
Chunky Split Pea & Ham	1 cup (8.4 oz)	170	3	1	10	12	24	4	5	20	410	1000	—	2

FOOD	PORTION	CALS	FAT	SAT FAT	CHOL	PROT	CARB	SUGAR	FIBER	CALCI	SOD	POTAS	FOLIC	VIT C
CAMPBELL'S (CONT.)														
Curly Noodle as prep	1 cup	80	2	1	15	4	11	1	1	20	480	—	—	0
Double Noodle Chicken as prep	1 cup	110	2	1	10	3	20	1	1	0	480	—	—	0
Goldfish Pasta Meatball as prep	1 cup	90	3	1	10	4	11	1	1	0	480	—	—	0
Healthy Kids Goldfish Pasta as prep	1 cup	80	2	1	5	3	12	1	1	0	480	540	—	0
Healthy Request Cream Of Chicken as prep	1 cup (8.4 oz)	80	3	1	5	2	12	7	1	0	410	750	—	0
Healthy Request Tomato as prep	1 cup	90	2	1	0	2	10	10	1	0	470	280	—	6
Italian Wedding Light as prep	1 cup (8.4 oz)	80	2	1	5	3	12	2	2	40	480	720	—	0
Light Chicken Gumbo as prep	1 cup (8.4 oz)	70	1	1	5	2	12	2	1	20	480	700	—	0
Low Sodium Chicken Broth	1 can	25	1	1	5	4	1	1	0	0	140	—	—	0
Mega Noodle as prep	1 cup	90	2	1	15	3	15	1	1	0	480	—	—	0
Microwavable Bowl Chicken Noodle	1 cup	70	2	1	15	4	10	0	tr	0	870	—	—	0
Minestrone as prep	1 cup (8.4 oz)	90	1	1	5	4	17	3	3	20	650	1050	—	0
Select Italian Sausage w/ Pasta & Pepperoni	1 cup	150	6	3	15	7	18	4	2	40	800	—	—	0
Select Mexican Chicken Tortilla	1 cup	130	3	1	10	8	19	3	3	40	850	—	—	0
Select Vegetable Beef	1 cup	110	2	1	15	8	16	2	3	20	910	—	—	0
Slow Kettle Burgundy Beef Stew w/ Baby Bella Mushrooms & Roasted Garlic	1 cup (8.4 oz)	160	4	2	20	11	19	5	4	40	700	—	—	4
Slow Kettle Portobello Mushroom & Madeira Bisque w/ Shallots	1 cup (8.4 oz)	230	17	6	25	6	14	7	4	80	770	—	—	0

FOOD	PORTION	CALS	FAT	SAT FAT	CHOL	PROT	CARB	SUGAR	FIBER	CALCI	SOD	POTAS	FOLIC	VIT C
CAMPBELL'S (CONT.)														
Slow Kettle Southwest Chicken Chile w/ Black Beans & Sweet Corn	1 cup (8.4 oz)	190	2	1	20	15	27	6	7	80	740	—	—	5
Slow Kettle Tuscan Chicken & White Bean w/ Asiago Cheese Thyme & Rosemary	1 cup (8.4 oz)	140	3	1	15	12	17	4	4	80	760	—	—	1
Soup At Hand 25% Less Sodium Chicken w/ Mini Noodles	1 pkg (10.75 oz)	80	2	1	10	4	11	2	2	0	730	—	—	2
Soup At Hand Vegetable Medley	1 pkg (10.75 oz)	100	2	1	<5	3	19	9	4	20	890	—	—	30
Soup At Hand Velvety Potato	1 pkg (10.75 oz)	160	7	1	<5	2	21	5	4	20	870	—	—	0
Tomato as prep	1 cup (8.4 oz)	90	0	0	0	2	20	12	1	0	480	690	—	6
V8 Carden Broccoli	1 cup (8.4 oz)	90	2	1	5	3	15	6	3	40	480	—	—	6
V8 Golden Butternut Squash	1 cup	140	2	1	5	3	28	6	3	—	750	100	—	—
V8 Sweet Red Pepper	1 cup	120	2	1	5	3	22	10	4	—	620	100	—	6
V8 Tomato Herb	1 cup	90	0	0	0	3	19	14	3	—	750	100	—	12
COLLEGE INN														
Beef Broth 99% Fat Free	1 cup (8.4 oz)	25	1	0	0	4	0	0	0	20	900	—	—	0
Beef Broth Fat Free Lower Sodium	1 cup (8.4 oz)	15	0	0	0	4	0	0	0	0	450	—	—	0
Bold Stock Rotisserie Chicken	1 cup (8.4 oz)	30	0	0	0	3	4	1	0	20	720	—	—	12
Bold Stock Tender Beef	1 cup (8.4 oz)	45	0	0	0	7	4	2	0	20	730	—	—	0
Chicken Broth 99% Fat Free	1 cup (8.5 oz)	15	1	0	0	1	3	1	0	0	930	—	—	0
Chicken Broth Light & Fat Free 50% Less Sodium	1 cup (8.4 oz)	5	0	0	0	1	0	0	0	0	450	—	—	0
Chicken Broth w/ Roasted Garlic	1 cup (8.5 oz)	20	0	0	0	1	3	1	0	0	1000	—	—	0
Chicken Broth w/ Roasted Vegetables & Herbs	1 cup (8.5 oz)	20	0	0	0	1	3	1	0	0	1060	—	—	0

FOOD	PORTION	CALS	FAT	SAT FAT	CHOL	PROT	CARB	SUGAR	FIBER	CALCI	SOD	POTAS	FOLIC	VIT C
COLLEGE INN (CONT.)														
Culinary Broth Thai Coconut Curry	1 cup (8.4 oz)	20	1	0	0	0	5	4	0	20	1010	—	—	0
Culinary Broth Wine & Herbs	1 cup (8.4 oz)	5	1	0	0	0	1	1	1	20	920	—	—	0
Garden Vegetable Broth	1 cup (8.4 oz)	25	1	0	0	1	6	4	0	0	590	—	—	0
Turkey Broth	1 cup (8.4 oz)	20	1	0	0	2	0	0	0	0	950	—	—	0
COMFORT CARE														
Hearty Beef Barley	1 cup (8 oz)	190	7	2	20	12	23	9	4	80	85	—	—	42
Savory Chicken	1 cup (8 oz)	200	7	2	15	13	25	9	5	80	70	—	—	42
Tomato Cheddar Jack	1 cup (8 oz)	90	2	1	5	8	13	7	5	150	140	—	—	30
DR. MCDOUGALL'S														
Chunky Tomato Gluten Free	1 cup (8.6 oz)	90	0	0	0	2	20	8	3	—	440	—	—	—
Lentil	1 cup (8.6 oz)	115	1	0	0	1	21	1	8	—	480	—	—	—
Organic Black Bean Lower Sodium	1 cup (8.6 oz)	150	1	0	0	8	28	3	6	80	290	—	—	7
Organic Tortilla	1 cup (8.6 oz)	100	1	0	0	5	20	2	4	40	530	—	—	10
Split Pea	1 cup (8.6 oz)	110	0	0	0	7	20	1	8	—	420	—	—	—
Vegetable Gluten Free Vegan	1 cup (3.3 oz)	230	13	8	90	4	25	24	0	100	55	—	—	0
FRONTERA														
Gourmet Mexican Classic Tortilla	1 cup (8.6 oz)	80	2	0	0	3	15	5	3	40	1060	—	—	21
Gourmet Mexican Roasted Vegetable	1 cup (8.6 oz)	80	2	0	0	3	14	5	2	60	720	—	—	54
GO APPETIT														
Carrot Bisque	8 oz	110	5	1	5	6	13	7	3	—	450	250	—	—
Gazpacho	8 oz	100	7	1	0	1	9	3	1	—	400	340	—	—
Mango Melange	8 oz	150	5	4	0	3	27	24	1	—	—	—	—	—
GOLD'S														
Borscht Unsalted	1 cup	70	0	0	0	1	13	11	tr	20	30	—	—	2
Schav	1 cup	15	1	—	15	1	1	—	1	20	880	—	—	21
HEALTHY CHOICE														
Bean & Ham	1 cup (8.7 oz)	180	3	1	10	11	28	3	6	80	480	—	—	0
Chicken & Dumplings	1 cup (8.8 oz)	150	3	1	25	8	22	2	3	40	480	—	—	4
Chicken w/ Rice	1 cup (8.4 oz)	110	2	1	10	5	17	tr	2	40	390	—	—	2
Garden Vegetable	1 cup (8.6 oz)	130	1	0	5	5	25	4	5	40	450	—	—	1
Italian Wedding	1 cup (8.6 oz)	120	3	1	10	9	16	1	3	60	430	—	—	1
New England Clam Chowder	1 cup (8.4 oz)	110	2	1	10	4	20	3	3	40	480	—	—	0

FOOD	PORTION	CALS	FAT	SAT FAT	CHOL	PROT	CARB	SUGAR	FIBER	CALCI	SOD	POTAS	FOLIC	VIT C
HEALTHY CHOICE (CONT.)														
Split Pea & Ham	1 cup (8.8 oz)	160	3	1	10	12	27	3	6	40	470	—	—	0
Tomato Basil	1 cup (8.8 oz)	100	0	0	0	2	22	10	3	20	450	—	—	0
HEALTH VALLEY														
Beef Broth Fat Free	1 cup	10	0	0	0	2	0	0	0	0	390	—	—	0
Chicken Broth Fat Free	1 cup	20	0	0	0	5	0	0	0	0	390	—	—	0
Chicken Broth Fat Free No Salt Added	1 cup	35	2	1	0	5	0	0	0	—	130	—	—	—
Chicken Broth Low Fat	1 cup	35	2	1	25	5	0	0	0	0	390	—	—	0
Clam Chowder Manhattan	1 cup	90	3	0	0	3	13	5	1	40	680	—	—	6
Clam Chowder New England	1 cup	110	4	2	10	5	15	5	0	100	680	—	—	1
Corn & Vegetable Fat Free	1 cup	70	0	0	0	5	17	8	7	40	135	—	—	6
Garden Vegetable Fat Free	1 cup	80	0	0	0	3	18	6	4	60	480	—	—	12
Lentil & Carrot Fat Free	1 cup	100	0	0	0	10	25	7	7	40	220	—	—	2
Organic Black Bean	1 cup	130	1	0	0	7	25	7	5	60	380	—	—	5
Organic Cream Of Mushroom	1 cup	90	5	3	0	1	11	0	0	20	660	—	—	1
Organic Minestrone	1 cup	100	2	0	0	4	20	3	5	40	480	—	—	6
Organic Minestrone No Salt Added	1 cup	70	0	0	0	3	17	5	3	40	45	—	—	9
Organic Mushroom Barley	1 cup	70	0	0	0	2	17	4	3	20	380	—	—	6
Organic Mushroom Barley No Salt Added	1 cup	70	0	0	0	2	17	4	3	20	25	—	—	6
Organic Split Pea No Salt Added	1 cup	110	0	0	0	10	23	5	8	20	45	—	—	1
Organic Tomato	1 cup	80	0	0	0	3	18	14	1	40	380	—	—	24
Organic Tomato No Salt Added	1 cup	80	0	0	0	3	18	14	1	40	35	—	—	24
Tomato Vegetable Fat Free	1 cup	80	0	0	0	6	17	9	5	40	240	—	—	9
Vegetable Broth Fat Free	1 cup	20	0	0	0	0	5	1	0	0	330	—	—	0

FOOD	PORTION	CALS	FAT	SAT FAT	CHOL	PROT	CARB	SUGAR	FIBER	CALCI	SOD	POTAS	FOLIC	VIT C
HORMEL														
Bean & Ham	1 pkg (7.5 oz)	190	4	1	10	9	29	2	7	60	720	—	—	0
Beef Vegetable	1 pkg (7.5 oz)	100	1	0	10	6	16	3	1	20	790	—	—	0
Chicken Noodle	1 pkg (7.5 oz)	100	3	1	25	7	12	0	0	20	790	—	—	0
Chicken w/ Rice	1 pkg (7.5 oz)	110	3	1	10	4	18	3	1	20	850	—	—	0
New England Clam Chowder	1 pkg (7.5 oz)	140	5	3	20	5	18	0	1	20	800	—	—	0
IMAGINE														
Lobster Bisque	1 cup	130	5	3	15	5	15	4	—	150	690	—	—	6
Organic Creamy Butternut Squash	1 cup	90	2	0	0	0	18	7	2	40	480	—	—	0
Organic Creamy Chicken	1 cup	70	2	0	0	3	12	1	1	20	680	—	—	5
Organic Creamy Sweet Corn	1 cup	120	3	1	0	4	20	9	3	20	450	—	—	0
Organic Sweet Potato	1 cup	110	2	0	0	2	23	2	1	20	400	—	—	21
Organic Bistro Cuban Black Bean Bisque	1 cup	170	4	0	0	8	30	4	6	40	480	—	—	9
Organic Broth Beef	1 cup	20	1	0	5	2	1	1	0	0	700	—	—	1
Organic Broth Free Range Chicken	1 cup	10	0	0	0	1	1	0	0	40	570	—	—	0
Organic Broth Vegetable	8 oz	20	0	0	0	2	2	2	0	20	550	—	—	0
LUCINI														
Roman Tomato Cream	1 cup (8.6 oz)	170	9	5	25	4	18	10	4	100	770	—	—	36
Umbrian Lentil	1 cup (8.6 oz)	160	5	1	0	7	23	6	9	80	770	—	—	15
MANISCHEWITZ														
Beef Broth	1 cup (8.4 oz)	150	1	0	0	1	1	1	0	0	790	—	—	0
Chicken Broth	1 cup (8.4 oz)	15	1	0	0	1	1	1	0	0	790	—	—	0
Chicken Broth Low Sodium	1 cup (8.4 oz)	15	1	0	0	1	1	1	0	0	420	—	—	0
MUIR GLEN														
Organic Garden Vegetable	1 cup	80	1	0	0	3	16	5	3	40	560	—	—	0
Organic Southwest Black Bean	1 cup	140	1	0	0	7	27	4	8	60	670	—	—	6
NEW ENGLAND COUNTRY SOUP														
Caribbean Black Bean	1 cup (8.8 oz)	210	3	0	0	10	38	4	8	80	230	—	—	30
Chicken Pomodoro	1 cup (8.6 oz)	140	6	2	15	7	16	3	2	40	260	—	—	9
Nana's Chicken	1 cup (8.6 oz)	120	4	1	10	7	2	2	4	60	350	—	—	5

FOOD	PORTION	CALS	FAT	SAT FAT	CHOL	PROT	CARB	SUGAR	FIBER	CALCI	SOD	POTAS	FOLIC	VIT C
NEW ENGLAND COUNTRY SOUP (CONT.)														
Sweet Chicken Curry	1 cup (8.8 oz)	160	4	1	20	9	27	9	3	40	75	—	—	5
Yankee White Bean	1 cup (9.3 oz)	380	9	5	35	26	52	41	12	200	340	—	—	12
ORIGINAL SOUPMAN														
Italian Wedding	1 cup	120	6	3	10	4	18	4	4	80	600	—	—	18
New England Clam Chowder	1 cup	290	19	11	90	14	16	1	1	100	930	—	—	18
Organic Butternut Squash	1 cup	250	13	8	50	3	33	12	3	60	560	—	—	15
Tomato Basil	1 cup	140	7	4	15	4	18	11	4	40	1110	—	—	30
Turkey Chili	1 cup	210	7	2	40	18	18	4	5	80	910	—	—	36
PACIFIC FOODS														
Beef Broth Organic	1 cup (8 oz)	20	1	0	5	2	1	1	0	20	570	—	—	0
Butternut Squash Organic	1 cup (8 oz)	90	2	0	0	2	17	4	3	40	550	—	—	2
Cashew Carrot Ginger Bisque	1 cup (8.4 oz)	130	5	4	0	2	20	8	4	40	670	—	—	0
Chicken Broth Free Range	1 cup (8 oz)	10	0	0	0	1	1	1	0	0	570	—	—	0
Chicken Broth Free Range Low Sodium Organic	1 cup (8 oz)	15	0	0	0	2	1	0	0	0	70	45	—	0
Cream Of Celery	1 cup (8.6 oz)	70	3	2	10	1	11	1	0	20	760	—	—	0
Curried Red Lentil	1 cup (8 oz)	140	5	4	0	5	19	8	5	20	720	—	—	2
French Onion Organic	1 cup (8 oz)	30	1	1	0	1	5	3	0	20	720	—	—	0
Minestrone w/ Chicken Meatballs	1 cup (8.8 oz)	130	4	1	10	6	19	3	3	40	700	—	—	0
Mushroom Broth Organic	1 cup (8 oz)	5	0	0	0	0	1	0	0	0	530	—	—	0
Organic Pho Vegetarian Soup Base	1 cup (8 oz)	25	0	0	0	1	5	5	0	0	650	—	—	0
Organic Broth Pho Beef	1 cup (8 oz)	35	0	0	5	3	5	5	0	20	660	—	—	0
Poblano Pepper & Corn Chowder	1 cup (8.7 oz)	190	10	6	35	3	22	2	1	40	700	—	—	4
Red Pepper & Tomato Light Sodium Organic	1 cup (8 oz)	110	2	2	10	5	16	12	1	150	360	—	—	2
Rosemary Potato Chowder	1 cup (8.7 oz)	230	8	5	30	1	36	0	2	20	730	—	—	5
Thai Sweet Potato	1 cup (8.6 oz)	160	6	4	0	3	25	3	3	40	660	—	—	9

FOOD	PORTION	CALS	FAT	SAT FAT	CHOL	PROT	CARB	SUGAR	FIBER	CALCI	SOD	POTAS	FOLIC	VIT C
PACIFIC FOODS (CONT.)														
Tomato Light Sodium Organic	1 cup (8 oz)	100	2	2	10	5	16	12	1	150	380	—	—	4
Vegetable Broth Organic	1 cup (8 oz)	15	0	0	0	0	3	2	1	20	530	—	—	0
PROGRESSO														
40% Less Sodium Italian Style Wedding	1 cup (8.7 oz)	90	2	1	10	5	11	2	1	20	480	—	—	0
50% Less Sodium Garden Vegetable	1 cup (8.8 oz)	100	0	0	0	3	22	4	3	20	450	—	—	0
High Fiber Chicken Tuscany	1 cup (8.7 oz)	130	3	2	15	9	20	2	7	60	690	700	—	0
High Fiber Creamy Tomato Basil	1 cup (8.8 oz)	130	4	1	5	3	26	13	7	20	690	520	—	2
Light Beef Pot Roast	1 cup (8.4 oz)	80	1	0	15	6	12	4	2	20	690	—	—	0
Light Chicken Vegetable Rotini	1 cup (8.3 oz)	70	2	1	15	6	10	2	2	0	700	—	—	0
Light Chicken Noodle	1 cup (8.3 oz)	70	2	1	15	5	10	1	1	0	690	270	—	0
Light Italian Style Vegetable	1 cup (8.6 oz)	60	0	0	0	3	12	3	4	40	700	—	—	5
Light Savory Vegetable Barley	1 cup (8.5 oz)	60	0	0	0	2	14	3	4	40	740	—	—	0
Light Vegetable	1 cup (8.4 oz)	60	0	0	0	3	14	4	4	20	470	600	—	0
Light Vegetable & Noodle	1 cup (8.7 oz)	60	1	0	5	2	13	2	4	20	690	420	—	0
Reduced Sodium Chicken Gumbo	1 cup (8.7 oz)	110	2	1	10	7	18	3	4	40	480	650	—	0
Reduced Sodium Chicken Noodle	1 cup (8.4 oz)	90	2	1	20	6	13	1	1	0	470	480	—	0
Rich & Hearty Beef Pot Roast	1 cup (8.7 oz)	120	2	1	15	8	20	4	2	20	830	—	—	0
Rich & Hearty Chicken & Homestyle Noodles	1 cup (8.6 oz)	100	3	1	25	7	14	2	1	0	690	340	—	0
Rich & Hearty Chicken Pot Pie	1 cup (8.6 oz)	170	6	2	15	8	21	3	2	20	940	—	—	0
Rich & Hearty Savory Beef Barley Vegetable	1 cup (8.6 oz)	130	1	1	15	8	22	4	3	20	970	—	—	0
Rich & Hearty Sirloin Steak & Vegetables	1 cup	130	2	1	15	8	21	5	2	20	870	—	—	0

FOOD	PORTION	CALS	FAT	SAT FAT	CHOL	PROT	CARB	SUGAR	FIBER	CALCI	SOD	POTAS	FOLIC	VIT C
PROGRESSO (CONT.)														
Rich & Hearty Slow Cooked Vegetable Beef	1 cup (8.6 oz)	120	1	0	15	6	20	6	3	40	840	—	—	0
Rich & Hearty Steak & Roasted Russet Potatoes	1 cup (8.6 oz)	140	2	0	15	8	23	3	2	20	990	—	—	5
Traditional Beef & Vegetable	1 cup (8.7 oz)	120	2	1	15	8	18	4	2	20	850	—	—	0
Traditional Beef Barley	1 cup (8.5 oz)	120	2	1	10	7	20	3	4	20	720	—	—	0
Traditional Chickarina	1 cup (8.3 oz)	120	5	2	20	8	12	1	2	20	950	—	—	1
Traditional Chicken & Wild Rice	1 cup (8.4 oz)	100	2	1	15	6	15	1	1	20	870	—	—	0
Traditional Chicken Noodle	1 cup (8.3 oz)	100	3	1	20	7	12	1	1	0	690	350	—	0
Traditional Italian Style Wedding	1 cup (8.4 oz)	100	4	2	10	6	12	1	1	20	840	—	—	0
Traditional Manhattan Clam Chowder	1 cup (8.4 oz)	100	2	0	10	3	17	4	2	20	970	—	—	0
Traditional New England Clam Chowder	1 cup (8.4 oz)	180	9	2	15	6	20	2	1	20	890	—	—	0
Traditional Potato Broccoli & Cheese	1 cup (8.8 oz)	180	10	3	10	5	18	2	2	60	920	—	—	0
Traditional Split Pea w/ Ham	1 cup (8.5 oz)	140	1	0	5	9	24	3	4	20	690	—	—	0
Traditional Turkey Noodle	1 cup (8.4 oz)	80	2	0	15	5	12	1	1	0	980	—	—	0
Vegetable Classics Creamy Mushroom	1 cup (8.1 oz)	130	3	3	10	2	9	2	1	0	820	—	—	0
Vegetable Classics French Onion	1 cup (8 oz)	50	2	1	<5	1	8	3	tr	20	850	—	—	—
Vegetable Classics Hearty Black Bean	1 cup (8.5 oz)	160	1	1	<5	8	29	3	8	60	690	—	—	0
Vegetable Classics Hearty Tomato	1 cup (8.6 oz)	110	1	0	0	2	23	9	3	40	980	—	—	5
Vegetable Classics Lentil	1 cup (8.5 oz)	160	2	1	0	9	30	2	5	20	810	—	—	0
Vegetable Classics Vegetable	1 cup (8.4 oz)	80	0	0	0	5	15	4	3	20	660	560	—	0
World Recipes Caldo De Pollo	1 cup (8.6 oz)	90	2	0	10	5	14	3	1	0	690	370	—	0

FOOD	PORTION	CALS	FAT	SAT FAT	CHOL	PROT	CARB	SUGAR	FIBER	CALCI	SOD	POTAS	FOLIC	VIT C
SNOW'S														
Clam Chowder	1 cup (8.4 oz)	200	15	4	15	5	13	3	1	40	900	—	—	4
SPOONFUL OF COMFORT														
Chicken Soup	1 serv (8 oz)	80	2	0	20	6	11	1	1	20	570	—	—	1
SWANSON														
50% Low Sodium Beef Broth	1 cup	15	0	0	0	3	1	1	0	0	440	—	—	0
Beef Broth	1 cup	15	0	0	0	2	1	0	0	0	890	—	—	0
Beef Stock	1 cup	30	0	0	0	4	3	3	0	20	500	—	—	0
Chicken Broth	1 cup	10	0	0	5	1	1	1	0	0	860	—	—	0
Chicken Stock	1 cup	20	0	0	0	4	1	1	0	0	510	—	—	0
Vegetable Broth	1 cup	15	0	0	0	0	3	2	tr	0	940	—	—	0
TABATCHNICK														
Garden Fresh Vegetable Broth	⅔ cup (5.5 oz)	10	0	0	0	0	2	1	0	0	550	—	—	0
Wisconsin Cheddar Cheese	⅔ cup (5.5 oz)	150	11	3	0	1	10	2	0	40	970	65	—	0
VALLEY FRESH														
Chicken Broth	1 cup	30	2	1	<5	2	1	1	—	—	1000	—	—	—
Chicken Broth 40% Less Sodium	1 cup	15	0	0	<5	2	1	1	—	—	600	—	—	—
FROZEN														
KETTLE CUISINE														
Angus Beef Steak Chili w/ Beans Gluten Free Dairy Free	1 pkg (10 oz)	250	12	5	55	19	17	9	4	20	760	—	—	24
Chicken w/ Rice Noodles Gluten Free	1 pkg (10 oz)	140	3	1	40	14	15	1	2	20	540	—	—	0
Roasted Vegetable Gluten Free Dairy Free	1 pkg (10 oz)	140	6	1	0	3	19	4	5	100	560	—	—	0
Thai Curry Chicken Gluten Free Dairy Free	1 pkg (10 oz)	330	11	8	25	13	44	2	4	20	560	—	—	0
Three Bean Chili Gluten Free	1 pkg (10 oz)	220	4	1	0	11	36	11	13	100	450	—	—	6
TABATCHNICK														
Cabbage	1 serv (7.5 oz)	90	1	0	0	2	21	11	1	40	160	240	—	15
Chicken Broth w/ Noodles & Dumplings	1 serv (7.25 oz)	150	6	1	65	5	19	1	tr	40	740	85	—	1
Corn Chowder	1 serv (7.5 oz)	130	5	2	10	4	21	4	2	60	390	270	—	6
Organic Vegetarian Chili	1 serv (7.5 oz)	180	4	0	0	12	28	3	8	40	360	670	—	15

FOOD	PORTION	CALS	FAT	SAT FAT	CHOL	PROT	CARB	SUGAR	FIBER	CALCI	SOD	POTAS	FOLIC	VIT C
TABATCHNICK (CONT.)														
Soup Singles Split Pea	1 bowl (10.9 oz)	210	1	0	0	19	50	1	20	10	540	125	—	1
Split Pea	1 serv (7.5 oz)	140	0	0	0	13	34	0	13	20	380	90	—	1
Vegetable	1 serv (7.5 oz)	90	2	0	0	3	17	3	4	40	350	170	—	6
Vegetable Low Sodium	1 serv (7.5 oz)	90	2	0	0	4	17	3	4	40	45	170	—	6
Wilderness Wild Rice	1 serv (7.5 oz)	80	1	0	0	3	16	1	1	0	220	140	—	15
Yankee Bean	1 serv (7.5 oz)	180	2	0	0	11	33	2	10	80	340	750	—	0
MIX														
beef broth cube	1 cube	6	tr	tr	tr	1	1	—	—	—	864	15	—	—
chicken broth cube	1 cube (4.8 g)	9	tr	tr	1	1	1	—	—	—	1152	18	—	—
ANNIE CHUN'S														
Noodle Bowl Chicken Noodle	1 pkg	260	2	0	0	8	52	1	2	20	990	—	—	2
Noodle Bowl Hot & Sour	1 pkg	280	3	0	0	8	55	1	2	40	910	—	—	0
Noodle Bowl Korean Kimchi	½ pkg	140	2	0	0	6	28	0	1	0	720	—	—	0
Ramen Soy Ginger as prep	1 pkg (4.9 oz)	230	1	0	0	12	45	tr	1	20	1000	—	—	0
Ramen Spring Vegetable as prep	1 pkg (4.9 oz)	230	1	0	0	8	48	2	2	40	1000	—	—	0
DR. MCDOUGALL'S														
Black Bean & Lime not prep	1 pkg (3.3 oz)	340	2	0	0	20	60	4	28	—	660	—	—	—
Chicken Noodle Light Sodium not prep	1 pkg (1.4 oz)	140	1	0	0	3	28	2	2	—	360	—	—	—
Chinese Chicken Noodle Light Sodium not prep	1 pkg (1.4 oz)	140	1	0	0	3	28	2	2	—	360	—	—	—
Minestrone & Pasta not prep	1 pkg (2.3 oz)	200	1	0	0	8	40	2	8	—	620	—	—	—
Tamale w/ Baked Chips not prep	1 pkg (2.4 oz)	200	2	0	0	8	36	2	6	—	640	—	—	—
Tortilla w/ Baked Chips not prep	1 pkg (2 oz)	200	2	0	0	10	34	2	6	—	620	—	—	—
White Bean & Pasta Light Sodium not prep	1 pkg (1.8 oz)	170	1	0	0	7	34	2	8	—	360	—	—	—
EDWARD & SONS														
Bouillon Cubes Not-Beef	½ cube	20	2	1	0	1	1	tr	0	—	920	—	—	—
Bouillon Cubes Not-Chicken	½ cube	15	2	1	0	1	1	0	0	—	800	—	—	—

FOOD	PORTION	CALS	FAT	SAT FAT	CHOL	PROT	CARB	SUGAR	FIBER	CALCI	SOD	POTAS	FOLIC	VIT C
EDWARD & SONS (CONT.)														
Veggie Low Sodium	½ cup	20	2	1	0	1	1	1	0	—	135	—	—	—
FANTASTIC														
Noodle Soup Spicy Thai as prep	2 cups	110	1	0	0	3	22	3	1	20	460	—	—	5
Noodle Soup Cup Vegetarian Chicken as prep	1 cup	90	1	0	0	4	19	0	1	0	590	—	—	0
HAMBEENS														
15 Bean as prep	½ cup	120	1	0	0	8	20	1	9	40	70	470	—	0
15 Bean Beef as prep	½ cup	120	1	0	0	8	20	1	9	40	310	480	—	0
15 Bean Cajun as prep	½ cup	120	1	0	0	8	20	1	9	40	100	490	—	0
15 Bean Chicken as prep	½ cup	120	1	0	0	8	20	1	9	40	250	470	—	0
Spanish American Black Bean as prep	½ cup	120	1	0	0	7	22	1	8	40	280	520	—	0
HERB OX														
Instant Chicken Bouillon	1 pkg (4 g)	5	0	0	0	0	tr	—	—	—	1100	—	—	—
KIKKOMAN														
Instant Tofu Miso	1 pkg (6 g)	15	0	0	0	tr	3	0	0	0	700	—	—	0
Instant Wakame Seaweed	1 pkg (10 g)	35	1	0	0	3	3	0	0	20	740	—	—	0
LEAHEY GARDENS														
No Beef Noodle as prep	1½ cups	89	1	0	0	7	16	tr	6	0	415	—	—	0
No Chicken Noodle as prep	1½ cups	94	1	0	0	7	16	tr	6	80	495	—	—	4
MANISCHEWITZ														
Lentil as prep	1 cup	150	0	0	0	7	29	2	12	40	530	—	—	0
Matzo Ball Soup as prep	1 cup	40	1	1	0	1	9	3	1	20	1290	—	—	0
Southwestern Black Bean as prep	1 cup	90	1	0	0	4	16	2	4	40	1340	—	—	1
Split Pea w/ Barley as prep	1 cup	110	0	0	0	7	21	2	3	0	780	—	—	0
Vegetable & Pasta as prep	1 cup	90	0	0	0	4	17	1	2	20	650	—	—	2
MISO-CUP														
Golden Vegetable as prep	1 cup	30	1	0	0	2	3	1	tr	20	780	—	—	0

FOOD	PORTION	CALS	FAT	SAT FAT	CHOL	PROT	CARB	SUGAR	FIBER	CALCI	SOD	POTAS	FOLIC	VIT C
MISO-CUP (CONT.)														
Japanese Restaurant Style as prep	1 cup	60	2	0	0	4	7	tr	tr	20	1170	—	—	0
Organic Traditional w/ Tofu as prep	1 cup	35	1	0	0	2	4	tr	tr	20	480	—	—	1
Reduced Sodium as prep	1 cup	25	1	0	0	2	3	tr	tr	20	270	—	—	1
Savory Seaweed as prep	1 cup	30	1	0	0	3	3	1	tr	0	690	—	—	0
NISSIN														
Chicken Vegetable as prep	1 pkg	290	13	7	<5	6	38	2	2	40	1430	—	—	0
White Cheddar as prep	1 pkg	290	13	6	0	6	38	1	2	40	1120	—	—	0
SILHOUETTE SOLUTION														
Mediterranean Tomato	1 pkg (1.16 oz)	110	3	1	30	15	8	4	1	300	440	620	100	24
Newbury Chicken Cream	1 pkg (1.3 oz)	110	3	1	30	15	8	1	1	250	520	620	80	15
STREIT'S														
Matzo Ball as prep	1 cup	50	0	0	0	tr	12	4	0	0	880	—	—	0
THAI KITCHEN														
Rice Noodle Bowl Lemongrass & Chili as prep	½ pkg	110	2	0	0	2	23	2	1	0	850	—	—	1
Rice Noodle Bowl Thai Ginger as prep	½ pkg	120	2	0	0	2	23	2	1	0	620	—	—	1
REFRIGERATED														
MOOSEWOOD														
Organic Creamy Potato & Corn Chowder	1 cup (8.4 oz)	170	6	1	15	5	28	5	3	60	410	—	—	9
Organic Hungarian Vegetable Noodle	1 cup (8.4 oz)	80	2	0	0	2	13	4	2	40	480	—	—	21
Organic Savannah Sweet Potato Bisque	1 cup (8.4 oz)	200	11	5	20	6	20	6	2	150	580	—	—	54
Organic Texas Two Bean Chili	1 cup (8.4 oz)	200	4	0	0	9	34	9	8	100	840	—	—	21
Organic Tuscan White Bean & Vegetable	1 cup (8.4 oz)	130	2	0	0	6	24	5	5	60	760	—	—	15

FOOD	PORTION	CALS	FAT	SAT FAT	CHOL	PROT	CARB	SUGAR	FIBER	CALCI	SOD	POTAS	FOLIC	VIT C
ORGANIC CLASSICS														
French Onion w/ Croutons	1 cup	140	6	1	0	3	17	8	2	40	790	—	—	9
Seafood Chowder	1 cup	160	6	3	50	11	17	4	1	100	800	—	—	9
TAKE-OUT														
ban mien fish head	1 serv (10 oz)	277	10	4	59	20	27	2	4	183	851	198	—	0
beef stew soup	1 cup (8.8 oz)	221	5	2	60	23	20	—	—	32	461	527	25	14
bird's nest	1 cup (8.6 oz)	112	3	1	27	13	8	1	0	15	1549	232	5	0
black bean turtle soup	1 cup (6.5 oz)	240	1	tr	0	15	45	1	10	102	442	801	159	0
broccoli cheese	1 cup	165	9	3	14	6	15	7	2	189	875	425	53	2
brunswick stew soup	1 cup (8.5 oz)	232	6	2	71	27	17	—	—	39	438	509	21	14
caldo de res beef soup	1 cup	143	5	2	22	12	12	3	2	36	784	674	24	11
chinese velvet corn	1¼ cups	135	0	0	1	—	—	—	—	—	708	—	—	—
corn & cheese chowder	¾ cup	215	12	7	66	9	21	—	3	220	386	337	12	7
duck soup	1 cup (8.6 oz)	412	37	12	88	16	2	tr	tr	22	268	351	15	tr
egg drop	1 cup	73	4	1	102	8	1	tr	0	22	730	220	15	0
gazpacho	1 cup	46	tr	—	0	1	5	—	—	28	63	—	—	—
greek lemon	¾ cup	63	2	1	83	4	7	—	2	22	386	45	8	4
hot & sour	1 serv (14 oz)	173	9	3	79	14	9	3	3	58	1314	119	9	1
matzo ball soup	1 cup	118	5	1	63	7	10	tr	1	31	757	190	19	0
minestrone	1 cup	233	13	4	9	9	22	4	4	45	700	588	87	9
miso w/ tofu	1 cup	84	3	1	0	6	8	2	2	65	989	362	58	5
onion soup gratinee	1 serv	492	27	16	77	25	38	6	4	637	1325	528	57	11
oxtail	1 cup	68	2	1	2	3	9	2	1	10	1166	81	10	0
pasta e fagioli	1 cup (8.8 oz)	194	5	1	3	9	30	—	—	62	790	522	49	12
ratatouille	1 cup (7.5 oz)	266	25	3	0	2	12	—	—	56	329	485	34	41
shark fin	1 bowl (10 oz)	164	9	2	84	15	9	—	00	—	1164	—	—	—
shrimp bisque	1 cup	263	14	4	129	22	13	10	tr	263	263	436	15	2
shrimp gumbo	1 cup (8.6 oz)	163	7	1	73	9	18	5	3	129	661	429	61	19
sopa de albondigas	1 cup	171	11	4	50	10	9	3	1	33	187	431	21	12
thai lemon grass	1 bowl	100	4	—	65	10	5	—	—	—	553	—	—	—
vietnamese pho beef noodle	1 serv (7.8 oz)	480	12	5	46	15	78	2	1	44	43	334	33	50
wonton soup	1 cup	183	7	2	53	14	14	tr	1	36	769	321	39	3
yookgaejang korean beef	1 cup (8.4 oz)	94	6	2	50	6	4	—	1	25	209	164	18	8
zupa koprowa polish dill soup	1 bowl	54	2	—	55	11	6	—	—	—	524	—	—	—
SOUR CREAM														
fat free	1 tbsp	12	0	0	1	1	3	tr	0	20	23	21	2	0
fat free	½ cup (4.5 oz)	95	0	0	12	4	20	1	0	160	180	165	14	0

FOOD	PORTION	CALS	FAT	SAT FAT	CHOL	PROT	CARB	SUGAR	FIBER	CALCI	SOD	POTAS	FOLIC	VIT C
reduced fat	½ cup (4.4 oz)	224	17	11	43	9	9	tr	0	175	87	262	14	1
reduced fat	1 tbsp (0.5 oz)	29	2	1	6	1	1	tr	0	23	11	34	2	tr
sour cream	1 tbsp (0.4 oz)	23	2	1	6	tr	tr	tr	0	13	10	17	1	tr
sour cream	½ cup (4 oz)	222	23	13	60	2	3	3	0	126	92	162	8	1
BREAKSTONE'S														
Sour Cream	2 tbsp (1 oz)	60	5	4	20	tr	1	1	0	20	10	—	—	0
CABOT														
Light	2 tbsp	35	3	2	10	1	2	0	0	40	25	—	—	0
No Fat	2 tbsp	20	0	0	0	1	3	2	0	40	40	—	—	0
Sour Cream	2 tbsp	50	5	3	15	1	1	0	0	20	35	—	—	0
DAISY														
No Fat	2 tbsp	20	0	0	0	2	1	1	0	40	15	—	—	0
Sour Cream	2 tbsp	60	5	4	0	1	1	1	0	20	15	—	—	0
FRIENDSHIP														
All Natural	2 tbsp (1 oz)	60	5	4	20	1	1	1	0	40	15	—	—	—
Light	1 tbsp (1 oz)	40	3	2	10	1	3	1	0	40	25	—	—	—
Nonfat	2 tbsp (1 oz)	25	0	0	0	2	4	2	0	40	20	—	—	—
GREEN VALLEY														
Sour Cream	2 tbsp	100	10	7	35	1	1	1	0	0	20	—	—	0
HOOD														
Fat Free	2 tbsp	20	0	0	0	1	4	2	0	60	25	—	—	0
Low Fat	2 tbsp	35	2	1	5	1	3	2	0	60	20	—	—	0
Sour Cream	2 tbsp	60	5	4	20	1	2	1	0	40	15	—	—	0
HORIZON ORGANIC														
Lowfat	2 tbsp	35	2	1	10	1	3	2	0	60	25	—	—	0
Sour Cream	2 tbsp	60	5	4	20	1	1	1	0	40	15	—	—	0
LAND O LAKES														
Fat Free	2 tbsp (1.1 oz)	20	0	0	0	1	3	2	0	40	50	—	—	0
Light	2 tbsp (1.1 oz)	40	3	2	5	1	2	2	0	40	20	—	—	0
Sour Cream	2 tbsp (1.1 oz)	60	6	4	20	1	2	2	0	40	40	—	—	0
NANCY'S														
Organic	2 tbsp	60	6	3	20	1	2	1	0	50	20	—	—	0
ORGANIC VALLEY														
Lowfat	2 tbsp	40	2	2	10	1	1	1	0	40	15	—	—	0
SOUR CREAM SUBSTITUTES														
imitation	½ cup (4 oz)	239	22	20	0	3	8	8	0	3	117	185	0	0
TOFUTTI														
Better Than Sour Cream	2 tbsp (1 oz)	85	5	2	0	1	9	2	0	—	160	—	—	—
VEGAN GOURMET														
Alternative Sour Cream	2 tbsp (1 oz)	50	5	1	0	0	3	0	2	40	25	—	—	0
SOURSOP														
fresh	1	416	2	—	0	6	105	—	—	88	87	1739	—	129
fresh cut up	1 cup	150	1	—	0	2	38	—	—	32	31	626	—	46

SOY

(see also CHEESE SUBSTITUTES, ICE CREAM AND FROZEN DESSERTS, MILK SUBSTITUTES, MISO, SMOOTHIES, SOY SAUCE, SOYBEANS, TEMPEH, TOFU, YOGURT FROZEN)

FOOD	PORTION	CALS	FAT	SAT FAT	CHOL	PROT	CARB	SUGAR	FIBER	CALCI	SOD	POTAS	FOLIC	VIT C
natto	½ cup (3.1 oz)	187	10	1	0	16	13	4	5	191	6	642	7	11
BOB'S RED MILL														
Protein Powder	1 tbsp	20	0	0	0	5	0	0	0	—	60	—	—	—
I.M. HEALTHY														
SoyNut Butter Chocolate	2 tbsp	190	14	2	0	6	12	9	3	20	0	—	—	0
SoyNut Butter Honey Creamy	2 tbsp	170	11	2	0	7	10	4	3	60	140	—	—	0
SoyNut Butter Original Chunky	2 tbsp	170	11	2	0	7	10	3	3	60	140	—	—	0
SoyNut Butter Original Creamy	2 tbsp	170	11	2	0	7	10	3	3	60	140	—	—	0
SoyNut Butter Unsweetened Creamy	2 tbsp	190	15	2	0	9	6	1	5	60	140	—	—	0
SIMPLE FOOD														
Soynut Butter Chocolate	2 tbsp	190	12	2	0	10	8	8	2	—	90	—	—	—
Soynut Butter No Sugar No Salt	2 tbsp	200	14	2	0	10	8	2	2	—	0	—	—	—
SOY WONDER														
Creamy Spread	2 tbsp	170	11	2	0	8	10	3	1	60	170	—	—	0
SOYBUTTER														
Spread	2 tbsp	200	15	3	0	7	8	4	2	20	120	—	—	0

SOY DRINKS

(see MILK SUBSTITUTES, SMOOTHIES)

SOY SAUCE

FOOD	PORTION	CALS	FAT	SAT FAT	CHOL	PROT	CARB	SUGAR	FIBER	CALCI	SOD	POTAS	FOLIC	VIT C
shoyu	1 tbsp	9	tr	tr	0	1	2	—	—	3	1029	32	3	0
soy sauce	1 tbsp	7	tr	tr	0	tr	1	—	—	1	1024	27	2	0
tamari	1 tbsp	11	tr	tr	0	2	1	—	—	4	1005	38	3	0
ANGOSTURA														
Lite Soy	1 tbsp (0.5 oz)	10	0	0	0	1	2	2	0	0	390	—	—	0
Soy Sauce	1 tbsp (0.5 oz)	10	0	0	0	1	1	1	0	0	670	—	—	0
DAVE'S GOURMET														
Soyabi Sauce	1 tbsp (0.6 oz)	30	2	—	—	0	4	3	—	0	340	—	—	0
HOUSE OF TSANG														
Ginger Soy Sauce	1 tbsp	20	0	0	0	0	4	3	0	0	760	49	—	0
Less Sodium	1 tbsp	5	0	0	0	0	0	0	0	0	300	19	—	0
KIKKOMAN														
Less Sodium	1 tbsp (0.5 oz)	10	0	0	0	1	1	—	—	—	575	—	—	—
Ponzu	1 tbsp (0.5 oz)	10	0	0	0	tr	2	2	—	—	400	—	—	—
Soy Sauce	1 tbsp (0.5 oz)	10	0	0	0	2	0	0	0	—	920	—	—	—
Sushi Sashimi	1 tbsp (0.5 oz)	15	0	0	0	1	2	2	—	—	870	—	—	—

FOOD	PORTION	CALS	FAT	SAT FAT	CHOL	PROT	CARB	SUGAR	FIBER	CALCI	SOD	POTAS	FOLIC	VIT C
LA CHOY														
Lite	1 tbsp (0.5 oz)	15	0	0	0	1	2	2	0	0	550	—	—	0
LEE KUM KEE														
Lite	1 tbsp (0.5 oz)	10	0	0	0	tr	1	1	—	—	600	—	—	—
MITSUKAN														
Ponzu Citrus Seasoned	1 tbsp (0.5 oz)	10	0	0	0	0	1	1	—	—	580	—	—	—
SAN-J														
Tamari Organic Gluten Free	2 pkg (0.5 oz)	10	0	0	0	2	tr	—	—	—	940	—	—	—
SOY VAY														
Wasabiyaki	1 tbsp	35	1	0	0	tr	6	5	0	0	420	—	—	0
TREE OF LIFE														
Organic Shoyu	1 tbsp (0.5 oz)	15	0	0	0	2	1	1	0	0	960	—	—	0
Organic Tamari Wheat Free	1 tbsp (0.5 oz)	15	0	0	0	2	1	1	0	0	940	—	—	0
SOYBEANS														
dried cooked	1 cup	298	15	2	0	29	17	—	—	175	1	886	93	3
dry roasted	½ cup	387	19	3	0	34	28	—	—	232	2	1173	176	4
green cooked	½ cup	127	6	1	0	11	10	—	4	—	13	485	100	—
roasted	½ cup	405	22	3	0	30	29	—	—	119	140	1264	182	2
roasted & toasted	1 cup	490	26	3	0	40	33	—	—	149	4	1588	244	2
roasted & toasted salted	1 cup	490	26	3	0	40	33	—	—	149	176	1588	244	2
sprouts raw	½ cup	43	2	tr	0	5	3	—	—	23	5	169	60	5
sprouts steamed	½ cup	38	2	tr	0	4	3	—	—	28	5	167	—	4
sprouts stir fried	1 cup	125	7	1	0	13	9	—	—	82	14	567	—	12
ARROWHEAD MILLS														
Organic Dried not prep	¼ cup	160	8	1	0	14	11	3	4	100	0	680	—	2
C&W														
In the Pod	½ cup	110	4	0	0	9	12	2	9	80	0	—	—	6
CRUNCHIES														
Freeze Dried Edamame	⅜ cup (1 oz)	124	6	1	0	11	9	2	3	80	0	—	—	0
Freeze Dried Edamame Grilled	⅜ cup (0.9 oz)	84	1	0	0	3	13	1	1	20	68	—	—	2
Freeze Dried Edamame Salted	¼ cup (0.9 oz)	90	4	0	0	8	7	0	3	100	130	—	—	18
EDEN														
Organic Blacksoy	½ cup	120	6	1	0	11	8	1	7	80	30	310	24	—
KOOLOOS														
Soy Nuts & Flaxseed BBQ	1 pkg (1 oz)	130	4	1	0	7	16	1	3	20	220	—	—	5

FOOD	PORTION	CALS	FAT	SAT FAT	CHOL	PROT	CARB	SUGAR	FIBER	CALCI	SOD	POTAS	FOLIC	VIT C
KOOLOOS (CONT.)														
Soy Nuts & Flaxseed Original	1 pkg (1 oz)	140	5	1	0	7	15	1	3	20	280	—	—	5
SEAPOINT FARMS														
Edamame Dry Roasted Goji Blend	¼ cup	120	3	0	0	11	15	5	7	40	140	—	—	4
Edamame Dry Roasted Lightly Salted	¼ cup	130	4	1	0	14	10	1	8	40	150	—	—	1
Edamame Dry Roasted Wasabi	¼ cup	130	5	1	0	14	9	1	7	40	130	—	—	1
Edamame In Pods	½ cup	100	3	0	0	8	9	1	4	40	30	—	—	6
Edamame In Pods Lightly Salted	½ cup	100	3	1	0	8	9	1	4	40	260	—	—	6
Edamame Shelled	½ cup	100	3	0	0	8	9	1	4	40	30	—	—	6
Organic Edamame In Pods	½ cup	100	3	0	0	8	9	1	4	40	30	—	—	6
Organic Edamame Shelled	½ cup	100	3	0	0	8	9	1	4	40	30	—	—	6
SOUTH BEACH														
Soy Nuts Dark Chocolate	1 pkg (0.7 oz)	100	6	3	0	3	9	6	2	—	0	—	—	—
SUNRICH NATURALS														
Edamame Fiesta Blend frzn	½ cup (3 oz)	90	3	0	0	6	12	1	3	60	10	—	—	18
Edamame In The Shell frzn	½ cup (3 oz)	120	5	1	0	10	9	3	4	100	10	—	—	15
Soy Honey Nutz	1 pkg (1 oz)	130	6	1	0	9	12	3	4	40	55	—	52	0

SPAGHETTI

(*see* PASTA, PASTA DINNERS, PASTA SALAD, SPAGHETTI SAUCE)

SPAGHETTI SAUCE

FOOD	PORTION	CALS	FAT	SAT FAT	CHOL	PROT	CARB	SUGAR	FIBER	CALCI	SOD	POTAS	FOLIC	VIT C
JARRED														
marinara sauce	1 cup	171	8	tr	0	4	25	—	—	44	1572	1061	—	32
spaghetti sauce	1 cup	272	12	2	0	12	40	—	—	70	1236	957	—	28
AMY'S														
Organic Family Marinara	½ cup (4.4 oz)	80	5	1	0	1	10	5	3	0	590	—	—	9
Organic Marinara Low Sodium	½ cup (4.4 oz)	40	1	0	0	1	7	5	1	20	100	—	—	5
BARILLA														
Arrabbiata Tomato & Spicy Pepper	½ cup	90	3	1	0	2	11	6	3	60	560	—	—	7
Garden Vegetable	½ cup	70	2	0	0	2	11	6	2	80	460	—	—	9

FOOD	PORTION	CALS	FAT	SAT FAT	CHOL	PROT	CARB	SUGAR	FIBER	CALCI	SOD	POTAS	FOLIC	VIT C
BARILLA (CONT.)														
Green & Black Olive	½ cup	80	3	0	0	2	10	5	4	20	770	—	—	9
Italian Baking Sauce	¼ cup (4.4 oz)	60	1	0	0	2	12	6	2	60	460	—	—	6
Mushroom & Garlic	½ cup	70	2	0	0	3	12	6	2	20	450	—	—	9
Toscana Tuscan Herb	½ cup (4.4 oz)	70	2	0	0	2	10	6	3	20	470	—	—	6
BELLA SUN LUCI														
Sun Dried Tomato Pesto w/ Whole Pine Nuts	¼ cup (1.9 oz)	270	27	3	<5	3	8	5	1	60	70	—	—	9
DAVE'S GOURMET														
Pasta Sauce Spicy Heirloom Marinara	½ cup (4.4 oz)	45	2	0	—	1	7	4	2	20	280	—	—	24
Pasta Sauce Wild Mushroom	½ cup (4.4 oz)	60	3	1	—	2	7	2	tr	40	270	—	—	21
DEI FRATELLI														
Arrabbiata	½ cup (4.2 oz)	50	2	0	0	2	8	5	2	40	300	—	—	15
Pizza Sauce	¼ cup (2.2 oz)	30	2	0	0	1	5	4	1	40	230	—	—	15
DEL MONTE														
Garlic & Onion	½ cup (4.4 oz)	70	1	0	0	2	14	6	2	20	490	320	—	27
W/ Mushrooms	½ cup (4.4 oz)	70	1	0	0	2	14	10	2	20	630	—	—	9
DELGROSSO														
Garden Style	½ cup (4.4 oz)	70	2	0	0	2	12	7	2	40	580	—	—	21
Mushroom	½ cup (4.4 oz)	70	2	0	0	3	11	8	3	20	510	—	—	6
New York Style	¼ cup (2.1 oz)	35	1	0	0	1	6	4	1	20	310	—	—	0
Original Meat Flavored	½ cup (4.4 oz)	80	2	1	5	3	12	8	3	40	500	—	—	9
Pizza Sauce Pepperoni	¼ cup (2.2 oz)	40	1	0	0	2	6	4	2	0	270	—	—	9
Three Cheese	½ cup (4.4 oz)	80	2	0	0	2	13	8	3	40	660	—	—	18
EDEN														
Organic No Salt	½ cup	80	3	0	0	3	12	6	3	40	10	530	—	12
Organic Pizza Pasta Sauce	½ cup	65	3	0	0	2	9	4	5	40	300	330	—	12
FRANCESCO RINALDI														
Alfredo	¼ cup (2.1 oz)	80	6	4	35	1	3	1	0	20	400	—	—	0
Chunky Eggplant Parmesan	½ cup (4.4 oz)	90	5	1	0	2	11	9	tr	60	650	—	—	0
Chunky Mushroom & Pepper	½ cup (4.4 oz)	80	3	0	0	2	13	9	2	20	660	—	—	0
Hearty Mushroom Pepper & Onion	½ cup (4.4 oz)	80	3	0	0	2	12	8	2	20	640	—	—	0

FOOD	PORTION	CALS	FAT	SAT FAT	CHOL	PROT	CARB	SUGAR	FIBER	CALCI	SOD	POTAS	FOLIC	VIT C
FRANCESCO RINALDI (CONT.)														
Hearty Sweet & Tasty Tomato	½ cup (4.4 oz)	100	5	1	0	2	16	15	tr	40	700	—	—	0
Hearty Three-Cheese	½ cup (4.4 oz)	80	2	1	0	3	15	14	tr	60	470	—	—	0
Organic Burgundy Marinara	½ cup (4.3 oz)	100	7	1	0	1	9	8	tr	80	820	—	—	0
Premium Vodka	¼ cup (2.1 oz)	60	4	2	10	2	4	4	0	20	290	—	—	0
Traditional Meat Flavored	½ cup (4.4 oz)	80	4	1	5	2	12	11	tr	20	650	—	—	0
Traditional No Salt Added	½ cup (4.4 oz)	70	3	0	0	2	12	6	2	0	40	—	—	0
Traditional Original	½ cup (4.4 oz)	80	3	0	0	2	12	11	tr	20	650	—	—	0
HUNT'S														
Pasta Sauce Four Cheese	½ cup (4.4 oz)	60	1	0	0	2	10	5	3	40	580	350	—	2
Pasta Sauce Garlic & Herb	½ cup (4.4 oz)	40	1	0	0	1	8	4	3	20	610	290	—	4
Pasta Sauce Meat	½ cup (4.4 oz)	60	1	0	0	2	10	6	3	20	610	300	—	4
Pasta Sauce Mushroom	½ cup (4.4 oz)	50	1	0	0	1	10	6	3	20	590	330	—	4
Tomato Sauce	¼ cup (2.2 oz)	20	0	0	0	tr	4	2	1	0	410	160	—	4
Tomato Sauce No Salt Added	¼ cup (2.2 oz)	20	0	0	0	tr	5	3	1	0	20	170	—	2
Traditional Pasta Sauce	½ cup (4.4 oz)	50	1	0	0	1	11	5	3	20	560	330	—	4
KNORR														
W/ Meat	4 oz	110	5	2	20	6	9	—	—	—	820	—	—	—
LUCINI														
Spicy Tuscan	½ cup (4.4 oz)	80	5	1	0	2	8	5	2	80	480	—	—	21
Tuscan Marinara w/ Roasted Garlic	½ cup (4.4 oz)	60	3	0	0	2	8	5	1	40	310	—	—	12
MOM'S														
Artichoke Heart & Asiago Cheese	½ cup (4.2 oz)	90	6	2	5	3	7	3	3	60	360	—	—	12
Fresh Garlic Basil	½ cup (4.2 oz)	30	3	0	0	2	7	4	2	40	420	—	—	15
Martini	½ cup (4.2 oz)	120	4	0	20	3	6	3	1	40	250	—	—	6
Puttanesca	½ cup (4.2 oz)	90	6	2	5	2	8	5	2	40	550	—	—	12
MUIR GLEN														
Organic Chunky Tomato	¼ cup	15	0	0	0	tr	4	2	tr	0	230	—	—	9
Organic Garlic Roasted Garlic	½ cup	60	1	0	0	2	12	4	2	20	380	—	—	9
Organic Pizza Sauce	¼ cup	40	2	0	0	1	6	3	1	0	290	—	—	12

FOOD	PORTION	CALS	FAT	SAT FAT	CHOL	PROT	CARB	SUGAR	FIBER	CALCI	SOD	POTAS	FOLIC	VIT C
MUIR GLEN (CONT.)														
Organic Tomato Sauce No Salt Added	¼ cup	25	0	0	0	1	5	3	1	0	10	—	—	6
NEWMAN'S OWN														
Bambolina	½ cup	90	5	1	0	2	13	12	tr	20	620	—	—	0
Five Cheese	½ cup	80	3	2	5	3	10	0	tr	0	610	—	—	0
Roasted Garlic & Green Peppers	½ cup	70	3	0	0	2	11	6	4	—	460	—	—	—
POMI														
Strained	½ cup (4.4 oz)	30	0	0	0	1	5	5	3	0	10	—	—	24
PREGO														
Heart Smart Traditional Italian	½ cup	100	3	1	0	2	15	9	3	20	430	380	—	2
Italian	½ cup	70	2	1	0	2	13	10	3	20	470	—	—	4
Italian Marinara	½ cup	100	5	1	0	2	11	7	4	20	550	370	—	2
Italian Meat	½ cup	130	4	1	5	2	19	12	3	20	570	—	—	2
Italian Roasted Red Pepper & Garlic	½ cup	90	4	1	0	2	13	9	3	20	530	400	—	2
Italian Three Cheese	½ cup	80	2	1	0	3	14	11	3	40	430	450	—	2
Italian Tomato Basil & Garlic	½ cup	80	3	1	0	2	12	9	3	20	420	400	—	4
Organic Mushroom	½ cup	90	3	0	0	2	13	9	4	20	540	—	—	5
Veggie Smart	½ cup (4.2 oz)	90	2	0	0	2	16	10	3	20	360	510	—	2
PROGRESSO														
Lobster Sauce	½ cup (4.3 oz)	100	7	1	5	3	6	3	2	20	430	—	—	0
Pesto Arrabbiata	2 tbsp (1 oz)	140	11	2	5	3	7	2	2	60	140	—	—	6
Pesto Basil & Roasted Garlic	2 tbsp (1 oz)	130	13	2	0	2	3	0	0	40	75	—	—	2
Red Clam	½ cup (4.4 oz)	60	1	0	10	4	8	4	1	20	350	—	—	0
White Clam	½ cup (4.4 oz)	150	10	2	20	9	5	tr	0	40	710	—	—	0
RACCONTO														
Essentials Heart Health Roasted Garlic	½ cup (4.4 oz)	90	5	1	0	2	10	5	2	40	430	—	—	4
RAGU														
Light Tomato & Basil No Sugar Added	½ cup (4.4 oz)	50	1	0	0	2	9	6	3	40	330	—	—	4
Old World Style Margherita	½ cup (4.4 oz)	70	2	1	0	2	10	6	2	40	410	—	—	2
Old World Style Meat	½ cup (4.4 oz)	70	3	1	0	2	9	6	2	20	460	310	—	2

FOOD	PORTION	CALS	FAT	SAT FAT	CHOL	PROT	CARB	SUGAR	FIBER	CALCI	SOD	POTAS	FOLIC	VIT C
RAGU (CONT.)														
Old World Style Sweet Tomato Basil	½ cup (4.4 oz)	60	2	0	0	2	10	6	3	20	410	—	—	2
Pizza Quick Fresh Italian	2 oz	35	1	0	0	1	5	—	—	—	270	—	—	—
RANDAZZO'S														
Alfredo	¼ cup (2.2 oz)	200	20	13	65	4	3	1	0	—	330	—	—	—
Fra Diavolo	½ cup (4.4 oz)	90	4	1	0	2	9	4	4	—	440	—	—	—
Puttanesca	½ cup (4.4 oz)	100	6	1	0	2	9	4	4	—	530	—	—	—
Vodka	½ cup (4.4 oz)	230	20	11	65	2	7	3	3	—	280	—	—	—
ROBERT ROTHCHILD FARM														
Artichoke	½ cup	80	5	0	0	2	8	7	0	0	90	—	—	0
S&W														
Tomato Sauce	¼ cup (2.1 oz)	20	0	0	0	1	4	2	1	0	260	—	—	2
SEEDS OF CHANGE														
Balsamic Olive & Onion	½ cup	80	2	1	0	3	14	8	2	20	650	—	—	2
Garden Vegetable	½ cup	70	1	0	0	2	14	8	2	10	550	—	—	5
Mushroom & Onion	½ cup	70	2	0	0	2	12	7	2	20	550	—	—	5
Three Cheese Marinara	½ cup	70	2	1	5	2	12	8	2	40	590	—	—	9
Traditional Herb	½ cup	70	0	0	0	2	16	9	2	20	550	—	—	6
TWO GUYS														
Jersey Tomato Sauce	½ cup (4.6 oz)	60	2	tr	0	2	10	4	2	50	190	—	—	12
VINO DE MILO														
Mediterranean Pinot Grigio	½ cup	90	4	1	0	2	12	1	2	40	320	—	—	15
Portobello Shiraz	½ cup	40	1	0	0	1	9	5	2	20	340	—	—	15
Tuscan Merlot	½ cup	80	3	0	0	—	2	13	2	20	470	—	—	15
WALDEN FARMS														
Alfredo Sauce Calorie Free	3 tbsp (1.6 oz)	0	0	0	0	0	0	0	0	0	200	—	—	0
WALNUT ACRES														
Organic Garlic Garlic	½ cup	125	1	0	0	2	10	6	1	20	280	—	—	15
Organic Marinara & Zinfandel	½ cup	125	1	0	0	2	9	6	1	20	330	—	—	9
Organic Roasted Garlic	½ cup	125	1	0	0	2	11	7	1	20	280	—	—	9
Organic Tomato & Basil	½ cup	125	1	0	0	2	9	7	1	20	330	—	—	9

FOOD	PORTION	CALS	FAT	SAT FAT	CHOL	PROT	CARB	SUGAR	FIBER	CALCI	SOD	POTAS	FOLIC	VIT C
MIX														
LONEY'S														
Carbonara as prep	¼ cup (2.1 oz)	33	3	2	9	tr	3	0	0	60	240	—	—	0
Rose as prep	¼ cup (2.1 oz)	29	3	0	0	1	6	1	0	80	240	—	—	1
REFRIGERATED														
BUITONI														
Alfredo	¼ cup (2.1 oz)	140	12	7	30	4	4	2	0	100	350	—	—	0
Alfredo Light	¼ cup (2.1 oz)	90	6	4	15	4	5	1	0	100	350	—	—	0
Marinara	½ cup (4.4 oz)	70	3	0	0	0	10	6	2	40	540	—	—	2
Pesto	¼ cup (2.2 oz)	270	23	4	10	6	6	4	1	200	450	—	—	4
Pesto Basil Reduced Fat	¼ cup (2.2 oz)	230	17	3	10	7	8	6	2	250	500	—	—	2
Vodka Sauce	½ cup (4.2 oz)	90	6	4	15	3	5	3	1	40	550	—	—	2
TAKE-OUT														
bolognese	5 oz	195	15	—	—	11	4	—	tr	36	—	—	—	7
# SPANISH FOOD														
FRESH														
TEXAS TAMALE COMPANY														
Tamales Beef	2 (3 oz)	160	12	3	25	8	8	0	2	20	580	—	—	0
Tamales Chicken	2 (3 oz)	130	7	1	15	9	8	1	1	40	620	—	—	1
Tamales Spinach	2 (3 oz)	140	8	4	20	5	12	0	0	100	310	—	—	4
FROZEN														
AMY'S														
Bowl Mexican Casserole	1 pkg (9.4 oz)	470	16	5	20	11	70	3	7	250	780	—	—	4
Burrito Black Bean	1 (6 oz)	280	8	1	0	9	44	4	4	80	580	—	—	24
Burrito Cheddar Cheese	1 (6 oz)	300	9	3	10	11	43	1	6	100	580	—	—	5
Burrito Southwestern	1 (5.5 oz)	300	10	4	15	12	43	2	6	150	680	—	—	5
Enchilada Black Bean Vegetable	1 (4.7 oz)	180	6	1	0	5	26	2	3	40	390	—	—	6
CEDARLANE														
Organic Burrito Low Fat Rice & Cheese	1 (6 oz)	260	1	0	0	13	48	2	7	100	490	—	—	15
Organic Enchilada Low Fat Black Bean & Tofu	1 (9 oz)	220	3	0	0	10	42	3	6	100	390	—	—	36
Roasted Chile Relleno	1 pkg (10 oz)	400	20	12	55	23	37	12	5	500	770	—	—	324
Zone Burrito Beans & Cheese	1 (6 oz)	350	13	5	15	27	37	3	8	100	380	—	—	6
CONTESSA														
Fajitas Shrimp	2 (8 oz)	230	4	1	45	11	37	4	5	100	940	—	—	36

FOOD	PORTION	CALS	FAT	SAT FAT	CHOL	PROT	CARB	SUGAR	FIBER	CALCI	SOD	POTAS	FOLIC	VIT C
CONTESSA (CONT.)														
Paella w/ Chicken & Seafood	1½ cups	200	3	0	50	17	28	3	2	20	780	—	—	5
Seafood Veracruz not prep	1¾ cups	180	2	1	35	15	27	4	6	60	920	—	—	21
DR. PRAEGER'S														
Burrito Bites	2 (2 oz)	130	3	0	0	5	20	1	4	20	210	—	—	0
EL MONTEREY														
Burrito Bean & Cheese	1 (5 oz)	280	8	2	5	10	43	1	5	50	560	—	—	1
Burrito Beef & Bean	1 (5 oz)	370	17	6	20	10	42	2	4	30	610	—	—	1
Burrito Half Pound Spicy Red Hot Beef & Bean	1 (8 oz)	600	29	10	35	17	68	3	7	50	1120	—	—	3
Burrito Supreme Breakfast Egg Cheese & Sausage	1 (4.5 oz)	300	13	5	75	10	34	1	1	30	630	—	—	1
Burrito Supreme Shredded Steak & Cheese	1 (5 oz)	290	9	3	20	12	41	1	1	70	590	—	—	3
Burrito XX Large Bean & Cheese	1 (10 oz)	590	17	4	10	21	88	2	5	100	950	—	—	2
Burrito XX Large Beef & Bean	1 (10 oz)	730	35	12	40	22	83	2	8	60	1180	—	—	2
Cruncheros Cheese & Beef	3 (4.5 oz)	330	16	6	20	10	35	1	2	150	560	—	—	1
Cruncheros Taco Beef & Cheese	4 (5.6 oz)	460	29	9	40	12	38	2	2	30	1040	—	—	3
Enchiladas Cheese w/ Sauce	1 serv (8 oz)	250	15	8	35	11	22	1	3	150	990	—	—	9
Enchiladas Shredded Beef w/ Sauce	1 serv (4 oz)	140	6	3	15	6	15	1	2	70	450	—	—	6
Quesadillas Chicken & Cheese	2 (6 oz)	380	15	6	35	17	43	1	2	200	930	—	—	12
Quesadillas Steak & Cheese	2 (6 oz)	400	15	7	55	21	42	2	1	250	860	—	—	3
Tamales Chicken	1 (4.5 oz)	240	12	3	25	8	27	1	2	100	750	—	—	4
Tamales Shredded Beef	1 (4.5 oz)	310	19	5	30	9	27	1	3	50	660	—	—	1
Taquitos Southwest Chicken In A Seasoned Batter	2 (2.8 oz)	175	8	3	10	6	20	0	1	50	330	—	—	4
Taquitos Corn Shredded Beef	3 (4.5 oz)	300	13	2	40	11	31	1	1	0	560	—	—	0

FOOD	PORTION	CALS	FAT	SAT FAT	CHOL	PROT	CARB	SUGAR	FIBER	CALCI	SOD	POTAS	FOLIC	VIT C
EL MONTEREY (CONT.)														
Taquitos Flour Char-Broiled Chicken Breast	3 (5 oz)	380	19	5	35	15	36	1	1	100	670	—	—	1
Taquitos Flour Chicken & Cheese	3 (4.5 oz)	350	18	4	15	10	36	1	2	50	650	—	—	2
Tornados Apple Cinnamon	1 (3 oz)	180	5	1	0	4	31	8	0	20	140	—	—	5
Tornados Sausage Egg & Cheese	1 (3 oz)	230	13	3	40	6	23	1	1	20	410	—	—	1
Tornados Shredded Beef	1 (3 oz)	210	10	2	15	7	23	1	1	20	400	—	—	6
Tornados Steak Egg & Cheese	1 (3 oz)	170	6	1	10	7	22	1	0	40	310	—	—	1
Tornados XXL Southwest Chicken	1 (4.2 oz)	210	10	3	15	7	28	1	1	70	530	—	—	12
FARM RICH														
Quesadillas	2 (3.1 oz)	200	10	5	25	11	19	1	1	200	400	—	—	12
GLUTENFREEDA														
Burrito Breakfast Beef	1 (3.9 oz)	199	8	3	27	10	23	1	2	70	150	—	—	6
Burrito Vegetarian Bean & Cheese	1 (3.9 oz)	196	7	2	12	6	29	0	3	70	188	—	—	2
HEALTH IS WEALTH														
Vegetarian Hot Tamale Munchees	6 (3 oz)	160	3	2	5	6	26	0	3	60	330	—	—	4
HELEN'S KITCHEN														
Cheese Enchiladas w/ Tofu Steaks In Spicy Red Sauce	½ pkg (5 oz)	150	9	1	10	5	20	3	5	180	300	—	—	9
JOSE OLE														
Burrito Chicken	1 (5 oz)	270	7	2	20	9	41	tr	2	40	630	—	—	0
Burrito Steak & Jalapeno	1 (5 oz)	300	9	3	15	11	43	tr	3	20	710	—	—	1
Chimichanga Chicken & Cheese	1 (5 oz)	330	12	3	20	11	44	tr	2	80	550	—	—	1
Chimichanga Shredded Beef	1 (5 oz)	350	15	5	25	13	39	1	2	100	510	—	—	5
Mini Burrito Chicken & Cheese	3	200	8	2	10	6	25	tr	1	40	440	—	—	1

FOOD	PORTION	CALS	FAT	SAT FAT	CHOL	PROT	CARB	SUGAR	FIBER	CALCI	SOD	POTAS	FOLIC	VIT C
JOSE OLE (CONT.)														
Mini Chimichanga Beef & Cheddar	3	240	12	3	10	8	25	tr	1	80	520	—	—	2
Mini Quesadilla Grilled Chicken	3	220	8	3	20	9	28	tr	1	100	600	—	—	0
Mini Tacos Beef & Cheese	4	200	11	4	20	7	19	tr	3	100	390	—	—	1
Mini Taquitos Beef & Cheese	4	180	8	2	5	7	21	tr	2	60	390	—	—	4
Soft Taco Beef & Cheese	1 (5 oz)	280	11	4	25	14	31	1	1	100	850	—	—	6
Taquitos Beef & Cheese Flour Tortilla	2	220	10	3	10	8	24	tr	1	80	430	—	—	2
Taquitos Buffalo Chicken Flour Tortilla	2	200	10	2	15	7	23	tr	tr	40	480	—	—	4
Taquitos Chicken & Cheese Flour Tortilla	2	220	10	3	15	8	25	1	1	60	430	—	—	0
Taquitos Chicken Flour Tortilla	3	180	8	1	10	6	23	0	2	10	430	—	—	0
Taquitos Pepperoni Pizza Flour Tortilla	2	240	14	4	15	7	23	1	1	40	490	—	—	0
Taquitos Shredded Beef Corn Tortilla	3	180	7	2	<5	7	21	0	2	60	440	—	—	4
LEAN CUISINE														
Simple Favorites Chicken Enchilada Suiza	1 pkg (9 oz)	290	5	2	20	10	51	8	3	150	560	340	—	0
MEALS TO LIVE														
White Chicken Burrito w/ Green Sauce	1 pkg (9 oz)	330	5	1	15	17	58	8	15	—	480	—	—	42
MOM MADE														
Fiesta Rice	1 pkg (7 oz)	200	1	0	0	8	38	2	5	40	190	—	—	12
Munchie Bean Burrito	1 (2.5 oz)	140	9	4	10	4	10	1	1	20	190	—	—	0
PATIO														
Burrito Bean & Cheese	1	280	8	3	5	8	44	4	5	40	630	—	—	0
Burrito Beef & Bean Mild	1	300	10	3	<5	10	44	6	5	20	740	—	—	0
Enchilada & Beef Tamale	1 meal	460	14	5	0	13	69	2	5	80	1210	—	—	0

FOOD	PORTION	CALS	FAT	SAT FAT	CHOL	PROT	CARB	SUGAR	FIBER	CALCI	SOD	POTAS	FOLIC	VIT C
PATIO (CONT.)														
Enchilada Beef	1 meal	380	12	4	5	11	55	2	5	80	1270	—	—	0
Enchilada Cheese	1 meal	390	13	4	10	12	58	2	10	100	1500	—	—	0
Enchilada Combo Dinner	1 meal	380	12	4	5	11	57	2	5	80	1250	—	—	0
STOUFFER'S														
Chicken Enchilada w/ Cheese Sauce & Rice	1 pkg (7.13 oz)	280	12	7	40	12	30	6	3	200	720	—	—	0
TYSON														
Meal Kit Chicken Fajita	1 (3.8 oz)	130	4	1	15	8	17	3	2	20	350	—	—	9
Meal Kit Quesadilla Chicken	1 (4 oz)	250	10	5	35	15	26	2	3	150	430	—	—	4
READY-TO-EAT														
taco shell corn	1 (6.5 inch)	98	5	1	0	2	13	tr	2	34	77	38	28	0
taco shell flour	1 (7 inch)	173	9	2	0	3	19	tr	1	44	168	46	24	0
FANTASTIC														
Spanish Paella	1 pkg (8 oz)	280	5	1	0	6	55	2	4	60	650	—	—	48
TAKE-OUT														
arroz con coco	1 cup	532	38	33	4	7	46	5	4	38	108	452	132	4
burrito w/beans	1 med (5 oz)	295	8	2	6	10	45	1	7	97	501	304	106	3
burrito w/ beans & rice	1 (3.5 oz)	221	5	1	2	7	37	tr	4	68	397	161	76	1
burrito w/ beef	1 sm (3.4 oz)	297	13	5	49	18	25	tr	1	74	460	253	48	0
burrito w/ beef & beans	1 med (5 oz)	331	13	4	34	17	36	1	6	89	524	364	89	3
burrito w/ beef beans & cheese	1 med (5 oz)	379	19	9	57	21	30	1	5	267	596	324	78	2
burrito w/ chicken & beans	1 med (5 oz)	295	9	2	37	18	34	1	5	80	498	302	84	3
burrito w/ pork & beans	1 med (5 oz)	320	12	4	34	18	35	1	6	82	494	376	84	3
chiles rellenos meat & cheese filled	1 (5 oz)	213	16	5	109	10	9	3	2	116	430	345	21	32
chimichanga w/ bean cheese lettuce & tomato	1 (4.1 oz)	271	18	5	17	8	22	2	3	150	301	300	48	7
chimichanga w/ beef & rice	1 (10 oz)	634	36	8	35	19	58	5	5	118	573	708	101	15
chimichanga w/ beef beans lettuce & tomato	1 (4.1 oz)	254	15	3	15	9	22	2	3	53	225	336	47	7

FOOD	PORTION	CALS	FAT	SAT FAT	CHOL	PROT	CARB	SUGAR	FIBER	CALCI	SOD	POTAS	FOLIC	VIT C
chimichanga w/ beef cheese lettuce & tomato	1 (4.1 oz)	337	24	8	37	13	19	1	1	182	348	208	35	4
chimichanga w/ chicken sour cream lettuce & tomato	1 (4 oz)	277	20	6	30	9	17	1	1	74	153	183	30	4
empanada fruit filled	1 (3.8 oz)	452	25	6	0	4	55	25	2	53	281	72	46	0
empanada meat & vegetable	1 (7.8 oz)	881	61	15	40	18	66	1	3	115	697	382	102	12
empanada sweet potato	1 (7.8 oz)	546	23	6	56	8	76	22	4	60	622	269	93	3
enchilada w/beans	1 (4.1 oz)	179	6	1	4	6	27	2	6	79	297	373	68	13
enchilada w/ beans & cheese	1 (4.6 oz)	233	11	5	21	9	25	2	5	199	381	403	62	15
enchilada w/ beef	1 (4 oz)	214	10	3	30	11	21	2	3	84	179	401	43	13
enchilada w/ beef & beans	1 (4 oz)	195	8	2	15	8	25	2	4	81	303	384	57	13
frijoles	1 cup	278	2	tr	0	18	49	6	9	88	606	793	322	10
frijoles w/ cheese	1 cup	225	8	4	37	11	29	—	—	189	882	605	112	2
nachos w/ beans & cheese	1 serv (9.4 oz)	616	33	13	56	25	57	2	13	433	990	608	142	8
nachos w/ beef beans cheese & sour cream	1 serv (19 oz)	1620	97	37	171	59	133	4	19	970	1846	1190	143	14
paella	1 serv (7 oz)	308	16	3	92	23	17	—	3	52	580	386	—	10
pupusa meat filled	1 (3.6 oz)	187	6	2	20	8	26	1	3	66	88	191	56	2
quesadilla w/ cheese	1 (5 oz)	498	28	14	60	20	40	1	3	498	1234	199	57	6
quesadilla w/ meat & cheese	1 (6.5 oz)	605	35	16	98	32	40	1	2	506	1268	372	61	6
taco de jueye w/ crab meat	1 (4.2 oz)	266	14	5	79	16	18	1	2	160	800	317	47	11
taco w/ beans lettuce tomato & salsa	1 (2.8 oz)	117	5	1	2	4	16	1	4	39	214	184	49	5
taco w/ chicken lettuce tomato & salsa	1 (2.5 oz)	114	5	1	22	8	10	1	1	32	134	139	27	4
taco w/ fish lettuce tomato & salsa	1 (2.7 oz)	101	4	1	39	8	10	1	1	52	190	179	32	5
tostada w/ beef lettuce tomato & salsa	1 (2.7 oz)	143	8	2	21	8	11	1	2	40	152	189	31	4

SPICES

(see individual names, HERBS/SPICES)

SPINACH

FOOD	PORTION	CALS	FAT	SAT FAT	CHOL	PROT	CARB	SUGAR	FIBER	CALCI	SOD	POTAS	FOLIC	VIT C
CANNED														
drained	1 cup	49	1	tr	0	6	7	1	5	272	58	740	210	31
FRESHLIKE														
Cut Leaf	½ cup	45	1	0	0	5	5	0	3	200	200	—	—	15
POPEYE														
Leaf Spinach	½ cup	30	0	0	0	3	4	tr	2	60	190	—	—	15
Leaf Spinach No Salt Added	½ cup	40	1	0	0	4	5	0	2	200	30	—	—	15
S&W														
Leaf	½ cup (4 oz)	30	0	0	0	2	4	0	2	100	360	—	—	15
FRESH														
baby raw	2 cups	20	0	0	0	1	5	0	3	30	80	—	—	8
cooked	1 cup	41	tr	tr	0	5	7	1	4	245	126	839	263	18
malabar cooked	1 cup	10	tr	—	0	1	1	—	1	55	24	113	50	3
mustard cooked	1 cup	29	tr	—	0	3	5	—	4	284	25	513	131	117
new zealand cooked	1 cup	22	tr	tr	0	2	4	—	—	86	193	184	14	29
raw	1 cup	7	tr	tr	0	1	1	tr	1	30	24	167	58	8
DOLE														
Baby Spinach	1½ cups (3 oz)	20	0	0	0	2	3	0	2	80	65	—	160	24
FRESH EXPRESS														
Baby Spinach	3 cups	20	0	0	0	2	3	0	2	80	65	470	160	24
Organic Baby Spinach	3 cups	35	0	0	0	2	9	0	4	60	135	—	—	12
READY PAC														
Microwave Spinach as prep	½ cup (3 oz)	20	0	0	0	2	3	0	1	80	60	—	80	6
FROZEN														
chopped cooked	1 cup	30	tr	tr	0	4	5	tr	4	145	92	287	115	2
BIRDS EYE														
Chopped	⅓ cup	20	0	0	0	2	2	1	2	60	115	—	—	6
Creamed	½ cup (4.4 oz)	90	4	3	10	3	9	3	4	150	500	—	—	5
C&W														
Baby Chopped	1 cup	30	0	0	0	2	3	tr	1	80	120	—	—	1
Creamed	½ cup	100	7	2	20	4	6	1	4	150	410	—	—	9
CASCADIAN FARM														
Organic Cut	⅓ cup	25	0	0	0	2	3	tr	1	80	160	250	—	5
CEDARLANE														
Organic Spanakopita Spinach & Feta Pie	½ pkg (5 oz)	260	8	4	20	12	38	3	2	200	650	—	—	15
HEALTH IS WEALTH														
Creamed	½ pkg (4.5 oz)	100	4	2	15	5	27	5	2	100	160	—	—	6

FOOD	PORTION	CALS	FAT	SAT FAT	CHOL	PROT	CARB	SUGAR	FIBER	CALCI	SOD	POTAS	FOLIC	VIT C
HEALTH IS WEALTH (CONT.)														
Spinach Munchees	6 (3oz)	180	7	1	0	7	25	1	3	100	320	—	—	6
SEABROOK FARMS														
Chopped	⅓ cup (2.9 oz)	20	0	0	0	2	2	1	2	60	115	—	—	6
Creamed	½ cup (4.4 oz)	100	5	2	10	4	10	3	2	100	390	—	—	2
STOUFFER'S														
Creamed	½ pkg (4.5 oz)	200	16	4	25	5	8	3	2	150	490	—	—	1
TABATCHNICK														
Creamed	1 serv (3.7 oz)	40	1	1	5	1	7	1	1	40	240	110	—	6
TANDOOR CHEF														
Palak Paneer	½ pkg (5 oz)	170	14	6	35	6	6	1	2	80	600	—	—	18
THE FILLO FACTORY														
Spanakopita Spinach & Cheese Fillo Appetizers	3 (3 oz)	190	9	5	20	6	20	1	1	100	280	—	—	1
VEGGIE PATCH														
Spinach Bites	3 (2.6 oz)	150	8	3	10	6	16	2	3	200	350	—	—	6
TAKE-OUT														
indian saag	1 serv	28	2	tr	0	2	2	—	1	—	44	—	—	—
spanakopita spinach pie	1 serv (3 oz)	148	11	5	60	5	8	1	1	117	289	215	58	6
SPINACH JUICE														
juice	7 oz	14	0	0	0	2	2	—	—	2	146	824	—	58
SPORTS DRINKS														
(*see* ENERGY DRINKS)														
SPOT														
baked	3 oz	134	5	2	—	20	0	0	0	15	32	541	—	—
SPROUTS														
kidney bean	½ cup	27	tr	tr	0	4	4	—	—	16	—	172	—	36
lentil sprouts	½ cup	40	tr	tr	0	3	8	—	—	9	4	122	38	6
mung bean	½ cup	16	tr	tr	0	2	3	—	—	7	3	77	32	7
mung bean canned	½ cup	8	tr	tr	0	1	1	—	—	9	—	17	6	tr
mung bean cooked	½ cup	13	tr	tr	0	1	3	—	—	7	6	63	—	7
pea	½ cup (2.1 oz)	74	tr	tr	0	5	16	—	—	22	12	229	86	6
radish	½ cup	8	tr	tr	0	1	1	—	—	10	1	16	18	6
BRASSICA														
BroccoSprouts	½ cup (1 oz)	16	0	0	0	1	2	—	1	26	3	—	0	20
LA CHOY														
Bean Sprouts	⅔ cup	15	0	0	0	tr	3	tr	1	0	60	—	—	36
TAKE-OUT														
mung bean stir fried	½ cup	31	tr	tr	0	3	7	—	—	8	—	—	—	—

FOOD	PORTION	CALS	FAT	SAT FAT	CHOL	PROT	CARB	SUGAR	FIBER	CALCI	SOD	POTAS	FOLIC	VIT C
SQUAB														
boneless baked	1 (4 oz)	242	14	4	129	26	0	0	0	19	243	283	7	3 .
SQUASH														
(*see also* SQUASH SEEDS, ZUCCHINI)														
CANNED														
crookneck sliced	½ cup	14	tr	tr	0	1	3	—	—	13	5	104	11	3
SUNSHINE														
Slice Yellow	½ cup	25	0	0	0	0	5	3	2	40	160	—	—	1
FRESH														
acorn cooked mashed	½ cup	41	tr	tr	0	1	11	—	3	32	3	321	14	8
acorn cubed baked	½ cup	57	tr	tr	0	1	15	—	2	45	4	446	19	11
butternut baked	½ cup	41	tr	tr	0	1	11	—	2	42	4	290	20	15
crookneck sliced cooked	½ cup	18	tr	tr	0	1	4	—	1	24	1	173	18	5
hubbard baked	½ cup	51	tr	tr	0	3	11	—	3	17	8	365	17	10
hubbard cooked mashed	½ cup	35	tr	tr	0	2	8	—	3	12	6	252	12	8
scallop sliced cooked	½ cup	14	tr	tr	0	1	3	—	1	14	1	126	19	10
spaghetti cooked	½ cup	23	tr	tr	0	1	5	—	2	17	14	91	6	3
GLORY														
Yellow Sliced	¾ cup	20	0	0	0	1	3	1	1	20	20	—	—	6
MANN'S														
Butternut Cubes	1 serv (3 oz)	40	0	0	0	1	10	2	2	40	0	—	—	18
FROZEN														
butternut cooked mashed	½ cup	47	tr	tr	0	1	12	—	3	23	2	160	—	4
crookneck sliced cooked	½ cup	24	tr	tr	0	1	5	—	—	19	6	243	12	7
C&W														
Butternut	½ cup	45	0	0	0	1	10	2	1	20	2	—	—	2
MCKENZIE'S														
Southland Butternut	½ cup	70	3	1	0	1	10	6	1	20	270	—	—	2
TAKE-OUT														
fritter	1 (0.8 oz)	81	5	1	15	2	8	1	1	29	79	81	13	1
squash pie	1 slice (5.4 oz)	291	12	4	66	6	40	24	2	88	259	240	35	3
SQUASH SEEDS														
kernels dried	¼ cup (1.1 oz)	180	16	3	0	10	3	tr	2	15	2	261	19	1
kernels roasted	¼ cup (1 oz)	169	14	3	0	9	4	tr	2	15	5	232	17	1
kernels roasted w/ salt	¼ cup (1 oz)	169	14	3	0	9	4	tr	2	15	76	232	17	1
whole roasted w/ salt	¼ cup (0.5 oz)	71	3	1	0	3	9	—	3	9	407	147	1	0

FOOD	PORTION	CALS	FAT	SAT FAT	CHOL	PROT	CARB	SUGAR	FIBER	CALCI	SOD	POTAS	FOLIC	VIT C
whole roasted w/o salt	¼ cup (0.5 oz)	71	3	1	0	3	9	—	3	9	3	147	1	0

SQUID

FOOD	PORTION	CALS	FAT	SAT FAT	CHOL	PROT	CARB	SUGAR	FIBER	CALCI	SOD	POTAS	FOLIC	VIT C
baked	1 cup	192	6	1	393	26	5	0	0	55	540	416	8	8
canned in its own ink	1 can (4 oz)	122	2	tr	308	21	4	0	0	43	360	260	5	4
dried	1 sm (1.5 oz)	147	2	1	371	25	5	0	0	51	255	392	8	7
pickled	1 oz	26	tr	tr	63	4	1	tr	0	9	431	68	1	1
steamed	1 cup	147	2	1	374	25	5	0	0	52	587	316	6	5
CONTESSA														
Calamari + Sauce	13 pieces + 2 tbsp sauce	160	6	2	55	5	21	1	1	20	370	—	—	0
MARGARITAVILLE														
Captain's Calamari Rings + Sauce	3 + 2 tbsp sauce	320	21	4	100	9	25	3	1	60	810	—	—	2
VAN DE KAMP'S														
Fried Calamari	15 pieces (4 oz)	270	13	4	105	10	26	0	1	60	650	—	—	0
TAKE-OUT														
arroz con calamares	1 cup	400	17	2	150	14	47	2	1	45	906	326	82	42
calamari breaded & fried	1 cup	296	12	3	378	26	17	1	1	87	584	411	22	6

SQUIRREL

FOOD	PORTION	CALS	FAT	SAT FAT	CHOL	PROT	CARB	SUGAR	FIBER	CALCI	SOD	POTAS	FOLIC	VIT C
roasted	3 oz	147	4	tr	103	26	0	0	0	2	102	300	—	—

STARFRUIT

FOOD	PORTION	CALS	FAT	SAT FAT	CHOL	PROT	CARB	SUGAR	FIBER	CALCI	SOD	POTAS	FOLIC	VIT C
fresh	1	42	tr	—	0	1	10	—	—	6	2	207	—	27

STRAWBERRIES

FOOD	PORTION	CALS	FAT	SAT FAT	CHOL	PROT	CARB	SUGAR	FIBER	CALCI	SOD	POTAS	FOLIC	VIT C
canned in heavy syrup	½ cup	117	tr	tr	0	1	30	28	2	17	5	109	36	40
fresh halves	1 cup	49	tr	tr	0	1	12	7	3	24	2	233	36	89
fresh whole	1 cup	46	tr	tr	0	1	11	7	3	23	1	220	35	85
fresh whole	1 pint	114	1	tr	0	2	27	17	7	57	4	546	86	210
frzn sweetened sliced	½ cup	122	tr	tr	0	1	33	31	2	14	4	125	19	53
frzn sweetened whole	1 cup	199	tr	tr	0	1	54	48	5	28	3	250	10	101
frzn whole unsweetened	1 cup	77	tr	tr	0	1	20	10	5	35	4	327	38	91
organic fresh whole	8 med	45	0	0	0	1	12	8	4	20	0	—	—	96
C&W														
Ultimate Sliced frzn	⅔ cup	50	0	0	0	0	12	8	1	20	5	—	—	42
CHUKAR CHERRIES														
Dried	¼ cup	120	0	0	0	tr	29	25	2	0	0	—	—	0

FOOD	PORTION	CALS	FAT	SAT FAT	CHOL	PROT	CARB	SUGAR	FIBER	CALCI	SOD	POTAS	FOLIC	VIT C
CRUNCHIES														
Freeze Dried	¼ cup (6 g)	20	0	0	0	0	5	3	1	0	0	—	—	36
CRUNCHY N'YUMMY														
Organic Freeze Dried	1 pkg (1 oz)	60	0	0	0	2	11	0	3	34	2	233	—	110
DOLE														
Sliced frzn	1 pkg (3 oz)	35	0	0	0	0	8	4	2	0	0	—	—	36
Squish'ems	1 pkg	70	0	0	0	0	16	15	1	0	0	110	—	60
Whole Fresh	1 cup (5.2 oz)	45	0	0	0	tr	11	7	3	20	0	—	—	84
Whole frzn	1 cup (4.9 oz)	50	0	0	0	1	13	61	3	20	0	—	—	60
EMILY'S														
Dark Chocolate Covered	6 (1.4 oz)	170	8	5	0	1	28	22	2	40	0	—	—	21
LITEHOUSE														
Glaze Sugar Free	3 tbsp	35	0	0	0	0	8	0	0	0	55	—	—	0
MARIE'S														
Glaze	2 tbsp	40	0	0	0	0	10	8	0	0	40	—	—	0
POLAR														
Strawberries In Syrup	½ cup	90	0	0	0	1	21	10	1	20	10	—	—	21
STONERIDGE ORCHARDS														
Dried	⅓ cup (1.4 oz)	140	0	0	0	0	35	32	0	0	15	—	—	12
STUFFING/DRESSING														
FRESH GOURMET														
All Natural Multi-Grain w/ Cranberries not prep	⅓ cup (1 oz)	110	3	0	0	3	19	3	1	0	360	—	—	0
Organic Seasoned not prep	⅓ cup (1 oz)	110	3	0	0	3	19	1	1	0	350	—	—	0
PEPPERIDGE FARM														
Cornbread	¾ cup	170	2	0	0	4	33	2	2	40	480	—	—	0
Country Style	¾ cup	140	1	0	0	5	27	2	2	0	380	—	—	0
Herb Seasoned	¾ cup	170	2	1	0	5	33	2	3	40	600	—	—	0
TAKE-OUT														
bread	1 cup	352	17	3	0	6	44	5	2	58	1028	142	66	0
cornbread	½ cup	179	9	2	0	3	22	0	3	26	455	62	97	1
kishke stuffed derma	1 piece (1.3 oz)	166	12	6	13	2	13	tr	1	5	145	30	21	1
oyster	1 cup	304	18	4	23	7	29	3	2	113	953	211	50	4
sausage	½ cup	292	11	2	12	8	40	—	1	17	258	96	3	2
STURGEON														
broiled	3 oz	115	4	1	65	18	0	0	0	14	59	310	14	0
roe raw	1 oz	59	3	—	—	7	tr	—	—	—	—	—	—	5
smoked	1 oz	49	1	tr	23	9	0	0	0	5	210	107	6	0

FOOD	PORTION	CALS	FAT	SAT FAT	CHOL	PROT	CARB	SUGAR	FIBER	CALCI	SOD	POTAS	FOLIC	VIT C
TAKE-OUT														
breaded & fried	4 oz	252	15	3	85	19	9	1	1	41	416	325	25	0
SUCKER														
white baked	3 oz	101	3	tr	45	18	0	0	0	76	44	414	—	—
SUGAR														
(*see also* FRUCTOSE, SYRUP)														
brown organic	1 tsp	17	0	0	0	0	4	4	0	—	0	—	—	—
brown packed	1 cup (7.7 oz)	828	0	0	0	0	214	214	—	167	86	762	1	0
brown unpacked	1 cup (5.1 oz)	547	0	0	0	0	141	140	0	123	57	502	1	0
cinnamon sugar	1 tsp	16	tr	tr	0	tr	4	4	tr	3	0	1	0	0
cube	1 (2 g)	9	0	0	0	0	2	2	0	0	0	0	0	0
maple	1 piece (1 oz)	99	tr	tr	0	tr	25	24	0	25	3	77	0	0
powdered	1 tbsp (0.3 oz)	31	0	0	0	0	8	8	—	0	0	0	0	0
powdered unsifted	1 cup (4.2 oz)	467	tr	—	0	tr	119	115	—	1	2	3	0	0
raw	1 pkg (5 g)	19	0	0	0	0	5	5	0	4	2	17	0	0
sugarcane stem	3 oz	54	0	0	0	1	14	—	3	2	—	—	—	1
white	1 cup (7 oz)	773	0	0	0	0	200	200	—	2	3	4	0	0
white	1 tbsp (0.4 oz)	49	0	0	0	0	13	13	0	0	0	0	0	0
white	1 tsp (4 g)	15	0	0	0	0	4	4	—	0	0	0	0	0
white	1 pkg (3 g)	12	0	0	0	0	3	3	0	0	0	0	0	0
BOB'S RED MILL														
Date Sugar	1 tsp	11	0	0	0	0	3	3	0	—	0	—	—	—
Turbinado	1 tsp	10	0	0	0	0	3	3	0	—	0	—	—	—
COCONUT WORLD														
Coconut Sugar	1 tsp (3 g)	10	0	0	0	0	3	3	0	0	0	—	—	0
DOMINO														
Dark Brown	1 tsp (4 g)	15	0	0	0	0	4	4	—	—	0	—	—	—
Demerara Raw Cane	1 tsp	15	0	0	0	0	4	4	0	—	0	—	—	—
Organic Cane Sugar	1 tsp	15	0	0	0	0	4	4	—	—	0	—	—	—
EQUINOX														
Organic Maple Flakes	2 tsp	15	0	0	0	0	4	4	—	—	0	—	—	—
MAPLE GROVE FARMS														
Granulated Maple	1 tsp (4 g)	15	0	0	0	0	4	3	—	—	0	—	—	—
SUGAR IN THE RAW														
Turbinado Sugar	1 pkg (5 g)	20	0	0	0	0	5	5	—	—	0	—	—	—
TREE OF LIFE														
Date Sugar	1 tsp (4 g)	10	0	0	0	0	3	3	0	0	0	—	—	0
Organic Cane Juice Dehydrated	1 tsp (3.5 g)	15	0	0	0	0	3	3	0	<20	10	—	—	tr
Turbinado	1 tsp (4 g)	15	0	0	0	0	4	4	0	0	0	—	—	0
WHOLESOME SWEETENERS														
Organic	1 tsp (4 g)	15	0	0	0	0	4	4	0	0	0	—	—	—

FOOD	PORTION	CALS	FAT	SAT FAT	CHOL	PROT	CARB	SUGAR	FIBER	CALCI	SOD	POTAS	FOLIC	VIT C
WHOLESOME SWEETENERS (CONT.)														
Organic Fair Trade Dark Brown Sugar	1 tsp (4 g)	15	0	0	0	0	4	4	0	0	0	—	—	—
Organic Fair Trade Powdered	¼ cup (1 oz)	120	0	0	0	0	30	30	0	0	0	—	—	—
Organic Fair Trade Sucanat	1 tsp (4 g)	15	0	0	0	0	4	4	0	0	0	—	—	—
Organic Turbinado	1 tsp (4 g)	15	0	0	0	0	4	4	0	0	0	—	—	—
SUGAR SUBSTITUTES														
EMERALD CITY														
Erythritol	1 tsp (4 g)	0	0	0	0	0	4	0	0	0	0	—	—	0
EMERALD FOREST														
Xylitol	1 tsp (4 g)	10	0	0	0	0	4	0	0	0	0	—	—	0
EQUAL														
Packet	1 pkg	0	0	0	0	0	tr	tr	—	—	0	—	—	—
FIBRELLE														
Fiber-Rich Sweetener	1 tsp (4 g)	5	0	0	0	0	4	0	2	—	0	—	—	—
FRUCTEVIA														
All Natural	1 tsp (4 g)	5	0	0	0	0	2	2	0	300	0	300	4	0
FRUIT SWEETNESS														
Sugar Substitute	1 serv (0.9 oz)	0	0	0	0	0	0	0	0	0	0	—	—	0
IDEAL														
Brown	1 tsp (1.5 g)	0	0	0	0	0	2	0	0	0	0	2	—	0
Confectionary	¼ cup (1 oz)	86	0	0	0	0	30	0	0	0	0	0	—	0
Packets	1 (1.5 g)	0	0	0	0	0	2	0	0	0	0	0	—	0
White Granulated	1 tsp (1.5 g)	0	0	0	0	0	2	0	0	0	0	0	—	0
NATURE'S FAMILY														
Sun Crystals	1 pkg (4.5 g)	4	0	0	0	0	1	tr	—	—	0	—	—	—
NEVELLA														
No Calorie Sweetener	1 tsp (0.5 g)	0	0	0	0	0	tr	0	0	—	0	0	—	—
NEWAY														
Sweet Sensation	¼ tsp	0	0	0	0	0	tr	0	0	—	0	—	—	—
PUREVIA														
All Natural	1 pkg (2 g)	0	0	0	0	0	2	tr	0	—	0	—	—	—
SPLENDA														
Brown Sugar Blend	½ tsp (2 g)	10	0	0	0	0	2	2	0	—	0	—	—	—
Flavors For Coffee	1 pkg (1 g)	0	0	0	0	0	tr	0	0	—	0	—	—	—
No Calorie Granulated	1 tsp (0.5 g)	0	0	0	0	0	tr	0	0	—	0	—	—	—
No Calorie Sweetener w/ Antioxidants	1 pkg	0	0	0	0	0	tr	0	—	—	0	—	—	12

FOOD	PORTION	CALS	FAT	SAT FAT	CHOL	PROT	CARB	SUGAR	FIBER	CALCI	SOD	POTAS	FOLIC	VIT C
SPLENDA (CONT.)														
No Calorie Sweetener w/ B Vitamins	1 pkg	0	0	0	0	0	tr	0	0	—	0	—	—	—
No Calorie Sweetener w/Fiber	1 pkg	0	0	0	0	0	2	0	1	—	0	—	—	—
STEEL'S														
Nature Sweet Brown Crystals	1 tsp (3 g)	6	0	0	0	0	3	0	0	0	0	—	—	0
Nature Sweet Crystals	1 tsp (4 g)	8	0	0	0	0	4	0	0	0	0	—	—	0
Sugar Free Vanilla Flavor	1 tbsp (0.5 oz)	23	0	0	0	0	11	0	0	0	0	—	—	0
STEVIA IN THE RAW														
100% Natural Sweetener	1 pkg (1 g)	0	0	0	0	0	0	0	0	—	0	—	—	—
STEVIVA														
Blend	1 tbsp (0.4 oz)	2	0	0	0	0	0	0	0	—	0	—	—	—
SUGAR TWIN														
Granulated Brown	1 tsp (0.4 g)	0	0	0	0	0	tr	0	0	—	0	0	—	—
Granulated White	1 tsp (0.4 g)	0	0	0	0	0	tr	0	0	—	0	0	—	—
Liquid	¼ tsp (1.3 g)	0	0	0	0	0	0	0	0	—	0	0	—	—
Packets	1 (0.8 g)	0	0	0	0	0	1	—	—	—	0	0	—	—
SUN CRYSTALS														
Natural Sweetener	1 pkg (5 g)	5	0	0	0	0	1	1	—	—	0	—	—	—
SUSTA														
Natural Sweetener	1 pkg (2 g)	5	0	0	0	0	2	tr	1	—	0	—	20	6
SUZANNE														
Somersweet Baking Blend	1 tsp (4 g)	5	0	0	0	0	4	0	2	0	0	—	—	0
SWEET FIBER														
All Natural	1 pkg	0	0	0	0	0	tr	tr	tr	—	0	—	—	—
SWEETE														
Sugar Free	1 pkg	0	0	0	0	0	tr	0	0	—	10	10	—	—
SWERVE														
Sweetener	1 tsp (5 g)	0	0	0	0	0	5	0	—	—	0	—	—	—
TRUVIA														
Calorie Free Sweetener	1 pkg (3.5 g)	0	0	0	0	0	3	0	0	—	0	—	—	—
WHEY LOW														
Gold	1 tsp	4	0	0	0	0	4	4	0	0	0	—	—	0
Granular	1 tsp	4	0	0	0	0	4	4	0	0	0	—	—	0
Maple Buzz	¼ cup	57	0	0	0	0	57	57	0	0	0	—	—	0
WHOLESOME SWEETENERS														
Organic Zero	1 pkg (6 g)	0	0	0	0	0	6	0	0	0	0	—	—	—

FOOD	PORTION	CALS	FAT	SAT FAT	CHOL	PROT	CARB	SUGAR	FIBER	CALCI	SOD	POTAS	FOLIC	VIT C
ZSWEET														
All Natural	1 pkg (1 g)	0	0	0	0	0	tr	0	0	—	0	—	—	—
SUGAR-APPLE														
fresh	1	146	tr	—	0	3	37	—	—	37	15	384	—	66
fresh cut up	1 cup	236	1	—	0	5	59	—	—	59	24	619	—	91
SUNCHOKE														
fresh raw sliced	½ cup	57	tr	0	0	2	13	—	—	10	—	—	—	3
SUNFISH														
pumpkinseed baked	3 oz	97	1	tr	73	21	0	0	0	87	87	381	—	—
SUNFLOWER														
seeds dry roasted w/ salt	¼ cup	186	16	2	0	6	8	1	3	22	131	272	76	tr
seeds dry roasted w/o salt	¼ cup	186	16	2	0	6	8	1	4	22	1	272	76	tr
seeds w/ hulls dried	¼ cup	66	6	1	0	3	2	tr	1	13	0	79	26	tr
ARROWHEAD MILLS														
Organic Seeds	¼ cup	170	15	2	0	7	6	1	3	100	0	210	—	0
BOB'S RED MILL														
Seeds Roasted & Salted	3 tbsp	186	15	2	0	6	6	1	5	—	104	—	—	—
DAKOTA GOURMET														
Seeds Honey Roasted	¼ cup (1 oz)	170	12	2	0	5	8	1	2	0	110	—	60	0
DAVID														
Kernels	¼ cup (1.1 oz)	190	15	2	0	9	4	tr	3	20	220	—	80	—
Seeds Reduced Sodium w/o Shell	¼ cup (1.1 oz)	190	14	2	0	9	7	tr	3	40	75	—	60	—
Seeds w/o Shell	¼ cup (1.1 oz)	190	15	2	0	9	5	tr	4	20	135	—	80	—
FRITO LAY														
Seeds	1 oz	190	16	2	0	6	5	tr	3	20	90	—	—	0
KAIA FOODS														
Seeds Sprouted Cocoa Mole	⅙ pkg (1 oz)	80	6	1	0	3	5	3	2	20	15	—	24	0
Sprouted Seeds Sweet Curry	⅙ pkg (1 oz)	80	6	1	0	3	4	2	2	20	10	—	32	0
LANCE														
Shelled Seeds	1 pkg (1.8 oz)	300	25	4	0	6	14	1	3	60	160	—	—	0
PLANTERS														
Kernels	1 oz	160	14	2	0	7	5	1	3	40	150	—	—	0
Seeds Roasted & Salted	¾ cup (1 oz)	160	14	2	0	5	7	0	3	20	45	—	—	0
SPITZ														
Seeds Salted	⅓ pkg (1 oz)	180	15	2	0	7	5	tr	3	20	530	—	—	0

FOOD	PORTION	CALS	FAT	SAT FAT	CHOL	PROT	CARB	SUGAR	FIBER	CALCI	SOD	POTAS	FOLIC	VIT C
SUNBUTTER														
Creamy	2 tbsp	200	16	2	0	7	7	3	4	20	120	—	—	0
Organic	2 tbsp	203	16	1	0	8	7	4	3	20	100	—	—	0
SUNGOLD														
Seeds Roasted Salted	1 oz	172	15	2	0	7	4	2	2	20	168	—	—	0
SUNRICH NATURALS														
Kernels Cocoa Sunnies	1 pkg (2 oz)	280	16	2	0	7	30	13	4	40	135	—	—	0
Kernels Honey Roasted	1 pkg (1 oz)	170	14	2	0	5	6	3	2	20	110	—	60	0
Kernels Lightly Salted	1 pkg (1 oz)	170	16	2	0	6	4	1	2	20	110	—	64	0
TREE OF LIFE														
Seeds Kernels Raw	¼ cup (1.3 oz)	210	18	2	0	8	7	1	2	40	15	—	—	0
SUSHI														
TAKE-OUT														
california roll	1 (1.2 oz)	48	1	tr	17	1	8	1	tr	8	163	27	—	0
crabmeat mayonnaise	1 (1.2 oz)	60	2	tr	3	2	10	—	tr	9	155	19	—	—
futomaki roll	1 (1.8 oz)	73	1	tr	22	2	14	3	1	12	228	30	—	0
ikura salmon roe & cucumber	1 (1.1 oz)	50	1	tr	22	3	7	1	1	7	141	23	—	1
inari	1 sm (1.2 oz)	46	1	0	0	1	9	—	0	13	79	20	4	0
kappa cucumber roll	1 (1.1 oz)	43	0	0	0	1	9	2	tr	4	106	24	—	0
kim bap	1 (1.2 oz)	56	2	0	10	2	8	—	0	5	68	34	3	1
nigiri	1 (0.7 oz)	27	0	0	6	1	5	—	0	4	30	25	1	0
prawn cooked	1 (1.1 oz)	36	0	0	0	1	8	—	1	13	105	17	—	0
preserved radish roll	1 (0.3 oz)	9	0	0	0	0	2	0	tr	1	45	6	—	0
saba raw mackerel	1 (0.8 oz)	33	1	1	2	1	5	1	tr	3	47	6	—	0
salmon slice	1 (1.2 oz)	59	1	1	3	2	10	1	tr	4	115	31	—	0
sashimi ahi	1 slice (0.3 oz)	10	0	0	4	2	0	0	0	1	3	40	tr	0
scallop cooked	1 (1.1 oz)	43	tr	tr	10	2	8	—	tr	6	130	23	—	0
seasoned baby octopus	1 (1.2 oz)	55	tr	tr	19	2	10	1	tr	5	150	24	—	0
seasoned jellyfish	1 (1.2 oz)	58	1	tr	1	2	11	2	tr	9	246	21	—	0
seaweed roll	1 (1.1 oz)	43	1	tr	1	1	9	1	1	5	188	18	—	0
sweet beancurd	1 (1.2 oz)	64	2	tr	0	2	10	3	1	24	147	11	—	0
tekka tuna maki	1 (0.6 oz)	25	0	0	0	1	5	—	0	7	24	38	2	0
torigai cockle	1 piece (1.1 oz)	41	0	0	0	3	7	—	tr	4	131	13	—	0
tuna roll	1 (0.6 oz)	19	0	0	0	1	4	0	tr	2	48	26	—	0
unagi grilled eel	1 (1 oz)	54	2	1	9	2	8	1	1	10	114	19	—	0
vegetable roll	1 (1.2 oz)	27	1	tr	0	1	5	tr	—	20	47	60	16	3
vinegared ginger	⅓ cup (1.6 oz)	48	tr	tr	0	1	12	4	—	8	6	189	5	2

FOOD	PORTION	CALS	FAT	SAT FAT	CHOL	PROT	CARB	SUGAR	FIBER	CALCI	SOD	POTAS	FOLIC	VIT C
wasabi	2 tsp (0.3 oz)	5	tr	0	0	tr	1	—	—	6	124	28	0	0
yellowtail roll	1 (0.6 oz)	25	1	tr	0	1	3	tr	—	12	32	14	3	1

SWAMP CABBAGE

FOOD	PORTION	CALS	FAT	SAT FAT	CHOL	PROT	CARB	SUGAR	FIBER	CALCI	SOD	POTAS	FOLIC	VIT C
chopped cooked w/o salt	1 cup	20	tr	tr	0	2	4	—	2	53	120	278	34	16

SWEET POTATO
(*see also* YAM)

FOOD	PORTION	CALS	FAT	SAT FAT	CHOL	PROT	CARB	SUGAR	FIBER	CALCI	SOD	POTAS	FOLIC	VIT C
baked w/ skin w/o salt	1 lg (6.3 oz)	162	tr	tr	0	4	37	12	6	68	65	855	11	35
baked w/ skin w/o salt	1 med (4 oz)	103	tr	tr	0	2	24	7	4	43	41	542	7	22
canned in syrup	½ cup	106	tr	tr	0	1	25	6	3	17	38	189	8	11
canned mashed	½ cup	129	tr	tr	0	3	30	7	2	38	96	268	14	7
leaves cooked w/o salt	1 cup	22	tr	tr	0	1	5	3	1	15	8	305	31	1
paste dulce de calabaza	1 oz	82	tr	tr	0	tr	21	20	tr	3	2	20	1	1
DINER'S CHOICE														
Mashed	⅔ cup	160	3	1	0	3	33	18	2	60	105	—	—	21
GLORY														
Casserole	½ cup	180	0	0	0	2	43	27	2	60	250	—	—	12
Cut Fresh	1 serv (5 oz)	140	0	0	0	2	36	8	4	20	50	—	—	18
Sweet Potatoes	⅔ cup	160	0	0	0	3	37	17	2	20	35	300	—	18
GREEN GIANT														
Candied	¾ cup	240	7	1	0	2	41	20	3	20	430	—	—	12
HEALTH IS WEALTH														
Southern Style	½ pkg (5 oz)	190	5	3	15	2	36	8	2	60	260	—	—	18
IAN'S														
Fries	7 pieces (2.5 oz)	70	3	1	0	1	13	4	1	20	25	—	—	9
JAKE & AMOS														
Sweet Potato Butter	1 tbsp (0.5 oz)	25	0	0	0	0	6	3	0	0	10	—	—	1
MANN'S														
Fresh Cubes	1 serv (3 oz)	60	0	0	0	1	15	3	3	20	10	290	12	18
Fries Fresh	1 serv (3 oz)	60	0	0	0	1	15	3	3	20	10	290	12	18
MRS. PAUL'S														
Candied	1 serv (5 oz)	300	1	1	0	1	73	47	3	150	130	—	—	5
PRINCELLA														
In Light Syrup	⅔ cup	160	0	0	0	0	39	20	3	20	35	—	—	5
Mashed	⅔ cup	120	0	0	0	1	28	15	3	20	30	—	—	5
ROYAL PRINCE														
Candied	½ cup	210	0	0	0	1	50	35	2	20	30	—	—	4

FOOD	PORTION	CALS	FAT	SAT FAT	CHOL	PROT	CARB	SUGAR	FIBER	CALCI	SOD	POTAS	FOLIC	VIT C
TRAPPEY'S														
Sugary Sam Cut Sweet	⅔ cup	160	0	0	0	0	39	20	3	20	35	—	—	5
TREE OF LIFE														
Organic Puree	½ cup (4.5 oz)	130	0	0	0	3	30	15	2	40	100	—	—	6
TAKE-OUT														
candied	1 serv (3.7 oz)	151	3	1	8	1	29	—	3	27	74	198	12	7
white fried batata blanca frita	1 serv (8 oz)	792	29	7	0	7	129	2	19	79	43	3780	79	63

SWEETBREAD (PANCREAS)

FOOD	PORTION	CALS	FAT	SAT FAT	CHOL	PROT	CARB	SUGAR	FIBER	CALCI	SOD	POTAS	FOLIC	VIT C
beef braised	3 oz	230	15	5	223	23	0	0	0	14	51	209	3	17
lamb braised	3 oz	199	13	6	340	19	0	0	0	10	44	247	11	17
pork braised	3 oz	186	9	3	268	24	0	0	0	14	36	143	4	5
veal braised	3 oz	218	12	4	—	25	0	0	0	15	58	236	3	5
RUMBA														
Beef	4 oz	260	23	8	250	14	0	0	0	0	110	—	—	36

SWISS CHARD

FOOD	PORTION	CALS	FAT	SAT FAT	CHOL	PROT	CARB	SUGAR	FIBER	CALCI	SOD	POTAS	FOLIC	VIT C
cooked	½ cup	18	tr	—	0	2	4	—	—	51	158	483	—	16
raw chopped	½ cup	3	tr	—	0	tr	1	—	—	9	38	68	—	5

SWORDFISH

FOOD	PORTION	CALS	FAT	SAT FAT	CHOL	PROT	CARB	SUGAR	FIBER	CALCI	SOD	POTAS	FOLIC	VIT C
cooked	3 oz	132	4	1	43	22	0	0	0	5	98	314	—	1
raw	3 oz	103	3	1	33	17	0	0	0	4	76	245	—	1

SYRUP

FOOD	PORTION	CALS	FAT	SAT FAT	CHOL	PROT	CARB	SUGAR	FIBER	CALCI	SOD	POTAS	FOLIC	VIT C
corn dark & light	¼ cup	240	tr	0	0	0	65	65	0	2	99	3	0	0
date syrup	1 tbsp	63	tr	—	—	tr	15	—	0	12	—	—	—	—
maple	1 cup (11.1 oz)	824	1	—	0	tr	212	191	—	211	27	643	1	0
maple	1 tbsp	52	0	—	0	0	13	12	—	13	2	41	0	0
raspberry	1 oz	76	0	0	0	tr	19	—	—	8	1	45	—	8
rose hip	1 oz	9	0	0	—	0	2	2	0	—	—	—	—	—
sorghum	1 cup (11.6 oz)	957	0	0	0	0	247	247	—	495	28	3300	—	—
sorghum	1 tbsp (0.7 oz)	61	0	0	0	0	16	16	—	31	2	210	—	—
sugar syrup	¼ cup	76	0	0	0	0	20	20	0	1	1	1	0	0
CARY'S														
Maple	¼ cup	210	0	0	0	0	53	50	—	40	5	—	—	—
Sugar Free	¼ cup	30	0	0	0	0	12	0	tr	—	115	—	—	—
DOMINO														
Agave Nectar Organic Light or Amber	1 tbsp (0.7 oz)	60	0	0	0	0	16	16	—	—	0	—	—	—
HERSHEY'S														
Caramel	2 tbsp (1.4 oz)	110	0	0	0	tr	27	21	—	20	125	—	—	0
Strawberry	2 tbsp (1.4 oz)	100	0	0	0	0	26	24	—	—	10	—	—	0
Strawberry Sugar Free	2 tbsp (1 oz)	10	0	0	0	0	4	—	—	0	55	—	—	0

FOOD	PORTION	CALS	FAT	SAT FAT	CHOL	PROT	CARB	SUGAR	FIBER	CALCI	SOD	POTAS	FOLIC	VIT C
LUNDBERG														
Organic Sweet Dreams Brown Rice	2 tbsp	110	0	0	0	1	31	25	0	—	30	—	—	—
MAPLE GROVE FARMS														
Apricot	¼ cup (2.1 oz)	170	0	0	0	0	42	40	—	—	5	—	—	—
Butter Flavor Sugar Free	¼ cup (2.1 oz)	30	0	0	0	0	11	0	—	—	100	—	—	—
Red Raspberry	¼ cup (2.1 oz)	230	0	0	0	0	46	45	—	—	5	—	—	—
MONIN														
Acai	1 oz	90	0	0	0	0	23	22	—	—	0	—	—	—
Amaretto	1 oz	97	0	0	0	0	24	24	—	—	0	—	—	—
Banana	1 oz	98	0	0	0	0	24	24	—	—	0	—	—	—
Coconut	1 oz	100	0	0	0	0	25	25	—	—	0	—	—	—
Organic Vanilla	1 oz	100	0	0	0	0	24	23	—	—	0	—	—	—
Pure Cane	1 oz	101	0	0	0	0	25	25	—	—	0	—	—	—
NATURE'S AGAVE														
Agave Nectar Organic Amber Clear or Raw	1 tbsp (0.7 oz)	60	0	0	0	0	16	16	—	—	0	—	—	—
NAVITAS NATURALS														
Yacon	2 tbsp	90	0	0	0	0	22	14	0	0	25	—	—	0
NESQUIK														
Strawberry Calcium Fortified	2 tbsp (1.4 oz)	110	0	0	0	0	27	27	0	100	0	—	—	0
NEWAY														
Sweet Sensation Luo Han Guo Syrup	1 tsp	8	0	0	0	0	2	0	0	—	0	—	—	—
SMUCKER'S														
Blackberry	¼ cup (2.1 oz)	200	0	0	0	0	51	44	—	—	0	—	—	—
Blueberry Sugar Free	¼ cup (2.1 oz)	25	0	0	0	0	8	0	1	—	60	—	—	—
Plate Scrapers Caramel	2 tbsp (1.4 oz)	100	0	0	0	1	25	20	0	0	110	—	—	0
Plate Scrapers Raspberry	2 tbsp (1.3 oz)	100	0	0	0	0	25	17	0	0	5	—	—	0
Plate Scrapers Vanilla	2 tbsp (1.4 oz)	110	1	0	0	1	24	19	0	40	125	—	—	0
Pure Maple	¼ cup (2.1 oz)	210	0	0	0	0	53	47	—	—	5	—	—	—
Red Raspberry	¼ cup (2.1 oz)	200	0	0	0	0	51	44	—	—	0	—	—	—
STEEL'S														
Maple Flavor No Sugar Added	3 tbsp (1.6 oz)	64	0	0	0	0	16	0	0	0	10	—	—	0
TREE OF LIFE														
Maple Grade A	¼ cup	200	0	0	0	0	53	53	—	60	10	—	—	—

FOOD	PORTION	CALS	FAT	SAT FAT	CHOL	PROT	CARB	SUGAR	FIBER	CALCI	SOD	POTAS	FOLIC	VIT C
WHOLESOME SWEETENERS														
Organic Blue Agave	1 tbsp (0.7 oz)	60	0	0	0	0	16	16	0	0	0	—	—	—
Organic Blue Agave Cinnamon	2 tbsp (1 oz)	120	0	0	0	0	16	16	0	0	0	—	—	—
Organic Blue Agave Maple	2 tbsp (1 oz)	120	0	0	0	0	16	16	0	0	0	—	—	—
Organic Corn Syrup	2 tbsp (1 oz)	120	0	0	0	0	30	30	0	0	30	—	—	—
TAHINI														
(*see* SESAME)														
TAMARIND														
dried sweetened pulpitas	½ cup	279	1	tr	0	3	73	68	5	74	28	622	7	1
dried sweetened pulpitas	1 piece (0.8 oz)	56	tr	tr	0	1	15	14	1	15	6	124	1	tr
fresh	1 (2 g)	5	tr	tr	0	tr	1	0	tr	1	1	13	0	tr
fresh cut up	1 cup	143	tr	tr	0	2	38	34	3	44	17	377	8	2
TAMARIND JUICE														
nectar	1 cup	143	tr	—	0	tr	37	32	1	25	18	68	3	18
TANGERINE														
CANNED														
in light syrup	1 cup	154	tr	tr	0	1	41	39	2	18	15	197	13	50
juice pack	1 cup	92	tr	tr	0	2	24	22	2	27	12	331	12	85
FRESH														
fresh	1 med (3.1 oz)	47	tr	tr	0	1	12	9	2	33	2	146	14	24
fresh	1 sm (2.7 oz)	40	tr	tr	0	1	10	8	1	28	2	126	12	20
fresh	1 lg (4.2 oz)	64	tr	tr	0	1	16	13	2	44	2	199	19	32
sections	1 cup	103	1	tr	0	2	26	21	4	72	4	324	31	52
NOBLE														
Florida Tangerines	1 (3.8 oz)	50	1	0	0	1	15	12	3	40	0	—	—	30
RIVER PRIDE														
Sweet	1 (3.8 oz)	50	1	0	0	1	15	12	3	40	0	—	—	30
TANGERINE JUICE														
canned sweetened	1 cup	124	1	tr	0	1	30	29	1	45	2	443	12	55
fresh	1 cup	106	tr	tr	0	1	25	24	1	44	2	440	12	77
ITALIAN VOLCANO														
Organic	8 oz	113	1	—	0	2	24	23	—	—	1	380	—	24
NATALIE'S ORCHID ISLAND JUICE														
100% Juice	8 oz	106	0	0	0	1	25	24	0	40	2	440	12	72
ODWALLA														
100% Juice	8 oz	110	0	0	0	1	25	25	0	40	0	450	—	78
SANTA CRUZ														
Organic Sparkling	8 oz	110	0	0	0	0	26	26	0	—	10	45	—	2

FOOD	PORTION	CALS	FAT	SAT FAT	CHOL	PROT	CARB	SUGAR	FIBER	CALCI	SOD	POTAS	FOLIC	VIT C
SSIPS														
Drink	1 box (7 oz)	120	0	0	0	0	31	30	—	—	10	—	—	—
TAPIOCA														
pearl dry	¼ cup (1.3 oz)	136	tr	tr	0	tr	34	1	tr	8	0	4	2	0
starch	1 oz	98	tr	—	—	17	24	—	—	3	1	6	—	0
LET'S DO ORGANIC														
Granulated	1 tbsp	35	0	0	0	0	9	0	0	0	0	—	—	0
Starch	1 tbsp	0	0	0	0	0	9	0	0	0	0	—	—	0
MON CHONG LOONG														
Starch	1 oz	110	0	0	0	0	26	0	0	20	0	—	—	0
TARO														
chips	10 (0.8 oz)	115	6	1	0	1	16	—	—	14	79	174	—	1
leaves cooked	½ cup	18	tr	tr	0	2	3	—	—	63	2	341	—	26
raw sliced	½ cup	56	tr	tr	0	1	14	—	—	22	6	307	—	2
shoots sliced cooked	½ cup	10	tr	tr	0	1	2	—	—	9	1	240	—	—
sliced cooked	½ cup (2.3 oz)	94	tr	tr	0	tr	23	—	—	12	10	319	—	3
tahitian sliced cooked	½ cup	30	tr	tr	0	3	5	—	—	101	37	423	—	26
TARPON														
fresh	3 oz	87	2	—	—	17	0	0	0	46	70	306	—	—
TARRAGON														
dried crumbled	1 tsp	2	tr	tr	0	tr	tr	—	0	7	0	18	2	tr
ground	1 tsp	5	tr	tr	0	tr	1	—	tr	18	1	48	4	1
TEA/HERBAL TEA														
(*see also* ICED TEA)														
HERBAL														
chamomile brewed	1 cup	2	tr	tr	0	0	tr	0	0	5	2	21	1	0
BAMBUSLAND														
Bamboo Tea Blueberry as prep	1 tea bag	0	0	0	0	0	1	0	0	—	0	—	—	—
Bamboo Tea Organic	1 tea bag	0	0	0	0	0	1	0	0	—	0	—	—	—
BIGELOW														
Cozy Chamomile	1 tea bag	0	0	0	0	0	0	0	0	—	0	25	—	—
CELESTIAL SEASONINGS														
Chamomile Honey Vanilla as prep	1 cup (8 oz)	0	0	0	0	0	0	0	0	—	0	—	—	—
Zinger Lemon as prep	1 cup	0	0	0	0	0	0	0	0	—	0	30	—	—
REGULAR														
brewed tea	1 cup (6 oz)	2	0	0	0	0	1	—	0	0	5	66	9	0

FOOD	PORTION	CALS	FAT	SATFAT	CHOL	PROT	CARB	SUGAR	FIBER	CALCI	SOD	POTAS	FOLIC	VIT C
DAILY DETOX														
Original	1 tea bag	0	0	0	0	0	0	0	0	—	0	—	—	—
EDEN														
Organic Bancha Green Tea	1 tea bag	0	0	0	0	0	0	0	0	0	0	0	—	0
Organic Hojicha Tea	1 tea bag	0	0	0	0	0	0	0	0	0	0	0	—	0
HANSEN'S														
Tea Stix Blackberry	½ pkg (2 g)	5	0	0	0	0	1	0	—	—	5	—	—	60
LIPTON														
Black Tea as prep	8 oz	0	0	0	0	0	0	0	0	—	0	25	—	—
Black Tea French Vanilla	1 tea bag	0	0	0	0	0	0	0	0	—	0	15	—	—
Black Tea Mint	1 tea bag	0	0	0	0	0	0	0	0	—	0	20	—	—
Black Tea Orange & Spice	1 tea bag	0	0	0	0	0	0	0	0	—	0	20	—	—
Black Tea Spiced Chai	1 tea bag	0	0	0	0	0	1	0	—	—	0	20	—	—
English Breakfast	1 tea bag	0	0	0	0	0	0	0	0	—	0	25	—	—
Green Tea as prep	1 cup (8 oz)	0	0	0	0	0	0	0	0	—	0	15	—	—
Green Tea Cranberry Pomegranate	1 tea bag	0	0	0	0	0	0	0	0	—	0	20	—	—
OREGON CHAI														
Chai Tea Latte Original Caffeine Free Concentrate	½ cup	78	0	0	0	0	18	17	—	—	8	—	—	—
Chai Tea Latte Original Concentrate	½ cup	78	0	0	0	0	19	18	—	0	8	—	—	0
Chai Tea Latte Spiced Original Mix	1 pkg	100	1	1	5	2	20	16	—	60	135	—	—	1
Chai Tea Latte Vanilla Mix	1 pkg	120	2	1	5	2	25	21	—	60	130	—	—	0
Organic Chai Cider Concentrate	½ cup	110	0	0	0	0	26	—	—	0	10	—	—	0
Organic Chai Nog Concentrate	½ cup	90	0	0	0	0	15	25	—	0	15	—	—	1
RED ROSE														
Black Tea	1 tea bag	0	0	0	0	0	0	0	0	—	0	—	—	—
English Breakfast Tea Bag as prep	1 cup	0	0	0	0	0	0	0	0	—	0	—	—	—

FOOD	PORTION	CALS	FAT	SAT FAT	CHOL	PROT	CARB	SUGAR	FIBER	CALCI	SOD	POTAS	FOLIC	VIT C
TASTEFULLY SIMPLE														
Oh My! Itty Bitty Chai Mix as prep w/water	1 pkg (1.2 oz)	140	3	3	0	2	25	22	0	80	60	—	—	0
TETLEY														
Classic Black as prep	1 tea bag	0	0	0	0	0	0	0	0	—	0	—	—	—
TAKE-OUT														
chai spiced latte	1 cup	130	3	1	0	2	23	18	0	80	45	—	—	0
TEMPEH														
tempeh	½ cup (2.9 oz)	160	9	2	0	15	8	—	—	92	7	342	20	0
LIGHTLIFE														
Organic Grilles Lemon	1 patty (2.7 oz)	140	6	2	0	11	11	2	0	—	280	—	—	—
Organic Grilles Tamari	1 patty (2.7 oz)	130	5	2	0	11	9	2	0	—	260	—	—	—
Organic Three Grain	1 serv (4 oz)	240	9	2	0	18	21	0	8	—	0	290	—	—
Organic Wild Rice	1 serv (4 oz)	280	11	2	0	19	14	0	10	—	10	240	—	—
WHITE WAVE														
Five Grain	⅓ block (2.7 oz)	160	6	1	0	12	15	1	7	60	10	—	—	0
WILDWOOD														
Organic Nori Seaweed	3 oz	170	7	1	0	13	16	2	4	100	0	0	—	2
TESTICLES														
prairie oysters cooked	1 pair (6.8 oz)	241	6	2	673	44	0	0	0	8	739	836	39	76
THYME														
dried crumbled	1 tsp	3	tr	tr	0	tr	1	tr	tr	19	1	8	3	1
fresh	1 tsp	1	tr	tr	0	tr	tr	—	tr	3	0	5	0	1
ground	1 tsp	4	tr	tr	0	tr	1	tr	1	26	1	11	4	1
TILAPIA														
BEACON LIGHT														
Boneless Fillet Farm Raised	1 (3 oz)	85	1	0	50	15	1	0	0	110	35	—	—	0
DR. PRAEGER'S														
Fillets Lightly Breaded	1 (4.5 oz)	220	9	tr	25	16	20	3	3	0	240	—	—	0
GORTON'S														
Grilled Fillets Roasted Garlic & Butter	1 (3 oz)	80	3	1	50	14	tr	—	—	—	150	280	—	—
HIGH LINER														
Loins	1 fillet (4 oz)	110	2	1	25	23	0	0	0	40	25	—	—	0

FOOD	PORTION	CALS	FAT	SAT FAT	CHOL	PROT	CARB	SUGAR	FIBER	CALCI	SOD	POTAS	FOLIC	VIT C
SEAPAK														
Tenders	2 (4 oz)	280	14	3	25	14	24	2	1	20	460	—	—	0
VAN DE KAMP'S														
Lightly Breaded Fillets	1 (4 oz)	240	11	3	35	16	17	tr	1	0	280	—	—	1
TAKE-OUT														
battered & fried	1 fillet (4 oz)	206	9	2	109	21	8	tr	tr	107	133	302	9	2
breaded & fried	1 fillet (4 oz)	300	14	3	142	26	16	2	1	138	708	359	13	2
broiled w/o fat	1 fillet (3.5 oz)	128	3	1	57	26	0	0	0	14	56	380	6	0
TILEFISH														
cooked	½ fillet (5.3 oz)	220	7	1	—	37	0	0	0	39	88	768	—	—
cooked	3 oz	125	4	1	—	21	0	0	0	22	50	435	—	—
raw	3 oz	81	2	tr	—	15	0	0	0	22	45	368	—	—
TOFU														
firm	¼ block (3 oz)	118	7	1	0	13	3	—	1	166	11	192	24	tr
firm	½ cup	183	11	2	0	20	5	—	2	258	17	298	37	tr
fresh fried	1 piece (0.5 oz)	35	3	tr	0	2	1	—	tr	48	2	19	4	0
fuyu salted & fermented	1 block (⅓ oz)	13	1	tr	0	1	1	—	tr	5	316	8	—	—
koyadofu dried frozen	1 piece (½ oz)	82	5	1	0	8	2	—	tr	62	1	3	16	tr
okara	½ cup	47	1	tr	0	2	8	—	1	49	6	130	—	0
regular	¼ block (4 oz)	88	6	1	0	9	2	—	1	122	8	141	17	tr
regular	½ cup	94	6	1	0	6	2	—	1	130	9	150	19	tr
AMY'S														
Organic Tofu Scramble w/ Hash Browns & Veggies	1 pkg (8.9 oz)	320	19	3	0	19	19	4	4	150	580	—	—	18
AZUMAYA														
Extra Firm	3 oz	70	4	0	0	8	2	0	1	150	20	—	—	0
Lite Extra Firm	⅕ pkg (2.8 oz)	60	2	0	0	7	3	0	1	300	30	—	—	0
Silken	⅕ pkg (3.2 oz)	40	2	0	0	4	1	0	tr	60	0	160	—	0
HOUSE														
Atsu-Age Cutlet	1 (2.5 oz)	100	5	1	0	11	2	0	5	200	10	—	—	0
Cut-Age Shredded Fried	1 serv (0.5 oz)	50	4	1	0	4	0	0	0	80	10	—	—	0
Ganmodoki Fritter Small	3 (1.6 oz)	120	9	2	0	7	2	0	0	150	105	—	—	0
Medium Firm	3 oz	60	3	0	0	7	1	0	tr	100	30	—	—	0
Organic Extra Firm	3 oz	90	5	1	0	11	0	0	0	150	20	—	—	0
Organic Firm	3 oz	60	3	0	0	8	0	0	0	100	20	—	—	0
Soft Silken	3 oz	50	3	0	0	5	2	0	tr	80	30	—	—	0
Steak Cajun	1 (3 oz)	40	1	0	0	12	1	0	tr	200	75	—	—	0

FOOD	PORTION	CALS	FAT	SAT FAT	CHOL	PROT	CARB	SUGAR	FIBER	CALCI	SOD	POTAS	FOLIC	VIT C
HOUSE (CONT.)														
Steak Grilled	1 (3 oz)	90	5	1	0	9	2	0	0	100	15	—	—	1
Sukui	3 oz	45	2	0	0	5	2	1	0	60	30	—	—	0
Tokusen Kinugoshi	1 piece (5 oz)	90	4	1	0	10	3	0	tr	40	30	—	—	0
Yaki Broiled	3 oz	90	5	1	0	9	2	0	0	100	15	—	—	1
NASOYA														
Extra Firm	⅕ pkg (2.8 oz)	80	4	1	0	8	2	0	1	60	0	—	—	0
Silken	⅕ pkg (3.2 oz)	160	1	0	0	4	1	0	0	60	0	—	—	0
Sprouted	3 oz	160	6	1	0	12	3	1	1	20	35	—	—	0
TOFUTOWN														
Tofu Tenders Havana Black Bean	½ pkg (5 oz)	210	8	1	0	15	18	13	2	100	690	—	—	0
Tofu Tenders Mediterranean Tahini	½ pkg (5 oz)	240	13	2	0	15	16	9	3	150	640	—	—	0
Tofu Tenders Sesame Ginger Teriyaki	½ pkg (5 oz)	240	9	0	0	15	24	16	3	100	680	—	—	0
TREE OF LIFE														
Organic Firm	½ block (3.2 oz)	110	5	0	0	11	4	0	2	150	5	—	—	0
WHITE WAVE														
Baked Garlic Herb Italian	1 piece (2 oz)	90	5	1	0	9	2	0	1	80	240	—	—	0
Baked Sesame Peanut Thai	1 piece (2 oz)	90	5	1	0	9	2	1	1	80	280	—	—	0
Baked Zesty Lemon Pepper	1 piece (2 oz)	90	5	1	0	9	3	1	1	80	200	—	—	0
Extra Firm	⅕ block (3.2 oz)	110	6	1	0	11	3	0	1	100	5	—	—	0
Organic Extra Firm	⅕ block (3.2 oz)	110	6	1	0	11	3	0	1	100	5	—	—	0
Organic Firm	⅓ block (3.2 oz)	110	6	1	0	11	3	0	1	80	5	—	—	0
Organic Soft	⅕ block (3.2 oz)	110	6	1	0	10	3	0	1	60	5	—	—	0
Reduced Fat	⅕ block (3.2 oz)	90	4	1	0	10	4	1	2	100	5	—	—	0
WILDWOOD														
Organic Baked Aloha	1 piece (3.5 oz)	180	5	1	0	20	15	2	3	100	239	0	—	1
Organic Calcium Rich Medium	3 oz	70	4	1	0	7	2	0	1	200	5	0	—	0
Organic Golden Pineapple Teriyaki	3 oz	160	12	2	0	13	5	3	1	0	230	0	—	0

FOOD	PORTION	CALS	FAT	SAT FAT	CHOL	PROT	CARB	SUGAR	FIBER	CALCI	SOD	POTAS	FOLIC	VIT C
WILDWOOD (CONT.)														
Organic High Protein Super Firm	3 oz	100	4	1	0	14	5	0	1	60	45	0	—	0
Organic Smoked Mild Szechuan	3 oz	150	6	1	0	14	11	4	2	0	368	0	—	0
TAKE-OUT														
breaded deep fried w/ soy sauce japanese style	1 piece (0.4 oz)	15	1	tr	1	0	1	0	tr	4	16	17	—	0
soy sauce marinated & grilled	1 serv (4 oz)	181	11	2	0	19	6	—	1	—	294	—	—	—
stir fried w/ vegetables	1 cup (7.6 oz)	186	10	1	0	5	21	—	3	99	782	334	45	6
TOMATILLO														
fresh	1 (1.2 oz)	11	tr	tr	0	tr	2	1	1	2	0	91	2	4
fresh chopped	½ cup (2.3 oz)	21	1	tr	0	1	4	3	1	5	1	177	5	8
TOMATO														
CANNED														
green pickled	½ cup (2.5 oz)	26	tr	tr	0	1	6	5	1	11	89	129	6	17
green whole pickled	1 (2.6 oz)	27	tr	tr	0	1	6	5	1	11	92	134	7	18
paste	1 can (6 oz)	139	1	tr	0	7	32	21	7	61	1343	1724	20	37
paste	¼ cup (2.3 oz)	54	tr	tr	0	3	12	8	3	24	517	664	8	14
paste no salt added	1 can (6 oz)	139	1	tr	0	7	32	21	7	61	167	1724	20	37
puree	1 can (28 oz)	312	2	tr	0	14	74	40	16	148	3280	3609	90	87
puree	1 cup (8.8 oz)	95	1	tr	0	4	22	12	5	45	998	1098	28	27
puree w/o salt	1 can (28 oz)	312	2	tr	0	14	74	40	16	148	230	3609	90	87
sauce	1 cup (8.6 oz)	59	tr	tr	0	3	13	10	4	32	1284	811	27	17
sauce no salt added	1 cup (8.6 oz)	102	tr	tr	0	3	21	13	4	34	27	905	22	32
stewed	1 cup (8.9 oz)	66	tr	tr	0	2	16	9	3	87	564	528	13	20
BELLA SUN LUCI														
Bruschetta w/ Italian Basil	¼ cup (1.9 oz)	190	17	3	<5	4	6	4	2	100	170	—	—	6
Sun Dried Halves w/ Italian Herbs	1 tbsp (0.7 oz)	70	5	1	0	1	6	3	1	20	10	—	—	6
Sun Dried Julienne Cut w/ Italian Herbs	1 tbsp (0.7 oz)	70	5	1	0	1	6	3	1	20	10	—	—	6
CENTO														
Crushed	¼ cup	35	0	0	0	2	7	4	2	0	20	180	0	4
Paste	2 tbsp (1.2 oz)	30	0	0	0	1	7	5	2	20	25	—	—	6
CONTADINA														
Paste Italian Herbs	2 tbsp	35	1	0	0	1	7	4	1	0	290	—	—	6

FOOD	PORTION	CALS	FAT	SAT FAT	CHOL	PROT	CARB	SUGAR	FIBER	CALCI	SOD	POTAS	FOLIC	VIT C
DEI FRATELLI														
Chopped Italian Tomatoes	½ cup (4.3 oz)	40	1	0	0	1	8	5	1	20	270	—	—	12
DEL MONTE														
Diced w/ Garlic & Onion	½ cup	40	1	0	0	2	8	6	tr	20	610	—	—	9
Organic Tomato Paste	2 tbsp	30	0	0	0	2	6	3	1	0	20	—	—	6
Petite Cut Garlic & Olive Oil	½ cup (4.4 oz)	40	1	0	0	1	9	6	1	20	450	280	—	9
HUNT'S														
Crushed	½ cup (4.2 oz)	45	0	0	0	2	9	4	3	0	230	370	—	6
Diced	½ cup (4.2 oz)	30	0	0	0	1	6	3	2	40	280	240	—	15
Diced Fire Roasted	½ cup (4.3 oz)	30	0	0	0	tr	6	3	2	20	280	260	—	4
Diced In Sauce	½ cup (4.3 oz)	35	0	0	0	1	7	3	2	40	310	300	—	12
Diced No Salt Added	½ cup (4.2 oz)	30	0	0	0	1	6	3	2	40	15	240	—	15
Diced Petite	½ cup (4.2 oz)	30	0	0	0	1	6	2	2	20	280	260	—	12
Diced w/ Roasted Garlic	½ cup (4.2 oz)	35	0	0	0	1	8	4	2	40	260	270	—	12
Stewed	½ cup (4.2 oz)	45	0	0	0	1	10	6	2	40	330	280	—	12
Stewed No Salt Added	½ cup (4.2 oz)	40	0	0	0	1	8	5	2	40	30	270	—	12
Whole	½ cup (4.2 oz)	25	0	0	0	1	5	3	2	20	180	250	—	15
Whole No Salt Added	½ cup (4.2 oz)	30	0	0	0	1	6	3	2	40	20	250	—	18
MUIR GLEN														
Organic Chunky Tomato & Herb	½ cup	60	1	0	0	2	11	5	2	20	350	—	—	9
Organic Diced Fire Roasted	½ cup	30	0	0	0	1	6	4	1	20	290	—	—	21
Organic Diced w/ Basil & Garlic	½ cup	30	0	0	0	1	6	4	1	20	290	—	—	21
POLAR														
Grape	½ cup	50	0	0	0	0	12	11	2	0	20	—	—	0
POMI														
Chopped	½ cup	20	0	0	0	1	4	4	3	0	10	—	—	15
PROGRESSO														
Crushed w/ Added Puree	¼ cup (2.1 oz)	20	0	0	0	1	4	2	1	40	95	—	—	9
Diced	½ cup (4.4 oz)	25	0	0	0	1	5	3	1	20	250	—	—	21
Puree	¼ cup (2.2 oz)	25	0	0	0	1	5	3	1	0	15	—	—	6
Whole Peeled w/ Basil	½ cup (4.2 oz)	20	0	0	0	1	4	3	1	20	260	—	—	9
REDPACK														
Crushed In Puree	¼ cup	20	0	0	0	0	4	2	1	0	120	—	—	6

FOOD	PORTION	CALS	FAT	SAT FAT	CHOL	PROT	CARB	SUGAR	FIBER	CALCI	SOD	POTAS	FOLIC	VIT C
REDPACK (CONT.)														
Crushed w/ Basil Garlic & Oregano	¼ cup (2.1 oz)	20	0	0	0	1	4	1	1	0	90	—	—	6
Diced In Juice	½ cup	25	0	0	0	1	5	3	1	40	220	—	—	9
Petite Diced Onion Celery & Green Pepper	½ cup	45	0	0	0	1	10	7	1	40	370	—	—	9
RIENZI														
Italian Cherry Tomatoes No Salt Added	⅓ can (4.5 oz)	30	0	0	0	1	6	4	1	20	60	—	—	21
S&W														
Crushed	¼ cup (2.1 oz)	20	0	0	0	1	4	2	1	20	125	—	—	6
Paste	2 tbsp (1.2 oz)	30	0	0	0	2	6	3	1	0	20	—	—	6
Petite Cut	½ cup (4.4 oz)	25	0	0	0	1	6	4	2	20	250	—	—	9
Puree	¼ cup (2.2 oz)	30	0	0	0	1	6	3	2	0	15	—	—	9
Ready-Cut Italian Recipe	½ cup (4.2 oz)	25	0	0	0	1	4	4	tr	40	190	—	—	9
Ready-Cut No Salt Added	½ cup (4.4 oz)	25	0	0	0	1	6	4	2	20	50	—	—	9
Stewed No Salt Added	½ cup (4.4 oz)	35	0	0	0	1	9	7	2	20	50	—	—	9
Stewed Original	½ cup (4.3 oz)	35	0	0	0	1	7	5	2	40	270	—	—	12
Whole Peeled	½ cup (4.4 oz)	25	0	0	0	1	6	4	2	20	250	—	—	9
DRIED														
sun dried	¼ cup (0.5 oz)	35	tr	tr	0	2	8	5	2	15	283	463	9	5
sun dried	1 piece (2 g)	5	tr	tr	0	tr	1	1	tr	2	42	69	1	1
sun dried in oil drained	1 piece (3 g)	6	tr	tr	0	tr	1	—	tr	1	8	47	1	3
sun dried in oil drained	¼ cup (1 oz)	59	4	1	0	1	6	—	2	13	73	430	6	28
tomato powder	1 oz	85	tr	tr	0	4	21	12	5	46	38	540	34	33
BELLA SUN LUCI														
Sun Dried w/ Italian Basil	⅐ pkg (0.5 oz)	35	0	0	0	2	6	4	1	0	35	—	—	5
Sun Dried w/ Zesty Peppers	⅐ pkg (0.5 oz)	35	0	0	0	2	6	4	1	0	35	—	—	5
FRESH														
bruschetta	¼ cup	50	3	0	0	2	6	4	tr	0	360	—	—	8
cherry	½ cup (2.6 oz)	13	tr	tr	0	1	3	2	1	7	1	64	11	10
cherry	1 (0.6 oz)	3	tr	tr	0	tr	1	tr	tr	2	1	40	3	2
grape tomatoes	20	30	0	0	0	1	6	4	1	0	0	250	—	27
green	1 lg (6.4 oz)	42	tr	tr	0	2	9	7	2	24	24	371	16	43
green	1 med (4.3 oz)	28	tr	tr	0	1	6	5	1	16	16	251	11	29
green	1 sm (3.2 oz)	21	tr	tr	0	1	5	4	1	12	12	186	8	21

FOOD	PORTION	CALS	FAT	SAT FAT	CHOL	PROT	CARB	SUGAR	FIBER	CALCI	SOD	POTAS	FOLIC	VIT C
green chopped	1 cup (6.3 oz)	41	tr	tr	0	2	9	7	2	23	23	367	16	42
orange	1 (4 oz)	18	tr	tr	0	1	4	—	1	6	47	235	32	18
orange chopped	1 cup (5.5 oz)	25	tr	tr	0	2	5	—	1	8	66	335	46	25
plum	1 (2.2 oz)	11	tr	tr	0	1	2	2	1	6	3	147	9	8
red	1 sm (3.2 oz)	16	tr	tr	0	1	4	2	1	9	5	216	14	12
red	1 med (4.3 oz)	22	tr	tr	0	1	5	3	2	12	6	292	18	16
red	1 lg (6.4 oz)	33	tr	tr	0	2	7	5	2	18	9	431	27	23
red chopped	½ cup (3.2 oz)	16	tr	tr	0	1	4	2	1	9	4	213	14	11
red slice	1 lg (0.9 oz)	5	tr	tr	0	tr	1	1	tr	3	4	64	4	3
roma	1 (2.2 oz)	11	tr	tr	0	1	2	2	1	6	3	147	9	8
yellow	1 (7.4 oz)	32	1	tr	0	2	6	—	2	23	49	547	64	19
yellow chopped	½ cup (2.4 oz)	10	tr	tr	0	1	2	—	1	8	16	179	21	6
EARTHBOUND FARMS														
Organic Roma	1 med (5.2 oz)	35	1	0	0	1	7	4	1	20	5	—	—	24
READY PAC														
Bruschetta	2 tbsp (1.6 oz)	70	7	1	0	0	3	1	1	0	250	—	—	5
TAKE-OUT														
aspic	½ cup (4 oz)	32	tr	tr	0	3	6	5	tr	11	242	216	19	21
broiled slices	2 (2.9 oz)	18	tr	tr	0	1	4	3	1	10	5	249	11	13
broiled whole	1 med (3.7 oz)	23	tr	tr	0	1	5	3	2	13	6	311	14	16
bruschetta on toasted italian bread	1 slice	106	3	0	0	4	18	2	tr	23	355	—	—	4
fried slices	2 (2.5 oz)	122	9	1	17	2	8	2	1	42	127	149	15	6
scalloped	½ cup (4 oz)	99	5	1	0	2	12	5	1	54	611	217	15	10
stewed	½ cup (1.8 oz)	40	1	tr	0	1	7	—	1	13	230	125	6	9
stuffed w/ rice	1 (5.2 oz)	110	3	1	0	2	20	3	2	19	396	270	40	18
stuffed w/ rice & meat	1 (5.2 oz)	142	6	2	18	7	15	3	2	21	437	320	33	15

TOMATO JUICE

FOOD	PORTION	CALS	FAT	SAT FAT	CHOL	PROT	CARB	SUGAR	FIBER	CALCI	SOD	POTAS	FOLIC	VIT C
tomato juice	1 cup (8.5 oz)	41	tr	tr	0	2	10	9	1	24	654	556	49	45
tomato juice w/o added salt	1 cup (8.5 oz)	41	tr	tr	0	2	10	9	1	24	24	556	49	45
CAMPBELL'S														
Healthy Request	8 oz	50	0	0	0	2	10	8	2	20	480	500	—	72
Low Sodium	8 oz	50	0	0	0	2	10	7	2	20	140	920	—	72
Organic	8 oz	50	0	0	0	2	10	7	2	20	680	430	—	72
DEI FRATELLI														
Tomato Juice	8 oz	40	0	0	0	2	10	0	1	20	450	—	—	48
LAKEWOOD														
Organic	8 oz	35	0	0	0	1	7	6	1	30	140	530	120	30
TREE OF LIFE														
Organic 100% Juice	8 oz	50	0	0	0	1	10	10	—	20	480	—	—	36

FOOD	PORTION	CALS	FAT	SAT FAT	CHOL	PROT	CARB	SUGAR	FIBER	CALCI	SOD	POTAS	FOLIC	VIT C
TONGUE														
beef simmered	3 oz	241	19	7	112	16	0	0	0	4	55	156	6	1
lamb braised	3 oz	234	17	7	161	18	0	0	0	9	57	134	3	6
pork braised	3 oz	230	16	5	124	20	0	0	0	16	93	201	3	1
veal braised	3 oz	172	9	4	202	22	0	0	0	8	54	138	8	5
RUMBA														
Beef	4 oz	250	18	8	95	17	4	0	0	0	75	—	—	5
TORTILLA														
corn	1 (6 in diam)	56	1	tr	0	1	12	—	1	44	40	39	4	0
corn w/o salt	1 (6 in diam)	56	1	tr	0	1	12	—	1	44	3	39	4	0
flour w/o salt	1 (8 in diam)	114	3	tr	0	3	20	—	1	44	167	46	4	0
FRENCH MEADOW BAKERY														
Fat Flush	1 (1 oz)	100	1	0	0	5	18	1	3	0	105	—	—	0
Gluten Free	1 (1.5 oz)	120	1	0	0	1	24	1	1	0	290	—	—	0
Hemp	1 (1.1 oz)	90	3	0	0	5	12	1	3	20	130	—	—	0
LA TORTILLA FACTORY														
Corn Chipotle	1 (1.4 oz)	90	1	0	0	5	14	0	1	60	210	—	—	0
Smart & Delicious 100 Calorie 100% Whole Wheat	1 (2 oz)	100	2	0	0	5	24	3	8	200	320	—	—	0
Smart & Delicious 100 Calorie Traditional	1 (2 oz)	100	2	0	0	5	24	0	8	200	320	—	—	0
Smart & Delicious Low Carb Whole Wheat	1 (2.2 oz)	80	3	0	0	8	18	1	12	60	300	35	—	0
White Corn	1 (1.4 oz)	90	1	0	0	5	14	0	1	60	190	—	—	0
RUDI'S ORGANIC BAKERY														
Spelt	1 (2 oz)	140	3	0	0	5	27	1	1	0	200	—	0	0
SALBA SMART														
Whole Wheat Omega-3 Enriched	1 (1.5 oz)	120	3	0	0	4	21	1	2	20	360	—	—	0
TUMARO'S														
Honey Wheat	1 (8 in)	110	2	0	0	3	23	1	2	100	135	—	—	0
Low In Carbs Garden Vegetable	1 (8 in)	100	3	0	0	7	12	1	8	80	115	—	—	0
Low In Carbs Green Onion	1 (8 in)	100	3	0	0	7	13	0	7	100	115	—	—	0
Low In Carbs Multi Grain	1 (8 in)	100	3	0	0	7	13	1	8	80	115	—	—	0
Low In Carbs Salsa	1 (8 in)	100	3	0	0	7	13	1	8	80	115	—	—	0
Pesto & Garlic	1 (8 in)	110	1	0	0	3	23	1	1	100	135	—	—	0
Premium White	1 (8 in)	120	2	0	0	3	23	1	tr	100	130	—	—	0

FOOD	PORTION	CALS	FAT	SAT FAT	CHOL	PROT	CARB	SUGAR	FIBER	CALCI	SOD	POTAS	FOLIC	VIT C
TUMARO'S (CONT.)														
Soy-full Heart 8 Grain 'N Soy	1 (1.4 oz)	100	0	0	0	6	14	1	4	100	60	—	—	0
Soy-full Heart Apple 'N Cinnamon	1 (1.4 oz)	90	3	0	0	6	13	1	4	150	65	—	—	0
Soy-full Heart Wheat Soy & Flax	1 (1.4 oz)	90	3	0	0	6	13	1	4	150	65	—	—	1
Spinach & Vegetables	1 (8 in)	110	2	0	0	3	23	1	1	100	140	—	—	1

TORTILLA CHIPS

(*see* CHIPS)

TRAIL MIX

FOOD	PORTION	CALS	FAT	SAT FAT	CHOL	PROT	CARB	SUGAR	FIBER	CALCI	SOD	POTAS	FOLIC	VIT C
BACK TO NATURE														
Bar Harbor Blend	1 oz	130	7	2	0	2	17	14	2	20	0	—	—	5
Harvest Blend	1 oz	150	10	1	0	5	12	7	3	40	5	—	—	0
Nantucket Blend	1 oz	130	7	1	0	3	15	11	3	40	25	—	—	4
Pacific Heights Blend	1 oz	160	11	3	0	4	13	9	3	40	40	—	—	2
BEAR NAKED														
Peak Chocolate Cherry	½ cup (1.1 oz)	120	5	1	0	2	21	11	2	0	0	45	—	0
Peak Pecan Apple Flax	½ cup (1.1 oz)	140	8	1	0	4	16	6	2	0	45	65	—	0
CRAISINS														
Cranberry & Chocolate	1 pkg (1.75 oz)	230	28	—	—	5	26	18	—	40	170	—	—	0
Fruit & Nuts	1 pkg (1.4 oz)	230	10	—	—	3	31	18	—	0	60	—	—	4
EMERALD														
Breakfast On The Go Berry Nut Blend	1 pkg (1.5 oz)	180	9	2	0	4	24	16	3	100	75	—	—	0
Breakfast On The Go Breakfast Nut Blend	1 pkg (1.5 oz)	180	7	2	0	3	27	20	3	100	75	—	—	0
Breakfast On The Go Smores Nut Blend	1 pkg (1.5 oz)	200	10	3	0	4	24	14	2	40	70	—	—	0
ENJOY LIFE														
Gluten Free Not Nuts! Beach Bash	1 oz	130	7	1	0	4	13	9	2	0	45	—	—	0
Gluten Free Not Nuts! Mountain Mambo	1 oz	140	8	2	0	5	12	9	2	0	45	—	—	0

FOOD	PORTION	CALS	FAT	SAT FAT	CHOL	PROT	CARB	SUGAR	FIBER	CALCI	SOD	POTAS	FOLIC	VIT C
FRITO LAY														
Nut & Fruit	1 oz	150	9	2	0	4	12	7	2	20	80	—	—	0
Original	3 tbsp	160	9	2	0	4	14	11	2	20	45	—	—	0
KOPALI														
Organic Mix	½ pkg (1 oz)	130	6	2	0	4	15	7	4	30	40	—	—	23
MRS. MAY'S														
Coconut Almond Crunch	1 oz	183	15	1	0	4	10	6	2	60	40	—	—	0
NAVITAS NATURALS														
3 Berry Cacao Nibs & Cashews	1 oz	110	5	2	0	3	16	8	4	20	45	—	—	24
Goji Cacao Nibs & Cashews	1 oz	120	6	2	0	4	13	7	3	20	70	—	—	4
Goji Golden Berry & Mulberry	1 oz	90	0	0	0	3	19	12	2	20	65	—	—	30
ORGANIC TRAILS														
Summit Blend	¼ cup	150	8	2	0	3	19	14	2	20	40	—	—	0
PLANTERS														
Berry Nut & Chocolate	3 tbsp (1 oz)	120	5	1	0	2	18	16	1	20	20	115	—	0
Daybreak Blend Berry & Almond	⅕ pkg (1.5 oz)	180	7	1	0	3	27	19	3	40	55	—	—	0
Energy Go-Paks	1 (1.5 oz)	250	20	3	0	6	14	6	3	40	135	—	—	0
Fruit & Nut	⅙ pkg (1 oz)	140	9	3	0	4	14	10	2	20	15	—	—	0
Sweet & Nutty	⅕ pkg (1.1 oz)	160	10	2	0	5	15	11	2	20	35	—	—	0
SUNRIDGE FARMS														
Cherry Pecan Vanilla Dream	¼ cup (1.4 oz)	200	12	3	0	5	20	13	3	60	10	—	—	30
Mountain Rainbow Mix	¼ cup (1 oz)	150	9	3	0	3	16	12	2	20	5	—	—	0
Organic Deluxe	¼ cup (1 oz)	140	8	1	0	4	13	9	2	20	10	—	—	1
SUNRISE														
Honey Coated	3 tbsp(1 oz)	137	6	1	1	5	14	9	4	30	67	—	—	0
W/ Fruit	3 tbsp (1 oz)	130	6	1	0	4	16	11	2	20	50	—	—	0
TREE FERN														
chopped cooked	½ cup	28	tr	—	0	tr	8	—	—	6	3	3	—	21
TRIPE														
beef simmered	3 oz	80	3	1	133	10	2	0	0	69	58	36	3	0
RUMBA														
Beef Tripe	4 oz	110	5	3	105	15	0	0	0	20	50	—	—	4
TAKE-OUT														
mondongo w/ potatoes	1 cup	300	11	3	148	24	26	5	6	123	1565	781	84	49
TRITICALE														
dry	½ cup (3.4 oz)	323	2	tr	0	13	69	—	—	36	5	319	70	0

FOOD	PORTION	CALS	FAT	SAT FAT	CHOL	PROT	CARB	SUGAR	FIBER	CALCI	SOD	POTAS	FOLIC	VIT C
TROUT														
baked	3 oz	162	7	1	63	23	0	0	0	47	57	393	13	tr
rainbow cooked	3 oz	129	4	1	62	22	0	0	0	73	29	539	—	3
seatrout baked	3 oz	113	4	1	90	18	0	0	0	19	63	372	—	—
TRUFFLES														
fresh	0.5 oz	4	tr	—	0	2	9	—	2	12	39	263	—	—
AUX DELICES DES BOIS														
Black Truffle Butter	0.5 oz	90	10	6	25	0	0	0	0	—	80	—	—	—
TUNA														
CANNED														
light in oil	3 oz	169	7	1	15	25	0	0	0	11	301	176	5	—
light in oil	1 can (6 oz)	399	14	3	30	50	0	0	0	23	606	354	9	—
light in water	1 can (5.8 oz)	192	1	tr	49	42	0	0	0	19	558	391	6	0
light in water	3 oz	99	1	tr	25	22	0	0	0	10	287	202	3	0
white in oil	1 can (6.2 oz)	331	14	—	55	47	0	0	0	8	704	593	8	—
white in oil	3 oz	158	7	—	26	23	0	0	0	4	336	283	4	—
white in water	3 oz	116	2	1	35	23	0	0	0	—	333	241	4	—
white in water	1 can (6 oz)	234	4	1	72	46	0	0	0	—	673	487	7	—
ARROYABE														
Bonito In Olive Oil	2 oz	109	5	0	0	16	0	0	0	20	290	—	—	0
BUMBLE BEE														
Sensations Lemon & Pepper w/ Crackers	1 pkg (3.6 oz)	200	8	4	25	19	13	2	0	40	460	—	—	1
Solid White Albacore In Water	¼ cup (2 oz)	60	1	0	25	13	0	0	0	—	180	105	—	—
CHICKEN OF THE SEA														
Albacore Solid White In Oil	2 oz	90	4	1	25	13	0	0	0	0	180	—	—	0
Albacore Solid White In Water	2 oz	80	4	0	25	11	0	0	0	0	180	—	—	0
Albarcore Chunk White In Water	½ can (2.5 oz)	50	1	0	25	11	0	0	0	0	180	—	—	0
Chunk Light 50% Less Sodium	2 oz	80	1	0	25	11	0	0	0	0	90	—	—	0
Chunk Light In Oil	2 oz	100	6	1	25	10	0	0	0	0	180	—	—	0
Chunk Light In Water	2 oz	50	1	0	25	11	0	0	0	0	180	—	—	0
Chunk White In Water Very Low Sodium	2 oz	50	1	0	25	12	0	0	0	0	35	—	—	0

FOOD	PORTION	CALS	FAT	SAT FAT	CHOL	PROT	CARB	SUGAR	FIBER	CALCI	SOD	POTAS	FOLIC	VIT C
GENOVA														
Tonno In Olive Oil	2 oz	110	6	1	25	13	0	0	0	0	250	—	—	0
POLAR														
Albacore Solid White In Water	2 oz	70	1	0	30	18	0	0	0	0	250	—	—	0
Chunk Light In Water	2 oz	60	1	0	25	13	0	0	0	0	250	—	—	0
PROGRESSO														
Albacore Solid White Olive Oil	¼ cup (2 oz)	90	3	1	20	16	0	0	0	0	330	—	—	0
Light Olive Oil drained	¼ cup (2 oz)	120	6	2	35	15	0	0	0	0	330	—	—	0
STARKIST														
Chunk Light In Water	¼ cup (2 oz)	60	5	0	30	13	0	0	0	0	250	—	—	0
Chunk Light In Water Flavor Pouch	1 pkg (3 oz)	90	1	0	45	19	0	0	0	—	380	—	—	—
Low Sodium Chunk White In Water	¼ cup (2 oz)	60	1	0	25	15	0	0	0	0	100	—	—	0
Solid Light In Water	2 oz	60	1	0	30	13	0	0	0	—	250	—	—	—
Solid White Albacore In Water	2 oz	70	1	0	25	15	0	0	0	—	250	—	—	—
Tuna Creations Hickory Smoked Flavor Pouch	2 oz	60	1	0	20	13	0	0	0	—	—	—	—	—
TONNINO														
Fillets In Olive Oil	2 oz	90	3	0	26	16	tr	0	0	0	260	—	—	0
Fillets In Olive Oil w/ Jalapeno	2 oz	80	5	0	20	13	1	0	tr	0	115	—	—	0
Fillets In Olive Oil w/ Oregano	2 oz	90	4	0	25	15	0	0	0	0	220	—	—	0
Fillets In Spring Water Wild Caught	2 oz	50	1	0	16	14	1	0	0	0	200	—	—	0
Ventresca In Olive Oil	2 oz	110	6	0	25	13	2	0	tr	0	190	—	—	0
TREE OF LIFE														
Wild Light Tongol Chunk In Spring Water No Salt Added	¼ cup (2.4 oz)	50	0	0	45	12	0	0	0	0	50	—	—	0
WILD PLANET														
Albacore Wild	2 oz	120	6	1	15	16	0	0	0	0	250	—	—	0

FOOD	PORTION	CALS	FAT	SAT FAT	CHOL	PROT	CARB	SUGAR	FIBER	CALCI	SOD	POTAS	FOLIC	VIT C
WILD PLANET (CONT.)														
Albacore Wild Fillet	2 oz	120	6	5	15	16	0	0	0	0	250	—	—	0
Albacore Wild No Salt	2 oz	120	6	1	15	16	0	0	0	0	100	—	—	0
Albacore Wild Smoked Troll Caught	2 oz	90	5	1	20	12	0	0	0	0	540	—	—	2
Skipjack Wild Light	2 oz	69	2	1	22	13	0	0	0	0	268	—	—	0
FRESH														
bluefin cooked	3 oz	157	5	1	42	25	0	0	0	—	43	275	—	—
bluefin raw	3 oz	122	4	1	32	20	0	0	0	—	33	214	—	—
skipjack baked	3 oz	112	1	tr	51	24	0	0	0	32	40	444	—	—
yellowfin baked	3 oz	118	1	tr	49	25	0	0	0	17	40	—	—	—
FROZEN														
SEAPAK														
Seasoned Ahi Steaks	1 (4.5 oz)	240	14	1	45	24	2	1	0	20	840	—	—	1
MIX														
STARKIST														
Lunch To-Go Chunk Light	1 pkg	310	9	3	40	20	27	8	2	—	720	—	—	—
TUNA HELPER														
Creamy Broccoli as prep	1 cup	310	11	3	12	6	39	2	2	100	912	280	80	—
Creamy Pasta as prep	1 cup	320	12	3	15	5	39	2	1	100	888	315	60	—
Tetrazzini as prep	1 cup	290	10	3	12	6	33	2	1	60	768	280	60	—
SHELF STABLE														
SEA FARE PACIFIC														
Albacore Wild Caught Jalapeno	⅓ pkg (2 oz)	160	13	3	15	11	0	0	0	0	200	—	—	0
Albacore Wild Caught Salt Free	⅓ pkg (2 oz)	100	6	2	20	16	0	0	0	0	30	—	—	0
Albacore Wild Caught Sea Salt	⅓ pkg (2 oz)	100	6	2	20	16	0	0	0	0	210	—	—	0
Albacore Wild Caught Smoked	⅓ pkg (2 oz)	100	6	2	10	16	0	0	0	0	210	—	—	0
TAKE-OUT														
tuna salad	1 cup	383	19	3	27	33	19	—	—	35	824	365	15	5
TURBOT														
european baked	3 oz	104	3	—	—	17	0	0	0	20	163	259	—	—

TURKEY

(see also JERKY, TURKEY DISHES, TURKEY SUBSTITUTES)

FOOD	PORTION	CALS	FAT	SAT FAT	CHOL	PROT	CARB	SUGAR	FIBER	CALCI	SOD	POTAS	FOLIC	VIT C
CANNED														
w/ broth	1 cup	220	9	3	89	32	0	0	0	16	630	302	8	3
HORMEL														
Chunk White & Dark	2 oz	70	3	1	45	11	0	0	0	0	270	—	—	0
Premium Chunk White	2 oz	60	2	1	35	11	0	0	0	0	230	—	—	0
VALLEY FRESH														
Chunk White	2 oz	80	2	1	55	16	0	0	0	0	150	—	—	0
FRESH														
breast roasted pre-basted w/ skin	3.5 oz	126	3	1	42	22	0	0	0	9	397	248	5	0
breast roasted w/ skin	4 oz	212	8	2	83	32	0	0	0	24	70	323	7	0
breast roasted w/o skin	4 oz	212	4	1	77	33	0	0	0	21	253	340	7	0
dark meat w/o skin roasted	3 oz	170	7	2	78	26	0	0	0	19	72	264	9	0
dark meat w/o skin roasted	1 cup (5 oz)	262	10	3	119	40	0	0	0	45	110	406	13	0
ground cooked	3 oz	193	11	3	84	22	0	0	0	20	88	221	6	0
leg w/ skin roasted	1 (19 oz)	1136	54	17	464	152	0	0	0	175	420	1529	49	0
light meat w/ skin roasted half turkey	2.3 lbs	2069	87	25	794	87	0	0	0	225	658	2996	61	0
light meat w/o skin roasted	4 oz	183	4	1	81	35	0	0	0	23	75	356	7	0
neck simmered	1 (5.3 oz)	274	11	4	186	41	0	0	0	56	84	226	12	0
skin roasted	1 oz	141	13	3	36	13	0	0	0	11	17	51	1	0
skin roasted from half turkey	8.7 oz	1096	98	26	281	49	0	0	0	87	132	396	10	0
tail cooked	1 (2 oz)	197	16	5	53	13	0	0	0	16	223	127	4	0
w/ skin roasted	½ turkey (4 lbs)	3857	181	53	1514	522	0	0	0	488	1269	5207	130	0
w/ skin roasted	1 serv (4.2 oz)	249	12	4	98	34	0	0	0	32	82	337	9	0
w/o skin roasted	1 cup (5 oz)	238	7	2	107	41	0	0	0	35	99	418	10	0
w/o skin roasted	1 serv (3.7 oz)	177	5	2	80	31	0	0	0	26	74	311	8	0
wing w/ skin roasted	1 (6.5 oz)	426	23	6	151	51	0	0	0	44	114	494	10	0
wing w/o skin roasted	1 (5.2 oz)	237	5	2	147	45	0	0	0	38	584	295	10	0
BUTTERBALL														
Burger Patties	1 (4 oz)	150	8	3	80	22	0	0	0	20	330	—	—	—
Cutlets	4 oz	120	1	0	70	28	0	0	0	—	55	—	—	—

FOOD	PORTION	CALS	FAT	SAT FAT	CHOL	PROT	CARB	SUGAR	FIBER	CALCI	SOD	POTAS	FOLIC	VIT C
BUTTERBALL (CONT.)														
Drumstick	4 oz	170	8	3	70	22	0	0	0	—	70	—	—	—
Ground 7% Fat	4 oz	150	8	4	80	22	0	0	0	—	95	—	—	—
Ground White	4 oz	130	4	1	75	26	0	0	0	—	75	—	—	—
Strips	4 oz	120	1	0	70	28	0	0	0	—	55	—	—	—
Thighs	4 oz	170	8	3	70	22	0	0	0	—	80	—	—	—
Wings	1 (6.3 oz)	380	25	7	115	36	0	0	0	—	90	—	—	—
EMPIRE														
Ground White	4 oz	160	8	3	65	23	0	0	0	40	125	—	—	0
FOSTER FARMS														
Breast Cutlets	4 oz	120	1	—	45	20	0	0	0	—	100	—	—	—
Necks	4 oz	150	6	—	90	23	0	0	0	40	105	—	—	—
Tails	4 oz	380	36	—	35	13	0	0	0	40	210	—	—	—
HONEYSUCKLE WHITE														
85% Lean Ground	4 oz	240	17	5	85	20	0	0	0	—	70	—	—	—
93% Lean Patties	1 (4 oz)	160	8	3	80	22	0	0	0	—	200	—	—	—
97% Lean Ground White	4 oz	130	2	1	65	26	0	0	0	—	70	—	—	—
99% Fat Free Breast Cutlets	4 oz	120	1	0	70	28	0	0	0	—	55	—	—	—
99% Fat Free Breast Tenderloin	4 oz	120	1	0	70	28	0	0	0	—	55	—	—	—
Drumettes	4 oz	180	8	2	75	24	0	0	0	—	75	—	—	—
Marinated Strips Asian Grill	4 oz	160	7	2	55	17	8	5	0	—	490	—	—	—
Necks	4 oz	150	6	2	90	23	0	0	0	—	105	—	—	—
Tenderloins Creamy Dijon Mustard	4 oz	140	4	0	50	21	0	0	0	—	500	—	—	—
Tenderloins Homestyle	4 oz	130	4	0	55	21	0	0	0	—	440	—	—	—
Tenderloins Teriyaki	4 oz	140	4	0	50	21	5	2	0	—	530	—	—	—
Thighs	4 oz	190	11	4	75	21	0	0	0	—	75	—	—	—
Whole Honey Roasted	4 oz	180	9	3	70	20	5	5	0	—	250	—	—	—
Wings	4 oz	220	14	4	80	23	0	0	0	—	60	—	—	—
PERDUE														
Breast Fillets Boneless Skinless cooked	3 oz	110	1	0	60	26	0	0	0	0	40	—	—	0
Drumsticks roasted	3 oz	140	7	2	125	21	0	0	0	0	250	—	—	6
Ground Breast cooked	3 oz	110	1	0	50	25	0	0	0	0	40	—	—	0
Patties cooked	1 (3 oz)	160	8	3	85	20	0	0	0	40	65	—	—	0

FOOD	PORTION	CALS	FAT	SAT FAT	CHOL	PROT	CARB	SUGAR	FIBER	CALCI	SOD	POTAS	FOLIC	VIT C
PERDUE (CONT.)														
Whole Dark Meat cooked	3 oz	190	11	4	90	21	0	0	0	0	70	—	—	0
Whole White Meat roasted	3 oz	150	7	3	65	23	0	0	0	0	50	—	—	0
Whole Breast Bone-In Seasoned	4 oz	140	7	2	75	20	1	0	0	20	410	—	—	0
SHADY BROOK														
Breast Tenderloin Lemon Garlic	4 oz	130	4	0	55	21	4	1	0	20	460	—	—	1
Breast Tenderloin Rotisserie	4 oz	130	4	0	50	21	4	1	0	20	700	—	—	1
Tenderloin Zesty Italian Herb	4 oz	130	4	0	50	21	4	2	0	20	490	—	—	2
FROZEN														
roast boneless seasoned light & dark meat roasted	3.5 oz	155	6	2	53	21	3	0	0	5	680	298	5	0
sticks breaded fried	1 (2.2 oz)	179	11	3	41	9	11	—	—	9	536	166	19	0
BUTTERBALL														
Boneless Roast	4 oz	130	5	2	65	22	0	0	0	—	460	—	—	—
Breast Boneless Roast	4 oz	110	3	1	45	21	1	0	0	—	500	—	—	—
Breast Tenderloin Teriyaki	4 oz	110	1	0	55	21	4	3	—	60	780	—	—	—
Breast Whole	4 oz	110	3	1	45	21	1	1	0	—	500	—	—	—
Breast Whole Smoked Cooked	3 oz	120	5	2	45	18	1	1	0	—	650	—	—	—
Whole Turkey	1 serv (4 oz)	170	10	4	70	20	0	0	0	—	320	—	—	—
Whole Turkey Baked	3 oz	130	7	2	45	17	0	0	0	—	580	—	—	—
HONEYSUCKLE WHITE														
Breast Boneless Roast	4 oz	170	7	3	60	21	0	0	0	—	700	—	—	—
JENNIE-O														
Burger	1 (4 oz)	160	9	2	100	19	0	0	0	60	90	—	—	2
ORGANIC PRAIRIE														
Whole Young	4 oz	90	10	3	70	23	0	0	0	0	70	—	—	0
READY-TO-EAT														
bologna	1 slice (1 oz)	59	4	1	21	3	1	1	tr	34	351	38	3	4
breast	1 slice (0.7 oz)	22	tr	tr	9	4	1	1	tr	2	213	63	1	1
ham	1 slice (1 oz)	35	1	tr	20	5	1	tr	tr	2	312	80	2	3
pastrami	2 oz	70	2	1	39	9	2	2	tr	6	559	197	3	9
salami	1 slice (1 oz)	48	3	1	21	5	tr	tr	0	11	281	60	3	0
APPLEGATE FARMS														
Organic Herb	2 oz	50	1	0	30	11	0	0	0	0	420	—	—	0

FOOD	PORTION	CALS	FAT	SAT FAT	CHOL	PROT	CARB	SUGAR	FIBER	CALCI	SOD	POTAS	FOLIC	VIT C
BOAR'S HEAD														
Breast Cracked Pepper Smoked	2 oz	60	1	0	30	13	1	1	0	0	460	—	—	0
BUTTERBALL														
Breast Honey Roasted Thick Sliced	1 slice (1 oz)	35	1	0	15	5	2	1	0	—	280	—	—	—
Breast Oven Roasted Extra Thin Slice	7 slices (2 oz)	70	2	1	25	10	3	2	0	—	580	—	—	—
Breast Smoked Thin Sliced	4 slices (1.9 oz)	70	2	1	25	7	4	2	0	0	560	—	—	0
Breast Strips Oven Roasted	½ pkg (3 oz)	90	1	1	40	18	2	—	—	—	750	—	—	—
Deep Fried Original Thick Sliced	1 slice (1 oz)	30	1	0	15	5	1	0	0	0	260	—	—	0
CARL BUDDIG														
Honey Roasted Sliced	2 oz	90	5	—	—	9	2	—	—	—	—	—	—	—
Turkey Sliced	2 oz	90	5	—	—	9	tr	—	—	—	—	—	—	—
FOSTER FARMS														
Breast Honey Roasted	1 slice (1 oz)	25	0	0	10	6	1	1	0	—	240	—	—	—
Breast Oven Roasted	1 slice (1 oz)	30	0	0	10	6	0	0	0	—	220	—	—	—
HEALTHY ONES														
Oven Roasted 97% Fat Free	7 slices (2 oz)	60	2	1	20	9	2	tr	—	0	460	—	—	0
HONEYSUCKLE WHITE														
Simply Done Whole Breast	4 oz	160	7	2	60	21	2	0	0	—	500	—	—	—
HORMEL														
Natural Choice Deli Turkey Honey	4 slices (2 oz)	60	1	0	25	10	3	3	0	0	440	—	—	0
Natural Choice Deli Turkey Oven Roasted	4 slices (2 oz)	60	1	0	25	10	3	3	0	0	440	—	—	0
Natural Choice Deli Turkey Smoked	4 slices (2 oz)	60	1	0	25	10	3	3	0	0	440	—	—	0
OSCAR MAYER														
Breast Smoked Shaved	2 oz	50	1	0	20	8	2	0	0	0	570	—	—	0
RUSSER														
Turkey Breast Honey Roasted	1 slice (1 oz)	25	1	0	10	5	1	1	0	0	190	—	—	0

FOOD	PORTION	CALS	FAT	SAT FAT	CHOL	PROT	CARB	SUGAR	FIBER	CALCI	SOD	POTAS	FOLIC	VIT C
SARA LEE														
Breast Cracked Pepper	4 slices (1.8 oz)	50	1	0	25	9	1	0	0	0	480	—	—	0
Breast Hardwood Smoked	4 slices (1.8 oz)	50	1	0	20	11	1	0	0	0	490	—	—	0
SHADY BROOK														
Hickory Smoked Breast Fat Free	2 oz	50	0	0	25	11	1	1	—	—	470	—	—	—
Turkey Ham Smoked	2 oz	60	2	1	30	9	0	0	0	—	590	—	—	—
TYSON														
Breast Oven Roasted	2 slices (1.6 oz)	40	1	0	15	8	1	0	0	0	560	—	—	0

TURKEY DISHES

FROZEN

FOOD	PORTION	CALS	FAT	SAT FAT	CHOL	PROT	CARB	SUGAR	FIBER	CALCI	SOD	POTAS	FOLIC	VIT C
gravy & turkey	1 cup (8.4 oz)	160	6	2	—	14	11	—	—	33	1328	—	—	—

TAKE-OUT

FOOD	PORTION	CALS	FAT	SAT FAT	CHOL	PROT	CARB	SUGAR	FIBER	CALCI	SOD	POTAS	FOLIC	VIT C
boneless breast w/ cranberry apple stuffing	1 serv (5 oz)	260	9	2	80	32	10	2	1	30	250	—	—	1
turkey a la king	1 cup (8.5 oz)	465	34	12	190	24	16	4	1	149	880	429	34	6
turkey creole w/o rice	1 cup	189	4	1	69	29	9	5	2	52	585	662	17	24
turkey croquette	1 (2 oz)	158	9	2	28	10	8	2	tr	45	226	126	11	1
turkey divan	1 cup	321	14	6	135	40	9	2	3	269	387	434	40	40
turkey fricassee	1 cup	322	18	5	85	29	8	tr	tr	20	693	295	22	0
turkey meatloaf	1 lg slice (5 oz)	243	9	3	122	29	11	3	1	73	658	312	29	5
turkey salad	1 cup	417	32	6	100	29	3	1	1	38	288	318	25	2
turkey tetrazzini	1 cup	369	18	6	49	19	29	2	2	130	657	204	59	5

TURKEY SUBSTITUTES

WORTHINGTON

FOOD	PORTION	CALS	FAT	SAT FAT	CHOL	PROT	CARB	SUGAR	FIBER	CALCI	SOD	POTAS	FOLIC	VIT C
Turkee Slices	3 slices (3.3 oz)	180	12	2	0	14	5	1	0	100	530	50	—	0

YVES

FOOD	PORTION	CALS	FAT	SAT FAT	CHOL	PROT	CARB	SUGAR	FIBER	CALCI	SOD	POTAS	FOLIC	VIT C
Meatless Ground Turkey	⅓ cup	60	1	0	0	12	8	0	2	40	330	230	—	0
Meatless Deli Turkey Slices	4 slices	100	2	0	0	16	5	tr	0	20	340	230	—	9

TURMERIC

FOOD	PORTION	CALS	FAT	SAT FAT	CHOL	PROT	CARB	SUGAR	FIBER	CALCI	SOD	POTAS	FOLIC	VIT C
ground	1 tsp	8	tr	tr	0	tr	1	tr	tr	4	1	56	1	1

TURNIPS

FOOD	PORTION	CALS	FAT	SAT FAT	CHOL	PROT	CARB	SUGAR	FIBER	CALCI	SOD	POTAS	FOLIC	VIT C
canned greens	½ cup	17	tr	tr	0	2	3	—	—	138	325	165	48	18
cooked mashed	½ cup (4.2 oz)	47	tr	tr	0	2	10	—	—	58	25	391	19	23
cubed cooked	½ cup (3 oz)	33	tr	tr	0	1	7	—	—	41	17	277	13	17
fresh greens chopped cooked	½ cup	15	tr	tr	0	1	3	—	2	99	21	146	85	20

FOOD	PORTION	CALS	FAT	SAT FAT	CHOL	PROT	CARB	SUGAR	FIBER	CALCI	SOD	POTAS	FOLIC	VIT C
frzn greens cooked	½ cup	24	tr	tr	0	3	4	—	2	125	12	184	32	18
greens raw chopped	½ cup	7	tr	tr	0	tr	2	—	1	53	11	83	54	17
raw cubed	½ cup (2.4 oz)	25	tr	tr	0	1	6	—	—	39	14	236	14	18
ALLENS														
Seasoned	½ cup	35	1	0	0	4	5	1	2	150	860	—	—	9
GLORY														
Greens Fresh	2 cups	20	0	0	0	1	5	tr	3	150	30	—	—	48
Greens Seasoned canned	½ cup	35	0	0	0	1	4	1	2	80	490	—	—	18
Root Cut Fresh	½ cup	20	0	0	0	1	4	2	1	20	45	—	—	15
Sensibly Seasoned Greens	½ cup	20	0	0	0	1	4	0	2	100	240	—	—	18

TURTLE

FOOD	PORTION	CALS	FAT	SAT FAT	CHOL	PROT	CARB	SUGAR	FIBER	CALCI	SOD	POTAS	FOLIC	VIT C
raw	3.5 oz	85	1	—	—	18	0	0	0	107	—	235	—	—

TUSK FISH

FOOD	PORTION	CALS	FAT	SAT FAT	CHOL	PROT	CARB	SUGAR	FIBER	CALCI	SOD	POTAS	FOLIC	VIT C
raw	3.5 oz	79	tr	—	—	17	0	0	0	17	113	328	tr	—

VANILLA

FOOD	PORTION	CALS	FAT	SAT FAT	CHOL	PROT	CARB	SUGAR	FIBER	CALCI	SOD	POTAS	FOLIC	VIT C
vanilla extract	1 tbsp (0.5 oz)	37	tr	tr	0	tr	2	2	0	1	1	19	0	0
vanilla extract	1 tsp (4.2 g)	12	0	0	0	0	1	1	0	0	0	6	0	0
vanilla extract alcohol free	1 tsp (4.2 g)	2	0	0	0	0	1	1	0	0	0	0	0	0
BOB'S RED MILL														
Organic Extract	1 tsp	0	0	0	0	0	0	0	0	—	0	—	—	—
NIELSEN-MASSEY														
Madagascar Bourbon Extract	1 tsp	11	tr	tr	tr	tr	tr	tr	tr	16	1	—	—	tr

VEAL

(*see also* VEAL DISHES)

FOOD	PORTION	CALS	FAT	SAT FAT	CHOL	PROT	CARB	SUGAR	FIBER	CALCI	SOD	POTAS	FOLIC	VIT C
breast braised	3 oz	226	14	6	96	23	0	0	0	8	55	231	11	—
chop breaded fried	1 med (6.5 oz)	290	12	4	142	35	13	0	tr	50	577	471	34	0
chop cooked	1 med (6.5 oz)	230	13	6	109	26	0	0	0	20	444	345	16	0
cubed braised	3 oz	160	4	1	123	30	0	0	0	25	79	291	14	0
cutlet cooked	3 oz	141	4	1	83	26	0	0	0	5	311	342	12	0
ground broiled	3 oz	146	6	3	88	21	0	0	0	14	71	286	9	0
leg roasted	3 oz	136	4	2	88	24	0	0	0	5	58	331	14	0
loin roasted	3 oz	184	10	4	88	21	0	0	0	16	79	276	13	0
patty breaded fried	1 (2.8 oz)	211	13	4	80	16	7	1	tr	31	329	224	16	0
shank braised	3 oz	162	5	2	105	27	0	0	0	28	79	259	14	—

VEAL DISHES

TAKE-OUT

FOOD	PORTION	CALS	FAT	SAT FAT	CHOL	PROT	CARB	SUGAR	FIBER	CALCI	SOD	POTAS	FOLIC	VIT C
cordon bleu	1 serv (8 oz)	490	35	19	172	33	4	2	1	153	552	497	25	4
marengo	1 serv (8.8 oz)	274	9	3	118	33	7	3	1	23	607	733	30	9

FOOD	PORTION	CALS	FAT	SAT FAT	CHOL	PROT	CARB	SUGAR	FIBER	CALCI	SOD	POTAS	FOLIC	VIT C
marsala	1 slice + sauce (3.4 oz)	268	19	9	69	12	6	2	tr	15	191	211	12	2
paprikash	1 serv (8.6 oz)	280	12	5	138	36	5	1	1	37	829	689	27	2
parmigiana	1 serv (6.4 oz)	362	21	8	146	27	15	3	2	187	790	515	31	4
picatta	1 piece + sauce (3.5 oz)	154	9	5	72	16	2	tr	tr	8	546	195	11	tr
scallopini	1 slice + sauce (3.4 oz)	238	17	5	64	18	2	1	tr	44	304	250	12	1
stew	1 serv (8.8 oz)	192	6	3	50	15	18	4	3	40	605	547	35	12

VEGETABLE JUICE

FOOD	PORTION	CALS	FAT	SAT FAT	CHOL	PROT	CARB	SUGAR	FIBER	CALCI	SOD	POTAS	FOLIC	VIT C
low sodium tomato & vegetable juice	1 cup	53	tr	tr	0	1	11	9	2	27	169	467	51	67
vegetable juice cocktail	8 oz	46	tr	tr	0	2	11	8	2	27	653	467	51	67
BOLTHOUSE FARMS														
Vedge Tomato Carrot Celery	8 oz	60	0	0	0	3	11	9	2	40	440	640	—	42
DEI FRATELLI														
Vegetable Juice	8 oz	45	2	0	0	2	11	9	1	20	600	—	—	48
GREEN TO GO														
100% Natural Organic as prep	1 pkg (0.3 oz)	32	tr	0	0	1	6	1	tr	23	12	93	—	28
LAKEWOOD														
Super Veggie	6 oz	40	0	0	0	2	9	6	4	40	135	455	100	45
MOTT'S														
100% Juice Veggie Blend	1 bottle (14 oz)	90	1	0	0	5	15	9	4	40	790	1240	—	60
V8														
100% Juice Low Sodium	8 oz	50	0	0	0	2	10	7	2	20	140	900	—	72
100% Vegetable Essential Antioxidants	8 oz	50	0	0	0	2	11	6	2	40	480	430	—	120
Calcium Enriched	8 oz	50	0	0	0	2	11	8	2	300	460	680	—	72
High Fiber	8 oz	60	0	0	0	2	13	8	5	40	480	470	—	72
Low Sodium Spicy Hot	8 oz	50	0	0	0	2	11	8	2	20	140	1000	—	60
Vegetable Juice Original	8 oz	50	0	0	0	0	10	8	2	40	420	470	—	72
WALNUT ACRES														
Organic Incredible Vegetable	8 oz	50	0	0	0	2	12	11	1	40	580	—	—	12

VEGETABLES MIXED

CANNED

FOOD	PORTION	CALS	FAT	SAT FAT	CHOL	PROT	CARB	SUGAR	FIBER	CALCI	SOD	POTAS	FOLIC	VIT C
mixed vegetables	½ cup	39	tr	tr	0	2	8	—	—	22	122	239	19	4

FOOD	PORTION	CALS	FAT	SAT FAT	CHOL	PROT	CARB	SUGAR	FIBER	CALCI	SOD	POTAS	FOLIC	VIT C
peas & carrots	½ cup (4.5 oz)	48	tr	tr	0	3	11	—	3	29	332	128	23	8
peas & onions	½ cup (2.1 oz)	31	tr	tr	0	2	5	—	1	10	265	58	16	2
succotash	½ cup	102	1	tr	0	4	23	—	—	15	325	243	59	9
DEL MONTE														
Savory Sides Homestyle Vegetable Medley	½ cup	70	3	0	0	1	11	3	2	40	380	—	—	5
Savory Sides Rio Grande Vegetables	½ cup	70	0	0	0	2	14	3	2	20	470	—	—	6
MCSWEET														
Giardiniera	5 pieces (1 oz)	25	0	0	0	0	6	5	tr	20	240	—	—	12
S&W														
Mixed	½ cup (4.4 oz)	45	0	0	0	2	10	3	2	40	360	—	—	6
Peas & Pearl Onions	½ cup (4.3 oz)	40	0	0	0	3	11	1	3	0	530	—	—	9
THE GRACIOUS GOURMET														
Tapenade Fennel Blood Orange	2 tbsp (1 oz)	50	5	1	0	0	3	1	tr	20	190	—	—	6
VEG-ALL														
Original Mixed	½ cup	40	0	0	0	1	8	2	2	20	290	—	—	5
DRIED														
CRUNCHIES														
Freeze Dried Power Veggies Buttered	½ cup (0.7 oz)	110	3	0	0	6	17	6	4	20	300	—	—	15
Freeze Dried Power Veggies Herb Spiced	½ cup (0.7 oz)	110	3	0	0	6	17	6	5	40	110	—	—	15
Freeze Dried Roasted Veggies	⅝ cup (1 oz)	100	1	0	0	4	21	10	2	30	35	—	—	90
Freeze Dried Roasted Veggies BBQ	½ cup (0.8 oz)	100	2	0	0	3	20	7	4	0	260	—	—	60
FUN-YUMS														
Fresh Crispy Mixed Veggies	1 serv (0.9 oz)	114	4	2	—	1	18	2	1	25	48	—	—	tr
FRESH														
DOLE														
Stir Fry Medley	1 cup (3 oz)	30	0	0	0	2	7	3	2	40	35	—	40	48
Vegetable Medley	3 oz	30	0	0	0	2	6	2	2	40	35	—	—	42
MANN'S														
Broccoli & Carrots	1 serv (3 oz)	25	0	0	0	2	5	3	2	40	25	260	48	48
Broccoli & Cauliflower	1 serv (3 oz)	25	0	0	0	2	4	2	2	40	25	270	56	60
California Stir Fry	1 serv (3 oz)	30	0	0	0	2	6	3	2	40	30	220	32	42

FOOD	PORTION	CALS	FAT	SAT FAT	CHOL	PROT	CARB	SUGAR	FIBER	CALCI	SOD	POTAS	FOLIC	VIT C
MANN'S (CONT.)														
Low Mein Stir Fry	1 serv (3 oz)	80	1	0	0	3	14	5	2	40	250	—	—	42
Medley	1 serv (3 oz)	25	0	0	0	2	5	3	2	20	25	270	44	48
READY PAC														
Carrots & Celery w/ Ranch Dressing	1 pkg (7 oz)	250	21	2	15	2	14	8	3	80	500	—	—	9
Ready Fixin's Chop Suey	1½ cups (3 oz)	15	0	0	0	1	2	1	1	60	45	—	—	27
FROZEN														
mixed vegetables cooked	½ cup	54	tr	tr	0	3	12	—	2	22	32	154	17	3
peas & carrots cooked	½ cup (2.8 oz)	38	tr	tr	0	3	8	3	3	18	54	126	21	7
peas & carrots creamed	½ cup (4.3 oz)	111	6	2	4	4	12	5	2	79	235	192	22	6
succotash cooked	½ cup	79	1	tr	0	4	17	—	—	13	38	225	28	5
BIRDS EYE														
Asparagus Gold & White Corn & Baby Carrots	⅔ cup	70	1	0	0	2	13	4	1	20	15	—	—	5
Italian Herb Harvest Vegetables	1¼ cups	90	6	4	15	2	6	3	2	40	150	—	—	30
Spring Vegetables In Citrus Sauce	1¼ cups	70	4	2	10	2	8	4	2	40	280	—	—	12
Steamfresh Asian Medley	1 cup (3.3 oz)	50	2	0	0	2	6	3	2	40	310	—	—	15
Steamfresh Broccoli Cauliflower & Carrots	¾ cup	30	0	0	0	1	5	2	2	20	30	—	—	18
Steamfresh Broccoli & Cauliflower	1 cup	30	0	0	0	1	4	2	2	20	25	—	—	30
Steamfresh Broccoli Carrots Sugar Snap Peas & Water Chestnuts	¾ cup (2.9 oz)	35	0	0	0	1	6	3	2	20	25	—	—	15
Steamfresh Mixed Vegetables	⅔ cup (3.2 oz)	40	0	0	0	2	12	4	2	20	20	—	—	5
C&W														
Early Harvest Peas & Baby Carrots	⅔ cup	60	0	0	0	3	10	4	3	20	150	—	—	5
Petite Peas & Pearl Onions	⅔ cup	60	0	0	0	4	11	4	3	20	160	—	—	6

FOOD	PORTION	CALS	FAT	SAT FAT	CHOL	PROT	CARB	SUGAR	FIBER	CALCI	SOD	POTAS	FOLIC	VIT C
CASCADIAN FARM														
Organic Peas & Carrots	⅔ cup	50	0	0	0	2	10	4	3	20	75	140	—	5
Organic Mixed Vegetables	⅔ cup	60	0	0	0	2	12	4	2	20	20	150	—	5
FRENCH MEADOW BAKERY														
Vegetarian Sweet N' Spicy Cuban Style Veggies	1 pkg (12 oz)	250	9	2	0	6	39	9	7	60	450	—	—	30
GREEN GIANT														
Garden Vegetable Medley as prep	½ cup	70	1	0	0	2	14	3	2	20	220	—	—	15
Mixed Vegetables as prep	½ cup	50	0	0	0	2	11	3	2	0	20	—	—	4
Southwestern Style as prep	½ cup	90	1	0	0	4	18	3	4	0	190	—	—	18
Steamers Basil Vegetable Medley as prep	¾ cup	45	1	0	0	2	10	5	2	20	270	320	—	15
Szechuan Vegetables as prep	½ cup	50	1	0	0	2	9	5	2	20	410	—	—	21
HEALTH IS WEALTH														
Veggie Munchees Vegan	6 (3 oz)	150	4	0	0	4	26	2	3	20	500	—	—	12
LA CHOY														
Chop Suey Vegetables	½ cup (2.2 oz)	15	0	0	0	tr	3	1	tr	0	640	—	—	15
Fancy Chinese Mixed Vegetables	½ cup (2.9 oz)	15	2	0	0	1	3	0	1	0	60	—	—	15
Stir Fry Vegetables	½ cup	15	0	0	0	tr	3	1	2	0	180	—	—	18
MCKENZIE'S														
Okra Tomatoes w/ Onions	1 serv (2.8 oz)	20	0	0	0	1	4	2	2	—	30	—	—	—
MELROSE MADE GOURMET														
Vegetable Souffle Fat Free	1 serv (4 oz)	70	0	0	0	12	5	2	3	80	530	—	—	24
SEAPOINT FARMS														
Organic Veggie Blends w/ Edamame Eat Your Greens	¾ cup	60	2	0	0	5	7	tr	3	60	30	—	—	24
Veggie Blends w/ Edamame Garden	¾ cup	60	2	0	0	4	7	2	3	40	25	—	—	27
Veggie Blends w/ Edamame Oriental	¾ cup	60	1	0	0	4	8	2	3	20	80	—	—	12

FOOD	PORTION	CALS	FAT	SAT FAT	CHOL	PROT	CARB	SUGAR	FIBER	CALCI	SOD	POTAS	FOLIC	VIT C
TAKE-OUT														
buddha's delight	1 serv (16 oz)	174	5	1	35	17	17	8	3	109	1368	668	161	64
fukujinzuke japanese pickled vegetables	1 tbsp (6 g)	8	0	0	0	0	2	—	0	3	180	7	tr	0
pakoras	4 (1.7 oz)	57	2	tr	0	2	7	1	2	14	530	119	61	2
ratatouille	1 serv (3.5 oz)	96	7	1	0	2	7	7	4	32	812	468	36	50
samosa	1 (2.4 oz)	206	11	5	12	4	22	1	2	25	311	148	—	1
stir fry mixed vegetables	1 serv (4 oz)	66	5	1	0	3	3	2	2	25	292	138	—	18
succotash	½ cup	111	1	tr	0	5	23	—	—	16	16	393	—	8

VENISON

(see also JERKY)

FOOD	PORTION	CALS	FAT	SAT FAT	CHOL	PROT	CARB	SUGAR	FIBER	CALCI	SOD	POTAS	FOLIC	VIT C
cubed stewed	1 cup (5 oz)	266	6	3	157	51	0	0	0	8	375	435	15	0
hamburger grilled	1 (3.3 oz)	174	8	4	91	25	0	0	0	13	73	339	7	0
loin steak lean only broiled	1 (2 oz)	81	1	tr	43	16	0	0	0	3	31	215	5	0
shoulder lean only braised	3 oz	162	3	2	96	31	0	0	0	5	44	266	9	0
tenderloin roasted	3 oz	127	2	1	75	25	0	0	0	4	48	369	8	0
top round lean only broiled	3 oz	129	2	1	72	27	0	0	0	3	38	320	8	0
TAKE-OUT														
meatloaf	1 lg slice (5 oz)	238	10	4	125	27	9	2	1	63	576	442	19	1
stew w/ potatoes & vegetables	1 cup (8.8 oz)	179	2	1	48	19	22	5	4	38	544	713	38	27

VINEGAR

FOOD	PORTION	CALS	FAT	SAT FAT	CHOL	PROT	CARB	SUGAR	FIBER	CALCI	SOD	POTAS	FOLIC	VIT C
balsamic	1 tbsp	14	0	0	0	tr	3	2	—	4	4	18	—	0
cider	1 tbsp	3	0	0	0	0	tr	tr	0	1	1	11	0	0
coconut	1 tbsp (0.5 oz)	1	tr	—	—	0	tr	—	—	3	—	—	—	—
red wine	1 tbsp	3	0	0	0	tr	tr	0	0	1	1	6	—	tr
white	1 tbsp	3	0	0	0	0	tr	tr	0	1	0	0	0	0
BARENGO														
Balsamic	1 tbsp (0.5 oz)	15	0	0	0	0	4	4	—	—	0	—	—	—
Red Wine	1 tbsp (0.5 oz)	0	0	0	0	0	0	0	0	—	0	—	—	—
CARAPELLI														
Balsamic	1 tbsp	15	0	0	0	0	4	0	0	0	0	—	—	0
Red Wine	1 tbsp	5	0	0	0	0	0	0	0	0	0	—	—	0
White Wine	1 tbsp	5	0	0	0	0	0	0	0	0	0	—	—	0
EDEN														
Organic Apple Cider	1 tbsp	0	0	0	0	0	0	0	0	0	0	—	—	0
Red Wine	1 tbsp	0	0	0	0	0	0	0	0	—	0	—	—	—
GEDNEY														
Apple Cider	1 tbsp	3	0	0	0	0	0	0	0	0	0	—	—	0
Distilled White	1 tbsp	3	0	0	0	0	0	0	0	0	0	—	—	0

FOOD	PORTION	CALS	FAT	SAT FAT	CHOL	PROT	CARB	SUGAR	FIBER	CALCI	SOD	POTAS	FOLIC	VIT C
GOURME MIST														
Balsamic Of Modena	1 sec spray	1	0	0	0	0	0	0	0	—	0	—	—	—
Balsamic Vinegar + Raspberry	1 sec spray	1	0	0	0	0	0	0	0	—	0	—	—	—
HEINZ														
Apple Cider	1 tbsp (0.5 oz)	0	0	0	0	0	0	0	0	0	0	—	—	0
Malt	1 (0.5 oz)	0	0	0	0	0	0	0	0	0	0	—	—	0
Red Wine	1 tbsp (1 oz)	0	0	0	0	0	0	0	0	0	0	—	—	0
Tarragon	1 tbsp (0.5 oz)	0	0	0	0	0	0	0	0	0	0	—	—	0
White	1 tbsp (0.5 oz)	0	0	0	0	0	0	0	0	0	0	—	—	0
HOLLAND HOUSE														
Malt	1 tbsp (0.5 oz)	0	0	0	0	0	0	0	0	—	0	—	—	—
Red Wine	1 tbsp (0.5 oz)	0	0	0	0	0	0	0	0	—	0	—	—	—
LATINO CHEF														
Lulo	1 tbsp	35	3	—	0	1	1	—	—	80	0	—	—	4
Passion Fruit	1 tbsp	40	3	—	—	0	2	1	tr	—	0	—	—	2
LUCINI														
Balsamic 10 Year Gran Reserve	1 tbsp (0.5 oz)	20	0	0	0	0	4	4	—	—	0	—	—	—
Balsamic Dark Cherry Infused	1 tbsp	30	0	0	0	0	7	7	—	—	3	—	—	—
Italian Wine Pinot Noir	1 tbsp (0.5 oz)	<1	0	0	0	0	0	0	0	—	2	—	—	—
MITSUKAN														
Rice	1 tbsp (0.5 oz)	0	0	0	0	0	0	0	0	—	0	—	—	—
Rice Seasoned	1 tbsp (0.5 oz)	25	0	0	0	0	5	5	—	—	420	—	—	—
NAKANO														
Natural Rice	1 tbsp (0.5 oz)	0	0	0	0	0	0	0	0	—	0	—	—	—
Red Wine Italian Herb Seasoned	1 tbsp (0.5 oz)	20	0	0	0	0	5	5	—	—	240	—	—	—
Rice Pesto Seasoned	1 tbsp (0.5 oz)	20	0	0	0	0	5	5	—	—	240	—	—	—
Rice Red Pepper Seasoned	1 tbsp (0.5 oz)	20	0	0	0	0	5	5	—	—	240	—	—	—
PROGRESSO														
Balsamic	2 tbsp (0.5 oz)	10	0	0	0	0	2	—	—	—	0	—	—	—
TREE OF LIFE														
Organic Apple Cider Raw Unfiltered	1 tbsp	0	0	0	0	0	tr	—	—	—	0	—	—	—

WAFFLES

FROZEN

FOOD	PORTION	CALS	FAT	SAT FAT	CHOL	PROT	CARB	SUGAR	FIBER	CALCI	SOD	POTAS	FOLIC	VIT C
AUNT JEMIMA														
Blueberry	2 (2.5 oz)	170	5	1	<5	4	27	5	tr	80	380	—	—	0
Buttermilk	2 (2.5 oz)	190	5	1	<5	5	29	3	tr	100	390	—	—	0

FOOD	PORTION	CALS	FAT	SAT FAT	CHOL	PROT	CARB	SUGAR	FIBER	CALCI	SOD	POTAS	FOLIC	VIT C
AUNT JEMIMA (cont.)														
Homestyle	2 (2.5 oz)	160	5	1	<5	4	25	2	tr	100	370	—	—	0
Low Fat	2 (2.5 oz)	160	3	0	<5	4	27	2	tr	100	460	—	—	0
EGGO														
Special K	3	190	1	0	0	8	37	5	1	150	400	190	60	0
KASHI														
Heart To Heart Honey Oat	2 (3 oz)	160	3	0	0	6	31	6	3	60	370	120	400	30
LIFESTREAM														
Organic Fig + Flax	2 (2.8 oz)	210	0	2	0	5	29	6	6	40	410	—	—	0
Organic Pomegran Plus	2 (2.8 oz)	190	5	1	0	5	31	6	5	20	370	—	—	0
NATURE'S PATH														
Buckwheat Wild Blueberry Organic	2 (2.5 oz)	190	7	1	0	2	33	5	1	20	330	—	—	0
Hemp Plus Organic	2 (2.5 oz)	200	8	1	0	4	30	5	5	60	290	170	—	0
Maple Cinn Organic	2 (2.5 oz)	180	6	1	0	4	28	6	4	20	380	—	—	0
Pomegran Plus Organic	2 (2.5 oz)	160	4	1	0	4	27	5	4	20	350	—	—	0
SMUCKER'S														
Snack'n Waffles Blueberry	1 (2 oz)	230	8	2	20	4	33	16	2	20	220	—	—	0
Snack'n Waffles Maple	1 (2 oz)	220	8	3	25	4	32	15	2	20	230	—	—	0
VAN'S														
Belgian Multigrain	2 (2.7 oz)	190	8	1	0	4	25	3	4	100	310	—	—	0
Mini Homestyle	4 (2.8 oz)	210	8	1	0	4	32	6	1	300	470	—	—	0
Organic Flax	2 (2.7 oz)	190	9	2	0	4	24	3	3	80	390	—	—	0
Organic Homestyle	2 (2.7 oz)	200	9	2	0	4	25	3	2	20	430	—	—	0
Original 97% Fat Free	2 (2.7 oz)	140	2	0	0	4	26	4	3	100	320	—	—	0
Original Buttermilk	2 (2.7 oz)	220	9	1	0	4	31	6	1	40	450	—	—	0
Wheat Free Buckwheat	2 (3 oz)	230	9	1	0	2	36	5	2	80	370	—	—	1
Wheat Free Flax	2 (3 oz)	210	8	1	0	3	33	4	1	80	380	—	—	2
MIX														
plain as prep 7 in diam	1 (2.6 oz)	218	11	2	52	6	25	—	—	191	383	119	34	tr

FOOD	PORTION	CALS	FAT	SAT FAT	CHOL	PROT	CARB	SUGAR	FIBER	CALCI	SOD	POTAS	FOLIC	VIT C
READY-TO-EAT														
KASHI														
GoLean Blueberry	2 (3 oz)	170	3	0	0	8	33	4	6	60	300	130	—	0
GoLean Original	2 (3 oz)	170	3	0	0	8	33	4	6	60	330	130	—	0
UNIQUE BELGIQUE														
Imported From Belgium	2 (2.3 oz)	230	12	6	55	4	27	15	1	20	300	—	—	0
TAKE-OUT														
belgian	1 (4.7 oz)	412	13	3	19	10	65	6	3	403	958	188	96	0
blueberry 9 in sq	1 (7 oz)	556	16	3	24	13	90	12	5	522	1232	274	124	4
round 10 in diam	1 (6.8 oz)	598	18	4	27	14	94	9	5	585	1390	272	139	0
square 9 in	1 (7 oz)	620	19	4	28	15	98	9	5	606	1440	282	144	0
whole wheat 9 in sq	1 (7 oz)	534	22	6	188	18	67	15	5	518	990	456	76	0
WALNUTS														
black chopped	¼ cup	193	18	1	0	8	3	tr	2	19	1	163	10	1
english chopped	¼ cup	191	19	2	0	4	4	1	2	29	1	129	29	tr
english ground	¼ cup	131	13	1	0	3	3	1	1	20	0	88	20	tr
english halves	14 (1 oz)	185	18	2	0	4	4	1	2	28	1	125	28	tr
english in shell	7 (1 oz)	183	18	2	0	4	4	1	2	27	1	123	27	tr
honey roasted	¼ cup	172	16	2	0	4	7	4	2	24	5	107	19	tr
BACK TO NATURE														
Unroasted Unsalted	1 oz	190	18	2	0	4	4	1	2	20	0	—	—	0
DIAMOND														
Chopped	¼ cup	200	20	2	0	5	4	1	2	20	0	—	—	0
PLANTERS														
Halves	1 oz	190	18	2	0	4	4	1	2	20	0	—	—	0
NUT-rition Omega-3 Mix	¼ cup (1.1 oz)	160	10	2	0	3	15	12	2	20	0	100	—	0
Recipe Ready Pieces	½ pkg (1 oz)	210	19	2	0	5	4	1	2	20	0	—	—	0
WASABI														
(*see* HORSERADISH)														
WATER														
ice cubes	3	0	0	0	0	0	0	0	0	2	2	1	0	0
tap water	8 oz	0	0	0	0	0	0	0	0	7	7	2	0	0
ACQUAFIBRE														
Fiber Enhanced All Flavors	1 bottle (11.15 oz)	5	0	0	0	0	0	0	5	—	1	—	—	—
ADIRONDACK														
Sparkling All Flavors	8 oz	0	0	0	0	0	0	0	0	—	0	—	—	—

FOOD	PORTION	CALS	FAT	SAT FAT	CHOL	PROT	CARB	SUGAR	FIBER	CALCI	SOD	POTAS	FOLIC	VIT C
ALOE BREEZE														
Organic All Flavors	8 oz	0	0	0	0	0	0	0	0	—	10	—	—	—
ALOE SPLASH														
All Flavors	8 oz	0	0	0	0	0	0	0	0	—	0	—	—	15
APPLE & EVE														
Water Fruits All Flavors	1 bottle (10 oz)	90	0	0	0	0	21	21	—	—	10	—	—	12
AQUA PACIFIC														
Water	1 liter	0	0	0	0	0	0	0	0	33	10	1	—	—
AQUAFINA														
Alive Wellness Berry Pomegranate	8 oz	10	0	0	0	0	2	2	0	—	65	—	—	—
ARIZONA														
Rescue Relax	8 oz	25	0	0	0	0	7	6	—	—	—	—	—	15
Vapor	8 oz	0	0	0	0	0	0	0	0	—	0	—	—	—
AROMA WATER														
All Flavors	8 oz	0	0	0	0	0	0	0	0	—	0	—	—	—
AYALA'S														
Herbal All Flavors	1 bottle	0	0	0	0	0	0	0	0	—	0	—	—	—
BOT														
Fortified All Flavors	1 bottle (12 oz)	40	0	0	0	0	10	9	0	—	0	—	—	—
CLEARLY CANADIAN														
Sparkling Blackberry	8 oz	90	0	0	0	0	22	22	—	—	10	—	—	—
Sparkling Cherry	8 oz	85	0	0	0	0	23	22	—	—	10	—	—	—
Sparkling Raspberry	8 oz	75	0	0	0	0	20	20	—	—	10	—	—	—
Sparkling Strawberry	8 oz	85	0	0	0	0	20	20	—	—	10	—	—	—
CRYSTAL GEYSER														
Spring Water	8 oz	0	0	0	0	0	0	0	0	—	0	—	—	—
DASANI														
Purified Water	8 oz	0	0	0	0	0	0	0	0	0	0	—	—	0
DOX														
Cardio Water	1 bottle (12 oz)	20	0	0	0	0	5	5	—	—	30	—	—	—
EDEN														
Springs Artesian	8 oz	0	0	0	0	0	0	0	0	—	0	—	—	—
EVIAN														
Spring Water	1 liter	0	0	0	0	0	0	0	0	78	6	1	—	—
EX														
Aqua Vitamins Raspberry	1 bottle (16.9 oz)	110	0	0	0	0	27	27	—	—	5	—	—	—

FOOD	PORTION	CALS	FAT	SAT FAT	CHOL	PROT	CARB	SUGAR	FIBER	CALCI	SOD	POTAS	FOLIC	VIT C
FIJI														
Natural Artesian	1 liter	0	0	0	0	0	0	0	0	17	0	0	—	—
FRUIT REFRESHERS														
Lemonade	8 oz	0	0	0	0	0	0	0	0	—	35	—	—	—
GEROLSTEINER														
Sparkling Mineral	8 oz	0	0	0	0	0	0	0	0	80	30	—	—	—
H 10 O														
Citrus Sport For Men	1 bottle (15.9 oz)	0	0	0	0	0	0	0	0	—	20	—	—	30
Peach Mango Tea For Women	1 bottle (15.9 oz)	0	0	0	0	0	0	0	0	—	20	—	40	—
H2ODWALLA														
Enhanced Tropical Orange	1 bottle (20 oz)	120	0	0	0	0	33	27	2	250	15	—	—	—
Organic Enhanced Blueberry Tea	1 bottle (20 oz)	120	0	0	0	0	29	27	—	—	20	—	—	90
Organic Enhanced Jasmine Lime	1 bottle (20 oz)	120	0	0	0	0	30	29	—	—	20	—	—	—
HAWAIIAN SPRINGS														
Naturally Pure	1 liter	0	0	0	0	0	0	0	0	7	0	—	—	—
HIGHLAND SPRING														
Spring Water	1 liter	0	0	0	0	0	0	0	0	41	9	1	—	—
IQ														
H2O Orange Mango	8 oz	40	0	0	0	0	10	9	—	—	0	—	—	—
ISLAND CHILL														
Artesian Water	1 liter	0	0	0	0	0	0	0	0	26	—	2	—	—
JANA														
Natural European Artesian	1 liter	0	0	0	0	0	0	0	0	63	0	—	—	—
JONES SODA														
24C Multi Vitamin Enhanced All Flavors	1 bottle	100	0	0	0	0	24	24	—	—	30	—	100	300
KLEAR SPLASH														
Mini Sip	1 pkg (4 oz)	0	0	0	0	0	0	0	0	—	0	—	—	—
LIFE WATER														
B-Strong	1 bottle (20 oz)	100	0	0	0	0	42	25	—	—	55	—	—	150
Enlighten	1 bottle (20 oz)	100	0	0	0	0	41	24	—	—	55	—	—	150
Zingseng	1 bottle (20 oz)	100	0	0	0	0	41	24	—	—	55	—	—	150
LIQUID SALVATION														
Ultra Hydrating	1 bottle	0	0	0	0	0	0	0	0	—	0	—	—	0

FOOD	PORTION	CALS	FAT	SAT FAT	CHOL	PROT	CARB	SUGAR	FIBER	CALCI	SOD	POTAS	FOLIC	VIT C
NESTLE														
Pure Life Splash All Flavors	8 oz	0	0	0	0	0	0	0	0	—	10	—	—	—
NUI														
All Natural Kid Water	10 oz	90	0	0	0	0	21	16	3	250	10	190	—	60
O WATER														
Hydrate Black Raspberry	8 oz	25	0	0	0	0	7	7	0	40	0	94	—	—
Replenish Lemon Lime	8 oz	25	0	0	0	0	7	7	0	40	0	94	—	—
Vitalize Peach Mango	8 oz	25	0	0	0	0	7	7	0	—	0	—	40	—
PROPEL														
Fitness Water All Flavors	1 bottle (24 oz)	30	0	0	0	0	6	6	—	—	220	—	—	21
R.W. KNUDSEN														
Organic Sparkling Essence Lemon	1 can (10.5 oz)	0	0	0	0	0	0	0	0	—	0	—	—	—
SAN BENEDETTO														
Sparkling Mineral Water	1 liter	0	0	0	0	0	0	0	0	48	7	1	—	—
SKINNY WATER														
Hi-Energy Acai Grape Blueberry	8 oz	0	0	0	0	0	0	0	0	70	10	99	—	—
Total-V Passionfruit Lemonade	8 oz	0	0	0	0	0	0	0	0	70	10	99	96	29
SNAPPLE														
Antioxidant Water Awaken Dragonfruit	8 oz	50	0	0	0	0	12	12	—	20	0	—	—	0
Antioxidant Water Restore Agave Melon	8 oz	60	0	0	0	0	13	13	—	20	0	—	—	—
Lyte Water	8 oz	0	0	0	0	0	0	0	—	—	—	—	—	—
SOBE														
All Flavors	8 oz	50	0	0	0	0	13	13	—	—	25	—	—	60
SONU														
Organic 10 Calories All Flavors	8 oz	10	0	0	0	0	4	3	0	20	5	10	—	66
Organic All Flavors	8 oz	45	0	0	0	0	13	13	0	20	5	10	—	66
SPARKLING ICE														
All Flavors	1 bottle (16 oz)	0	0	0	0	0	0	0	0	—	0	—	—	—

FOOD	PORTION	CALS	FAT	SAT FAT	CHOL	PROT	CARB	SUGAR	FIBER	CALCI	SOD	POTAS	FOLIC	VIT C
SPECIAL K2O														
Protein Water All Flavors	1 bottle (16.6 oz)	50	0	0	0	5	8	8	—	100	30	—	—	—
THORPEDO														
Ultra Low GI Energy Water	8 oz	45	0	0	0	0	11	10	0	—	60	30	80	—
TIPPERARY														
Mineral Water	1 liter	0	0	0	0	0	0	0	0	37	25	17	—	—
TRIM WATER														
Purified	1 bottle (20 oz)	10	0	0	0	0	3	3	0	—	65	—	—	—
TWIST														
Organics All Flavors	8 oz	10	0	0	0	0	2	2	0	0	0	—	—	0
VICTORIA'S KITCHEN														
Almond Water	8 oz	55	0	0	0	0	15	15	0	—	0	—	—	—
VITAMIN + FIBER WATER														
All Fruit Flavors	8 oz	50	0	0	0	0	13	12	3	—	10	—	—	60
VITAMINWATER														
XXX Acai Blueberry Pomegranate	8 oz	50	0	0	0	0	13	13	—	—	0	—	—	60
VOLVIC														
Mineral Water	1 liter	0	0	0	0	0	0	0	0	12	12	6	—	—
Natural Lemon	8 oz	0	0	0	0	0	1	1	0	—	0	—	—	—
WATERPLUS														
Antioxidants Acai Berry	8 oz	50	0	0	0	0	13	13	—	—	0	—	—	—
Electrolytes Fruit Punch	8 oz	50	0	0	0	0	13	13	—	40	0	—	—	—
Extra-C Orange Tangerine	8 oz	50	0	0	0	0	13	13	0	—	0	—	—	60
Vitamins Dragonfruit Kiwi	8 oz	50	0	0	0	0	13	13	—	—	0	—	—	—
WATER CHESTNUTS														
chinese sliced canned	½ cup	35	tr	—	0	1	9	—	—	3	6	82	—	1
fresh sliced	½ cup	66	tr	—	0	1	15	—	—	7	9	362	—	3
LA CHOY														
Sliced	½ cup	25	0	0	0	1	5	2	1	0	10	—	—	0
POLAR														
Sliced	2 tbsp	10	0	0	0	1	3	1	1	<20	15	—	—	tr
WATERCRESS														
cooked w/o fat	1 cup	15	tr	tr	0	3	2	tr	1	163	427	449	10	41
raw chopped	1 cup	4	tr	tr	0	1	tr	tr	tr	41	14	112	3	15

FOOD	PORTION	CALS	FAT	SAT FAT	CHOL	PROT	CARB	SUGAR	FIBER	CALCI	SOD	POTAS	FOLIC	VIT C
WATERMELON														
cut up	1 cup	46	tr	tr	0	1	12	10	1	11	2	172	5	13
seeds dried	¼ cup	150	13	3	0	8	4	—	—	15	27	175	16	0
wedge	1 med (10 oz)	86	tr	tr	0	2	22	18	1	20	3	320	9	23
wedge	1 sm (2.5 oz)	21	tr	tr	0	tr	5	4	tr	5	1	80	2	6
wedge	1 lg (20 oz)	172	1	tr	0	3	43	35	2	40	6	641	17	46
whole melon	1 (9 lb)	1227	6	1	0	25	309	254	16	286	41	4581	123	331
JAKE & AMOS														
Pickled Sweet Rind	2 tbsp (1 oz)	70	0	0	0	0	17	12	0	20	40	—	—	4
MINI ME														
Personal Seedless	2 cups (10 oz)	80	0	0	0	1	27	25	2	20	0	—	—	15
WATERMELON JUICE														
juice	8 oz	71	tr	tr	0	1	18	15	1	17	2	267	7	19
ARIZONA														
Fruit Juice Cocktail	8 oz	100	0	0	0	0	25	24	0	0	10	—	—	15
EARTHWISE														
Watermelon Supreme	8 oz	100	0	0	0	0	26	25	0	0	10	—	—	1
IZZE														
Esque Sparkling Watermelon	1 bottle (12 oz)	50	0	0	0	0	14	14	—	—	10	—	—	—
WHALE														
beluga dried	1 oz	93	2	tr	35	20	0	0	0	6	63	228	3	0
beluga raw	3.5 oz	111	1	tr	80	27	0	0	0	7	78	283	4	0
WHEAT														
sprouted	1 cup (3.8 oz)	214	1	tr	0	8	46	—	1	30	17	183	41	3
starch	3.5 oz	348	tr	—	—	tr	86	—	—	0	2	16	—	0
AMAZING GRASS														
Organic Wheat Grass	1 tbsp (0.3 oz)	35	0	0	0	2	4	—	2	35	2	230	80	17
ARROWHEAD MILLS														
Whole Grain Wheat	¼ cup (1.6 oz)	150	1	0	0	7	31	0	5	20	0	150	—	0
BOB'S RED MILL														
Vital Wheat Gluten	¼ cup	120	1	0	0	23	6	0	0	—	9	—	—	—
NEAR EAST														
Taboule Wheat Salad as prep	⅔ cup (3.5 oz)	120	3	tr	0	3	24	1	5	0	270	—	—	9
WHITE WAVE														
Seitan Chicken Meat Of Wheat	3 oz	130	0	0	0	24	9	0	3	60	270	—	—	0
Seitan Traditional	3 oz	90	1	0	0	18	3	0	1	0	380	—	—	0

FOOD	PORTION	CALS	FAT	SAT FAT	CHOL	PROT	CARB	SUGAR	FIBER	CALCI	SOD	POTAS	FOLIC	VIT C
WHITE WAVE (CONT.)														
Seitan Vegetarian Stir Fry Strips	3 oz	110	2	0	0	22	2	0	1	20	420	—	—	0
WHEAT GERM														
plain	¼ cup	108	3	1	0	8	14	2	4	13	1	267	99	2
BOB'S RED MILL														
Wheat Germ	2 tbsp	59	2	0	0	4	7	3	2	—	2	—	—	—
HODGSON MILL														
Untoasted	2 tbsp	55	1	0	0	4	7	0	4	0	0	40	40	0
KRETSCHMER														
Original Toasted	¼ cup (0.6 oz)	35	1	0	0	3	10	—	7	—	0	210	—	—
MOTHER'S														
Wheat Germ	2 tbsp (0.5 oz)	50	1	0	0	4	6	1	2	—	0	140	80	—
TREE OF LIFE														
Toasted	3 tbsp (0.8 oz)	100	3	1	0	9	12	3	3	0	0	—	—	0
WHEY														
acid dry	1 tbsp	10	tr	tr	0	tr	2	2	0	60	28	66	1	0
sweet dry	1 tbsp	26	tr	tr	0	1	6	6	0	60	81	156	1	tr
sweet fluid	½ cup	33	tr	tr	2	1	6	6	0	58	66	198	1	tr
whey cheese	1 oz	126	8	5	—	4	9	0	0	97	146	—	—	tr
ACTION WHEY														
Dream Shake All Flavors	1 scoop (0.8 oz)	90	3	2	40	15	3	2	1	157	50	100	—	—
BOB'S RED MILL														
Protein Concentrate	¼ cup	80	1	1	30	16	1	1	0	—	40	—	—	—
Sweet Dairy	1 tbsp	30	0	0	1	1	6	5	0	—	70	—	—	—
PREMIER														
100% Whey Isolate	2 scoops (1.5 oz)	160	2	1	5	30	8	1	2	150	55	390	—	—
WELLEMENTS														
Whey Protein Chocolate	1 scoop (1 oz)	120	2	1	42	22	4	tr	0	—	55	170	—	—
Whey Protein Vanilla	1 scoop (1 oz)	120	2	1	39	22	4	tr	0	—	55	170	—	—
WHIPPED TOPPINGS														
dairy fat free pressurized	¼ cup (0.6 oz)	24	1	tr	0	tr	4	3	tr	17	12	17	3	0
nondairy fat free frzn	¼ cup (0.7 oz)	28	1	1	3	1	5	3	tr	20	14	20	3	0
nondairy frzn	¼ cup (0.7 oz)	60	5	4	0	tr	4	4	0	1	5	3	0	0
nondairy lowfat frzn	¼ cup (0.7 oz)	42	2	2	0	1	4	4	0	13	14	19	1	0
nondairy pressurized	¼ cup (0.6 oz)	46	4	3	0	tr	3	3	0	1	11	3	0	0

FOOD	PORTION	CALS	FAT	SAT FAT	CHOL	PROT	CARB	SUGAR	FIBER	CALCI	SOD	POTAS	FOLIC	VIT C
COOL WHIP														
Chocolate	2 tbsp	25	2	2	—	0	2	2	—	—	0	—	—	—
Free	2 tbsp	15	0	0	0	0	3	1	—	—	5	—	—	—
Regular	2 tbsp	25	2	2	—	0	2	1	—	—	0	—	—	—
Strawberry	2 tbsp	25	2	2	—	0	2	1	—	—	0	—	—	—
HOOD														
Light Sugar Free Whipped Cream	2 tbsp	10	1	0	<5	0	tr	0	0	0	5	—	—	0
Whipped Light Cream	2 tbsp	20	2	1	5	0	tr	tr	0	0	0	—	—	0
SOYATOO														
Rice Whip	2 tbsp (6 g)	10	1	1	0	0	1	1	0	—	0	—	—	—
Soy Whip	2 tbsp (6 g)	10	1	1	0	0	1	1	0	—	0	—	—	—
TRUWHIP														
Whipped Topping	2 tbsp (0.4 oz)	30	2	2	0	0	3	2	0	0	0	—	—	0
WHITE BEANS														
canned	1 cup (9.2 oz)	299	1	tr	0	19	56	1	13	191	13	1189	170	0
dried small cooked w/o salt	1 cup (6.3 oz)	254	1	tr	0	16	46	—	19	131	4	829	245	0
WHITEFISH														
baked	3 oz	146	6	1	65	21	0	0	0	28	55	345	14	0
fillet grilled no added fat	1 (5.4 oz)	265	12	2	119	38	0	0	0	51	100	625	26	0
smoked boneless	1 oz	31	tr	tr	9	7	0	0	0	5	289	120	2	0
WHITING														
broiled w/o fat	3 oz	99	1	tr	71	20	0	0	0	53	112	369	13	0
fillet broiled w/o fat	1 (2.5 oz)	84	1	tr	60	17	0	0	0	45	95	312	11	0
fillet steamed w/o fat	1 (2.6 oz)	84	1	tr	63	17	0	0	0	45	61	198	10	0
hake raw	3.5 oz	84	1	—	—	17	0	0	0	41	101	294	—	—
TAKE-OUT														
fillet battered & fried	1 (3.1 oz)	157	7	1	66	15	6	tr	tr	57	110	215	19	0
fillet breaded & fried	1 (3.1 oz)	191	10	2	75	17	7	1	tr	62	350	233	18	0
WILD RICE														
cooked	1 cup (5.8 oz)	166	1	tr	0	7	35	1	3	5	5	166	43	0
GOURMET HOUSE														
Cracked as prep	1 cup	170	0	0	0	6	35	0	2	—	0	120	—	0
Quick Cooking not prep	½ cup	170	0	0	0	6	25	0	2	0	0	120	—	0
Thai Jasmine as prep	¾ cup	160	0	0	0	3	36	0	0	0	0	—	80	0

FOOD	PORTION	CALS	FAT	SAT FAT	CHOL	PROT	CARB	SUGAR	FIBER	CALCI	SOD	POTAS	FOLIC	VIT C
LUNDBERG														
Organic Quick not prep	¼ cup	150	1	0	0	6	33	1	2	0	0	—	—	0
WINE														
chianti	1 serv (5 oz)	125	0	0	0	tr	4	1	0	12	6	187	1	0
chinese cooking	1 bottle (15 oz)	559	0	0	0	0	3	0	0	4	43	30	—	0
cooking	¼ cup (2 oz)	29	0	0	0	tr	4	1	0	5	363	51	1	0
haiku	1 serv	93	0	0	0	tr	3	—	0	3	2	17	—	—
japanese plum	3 oz	139	tr	—	0	tr	16	—	0	1	—	—	—	0
japanese sake	2 oz	78	0	0	0	tr	3	0	0	3	1	15	0	0
kir	1 serv	78	0	0	0	tr	3	—	0	8	4	71	tr	—
liebfraumilch	4 oz	86	—	—	—	—	—	—	—	—	—	—	—	—
madeira	3.5 oz	169	0	—	—	0	10	10	0	8	—	—	—	—
marsala	4 oz	80	—	—	—	—	—	—	—	—	—	—	—	—
merlot	4 oz	95	—	—	—	—	—	—	—	—	—	—	—	—
muscat	1 serv (5 oz)	123	0	00	0	tr	8	—	—	—	—	—	—	—
nonalcoholic	1 serv (5 oz)	9	0	0	0	1	2	2	0	13	10	128	1	0
port	1 serv (3.5 oz)	165	0	0	0	tr	14	8	0	8	9	95	0	0
red barbera	1 serv (5 oz)	125	0	0	0	tr	4	—	—	—	—	—	—	—
red burgundy	1 serv (5 oz)	127	0	0	0	tr	5	—	—	—	—	—	—	—
red cabernet franc	1 serv (5 oz)	122	0	0	0	tr	4	—	—	—	—	—	—	—
red claret	1 serv (5 oz)	122	0	0	0	tr	4	—	—	—	—	—	—	—
red gamay	1 serv (5 oz)	115	0	0	0	tr	4	—	—	—	—	—	—	—
red mourvedre	1 serv (5 oz)	129	0	0	0	tr	4	—	—	—	—	—	—	—
red pinot noir	1 serv (5 oz)	121	0	0	0	tr	3	—	—	—	—	—	—	—
red syrah	1 serv (5 oz)	122	0	0	0	tr	4	—	—	—	—	—	—	—
red zinfandel	1 serv (5 oz)	129	0	0	0	tr	4	—	—	—	—	—	—	—
sake screwdriver	1 serv	175	tr	tr	0	2	23	—	tr	24	3	389	56	93
sangria	1 serv	88	tr	0	0	tr	6	—	tr	7	4	95	5	7
sangria blanco	1 serv	155	tr	tr	0	1	24	—	3	70	13	267	23	27
sherry	2 oz	84	0	0	0	tr	5	—	—	—	—	—	—	—
vermouth dry	3.5 oz	105	0	0	0	—	1	—	—	—	—	—	—	—
vermouth sweet	3.5 oz	167	0	0	0	—	12	—	—	—	—	—	—	—
wassail wine	1 serv	142	tr	tr	0	1	22	—	2	50	6	190	17	23
white	1 serv (5 oz)	121	0	0	0	tr	4	1	0	13	7	104	0	0
white fume blanc	1 serv (5 oz)	121	0	0	0	tr	3	—	—	—	—	—	—	—
white pinot blanc	1 serv (5 oz)	119	0	0	0	tr	3	—	—	—	—	—	—	—
white pinot grigio	1 serv (5 oz)	122	0	0	0	tr	3	—	—	—	—	—	—	—
white riesling	1 serv (5 oz)	118	0	0	0	tr	6	—	—	—	—	—	—	—
white sauvignon blanc	1 serv (5 oz)	119	0	0	0	tr	3	—	—	—	—	—	—	—
wine cooler	1 (7 oz)	116	tr	tr	0	tr	14	11	0	13	15	103	2	4
wine spritzer	1 serv (7 oz)	73	0	0	0	tr	2	1	0	10	16	88	1	0

FOOD	PORTION	CALS	FAT	SAT FAT	CHOL	PROT	CARB	SUGAR	FIBER	CALCI	SOD	POTAS	FOLIC	VIT C
ALMADEN														
Merlot	5 oz	115	0	0	0	—	5	—	—	—	—	—	—	—
BARTLES & JAYMES														
Wine Cooler Classic Original	1 bottle (12 oz)	190	0	0	0	—	29	—	—	—	—	—	—	—
BERINGER														
Chardonnay	5 oz	125	0	0	0	—	0	—	—	—	—	—	—	—
CARLO ROSSI														
Cabernet Sauvignon	5 oz	125	0	0	0	—	5	0	0	—	tr	—	—	—
FRANZIA VINTER														
Select Merlot	5 oz	105	0	0	0	—	0	—	—	—	—	—	—	—
HOLLAND HOUSE														
Cooking Wine Marsala	2 tbsp (1 oz)	45	0	0	0	0	4	4	—	—	190	—	—	—
Cooking Wine Red	2 tbsp (1 oz)	20	0	0	0	0	1	0	—	—	190	—	—	—
Cooking Wine Sherry	2 tbsp (1 oz)	45	0	0	0	0	2	2	—	—	190	—	—	—
Cooking Wine Vermouth	2 tbsp (1 oz)	35	0	0	0	0	2	2	—	—	190	—	—	—
Cooking Wine White	2 tbsp (1 oz)	20	0	0	0	0	0	0	0	—	190	—	—	—
KEDEM														
Cooking Red	2 tbsp (1 oz)	30	0	0	0	0	1	—	—	—	150	—	—	—
Cooking Sherry	2 tbsp (1 oz)	40	0	0	0	0	1	1	—	—	170	—	—	—
Cooking Wine Marsala	2 tbsp (1 oz)	40	0	0	0	0	1	1	—	—	170	—	—	—
TWIN VALLEY														
Cabernet Sauvignon	5 oz	120	0	0	0	—	5	—	—	—	—	—	—	—
WINGED BEANS														
dried cooked w/o salt	1 cup	253	10	1	0	18	26	—	3	244	22	482	17	0
WRAPS														
(*see* BREAD, SANDWICHES)														
YACON														
NAVITAS NATURALS														
Slices Dried	1 oz	90	0	0	0	1	22	12	1	20	10	—	—	6
YAM														
(*see also* SWEET POTATO)														
CANNED														
GLORY														
Candied	½ cup	210	0	0	0	1	52	38	1	40	240	—	—	9

FOOD	PORTION	CALS	FAT	SAT FAT	CHOL	PROT	CARB	SUGAR	FIBER	CALCI	SOD	POTAS	FOLIC	VIT C
S&W														
Candied	½ cup (4.9 oz)	170	0	0	0	2	46	21	4	20	360	210	—	5
FRESH														
mountain yam hawaii cooked w/o salt	1 cup	119	tr	tr	0	3	29	—	—	12	17	718	17	0
yam cooked w/o salt	1 cup	158	tr	tr	0	2	38	1	5	19	11	911	22	17
EARTHBOUND FARMS														
Organic	1 med (4.6 oz)	130	0	0	0	2	33	7	4	20	45	—	—	18
HOUSE														
Black Ita Konnyaku Yam Cake	1 serv (2 oz)	5	0	0	0	0	1	0	tr	60	0	—	—	0

YARDLONG BEANS

FOOD	PORTION	CALS	FAT	SAT FAT	CHOL	PROT	CARB	SUGAR	FIBER	CALCI	SOD	POTAS	FOLIC	VIT C
sliced cooked w/o salt	1 cup	49	tr	tr	0	3	10	—	—	46	4	302	47	17

YAUTIA

(*see* MALANGA)

YEAST

FOOD	PORTION	CALS	FAT	SAT FAT	CHOL	PROT	CARB	SUGAR	FIBER	CALCI	SOD	POTAS	FOLIC	VIT C
baker's compressed	1 cake (0.6 oz)	18	tr	tr	0	1	3	0	1	3	5	102	133	0
baker's dry	1 pkg (7 g)	21	tr	tr	0	3	3	0	2	4	4	140	164	0
baker's dry	1 tbsp	35	1	tr	0	5	5	0	3	8	6	240	281	0
brewer's dry	1 tbsp	35	1	tr	0	5	5	0	3	8	6	240	281	0
BOB'S RED MILL														
Active Dry	1 tbsp	25	1	0	0	0	5	0	2	—	0	—	—	—

YELLOW BEANS

FOOD	PORTION	CALS	FAT	SAT FAT	CHOL	PROT	CARB	SUGAR	FIBER	CALCI	SOD	POTAS	FOLIC	VIT C
fresh cooked w/o salt	1 cup	44	tr	tr	0	2	10	2	4	58	4	374	41	12
fresh raw	1 cup	34	tr	tr	0	2	8	—	4	41	7	230	41	18

YELLOWTAIL

FOOD	PORTION	CALS	FAT	SAT FAT	CHOL	PROT	CARB	SUGAR	FIBER	CALCI	SOD	POTAS	FOLIC	VIT C
baked	4 oz	199	7	—	75	32	0	0	0	31	53	572	4	3

YOGURT

(*see also* YOGURT DRINKS, YOGURT FROZEN)

FOOD	PORTION	CALS	FAT	SAT FAT	CHOL	PROT	CARB	SUGAR	FIBER	CALCI	SOD	POTAS	FOLIC	VIT C
plain lowfat	8 oz	143	4	2	14	12	16	16	0	415	159	531	25	2
plain nonfat	8 oz	127	tr	tr	5	13	17	17	0	452	175	579	27	2
plain whole milk	8 oz	138	7	5	30	8	11	11	0	275	104	352	16	1
tofu yogurt	1 cup	246	5	1	0	9	42	3	1	309	92	123	16	7
BETTER WHEY														
All Fruit Flavors	1 pkg (6 oz)	145	1	0	5	15	23	14	3	300	80	—	—	0
Plain	1 pkg (6 oz)	130	1	0	5	17	17	7	3	350	95	—	—	0
BREYERS														
Creme Savers All Flavors	1 pkg (6 oz)	160	2	1	10	6	31	26	0	300	170	200	—	1

FOOD	PORTION	CALS	FAT	SAT FAT	CHOL	PROT	CARB	SUGAR	FIBER	CALCI	SOD	POTAS	FOLIC	VIT C
BREYERS (CONT.)														
Fruit On The Bottom Black Cherry	1 pkg (6 oz)	160	1	1	10	5	32	28	tr	150	80	190	—	1
Fruit On The Bottom Chocolate Raspberry	1 pkg (6 oz)	170	1	1	10	5	34	27	tr	200	75	200	—	1
Fruit On The Bottom Mixed Berry	1 pkg (6 oz)	160	1	1	10	5	31	26	tr	150	75	190	—	5
Fruit On The Bottom Peach Mango Orange	1 pkg (6 oz)	160	1	1	10	5	31	27	tr	150	75	210	—	5
Fruit On The Bottom Pineapple	1 pkg (6 oz)	150	1	1	10	5	31	27	tr	150	75	190	—	2
Fruit On The Bottom Strawberry	1 pkg (6 oz)	150	1	1	10	5	31	26	tr	150	70	190	—	5
Inspirations Cherry Chocolate Chip	1 pkg (4 oz)	140	3	3	5	4	23	20	0	100	65	150	—	1
Inspirations Mint Chocolate Chip	1 pkg (4 oz)	140	4	3	5	4	23	19	0	100	65	140	—	1
Inspirations Vanilla Bean	1 pkg (4 oz)	110	1	1	5	4	21	17	0	100	60	150	—	1
Light Blueberry	1 pkg (4 oz)	50	0	0	<5	4	8	5	tr	150	70	160	—	1
Smooth & Creamy Peaches 'N Cream	1 pkg (4 oz)	120	1	1	10	3	24	19	0	0	50	0	—	0
Smooth & Creamy Strawberry	1 pkg (4 oz)	110	1	1	10	3	23	18	0	100	50	0	—	0
CABOT														
Greek	1 pkg (6 oz)	210	17	11	55	7	9	6	0	200	80	—	—	0
Greek 2%	1 pkg (6 oz)	160	3	2	20	13	25	24	0	250	80	—	—	6
Non Fat Berry Banana	1 cup	130	0	0	5	8	24	19	0	250	115	—	—	15
Non Fat Black Cherry	1 cup	130	0	0	5	8	24	19	0	250	115	—	—	15
Non Fat French Vanilla	1 cup	130	0	0	5	8	24	19	—	250	115	—	—	15
Non Fat Plain	1 cup	100	0	0	5	10	19	13	0	300	135	—	—	18
Non Fat Raspberry	1 cup	130	0	0	5	8	24	19	0	250	115	—	—	15
CHOBANI														
Champions Honey-nana	1 pkg (3.5 oz)	100	2	1	5	8	14	13	0	100	40	—	—	0

FOOD	PORTION	CALS	FAT	SAT FAT	CHOL	PROT	CARB	SUGAR	FIBER	CALCI	SOD	POTAS	FOLIC	VIT C
CHOBANI (CONT.)														
Greek Yogurt Nonfat Blueberry	1 pkg (6 oz)	140	0	0	0	14	20	20	tr	200	65	—	—	0
Greek Yogurt Nonfat Caramel	1 pkg (6 oz)	140	0	0	0	16	13	13	0	200	75	—	—	0
Greek Yogurt Nonfat Honey	1 pkg (6 oz)	150	0	0	0	16	20	20	0	200	75	—	—	0
Greek Yogurt Nonfat Peach	1 pkg (6 oz)	140	0	0	0	14	20	19	tr	200	65	—	—	1
Greek Yogurt Nonfat Plain	1 pkg (6 oz)	100	0	0	0	18	7	7	0	200	80	—	—	0
Greek Yogurt Nonfat Pomegranate	1 pkg (6 oz)	140	0	0	0	14	21	19	0	150	75	—	—	0
Greek Yogurt Nonfat Raspberry	1 pkg (6 oz)	140	0	0	0	14	22	19	1	150	65	—	—	2
Greek Yogurt Nonfat Strawberry	1 pkg (6 oz)	140	0	0	0	14	20	19	tr	200	65	—	—	1
Greek Yogurt Nonfat Vanilla	1 pkg (6 oz)	120	0	0	0	16	13	13	0	200	75	—	—	0
DANNON														
Activia Blueberry	1 pkg (4 oz)	110	2	2	10	5	19	17	0	150	65	220	—	0
Activia Cherry	1 pkg (4 oz)	110	2	2	10	5	19	18	0	150	75	210	—	0
Activia Harvest Picks Strawberry	1 pkg (4 oz)	110	4	3	10	4	16	15	—	150	60	200	—	—
Activia Peach	1 pkg (4 oz)	110	2	2	10	5	19	17	0	150	70	230	—	0
Activia Prune	1 pkg (4 oz)	110	2	2	10	5	19	17	0	150	75	230	—	0
Activia Strawberry	1 pkg (4 oz)	120	2	1	5	4	22	19	0	150	65	160	—	0
Activia Strawberry Banana	1 pkg (4 oz)	110	2	1	5	4	19	17	0	150	75	210	—	0
Activia Vanilla	1 pkg (4 oz)	110	2	2	10	5	19	17	0	150	70	230	—	0
Activia Light Blueberry	1 pkg (4 oz)	70	0	0	<5	4	13	9	2	150	65	200	—	0
Activia Light Peach	1 pkg (4 oz)	70	0	0	<5	4	12	8	2	150	65	210	—	0
Activia Light Raspberry	1 pkg (4 oz)	70	0	0	<5	4	13	8	2	150	75	210	—	0
Activia Light Strawberry	1 pkg (4 oz)	70	0	0	<5	4	13	8	2	150	70	210	—	0
Activia Light Vanilla	1 pkg (4 oz)	70	0	0	<5	5	14	7	3	150	70	210	—	0
All Natural Coffee	1 pkg (6 oz)	150	3	2	10	7	25	25	0	250	100	370	—	2
All Natural Lemon	1 pkg (6 oz)	150	3	2	10	7	25	25	0	250	100	330	—	2
All Natural Plain	1 pkg (6 oz)	100	3	2	10	8	12	12	0	300	115	390	—	2
All Natural Vanilla	1 pkg (6 oz)	150	3	2	10	7	25	25	0	250	100	330	—	1

FOOD	PORTION	CALS	FAT	SAT FAT	CHOL	PROT	CARB	SUGAR	FIBER	CALCI	SOD	POTAS	FOLIC	VIT C
EHRMANN														
Bavarian Lowfat Cherry	1 pkg	140	2	1	5	7	25	24	0	150	80	190	—	0
Bavarian Lowfat Peach	1 pkg	140	2	1	5	7	25	24	0	150	80	190	—	0
Bavarian Lowfat Strawberry	1 pkg	140	2	1	5	7	25	24	0	150	80	180	—	0
EMMI														
Apricot Low-fat	1 pkg (6 oz)	170	3	2	15	9	27	25	0	300	170	340	—	1
Green Apple Low-fat	1 pkg (6 oz)	170	3	2	15	9	27	26	0	300	160	340	—	1
Pink Grapefruit Low-fat	1 pkg (6 oz)	170	3	2	15	9	27	26	0	300	160	340	—	5
Plain Low-fat	1 pkg (6 oz)	170	3	2	15	10	10	10	0	350	150	310	—	2
FAGE														
Total Cherry	1 pkg (5.3 oz)	170	6	5	15	11	17	16	0	100	45	—	—	0
Total Peach	1 pkg (5.3 oz)	170	6	5	15	11	17	16	0	100	45	—	—	0
Total Plain	1 pkg (5.3 oz)	190	10	7	25	18	8	8	0	200	70	—	—	0
Total Strawberry	1 pkg (5.3 oz)	170	6	5	15	11	17	16	0	100	45	—	—	0
Total 0% Cherry	1 pkg (5.3 oz)	130	0	0	0	13	19	16	0	150	50	—	—	0
Total 0% Cherry Pomegranate	1 pkg (5.3 oz)	130	0	0	0	13	19	16	0	150	50	—	—	0
Total 0% Honey	1 pkg (5.3 oz)	120	0	0	0	13	17	16	0	150	50	—	—	0
Total 0% Mango Guanabana	1 pkg (5.3 oz)	120	0	0	0	13	18	17	0	150	45	—	—	0
Total 0% Peach	1 pkg (5.3 oz)	120	0	0	0	13	17	16	0	150	45	—	—	0
Total 0% Plain	1 pkg (5.3 oz)	100	0	0	0	18	7	7	0	200	65	—	—	0
Total 2% Cherry	1 pkg (5.3 oz)	140	3	2	5	12	17	16	0	100	40	—	—	0
Total 2% Plain	1 pkg (5.3 oz)	150	4	3	10	20	8	8	0	200	65	—	—	0
Total 2% Strawberry	1 pkg (5.3 oz)	140	3	2	5	12	17	16	0	100	40	—	—	0
FIBER ONE														
Creamy Nonfat Vanilla	1 pkg (4 oz)	80	0	0	<5	4	19	10	5	100	65	180	—	—
FRIENDSHIP														
Plain	1 cup	150	3	2	15	12	18	17	1	400	190	—	—	—
GREEN VALLEY														
Organic Lactose Free Blueberry	1 pkg (6 oz)	140	2	1	10	7	23	16	0	250	70	—	—	0
Organic Lactose Free Honey	1 pkg (6 oz)	140	2	2	10	7	24	14	0	250	100	—	—	0
Organic Lactose Free Plain	1 pkg (6 oz)	100	3	2	10	8	11	4	0	300	85	—	—	0
Organic Lactose Free Vanilla	1 pkg (6 oz)	120	3	2	10	7	17	9	0	300	60	—	—	0

FOOD	PORTION	CALS	FAT	SAT FAT	CHOL	PROT	CARB	SUGAR	FIBER	CALCI	SOD	POTAS	FOLIC	VIT C
HORIZON ORGANIC														
Kids Strawberry	1 pkg (4 oz)	110	1	1	5	4	20	20	1	150	75	—	—	1
Lowfat Blended Blueberry	1 pkg (6 oz)	160	2	1	10	7	30	29	2	250	110	—	—	1
Tube Lowfat Blueberry	1 (2 oz)	70	1	1	5	2	12	11	0	80	40	—	—	0
Whole Milk Plain	1 cup	160	7	5	30	10	14	14	0	350	150	—	—	2
KAROUN														
Plain Lowfat	1 cup (8 oz)	180	5	3	25	11	16	15	0	400	170	530	—	2
Plain Whole Milk	1 cup (8 oz)	210	12	7	50	11	15	14	0	400	170	490	—	2
LA YOGURT														
Lowfat Blueberries 'N' Cream	1 pkg (6 oz)	200	2	1	10	7	39	36	0	200	90	290	—	1
Lowfat Fruit On The Bottom Cherry	1 pkg (8 oz)	230	3	2	10	6	47	46	tr	200	85	310	—	2
Lowfat Fruit On The Bottom Probiotic Peach	1 pkg (6 oz)	160	2	1	5	6	31	29	0	250	100	330	—	2
Lowfat Fruit On The Bottom Strawberry	1 pkg (8 oz)	220	2	2	10	9	43	41	tr	300	140	470	—	4
Lowfat Peaches 'N' Cream	1 pkg (6 oz)	200	2	1	10	7	39	37	0	200	90	310	—	2
Lowfat Pina Colada	1 pkg (6 oz)	160	2	1	5	5	30	26	0	200	90	250	—	4
Lowfat Probiotic Pina Colada	1 pkg (6 oz)	160	2	2	5	5	30	26	0	300	90	250	—	60
Lowfat Probiotic Plain	1 pkg (6 oz)	100	2	2	10	9	12	11	0	300	130	410	—	2
Lowfat Probiotic Vanilla	1 pkg (6 oz)	150	2	2	10	8	26	25	0	300	120	370	—	2
Lowfat Vanilla 'N' Cream	1 pkg (6 oz)	200	2	1	10	7	39	37	0	200	90	280	—	1
Nonfat Banana Cream	1 pkg (6 oz)	100	0	0	0	6	18	14	0	200	90	240	—	1
Nonfat Probiotic Cherry	1 pkg (6 oz)	100	0	0	0	6	17	13	0	200	90	280	—	2
Nonfat Probiotic Peach	1 pkg (6 oz)	90	0	0	0	6	16	12	0	200	85	280	—	2
Nonfat Probiotic Raspberry	1 pkg (6 oz)	90	0	0	0	6	15	11	0	200	85	250	—	1
Nonfat Probiotic Vanilla	1 pkg (6 oz)	90	0	0	0	6	15	10	0	200	85	240	—	1
Sabor Latino Lowfat Dulce De Leche	1 pkg (6 oz)	190	2	1	10	7	36	31	0	250	105	300	—	2

FOOD	PORTION	CALS	FAT	SAT FAT	CHOL	PROT	CARB	SUGAR	FIBER	CALCI	SOD	POTAS	FOLIC	VIT C
LA YOGURT (CONT.)														
Sabor Latino Lowfat Guava	1 pkg (6 oz)	190	2	1	10	7	37	32	0	250	110	310	—	9
Sabor Latino Lowfat Horchata	1 pkg (6 oz)	210	2	1	10	7	41	36	0	250	105	300	—	2
Sabor Latino Lowfat Papaya	1 pkg (6 oz)	190	2	1	10	7	37	32	0	250	105	310	—	4
LAND O LAKES														
Strawberry Light	1 pkg (8 oz)	80	0	0	0	8	38	31	0	250	135	—	—	0
Strawberry Lowfat	1 pkg (8 oz)	190	2	2	10	8	36	29	0	250	125	—	—	0
LIBERTE														
Plain Lowfat	1 pkg (6 oz)	110	4	2	15	9	10	7	0	300	110	—	—	2
Six Grains Peach	1 pkg (6 oz)	150	3	2	10	8	23	18	1	250	90	—	—	2
Six Grains Pear	1 pkg (6 oz)	160	3	2	10	8	23	18	1	250	90	—	—	2
LOWELL														
Multi Grain Peach & Whole Grain	1 pkg (6 oz)	170	5	3	20	6	26	21	1	200	80	—	—	1
MOUNTAIN HIGH														
Black Cherry Classic Lowfat	1 pkg (6 oz)	140	2	1	10	7	24	23	0	250	105	—	—	—
Blueberry Classic Lowfat	1 pkg (6 oz)	140	2	1	10	7	24	23	0	250	105	—	—	—
Lemon Lowfat	1 pkg (8 oz)	190	2	2	10	10	34	33	0	350	150	470	—	2
Mountain Berry Classic Lowfat	1 pkg (6 oz)	150	2	1	10	7	26	25	0	250	110	—	—	—
Plain Fat Free	1 pkg (8 oz)	120	0	0	5	12	18	17	0	450	180	570	—	4
Plain Lowfat	1 pkg (8 oz)	140	3	2	15	11	18	16	0	400	170	560	—	4
Plain Original	1 pkg (8 oz)	180	8	5	35	11	17	15	0	400	160	530	—	2
Strawberry Classic Lowfat	1 pkg (6 oz)	140	2	1	10	7	24	23	0	250	105	—	—	—
Vanilla Fat Free	1 pkg (8 oz)	160	0	0	<5	11	30	28	0	400	160	520	—	4
Vanilla Lowfat	1 pkg (8 oz)	180	3	2	15	10	29	28	0	400	160	500	—	2
Vanilla Original	1 pkg (8 oz)	210	7	5	30	10	28	27	0	350	150	480	—	2
NANCY'S														
Lowfat Lemon	1 pkg (8 oz)	150	3	3	20	11	16	16	0	400	170	—	—	2
Lowfat Maple	1 pkg (8 oz)	180	3	2	15	10	26	26	0	400	160	—	—	2
Lowfat Peach	1 pkg (8 oz)	170	3	2	15	10	26	26	0	350	150	—	—	4
Lowfat Plain	1 pkg (8 oz)	150	3	3	20	11	16	16	0	400	170	—	—	2
Lowfat Vanilla	1 pkg (8 oz)	140	3	2	15	10	15	15	0	350	160	—	—	2
Organic Whole Milk Fruit On The Top Blackberry	1 pkg (8 oz)	220	5	3	20	8	38	37	2	250	110	—	—	12
Organic Whole Milk Fruit On The Top Cherry	1 pkg (8 oz)	220	6	3	20	8	36	32	1	250	110	—	—	6

FOOD	PORTION	CALS	FAT	SAT FAT	CHOL	PROT	CARB	SUGAR	FIBER	CALCI	SOD	POTAS	FOLIC	VIT C
NANCY'S (CONT.)														
Organic Whole Milk Fruit On The Top Peach	1 pkg (8 oz)	220	5	3	20	8	38	38	tr	250	110	—	—	5
Organic Whole Milk Honey	1 pkg (8 oz)	170	8	4	30	10	17	17	0	350	160	—	—	2
Organic Whole Milk Plain	1 pkg (8 oz)	130	6	4	25	8	11	12	0	250	125	—	—	2
Organic Soy Kiwi Lime	1 pkg (6 oz)	160	3	0	0	5	31	21	4	150	20	—	—	114
Organic Soy Mango	1 (6 oz)	170	3	0	0	4	33	23	3	150	20	—	—	84
Organic Soy Plain	1 pkg (6 oz)	150	3	0	0	5	25	15	2	150	20	—	—	78
Organic Soy Vanilla	1 pkg (6 oz)	120	3	0	0	4	19	10	3	150	20	—	—	66
OIKOS														
Blueberry	1 pkg (5.3 oz)	120	0	0	0	13	16	15	0	150	70	190	—	0
Caramel	1 pkg (4 oz)	110	0	0	0	10	17	16	0	150	60	140	—	0
Chocolate	1 pkg (4 oz)	110	0	0	0	10	17	16	tr	150	55	140	—	0
Honey	1 pkg (5.3 oz)	120	0	0	0	13	18	17	0	150	50	190	—	0
Plain	1 pkg (5.3 oz)	80	0	0	0	15	6	6	0	200	60	230	—	0
Strawberry	1 pkg (5.3 oz)	110	0	0	0	13	16	7	0	150	80	190	—	0
Super Fruits	1 pkg (5.3 oz)	130	0	0	0	13	18	16	0	150	80	—	—	0
Vanilla	1 pkg (5.3 oz)	110	0	0	0	15	12	11	0	200	60	220	—	0
OLYMPUS														
Greek Strained Strawberry 1% Lowfat	1 pkg (6 oz)	155	15	1	3	12	23	22	tr	170	40	—	—	1
RACHEL'S														
Essence Berry Jasmine w/ Zinc	1 pkg (6 oz)	160	3	2	10	8	28	26	2	250	115	—	—	2
Essence Plum Honey Lavender	1 pkg (6 oz)	160	3	2	10	8	28	26	2	250	115	—	—	2
Essence Pomegranate Acai	1 pkg (6 oz)	170	3	2	10	8	29	27	2	250	125	—	—	5
Exotic Kiwi Passion Fruit Lime	1 pkg (6 oz)	160	3	2	10	8	28	26	2	250	135	—	—	6
Exotic Orange Strawberry Mango	1 pkg (6 oz)	160	3	2	10	8	28	27	2	250	120	—	—	5
Exotic Pomegranate Blueberry	1 pkg (6 oz)	170	3	2	10	8	29	27	2	250	135	—	—	2

FOOD	PORTION	CALS	FAT	SAT FAT	CHOL	PROT	CARB	SUGAR	FIBER	CALCI	SOD	POTAS	FOLIC	VIT C
SIGGI'S														
Icelandic Skyr Vanilla 0% Milkfat	1 pkg (6 oz)	120	0	0	5	16	12	10	0	200	65	—	—	0
SILK														
Live! Blueberry	1 pkg (6 oz)	150	2	0	0	4	29	21	1	300	25	—	—	0
Soy Blueberry	1 pkg (6 oz)	150	2	0	0	4	29	21	1	300	25	—	—	30
Soy Key Lime	1 pkg (6 oz)	150	2	0	0	4	30	21	1	300	25	—	—	30
Soy Plain	1 cup (8 oz)	150	4	1	0	6	22	12	1	400	30	—	—	30
Soy Vanilla	1 pkg (6 oz)	150	3	0	0	5	25	18	1	300	20	—	—	30
Strawberry	1 pkg (6 oz)	160	2	0	0	4	31	22	1	300	25	—	—	30
SODELICIOUS														
Coconut Milk Plain	1 pkg (6 oz)	130	7	6	0	1	16	12	3	300	10	—	—	0
Coconut Milk Vanilla	1 pkg (6 oz)	150	6	6	0	1	22	19	2	250	5	—	—	0
Dairy Free Cinnamon Bun	1 pkg (6 oz)	160	3	0	0	6	29	24	3	300	25	—	—	0
Dairy Free Raspberry	1 pkg (6 oz)	150	3	0	0	6	29	22	3	300	35	—	—	1
STONYFIELD FARM														
0% Fat Chocolate Underground	1 pkg (6 oz)	150	0	0	<5	7	30	29	1	250	105	320	—	0
0% Fat Fruit On The Bottom Blueberry	1 pkg (6 oz)	120	0	0	0	6	22	20	0	250	100	330	—	0
0% Fat Fruit On The Bottom Pomegranate Raspberry	1 pkg (6 oz)	120	0	0	0	6	22	22	0	250	130	330	—	0
0% Fat Fruit On The Bottom Strawberry	1 pkg (6 oz)	110	0	0	0	6	22	21	0	250	125	350	—	0
0% Fat Smooth & Creamy Black Cherry	1 pkg (6 oz)	100	0	0	<5	7	18	17	0	300	120	380	—	0
0% Fat Smooth & Creamy French Vanilla	1 pkg (6 oz)	100	0	0	<5	7	17	17	0	300	115	380	—	0
0% Fat Smooth & Creamy Key Lime	1 pkg (6 oz)	100	0	0	<5	7	17	16	0	300	125	380	—	0
0% Fat Smooth & Creamy Lemon	1 pkg (6 oz)	100	0	0	<5	7	18	17	0	300	120	360	—	0
0% Fat Smooth & Creamy Peach	1 pkg (6 oz)	100	0	0	<5	7	18	17	0	250	115	370	—	0
0% Fat Smooth & Creamy Plain	1 pkg (6 oz)	80	0	0	0	8	11	11	0	300	120	400	—	0

FOOD	PORTION	CALS	FAT	SAT FAT	CHOL	PROT	CARB	SUGAR	FIBER	CALCI	SOD	POTAS	FOLIC	VIT C
STONYFIELD FARM (CONT.)														
0% Fat Smooth & Creamy Pomegranate Berry	1 pkg (6 oz)	100	0	0	<5	7	17	16	0	300	120	400	—	0
0% Fat Smooth & Creamy Strawberry	1 pkg (6 oz)	100	0	0	<5	7	18	17	0	300	120	380	—	0
Lowfat Cherry Vanilla	1 pkg (6 oz)	130	2	1	5	7	23	21	0	250	110	370	—	0
Lowfat Fruit On The Bottom Blueberry	1 pkg (6 oz)	120	2	1	5	6	21	20	tr	250	90	310	—	0
Lowfat Fruit On The Bottom Peach	1 pkg (6 oz)	130	2	1	5	6	22	22	0	250	110	330	—	0
Lowfat Fruit On The Bottom Strawberry	1 pkg (6 oz)	120	2	1	5	6	21	20	tr	250	120	330	—	0
Lowfat Plain	1 pkg (6 oz)	90	2	1	5	7	11	11	0	300	110	380	—	0
O'Soy Chocolate	1 pkg (6 oz)	160	3	1	0	8	25	22	2	150	35	310	—	0
O'Soy Fruit On The Bottom Peach	1 pkg (6 oz)	170	3	0	0	7	30	28	2	150	45	290	—	0
O'Soy Fruit On The Bottom Strawberry	1 pkg (6 oz)	170	3	0	0	7	29	26	2	150	55	300	—	0
O'Soy Vanilla	1 pkg (6 oz)	150	3	0	0	7	24	21	1	150	40	310	—	0
Whole Milk Cream Top French Vanilla	1 pkg (6 oz)	170	6	4	25	6	23	22	0	250	95	310	—	0
Whole Milk Cream Top White Chocolate Raspberry	1 pkg (6 oz)	170	6	4	25	6	23	23	0	250	105	320	—	0
STRAUS														
Organic Blueberry Pomegranate	1 cup (8 oz)	220	6	4	30	11	31	25	0	300	110	—	—	1
Organic Cinnamon Nonfat	1 cup (8 oz)	190	0	0	10	13	33	26	1	450	140	—	—	1
Organic Maple Whole Milk	1 cup (8 oz)	210	6	4	35	10	28	23	0	300	120	—	—	0
Organic Plain Lowfat	1 cup (8 oz)	150	2	1	15	14	21	10	0	400	140	—	—	1
Organic Plain Nonfat	1 cup (8 oz)	120	0	0	10	14	17	10	1	450	160	—	—	0
Organic Vanilla Nonfat	1 cup (8 oz)	190	0	0	10	13	34	25	0	450	140	—	—	0

FOOD	PORTION	CALS	FAT	SAT FAT	CHOL	PROT	CARB	SUGAR	FIBER	CALCI	SOD	POTAS	FOLIC	VIT C
THE GREEK GODS														
Honey	1 pkg (6 oz)	250	14	9	40	6	23	22	0	200	95	—	—	1
Plain Nonfat	1 pkg (6 oz)	60	0	0	0	6	10	7	2	250	105	—	—	1
Plain Traditional	1 pkg (4 oz)	130	11	7	30	4	5	5	0	150	70	—	—	1
Pomegranate	1 pkg (6 oz)	230	17	11	65	6	14	12	0	200	95	—	—	1
Vanilla Cinnamon Orange Reduced Fat	1 pkg (6 oz)	170	6	4	25	7	24	23	0	250	320	—	—	1
VOSKOS														
Greek Yogurt Exotic Fig	1 pkg (8 oz)	160	0	0	0	11	28	22	0	100	65	170	—	0
Greek Yogurt Plain Low Fat	1 pkg (8 oz)	160	3	2	20	23	9	7	0	250	100	295	—	0
Greek Yogurt Plain Non Fat	1 pkg (8 oz)	140	0	0	0	24	9	8	0	200	90	350	—	0
Greek Yogurt Plain Original	1 pkg (8 oz)	280	20	12	80	9	15	10	0	300	100	375	—	0
Greek Yogurt Wild Blueberry	1 pkg (8 oz)	120	0	0	10	13	16	14	0	150	55	170	—	0
Organic Vanilla Bean	1 pkg (5.3 oz)	130	0	0	0	12	20	17	0	150	45	175	—	0
WALLABY														
Lowfat Banana Vanilla	1 pkg (6 oz)	140	3	2	15	6	24	20	0	250	75	—	—	0
Lowfat Lemon	1 pkg (6 oz)	140	3	2	15	6	23	19	0	250	75	—	—	2
Lowfat Maple	1 pkg (6 oz)	140	3	2	15	6	24	20	0	250	75	—	—	1
Lowfat Plain	1 pkg (8 oz)	140	4	3	25	11	15	9	0	400	120	—	—	0
Lowfat Raspberry	1 pkg (6 oz)	140	3	2	15	7	23	19	0	250	75	—	—	2
Lowfat Vanilla	1 pkg (6 oz)	140	3	2	15	6	24	20	0	250	75	—	—	0
Original Guava	1 pkg (6 oz)	170	2	1	10	5	33	27	0	200	80	260	—	0
WHOLESOY & CO.														
Apricot Mango	1 pkg (6 oz)	160	4	0	0	6	30	19	2	300	35	—	—	6
Cherry	1 pkg (6 oz)	170	4	0	0	6	31	19	2	300	20	—	—	0
Lemon	1 pkg (6 oz)	160	4	0	0	6	29	18	2	300	15	—	—	1
Organic Soy Plain	1 pkg (6 oz)	150	3	0	0	6	27	12	2	300	25	—	—	0
Plain	1 pkg (6 oz)	150	5	1	0	8	19	13	1	350	15	—	—	1
Strawberry	1 pkg (6 oz)	160	4	0	0	6	30	21	2	300	20	—	—	4
Vanilla	1 pkg (6 oz)	160	4	1	0	7	23	18	1	350	15	—	—	1
WILDWOOD														
Organic Soyogurt Low Fat Peach	1 pkg (6 oz)	160	3	0	0	5	29	20	5	200	40	260	40	1
Organic Soyogurt Low Fat Vanilla	1 pkg (6 oz)	160	3	0	0	5	30	21	5	200	40	240	—	0
Organic Soyogurt Plain Unsweetened	1 pkg (6 oz)	110	4	1	0	6	14	4	4	250	45	300	—	0

FOOD	PORTION	CALS	FAT	SAT FAT	CHOL	PROT	CARB	SUGAR	FIBER	CALCI	SOD	POTAS	FOLIC	VIT C
YOFARM														
YoSmooth Apricot	1 pkg	220	6	4	20	6	36	31	—	200	90	—	—	—
YoSmooth Peach	1 pkg	220	6	4	20	6	35	30	—	200	100	—	—	—
YoSmooth Raspberry	1 pkg	230	6	4	20	6	36	31	—	200	95	—	—	—
YOPLAIT														
Delights Chocolate Raspberry	1 pkg (4 oz)	100	2	1	5	5	18	13	0	150	90	200	—	0
Delights Lemon Torte	1 pkg (4 oz)	100	2	1	5	5	16	12	0	150	80	180	—	0
Delights Triple Berry Creme	1 pkg (4 oz)	100	2	1	5	5	16	12	0	150	80	180	—	0
Light Strawberry	1 pkg (4 oz)	50	0	0	<5	4	8	5	tr	150	70	170	—	2
Orginal Coconut Cream	1 pkg (6 oz)	190	3	2	10	5	34	27	0	200	85	260	—	0
Orginal Passion Fruit	1 pkg (6 oz)	170	2	1	10	5	33	27	0	200	80	260	—	0
Original Lemon Burst	1 pkg (6 oz)	180	2	1	10	5	36	31	0	200	80	250	—	0
Original Pina Colada	1 pkg (6 oz)	170	2	2	10	5	33	28	0	200	95	250	—	0
Whips All Chocolate Flavors	1 pkg (6 oz)	160	4	3	10	5	26	23	0	100	105	230	—	0
Whips All Fruit Flavors	1 pkg (4 oz)	140	3	2	10	5	25	21	0	150	75	220	—	0
Yo Plus All Flavors	1 pkg (4 oz)	110	2	1	10	4	21	16	3	150	70	190	—	0

YOGURT DRINKS

(*see also* SMOOTHIES)

FOOD	PORTION	CALS	FAT	SAT FAT	CHOL	PROT	CARB	SUGAR	FIBER	CALCI	SOD	POTAS	FOLIC	VIT C
lassi	7 oz	78	5	3	19	0	8	8	0	79	—	96	—	—
DAHLICIOUS														
Lassi Green Tea	1 bottle	110	0	0	0	7	21	19	2	250	100	330	—	1
Lassi Mango	1 bottle	130	0	0	0	8	27	24	2	250	100	400	—	12
Lassi Plain	1 bottle	110	0	0	0	7	21	19	2	250	100	320	—	1
DANNON														
Activia Mixed Berry	1 bottle (6 oz)	160	3	2	10	6	27	25	1	200	60	200	—	0
Activia Peach	1 bottle (6 oz)	170	3	2	10	6	27	25	1	200	65	210	—	0
Activia Vanilla	1 bottle (6 oz)	160	3	2	10	6	27	25	1	200	60	200	—	0
Danactive Blueberry	1 bottle (3.1 oz)	80	2	1	5	3	14	13	0	80	40	135	—	0
Danactive Strawberry	1 bottle (3.1 oz)	80	2	1	5	3	14	13	0	80	40	135	—	0
Danactive Vanilla	1 bottle (3.1 oz)	80	2	1	5	3	14	13	0	80	40	130	—	0

FOOD	PORTION	CALS	FAT	SAT FAT	CHOL	PROT	CARB	SUGAR	FIBER	CALCI	SOD	POTAS	FOLIC	VIT C
DANNON (CONT.)														
Danimals Smoothies Rockin' Raspberry	1 bottle (3.1 oz)	70	1	0	<5	2	15	14	0	250	35	100	0	0
Danimals Smoothies Strawberry Explosion	1 bottle (3.1 oz)	70	1	0	<5	2	15	14	0	250	35	100	0	0
Danimals Smoothies Strikin' Strawberry Kiwi	1 bottle (3.1 oz)	70	1	0	<5	2	15	14	0	250	30	100	0	0
Light & Fit Smoothie Mixed Berry & Pomegranate	1 bottle (7 oz)	70	0	0	<5	4	13	12	0	200	70	230	—	0
Light & Fit Smoothie Peach	1 bottle (7 oz)	70	0	0	<5	4	13	12	0	200	90	230	—	0
Light & Fit Smoothie Strawberry Banana	1 bottle (7 oz)	70	0	0	<5	4	14	12	0	200	75	230	—	0
GOPI														
Lassi	8 oz	126	10	6	37	6	4	4	0	110	600	—	—	1
KAROUN														
Yogurt Drink	8 oz	126	10	6	37	6	4	4	0	110	600	—	—	1
LIFEWAY														
Lassi Mango	8 oz	160	2	2	10	11	25	21	3	300	125	—	—	2
Lassi Strawberry	8 oz	160	2	2	10	11	25	21	3	300	125	—	—	2
PROMISE														
Activ All Flavors	1 bottle (3.5 oz)	70	4	0	0	1	9	8	tr	40	20	—	—	2
YO ON THE GO														
All Flavors	1 box (8 oz)	180	3	2	0	6	31	29	0	200	80	240	120	18
YO-GOAT														
All Flavors	8 oz	160	8	6	30	7	11	12	0	300	115	—	—	1
Plain	8 oz	150	9	6	30	9	11	40	0	300	115	—	—	1
YOPLAIT														
Kids All Flavors	1 bottle (3.1 oz)	70	2	1	5	2	11	10	—	200	40	—	—	0
YOGURT FROZEN														
chocolate soft serve	1 cup	230	9	5	7	6	36	—	3	212	141	376	16	tr
vanilla soft serve	1 cup	236	8	5	3	6	35	35	0	206	125	304	9	1
BEN & JERRY'S														
Greek Banana Peanut Butter	½ cup (3.5 oz)	210	8	3	25	6	30	26	tr	150	100	—	—	1
Greek Blueberry Vanilla Graham	½ cup (3.5 oz)	200	7	3	25	6	29	23	0	200	105	—	—	0

FOOD	PORTION	CALS	FAT	SAT FAT	CHOL	PROT	CARB	SUGAR	FIBER	CALCI	SOD	POTAS	FOLIC	VIT C
BEN & JERRY'S (CONT.)														
Greek Raspberry Fudge Chunk	½ cup (3.4 oz)	200	7	5	25	6	29	25	tr	150	65	—	—	1
Greek Strawberry Shortcake	½ cup (3.5 oz)	180	5	3	30	6	28	23	0	150	75	—	—	6
DIPPIN' DOTS														
Strawberry Cheesecake	½ cup	100	0	0	0	4	21	17	1	80	80	—	—	0
HAAGEN-DAZS														
Lowfat Coffee	½ cup (3.7 oz)	200	5	3	65	8	31	20	0	200	50	—	—	0
Lowfat Tart Natural	½ cup (3.6 oz)	180	3	1	45	9	30	21	0	200	45	—	—	1
Lowfat Vanilla	½ cup (3.7 oz)	200	5	3	65	9	31	21	0	250	55	—	—	0
Lowfat Wildberry	½ cup (3.7 oz)	180	2	1	35	7	34	27	0	150	40	—	—	4
HOOD														
Fat Free Old Fashioned Vanilla	½ cup	110	0	0	0	3	24	15	tr	100	75	—	—	0
Fat Free Strawberry	½ cup	100	0	0	0	2	23	15	tr	100	70	—	—	2
Vanilla Swiss Almond	½ cup	150	5	2	10	3	25	17	tr	80	85	—	—	0
JULIE'S														
Organic Blackberry	½ cup	190	12	7	70	3	20	15	1	100	45	—	—	0
Organic Peanut Butter Fudge	½ cup	260	17	8	70	4	24	22	tr	100	125	—	—	0
Organic Strawberry	½ cup	200	12	7	70	3	22	20	0	100	50	—	—	0
Organic Vanilla	½ cup	220	15	9	85	4	20	18	0	100	55	—	—	0
STONYFIELD FARM														
Fat Free After Dark Chocolate	1 serv (4 oz)	100	0	0	<5	4	21	18	1	150	55	180	—	0
Fat Free Gotta Have Vanilla	1 serv (4 oz)	100	0	0	<5	4	20	19	0	150	65	220	—	0
Fat Free Vanilla Fudge Swirl	1 serv (4 oz)	120	0	0	<5	4	25	23	0	150	65	180	—	0
Low Fat Creme Caramel	1 serv (4 oz)	130	2	1	5	4	26	25	0	150	95	170	—	0
Lowfat Cookies 'N Cream	1 serv (4 oz)	130	2	1	<5	4	25	20	0	150	110	210	—	0
TURKEY HILL														
Fudge Ripple	½ cup	100	0	0	0	3	21	16	0	250	65	—	—	0
Neapolitan	½ cup	90	0	0	0	3	19	14	1	250	55	—	—	0
Smoothie Orange Cream Swirl	½ cup	100	0	0	0	2	22	18	0	150	40	—	—	0

FOOD	PORTION	CALS	FAT	SAT FAT	CHOL	PROT	CARB	SUGAR	FIBER	CALCI	SOD	POTAS	FOLIC	VIT C
TURKEY HILL (CONT.)														
Smoothie Peach Mango	½ cup	90	0	0	0	2	21	17	0	150	50	—	—	4
Vanilla Bean	½ cup	100	0	0	0	3	19	14	0	250	60	—	—	0

YOUNGBERRY JUICE

CERES

FOOD	PORTION	CALS	FAT	SAT FAT	CHOL	PROT	CARB	SUGAR	FIBER	CALCI	SOD	POTAS	FOLIC	VIT C
100% Juice	8 oz	120	0	0	0	0	30	26	0	20	10	210	—	60

ZUCCHINI

FOOD	PORTION	CALS	FAT	SAT FAT	CHOL	PROT	CARB	SUGAR	FIBER	CALCI	SOD	POTAS	FOLIC	VIT C
baby raw	1 (0.5 oz)	3	tr	tr	0	tr	1	—	tr	3	0	73	3	6
canned italian style	1 cup	66	tr	tr	0	2	16	—	—	39	849	622	68	5
fresh	1 sm (4.1 oz)	19	tr	tr	0	1	4	2	1	18	12	309	34	20
pickled	¼ cup	16	tr	tr	0	tr	4	3	1	7	71	88	8	8
raw sliced	1 cup	19	tr	tr	0	1	4	2	1	17	11	296	33	19
sliced cooked w/o salt	1 cup	29	tr	tr	0	1	7	3	3	23	5	455	31	8
C&W														
Yellow & Green	⅔ cup	20	0	0	0	1	3	2	tr	20	5	—	—	0
TAKE-OUT														
breaded & fried	6 slices (3 oz)	141	11	1	2	2	10	3	1	20	105	157	19	7
indian pakora	1 serv	46	2	tr	1	2	7	—	2	—	141	—	—	—
sticks breaded & fried	6 (2 oz)	90	7	1	2	1	6	2	1	14	67	107	15	5

Part Two

RESTAURANT CHAINS

Bigger Isn't Always Better

*Supersizing, add-ons, toppings, extras, stuffed, doubles,
and "buy one, get one free" may cost little,
but the extra calories, fat, and sodium
you'll be tempted to eat are no bargain.*

FOOD	PORTION	CALS	FAT	SAT FAT	CHOL	PROT	CARB	SUGAR	FIBER	CALCI	SOD	POTAS	FOLIC	VIT C
A&W														
BEVERAGES														
Coke	1 sm (11 oz)	145	0	0	0	0	37	37	0	0	23	—	—	0
Diet Coke	1 sm (11 oz)	0	0	0	0	0	0	0	0	0	25	—	—	0
Diet Root Beer	1 sm (15 oz)	0	0	0	0	0	0	0	0	0	40	—	—	0
Float Diet Root Beer	1 sm (14 oz)	170	5	3	40	2	30	17	0	80	100	—	—	0
Float Root Beer	1 sm (14 oz)	330	5	3	40	2	70	57	0	80	100	—	—	0
Milkshake Chocolate	1 med	700	29	18	125	11	100	60	2	300	200	—	—	0
Milkshake Strawberry	1 med	670	29	18	115	11	90	52	0	400	180	—	—	0
Milkshake Vanilla	1 med	720	31	19	135	12	97	57	0	450	210	—	—	0
Root Beer	1 sm (15 oz)	220	0	0	0	0	57	29	0	0	40	—	—	0
DESSERTS														
Cone Vanilla	1 med	260	7	4	25	1	41	29	1	200	145	—	—	0
Freeze A&W Root Beer	1 med	480	10	6	40	25	89	42	0	300	230	—	—	0
Polar Swirl M&M	1 med	710	25	16	55	15	107	93	2	450	290	—	—	0
Polar Swirl Oreo	1 med	690	24	11	50	14	107	79	3	400	570	—	—	0
Polar Swirl Reese's	1 med	740	31	14	55	18	97	85	3	400	380	—	—	0
Sundae Caramel	1 med	340	9	4	35	8	57	13	0	200	250	—	—	0
Sundae Chocolate	1 med	320	8	4	30	8	53	15	0	200	180	—	—	0
Sundae Hot Fudge	1 med	350	11	8	30	8	54	15	4	200	140	—	—	0
Sundae Strawberry	1 med	300	8	4	30	7	47	12	0	200	140	—	—	0
Sundae Vanilla	1 med	310	8	4	30	7	52	18	0	200	140	—	—	0
MAIN MENU SELECTIONS														
Cheese Curds	1 serv	570	40	21	105	27	27	3	2	800	1220	—	—	0
Cheese Dog	1	320	20	7	40	11	25	4	1	60	910	—	—	1
Cheeseburger Original Bacon	1	570	33	10	90	27	41	9	2	200	1200	—	—	6
Cheeseburger Original Bacon Double	1	800	48	17	165	45	47	10	2	300	1600	—	—	6
Cheeseburger Original Double	1	720	42	15	150	41	46	10	2	300	1370	—	—	6
Chicken Strips	3	500	29	5	55	28	32	2	7	60	1050	—	—	0
Chili Bowl	1 serv	190	6	2	20	12	22	9	5	80	640	—	—	1
Coney Chili Dog	1	310	18	7	40	13	24	5	2	60	870	—	—	1
Coney Chili Dog Cheese	1	350	21	8	45	13	27	5	2	80	1070	—	—	1
Fries	1 lg	430	18	5	0	5	61	1	6	0	640	—	—	27
Fries Cheese	1 serv	380	19	5	5	4	50	0	4	40	870	—	—	18
Fries Chili	1 serv	370	16	5	10	8	49	2	5	20	780	—	—	18
Fries Chili & Cheese	1 serv	400	19	8	10	8	51	2	5	40	990	—	—	18

FOOD	PORTION	CALS	FAT	SAT FAT	CHOL	PROT	CARB	SUGAR	FIBER	CALCI	SOD	POTAS	FOLIC	VIT C
Hot Dog Plain	1	280	17	6	35	11	22	4	1	40	710	—	—	0
Onion Rings	1 serv	350	18	4	0	5	45	3	2	20	710	—	—	0
Papa Burger	1	720	42	15	145	41	46	10	2	300	1390	—	—	6
Sandwich Crispy Chicken	1	590	29	5	65	31	54	8	3	100	1170	—	—	6
Sandwich Grilled Chicken	1	440	19	4	90	31	54	9	2	80	860	—	—	6
SAUCES														
Dipping Sauce BBQ	1 serv (1 oz)	40	0	0	0	0	10	6	0	0	230	—	—	0
Dipping Sauce Honey Mustard	1 serv (1 oz)	100	6	2	0	0	12	6	0	0	170	—	—	0
Dipping Sauce Ranch	1 serv (1 oz)	160	17	3	15	0	2	1	0	0	240	—	—	0
Dipping Sauce Sweet & Sour	1 serv (1 oz)	45	0	0	0	0	12	7	0	0	120	—	—	1

ARBY'S

FOOD	PORTION	CALS	FAT	SAT FAT	CHOL	PROT	CARB	SUGAR	FIBER	CALCI	SOD	POTAS	FOLIC	VIT C
BEVERAGES														
Dr Pepper	1 (16 oz)	180	0	0	0	0	52	52	0	—	60	—	—	—
Jamocha Shake	1 reg	498	13	8	34	13	81	78	0	510	393	—	—	5
Pepsi	1 (16 oz)	130	0	0	0	0	34	34	0	—	30	—	—	—
Shake Chocolate	1 reg	507	13	8	34	13	83	81	0	510	257	—	—	6
Shake Orange Cream	1 (17 oz)	637	17	10	41	15	105	100	0	20	423	—	—	0
Shake Strawberry	1 reg	498	13	8	34	13	81	77	0	510	363	—	—	6
Shake Strawberry Banana Swirl	1 (17 oz)	567	16	9	39	15	87	79	0	580	425	—	—	7
Shake Vanilla	1 reg	437	13	8	34	13	66	65	0	510	350	—	—	6
Sierra Mist	1 (16 oz)	100	0	0	0	0	27	27	0	—	25	—	—	—
BREAKFAST SELECTIONS														
Biscuit	1	273	15	4	1	5	28	3	1	30	786	—	—	0
Biscuit Bacon	1	340	21	6	13	9	29	3	1	30	1028	—	—	0
Biscuit Bacon Egg & Cheese	1	461	28	8	169	17	30	4	1	150	1446	—	—	0
Biscuit Chicken	1	417	23	5	17	15	39	3	1	120	1240	—	—	0
Biscuit Ham	1	316	17	4	13	13	29	4	1	40	1240	—	—	1
Biscuit Ham Egg & Cheese	1	437	23	6	169	20	31	4	1	150	1658	—	—	1
Biscuit Sausage	1	436	31	9	32	10	26	3	1	30	1160	—	—	0
Biscuit Sausage Egg & Cheese	1	557	38	11	187	18	30	3	1	150	1579	—	—	0
Biscuit Sausage Gravy	1	961	68	14	12	7	107	19	1	30	3755	—	—	0
Breakfast Syrup	1 serv (1 oz)	78	0	0	0	0	20	11	0	0	25	—	—	—
Cinnamon Roll Original Gourmet	1	507	10	4	7	10	73	31	4	180	373	—	—	4

FOOD	PORTION	CALS	FAT	SAT FAT	CHOL	PROT	CARB	SUGAR	FIBER	CALCI	SOD	POTAS	FOLIC	VIT C
Croissant	1	190	10	6	30	3	21	2	1	20	190	—	—	1
Croissant Bacon & Egg	1	337	22	10	187	11	23	3	1	40	651	—	—	2
Croissant Bacon Egg & Cheese	1	378	22	10	198	14	23	3	1	140	850	—	—	1
Croissant Ham & Cheese	1	274	12	7	53	13	22	3	1	120	842	—	—	1
Croissant Ham Egg & Cheese	1	434	24	10	343	22	26	4	1	150	1282	—	—	1
Croissant Sausage & Egg	1	433	32	13	206	12	23	3	1	40	784	—	—	1
Croissant Sausage Egg & Cheese	1	475	32	13	216	15	23	3	1	140	982	—	—	1
French Toastix	1 serv	312	13	2	0	6	44	11	1	50	492	—	—	—
Muffin Blueberry	1	320	12	2	20	4	49	26	1	20	490	—	—	—
Pecan Sticky Bun	1	688	22	5	7	12	91	45	5	190	420	—	—	5
Sourdough Bacon Egg & Cheese	1	437	16	5	174	20	40	5	2	300	1220	—	—	0
Sourdough Egg & Cheese	1	392	12	3	166	17	40	5	2	300	1058	—	—	0
Sourdough Ham Egg & Cheese	1	679	35	11	354	34	42	6	2	320	2104	—	—	1
Sourdough Sausage Egg & Cheese	1	514	27	8	186	19	40	5	2	200	1232	—	—	0
Twist Chocolate	1	250	12	4	5	4	34	12	2	40	110	—	—	—
Twist Cinnamon	1	260	14	5	5	3	33	11	1	40	190	—	—	—
Wrap Bacon Egg & Cheese	1	515	29	8	165	16	50	2	2	230	1367	—	—	1
Wrap Ham Egg & Cheese	1	568	31	10	183	24	51	3	2	310	1929	—	—	2
Wrap Sausage Egg & Cheese	1	689	45	15	202	21	50	2	2	310	1849	—	—	1
CHILDREN'S MENU SELECTIONS														
Kids Meal Chicken Tenders	1 serv	289	14	2	32	19	21	0	1	170	907	—	—	1
Kids Meal Junior Roast Beef Sandwich	1	272	10	4	29	16	34	5	2	60	740	—	—	0
Market Fresh Mini Ham & Cheese Sandwich	1	228	5	1	23	14	28	6	2	160	916	—	—	1
Market Fresh Mini Turkey & Cheese Sandwich	1	235	4	1	33	17	28	6	2	160	798	—	—	0
DESSERTS														
Cookie Chocolate Chip	1 (1.6 oz)	202	10	4	15	2	26	16	1	10	213	—	—	—

FOOD	PORTION	CALS	FAT	SAT FAT	CHOL	PROT	CARB	SUGAR	FIBER	CALCI	SOD	POTAS	FOLIC	VIT C
Turnover Apple	1	377	16	5	0	4	65	41	2	10	201	—	—	2
Turnover Cherry	1	377	15	5	0	4	65	41	2	10	201	—	—	2
SALAD DRESSINGS AND SAUCES														
Arby's Sauce	1 serv (0.5 oz)	15	0	0	0	0	4	1	0	0	177	—	—	1
Dipping Sauce BBQ	1 pkg (1 oz)	40	0	0	0	0	11	8	0	10	343	—	—	1
Dipping Sauce Bronco Berry	1 serv (2 oz)	122	0	0	0	0	30	28	0	0	36	—	—	3
Dipping Sauce Buffalo	1 serv (1 oz)	10	1	0	0	0	2	1	0	—	790	—	—	—
Dipping Sauce Cool Ranch Sour Cream	1 serv (1.5 oz)	158	16	4	0	1	2	1	0	20	277	—	—	—
Dipping Sauce Honey Mustard	1 serv (1 oz)	129	12	2	9	0	6	5	0	0	151	—	—	0
Dressing Buttermilk Ranch	1 serv (2.2 oz)	325	34	5	28	1	4	2	0	40	657	—	—	1
Dressing Buttermilk Ranch Light	1 serv (2 oz)	112	6	1	1	1	13	5	1	40	472	—	—	1
Dressing Santa Fe Ranch	1 pkg (2.2 oz)	296	31	5	21	1	4	1	0	20	692	—	—	4
Horsey Sauce	1 pkg (0.5 oz)	62	5	1	5	0	3	0	0	0	173	—	—	0
Ketchup	1 pkg	13	0	0	0	0	3	3	0	—	158	—	—	—
Sauce Cheddar Cheese	1 serv (0.7 oz)	30	2	1	1	0	2	0	0	10	181	—	—	—
Sauce Spicy Three Pepper	1 serv (0.5 oz)	22	1	0	0	0	3	3	0	0	140	—	—	1
Sauce Tangy Southwest	1 serv (2 oz)	333	35	5	29	1	5	4	0	0	371	—	—	2
SALADS														
Chicken Club	1 serv	487	25	8	178	32	31	3	4	370	1220	—	—	30
Martha's Vineyard	1 serv	277	8	4	72	26	24	17	4	190	451	—	—	33
Santa Fe	1 serv	477	21	6	53	29	42	6	6	360	1131	—	—	35
SANDWICHES														
Arby's Melt	1	302	12	4	30	16	36	5	2	60	921	—	—	0
Beef'N Cheddar	1	445	21	6	51	22	44	8	2	80	1274	—	—	2
Chicken Bacon & Swiss Crispy	1	624	29	7	68	36	52	13	2	190	1320	—	—	1
Chicken Bacon & Swiss Grilled	1	462	17	4	25	38	38	9	2	180	1333	—	—	2
Chicken Cordon Bleu Crispy	1	650	31	6	74	40	49	11	2	190	1548	—	—	1
Chicken Cordon Bleu Grilled	1	488	19	4	32	42	35	7	2	180	1561	—	—	2
Chicken Fillet Crispy	1	576	30	5	52	30	50	11	3	90	901	—	—	10

FOOD	PORTION	CALS	FAT	SAT FAT	CHOL	PROT	CARB	SUGAR	FIBER	CALCI	SOD	POTAS	FOLIC	VIT C
Chicken Fillet Grilled	1	414	17	3	9	32	36	7	3	90	913	—	—	11
Chicken Salad w/ Pecans	1	769	39	10	74	30	79	17	9	180	1240	—	—	30
Corned Beef Reuben	1	606	33	9	83	34	55	6	3	360	1849	—	—	3
Fish	1	543	25	6	55	21	61	9	3	60	956	—	—	10
French Dip	1	391	16	6	58	26	37	2	3	40	1282	—	—	6
French Dip & Swiss	1	473	18	7	79	32	28	2	3	250	1679	—	—	6
Ham & Swiss Melt	1	275	6	2	27	18	35	6	1	160	1118	—	—	1
Roast Beef Cheddar	1	521	27	9	64	27	45	9	2	80	1573	—	—	2
Roast Beef Regular	1	320	14	5	44	21	34	5	2	60	953	—	—	0
Roast Beef Super	1	398	19	6	44	21	40	10	2	70	1060	—	—	6
Roast Beef Swiss	1	777	41	13	89	37	73	16	5	360	1743	—	—	6
Roast Ham Swiss	1	705	31	8	63	36	75	19	5	370	2103	—	—	11
Roast Turkey & Swiss	1	725	30	8	91	45	75	17	5	360	1788	—	—	10
Roast Turkey Ranch & Bacon	1	834	38	11	109	49	75	17	5	330	2258	—	—	11
Roast Turkey Reuben	1	611	30	8	94	44	56	6	3	370	1429	—	—	4
Sourdough Melt Beef	1	355	14	5	30	18	40	4	2	90	1047	—	—	0
Sourdough Melt Ham	1	380	13	3	31	19	39	5	2	190	1280	—	—	1
Spicy Cajun Fish	1	603	32	7	68	21	61	9	3	70	883	—	—	10
Sub Toasted Classic Italian	1	828	46	13	89	37	69	5	3	300	2496	—	—	13
Sub Toasted French Dip & Swiss	1	622	20	7	79	37	68	2	3	210	3397	—	—	0
Sub Toasted Philly Beef	1	739	37	9	85	32	64	4	3	210	1881	—	—	4
Sub Toasted Turkey Bacon Club	1	619	18	4	82	42	65	4	3	220	2052	—	—	10
Swiss Melt	1	303	12	4	29	16	37	6	2	60	919	—	—	0
Ultimate BLT	1	779	45	11	51	23	75	18	6	170	1571	—	—	17
Wrap Chicken Salad w/ Pecans	1	638	38	10	74	30	48	3	8	50	1199	—	—	30
Wrap Corned Beef Reuben	1	577	29	8	83	38	42	6	1	200	1721	—	—	4
Wrap Roast Turkey Ranch & Bacon	1	700	37	11	109	49	44	3	4	190	2215	—	—	8

FOOD	PORTION	CALS	FAT	SAT FAT	CHOL	PROT	CARB	SUGAR	FIBER	CALCI	SOD	POTAS	FOLIC	VIT C
Wrap Roast Turkey Reuben	1	581	27	6	94	48	43	6	1	210	1301	—	—	4
Wrap Southwest Chicken	1	567	29	9	88	36	42	3	4	240	1451	—	—	8
Wrap Ultimate BLT	1	648	44	11	51	23	45	4	5	40	1530	—	—	17
SIDES														
Bites Jalapeno	5	305	21	9	28	5	29	3	2	30	526	—	—	1
Bites Loaded Potato	5	353	22	7	13	11	27	0	2	180	800	—	—	13
Cheddar Fries	1 med	465	28	6	2	6	51	0	5	70	1311	—	—	6
Chicken Tenders	3 pieces	379	18	3	42	25	28	0	2	220	1188	—	—	1
Croutons Cheese & Garlic	1 pkg	77	5	1	1	2	7	0	0	0	116	—	—	0
Curly Fries	1 lg	631	37	7	0	8	73	0	7	80	1476	—	—	10
Curly Fries	1 sm	338	20	4	0	4	39	0	4	40	791	—	—	5
Fruit Cup	1 serv	35	0	0	0	0	9	8	1	0	0	—	—	4
Homestyle Fries	1 sm	302	20	4	0	3	44	1	3	30	549	—	—	7
Homestyle Fries	1 lg	566	37	7	0	6	82	1	6	50	1029	—	—	13
Mozzarella Sticks	8 pieces	849	56	26	90	36	75	9	4	760	2730	—	—	1
Onion Petals	1 reg	331	23	4	1	4	35	7	2	20	332		—	1
Popcorn Chicken	1 reg	365	18	1	40	24	27	0	2	210	1145	—	—	1
Potato Cakes	2	246	18	4	0	2	26	0	2	20	391	—	—	2
Seasoned Tortilla Strips	1 serv	71	3	0	0	1	9	0	1	20	25	—	—	—

AU BON PAIN

FOOD	PORTION	CALS	FAT	SAT FAT	CHOL	PROT	CARB	SUGAR	FIBER	CALCI	SOD	POTAS	FOLIC	VIT C
BAKED SELECTIONS														
Bagel Asiago Cheese	1	360	4	3	10	15	64	4	3	—	590	—	—	—
Bagel Cinnamon Raisin	1	320	1	0	0	11	67	4	3	—	440	—	—	—
Bagel Everything	1	350	5	0	0	13	64	4	3	—	990	—	—	—
Bagel Honey 9 Grain	1	330	2	0	0	13	68	4	6	—	540	—	—	—
Bagel Jalapeno Double Cheddar	1	350	10	6	30	17	55	4	2	—	650	—	—	—
Bagel Onion Dill	1	350	1	0	0	13	72	5	4	—	530	—	—	—
Bagel Plain	1	290	1	0	0	11	59	4	2	—	440	—	—	—
Bagel Poppy Seed	1	290	1	0	0	11	59	4	2	—	440	—	—	—
Bagel Sesame Seed	1	330	5	1	0	12	61	4	3	—	440	—	—	—
Baguette Artisan Honey Multigrain Salad Size	1 (3.5 oz)	240	3	0	0	8	47	1	4	—	460	—	—	—

FOOD	PORTION	CALS	FAT	SAT FAT	CHOL	PROT	CARB	SUGAR	FIBER	CALCI	SOD	POTAS	FOLIC	VIT C
Baguette Artisan Honey Multigrain Sandwich Size	1 (4.7 oz)	310	3	0	0	10	62	1	6	—	610	—	—	—
Baguette Artisan Salad Size	1 (3.5 oz)	210	1	0	0	7	44	1	2	—	460	—	—	—
Baguette Artisan Sandwich Size	1 (4.7 oz)	290	1	0	0	10	59	1	2	—	610	—	—	—
Blondie	1	330	19	6	35	7	61	25	3	—	350	—	—	—
Bread Artisan Multigrain	1 serv (4 oz)	260	3	0	0	9	51	0	4	—	610	—	—	—
Bread Artisan Sundried Tomato	1 serv (4 oz)	240	1	0	0	8	49	2	2	—	570	—	—	—
Bread Cheese	1 serv (4.8 oz)	290	8	4	2	14	55	1	3	—	730	—	—	—
Bread Country White	1 serv (4 oz)	240	1	0	0	6	50	1	2	—	590	—	—	—
Bread Bowl	1 (9.24 oz)	640	3	0	0	28	127	3	6	—	1830	—	—	—
Bread Stick Rosemary Garlic	1 (2.3 oz)	200	5	1	0	6	33	2	2	—	1430	—	—	—
Brownie Chocolate Chip	1	380	17	5	75	5	62	41	1	—	390	—	—	—
Brownie Hazelnut Mocha	1	430	21	5	65	6	58	31	3	—	360	—	—	—
Brownie Rocky Road	1	410	17	5	70	6	62	31	2	—	430	—	—	—
Ciabatta	1 sm	180	1	0	0	7	37	2	2	—	380	—	—	—
Cinnamon Roll	1	350	12	7	40	7	53	21	2	—	240	—	—	—
Cookie Chocolate Chip	1 (2 oz)	260	12	6	25	2	37	22	1	—	220	—	—	—
Cookie Confetti	1 (2.4 oz)	310	14	5	25	3	42	25	1	—	290	—	—	—
Cookie English Toffee	1 (2 oz)	210	11	4	20	2	26	15	1	—	240	—	—	—
Cookie Gingerbread	1 (2.7 oz)	300	9	4	10	4	50	21	1	—	140	—	—	—
Cookie Hazelnut Fudge	1 (2.25 oz)	290	16	6	40	4	34	25	3	—	150	—	—	—
Cookie Oatmeal Raisin	1 (2 oz)	230	8	4	35	3	36	23	2	—	190	—	—	—
Cookie Shortbread	1 (2.3 oz)	310	9	0	25	3	34	10	1	—	270	—	—	—
Creme De Fleur	1 serv	550	26	15	110	12	71	32	1	—	540	—	—	—
Croissant Almond	1	560	36	13	110	12	52	16	4	—	270	—	—	—
Croissant Apple	1	230	10	6	25	4	31	11	2	—	230	—	—	—
Croissant Chocolate	1	330	17	10	30	6	42	16	3	—	180	—	—	—
Croissant Plain	1 (2.8 oz)	260	15	8	55	5	28	3	1	—	190	—	—	—

FOOD	PORTION	CALS	FAT	SAT FAT	CHOL	PROT	CARB	SUGAR	FIBER	CALCI	SOD	POTAS	FOLIC	VIT C
Croissant Raspberry Cheese	1	330	16	10	60	7	41	16	1	—	280	—	—	—
Croissant Sweet Cheese	1	320	16	10	60	4	39	15	1	—	280	—	—	—
Danish Cherry	1	370	19	9	85	7	44	15	1	—	290	—	—	—
Danish Sweet Cheese	1	380	20	10	90	7	44	16	1	—	300	—	—	—
Focaccia	1 piece (4.4 oz)	310	4	1	0	11	57	2	3	—	640	—	—	—
Lavash	1 (4 oz)	320	1	0	0	15	62	1	2	—	190	—	—	—
Macaroon Chocolate Dipped Cranberry Almond	1	320	16	8	0	4	42	33	3	—	190	—	—	—
Mini Loaf Bacon & Cheese	1 (4.8 oz)	540	31	8	95	13	50	20	1	—	790	—	—	—
Muffin Blueberry	1	510	19	2	20	9	76	33	5	—	550	—	—	—
Muffin Carrot Walnut	1	520	25	5	55	8	66	38	4	—	800	—	—	—
Muffin Corn	1	460	16	3	60	9	69	29	2	—	550	—	—	—
Muffin Cranberry Walnut	1	500	24	2	20	10	61	26	5	—	460	—	—	—
Muffin Double Chocolate Chunk	1	590	20	6	25	10	83	46	5	—	480	—	—	—
Muffin Pumpkin	1	490	17	3	65	9	75	35	2	—	520	—	—	—
Muffin Raisin Bran	1	410	9	2	30	10	74	40	9	—	590	—	—	—
Muffin Low Fat Triple Berry	1	290	2	1	25	5	61	31	2	—	310	—	—	—
Pastry Hazelnut Creme	1	540	34	16	85	10	50	20	3	—	380	—	—	—
Poundcake Cappuccino	1 slice (5.2 oz)	530	26	5	85	3	68	43	1	—	490	—	—	—
Poundcake Chocolate	1 slice (4.7 oz)	500	29	6	100	7	58	35	3	—	580	—	—	—
Poundcake Lemon	1 slice (4.9 oz)	520	27	6	85	5	64	40	0	—	460	—	—	—
Poundcake Marble	1 slice (4.7 oz)	490	27	5	90	6	59	35	1	—	520	—	—	—
Roll Pecan	1	630	32	11	30	10	80	38	3	—	330	—	—	—
Roll Soft	1 (4.7 oz)	410	11	4	20	11	65	9	3	—	700	—	—	—
Scone Cinnamon	1	430	24	14	130	9	48	16	1	—	360	—	—	—
Scone Orange	1	410	20	11	130	9	51	16	2	—	370	—	—	—
Shortbread Chocolate Dipped	1	350	20	9	25	3	38	14	1	—	280	—	—	—
Toasts Basil Pesto Cheese	3 pieces (2 oz)	140	2	0	0	5	26	1	1	—	330	—	—	—

FOOD	PORTION	CALS	FAT	SAT FAT	CHOL	PROT	CARB	SUGAR	FIBER	CALCI	SOD	POTAS	FOLIC	VIT C
Tulip Blueberry	1	370	20	4	65	4	44	25	1	—	300	—	—	—
Tulip Chocolate Raspberry	1	430	21	5	70	5	55	34	1	—	410	—	—	—
Tulip Key Lime	1	440	22	5	70	5	55	33	1	—	360	—	—	—
BEVERAGES														
Blast Caramel	1 med (16 oz)	540	17	12	60	6	104	99	0	—	105	—	—	—
Blast Coffee	1 med (16 oz)	440	21	15	75	8	71	67	0	—	115	—	—	—
Blast Mocha	1 med (16 oz)	440	17	12	60	7	80	74	2	—	95	—	—	—
Blast Vanilla	1 med (12 oz)	540	17	12	60	6	104	99	0	—	100	—	—	—
Caffe Americano	1 sm (12 oz)	5	0	0	0	0	1	1	0	—	15	—	—	—
Cappuccino	1 sm (12 oz)	120	7	4	20	6	10	10	0	—	85	—	—	—
Caramel Macchiato	1 sm (12 oz)	350	10	6	30	10	53	50	0	—	160	—	—	—
Chocolate Milk	1 (12 oz)	320	9	5	25	10	54	51	3	—	100	—	—	—
Hot Chocolate	1 sm (12 oz)	350	11	7	30	12	58	54	3	—	125	—	—	—
Iced Caramel Macchiato	1 sm (12 oz)	290	7	5	25	7	49	46	0	—	125	—	—	—
Iced Tea Peach	1 med (22 oz)	120	0	0	0	0	30	30	0	—	35	—	—	—
Latte Caffe	1 sm (12 oz)	200	11	7	45	11	17	17	0	—	170	—	—	—
Latte Chai	1 sm (12 oz)	290	11	7	30	11	38	26	0	—	130	—	—	—
Latte Iced Caffe	1 sm (12 oz)	110	6	4	20	6	19	10	0	—	80	—	—	—
Latte Iced Chai	1 sm (12 oz)	190	5	4	15	5	31	18	0	—	65	—	—	—
Latte Iced Mocha	1 sm (12 oz)	210	11	7	35	6	27	26	1	—	70	—	—	—
Latte Iced Vanilla	1 sm (12 oz)	240	5	3	15	5	44	44	0	—	65	—	—	—
Latte Iced White Chocolate	1 sm (12 oz)	250	11	7	35	5	35	32	0	—	135	—	—	—
Latte Mocha	1 sm (12 oz)	300	16	10	60	11	35	33	1	—	160	—	—	—
Latte Vanilla	1 sm (12 oz)	320	9	6	30	9	50	50	0	—	120	—	—	—
Latte White Chocolate	1 sm (12 oz)	310	14	9	45	9	41	38	0	—	180	—	—	—
Lemonade	1 med (22 oz)	300	0	0	0	0	72	72	0	—	0	—	—	—
Orange Juice	1 (8 oz)	110	0	0	0	2	26	26	1	—	0	—	—	—
Smoothie Peach	1 med (16 oz)	310	1	0	10	4	69	41	4	—	115	—	—	—
Smoothie Strawberry	1 med (16 oz)	310	1	0	10	4	66	43	3	—	110	—	—	—
MAIN MENU SELECTIONS														
Fruit Cup	1 sm (6 oz)	70	0	0	0	1	16	15	1	—	10	—	—	—
Harvest Rice Bowl Cajun Shrimp	1 (20 oz)	520	17	8	145	16	69	8	2	—	1660	—	—	—
Harvest Rice Bowl Cajun Shrimp w/ Brown Rice	1 (20 oz)	560	20	7	145	14	73	8	5	—	1660	—	—	—
Harvest Rice Bowl Mayan Chicken	1 (19.25 oz)	490	14	3	70	25	67	5	4	—	1430	—	—	—

FOOD	PORTION	CALS	FAT	SAT FAT	CHOL	PROT	CARB	SUGAR	FIBER	CALCI	SOD	POTAS	FOLIC	VIT C
Harvest Rice Bowl Mayan Chicken w/ Brown Rice	1 (19.25 oz)	540	16	3	70	23	71	5	7	—	1430	—	—	—
Harvest Rice Bowl Steak Teriyaki	1 (19.25 oz)	530	15	3	60	30	72	11	2	—	1520	—	—	—
Harvest Rice Bowl Steak Teriyaki w/ Brown Rice	1 (19.25 oz)	570	18	3	60	28	76	11	5	—	1520	—	—	—
Macaroni & Cheese	1 med (12 oz)	440	26	17	95	19	31	4	2	—	1280	—	—	—
Stew Beef	1 med (12 oz)	300	16	3	55	18	25	4	3	—	1070	—	—	—
Stew Chicken Vegetable	1 med (12 oz)	290	17	5	40	11	26	5	3	—	930	—	—	—
SALAD DRESSINGS AND SPREADS														
Artichoke Aioli	1 serv (1 oz)	130	14	2	10	1	1	0	0	—	180	—	—	—
Basil Pesto	1 serv (1 oz)	140	15	3	5	2	1	0	0	—	160	—	—	—
Chili Dijon	1 serv (1 oz)	120	12	2	10	1	3	2	1	—	130	—	—	—
Cream Cheese Honey Pecan	1 serv (2 oz)	120	10	7	35	4	5	4	0	—	340	—	—	—
Cream Cheese Honey Walnut	1 serv (2 oz)	140	9	6	30	3	12	12	0	—	150	—	—	—
Cream Cheese Lite	1 serv (2 oz)	120	9	6	30	4	5	3	0	—	280	—	—	—
Cream Cheese Plain	1 serv (2 oz)	170	16	11	50	3	4	3	0	—	290	—	—	—
Cream Cheese Strawberry	1 serv (2 oz)	180	15	10	45	3	9	8	0	—	250	—	—	—
Cream Cheese Sundried Tomato	1 serv (2 oz)	120	10	7	35	4	5	4	0	—	340	—	—	—
Cream Cheese Vegetable	1 serv (2 oz)	170	16	10	45	3	3	2	0	—	270	—	—	—
Dressing Balsamic Vinaigrette	1 serv (2.25 oz)	190	16	3	0	9	11	10	0	—	430	—	—	—
Dressing Blue Cheese	1 serv (1.75 oz)	230	24	5	20	2	2	1	0	—	550	—	—	—
Dressing Caesar	1 serv (2 oz)	280	28	5	20	2	4	3	0	—	400	—	—	—
Dressing Fat Free Raspberry Vinaigrette	1 serv (2.25 oz)	70	0	0	0	0	17	16	0	—	150	—	—	—
Dressing Light Honey Mustard	1 serv (2.25 oz)	180	11	2	10	1	21	19	1	—	590	—	—	—
Dressing Light Olive Oil Vinaigrette	1 serv (2.25 oz)	130	10	2	0	0	9	7	0	—	630	—	—	—
Dressing Light Ranch	1 serv (2.25 oz)	150	15	3	15	2	3	2	0	—	470	—	—	—
Dressing Thai Peanut	1 serv (2.25 oz)	230	13	2	0	5	24	22	1	—	840	—	—	—

FOOD	PORTION	CALS	FAT	SAT FAT	CHOL	PROT	CARB	SUGAR	FIBER	CALCI	SOD	POTAS	FOLIC	VIT C
Guacamole	1 serv (1 oz)	60	6	1	0	1	2	0	2	—	125	—	—	—
Honey Mustard	1 serv (2.5 oz)	210	13	2	15	1	23	21	1	—	650	—	—	—
Hummus Roasted Red Pepper	1 serv (2 oz)	80	5	0	0	2	6	0	2	—	250	—	—	—
Mayonnaise	1 serv (1 oz)	200	22	3	20	0	0	0	0	—	150	—	—	—
Mayonnaise Herb	1 serv (1 oz)	210	23	4	20	0	1	1	0	—	210	—	—	—
Mayonnaise Jalapeno	1 serv (1 oz)	140	15	2	15	2	0	0	0	—	260	—	—	—
Mayonnaise Tarragon Sauce	1 serv (2 oz)	420	45	7	40	0	2	2	0	—	420	—	—	—
Mustard	1 tsp	0	0	0	0	0	0	0	0	—	70	—	—	—
Spread Herb Bagel	1 serv (2 oz)	130	11	7	35	4	5	4	0	—	470	—	—	—
Spread Sundried Tomato	1 serv (0.53 oz)	70	6	1	0	1	4	1	0	—	85	—	—	—
SALADS														
Caesar Asiago	1 serv	210	12	6	25	11	18	4	3	—	470	—	—	—
Caesar Asiago Grilled Chicken	1 (8.5 oz)	340	13	6	65	29	19	4	3	—	680	—	—	—
Caesar Asiago Side	1 (3.2 oz)	120	6	3	15	6	12	2	2	—	260	—	—	—
Chef's	1 serv	230	14	7	60	22	7	5	3	—	1090	—	—	—
Garden	1 (7 oz)	80	2	0	0	4	14	3	4	—	210	—	—	—
Garden Side	1 (3.6 oz)	50	1	0	0	2	10	2	3	—	70	—	—	—
Mediterranean Chicken	1 (9.75 oz)	330	16	5	60	24	12	1	2	—	1170	—	—	—
Riviera	1 (9.5 oz)	260	7	3	15	7	46	31	5	—	250	—	—	—
Thai Peanut Chicken	1 (11 oz)	250	8	0	40	22	22	7	4	—	290	—	—	—
Tuna Garden	1 (10.5 oz)	350	25	4	55	21	14	4	4	—	470	—	—	—
Turkey Medallion Cobb	1 (11 oz)	340	19	8	260	27	15	3	3	—	980	—	—	—
Turkey Spinach Sonoma	1 (12.3 oz)	310	13	7	65	29	22	9	5	—	1310	—	—	—
SANDWICHES														
Arizona Chicken	1 (12 oz)	750	29	9	120	49	61	6	4	—	1480	—	—	—
Baguette Turkey & Swiss	1 (12.3 oz)	770	38	10	95	41	65	4	3	—	2120	—	—	—
Baja Turkey	1 (13 oz)	700	32	9	90	41	61	6	4	—	1970	—	—	—
Breakfast Asiago Bagel Prosciutto & Egg	1 (9.6 oz)	660	25	8	185	40	67	4	3	—	1580	—	—	—
Breakfast Asiago Bagel Sausage Egg & Cheddar	1 (10.2 oz)	770	45	21	215	36	55	4	0	—	1450	—	—	—
Breakfast Bagel & Bacon	1 (4.2 oz)	340	6	2	15	15	56	4	0	—	630	—	—	—
Breakfast Egg On A Bagel	1 (6.8 oz)	370	4	1	115	21	62	5	2	—	790	—	—	—

FOOD	PORTION	CALS	FAT	SAT FAT	CHOL	PROT	CARB	SUGAR	FIBER	CALCI	SOD	POTAS	FOLIC	VIT C
Breakfast Egg On A Bagel w/ Bacon	1 (7.2 oz)	410	8	3	130	25	58	4	0	—	980	—	—	—
Breakfast Egg On A Bagel w/ Bacon Cheese	1 (7.9 oz)	500	15	6	150	30	59	4	0	—	1120	—	—	—
Breakfast Egg On A Bagel w/ Cheese	1 (7.6 oz)	450	10	5	135	26	62	5	2	—	920	—	—	—
Breakfast Onion Dill Bagel Smoked Salmon & Wasabi	1 (7.1 oz)	490	11	4	45	18	77	6	3	—	1250	—	—	—
Caprese	1 (11.8 oz)	700	35	15	65	28	65	3	4	—	1120	—	—	—
Chicken Mozzarella	1 (14.5 oz)	800	27	8	105	50	71	6	2	—	1360	—	—	—
Chicken Pesto	1 (12.5 oz)	700	23	5	80	44	62	5	2	—	1340	—	—	—
Chicken Tarragon	1 (11 oz)	720	29	4	85	40	61	5	1	—	1190	—	—	—
Ciabatta Bacon & Egg Melt	1 (7 oz)	400	15	6	155	26	40	2	2	—	1160	—	—	—
Ciabatta Ham & Cheddar	1 (12 oz)	650	20	9	95	40	80	19	4	—	2330	—	—	—
Club Smoked Turkey	1 (11.6 oz)	780	43	13	115	43	56	4	2	—	2330	—	—	—
Croissant Ham & Cheese	1 (4.2 oz)	350	18	10	60	14	34	4	1	—	550	—	—	—
Croissant Spinach & Cheese	1	250	14	8	35	8	25	3	2	—	280	—	—	—
Hot BBQ Chicken On Farmhouse Roll	1 (14.3 oz)	970	44	12	130	50	78	14	4	—	1630	—	—	—
Hot Eggplant & Mozzarella	1 (12.4 oz)	710	37	13	60	26	68	5	6	—	1440	—	—	—
Hot Steakhouse On Ciabatta	1 (13 oz)	800	41	11	100	43	70	8	4	—	1850	—	—	—
Melt Tuna	1 (12.5 oz)	760	41	10	100	40	60	6	4	—	1240	—	—	—
Melt Turkey	1 (12.2 oz)	890	47	15	120	45	70	18	3	—	2360	—	—	—
Portobello & Goat Cheese	1 (10 oz)	610	33	10	35	18	61	4	6	—	1290	—	—	—
Portobello Egg & Cheddar	1 (8.5 oz)	590	37	21	200	22	42	2	3	—	1050	—	—	—
Prosciutto Mozzarella	1 (12.7 oz)	880	49	17	110	40	71	5	4	—	2270	—	—	—
Spicy Tuna	1 (10.3 oz)	640	34	5	65	28	57	3	6	—	1100	—	—	—
The Montana	1 (12.5 oz)	560	23	12	105	40	62	5	4	—	1370	—	—	—
Turkey & Cranberry Chutney	1 (10.9 oz)	680	24	4	60	30	63	25	3	—	1970	—	—	—

FOOD	PORTION	CALS	FAT	SAT FAT	CHOL	PROT	CARB	SUGAR	FIBER	CALCI	SOD	POTAS	FOLIC	VIT C
Wrap Chicken Caesar Asiago	1	700	25	8	75	42	69	6	3	—	930	—	—	—
Wrap Chopped Turkey Club	1 (12 oz)	660	27	8	165	35	70	5	4	—	1200	—	—	—
Wrap Mediterranean	1 (12.8 oz)	670	28	6	20	24	80	5	7	—	1240	—	—	—
Wrap Southwest Tuna	1 (14 oz)	900	51	12	110	46	72	6	5	—	980	—	—	—
Wrap Thai Peanut Chicken	1 (14.5 oz)	660	19	2	40	38	84	10	4	—	770	—	—	—
Wrap Turkey Spinach Sonoma	1 (12 oz)	630	19	6	45	35	80	12	5	—	1070	—	—	—
Wrap Hot Cajun Shrimp	1 (14.9 oz)	700	24	8	90	20	95	8	4	—	1680	—	—	—
Wrap Hot Mayan Chicken	1 (13.5 oz)	630	19	3	40	24	92	6	5	—	1400	—	—	—
Wrap Hot Steak Teriyaki	1 (13.5 oz)	660	19	4	40	28	93	9	5	—	1780	—	—	—
SOUPS														
Baked Stuffed Potato	1 med (12 oz)	350	21	10	60	9	30	6	2	—	990	—	—	—
Broccoli Cheddar	1 med (12 oz)	310	21	10	50	11	20	7	2	—	1000	—	—	—
Carrot Ginger	1 mcd (12 oz)	130	5	0	0	7	21	10	3	—	920	—	—	—
Chicken Florentine	1 med (12 oz)	240	13	6	35	8	25	4	1	—	1030	—	—	—
Chicken & Dumplings	1 med (12 oz)	210	7	3	50	11	28	6	2	—	1280	—	—	—
Chicken Noodle	1 med (12 oz)	130	3	1	15	9	20	2	2	—	1000	—	—	—
Clam Chowder	1 med (12 oz)	320	18	7	55	9	27	8	1	—	1020	—	—	—
Corn & Green Chili Bisque	1 med (12 oz)	250	14	7	35	5	29	6	3	—	1540	—	—	—
Corn Chowder	1 med (12 oz)	350	18	8	50	9	40	10	3	—	1120	—	—	—
Curried Rice & Lentil	1 med (12 oz)	150	2	0	0	9	30	4	8	—	1260	—	—	—
French Moroccan Tomato Lentil	1 med (12 oz)	180	2	0	0	10	32	7	8	—	1050	—	—	—
French Onion	1 med (12 oz)	130	5	3	10	4	19	6	2	—	1310	—	—	—
Garden Vegetable	1 med (12 oz)	80	2	0	0	3	14	5	3	—	1010	—	—	—
Harvest Pumpkin	1 med (12 oz)	190	10	5	25	8	26	6	2	—	1110	—	—	—
Hearty Cabbage	1 med (12 oz)	110	5	1	10	4	14	4	3	—	910	—	—	—
Italian Wedding	1 med (12 oz)	170	7	3	15	8	10	4	2	—	1300	—	—	—
Jamaican Black Bean	1 med (12 oz)	180	1	0	0	16	45	4	25	—	460	—	—	—
Mediterranean Pepper	1 med (12 oz)	100	3	0	0	5	18	3	5	—	580	—	—	—
Old Fashioned Tomato Rice	1 med (12 oz)	120	1	0	0	4	24	7	3	—	340	—	—	—

FOOD	PORTION	CALS	FAT	SAT FAT	CHOL	PROT	CARB	SUGAR	FIBER	CALCI	SOD	POTAS	FOLIC	VIT C
Pasta E Fagioli	1 med (12 oz)	240	8	2	5	11	36	3	9	—	930	—	—	—
Portuguese Kale	1 med (12 oz)	120	5	1	5	5	15	2	3	—	1130	—	—	—
Potato Cheese	1 med (12 oz)	250	14	8	50	7	25	4	2	—	1340	—	—	—
Potato Leek	1 med (12 oz)	300	20	11	60	5	28	2	2	—	1000	—	—	—
Red Beans Italian Sausage & Rice	1 med (12 oz)	200	5	2	10	15	28	3	16	—	1140	—	—	—
Southern Black Eyed Pea	1 med (12 oz)	180	2	0	5	12	31	4	12	—	950	—	—	—
Southwest Tortilla	1 med (12 oz)	200	11	3	10	4	24	5	4	—	1290	—	—	—
Southwest Vegetable	1 med (12 oz)	160	3	0	0	4	17	3	3	—	370	—	—	—
Split Pea	1 med (12 oz)	210	2	0	5	18	42	3	15	—	1190	—	—	—
Thai Coconut Curry	1 med (12 oz)	150	7	2	0	3	20	4	2	—	1150	—	—	—
Tomato Basil Bisque	1 med (12 oz)	210	8	5	25	6	29	18	5	—	490	—	—	—
Tomato Cheddar	1 med (12 oz)	240	15	6	25	12	17	7	2	—	1040	—	—	—
Tomato Florentine	1 med (12 oz)	120	3	1	5	5	19	6	2	—	1390	—	—	—
Tuscan Vegetable	1 med (12 oz)	170	5	2	10	7	24	3	3	—	1170	—	—	—
Vegetable Beef Barley	1 med (12 oz)	140	3	2	20	9	21	4	4	—	1000	—	—	—
Vegetarian Chili	1 med (12 oz)	230	3	0	0	12	40	7	11	—	1000	—	—	—
Vegetarian Lentil	1 med (12 oz)	140	2	0	0	10	32	4	11	—	1260	—	—	—
Vegetarian Minestrone	1 med (12 oz)	120	2	0	0	5	21	6	4	—	1120	—	—	—
Wild Mushroom Bisque	1 med (12 oz)	190	9	2	10	5	23	6	2	—	1010	—	—	—
YOGURT														
Blueberry w/ Fruit	1 sm (7.5 oz)	220	2	2	10	6	44	37	0	—	120	—	—	—
Blueberry w/ Granola & Fruit	1 sm (8.5 oz)	310	6	2	10	10	56	36	2	—	130	—	—	—
Strawberry w/ Blueberries	1 sm (7.5 oz)	220	2	2	10	6	44	37	0	—	120	—	—	—
Strawberry w/ Granola & Blueberries	1 sm (8.5 oz)	310	6	2	10	10	56	36	2	—	130	—	—	—
Vanilla w/ Blueberries	1 sm (7.5 oz)	190	2	1	10	10	32	30	0	—	160	—	—	—
Vanilla w/ Granola & Blueberries	1 sm (8.5 oz)	310	6	2	10	10	56	36	2	—	130	—	—	—

AUNTIE ANNE'S

FOOD	PORTION	CALS	FAT	SAT FAT	CHOL	PROT	CARB	SUGAR	FIBER	CALCI	SOD	POTAS	FOLIC	VIT C
BEVERAGES														
Dutch Ice Blue Raspberry	1 (14 oz)	165	0	0	0	0	38	35	0	20	20	—	—	0
Dutch Ice Grape	1 (14 oz)	180	0	0	0	0	43	41	0	0	20	—	—	0
Dutch Ice Kiwi Banana	1 (14 oz)	190	0	0	0	0	44	41	0	10	30	—	—	2

FOOD	PORTION	CALS	FAT	SAT FAT	CHOL	PROT	CARB	SUGAR	FIBER	CALCI	SOD	POTAS	FOLIC	VIT C
Dutch Ice Lemonade	1 (14 oz)	315	0	0	0	0	77	77	0	0	0	—	—	7
Dutch Ice Lemonade Strawberry	1 (14 oz)	330	0	0	0	0	81	81	0	0	0	—	—	6
Dutch Ice Mocha	1 (14 oz)	400	10	9	0	0	74	52	0	0	100	—	—	0
Dutch Ice Orange Creme	1 (14 oz)	280	0	0	0	0	64	59	0	10	35	—	—	11
Dutch Ice Pina Colada	1 (14 oz)	220	0	0	0	0	53	50	0	0	15	—	—	10
Dutch Ice Strawberry	1 (14 oz)	220	0	0	0	0	50	48	0	10	40	—	—	4
Dutch Ice Watermelon	1 (14 oz)	200	0	0	0	0	50	48	0	0	35	—	—	0
Dutch Ice Wild Cherry	1 (14 oz)	210	0	0	0	0	48	45	0	0	25	—	—	0
Dutch Latte Caramel	1 (14 oz)	350	15	11	55	4	49	39	0	150	55	—	—	0
Dutch Latte Coffee	1 (14 oz)	290	14	9	50	4	38	33	0	150	135	—	—	0
Dutch Latte Mocha	1 (14 oz)	160	17	11	55	5	47	37	0	150	135	—	—	0
Dutch Shake Chocolate	1 (14 oz)	580	27	18	105	10	75	67	0	300	380	—	—	0
Dutch Shake Coffee	1 (14 oz)	590	27	18	105	10	77	70	0	300	304	—	—	0
Dutch Shake Strawberry	1 (14 oz)	610	27	18	105	10	78	74	0	300	304	—	—	0
Dutch Shake Vanilla	1 (14 oz)	510	27	17	105	10	58	54	0	300	300	—	—	0
Dutch Smoothie Blue Raspberry	1 (14 oz)	230	8	5	30	3	34	33	0	100	100	—	—	0
Dutch Smoothie Grape	1 (14 oz)	230	8	5	30	3	36	35	0	80	100	—	—	0
Dutch Smoothie Kiwi Banana	1 (14 oz)	240	8	5	30	3	38	35	0	100	100	—	—	1
Dutch Smoothie Lemonade	1 (14 oz)	300	8	5	30	3	53	53	0	80	80	—	—	4
Dutch Smoothie Mocha	1 (14 oz)	330	13	9	30	3	50	39	0	80	130	—	—	0
Dutch Smoothie Orange Creme	1 (14 oz)	280	8	5	30	3	46	44	0	100	100	—	—	5
Dutch Smoothie Pina Colada	1 (14 oz)	260	8	5	30	3	44	41	0	80	90	—	—	5
Dutch Smoothie Strawberry	1 (14 oz)	250	8	5	30	3	40	39	0	100	100	—	—	1
Dutch Smoothie Wild Cherry	1 (14 oz)	250	8	5	30	3	41	39	0	80	90	—	—	0

FOOD	PORTION	CALS	FAT	SAT FAT	CHOL	PROT	CARB	SUGAR	FIBER	CALCI	SOD	POTAS	FOLIC	VIT C
Lemonade	1 (22 oz)	180	0	0	0	0	43	43	0	0	0	—	—	7
Lemonade Strawberry	1 (22 oz)	190	0	0	0	0	48	48	0	0	0	—	—	6
DIPPING SAUCES														
Caramel Dip	1 serv (1.5 oz)	135	3	2	5	1	27	21	0	20	110	—	—	0
Cheese Sauce	1 serv (1.25 oz)	100	8	4	10	3	4	3	0	100	510	—	—	0
Cream Cheese Light	1 serv (1.25 oz)	70	6	4	25	3	1	1	0	20	140	—	—	0
Hot Salsa Cheese	1 serv (1.25 oz)	100	8	4	10	2	4	4	0	100	550	—	—	1
Marinara Sauce	1 serv (1.25 oz)	10	0	0	0	0	4	2	0	0	180	—	—	0
Sweet	1 serv (1.4 oz)	40	0	0	0	0	10	10	0	0	0	—	—	0
Sweet Mustard	1 serv (1.25 oz)	60	2	1	40	tr	8	8	0	0	120	—	—	0
PRETZELS														
Almond	1	400	8	5	20	9	72	15	2	20	400	—	—	0
Almond w/o Butter	1	350	2	1	0	9	72	15	2	20	390	—	—	0
Cinnamon Raisin w/o Butter	1	350	2	0	0	9	74	16	2	20	410	—	—	0
Cinnamon Sugar	1	450	9	5	25	8	83	26	3	30	430	—	—	0
Garlic	1	350	5	3	10	9	68	9	2	20	850	—	—	0
Garlic w/o Butter	1	320	1	0	0	9	66	9	2	20	830	—	—	0
Glazin' Raisin	1	510	4	2	10	11	107	38	4	30	480	—	—	0
Glazin' Raisin w/o Butter	1	470	1	0	0	11	104	37	3	30	460	—	—	0
Jalapeno	1	310	5	3	10	8	59	9	2	20	940	—	—	0
Jalapeno w/o Butter	1	270	1	0	0	8	58	8	2	20	780	—	—	0
Original	1	370	4	2	10	10	72	10	3	30	930	—	—	0
Original w/o Butter	1	340	1	0	0	10	72	10	3	30	900	—	—	0
Pretzel Dog	1	290	16	7	40	10	25	3	1	0	600	—	—	0
Sesame	1	410	12	4	15	12	64	9	7	20	860	—	—	0
Sesame w/o Butter	1	350	6	1	0	11	63	9	3	20	840	—	—	0
Sour Cream & Onion	1	340	5	3	10	9	66	10	2	40	930	—	—	0
Sour Cream & Onion w/o Butter	1	310	1	0	0	9	66	9	2	30	920	—	—	0
Stix	6	370	4	2	10	10	72	10	3	30	930	—	—	0
Stix w/o Butter	6	340	1	0	0	10	72	10	3	30	900	—	—	0
Whole Wheat	1	370	5	2	10	11	72	10	7	30	1120	—	—	0
Whole Wheat w/o Butter	1	350	2	0	0	11	72	10	7	30	1100	—	—	0
BABS DELI														
BAGELS														
Apple Cinnamon	1	332	2	0	0	12	70	6	4	—	472	—	—	—
Banana Nut	1	340	2	0	0	12	68	4	4	—	460	—	—	—

FOOD	PORTION	CALS	FAT	SAT FAT	CHOL	PROT	CARB	SUGAR	FIBER	CALCI	SOD	POTAS	FOLIC	VIT C
Blueberry	1	330	2	0	0	12	68	2	4	—	482	—	—	—
Blueberry Cobbler	1	392	8	4	12	10	70	4	2	—	440	—	—	—
Cheddar Herb	1	352	6	4	16	14	60	2	2	—	604	—	—	—
Cheddar Nacho	1	352	6	4	16	14	60	2	4	—	702	—	—	—
Chocolate Chip	1	348	2	2	0	12	68	4	4	—	472	—	—	—
Cinnamon Apple Pie	1	386	8	4	12	10	68	4	2	—	420	—	—	—
Cinnamon Bun	1	400	8	4	12	10	70	4	2	—	440	—	—	—
Cinnamon Danish	1	396	8	4	12	10	72	2	4	—	428	—	—	—
Cinnamon Raisin	1	336	2	0	0	12	70	2	4	—	464	—	—	—
Cinnamon Sugar	1	350	2	0	0	12	74	2	2	—	482	—	—	—
Cranberry Walnut	1	352	2	0	0	12	72	6	4	—	470	—	—	—
Egg	1	328	2	0	4	12	66	2	2	—	492	—	—	—
Everything	1	336	2	0	0	12	68	2	4	—	778	—	—	—
French Toast	1	372	4	4	0	12	74	4	2	—	464	—	—	—
Garlic	1	330	2	0	0	12	68	2	4	—	492	—	—	—
Honey Oat	1	320	2	0	0	12	68	2	2	—	446	—	—	—
Jalapeno	1	350	6	4	16	14	30	2	2	—	688	—	—	—
Onion	1	336	2	0	0	12	70	2	4	—	492	—	—	—
Plain	1	334	2	0	0	12	68	2	4	—	502	—	—	—
Poppy	1	344	2	0	0	12	68	2	4	—	490	—	—	—
Pumpernickel	1	332	2	0	0	12	68	2	4	—	492	—	—	—
Quiche Lorraine	1	354	8	4	20	16	54	2	2	—	125	—	—	—
Salt	1	324	2	0	0	12	66	2	2	—	1936	—	—	—
Sesame	1	358	4	0	0	14	66	2	4	—	476	—	—	—
Spinach	1	356	2	0	0	14	72	2	4	—	274	—	—	—
Strawberry	1	342	2	0	0	12	72	4	4	—	470	—	—	—
Strawberry White Chocolate	1	364	4	2	0	12	72	8	4	—	478	—	—	—
Swiss Melt	1	368	8	4	20	18	58	2	2	—	470	—	—	—
Tomato Basil	1	322	2	0	0	12	66	2	4	—	560	—	—	—
Vegetable	1	318	2	0	0	12	66	2	4	—	482	—	—	—
Wheat	1	330	2	0	0	12	78	2	4	—	476	—	—	—
White Chocolate Swirl	1	396	8	4	12	10	70	4	2	—	448	—	—	—
BEVERAGES														
Americano	1 (16 oz)	12	0	0	0	0	2	0	0	—	28	—	—	—
Cafe Caramello	1 (16 oz)	212	8	5	26	2	31	26	0	—	40	—	—	—
Cappuccino 2% Milk	1 (16 oz)	195	7	4	26	13	20	0	0	—	212	—	—	—
Cappuccino Fat Free Milk	1 (16 oz)	133	1	1	7	12	18	0	0	—	193	—	—	—
Coffee Black Forest	1 (16 oz)	198	5	3	16	1	37	29	1	—	35	—	—	—

FOOD	PORTION	CALS	FAT	SAT FAT	CHOL	PROT	CARB	SUGAR	FIBER	CALCI	SOD	POTAS	FOLIC	VIT C
Icepresso Caramel Decadence	1 (16 oz)	300	12	12	0	6	42	28	2	—	300	—	—	—
Icepresso Classic	1 (16 oz)	300	5	1	0	8	52	44	0	—	240	—	—	—
Icepresso Java Chip	1 (16 oz)	360	18	14	0	6	48	38	2	—	190	—	—	—
Icepresso Latte	1 (16 oz)	300	12	12	0	6	42	28	2	—	300	—	—	—
Icepresso Mocha	1 (16 oz)	300	12	12	0	6	42	28	2	—	300	—	—	—
Icepresso Strawberry	1 (16 oz)	340	12	12	0	2	56	48	0	—	120	—	—	—
Italiano 2% Milk	1 (16 oz)	131	5	3	18	9	13	0	0	—	139	—	—	—
Italiano Fat Free Milk	1 (16 oz)	89	1	0	5	8	12	0	0	—	126	—	—	—
Jittery Monkey	1 (16 oz)	482	11	7	39	13	82	52	1	—	230	—	—	—
Jittery Monkey Fat Free Milk	1 (16 oz)	429	6	4	22	12	80	52	1	—	214	—	—	—
Latte 2% Milk	1 (16 oz)	212	7	5	28	14	22	0	0	—	229	—	—	—
Latte 2% Milk Cinnamon Toast	1 (16 oz)	299	7	4	25	13	45	26	0	—	205	—	—	—
Latte Cinnamon Toast Fat Free Milk	1 (16 oz)	240	1	1	6	11	44	26	0	—	187	—	—	—
Latte Creme Caramel 2% Milk	1 (16 oz)	303	7	4	25	13	47	27	0	—	205	—	—	—
Latte Creme Caramel Fat Free Milk	1 (16 oz)	244	1	1	6	11	45	27	0	—	187	—	—	—
Latte Fat Free Milk	1 (16 oz)	145	1	1	7	13	20	0	0	—	209	—	—	—
Latte Oregon Chai Tea 2% Milk	1 (16 oz)	274	5	3	18	9	48	34	0	—	150	—	—	—
Latte Oregon Chai Tea Fat Free Milk	1 (16 oz)	231	1	0	5	8	47	34	0	—	137	—	—	—
Latte Raspberry Cheesecake 2% Milk	1 (16 oz)	319	7	4	25	13	51	30	0	—	209	—	—	—
Latte Raspberry Cheesecake Fat Free Milk	1 (16 oz)	259	1	1	6	11	50	30	0	—	191	—	—	—
Latte Vanilla Creme 2% Milk	1 (16 oz)	275	7	4	26	13	39	19	0	—	210	—	—	—
Mocha Whipped Cream 2% Milk	1 (16 oz)	454	12	7	42	15	71	39	2	—	272	—	—	—
Mocha Whipped Cream Fat Free Milk	1 (16 oz)	392	6	4	23	14	70	39	2	—	253	—	—	—
Turtle Mocha Fat Free Milk	1 (16 oz)	522	12	7	45	12	90	62	1	—	225	—	—	—

FOOD	PORTION	CALS	FAT	SAT FAT	CHOL	PROT	CARB	SUGAR	FIBER	CALCI	SOD	POTAS	FOLIC	VIT C
MUFFINS														
My Favorite Banana Nut	2 mini	195	11	2	21	4	21	12	1	—	121	—	—	—
My Favorite Blueberry	2 mini	168	8	2	24	2	22	12	0	—	136	—	—	—
My Favorite Blueberry Cheesecake	2 mini	199	12	5	38	3	20	9	0	—	145	—	—	—
My Favorite Boston Cream Pie	2 mini	176	7	2	22	2	26	17	0	—	144	—	—	—
My Favorite Cherry Cheesecake	2 mini	170	10	4	30	2	19	10	0	—	124	—	—	—
My Favorite Chocolate Cheesecake	2 mini	202	12	5	20	2	22	11	0	—	133	—	—	—
My Favorite Chocolate Chip	2 mini	211	11	3	25	3	27	16	1	—	142	—	—	—
My Favorite Cinnamon Crumb Cake	2 mini	212	13	5	37	3	21	11	0	—	135	—	—	—
My Favorite Cinnamon Swirl Cheesecake	2 mini	214	11	3	25	2	28	15	0	—	142	—	—	—
My Favorite Deep Dish Apple	2 mini	177	8	2	19	2	25	14	0	—	113	—	—	—
My Favorite Double Chocolate	2 mini	210	9	3	0	2	28	17	1	—	139	—	—	—
My Favorite Fat Free Blueberry	2 mini	108	0	0	0	2	26	12	1	—	192	—	—	—
My Favorite Fat Free Cherry Pie	2 mini	109	0	0	0	2	26	14	0	—	188	—	—	—
My Favorite Fat Free Chocolate Marble	2 mini	125	0	0	0	2	29	15	1	—	256	—	—	—
My Favorite Fat Free Cinnamon Bun	2 mini	168	0	0	0	1	42	11	0	—	176	—	—	—
My Favorite Fat Free Raspberry Amaretto	2 mini	127	0	0	0	2	31	18	1	—	186	—	—	—
My Favorite Golden Corn Bread	2 mini	197	9	2	24	3	26	12	1	—	135	—	—	—
My Favorite Lemon Poppyseed	2 mini	201	10	3	28	3	25	14	0	—	161	—	—	—

FOOD	PORTION	CALS	FAT	SAT FAT	CHOL	PROT	CARB	SUGAR	FIBER	CALCI	SOD	POTAS	FOLIC	VIT C
My Favorite Pumpkin Spice	2 mini	181	8	3	23	2	26	10	0	—	128	—	—	—
SALADS														
Calypso Chicken	1 (13.6 oz)	637	49	8	50	20	34	16	3	—	1229	—	—	—
Calypso Chicken w/ Lite Italian	1 (13.6 oz)	317	17	2	50	20	22	10	3	—	1823	—	—	—
Chicken Caesar	1 (11.5 oz)	524	41	9	83	23	15	3	3	—	1583	—	—	—
Chicken Caesar w/ Lite Italian	1 (11.5 oz)	268	12	3	56	20	17	9	3	—	1996	—	—	—
Classic Caesar	1 (8.4 oz)	414	36	7	33	9	12	1	3	—	1053	—	—	—
Classic Caesar Cafe	1 (4.3 oz)	225	19	4	16	5	9	1	2	—	573	—	—	—
Classic Caesar w/ Lite Italian	1 (8.4 oz)	158	8	2	6	6	14	7	3	—	1466	—	—	—
Garden Mix	1 (12.4 oz)	197	9	2	211	9	18	5	4	—	1352	—	—	—
Garden Mix Cafe	1 (6.5 oz)	100	5	1	105	5	9	3	2	—	684	—	—	—
Grilled Chicken Club	1 (17.9 oz)	820	69	21	104	35	16	5	3	—	2216	—	—	—
Grilled Chicken Club w/ Lite Italian	1 (17.9 oz)	500	31	14	104	35	18	7	3	—	2589	—	—	—
Mediterranean Bread	1 (18.8 oz)	973	73	22	75	30	52	1	5	—	2371	—	—	—
Mediterranean Bread w/ Lite Italian	1 (18.8 oz)	626	32	15	75	30	55	7	5	—	2775	—	—	—
Tuna Salad Plate Low Carb	1 serv (8.9 oz)	356	25	4	58	28	3	0	1	—	652	—	—	—
SANDWICHES														
Breakfast BLT	1	704	31	14	91	22	83	5	4	—	1371	—	—	—
Breakfast Lox & Cream Cheese	1	602	21	14	58	29	78	3	4	—	1456	—	—	—
Breakfast Morning Classic	1	486	11	5	256	23	73	2	3	—	861	—	—	—
Breakfast Northern Omelette	1	699	31	12	296	31	73	2	3	—	1192	—	—	—
Breakfast So Tradition w/ Bacon	1	566	18	8	271	27	73	2	3	—	1151	—	—	—
Breakfast So Tradition w/ Ham	1	547	15	6	283	29	73	2	3	—	1362	—	—	—
Breakfast So Tradition w/ Sausage	1	696	31	12	296	31	73	2	3	—	1191	—	—	—
Build Your Own Ham	1	495	9	3	53	27	77	1	4	—	1734	—	—	—
Build Your Own Roast Beef	1	480	6	2	46	29	77	1	4	—	1689	—	—	—

FOOD	PORTION	CALS	FAT	SAT FAT	CHOL	PROT	CARB	SUGAR	FIBER	CALCI	SOD	POTAS	FOLIC	VIT C
Build Your Own Tuna	1	547	14	2	29	27	77	1	4	—	1039	—	—	—
Build Your Own Turkey	1	465	3	0	61	32	77	1	4	—	1567	—	—	—
Enchilada Bagellata	1	522	11	7	30	22	84	3	4	—	895	—	—	—
Gourmet Classic Turkey	1	552	14	2	66	32	74	1	4	—	1450	—	—	—
Gourmet Holey Guacamole	1	476	5	1	61	33	76	2	4	—	1449	—	—	—
Gourmet Kick-N Roast Beef	1	579	15	2	74	29	79	1	4	—	1802	—	—	—
Gourmet Mediterranean Veg-Out	1	506	9	1	0	20	90	3	8	—	818	—	—	—
Overstuffed Classic Reuben	1	962	43	17	156	60	57	3	4	—	3017	—	—	—
Overstuffed Corned Beef	1	661	19	6	97	43	77	1	3	—	2770	—	—	—
Overstuffed Ham & Cheese	1	889	36	16	147	60	79	1	4	—	2893	—	—	—
Overstuffed Manhattan Club	1	1122	40	15	178	69	120	6	6	—	2992	—	—	—
Overstuffed Pastrami	1	661	19	6	97	43	77	1	3	—	2770	—	—	—
Overstuffed TD Classic California	1	759	12	6	80	49	113	2	8	—	2089	—	—	—
Overstuffed TD Classic Club	1	1110	43	13	158	61	122	2	5	—	3062	—	—	—
Overstuffed TD Clubhouse	1	1079	37	14	171	69	117	2	5	—	2957	—	—	—
Pizzaah Bruschetta	1 piece	162	12	7	38	7	7	0	3	—	175	—	—	—
Pizzaah Cheese	1 piece	189	7	4	22	10	23	1	3	—	268	—	—	—
Pizzaah Grilled Chicken Bruschetta	1 piece	343	21	12	78	17	24	1	3	—	625	—	—	—
Pizzaah Sausage	1 piece	211	17	7	42	11	6	1	2	—	306	—	—	—
Pizzaah Veggie	1 piece	238	10	4	22	12	32	1	7	—	272	—	—	—
Specialty All American Duo	1	752	28	13	107	46	78	1	4	—	1767	—	—	—
Specialty Big Apple Club	1	797	37	13	110	41	75	2	4	—	2438	—	—	—
Specialty Chicken Caesar	1	611	19	5	64	31	78	3	4	—	1459	—	—	—
Specialty Roma Italian	1	764	34	14	109	40	76	1	4	—	2393	—	—	—

FOOD	PORTION	CALS	FAT	SAT FAT	CHOL	PROT	CARB	SUGAR	FIBER	CALCI	SOD	POTAS	FOLIC	VIT C
Specialty Turkey Club	1	782	34	12	113	43	75	2	4	—	2355	—	—	—
Toasted Cafe Chicken Melt	1	815	32	14	133	51	80	6	4	—	1767	—	—	—
Toasted Deli Style Turkey	1	732	25	11	115	48	76	3	4	—	1602	—	—	—
Toasted Roast Beef Parmesan Grinder	1	583	15	7	66	36	76	4	4	—	1896	—	—	—
Toasted Spicy Italian Sub	1	770	34	14	109	40	77	1	4	—	2505	—	—	—
Toasted Tuna Melt	1	641	23	8	54	32	75	2	4	—	1310	—	—	—
SOUPS														
Beef Barley Mushroom	1 serv (8 oz)	100	3	—	—	6	12	—	—	—	1040	—	—	—
Boston Clam Chowder	1 serv (8 oz)	210	13	—	—	2	20	—	—	—	900	—	—	—
Chicken & Wild Rice	1 serv (8 oz)	190	9	—	—	5	22	—	—	—	960	—	—	—
Chicken Gumbo	1 serv (8 oz)	130	3	—	—	8	19	—	—	—	920	—	—	—
Cream Of Potato	1 serv (8 oz)	240	14	—	—	4	24	—	—	—	1080	—	—	—
Hearty Vegetable Beef	1 serv (8 oz)	100	1	—	—	5	16	—	—	—	880	—	—	—
New England Clam Chowder	1 serv (8 oz)	220	13	—	—	6	21	—	—	—	1100	—	—	—
Split Pea w/ Ham	1 serv (8 oz)	90	2	—	—	5	15	—	—	—	950	—	—	—
Wisconsin Cheese	1 serv (8 oz)	210	11	—	—	8	20	—	—	—	1050	—	—	—
SPREADS														
Cream Cheese	2 tbsp	90	9	6	25	1	2	1	0	—	200	—	—	—
Cream Cheese Cheddar Jalapeno	2 tbsp	90	8	5	25	1	2	2	0	—	150	—	—	—
Cream Cheese Garden Vegetable	2 tbsp	90	9	6	25	1	2	1	0	—	140	—	—	—
Cream Cheese Lite	2 tbsp	60	5	3	15	2	3	3	0	—	170	—	—	—
Cream Cheese Onion Chive	2 tbsp	80	8	5	25	1	2	1	0	—	110	—	—	—
Cream Cheese Strawberry	2 tbsp	90	5	0	20	1	5	5	0	—	65	—	—	—
Cream Cheese Whipped	2 tbsp	70	7	5	20	1	1	1	0	—	65	—	—	—
Cream Cheese Whipped Brown Sugar Cinnamon	2 tbsp	70	5	4	15	tr	5	3	0	—	80	—	—	—
Cream Cheese Whipped Reduced Fat Spring Veggie	2 tbsp	60	5	4	15	1	2	1	0	—	100	—	—	—

FOOD	PORTION	CALS	FAT	SAT FAT	CHOL	PROT	CARB	SUGAR	FIBER	CALCI	SOD	POTAS	FOLIC	VIT C
BAHAMA BREEZE														
BEVERAGES														
Beer Light	1 serv (12 oz)	103	0	0	0	—	6	—	—	—	14	—	—	—
Beer Regular	1 serv (12 oz)	153	0	0	0	—	13	—	—	—	14	—	—	—
Berries In Paradise	1 serv	110	0	0	0	—	24	—	—	—	15	—	—	—
Captain Berry Island	1 serv	110	0	0	0	—	24	—	—	—	15	—	—	—
Island Refresher	1 serv	370	7	5	—	—	73	—	—	—	30	—	—	—
Lemon Breeze	1 serv	410	0	0	0	—	103	—	—	—	0	—	—	—
Mango Beach	1 serv	300	8	7	—	—	56	—	—	—	20	—	—	—
Mango Mango Man	1 serv	300	8	7	—	—	56	—	—	—	20	—	—	—
Raspberry Surfer	1 serv	210	0	0	0	—	52	—	—	—	10	—	—	—
Shake Banana	1 serv	590	30	18	—	—	69	—	—	—	115	—	—	—
Shake Chocolate	1 serv	700	32	20	—	—	92	—	—	—	170	—	—	—
Shake Chocolate Banana	1 serv	760	31	19	—	—	108	—	—	—	70	—	—	—
Shake Mango	1 serv	450	25	15	—	—	47	—	—	—	115	—	—	—
Shake Raspberry	1 serv	560	29	18	—	—	64	—	—	—	170	—	—	—
Shake Strawberry	1 serv	530	32	20	—	—	50	—	—	—	190	—	—	—
Shake Strawberry Banana	1 serv	600	28	17	—	—	77	—	—	—	130	—	—	—
Shake Vanilla	1 serv	560	30	18	—	—	62	—	—	—	200	—	—	—
Slushies Kiwi	1 serv	120	0	0	0	—	29	—	—	—	30	—	—	—
Slushies Mango	1 serv	180	0	0	0	—	45	—	—	—	5	—	—	—
Slushies Strawberry	1 serv	240	0	0	0	—	58	—	—	—	40	—	—	—
Strawberry Beach	1 serv	370	7	6	—	—	74	—	—	—	30	—	—	—
Virgin Bahama Rita	1 serv	160	0	0	0	—	39	—	—	—	0	—	—	—
Virgin Ultimate Pina Colada	1 serv	340	9	8	—	—	65	—	—	—	20	—	—	—
Wine	1 serv (5 oz)	122	0	0	0	—	4	—	—	—	7	—	—	—
CHILDREN'S MENU SELECTIONS														
Bowtie Mac N' Cheese	1 serv	790	46	27	—	—	74	—	—	—	1100	—	—	—
Cheese Pizza	1 sm	750	23	10	—	—	101	—	—	—	1620	—	—	—
Crispy Chicken	1 serv	420	24	3	—	—	23	—	—	—	1580	—	—	—
French Fries	1 serv	265	13	1	—	—	34	—	—	—	470	—	—	—
Fresh Fruit Salad	1 serv	40	0	0	0	—	10	—	—	—	0	—	—	—
DESSERTS														
Bananas Supreme	1 serv	940	45	19	—	—	122	—	—	—	560	—	—	—
Chocolate Island	1 serv	1380	83	44	—	—	142	—	—	—	440	—	—	—
Dulce De Leche Cheesecake	1 serv	940	56	33	—	—	94	—	—	—	710	—	—	—

FOOD	PORTION	CALS	FAT	SAT FAT	CHOL	PROT	CARB	SUGAR	FIBER	CALCI	SOD	POTAS	FOLIC	VIT C
Rebecca's Key Lime Pie	1 serv	990	34	17	—	—	154	—	—	—	630	—	—	—
Warm Chocolate Pineapple Upside Down Cake	1 serv	1140	58	18	—	—	144	—	—	—	940	—	—	—
MAIN MENU SELECTIONS														
Bahamian Grilled Chicken Kabobs w/ Yellow Rice	1 serv	770	11	3	—	—	98	—	—	—	2480	—	—	—
Breeze Wood Grilled Chicken Breast w/ Citrus Butter Sauce	1 serv	680	39	10	—	—	18	—	—	—	2130	—	—	—
Breeze Wood Grilled Chicken Breast w/ Citrus Butter Sauce Lighter Portion	1 serv	390	23	8	—	—	11	—	—	—	1230	—	—	—
Broccoli	1 serv	120	9	6	—	—	6	—	—	—	125	—	—	—
Burger Wood Grilled Angus	1 serv	680	39	16	—	—	39	—	—	—	830	—	—	—
Chicken Santiago	1 serv	1180	58	8	—	—	85	—	—	—	4560	—	—	—
Chicken Santiago Lighter Portion	1 serv	1020	55	6	—	—	85	—	—	—	3680	—	—	—
Cinnamon Mashed Sweet Potatoes	1 serv	260	9	4	—	—	44	—	—	—	430	—	—	—
Coconut Shrimp Dinner	1 serv	794	50	11	—	—	60	—	—	—	347	—	—	—
Crab Claws St. Thomas	1 serv	710	64	39	—	—	13	—	—	—	1180	—	—	—
Crab Shrimp & Avocado Stack w/ Honey Red Pepper Drizzle	1 serv	250	6	1	—	—	20	—	—	—	840	—	—	—
Creole Baked Goat Cheese	1 serv	380	33	20	—	—	0	—	—	—	620	—	—	—
Crispy Yuca	1 serv	620	36	3	—	—	73	—	—	—	570	—	—	—
Filet Mignon w/ Onion Rings	1 serv	450	23	8	—	—	10	—	—	—	400	—	—	—
Fire Roasted Jerk Shrimp	1 serv	260	14	6	—	—	2	—	—	—	870	—	—	—
French Fries	1 serv	530	26	2	—	—	67	—	—	—	940	—	—	—
Garlic Mashed Potatoes	1 serv	290	20	12	—	—	24	—	—	—	780	—	—	—
Herb Cheese Toast	1 slice	120	5	2	—	—	15	—	—	—	180	—	—	—
Island Flatbread Grilled Chicken	1	515	22	9	—	—	43	—	—	—	1445	—	—	—

FOOD	PORTION	CALS	FAT	SAT FAT	CHOL	PROT	CARB	SUGAR	FIBER	CALCI	SOD	POTAS	FOLIC	VIT C
Island Flatbread Shrimp	1	480	20	9	—	—	43	—	—	—	1280	—	—	—
Island Flatbread Vine Ripened Tomato	1	430	20	9	—	—	43	—	—	—	1040	—	—	—
Island Onion Rings	1 serv	1910	116	17	—	—	186	—	—	—	2140	—	—	—
Jamaican Grilled Chicken Breast	1 serv	310	4	2	—	—	2	—	—	—	1900	—	—	—
Jamaican Grilled Chicken Breast Lighter Portion	1 serv	160	2	1	—	—	1	—	—	—	940	—	—	—
Linguine Calypso Shrimp Lighter Portion	1 serv	790	43	23	—	—	58	—	—	—	2430	—	—	—
Margarita Chicken w/ Roasted Corn Salsa	1 serv	470	6	2	—	—	30	—	—	—	1240	—	—	—
Margarita Chicken w/ Roasted Corn Salsa Lighter Portion	1 serv	310	5	1	—	—	24	—	—	—	790	—	—	—
Pasta Jerk Chicken	1 serv	1430	87	46	—	—	107	—	—	—	1500	—	—	—
Pasta Jerk Chicken Lighter Portion	1 serv	780	39	21	—	—	72	—	—	—	860	—	—	—
Pasta Lobster & Shrimp	1 serv	1080	42	18	—	—	82	—	—	—	2830	—	—	—
Pasta Pan-Seared Salmon	1 serv	1550	99	45	—	—	96	—	—	—	1860	—	—	—
Pasta Pan-Seared Salmon Lighter Portion	1 serv	910	55	23	—	—	68	—	—	—	1020	—	—	—
Plantains	1 serv	270	6	1	—	—	53	—	—	—	0	—	—	—
Quesadilla Fresh Vegetable	1	435	48	26	—	—	70	—	—	—	1910	—	—	—
Quesadilla Fresh Vegetable & Chicken	1	480	24	13	—	—	11	—	—	—	1490	—	—	—
Roasted Cuban Bread	1 serv	590	23	10	—	—	77	—	—	—	1030	—	—	—
Sandwich Cuban	1	1130	59	24	—	—	69	—	—	—	2450	—	—	—
Sandwich Oak Grilled Chicken	1	530	19	3	—	—	45	—	—	—	1330	—	—	—
Sandwich Sun Drenched Portobello & Veg	1	670	22	9	—	—	90	—	—	—	1170	—	—	—
Seafood Paella	1 serv	800	23	5	—	—	54	—	—	—	2910	—	—	—

FOOD	PORTION	CALS	FAT	SAT FAT	CHOL	PROT	CARB	SUGAR	FIBER	CALCI	SOD	POTAS	FOLIC	VIT C
Smothered Pork Tenderloin w/ Lemon Butter	1 serv	900	59	35	—	—	9	—	—	—	1970	—	—	—
Spinach Dip w/ Island Chips	1 serv	680	60	38	—	—	17	—	—	—	1180	—	—	—
Tacos Key West Fish	1 serv	550	26	5	—	—	30	—	—	—	1130	—	—	—
Tostones w/ Chicken	1 serv	1250	63	17	—	—	121	—	—	—	2400	—	—	—
West Indies Patties	1 serv	1150	68	24	—	—	102	—	—	—	1620	—	—	—
West Indies Ribs	1 serv	810	55	19	—	—	7	—	—	—	570	—	—	—
Wings Habanero	1 serv	920	53	13	—	—	11	—	—	—	2800	—	—	—
Wings Jamaican Grilled	1 serv	960	60	18	—	—	2	—	—	—	2570	—	—	—
Wood Grilled Top Sirloin w/ Cheese & Peppers	1 serv	440	21	10	—	—	4	—	—	—	570	—	—	—
Yellow Rice	1 serv	220	3	1	—	—	44	—	—	—	670	—	—	—
Yellow Rice & Black Beans	1 serv	280	3	1	—	—	55	—	—	—	1220	—	—	—
SALAD DRESSINGS AND TOPPINGS														
Citrus Mustard	1 serv	95	4	1	—	—	16	—	—	—	190	—		—
Dip Cilantro Vinaigrette	1 serv	110	6	1	—	—	12	—	—	—	840	—	—	—
Dipping Sauce Tangy	1 serv	50	1	0	—	—	12	—	—	—	190	—	—	—
Dressing Blue Cheese	1 serv	175	18	4	—	—	15	—	—	—	190	—	—	—
Dressing Caesar	1 serv	200	21	4	—	—	1	—	—	—	370	—	—	—
Dressing Ranch	1 serv	130	14	2	—	—	2	—	—	—	260	—	—	—
Dressing Tropical Island Vinaigrette	1 serv	60	4	1	—	—	15	—	—	—	600	—	—	—
Guava BBQ Sauce	1 serv	50	0	0	0	—	12	—	—	—	190	—	—	—
Homemade Croutons	12	500	29	14	—	—	47	—	—	—	740	—	—	—
Salsa Apple Mango	1 serv	20	0	0	0	—	5	—	—	—	15	—	—	—
Salsa Black Bean & Corn	1 serv	70	2	1	—	—	10	—	—	—	140	—	—	—
Salsa Mango Pineapple	1 serv	60	0	0	0	—	15	—	—	—	160	—	—	—
Salsa Tomato	1 serv	30	1	0	—	—	4	—	—	—	270	—	—	—
Sauce Chili Horseradish	1 serv	130	11	2	—	—	8	—	—	—	430	—	—	—
Sour Cream	1 serv	90	8	5	—	—	3	—	—	—	40	—	—	—
Sour Cream Ancho Chili	1 serv	70	6	4	—	—	4	—	—	—	290	—	—	—

FOOD	PORTION	CALS	FAT	SAT FAT	CHOL	PROT	CARB	SUGAR	FIBER	CALCI	SOD	POTAS	FOLIC	VIT C
SALADS														
Breeze No Dressing	1 serv	90	5	1	—	—	6	—	—	—	50	—	—	—
Caesar No Dressing	1 serv	70	3	2	—	—	6	—	—	—	210	—	—	—
Crispy Chicken Club w/ BBQ Drizzle	1 serv	880	52	12	—	—	47	—	—	—	3060	—	—	—
Fresh Fruit	1 serv	130	0	0	0	—	32	—	—	—	0	—	—	—
Grilled Chicken Ceasar w/ Croutons w/o Dressing	1 serv	490	20	9	—	—	22	—	—	—	1520	—	—	—
Grilled Chicken Cobb	1 serv	600	38	12	—	—	4	—	—	—	1630	—	—	—
Grilled Fresh Salmon Tostada w/ Chimichurri Sauce w/o Dressing	1 serv	1045	57	22	—	—	52	—	—	—	1930	—	—	—
Tropical Fruit & Grilled Chicken On Greens w/o Dressing	1 serv	430	11	3	—	—	40	—	—	—	670	—	—	—
Vine Ripened Tomato	1 serv	60	1	0	—	—	12	—	—	—	490	—	—	—
SOUPS														
Bahamian Seafood Chowder	1 serv	600	47	24	—	—	27	—	—	—	1710	—	—	—
Chicken Tortilla	1 serv	290	12	2	—	—	26	—	—	—	1910	—	—	—
Cuban Black Bean	1 serv	320	4	1	—	—	52	—	—	—	1210	—	—	—

BAJA FRESH

CHILDREN'S MENU SELECTIONS

FOOD	PORTION	CALS	FAT	SAT FAT	CHOL	PROT	CARB	SUGAR	FIBER	CALCI	SOD	POTAS	FOLIC	VIT C
Kid's Mini Burrito Bean & Cheese	1 serv	540	14	7	25	18	84	—	11	—	1050	—	—	—
Kid's Mini Burrito Bean & Cheese w/ Chicken	1 serv	590	15	7	50	28	84	—	12	—	1200	—	—	—
Kid's Mini Quesadilla Cheese	1 serv	610	26	13	50	19	72	—	5	—	940	—	—	—
Kid's Mini Quesadilla Cheese w/ Chicken	1 serv	650	27	13	75	28	72	—	5	—	1090	—	—	—
Kid's Taquitos Chicken	1 serv	630	33	7	70	18	60	—	4	—	990	—	—	—

FOOD	PORTION	CALS	FAT	SAT FAT	CHOL	PROT	CARB	SUGAR	FIBER	CALCI	SOD	POTAS	FOLIC	VIT C
MAIN MENU SELECTIONS														
Black Beans	1 serv	360	3	1	5	23	61	—	26	—	1120	—	—	—
Burrito Baja Breaded Fish	1 serv	850	44	16	80	40	78	—	7	—	1900	—	—	—
Burrito Baja Carnitas	1 serv	830	45	18	115	45	67	—	8	—	2280	—	—	—
Burrito Baja Chicken	1 serv	790	38	15	120	52	65	—	8	—	2140	—	—	—
Burrito Baja Mahi Mahi	1 serv	780	38	15	115	51	66	—	7	—	1840	—	—	—
Burrito Baja Shrimp	1 serv	760	37	15	295	47	66	—	7	—	2230	—	—	—
Burrito Baja Steak	1 serv	850	46	18	125	49	67	—	7	—	2260	—	—	—
Burrito Bare Carnitas	1 serv	600	14	4	70	37	99	—	20	—	2480	—	—	—
Burrito Bare Chicken	1 serv	640	7	1	75	45	97	—	20	—	2330	—	—	—
Burrito Bare Steak	1 serv	700	15	5	80	41	99	—	19	—	2450	—	—	—
Burrito Bare Veggie & Cheese	1 serv	580	10	4	15	19	101	—	20	—	1950	—	—	—
Burrito Bean & Cheese Breaded Fish	1 serv	1030	41	18	95	54	108	—	20	—	1990	—	—	—
Burrito Bean & Cheese Carnitas	1 serv	1010	42	20	130	59	98	—	21	—	2370	—	—	—
Burrito Bean & Cheese Chicken	1 serv	970	35	18	135	67	96	—	21	—	2230	—	—	—
Burrito Bean & Cheese Mahi Mahi	1 serv	960	35	18	130	65	96	—	20	—	1930	—	—	—
Burrito Bean & Cheese No Meat	1 serv	840	33	17	65	39	96	—	20	—	1790	—	—	—
Burrito Bean & Cheese Shrimp	1 serv	950	34	17	310	61	96	—	20	—	2320	—	—	—
Burrito Bean & Cheese Steak	1 serv	1030	43	21	140	64	97	—	20	—	2350	—	—	—
Burrito Dos Manos Breaded Fish	1 serv	890	33	13	70	39	107	—	13	—	2025	—	—	—
Burrito Dos Manos Carnitas	1 serv	780	30	14	73	34	95	—	14	—	2115	—	—	—
Burrito Dos Manos Chicken	1 serv	760	26	12	75	38	94	—	14	—	2040	—	—	—
Burrito Dos Manos Mahi Mahi	1 serv	780	26	12	83	42	95	—	13	—	1915	—	—	—
Burrito Dos Manos Shrimp	1 serv	780	26	12	223	41	95	—	13	—	2220	—	—	—

FOOD	PORTION	CALS	FAT	SAT FAT	CHOL	PROT	CARB	SUGAR	FIBER	CALCI	SOD	POTAS	FOLIC	VIT C
Burrito Dos Manos Steak	1 serv	795	30	14	78	36	95	—	13	—	2105	—	—	—
Burrito Grilled Veggie	1 serv	506	33	17	65	32	94	—	16	—	1880	—	—	—
Burrito Mexicano Breaded Fish	1 serv	850	19	4	30	37	129	—	18	—	2040	—	—	—
Burrito Mexicano Carnitas	1 serv	830	20	6	70	42	119	—	19	—	2420	—	—	—
Burrito Mexicano Chicken	1 serv	790	13	4	75	50	117	—	20	—	2270	—	—	—
Burrito Mexicano Mahi Mahi	1 serv	790	13	4	70	49	117	—	18	—	1970	—	—	—
Burrito Mexicano Shrimp	1 serv	770	13	4	245	44	117	—	18	—	2370	—	—	—
Burrito Mexicano Steak	1 serv	860	21	7	118	47	118	—	18	—	2400	—	—	—
Burrito Ultimo Breaded Fish	1 serv	940	42	19	95	41	96	—	8	—	1950	—	—	—
Burrito Ultimo Carnitas	1 serv	920	44	21	130	46	86	—	9	—	2330	—	—	—
Burrito Ultimo Chicken	1 serv	880	36	18	140	54	84	—	9	—	2190	—	—	—
Burrito Ultimo Mahi Mahi	1 serv	880	36	18	130	52	84	—	8	—	1890	—	—	—
Burrito Ultimo Shrimp	1 serv	860	36	18	310	48	85	—	8	—	2280	—	—	—
Burrito Ultimo Steak	1 serv	950	44	21	140	50	85	—	8	—	2310	—	—	—
Chips & Guacamole	1 serv	1340	83	8	0	21	141	—	20	—	950	—	—	—
Chips & Salsa Baja	1 serv	810	37	4	0	13	98	—	14	—	1140	—	—	—
Fajitas Corn Tortillas Breaded Fish	1 serv	1060	37	9	85	51	130	—	22	—	2180	—	—	—
Fajitas Corn Tortillas Carnitas	1 serv	920	34	11	120	50	108	—	23	—	2610	—	—	—
Fajitas Corn Tortillas Chicken	1 serv	860	24	7	130	61	105	—	24	—	2400	—	—	—
Fajitas Corn Tortillas Mahi Mahi	1 serv	840	23	7	110	57	105	—	22	—	1960	—	—	—
Fajitas Corn Tortillas Shrimp	1 serv	840	23	7	390	55	106	—	22	—	2570	—	—	—
Fajitas Corn Tortillas Steak	1 serv	960	36	12	135	58	107	—	22	—	2600	—	—	—

FOOD	PORTION	CALS	FAT	SAT FAT	CHOL	PROT	CARB	SUGAR	FIBER	CALCI	SOD	POTAS	FOLIC	VIT C
Fajitas Flour Tortillas Breaded Fish	1 serv	1340	46	12	85	59	172	—	25	—	3020	—	—	—
Fajitas Flour Tortillas Carnitas	1 serv	1190	43	14	120	58	150	—	26	—	3450	—	—	—
Fajitas Flour Tortillas Chicken	1 serv	1140	33	10	130	69	147	—	27	—	3240	—	—	—
Fajitas Flour Tortillas Mahi Mahi	1 serv	1120	32	10	110	64	147	—	25	—	2800	—	—	—
Fajitas Flour Tortillas Shrimp	1 serv	1120	32	10	390	62	148	—	25	—	3410	—	—	—
Fajitas Flour Tortillas Steak	1 serv	960	36	12	135	58	170	—	22	—	2600	—	—	—
Guacamole Side	1 (3 oz)	110	13	1	0	2	5	—	2	—	270	—	—	—
Nachos Breaded Fish	1 serv	2090	116	41	185	78	176	—	31	—	2740	—	—	—
Nachos Carnitas	1 serv	2060	117	43	220	83	166	—	32	—	3120	—	—	—
Nachos Cheese	1 serv	1890	108	40	155	63	163	—	31	—	2530	—	—	—
Nachos Chicken	1 serv	2020	110	41	230	91	164	—	32	—	2980	—	—	—
Nachos Mahi Mahi	1 serv	2020	110	41	220	90	164	—	31	—	2600	—	—	—
Nachos Shrimp	1 serv	2000	110	41	395	85	164	—	31	—	3060	—	—	—
Nachos Steak	1 serv	2120	118	44	163	96	163	—	31	—	2990	—	—	—
Pico De Gallo Side	1 serv (8 oz)	50	1	0	0	2	12	—	3	—	890	—	—	—
Pinto Beans	1 serv	320	1	0	5	19	56	—	21	—	840	—	—	—
Pronto Guacamole Side	1 serv (6 oz)	560	34	3	0	9	60	—	8	—	370	—	—	—
Quesadilla Breaded Fish	1 serv	1400	86	38	170	62	96	—	8	—	2350	—	—	—
Quesadilla Carnitas	1 serv	1370	87	40	205	67	86	—	9	—	2730	—	—	—
Quesadilla Cheese	1 serv	1200	78	37	140	47	84	—	8	—	2140	—	—	—
Quesadilla Chicken	1 serv	1330	80	37	215	75	84	—	9	—	2590	—	—	—
Quesadilla Mahi Mahi	1 serv	1330	79	37	205	73	84	—	8	—	2290	—	—	—
Quesadilla Shrimp	1 serv	1310	79	37	385	69	84	—	8	—	2680	—	—	—
Quesadilla Steak	1 serv	1430	87	41	240	80	84	—	8	—	2600	—	—	—
Quesadilla Veggie	1 serv	1260	78	37	145	48	96	—	11	—	2310	—	—	—
Rice	1 serv	280	4	1	0	5	55	—	4	—	980	—	—	—
Rice & Beans Plate	1 serv	420	5	2	10	18	72	—	18	—	1320	—	—	—
Salsa Baja Side	1 serv (8 oz)	70	3	0	0	2	7	—	4	—	970	—	—	—
Salsa Roja Side	1 serv (8 oz)	70	1	0	0	3	13	—	4	—	1080	—	—	—
Salsa Verde Side	1 serv (8 oz)	50	0	0	0	2	11	—	3	—	1170	—	—	—
Soup Tortilla w/ Chicken	1 serv (13.6 oz)	320	14	4	40	17	29	—	4	—	2760	—	—	—

FOOD	PORTION	CALS	FAT	SAT FAT	CHOL	PROT	CARB	SUGAR	FIBER	CALCI	SOD	POTAS	FOLIC	VIT C
Soup Tortilla w/o Chicken	1 serv (12.4 oz)	270	14	4	45	8	29	—	4	—	2600	—	—	—
Taco Grilled Mahi Mahi	1 serv	230	9	2	20	12	26	—	4	—	300	—	—	—
Taco Baja Breaded Fish	1 serv	250	13	2	15	8	27	—	2	—	420	—	—	—
Taco Baja Chicken	1 serv	210	5	1	25	12	28	—	2	—	230	—	—	—
Taco Baja Shrimp	1 serv	200	5	1	90	11	28	—	2	—	280	—	—	—
Taco Baja Steak	1 serv	230	8	2	25	11	28	—	2	—	260	—	—	—
Taco Soft Breaded Fish	1 serv	240	11	5	20	10	23	—	2	—	490	—	—	—
Taco Soft Carnitas	1 serv	250	12	5	35	13	21	—	2	—	640	—	—	—
Taco Soft Chicken	1 serv	230	10	5	35	16	20	—	2	—	590	—	—	—
Taco Soft Mahi Mahi	1 serv	240	10	5	40	17	20	—	2	—	490	—	—	—
Taco Soft Shrimp	1 serv	230	10	5	105	15	21	—	2	—	640	—	—	—
Taco Soft Steak	1 serv	260	13	6	40	15	21	—	2	—	640	—	—	—
Taquitos Chicken w/ Beans	3	780	40	12	85	39	68	—	17	—	1810	—	—	—
Taquitos Chicken w/ Rice	3	740	40	11	85	30	66	—	8	—	1770	—	—	—
Veggie Mix	1 serv	110	0	0	0	3	24	—	6	—	330	—	—	—
SALAD DRESSINGS														
Chipotle Vinaigrette	1 serv (2.5 oz)	110	9	1	0	0	0	0	0	—	490	—	—	—
Fat Free Salsa Verde	1 serv (2.5 oz)	15	0	0	0	0	3	—	1	—	370	—	—	—
Olive Oil Vinaigrette	1 serv (2.5 oz)	290	31	5	0	0	2	—	0	—	290	—	—	—
Ranch	1 serv (2.5 oz)	260	26	6	50	2	4	—	0	—	470	—	—	—
SALADS														
Baja Ensalada Chicken	1 serv	310	7	2	18	46	18	—	7	—	1210	—	—	—
Baja Ensalada Shrimp	1 serv	230	6	2	250	28	18	—	6	—	1110	—	—	—
Baja Ensalada Steak	1 serv	450	18	7	150	54	18	—	6	—	1240	—	—	—
Chipotle w/ Carnitas	1 serv	640	30	10	95	38	56	—	10	—	1280	—	—	—
Chipotle w/ Chicken	1 serv	590	22	6	105	47	54	—	11	—	1110	—	—	—
Chipotle w/ Steak	1 serv	700	31	11	135	54	54	—	9	—	1140	—	—	—
Side By Side Carnitas	1 serv	570	40	13	140	46	16	—	8	—	1560	—	—	—
Side By Side Chicken	1 serv	500	27	8	150	60	12	—	9	—	1310	—	—	—
Side By Side Steak	1 serv	620	42	14	160	55	14	—	6	—	1550	—	—	—

FOOD	PORTION	CALS	FAT	SAT FAT	CHOL	PROT	CARB	SUGAR	FIBER	CALCI	SOD	POTAS	FOLIC	VIT C
Side Salad	1 (6.5 oz)	130	6	2	5	5	16	—	4	—	430	—	—	—
Tostada Breaded Fish	1 serv	1200	61	15	71	47	111	—	25	—	2140	—	—	—
Tostada Carnitas	1 serv	1180	62	17	100	52	100	—	26	—	2520	—	—	—
Tostada Chicken	1 serv	1140	55	14	115	60	98	—	27	—	2370	—	—	—
Tostada Mahi Mahi	1 serv	1130	55	14	105	59	99	—	25	—	2070	—	—	—
Tostada No Meat	1 serv	1010	53	13	40	32	98	—	25	—	1930	—	—	—
Tostada Shrimp	1 serv	1120	55	14	285	55	99	—	25	—	2460	—	—	—
Tostada Steak	1 serv	1230	63	17	140	65	98	—	25	—	2380	—	—	—

BASKIN-ROBBINS

BEVERAGES

FOOD	PORTION	CALS	FAT	SAT FAT	CHOL	PROT	CARB	SUGAR	FIBER	CALCI	SOD	POTAS	FOLIC	VIT C
Cappuccino Blast w/ Whipped Cream	1 sm (16 oz)	330	14	9	55	6	48	42	0	200	110	—	—	1
Shake Chocolate Chip	1 sm (16 oz)	660	32	20	115	14	78	74	1	500	230	—	—	2
Shake Chocolate Chip Cookie Dough	1 sm (16 oz)	750	31	20	105	14	99	88	1	450	310	—	—	2
Shake Mint Chocolate Chip	1 sm (16 oz)	680	33	20	110	14	83	79	1	450	240	—	—	4
Shake Vanilla	1 sm (16 oz)	670	33	21	130	13	80	73	0	450	370	—	—	2

FROZEN YOGURT

FOOD	PORTION	CALS	FAT	SAT FAT	CHOL	PROT	CARB	SUGAR	FIBER	CALCI	SOD	POTAS	FOLIC	VIT C
Cherries Jubilee	1 scoop (4 oz)	240	12	7	45	4	30	26	1	150	80	—	—	1
Vanilla Fat Free	1 scoop (4 oz)	150	0	0	0	6	32	31	0	200	105	—	—	1

ICE CREAM

FOOD	PORTION	CALS	FAT	SAT FAT	CHOL	PROT	CARB	SUGAR	FIBER	CALCI	SOD	POTAS	FOLIC	VIT C
Butter Almond Crunch Reduced Fat No Sugar Added	1 scoop (4 oz)	220	11	5	25	7	31	7	4	200	140	—	—	1
Butter Pecan	1 scoop (4 oz)	280	18	9	50	5	24	24	1	150	95	—	—	1
Cabana Berry Banana Reduced Fat No Sugar Added	1 scoop (4 oz)	150	6	4	20	4	27	7	3	150	70	—	—	30
Chocolate	1 scoop (4 oz)	260	14	9	50	5	33	31	0	150	130	—	—	1
Chocolate Chip	1 scoop (4 oz)	270	16	10	55	5	28	26	1	150	95	—	—	1
Chocolate Chip Cookie Dough	1 scoop (4 oz)	310	15	10	50	5	36	30	0	150	135	—	—	1
Chocolate Overload Reduced Fat No Sugar Added	1 scoop (4 oz)	190	8	5	20	6	37	7	5	150	110	—	—	1
Gold Medal Ribbon	1 scoop (4 oz)	260	13	8	45	5	34	33	0	150	150	—	—	1

FOOD	PORTION	CALS	FAT	SAT FAT	CHOL	PROT	CARB	SUGAR	FIBER	CALCI	SOD	POTAS	FOLIC	VIT C
Mint Chocolate Chip	1 scoop (4 oz)	270	16	10	55	5	28	26	1	150	95	—	—	1
Nutty Coconut	1 scoop (4 oz)	300	20	9	45	6	28	27	1	150	90	—	—	1
Oreo Cookies 'N Cream	1 scoop (4 oz)	280	15	9	50	5	32	27	1	150	150	—	—	1
Peanut Butter 'N Chocolate	1 scoop (4 oz)	320	20	9	45	7	31	28	1	150	180	—	—	1
Pistachio Almond	1 scoop (4 oz)	290	19	9	50	7	25	23	1	150	85	—	—	1
Pralines 'N Cream	1 scoop (4 oz)	280	14	8	45	5	35	31	1	150	170	—	—	1
Reese's Peanut Butter Cup	1 scoop (4 oz)	300	18	10	50	6	31	29	1	150	130	—	—	1
Rocky Road	1 scoop (4 oz)	290	15	8	45	5	36	32	5	150	120	—	—	tr
Sundae Caramel Soft Serve	1 (10 oz)	580	21	13	70	13	89	78	1	450	470	—	—	4
Sundae Hot Fudge Soft Serve	1 (10 oz)	610	25	18	65	14	86	75	1	500	430	—	—	4
Sundae Strawberry Soft Serve	1 (10 oz)	450	18	11	65	12	59	57	1	450	310	—	—	12
Tax Crunch	1 scoop (4 oz)	330	20	11	45	5	32	28	1	150	115	—	—	1
Vanilla	1 scoop (4 oz)	260	16	10	65	4	26	26	0	150	70	—	—	1
Vanilla Soft Serve	1 serv (6 oz)	280	11	7	40	8	37	36	0	300	200	—	—	2
Very Berry Strawberry	1 scoop (4 oz)	320	11	7	40	4	28	27	0	150	70	—	—	12
ICES														
Sherbet Rainbow	1 scoop (4 oz)	160	2	2	10	1	34	34	0	40	40	—	—	1
Sorbet Lemon	1 scoop (4 oz)	130	0	0	0	0	33	33	0	0	15	—	—	5
Sorbet Mango	1 scoop (4 oz)	120	0	0	0	0	32	30	0	0	10	—	—	4
Sorbet Strawberry	1 scoop (4 oz)	130	0	0	0	0	34	34	0	0	10	—	—	9
BEAR ROCK CAFE														
SANDWICHES														
Colorado Turkey Club	1	855	37	17	126	38	95	12	5	358	2310	—	—	14
Coop's Chicken Salad Croissant	1	439	31	6	44	24	46	12	5	86	375	—	—	10
Garden Grill Ciabatta	1	406	25	7	33	12	55	7	4	93	907	—	—	93
Giant Panda Wrap	1	556	23	4	58	31	68	21	23	151	2045	—	—	25
Hoot Owl	1	641	42	12	92	34	32	3	2	159	1618	—	—	9
Rising Sunflower	1	596	35	9	86	35	35	6	2	231	1694	—	—	32
Roast Turkey & Bacon	1	522	30	6	71	32	31	2	2	15	1656	—	—	8
Rockslide Focaccia	1	958	62	17	129	43	57	2	3	417	2546	—	—	11
The Moose	1	976	54	18	142	54	64	17	7	633	2565	—	—	8

BEN & JERRY'S

FOOD	PORTION	CALS	FAT	SAT FAT	CHOL	PROT	CARB	SUGAR	FIBER	CALCI	SOD	POTAS	FOLIC	VIT C
FROZEN YOGURT														
Low Fat Cherry Garcia	½ cup	170	3	2	20	4	32	22	tr	200	65	—	—	0
Low Fat Chocolate Fudge Brownie	½ cup	190	3	2	15	5	35	23	1	150	100	—	—	0
Low Fat Half Baked	½ cup	190	3	2	20	5	35	23	tr	150	100	—	—	0
Phish Food	½ cup	220	5	4	15	4	41	22	1	150	95	—	—	0
ICE CREAM														
Bar Cherry Garcia	1	270	19	12	35	4	29	23	1	100	45	—	—	0
Bar Half Baked	1	340	16	10	40	5	46	36	2	100	125	—	—	0
Bar Vanilla	1	300	20	13	45	4	26	23	1	150	60	—	—	0
Bar Vanilla Almond	1	340	23	13	65	5	30	22	2	150	135	—	—	0
Black & Tan	½ cup	230	13	9	50	4	24	21	1	150	55	—	—	0
Brownie Batter	½ cup	310	18	10	70	5	32	26	1	150	115	—	—	0
Butter Pecan	½ cup	280	21	10	65	4	20	18	1	150	105	—	—	0
Cherry Garcia	½ cup	250	14	10	60	4	26	22	tr	150	50	—	—	0
Chocolate	½ cup	260	16	11	50	4	25	22	2	150	50	—	—	0
Chocolate Chip Cookie Dough	½ cup	270	15	10	65	4	32	24	0	150	85	—	—	0
Chocolate Fudge Brownie	½ cup	260	13	9	35	5	32	25	2	100	80	—	—	0
Chubby Hubby	½ cup	330	20	11	55	7	31	24	1	150	150	—	—	1
Chunky Monkey	½ cup	300	18	10	55	5	30	28	1	150	45	—	—	1
Coffee	½ cup	240	15	10	75	4	21	19	0	150	60	—	—	0
Coffee Heath Bar Crunch	½ cup	290	18	11	65	4	29	27	0	150	—	—	—	0
Dave Matthews Band Magic Brownies	½ cup	250	13	8	60	4	29	23	0	100	75	—	—	0
Dublin Mudslide	½ cup	270	16	10	65	4	28	23	tr	150	80	—	—	0
Everything But The	½ cup	310	19	12	50	5	30	27	1	150	85	—	—	0
Fossil Fuel	½ cup	280	17	11	60	4	30	26	1	150	60	—	—	0
Fudge Central	½ cup	300	18	12	55	4	31	27	1	150	60	—	—	0
Half Baked	½ cup	280	14	9	50	5	34	26	tr	100	90	—	—	0
In A Crunch	½ cup	350	23	10	55	6	30	22	1	150	150	—	—	0
Karamel Sutra	½ cup	280	15	10	50	4	32	27	1	150	75	—	—	0
Marsha Marsha Marshmallow	½ cup	300	17	10	30	4	33	24	1	100	60	—	—	0
Mint Chocolate Cookie	½ cup	260	16	9	65	4	26	21	0	150	100	—	—	0
Neapolitan Dynamite	½ cup	250	13	9	45	4	29	26	1	100	70	—	—	0

FOOD	PORTION	CALS	FAT	SAT FAT	CHOL	PROT	CARB	SUGAR	FIBER	CALCI	SOD	POTAS	FOLIC	VIT C
New York Super Fudge Chunk	½ cup	310	20	11	40	5	29	25	2	100	55	—	—	0
Oatmeal Cookie Chunk	½ cup	270	15	9	55	4	31	24	tr	100	120	—	—	0
Organic Chocolate Fudge Brownie	½ cup	270	13	9	35	4	30	26	2	100	55	—	—	0
Organic Strawberry	½ cup	210	12	8	55	3	21	19	0	100	40	—	—	9
Organic Sweet Cream & Cookies	½ cup	250	15	9	60	4	24	19	0	100	95	—	—	0
Organic Vanilla	½ cup	220	14	10	65	3	18	16	0	100	50	—	—	0
Peanut Butter Cup	½ cup	360	26	13	60	7	27	23	1	150	125	—	—	0
Phish Food	½ cup	280	13	9	30	4	37	22	1	100	85	—	—	0
Pistachio Pistachio	½ cup	260	17	10	65	5	21	18	tr	150	55	—	—	0
Sandwich Wich Ice Cream Cookie	1	350	18	13	55	4	45	30	1	80	220	—	—	0
Strawberry	½ cup	230	13	9	65	4	26	25	0	150	50	—	—	12
The Godfather	½ cup	270	14	9	30	4	32	24	2	100	50	—	—	4
Turtle Soup	½ cup	280	15	10	60	4	30	25	1	150	100	—	—	0
Uncanny Cashew	½ cup	290	19	13	70	4	27	22	0	150	130	—	—	0
Vanilla Caramel Fudge	½ cup	280	15	10	70	4	31	25	0	150	105	—	—	0
Vanilla Heath Bar Crunch	½ cup	290	18	11	65	4	29	27	0	150	120	—	—	0
Vermonty Python	½ cup	310	19	11	60	4	30	26	1	150	90	—	—	0
SORBETS														
Berried Treasure	½ cup	110	0	0	0	0	29	24	1	0	5	—	—	4
Jamaican Me Crazy	½ cup	130	0	0	0	0	33	28	4	0	10	—	—	4
Strawberry Kiwi Swirl	½ cup	110	0	0	0	0	28	24	1	0	10	—	—	5

BILLY'S BURGER HUT

BEVERAGES

FOOD	PORTION	CALS	FAT	SAT FAT	CHOL	PROT	CARB	SUGAR	FIBER	CALCI	SOD	POTAS	FOLIC	VIT C
Shake Chocolate	1 (20 oz)	420	10	4	30	9	63	50	0	250	260	—	—	—
Shake Vanilla	1 (20 oz)	320	10	4	25	8	49	44	0	250	157	—	—	—

MAIN MENU SELECTIONS

FOOD	PORTION	CALS	FAT	SAT FAT	CHOL	PROT	CARB	SUGAR	FIBER	CALCI	SOD	POTAS	FOLIC	VIT C
Big Billy's Roast Beef Sub	1	843	54	27	151	51	62	12	3	75	2860	—	—	—
Billyburger	1	426	22	12	63	20	35	6	3	100	1076	—	—	—
Billyburger w/ Cheese	1	498	35	19	57	23	35	8	4	200	1276	—	—	—
Billy's Best Red Potato Salad	1 serv	190	9	2	80	2	12	4	3	20	650	—	—	10

FOOD	PORTION	CALS	FAT	SAT FAT	CHOL	PROT	CARB	SUGAR	FIBER	CALCI	SOD	POTAS	FOLIC	VIT C
Billy's Biggest Burger ½ Pounder w/ Everything	1	852	58	—	140	70	61	15	4	200	2229	—	—	—
Billy's Famous 7 Layer Salad	1 serv	558	49	11	119	10	18	9	2	100	680	—	—	15
Billy's Seafood Sandwich	1	399	18	10	42	21	43	9	3	100	890	—	—	—
Caesar Side Salad	1 serv	360	28	4	70	11	12	1	4	180	610	—	—	39
Chili w/ Cheese & Onion	1 serv	380	12	6	64	33	35	8	7	80	1004	—	—	—
Cowboy Cobb Salad	1 serv	735	45	14	239	29	25	10	9	140	1450	—	—	40
Cowboy Coleslaw	1 serv	180	9	2	10	1	11	4	3	20	250	—	—	6
French Fries	1 reg	230	12	4	0	5	25	7	1	10	253	—	—	—
Onion Rings	1 serv	250	10	6	0	2	37	6	1	40	955	—	—	—
Super Billy Burger w/ Bacon	1	663	41	21	98	35	39	9	4	150	1869	—	—	—

BLIMPIE

DESSERTS

FOOD	PORTION	CALS	FAT	SAT FAT	CHOL	PROT	CARB	SUGAR	FIBER	CALCI	SOD	POTAS	FOLIC	VIT C
Cookie Chocolate Chunk	1 (1.5 oz)	200	10	5	15	2	25	16	0	0	150	—	—	0
Cookie Oatmeal Raisin	1 (1.5 oz)	180	7	3	10	2	27	16	tr	0	150	—	—	0
Cookie Peanut Butter	1 (1.5 oz)	210	13	5	10	3	21	13	tr	0	170	—	—	0
Cookie Sugar	1 (2.5 oz)	320	16	6	35	3	42	23	0	0	240	—	—	0
Cookie White Chocolate Macadamia Nut	1 (1.5 oz)	200	11	5	15	2	25	16	0	0	110	—	—	0

SALAD DRESSINGS AND SAUCES

FOOD	PORTION	CALS	FAT	SAT FAT	CHOL	PROT	CARB	SUGAR	FIBER	CALCI	SOD	POTAS	FOLIC	VIT C
Dressing Blue Cheese	1 serv (1.5 oz)	230	24	5	25	2	2	2	—	20	440	—	—	0
Dressing Buttermilk Ranch	1 serv (1.5 oz)	230	24	4	10	1	2	1	—	0	380	—	—	0
Dressing Buttermilk Ranch Light	1 serv (1.5 oz)	70	4	1	0	1	8	3	—	0	310	—	—	0
Dressing Creamy Caesar	1 serv (1.5 oz)	210	21	4	10	1	2	1	—	0	520	—	—	0
Dressing Creamy Italian	1 serv (1.5 oz)	180	18	3	0	0	4	3	0	0	420	—	—	0
Dressing Dijon Honey Mustard	1 serv (1.5 oz)	180	17	3	15	1	8	7	—	0	240	—	—	0
Dressing Italian Fat Free	1 serv (1.5 oz)	25	0	—	0	0	5	3	0	0	390	—	—	0

FOOD	PORTION	CALS	FAT	SAT FAT	CHOL	PROT	CARB	SUGAR	FIBER	CALCI	SOD	POTAS	FOLIC	VIT C
Dressing Italian Light	1 serv (1.5 oz)	20	1	0	0	0	2	2	—	0	770	—	—	0
Dressing Peppercorn	1 serv (1.5 oz)	240	26	5	20	1	1	1	0	0	450	—	—	0
Dressing Thousand Island	1 serv (1.5 oz)	210	20	3	15	0	6	6	0	0	350	—	—	0
Guacamole	1 serv (1 oz)	45	4	1	0	0	2	0	1	0	135	—	—	2
Mayonnaise	1 serv (1 oz)	200	22	3	20	0	0	0	0	0	200	—	—	0
Mustard Yellow Deli	1 serv (0.5 oz)	15	0	0	—	0	0	0	0	0	170	—	—	0
Oil Blend	1 serv (0.5 oz)	130	14	2	—	0	0	0	0	0	0	—	—	0
Sauce Blimpie Special	1 serv (0.5 oz)	40	5	0	0	0	0	—	—	0	0	—	—	0
Sauce Red Hot Original	1 serv (1 oz)	10	0	0	0	0	2	0	0	0	760	—	—	0
SALADS														
Antipasto	1 serv (11.6 oz)	254	14	6	60	20	12	6	4	250	1630	—	—	24
Buffalo Chicken	1 serv (7.7 oz)	220	9	5	60	25	10	5	4	200	840	—	—	30
Chicken Caesar	1 serv (9.4 oz)	190	8	4	65	25	6	3	3	150	460	—	—	24
Cole Slaw	1 side (4 oz)	160	9	2	5	1	20	17	2	40	240	—	—	5
Garden	1 serv (6.5 oz)	30	0	0	0	2	6	3	3	40	15	—	—	24
Macaroni	1 side (5 oz)	330	22	5	15	5	28	8	2	0	790	—	—	0
Northwest Potato	1 side (5 oz)	260	17	4	25	3	22	3	3	0	390	—	—	0
Potato	1 side (4.7 oz)	230	12	3	10	3	28	8	3	0	490	—	—	0
Tuna	1 serv (9.4 oz)	270	19	3	55	18	6	3	3	40	370	—	—	24
Ultimate Club	1 serv (10.1 oz)	280	14	7	65	23	10	5	3	350	1070	—	—	24
SANDWICHES														
6 Inch Sub Blimpie Best	1 (10.4 oz)	450	17	6	50	24	49	10	3	150	1330	—	—	9
6 Inch Sub Blimpie Best Super Stacked	1 (12.8 oz)	550	22	8	90	36	52	12	3	150	2090	—	—	9
6 Inch Sub Blimpie Trio Super Stacked	1 (13.5 oz)	510	15	5	90	40	51	11	3	200	1760	—	—	9
6 Inch Sub BLT	1 (7.2 oz)	430	22	5	25	15	43	6	2	20	960	—	—	6
6 Inch Sub BLT Super Stacked	1 (8.4 oz)	640	41	9	55	22	43	6	2	20	1440	—	—	6
6 Inch Sub Chicken Cheddar Bacon Ranch	1 (12.1 oz)	600	29	10	85	36	48	8	3	200	1570	—	—	9
6 Inch Sub Chicken Teriyaki	1 (8.7 oz)	450	12	5	65	33	52	13	2	150	1280	—	—	2
6 Inch Sub Club	1 (10.2 oz)	410	13	4	45	23	49	9	3	200	1050	—	—	9
6 Inch Sub Cuban	1 (8.2 oz)	410	11	5	65	29	43	6	1	200	1630	—	—	0

FOOD	PORTION	CALS	FAT	SAT FAT	CHOL	PROT	CARB	SUGAR	FIBER	CALCI	SOD	POTAS	FOLIC	VIT C
6 Inch Sub French Dip	1 (13.4 oz)	410	11	5	65	30	46	3	1	200	1650	—	—	0
6 Inch Sub Ham & Swiss	1 (10 oz)	420	14	5	45	23	49	10	3	200	1020	—	—	9
6 Inch Sub Hot Pastrami	1 (7.2 oz)	430	16	7	65	30	42	5	1	200	1350	—	—	0
6 Inch Sub Hot Pastrami Super Stacked	1 (10.1 oz)	570	23	10	110	46	43	7	1	200	2110	—	—	0
6 Inch Sub Meatball	1 (10 oz)	580	31	13	75	27	50	6	4	250	1960	—	—	2
6 Inch Sub Reuben	1 (9.2 oz)	530	20	6	70	34	52	7	3	250	1740	—	—	4
6 Inch Sub Roast Beef & Provolone	1 (10.8 oz)	430	14	5	55	28	46	7	3	150	980	—	—	9
6 Inch Sub Roast Beef & Provolone On Wheat	1 (11.3 oz)	430	16	5	60	32	44	6	6	150	1000	—	—	9
6 Inch Sub Tuna	1 (8.9 oz)	470	21	3	55	24	43	5	2	20	770	—	—	6
6 Inch Sub Turkey & Provolone	1 (10.8 oz)	410	13	4	40	24	49	8	3	150	1310	—	—	9
6 Inch Sub Turkey & Provolone On Wheat	1 (11.3 oz)	420	14	5	45	27	47	8	6	150	1350	—	—	9
6 Inch Sub VegiMax	1 (10.2 oz)	520	20	6	15	28	56	8	5	200	1270	—	—	6
Blimpie Burger	1 (6 oz)	460	24	10	70	21	42	4	1	20	1280	—	—	0
Blimpie Dog	1 (6.3 oz)	510	29	12	55	17	45	7	1	20	1420	—	—	6
Ciabatta Buffalo Chicken	1 (11.3 oz)	540	23	7	65	31	49	5	3	200	1970	—	—	15
Ciabatta French Dip	1 (13.8 oz)	430	11	5	65	31	49	2	2	250	1820	—	—	9
Ciabatta Grilled Chicken Caesar	1 (10.1 oz)	580	20	5	65	34	62	4	3	200	1480	—	—	18
Ciabatta Mediterranean	1 (10.1 oz)	450	8	3	35	26	65	6	3	200	1720	—	—	36
Ciabatta Roast Beef Turkey & Cheddar	1 (10 oz)	520	24	8	65	25	51	6	3	200	1780	—	—	18
Ciabatta Sicilian	1 (10 oz)	590	22	6	60	29	66	9	3	200	2170	—	—	27
Ciabatta Spicy Chicken & Pepperoni	1 (10.1 oz)	710	34	11	80	33	65	4	3	250	2070	—	—	15
Ciabatta Tuscan	1 (9.9 oz)	570	20	6	50	28	65	6	3	200	2030	—	—	27
Ciabatta Ultimate Club	1 (7.4 oz)	520	24	7	65	27	47	5	2	250	1600	—	—	9
Wrap Chicken Caesar	1 (9.7 oz)	220	8	0	60	30	56	5	4	400	1480	—	—	6
Wrap Southwestern	1 (10 oz)	530	22	6	55	23	61	10	4	250	1770	—	—	6

FOOD	PORTION	CALS	FAT	SAT FAT	CHOL	PROT	CARB	SUGAR	FIBER	CALCI	SOD	POTAS	FOLIC	VIT C
SOUPS														
Bean w/ Ham	1 serv (8.6 oz)	140	1	0	0	8	23	2	11	80	1070	—	—	1
Chicken Noodle	1 serv (8.6 oz)	130	4	1	30	7	18	5	2	20	1040	—	—	2
Chicken w/ White & Wild Rice	1 serv (8.6 oz)	250	10	3	30	14	15	4	4	60	1030	—	—	2
Cream Of Broccoli w/ Cheese	1 serv (8.6 oz)	250	19	11	55	7	13	2	tr	150	1040	—	—	15
Cream Of Potato	1 serv (8.6 oz)	190	9	3	<5	5	24	3	3	100	860	—	—	1
Garden Vegetable	1 serv (8.6 oz)	80	1	0	0	5	14	5	3	0	620	—	—	1
Grande Chili w/ Bean & Beef	1 serv (8.6 oz)	310	9	4	20	20	31	9	9	60	1440	—	—	15
Tomato Basil w/ Raviolini	1 serv (8.6 oz)	110	1	0	10	4	22	5	0	20	720	—	—	0
Vegetable Beef	1 serv (8.6 oz)	80	2	1	5	4	13	3	2	60	1010	—	—	1

BOB EVANS

FOOD	PORTION	CALS	FAT	SAT FAT	CHOL	PROT	CARB	SUGAR	FIBER	CALCI	SOD	POTAS	FOLIC	VIT C
BREAKFAST SELECTIONS														
Bacon	1 piece	36	4	2	5	1	0	0	0	—	54	—	—	—
Benedict Ham & Cheese	1 serv	826	52	19	564	44	44	8	0	—	3137	—	—	—
Country Benedict Sausage	1 serv	936	66	24	536	44	40	6	0	—	2098	—	—	—
Country Benedict Spinach Bacon & Tomato	1 serv	729	48	16	494	30	42	8	1	—	1885	—	—	—
Country Biscuit Breakfast	1 serv	659	45	16	269	24	40	6	1	—	1703	—	—	—
Egg Hardcooked	1	60	4	2	190	6	1	0	0	—	55	—	—	—
Egg Over Easy	1	101	8	2	229	7	1	1	0	—	68	—	—	—
Egg Scrambled	1 serv	255	17	5	723	20	2	0	0	—	213	—	—	—
Egg Beaters	1 serv	173	12	2	5	28	3	2	0	—	581	—	—	—
French Toast	1 slice	131	2	0	25	3	13	3	1	—	175	—	—	—
French Toast Stuffed Plain	1 serv	599	20	12	99	11	53	21	3	—	689	—	—	—
Fruit & Yogurt Plate	1 serv	403	2	1	5	9	93	80	9	—	109	—	—	—
Grits	1 serv	178	7	2	9	3	28	0	2	—	172	—	—	—
Ham Smoked	1 slice	87	2	1	52	14	2	1	0	—	1131	—	—	—
Hotcake Blueberry	1	328	9	2	0	6	55	17	2	—	749	—	—	—
Hotcake Buttermilk	1	318	9	2	0	6	53	16	2	—	746	—	—	—
Hotcake Cinnamon	1	417	15	4	0	6	66	27	2	—	749	—	—	—
Hotcake Multigrain	1	322	10	3	0	7	52	16	3	—	773	—	—	—
Mush	1 serv	79	3	1	0	1	11	5	2	—	466	—	—	—
Oatmeal	1 serv	172	3	0	0	6	32	1	4	—	394	—	—	—

FOOD	PORTION	CALS	FAT	SAT FAT	CHOL	PROT	CARB	SUGAR	FIBER	CALCI	SOD	POTAS	FOLIC	VIT C
Omelette Bacon & Cheese	1 serv	825	66	25	826	40	6	2	1	—	1603	—	—	—
Omelette Border Scramble	1	756	58	20	846	42	15	6	3	—	1059	—	—	—
Omelette Egg Beaters Bacon & Cheese	1 serv	615	47	20	108	57	7	4	1	—	1972	—	—	—
Omelette Egg Beaters Border Scramble	1 serv	517	37	14	72	48	16	8	3	—	1411	—	—	—
Omelette Egg Beaters Farmer's Market	1 serv	569	41	19	92	49	14	7	2	—	2108	—	—	—
Omelette Egg Beaters Garden Harvest	1 serv	444	31	14	64	40	14	7	2	—	1610	—	—	—
Omelette Egg Beaters Ham & Cheddar	1 serv	426	29	12	80	51	5	3	1	—	1789	—	—	—
Omelette Egg Beaters Sausage & Cheddar	1 serv	502	40	15	73	49	4	2	1	—	1295	—	—	—
Omelette Egg Beaters Three Cheese	1 serv	435	34	16	78	43	5	3	1	—	1394	—	—	—
Omelette Farmer's Market	1	778	60	24	810	42	13	5	2	—	1739	—	—	—
Omelette Garden Harvest	1 serv	654	50	20	782	33	13	5	2	—	1241	—	—	—
Omelette Ham & Cheddar	1 serv	634	48	17	798	44	3	0	1	—	1419	—	—	—
Omelette Sausage & Cheddar	1 serv	741	61	21	847	42	3	0	1	—	942	—	—	—
Omelette Three Cheese	1 serv	645	52	21	796	35	4	0	1	—	1025	—	—	—
Omelette Western	1 serv	654	48	17	798	44	8	3	2	—	1420	—	—	—
Pot Roast Hash	1 serv	652	39	14	533	38	34	5	4	—	1084	—	—	—
Sausage Gravy Bowl	1 serv	268	17	11	17	7	21	1	0	—	1238	—	—	—
Sausage Link	1	125	11	3	14	5	0	0	0	—	184	—	—	—
Skillet Sunshine	1 serv	842	60	18	819	37	36	2	4	—	1474	—	—	—
Waffles Sweet Cream	1 serv	598	12	7	149	15	100	30	3	—	1288	—	—	—
CHILDREN'S MENU SELECTIONS														
Hotcakes	1 serv	501	17	6	0	9	79	26	2	—	1071	—	—	—
Kid's Macaroni & Cheese	1 serv	320	11	3	23	11	45	11	2	—	778	—	—	—
Kid's Pasta	1 serv	113	5	1	12	3	15	4	1	—	857	—	—	—

FOOD	PORTION	CALS	FAT	SAT FAT	CHOL	PROT	CARB	SUGAR	FIBER	CALCI	SOD	POTAS	FOLIC	VIT C
Mini Cheeseburgers	1 serv	306	19	7	40	12	21	4	1	—	525	—	—	—
Smiley Face Potatoes	1 serv	524	31	6	2	5	57	2	3	—	646	—	—	—
Sundae Reese's I'm Smiling	1 serv	330	17	9	26	5	41	32	1	—	130	—	—	—
MAIN MENU SELECTIONS														
Seniors Chicken Parmesan	1 serv	522	26	9	127	38	33	7	3	—	2404	—	—	—
Seniors Garden Vegetable Alfredo	1 serv	363	23	9	36	11	29	7	5	—	1322	—	—	—
Seniors Garden Vegetable Alfredo Chicken	1 serv	452	26	10	74	26	29	7	5	—	1678	—	—	—
Seniors Steak Tips & Noodles	1 serv	422	22	6	101	33	23	3	2	—	2251	—	—	—
Seniors Stir-Fry Chicken	1 serv	368	13	2	37	21	44	16	5	—	1385	—	—	—
SOUPS														
Bean	1 cup	144	3	1	8	10	19	1	3	—	778	—	—	—
Cheddar Baked Potato	1 cup	294	20	8	34	10	19	3	1	—	1168	—	—	—
Sausage Chili	1 cup	268	17	6	42	16	18	2	7	—	687	—	—	—
Vegetable Beef	1 cup	135	5	2	14	6	17	2	3	—	370	—	—	—
BOJANGLES														
Biscuit	1	243	12	3	2	4	29		2	—	663	—	—	—
Biscuit Sandwich Bacon	1	290	17	5	10	8	26	—	1	—	810	—	—	—
Biscuit Sandwich Bacon Egg Cheese	1	550	42	14	160	17	27	—	1	—	1250	—	—	—
Biscuit Sandwich Cajun Filet	1	454	21	6	41	20	46	—	1	—	949	—	—	—
Biscuit Sandwich Country Ham	1	270	15	4	20	9	26	—	1	—	1010	—	—	—
Biscuit Sandwich Egg	1	400	30	6	120	8	26	—	1	—	630	—	—	—
Biscuit Sandwich Sausage	1	350	23	7	20	9	26	—	1	—	810	—	—	—
Biscuit Sandwich Smoked Sausage	1	380	26	9	20	10	27	—	1	—	940	—	—	—
Biscuit Sandwich Steak	1	649	49	13	34	14	37	—	1	—	1126	—	—	—
Botato Rounds	1 serv	235	11	4	13	3	31	—	3	—	328	—	—	—
Buffalo Bites	1 serv	180	5	2	105	27	5	—	0	—	720	—	—	—
Cajun Pintos	1 serv	110	0	0	0	6	18	—	6	—	480	—	—	—

FOOD	PORTION	CALS	FAT	SAT FAT	CHOL	PROT	CARB	SUGAR	FIBER	CALCI	SOD	POTAS	FOLIC	VIT C
Cajun Spiced Breast	1 serv	278	17	—	75	18	12	—	tr	—	565	—	—	—
Cajun Spiced Leg	1 serv	264	16	—	96	19	11	—	tr	—	530	—	—	—
Cajun Spiced Thigh	1 serv	310	23	—	67	15	11	—	tr	—	465	—	—	—
Cajun Spiced Wing	1 serv	355	25	—	94	21	11	—	tr	—	630	—	—	—
Chicken Supremes	1 serv	337	16	6	58	21	26	—	1	—	629	—	—	—
Corn On The Cob	1 serv	140	2	0	0	5	34	—	2	—	20	—	—	—
Dirty Rice	1 serv	166	6	2	10	5	24	—	1	—	762	—	—	—
Green Beans	1 serv	25	0	0	0	0	5	—	2	—	710	—	—	—
Macaroni & Cheese	1 serv	198	14	5	26	7	12	—	tr	—	418	—	—	—
Marinated Cole Slaw	1 serv	136	3	0	0	1	26	—	3	—	454	—	—	—
Potatoes w/o Gravy	1 serv	80	1	0	0	2	16	—	1	—	380	—	—	—
Sandwich Cajun Filet w/ Mayo	1	437	22	7	55	22	41	—	3	—	506	—	—	—
Sandwich Cajun Filet w/o Mayo	1	337	11	5	45	22	41	—	3	—	401	—	—	—
Sandwich Grilled Filet w/ Mayo	1	335	16	5	61	23	25	—	2	—	645	—	—	—
Sandwich Grilled Filet w/o Mayo	1	235	5	3	51	23	25	—	2	—	540	—	—	—
Seasoned Fries	1 serv	344	19	5	13	5	39	—	4	—	480	—	—	—
Southern Style Breast	1 serv	261	16	—	76	16	12	—	tr	—	702	—	—	—
Southern Style Leg	1 serv	254	15	—	94	19	11	—	tr	—	446	—	—	—
Southern Style Thigh	1 serv	308	21	—	78	16	14	—	tr	—	630	—	—	—
Southern Style Wing	1 serv	337	21	—	86	17	19	—	tr	—	684	—	—	—
Sweet Biscuit Bo Berry	1	320	18	4	tr	4	37	—	1	—	560	—	—	—
Sweet Biscuit Cinnamon	1	320	18	4	tr	4	37	—	1	—	560	—	—	—

BOSTON MARKET

DESSERTS

FOOD	PORTION	CALS	FAT	SAT FAT	CHOL	PROT	CARB	SUGAR	FIBER	CALCI	SOD	POTAS	FOLIC	VIT C
Apple Pie	1 slice	420	20	4	0	3	56	24	2	—	650	—	—	—
Brownie Chocolate Chip Fudge	1	580	23	5	90	9	81	61	3	—	390	—	—	—
Chocolate Cake	1 serv	600	32	7	65	5	75	55	2	—	210	—	—	—
Cookie Chocolate Chip	1	370	19	9	20	4	49	28	2	—	340	—	—	—
Cornbread	1 piece	180	5	2	10	2	31	12	0	—	320	—	—	—

FOOD	PORTION	CALS	FAT	SAT FAT	CHOL	PROT	CARB	SUGAR	FIBER	CALCI	SOD	POTAS	FOLIC	VIT C
MAIN MENU SELECTIONS														
Broccoli w/ Garlic Butter	1 serv	80	6	2	0	3	6	2	3	—	230	—	—	—
Butternut Squash	1 serv	140	5	3	10	2	25	9	2	—	35	—	—	—
Carver Boston Chicken	1	700	29	7	90	44	68	4	3	—	1560	—	—	—
Carver Boston Meatloaf	1	940	45	18	155	49	96	11	6	—	2080	—	—	—
Carver Boston Sirloin Dip	1	1000	51	15	200	67	70	4	3	—	1690	—	—	—
Carver Boston Turkey	1	770	27	8	125	66	68	3	3	—	1810	—	—	—
Carver Boston Turkey Dip	1	770	27	8	125	66	67	2	3	—	1890	—	—	—
Cinnamon Apples	1 serv	210	3	0	0	0	47	42	3	—	15	—	—	—
Cranberry Walnut Relish	1 serv	140	2	0	0	1	30	27	2	—	0	—	—	—
Creamed Spinach	1 serv	280	23	15	70	9	12	1	4	—	580	—	—	—
Dip Spinach Artichoke	1 serv	100	8	4	15	3	3	1	1	—	220	—	—	—
Family Meals Boneless Turkey Breast	1 serv (5 oz)	180	3	1	70	38	0	0	0	—	620	—	—	—
Family Meals Roasted Turkey	1 serv (5 oz)	180	3	1	72	38	0	0	0	—	635	—	—	—
Family Meals Rotisserie Chicken	1 serv (6 oz)	290	14	4	175	39	4	1	0	—	710	—	—	—
Family Meals Spiral Sliced Ham	1 serv (8 oz)	450	26	10	140	40	13	5	0	—	2230	—	—	—
Family Meals Whole Turkey	1 serv (6.7 oz)	310	18	5	135	40	0	0	0	—	940	—	—	—
Fresh Vegetable Stuffing	1 serv	190	8	1	0	3	25	4	2	—	580	—	—	—
Garden Fresh Coleslaw	1 serv	170	9	2	10	2	21	19	2	—	270	—	—	—
Garlic Dill New Potatoes	1 serv	140	3	1	0	3	24	2	3	—	120	—	—	—
Green Bean Casserole	1 serv	60	2	1	5	2	9	2	2	—	620	—	—	—
Green Beans	1 serv	60	4	2	0	2	7	1	3	—	180	—	—	—
Individual Meals 1 Thigh & 1 Drumstick	1 serv	300	17	5	180	32	6	1	0	—	630	—	—	—

FOOD	PORTION	CALS	FAT	SAT FAT	CHOL	PROT	CARB	SUGAR	FIBER	CALCI	SOD	POTAS	FOLIC	VIT C
Individual Meals ¼ White Rotisserie Chicken	1 serv	290	11	4	170	45	4	1	0	—	780	—	—	—
Individual Meals ¼ White Rotisserie Chicken No Skin	1 serv	210	2	1	135	42	6	0	0	—	640	—	—	—
Individual Meals 3 Piece Dark	1 serv	380	19	6	250	45	7	1	0	—	880	—	—	—
Individual Meals 3 Piece Dark Skinless	1 serv	240	8	3	205	37	7	1	0	—	650	—	—	—
Individual Meals Award Winning Roasted Sirloin	1 serv	290	15	6	125	39	0	0	0	—	440	—	—	—
Individual Meals Meatloaf	1	480	33	13	125	29	23	6	2	—	970	—	—	—
Individual Meals Roasted Turkey	1 serv	180	3	1	72	38	0	0	0	—	635	—	—	—
Macaroni & Cheese	1 serv	330	12	7	30	14	39	9	1	—	1290	—	—	—
Mashed Potatoes	1 serv	210	9	6	25	4	29	2	3	—	660	—	—	—
Pot Pie Pastry Topped Chicken	1	780	47	17	125	29	60	4	4	—	930	—	—	—
Poultry Gravy	1 serv (4 oz)	15	1	0	0	1	4	1	0	—	570	—	—	—
Seasonal Fresh Fruit Salad	1 serv	60	0	0	0	1	15	13	1	—	20	—	—	—
Spinach w/ Garlic Butter Sauce	1 serv	130	9	6	20	5	9	1	5	—	200	—	—	—
Squash Casserole	1 serv	320	24	11	50	9	21	8	3	—	1380	—	—	—
Steamed Fresh Vegetables	1 serv	60	2	0	0	2	8	3	3	—	40	—	—	—
Sweet Corn	1 serv	170	4	1	0	6	37	10	2	—	95	—	—	—
Sweet Potato Casserole	1 serv	460	17	6	20	4	77	39	3	—	210	—	—	—
SALADS														
Entree Caesar	1	500	45	11	45	13	12	8	3	—	1190	—	—	—
Entree Caesar w/o Dressing	1	140	8	5	15	11	8	6	2	—	280	—	—	—
Entree Market Chopped	1	580	48	9	10	10	30	15	9	—	1990	—	—	—
Entree w/o Dressing	1	210	9	4	10	10	28	14	9	—	280	—	—	—
Side Caesar	1	400	40	8	30	5	7	4	2	—	980	—	—	—
Side Caesar w/o Dressing	1	40	2	2	5	3	3	2	1	—	75	—	—	—

FOOD	PORTION	CALS	FAT	SAT FAT	CHOL	PROT	CARB	SUGAR	FIBER	CALCI	SOD	POTAS	FOLIC	VIT C
Side Market Chopped	1	440	43	7	5	4	12	7	3	—	1790	—	—	—
Side Market Chopped w/o Dressing	1	80	4	1	5	3	10	5	3	—	85	—	—	—
SOUPS														
Chicken Noodle	1 serv	170	5	2	60	13	17	1	1	—	210	—	—	—
Chicken Tortilla w/ Toppings	1 serv	340	22	7	45	12	24	2	1	—	1310	—	—	—
Tortilla Soup w/o Toppings	1 serv	80	5	1	15	5	7	2	1	—	900	—	—	—

BOSTON PIZZA

FOOD	PORTION	CALS	FAT	SAT FAT	CHOL	PROT	CARB	SUGAR	FIBER	CALCI	SOD	POTAS	FOLIC	VIT C
CHILDREN'S MENU SELECTIONS														
Baked Salmon w/ Caesar Salad	1 serv	330	14	—	—	23	13	—	tr	—	330	—	—	—
Bug N' Cheese	1 serv	500	13	—	—	21	73	—	3	—	710	—	—	—
Chicken Fingers w/ Fries	1 serv	390	19	—	—	26	28	—	2	—	570	—	—	—
Pizza Pint Size	1	390	7	—	—	19	64	—	tr	—	520	—	—	—
Quesadilla Bacon Double Cheeseburger w/ Caesar Salad	1 serv	540	27	—	—	26	49	—	3	—	1660	—	—	—
Reduced Size Fruit Cup	1 serv	80	0	0	0	0	18	—	tr	—	0	—	—	—
Sandwich Grilled Chicken w/ Garden Greens	1 serv	600	38	—	—	10	45	—	3	—	1000	—	—	—
Super Spaghetti	1 serv	440	13	—	—	12	68	—	5	—	690	—	—	—
Wrap Ham & Cheese w/ Fries	1 serv	550	28	—	—	16	60	—	4	—	790	—	—	—
DESSERTS														
Blondie Maple	1	850	43	—	—	7	111	—	1	—	350	—	—	—
Blondie Maple Bite Size	1	430	21	—	—	4	58	—	tr	—	170	—	—	—
Brownie Chocolate Addiction	1	490	13	—	—	5	92	—	2	—	170	—	—	—
Brownie Chocolate Addiction Bite Size	1	200	7	—	—	2	35	—	1	—	90	—	—	—
Cheesecake New York	1 slice	620	33	—	—	11	80	—	0	—	440	—	—	—
Cheesecake Vanilla Bean	1 slice	770	52	—	—	9	70	—	1	—	320	—	—	—
Chocolate Explosion	1 serv	890	50	—	—	11	103	—	4	—	510	—	—	—

FOOD	PORTION	CALS	FAT	SAT FAT	CHOL	PROT	CARB	SUGAR	FIBER	CALCI	SOD	POTAS	FOLIC	VIT C
Tarte Au Sucre	1 serv	310	21	—	—	4	71	—	1	—	9500	—	—	—
MAIN MENU SELECTIONS														
Angus Beef Sirloin Steak w/ Spaghetti	1 serv	1260	70	—	—	72	83	—	8	—	1560	—	—	—
Baked 3 Cheese Penne	1 half order	460	14	—	—	21	62	—	4	—	1030	—	—	—
Baked Seven Cheese Ravioli	1 half order	310	14	—	—	17	28	—	2	—	1000	—	—	—
Baked Shrimp & Feta Penne	1 half order	480	19	—	—	28	54	—	4	—	690	—	—	—
Boston's Lasagne	1 half order	340	10	—	—	18	45	—	3	—	860	—	—	—
Boston's Smokey Mountain Spaghetti	1 order	1290	47	—	—	59	161	—	13	—	2650	—	—	—
Chicken & Mushroom	1 half order	710	38	—	—	23	72	—	4	—	680	—	—	—
Chicken Parmesan Fettuccini w/ Seasonal Vegetables	1 serv	1060	74	—	—	47	55	—	9	—	1190	—	—	—
Fries	1 serv	430	25	—	—	7	45	—	5	—	640	—	—	—
Garlic Mashed Potatoes	1 serv	730	60	—	—	6	42	—	5	—	1800	—	—	—
Garlic Toast	1 slice	150	6	—	—	3	20	—	1	—	330	—	—	—
Homestyle Lasagna	1 order	590	33	—	—	39	37	—	4	—	1910	—	—	—
Jambalaya Fettuccini	1 half order	860	51	—	—	33	71	—	6	—	2170	—	—	—
Lemon Baked Salmon w/ Fries	1 serv	1150	74	—	—	50	61	—	9	—	2330	—	—	—
Mama Meata Penne	1 half order	940	62	—	—	35	66	—	7	—	1890	—	—	—
Mushroom Chicken w/ Garlic Mashed Potatoes	1 serv	1030	62	—	—	68	53	—	9	—	1450	—	—	—
Pad Thai w/ Chicken	1 serv	2110	47	—	—	77	356	—	21	—	30	—	—	—
Pad Thai w/ Shrimp	1 serv	2090	45	—	—	77	358	—	22	—	390	—	—	—
Pollo Pomodoro Spaghetti	1 serv	520	14	—	—	26	73	—	7	—	1060	—	—	—
Salmon Filet Lemon Baked	1 serv	430	13	—	—	51	33	—	10	—	250	—	—	—
Scallop & Prawn Fettuccini	1 half order	710	41	—	—	21	67	—	5	—	660	—	—	—

FOOD	PORTION	CALS	FAT	SAT FAT	CHOL	PROT	CARB	SUGAR	FIBER	CALCI	SOD	POTAS	FOLIC	VIT C
Seasoned Vegetables	1 serv	70	0	—	—	0	10	—	4	—	760	—	—	—
Shrimp Skewers Lime & Parmesan	1 serv	190	7	—	—	15	20	—	3	—	1020	—	—	—
Sicilian Penne	1 half order	720	48	—	—	20	55	—	5	—	740	—	—	—
Sirloin Steak w/ Prawns & Fries	1 serv	1480	104	—	—	78	58	—	9	—	2140	—	—	—
Slow Roasted Pork Back Ribs w/ Fries	1 serv	1680	123	—	—	68	78	—	8	—	2080	—	—	—
Spaghetti w/ Alfredo Sauce	1 half order	440	11	—	—	15	70	—	3	—	710	—	—	—
Spaghetti w/ Bolognese	1 half order	400	5	—	—	15	73	—	5	—	670	—	—	—
Spaghetti w/ Creamy Tomato Sauce	1 half order	410	11	—	—	14	66	—	4	—	410	—	—	—
Spaghetti w/ Pomodoro Sauce	1 half order	450	14	—	—	13	68	—	5	—	720	—	—	—
Spicy Italian Penne	1 half order	980	61	—	—	30	81	—	5	—	1440	—	—	—
Starter Baked Raviolo Bites	1 serv	450	22	—	—	20	45	—	4	—	1410	—	—	—
Starter Basket Garlic Twist	1 serv	1140	39	—	—	32	165	—	tr	—	2910	—	—	—
Starter Basket Three Cheese Toast	1 serv	730	34	—	—	33	72	—	0	—	1580	—	—	—
Starter Boston's Poutine	1 serv	740	45	—	—	23	53	—	7	—	1860	—	—	—
Starter Bruschetta Sun Dried Tomato	1 serv	470	21	—	—	10	59	—	5	—	1130	—	—	—
Starter Cactus Cuts Potatoes & Dip	1 serv	1150	89	—	—	15	72	—	7	—	1430	—	—	—
Starter Chicken Fingers	1 serv	360	14	—	—	46	12	—	0	—	520	—	—	—
Starter Chicken Fingers Buffalo Style	1 serv	370	14	—	—	46	14	—	1	—	2080	—	—	—
Starter Cracked Pepper Dry Ribs	1 serv	380	41	—	—	69	3	—	1	—	1880	—	—	—
Starter Nachos Cactus w/ Cactus Dip	1 serv	1830	128	—	—	59	111	—	12	—	3160	—	—	—

FOOD	PORTION	CALS	FAT	SAT FAT	CHOL	PROT	CARB	SUGAR	FIBER	CALCI	SOD	POTAS	FOLIC	VIT C
Starter Nachos Spicy Chicken w/ Sour Cream & Salsa	1 serv	1430	72	—	—	73	126	—	12	—	2330	—	—	—
Starter Nachos Taco Beef w/ Sour Cream & Salsa	1 serv	1560	86	—	—	73	129	—	13	—	2180	—	—	—
Starter Nachos w/ Sour Cream & Salsa	1 serv	1320	71	—	—	53	126	—	12	—	1790	—	—	—
Starter Panzerotti Roll	1	820	32	—	—	41	94	—	3	—	1370	—	—	—
Starter Pizza Bread Bandera w/ Santa Fe Ranch Dip	1 serv	960	54	—	—	32	89	—	tr	—	1880	—	—	—
Starter Pizza Bread w/o Sauce	1 serv	500	12	—	—	15	84	—	0	—	660	—	—	—
Starter Potato Skins	1 serv	650	46	—	—	22	39	—	tr	—	1390	—	—	—
Starter Quesadilla Oven Roasted Chicken	1 serv	900	39	—	—	43	96	—	6	—	1850	—	—	—
Starter Quesadilla Southwest w/ Sour Cream & Salsa	1 serv	770	27	—	—	55	77	—	4	—	1740	—	—	—
Starter Shrimp Stuffed Mushroom Caps	1 serv	490	41	—	—	23	12	—	2	—	1150	—	—	—
Starter Team Platter w/ Dips & Sauces	1 serv	3030	205	—	—	153	144	—	12	—	3930	—	—	—
Starter Thai Chicken Bites	1 serv	540	15	—	—	46	55	—	2	—	1540	—	—	—
Starter Wings Breaded BBQ	1 serv	930	52	—	—	72	28	—	tr	—	3770	—	—	—
Starter Wings Breaded Honey Garlic	1 serv	940	52	—	—	72	31	—	0	—	3470	—	—	—
Starter Wings Breaded Mild	1 serv	880	52	—	—	72	17	—	0	—	3380	—	—	—
Starter Wings Breaded Teriyaki	1 serv	940	52	—	—	73	30	—	tr	—	3720	—	—	—
Starter Wings Breaded Thai	1 serv	1110	52	—	—	73	73	—	2	—	4720	—	—	—
Starter Wings Oven Roasted BBQ	1 serv	670	42	—	—	54	19	—	tr	—	410	—	—	—

FOOD	PORTION	CALS	FAT	SAT FAT	CHOL	PROT	CARB	SUGAR	FIBER	CALCI	SOD	POTAS	FOLIC	VIT C
Starter Wings Oven Roasted Honey Garlic	1 serv	700	42	—	—	54	26	—	2	—	125	—	—	—
Starter Wings Oven Roasted Hot	1 serv	620	42	—	—	53	9	—	tr	—	1060	—	—	—
Starter Wings Oven Roasted Teriyaki	1 serv	670	42	—	—	54	20	—	tr	—	360	—	—	—
Starter Wings Oven Roasted Thai Chili	1 serv	770	40	—	—	52	50	—	1	—	1030	—	—	—
The Ribber w/ Spaghetti	1 serv	970	43	—	—	49	96	—	5	—	1540	—	—	—
Tortellini w/ Alfredo Sauce	1 half order	340	15	—	—	12	37	—	1	—	880	—	—	—
Tortellini w/ Bolognese	1 half order	300	9	—	—	13	40	—	3	—	840	—	—	—
Tortellini w/ Creamy Tomato Sauce	1 half order	310	14	—	—	11	33	—	2	—	580	—	—	—
Tortellini w/ Pomodoro Sauce	1 half order	340	18	—	—	10	35	—	3	—	880	—	—	—
Veal Parmesan w/ Spaghetti	1 serv	1020	72	—	—	44	106	—	9	—	1920	—	—	—
PIZZA														
Bacon Double Cheeseburger Individual	1 pie	1140	54	—	—	73	94	—	2	—	2600	—	—	—
Bacon Double Cheeseburger Slice	1 med	280	12	—	—	18	25	—	tr	—	660	—	—	—
BBQ Chicken Individual	1 pie	730	24	—	—	37	93	—	1	—	1270	—	—	—
BBQ Chicken Slice	1 med	190	6	—	—	10	25	—	0	—	350	—	—	—
Boston Royal Individual	1 pie	840	27	—	—	53	98	—	3	—	1520	—	—	—
Boston Royal Slice	1 med	210	6	—	—	13	26	—	tr	—	410	—	—	—
Californian Slice	1 med	280	15	—	—	11	24	—	0	—	280	—	—	—
Clubhouse Individual	1 pie	1040	56	—	—	44	94	—	3	—	1070	—	—	—
Deluxe Individual	1 pie	850	29	—	—	55	94	—	2	—	1550	—	—	—
Deluxe Slice	1 med	220	7	—	—	14	25	—	tr	—	420	—	—	—
Great White North Slice	1 med	240	9	—	—	16	24	—	0	—	400	—	—	—
Hawaiian Individual	1 pie	780	20	—	—	49	101	—	2	—	1150	—	—	—

FOOD	PORTION	CALS	FAT	SAT FAT	CHOL	PROT	CARB	SUGAR	FIBER	CALCI	SOD	POTAS	FOLIC	VIT C
Hawaiian Slice	1 med	210	5	—	—	13	27	—	0	—	320	—	—	—
Indy California	1 (11.3 oz)	440	12	—	—	16	69	—	7	—	490	—	—	—
La Quebecoise Individual	1 pie	770	27	—	—	42	93	—	3	—	1650	—	—	—
La Quebecoise Slice	1 med	200	7	—	—	11	25	—	tr	—	460	—	—	—
Meateor Individual	1 pie	950	37	—	—	63	91	—	1	—	1640	—	—	—
Meateor Slice	1 med	260	10	—	—	17	25	—	0	—	460	—	—	—
Pepperoni Individual	1 pie	750	27	—	—	40	89	—	2	—	1650	—	—	—
Pepperoni Slice	1 med	200	7	—	—	10	24	—	0	—	450	—	—	—
Pepperoni & Mushroom Individual	1 pie	750	27	—	—	41	90	—	2	—	1650	—	—	—
Pepperoni & Mushroom Slice	1 med	200	7	—	—	10	24	—	tr	—	460	—	—	—
Popeye Individual	1 pie	720	22	—	—	41	93	—	2	—	1170	—	—	—
Popeye Slice	1 med	200	7	—	—	11	25	—	tr	—	320	—	—	—
Rustic Italian Individual	1 pie	950	39	—	—	49	102	—	3	—	4270	—	—	—
Rustic Italian Slice	1 med	260	10	—	—	13	28	—	tr	—	1250	—	—	—
Spicy Perogy Individual	1 pie	980	45	—	—	46	99	—	2	—	1090	—	—	—
Spicy Perogy Slice	1 med	280	13	—	—	13	28	—	0	—	330	—	—	—
Szechuan Individual	1 pie	750	17	—	—	39	99	—	1	—	800	—	—	—
Szechuan Slice	1 med	200	4	—	—	10	27	—	0	—	210	—	—	—
Tandoori Individual	1 pie	730	24	—	—	40	90	—	2	—	940	—	—	—
Tandoori Slice	1 med	200	6	—	—	11	25	—	tr	—	260	—	—	—
Thai Chicken Individual	1 pie	840	28	—	—	45	108	—	4	—	1090	—	—	—
Thai Chicken Slice	1 med	240	8	—	—	12	30	—	1	—	300	—	—	—
The Basic Individual	1 pie	620	16	—	—	34	88	—	1	—	1140	—	—	—
The Basic Slice	1 med	160	4	—	—	9	24	—	0	—	310	—	—	—
Tropical Chicken Individual	1 pie	970	39	—	—	59	97	—	tr	—	1690	—	—	—
Tropical Chicken Slice	1 med	260	10	—	—	15	26	—	0	—	450	—	—	—
Tuscan Individual	1 pie	940	37	—	—	50	106	—	5	—	1650	—	—	—
Tuscan Slice	1 med	250	10	—	—	13	29	—	1	—	460	—	—	—
Ultimate Pepperoni Individual	1 pie	870	37	—	—	46	89	—	2	—	2010	—	—	—

FOOD	PORTION	CALS	FAT	SAT FAT	CHOL	PROT	CARB	SUGAR	FIBER	CALCI	SOD	POTAS	FOLIC	VIT C
Ultimate Pepperoni Slice	1 med	230	9	—	—	12	24	—	tr	—	550	—	—	—
Vegetarian Individual	1 pie	680	16	—	—	37	101	—	4	—	1160	—	—	—
Vegetarian Slice	1 med	180	4	—	—	9	26	—	1	—	320	—	—	—
Zorba The Greek Individual	1 pie	800	29	—	—	43	97	—	4	—	1400	—	—	—
Zorba The Greek Slice	1 med	210	8	—	—	11	26	—	1	—	390	—	—	—
SALAD DRESSINGS AND TOPPINGS														
House Dressing	1 serv (2 oz)	270	28	—	—	1	4	—	tr	—	210	—	—	—
Ketchup	1 serv (2 oz)	60	1	—	—	1	15	—	tr	—	460	—	—	—
Salsa	1 serv (2 oz)	20	1	—	—	1	3	—	tr	—	350	—	—	—
Sour Cream	1 serv (2 oz)	100	9	—	—	2	3	—	0	—	0	—	—	—
SALADS														
Chipotle Chicken & Bacon	1 serv	630	41	—	—	28	40	—	6	—	1040	—	—	—
Crispy Chicken Pecan	1 serv	1100	86	—	—	62	25	—	6	—	1310	—	—	—
Entree Caesar	1 serv	500	38	—	—	13	29	—	4	—	920	—	—	—
Entree Spinach	1 serv	450	41	—	—	13	9	—	3	—	890	—	—	—
Garden Greens w/ House Dressing	1 serv	310	29	—	—	3	13	—	4	—	230	—	—	—
Garden Greens w/ Low Fat Raspberry Vinaigrette	1 serv	130	6	—	—	2	19	—	3	—	160	—	—	—
Side Caesar	1 serv	170	11	—	—	5	13	—	1	—	300	—	—	—
Starter Spinach	1 serv	250	22	—	—	9	6	—	2	—	510	—	—	—
Taco Salad Beef w/o Sour Cream & Salsa	1 serv	610	33	—	—	31	50	—	6	—	830	—	—	—
Taco Salad Chicken w/o Sour Cream & Salsa	1 serv	480	19	—	—	31	48	—	6	—	990	—	—	—
Thai Chicken Salad	1 serv	1060	40	—	—	61	117	—	12	—	1020	—	—	—
SANDWICHES														
Beef Dip w/ Fries & Au Jus	1 serv	1340	62	—	—	77	118	—	5	—	3330	—	—	—
Boston Brute w/ Caesar Salad & Au Jus	1 serv	820	30	—	—	40	99	—	4	—	2660	—	—	—
Boston Cheesesteak w/ Caesar Salad & Au Jus	1 serv	1300	66	—	—	86	90	—	3	—	3350	—	—	—

FOOD	PORTION	CALS	FAT	SAT FAT	CHOL	PROT	CARB	SUGAR	FIBER	CALCI	SOD	POTAS	FOLIC	VIT C
Buffalo Chicken w/ Fries	1 serv	1220	53	—	—	55	130	—	7	—	4200	—	—	—
Chicken Parmesan w/ Fries	1 serv	1370	81	—	—	53	107	—	7	—	1810	—	—	—
Ciabatta Chicken w/ Caesar Salad	1 serv	920	53	—	—	40	73	—	4	—	1130	—	—	—
New York Steak w/ Garden Greens & Au Jus	1 serv	660	39	—	—	43	32	—	2	—	870	—	—	—
Stromboli Bacon Double Cheeseburger w/ Caesar Salad	1 serv	910	38	—	—	34	111	—	3	—	4230	—	—	—
Stromboli Chicken Santa Fe w/ Caesar Salad	1 serv	750	22	—	—	33	106	—	4	—	940	—	—	—
Stromboli Smoked Ham & Chicken w/ Caesar Salad	1 serv	880	31	—	—	52	99	—	1	—	820	—	—	—
Wrap Thai Chicken	1	570	9	—	—	26	98	—	6	—	1260	—	—	—
SOUPS														
Baked French Onion	1 serv	330	14	—	—	17	40	—	3	—	2480	—	—	—
Clam Chowder	1 serv	260	14	—	—	9	18	—	0	—	910	—	—	—

BRUEGGER'S BAGELS

FOOD	PORTION	CALS	FAT	SAT FAT	CHOL	PROT	CARB	SUGAR	FIBER	CALCI	SOD	POTAS	FOLIC	VIT C
BAGELS														
Asiago Parmesan	1	330	4	2	5	14	62	8	4	100	640	—	—	0
Baked Apple	1	370	3	0	0	12	77	19	5	40	660	—	—	0
Blueberry	1	330	2	0	0	11	67	14	4	20	530	—	—	0
Chocolate Chip	1	350	5	2	0	12	64	14	4	40	570	—	—	0
Cinnamon Sugar	1	330	2	0	0	11	69	17	4	40	510	—	—	0
Cranberry Orange	1	330	2	0	0	11	68	17	4	20	510	—	—	1
Everything	1	320	2	0	0	12	64	8	4	40	740	—	—	0
Garlic	1	320	2	0	0	12	65	8	4	40	560	—	—	0
Honey Grain	1	330	3	0	0	13	65	10	5	40	510	—	—	0
Jalapeno Bagel	1	320	2	0	0	12	64	8	4	20	560	—	—	4
Multi-Grain	1	350	4	0	0	12	68	10	6	20	540	—	—	0
Onion	1	320	2	0	0	12	64	8	4	20	560	—	—	1
Plain	1	320	2	0	0	12	64	8	4	20	560	—	—	0
Poppy	1	320	3	0	0	12	64	8	4	40	560	—	—	0
Pumpernickel	1	330	3	0	0	12	67	11	12	20	620	—	—	0
Pumpkin	1	330	2	0	0	11	68	13	6	40	500	—	—	6
Rosemary Olive Oil	1	350	7	1	0	12	64	10	4	20	540	—	—	0
Salt	1	320	2	0	0	12	64	8	4	20	1610	—	—	0

FOOD	PORTION	CALS	FAT	SAT FAT	CHOL	PROT	CARB	SUGAR	FIBER	CALCI	SOD	POTAS	FOLIC	VIT C
Sesame	1	360	3	0	0	13	68	11	4	20	660	—	—	0
Sourdough	1	340	2	0	0	13	68	8	4	20	640	—	—	0
Square Asiago Parmesan	1	360	5	2	5	15	66	11	4	100	740	—	—	0
Square Everything	1	320	2	0	0	12	64	8	4	40	740	—	—	0
Square Plain	1	350	3	0	0	13	70	11	4	20	670	—	—	0
Square Sesame	1	360	3	0	0	13	68	11	4	20	660	—	—	0
Sun Dried Tomato	1	320	2	0	0	12	64	11	4	40	640	—	—	1
Whole Wheat	1	390	6	1	0	16	73	8	9	20	680	—	16	0
DESSERTS														
Brownie Chocolate Chunk	1	330	18	7	55	4	40	27	2	20	150	—	—	0
Cake Lemon Pound	1 slice	320	13	7	75	5	48	25	tr	40	170	—	—	0
Cookie Chocolate Chip	1	500	22	12	40	5	71	43	3	20	300	—	—	0
Cookie Oatmeal Raisin	1	460	19	9	40	5	71	39	3	40	240	—	—	1
Cookie Peanut Butter	1	480	23	9	40	8	63	38	2	20	300	—	—	0
Cookie Triple Chocolate Chunk	1	560	28	16	35	6	71	44	3	40	350	—	—	0
Cookie White Chocolate Macadamia	1	580	31	16	35	6	70	46	1	40	360	—	—	0
Luscious Lemon Bar	1	300	16	9	95	3	36	24	0	0	120	—	—	0
Marshmallow Chew	1	280	6	3	10	2	55	29	0	0	330	—	—	0
Muffin Blueberry	1	450	19	4	65	8	64	29	3	100	290	—	—	2
Muffin Chocolate	1	460	24	6	30	6	57	38	3	60	250	—	—	0
Oreo Dream Bar	1	470	28	14	60	5	49	35	2	80	270	—	—	0
Pecan Chocolate Chunk	1 slice	310	19	6	40	3	32	16	1	40	160	—	—	0
Raspberry Sammies	1 slice	340	16	10	45	3	44	21	1	0	170	—	—	0
Seven Layer Bar	1	650	43	23	10	10	58	42	5	150	280	—	—	0
Toffee Almond Bar	1	400	19	8	50	4	53	34	1	40	340	—	—	0
SALADS														
Caesar w/ Dressing	1 serv	270	17	5	40	9	22	5	2	200	900	—	—	9
Tossed Chicken Caesar w/ Dressing	1 serv	370	20	5	85	27	23	5	2	200	1420	—	—	9

FOOD	PORTION	CALS	FAT	SAT FAT	CHOL	PROT	CARB	SUGAR	FIBER	CALCI	SOD	POTAS	FOLIC	VIT C
Tossed Mandarin Medley	1 serv	340	17	5	20	8	36	27	4	60	660	—	—	15
Tossed Sesame Chicken	1 serv	480	28	3	45	22	30	18	2	40	780	—	—	9
SANDWICHES														
BLT w/ Mayo	1	570	23	5	35	20	72	10	5	20	1060	—	—	6
Chicken Breast	1	660	11	3	95	47	87	26	5	40	780	—	—	6
Chicken Fajita	1	530	11	5	80	30	81	16	6	80	1040	—	—	36
Chicken Salad w/ Mayo	1	630	26	4	80	28	73	11	5	40	1080	—	—	6
Cranberry Gobbler	1	620	21	6	55	32	78	17	5	200	1430	—	—	2
Cuban Chicken	1	680	25	7	85	44	74	10	4	250	2180	—	—	2
Denver Egg	1	460	18	6	205	30	74	11	5	250	1150	—	—	24
Egg Cheese	1	420	18	6	195	23	71	9	4	150	1090	—	—	0
Egg Cheese Bacon	1	460	23	8	210	28	65	9	4	250	980	—	—	0
Egg Cheese Ham	1	460	18	6	210	31	73	11	4	250	1270	—	—	1
Egg Cheese Sausage	1	640	38	13	235	32	72	10	5	250	1130	—	—	0
Ham	1	460	7	1	30	27	76	12	5	60	2110	—	—	9
Herby Turkey	1	560	14	7	45	30	78	10	5	100	1310	—	—	9
Leonardo Da Veggie	1	480	12	6	30	21	74	11	5	200	870	—	—	15
Radishy Roast Beef	1	560	18	6	60	35	73	11	5	200	1270	—	—	5
Roadhouse Chicken	1	710	19	8	100	50	84	22	4	300	1600	—	—	2
Roast Beef	1	730	36	5	65	30	71	10	5	20	1280	—	—	6
Santa Fe Turkey	1	490	9	4	50	30	75	12	5	60	1450	—	—	21
Smoked Salmon	1	490	10	5	45	28	74	10	5	60	770	—	—	6
Softwich BLT w/ Mayo	1	600	25	6	40	22	73	14	5	20	1220	—	—	6
Softwich Chicken Breast	1	630	11	3	95	47	81	21	5	40	800	—	—	9
Softwich Chicken Fajita	1	570	10	4	20	39	81	18	6	80	1180	—	—	30
Softwich Chicken Salad	1	670	27	4	95	32	76	15	5	40	1220	—	—	12
Softwich Cranberry Gobbler	1	730	28	10	80	40	80	20	5	350	1750	—	—	2
Softwich Cuban Chicken	1	810	32	10	125	56	77	15	4	450	2740	—	—	4
Softwich Garden Veggie	1	380	3	0	0	15	76	15	6	40	680	—	—	36
Softwich Ham	1	510	6	2	40	29	85	25	5	40	1770	—	—	12
Softwich Herby Turkey	1	580	14	7	50	33	80	13	5	100	1490	—	—	9
Softwich Hummus	1	540	13	2	0	20	85	13	11	20	930	—	—	9

FOOD	PORTION	CALS	FAT	SAT FAT	CHOL	PROT	CARB	SUGAR	FIBER	CALCI	SOD	POTAS	FOLIC	VIT C
Softwich Leonardo De Veggie	1	550	15	8	40	25	79	16	6	300	1160	—	—	42
Softwich Mediterranean	1	790	33	15	45	30	90	13	11	350	1280	—	—	9
Softwich Peanut Chicken	1	590	12	3	60	36	82	18	5	80	1810	—	—	4
Softwich Radishy Roast Beef	1	670	26	10	90	43	75	14	5	350	1540	—	—	6
Softwich Roadhouse Chicken	1	670	19	8	100	50	74	13	4	300	1620	—	—	2
Softwich Roast Beef	1	750	40	6	75	33	72	10	5	40	1350	—	—	9
Softwich Roasted Turkey	1	550	15	2	45	32	74	13	5	40	1450	—	—	9
Softwich Smoked Salmon	1	520	11	5	50	30	76	14	5	60	800	—	—	9
Softwich Supreme Club w/o Mayo	1	880	39	14	120	55	79	18	5	40	2780	—	—	12
Softwich Tuna Salad	1	720	34	5	45	26	76	14	5	20	1170	—	—	9
Softwich Western Wheat	1	820	58	13	225	30	76	14	8	300	1480	—	—	27
Supreme Club w/o Mayo	1	470	9	2	35	28	72	11	5	40	1460	—	—	6
Tuna Salad	1	620	27	4	35	23	73	10	5	20	990	—	—	6
Turkey	1	510	14	2	35	26	70	9	5	40	1290	—	—	6
Wrap Classic w/ Bacon	1	520	45	15	405	36	52	4	4	350	1120	—	—	1
Wrap Classic w/ Ham	1	510	41	14	420	40	54	5	4	400	1630	—	—	1
Wrap Classic w/ Sausage	1	660	60	21	435	38	52	3	4	400	1210	—	—	0
Wrap Rio Grande Bacon	1	560	49	16	415	34	55	6	4	100	1380	—	—	5
Wrap Rio Grande Ham	1	630	34	10	400	31	55	7	4	100	1450	—	—	5
Wrap Rio Grande Sausage	1	510	47	15	400	27	53	4	4	100	960	—	—	4
Wrap Sesame Chicken Salad	1	770	36	5	45	31	80	18	5	20	1100	—	—	5
Wrap Tossed Chicken Caesar	1	660	28	7	85	36	73	5	5	750	1740	—	—	2
Wrap Tossed Mandarin Medley Salad	1	630	25	7	20	17	87	26	7	40	980	—	—	12
SOUPS														
Chicken Pot Pie	1 cup	250	19	10	80	10	12	2	2	60	1100	—	—	4

FOOD	PORTION	CALS	FAT	SAT FAT	CHOL	PROT	CARB	SUGAR	FIBER	CALCI	SOD	POTAS	FOLIC	VIT C
Chicken Spaetzle	1 cup	120	5	2	25	9	12	2	1	20	1050	—	—	2
Chicken Wild Rice	1 cup	260	19	11	75	2	16	2	1	40	1170	—	—	4
Creamy Tomato	1 cup	150	9	4	15	5	16	11	3	40	820	—	—	9
Hearty Mushroom Barley	1 cup	110	2	0	0	5	18	3	4	40	790	—	—	6
Italian Wedding	1 cup	160	8	4	20	8	15	2	2	80	680	—	—	5
Minestrone	1 cup	120	2	1	0	7	21	3	5	80	780	—	—	6
Moroccan Stew	1 cup	140	3	0	0	4	26	8	4	60	330	—	—	30
New England Clam	1 cup	300	18	8	55	10	23	tr	1	150	840	—	—	9
Sweet Potato Cheddar	1 cup	200	11	5	20	6	20	6	2	150	580	—	—	54
SPREADS														
Cream Cheese Bacon Scallion	1 scoop (1.5 oz)	140	12	7	40	3	5	2	0	60	150	—	—	0
Cream Cheese Cucumber Dill	1 scoop (1.5 oz)	140	13	6	35	3	3	1	0	60	120	—	—	0
Cream Cheese Garden Veggie	1 scoop (1.5 oz)	130	11	6	35	3	5	2	1	60	140	—	—	5
Cream Cheese Honey Walnut	1 scoop (1.5 oz)	150	12	6	35	3	8	3	tr	60	125	—	—	0
Cream Cheese Jalapeno	1 scoop (1.5 oz)	140	13	8	45	3	4	2	0	60	150	—	—	0
Cream Cheese Light Garden Veggie	1 scoop (1.5 oz)	90	6	4	25	6	3	2	0	60	105	—	—	2
Cream Cheese Light Herb Garlic	1 scoop (1.5 oz)	100	6	4	25	6	4	2	0	80	125	—	—	0
Cream Cheese Light Plain	1 scoop (1.5 oz)	100	6	3	25	3	4	3	tr	80	125	—	—	0
Cream Cheese Olive Pimento	1 scoop (1.5 oz)	140	13	6	45	3	3	1	0	60	130	—	—	0
Cream Cheese Onion & Chive	1 scoop (1.5 oz)	140	13	8	35	3	3	2	0	40	105	—	—	4
Cream Cheese Plain	1 scoop (1.5 oz)	130	11	7	40	3	6	2	tr	60	125	—	—	0
Cream Cheese Pumpkin	1 scoop (1.5 oz)	120	11	7	45	3	4	3	0	60	135	—	—	0
Cream Cheese Strawberry	1 scoop (1.5 oz)	140	13	7	30	3	4	2	0	20	100	—	—	1
Cream Cheese Wildberry	1 scoop (1.5 oz)	140	12	7	40	3	5	3	0	60	120	—	—	0
Hummus	1 scoop (2 oz)	110	6	1	0	5	10	0	0	20	120	—	—	0

BURGER KING

BEVERAGES

FOOD	PORTION	CALS	FAT	SAT FAT	CHOL	PROT	CARB	SUGAR	FIBER	CALCI	SOD	POTAS	FOLIC	VIT C
Apple Juice	1 (6.67 oz)	90	0	0	0	0	23	21	—	—	15	—	—	60
BK Joe Regular	1 sm	5	0	0	0	1	1	0	—	—	15	—	—	—

FOOD	PORTION	CALS	FAT	SAT FAT	CHOL	PROT	CARB	SUGAR	FIBER	CALCI	SOD	POTAS	FOLIC	VIT C
BK Joe Turbo	1 sm (12 oz)	10	0	0	0	1	1	0	—	—	20	—	—	—
Chocolate Milk 1% Low Fat	1 (9 oz)	180	3	2	15	9	31	29	1	—	140	—	—	—
Coke Classic	1 sm (16 oz)	140	0	0	0	0	39	39	—	—	0	—	—	—
Diet Coke	1 sm (16 oz)	0	0	0	0	0	0	0	0	—	15	—	—	—
Dr Pepper	1 sm (16 oz)	140	0	0	0	0	39	39	—	—	35	—	—	—
Iced Coffee Mocha BK Joe	1 (16 oz)	380	10	6	40	6	66	63	1	—	290	—	—	—
Icee Coco Cola	1 sm (16 oz)	110	0	0	0	0	31	31	—	—	10	—	—	0
Icee Minute Maid Cherry	1 sm (16 oz)	110	0	0	0	0	31	31	—	—	5	—	—	0
Milk 1% Low Fat	1	110	3	2	10	8	13	12	0	—	130	—	—	—
Minute Maid Orange Juice	8 oz	140	0	0	0	2	33	30	—	—	20	—	—	42
Shake Chocolate	1 sm (16 oz)	470	14	9	55	8	75	72	1	—	320	—	—	—
Shake Oreo Sundae Chocolate	1 sm (16 oz)	680	24	15	55	9	105	95	2	—	480	—	—	—
Shake Oreo Sundae Strawberry	1 sm (16 oz)	660	23	15	55	9	103	94	1	—	380	—	—	—
Shake Oreo Sundae Vanilla	1 sm (16 oz)	610	24	16	60	9	87	78	1	—	400	—	—	—
Shake Strawberry	1 sm (16 oz)	460	14	9	55	7	73	71	0	—	240	—	—	—
Shake Vanilla	1 sm (16 oz)	400	15	9	60	8	57	55	0	—	240	—	—	—
Sprite	1 sm (16 oz)	140	0	0	0	0	39	39	—	—	30	—	—	—
Water Nestle Pure Life	1 bottle (16 oz)	0	0	0	0	0	0	0	0	—	0	—	—	—
BREAKFAST SELECTIONS														
Biscuit Bacon Egg & Cheese	1	410	25	8	150	16	31	4	1	—	1320	—	—	—
Biscuit Ham Egg & Cheese	1	390	22	7	145	16	31	4	1	—	1410	—	—	—
Biscuit Sausage	1	390	26	8	35	12	28	2	1	—	1020	—	—	—
Biscuit Sausage Egg & Cheese	1	530	37	12	175	20	31	4	1	—	1490	—	—	—
Croissan'wich Bacon Egg & Cheese	1	340	20	7	155	15	26	5	tr	—	890	—	—	—
Croissan'wich Double w/ Bacon Egg & Cheese	1	430	27	10	175	21	27	6	tr	—	1250	—	—	—
Croissan'wich Double w/ Ham Bacon Egg & Cheese	1	420	24	9	180	24	27	7	1	—	1600	—	—	—

FOOD	PORTION	CALS	FAT	SAT FAT	CHOL	PROT	CARB	SUGAR	FIBER	CALCI	SOD	POTAS	FOLIC	VIT C
Croissan'wich Double w/ Ham Egg & Cheese	1	420	23	9	185	27	27	7	1	—	2210	—	—	—
Croissan'wich Double w/ Ham Sausage Egg & Cheese	1	550	37	14	205	28	27	6	1	—	2040	—	—	—
Croissan'wich Double w/ Sausage Bacon Egg & Cheese	1	550	39	14	200	25	27	6	1	—	1420	—	—	—
Croissan'wich Double w/ Sausage Egg & Cheese	1	680	51	18	220	29	26	6	1	—	1590	—	—	—
Croissan'wich Egg & Cheese	1	300	17	6	145	12	26	5	tr	—	740	—	—	—
Croissan'wich Ham Egg & Cheese	1	340	18	6	160	18	26	6	1	—	1230	—	—	—
Croissan'wich Sausage & Cheese	1	370	25	9	50	14	23	4	tr	—	810	—	—	—
Croissan'wich Sausage Egg & Cheese	1	470	32	11	180	19	26	5	tr	—	1060	—	—	—
French Toast Sticks	3 pieces	240	13	3	0	4	26	6	1	—	260	—	—	—
Hash Browns	1 lg	620	40	11	0	5	60	1	6	—	1200	—	—	—
Hash Browns	1 sm	260	17	5	0	2	25	0	2	—	500	—	—	—
Omelet Sandwich Enormous	1	730	45	16	330	37	44	8	2	—	1940	—	—	—
Omelet Sandwich Ham	1	290	13	5	85	13	33	8	1	—	870	—	—	—
DESSERTS														
Cini-minis	1 serv	390	18	5	20	7	51	19	2	—	560	—	—	—
Dutch Apple Pie	1 serv	300	13	3	0	2	45	23	1	—	270	—	—	—
Hershey Sundae Pie	1	310	19	12	10	3	32	22	1	—	220	—	—	—
MAIN MENU SELECTIONS														
BK Chicken Fries	6 pieces	260	15	4	35	12	18	1	2	—	650	—	—	—
BK Stacker Double	1	610	39	16	125	34	32	5	1	—	1100	—	—	—
BK Stacker Quad	1	1000	68	30	240	62	34	6	1	—	1800	—	—	—
BK Stacker Triple	1	800	54	23	185	48	33	5	1	—	1450	—	—	—
BK Veggie Burger	1	420	16	3	10	23	46	8	7	—	1100	—	—	—
Cheeseburger	1	330	16	7	55	17	31	6	1	—	780	—	—	—
Cheeseburger Double	1	500	29	14	105	30	31	6	1	—	1030	—	—	—

FOOD	PORTION	CALS	FAT	SAT FAT	CHOL	PROT	CARB	SUGAR	FIBER	CALCI	SOD	POTAS	FOLIC	VIT C
Chicken Sandwich Original	1	660	40	8	70	24	52	5	4	—	1440	—	—	—
Chicken Sandwich Tendercrisp	1	790	44	8	70	33	68	9	5	—	1640	—	—	—
Chicken Sandwich Tendergrill	1	510	19	4	75	37	49	7	4	—	1180	—	—	—
Chicken Tenders	5 pieces	210	12	3	35	12	13	0	0	—	600	—	—	—
Chick'n Crisp Spicy Sandwich	1	480	31	5	45	15	36	4	1	—	870	—	—	—
Double Cheeseburger	1	410	21	9	85	25	30	6	1	—	600	—	—	—
French Fries No Salt Added	1 sm	230	13	3	0	2	26	1	2	—	240	—	—	—
French Fries Salted	1 lg	500	28	6	0	5	57	1	5	—	820	—	—	—
French Fries Salted	1 sm	230	13	3	0	2	26	1	2	—	380	—	—	—
Hamburger	1	290	12	5	40	15	30	6	1	—	560	—	—	—
Onion Rings	1 lg	440	22	5	0	6	53	6	5	—	620	—	—	—
Onion Rings	1 sm	140	7	2	0	2	18	2	2	—	210	—	—	—
Sandwich BK Big Fish	1	640	32	6	65	24	67	9	3	—	1450	—	—	—
The Angus Steak Burger	1	640	33	10	185	33	55	10	3	—	1260	—	—	—
Whopper	1	670	39	11	95	28	51	11	3	—	1020	—	—	—
Whopper w/ Cheese	1	760	47	16	115	33	52	11	3	—	1450	—	—	—
Whopper Double	1	900	57	19	175	47	51	11	3	—	1090	—	—	—
Whopper Double w/ Cheese	1	990	64	25	195	52	52	11	3	—	1520	—	—	—
Whopper Jr.	1	370	21	6	50	15	31	6	2	—	570	—	—	—
Whopper Jr. w/ Cheese	1	410	24	8	60	18	32	6	2	—	780	—	—	—
Whopper Triple	1	1130	74	27	255	67	51	11	3	—	1160	—	—	—
Whopper Triple w/ Cheese	1	1230	82	32	275	71	52	11	3	—	1590	—	—	—
SALAD DRESSINGS AND TOPPINGS														
Breakfast Syrup	1 serv (1 oz)	80	0	0	0	0	21	14	0	—	20	—	—	—
Croutons Garlic Parmesan	1 serv	60	2	0	0	1	9	1	0	—	120	—	—	—
Dipping Sauce Barbecue	1 serv (1 oz)	40	0	0	0	0	11	10	0	—	310	—	—	—
Dipping Sauce Honey Mustard	1 serv (1 oz)	90	6	1	10	0	8	7	0	—	180	—	—	—
Dipping Sauce Ranch	1 serv (1 oz)	140	15	3	5	1	1	1	0	—	95	—	—	—

FOOD	PORTION	CALS	FAT	SAT FAT	CHOL	PROT	CARB	SUGAR	FIBER	CALCI	SOD	POTAS	FOLIC	VIT C
Dipping Sauce Sweet And Sour	1 serv (1 oz)	40	0	0	0	0	11	10	0	—	55	—	—	—
Dressing Ken's Creamy Caesar	1 serv (2 oz)	210	21	4	25	3	4	3	0	—	610	—	—	—
Dressing Ken's Fat Free Ranch	1 serv (2 oz)	60	0	0	0	0	15	5	2	—	740	—	—	—
Dressing Ken's Honey Mustard	1 serv (2 oz)	270	23	3	20	1	15	14	0	—	520	—	—	—
Dressing Ken's Ranch	1 serv (2 oz)	190	20	3	20	1	2	1	0	—	560	—	—	—
Jam Grape	1 serv	30	0	0	0	0	7	6	0	—	0	—	—	—
Jam Strawberry	1 serv	30	0	0	0	0	7	6	0	—	0	—	—	—
Ketchup	1 pkg	10	0	0	0	0	3	2	0	—	125	—	—	—
Mayonnaise	1 pkg	80	9	1	10	0	1	0	0	—	75	—	—	—
SALADS														
Chicken Garden Tendercrisp	1	410	22	6	70	29	26	5	5	—	1080	—	—	—
Chicken Garden Tendergrill w/o Dressing or Croutons	1	240	9	4	80	33	8	3	4	—	720	—	—	—
Side Garden w/o Dressing	1	15	0	0	0	1	3	1	1	—	0	—	—	—

BURGERVILLE

FOOD	PORTION	CALS	FAT	SAT FAT	CHOL	PROT	CARB	SUGAR	FIBER	CALCI	SOD	POTAS	FOLIC	VIT C
BEVERAGES														
Barq's Root Beer	1 (20 oz)	180	0	0	0	0	49	—	0	—	39	—	—	—
Coca-Cola	1 (20 oz)	161	0	0	0	0	44	—	0	—	10	—	—	—
Diet Coke	1 (20 oz)	0	0	0	0	0	0	—	0	—	16	—	—	—
Hot Chocolate Ghirardelli	1 (12 oz)	230	0	0	10	4	38	—	2	—	190	—	—	—
House Coffee	1 (10 oz)	5	0	0	0	0	1	—	0	—	5	—	—	—
Iced Tea	1 (20 oz)	0	0	0	0	0	0	—	0	—	0	—	—	—
Iced Tea Nestea Raspberry	1 (20 oz)	127	0	0	0	0	34	—	0	—	15	—	—	—
Lemonade Odwalla	1 (20 oz)	240	0	0	0	0	65	—	0	—	120	—	—	—
Milk 2%	1 (8 oz)	121	5	3	18	8	12	—	0	—	122	—	—	—
Orange Juice Odwalla	1 (10 oz)	138	0	0	0	3	31	—	1	—	31	—	—	—
Pibb Xtra	1 (20 oz)	163	0	0	0	0	42	—	0	—	40	—	—	—
Sprite	1 (20 oz)	158	0	0	0	0	42	—	0	—	34	—	—	—
BREAKFAST SELECTIONS														
Bagel	1	310	1	1	0	12	63	—	2	—	700	—	—	—
Bagel Bacon And Egg	1	490	16	5	250	23	64	—	2	—	1070	—	—	—
Bagel Ham And Egg	1	490	13	4	260	28	65	—	2	—	1380	—	—	—

FOOD	PORTION	CALS	FAT	SAT FAT	CHOL	PROT	CARB	SUGAR	FIBER	CALCI	SOD	POTAS	FOLIC	VIT C
Bagel Sausage And Egg	1	640	31	10	280	27	64	—	2	—	1100	—	—	—
Breakfast Platter w/ Bacon	1 serv	730	49	12	460	25	55	—	1	—	1060	—	—	—
Breakfast Platter w/ Ham	1 serv	725	46	10	500	30	56	—	1	—	1570	—	—	—
Breakfast Platter w/ Sausage	1 serv	880	64	17	520	29	56	—	1	—	1090	—	—	—
Hash Browns	1 serv	230	15	4	0	2	22	—	0	—	410	—	—	—
Toaster Biscuit	1	320	9	2	0	5	31	—	1	—	210	—	—	—
Toaster Biscuit Bacon And Egg	1	450	29	7	580	16	32	—	1	—	580	—	—	—
Toaster Biscuit Ham And Egg	1	440	26	6	260	21	33	—	1	—	890	—	—	—
Toaster Biscuit Sausage And Egg	1	600	44	12	280	20	32	—	1	—	610	—	—	—
DESSERTS														
Cone Vanilla	1	250	11	7	50	5	32	—	0	—	100	—	—	—
Cone YoCream Frozen Yogurt	1	190	0	0	0	4	39	—	0	—	110	—	—	—
Cookie Chocolate Chunk	1	320	14	5	20	4	48	—	0	—	340	—	—	—
Cookie Oatmeal Raisin	1	290	8	3	30	4	50	—	1	—	270	—	—	—
Cookie Sugar	1	305	15	4	20	3	39	—	1	—	250	—	—	—
Cookie White Chocolate Macadamia	1	340	16	6	20	4	46	—	0	—	360	—	—	—
Strawberry Shortcake	1 serv	440	15	6	25	6	72	—	3	—	500	—	—	—
Sundae Caramel	1	380	15	10	65	6	56	—	0	—	160	—	—	—
Sundae Fresh Strawberry	1	340	14	9	60	6	48	—	1	—	110	—	—	—
Sundae Hot Fudge	1	380	18	13	60	7	51	—	0	—	160	—	—	—
Sundae Triple Berry	1	340	14	9	60	6	46	—	0	—	110	—	—	—
Sundae YoCream Caramel	1	260	1	1	5	4	56	—	0	—	150	—	—	—
Sundae YoCream Hot Fudge	1	260	4	4	0	5	51	—	0	—	150	—	—	—
Sundae YoCream Strawberry	1	220	0	0	0	4	48	—	1	—	100	—	—	—
Sundae YoCream Triple Berry	1	200	0	0	0	4	43	—	0	—	100	—	—	—
MAIN MENU SELECTIONS														
Apple Slices	1 serv	29	0	0	0	0	9	—	2	—	0	—	—	—
Cheeseburger	1	350	19	7	35	14	29	—	2	—	730	—	—	—

FOOD	PORTION	CALS	FAT	SAT FAT	CHOL	PROT	CARB	SUGAR	FIBER	CALCI	SOD	POTAS	FOLIC	VIT C
Cheeseburger Colossal	1	520	30	9	75	30	31	—	5	—	1160	—	—	—
Cheeseburger Double Beef	1	430	25	—	55	22	29	—	2	—	790	—	—	—
Cheeseburger Tillamook	1	630	40	14	105	34	31	—	5	—	1080	—	—	—
Cheeseburger Tillamook Pepper Bacon	1	690	46	16	120	39	28	—	5	—	1170	—	—	—
Chicken Strips	5	320	14	6	30	23	26	—	0	—	746	—	—	—
French Fries	1 serv	410	18	4	0	6	57	—	6	—	240	—	—	—
Gardenburger Spicy Black Bean	1	550	32	7	40	24	45	—	10	—	1140	—	—	—
Gardenburger The Original	1	450	19	4	30	18	52	—	8	—	1490	—	—	—
Halibut	3 pieces	320	16	4	10	21	24	—	0	—	720	—	—	—
Hamburger	1	300	15	4	25	12	29	—	2	—	510	—	—	—
Hamburger Burgerville Classic	1	510	30	8	65	27	30	—	5	—	910	—	—	—
Onion Rings Walla Walla	1 serv	810	48	0	0	12	83	—	1	—	1260	—	—	—
Sandwich Crispy Chicken	1	490	19	4	40	21	59	—	3	—	1300	—	—	—
Sandwich Deluxe Crispy Chicken	1	590	30	10	80	27	56	—	3	—	1430	—	—	—
Sandwich Halibut	1	480	27	5	20	18	41	—	2	—	880	—	—	—
Sandwich Low Fat Grilled Chicken	1	320	5	1	24	24	44	—	3	—	880	—	—	—
Sandwich Nine Grain Turkey Club	1	550	32	8	55	27	38	—	3	—	970	—	—	—
Sweet Potato Fries	1 serv	530	29	0	0	4	60	—	3	—	510	—	—	—
Turkey Burger Seasoned	1	540	29	7	60	36	33	—	5	—	900	—	—	—
Yukon Golds	1 serv	450	21	0	0	5	59	—	5	—	590	—	—	—
SALAD DRESSINGS AND TOPPINGS														
Burgerville Spread Cup	1	280	30	4	20	0	4	—	0	—	360	—	—	—
Cream Cheese	1 serv	100	10	7	30	2	1	—	0	—	100	—	—	—
Cream Cheese Light	1 serv	70	5	4	15	3	2	—	0	—	150	—	—	—
Dip BBQ Sauce	1 serv	60	1	0	0	1	13	—	0	—	560	—	—	—
Dressing Blue Cheese	1 serv	240	24	2	15	1	3	—	0	—	340	—	—	—
Dressing Caesar	1 serv	220	22	2	25	1	2	—	0	—	250	—	—	—

FOOD	PORTION	CALS	FAT	SAT FAT	CHOL	PROT	CARB	SUGAR	FIBER	CALCI	SOD	POTAS	FOLIC	VIT C
Dressing Honey Mustard	1 serv	210	20	2	15	0	6	—	0	—	200	—	—	—
Dressing Ranch	1 serv	195	21	2	15	0	2	—	0	—	315	—	—	—
Sauce Sweet And Sour	1 serv	90	4	0	0	0	12	—	0	—	120	—	—	—
Tartar Cup	1	260	28	4	0	0	2	—	0	—	360	—	—	—
Vinaigrette Honey Lime	1 serv	250	23	3	0	0	10	—	0	—	440	—	—	—
Vinaigrette Raspberry	1 serv	45	2	0	0	0	6	—	0	—	260	—	—	—
SALADS														
Grilled Chicken	1	430	27	8	75	32	16	—	7	—	650	—	—	—
Rogue River Smokey Blue	1	290	11	6	25	9	38	—	4	—	200	—	—	—
Side Salad	1	50	3	2	10	3	4	—	2	—	75	—	—	—
Wild Smoked Salmon & Hazelnuts	1	440	28	7	35	30	19	—	7	—	1000	—	—	—

CARL'S JR.

FOOD	PORTION	CALS	FAT	SAT FAT	CHOL	PROT	CARB	SUGAR	FIBER	CALCI	SOD	POTAS	FOLIC	VIT C
BEVERAGES														
Malt Chocolate	1 (15 oz)	780	35	24	105	17	98	79	1	—	360	—	—	—
Malt Oreo Cookie	1 (15 oz)	790	39	25	105	18	91	72	1	—	420	—	—	—
Malt Strawberry	1 (15 oz)	770	35	24	105	17	97	83	0	—	310	—	—	—
Malt Vanilla	1 (15 oz)	760	35	24	105	17	99	84	0	—	300	—	—	—
Shake Chocolate	1 (14 oz)	710	33	23	100	14	85	71	1	—	290	—	—	—
Shake Oreo Cookie	1 (14 oz)	720	37	24	100	16	79	64	1	—	350	—	—	—
Shake Strawberry	1 (14 oz)	700	33	23	100	14	84	75	0	—	240	—	—	—
Shake Vanilla	1 (14 oz)	710	33	23	100	14	86	76	0	—	230	—	—	—
BREAKFAST SELECTIONS														
Breakfast Burger	1	830	47	15	275	37	65	13	3	—	1580	—	—	—
Burrito Bacon & Egg	1	570	33	11	515	30	37	1	1	—	990	—	—	—
Burrito Loaded Breakfast	1	820	51	16	595	38	52	3	2	—	1530	—	—	—
Burrito Steak & Egg	1	660	36	13	545	40	44	4	2	—	1690	—	—	—
French Toast Dips w/o Syrup	5	430	18	3	0	9	58	15	1	—	530	—	—	—
Hash Brown Nuggets	1 serv	330	21	5	0	3	32	1	3	—	460	—	—	—
Sandwich Sourdough Breakfast	1 serv	460	21	9	280	28	39	4	2	—	1050	—	—	—
Sunrise Croissant Sandwich	1	560	41	16	290	20	27	5	1	—	970	—	—	—

FOOD	PORTION	CALS	FAT	SAT FAT	CHOL	PROT	CARB	SUGAR	FIBER	CALCI	SOD	POTAS	FOLIC	VIT C
DESSERTS														
Cheesecake Strawberry Swirl	1 serv	290	17	9	55	6	30	20	0	—	230	—	—	—
Chocolate Cake	1 serv	300	12	3	30	3	48	37	1	—	350	—	—	—
Cookie Chocolate Chip	1	350	18	7	20	3	46	27	1	—	330	—	—	—
MAIN MENU SELECTIONS														
Burger Jalapeno	1	720	45	8	90	27	50	10	3	—	1320	—	—	—
Burger Teriyaki	1	660	34	11	80	28	61	19	3	—	1070	—	—	—
Cheeseburger Double Western Bacon	1	970	52	21	155	62	71	15	3	—	1820	—	—	—
Cheeseburger Western Bacon	1	710	33	12	85	32	70	15	3	—	1480	—	—	—
Chicken Breast Strips	3	420	25	4	50	23	28	1	1	—	1210	—	—	—
Chicken Stars	4	170	11	3	25	9	10	0	1	—	320	—	—	—
CrissCut Fries	1 serv	410	24	5	0	5	43	0	4	—	950	—	—	—
Famous Star w/ Cheese	1	660	39	12	85	27	53	10	3	—	1260	—	—	—
Fish & Chips	1 serv	630	28	5	10	26	68	4	3	—	990	—	—	—
French Fries	1 sm	290	14	3	0	5	37	0	3	—	180	—	—	—
Fried Zucchini	1 serv	320	19	5	0	6	31	0	0	—	850	—	—	—
Hamburger Big	1	470	17	6	60	24	54	13	3	—	1000	—	—	—
Hamburger Kid's	1	460	17	6	60	24	53	13	2	—	1060	—	—	—
Onion Rings	1 serv	430	21	4	0	6	53	5	2	—	550	—	—	—
Sandwich Bacon Swiss Crispy Chicken	1	720	35	8	85	35	64	9	3	—	1750	—	—	—
Sandwich Carl's Catch Fish	1	660	31	5	30	22	75	14	3	—	1290	—	—	—
Sandwich Charbroiled BBQ Chicken	1	360	5	1	60	34	48	12	4	—	1150	—	—	—
Sandwich Charbroiled Chicken Club	1	550	25	7	95	40	43	9	4	—	1410	—	—	—
Sandwich Charbroiled Santa Fe Chicken	1	610	32	8	100	37	43	10	4	—	1540	—	—	—
Sandwich Spicy Chicken	1	560	30	6	40	15	59	7	2	—	1480	—	—	—
Six Dollar Burger The Bacon Cheese	1	1070	76	30	170	46	50	10	3	—	1010	—	—	—
Six Dollar Burger The Guacamole Bacon	1	1140	86	29	160	43	54	11	6	—	2010	—	—	—

FOOD	PORTION	CALS	FAT	SAT FAT	CHOL	PROT	CARB	SUGAR	FIBER	CALCI	SOD	POTAS	FOLIC	VIT C
Six Dollar Burger The Jalapeno	1	1030	74	27	150	39	52	11	3	—	2050	—	—	—
Six Dollar Burger The Low Carb	1	490	37	15	130	33	6	4	2	—	1290	—	—	—
Six Dollar Burger The Original	1	1010	68	27	150	40	60	18	3	—	1980	—	—	—
Six Dollar Burger The Western Bacon	1	1130	66	28	150	47	83	19	4	—	2540	—	—	—
Super Star w/ Cheese	1	930	59	21	160	47	54	10	3	—	1600	—	—	—
SALAD DRESSINGS														
Balsamic Low Fat	1 serv (2 oz)	35	15	2	0	0	5	3	0	—	480	—	—	—
Blue Cheese	1 serv (2 oz)	320	34	7	20	2	1	1	0	—	410	—	—	—
House	1 serv (2 oz)	220	22	4	20	1	2	2	0	—	440	—	—	—
Italian Fat Free	1 serv (2 oz)	15	0	0	0	0	4	2	0	0	770	—	—	0
Thousand Island	1 serv (2 oz)	240	23	4	20	0	7	3	0	—	460	—	—	—
SALADS														
Charbroiled Chicken	1	260	7	4	75	34	16	8	5	—	710	—	—	—
Side	1	50	3	2	5	3	5	3	2	—	60	—	—	—
CARVEL														
Brown Bonnet	1	370	21	16	55	3	40	29	0	100	105	—	—	1
Cake Ice Cream	1 slice	270	14	9	35	4	33	23	1	100	135	—	—	1
Carvelanche Cake Mix	1 reg (16 oz)	720	27	16	85	13	106	74	0	400	540	—	—	5
Carvelanche Cookies & Cream	1 reg (16 oz)	550	30	17	120	7	64	49	0	200	280	—	—	2
Carvelanche Triple Fudge Cake Mix	1 reg (16 oz)	900	41	22	65	16	134	101	4	350	300	—	—	2
Chipsters	1	330	16	8	40	4	44	25	4	80	220	—	—	1
Cone Cake Chocolate	1 sm	260	13	8	35	6	32	25	1	150	135	—	—	1
Cone Cake Chocolate	1 lg	600	30	18	80	13	71	59	3	350	310	—	—	4
Cone Cake Vanilla	1 sm	280	16	10	75	4	31	24	0	150	135	—	—	1
Cone Cake Vanilla	1 lg	650	36	24	180	9	68	57	0	300	300	—	—	4
Cone Sugar Chocolate	1 sm	300	13	35	40	7	40	29	1	150	160	—	—	1
Cone Sugar Vanilla	1 sm	320	15	10	75	5	39	28	0	150	160	—	—	1
Cone Waffle Chocolate	1 lg	660	30	18	80	15	86	65	3	350	340	—	—	4

FOOD	PORTION	CALS	FAT	SAT FAT	CHOL	PROT	CARB	SUGAR	FIBER	CALCI	SOD	POTAS	FOLIC	VIT C
Cone Waffle Chocolate	1 sm	330	13	35	47	7	47	31	2	150	160	—	—	1
Cone Waffle Vanilla	1 lg	710	36	25	180	10	83	63	1	300	330	—	—	4
Cone Waffle Vanilla	1 sm	350	16	11	75	5	46	30	1	150	160	—	—	1
Dashers Banana Barge	1	940	46	24	110	17	121	86	7	300	250	—	—	30
Dashers Bananas Foster	1	600	24	19	100	6	90	60	2	250	350	—	—	6
Dashers Fudge Brownie	1	810	42	20	120	9	98	80	4	150	400	—	—	2
Dashers Mint Chocolate Chip	1	720	39	23	110	8	85	63	2	200	350	—	—	2
Dashers Peanut Butter Cup	1	1090	63	20	55	20	97	79	4	200	630	—	—	2
Dashers Strawberry Shortcake	1	590	29	17	100	8	78	59	2	200	170	—	—	36
Flying Saucer 98% Fat Free Chocolate	1	180	3	1	0	5	34	19	1	100	160	—	—	0
Flying Saucer 98% Fat Free Vanilla	1	180	3	0	0	5	35	20	1	100	170	—	—	1
Flying Saucer Chocolate	1	230	10	5	20	4	33	20	1	80	125	—	—	1
Flying Saucer Deluxe Sprinkles	1	330	15	7	40	4	47	26	1	60	120	—	—	1
Flying Saucer Vanilla	1	240	11	6	45	4	33	19	1	80	170	—	—	1
Ice Cream Chocolate	1 sm (4 oz)	250	13	8	35	6	29	25	0	150	130	—	—	1
Ice Cream Vanilla	1 sm (4 oz)	240	14	9	70	3	25	21	0	100	115	—	—	1
Ice Cream No Fat Chocolate	1 sm (4 oz)	160	0	0	0	3	37	33	0	100	55	—	—	0
Ice Cream No Fat Vanilla	1 sm (4 oz)	160	0	0	0	5	33	29	0	200	75	—	—	1
Sherbet All Flavors	1 sm (4 oz)	180	2	1	5	1	39	30	0	60	70	—	—	0
Sinful Love Bar	1	460	29	15	25	4	47	28	5	100	220	—	—	0
Sprinkle Cup	1	230	15	9	45	2	28	20	1	80	75	—	—	1
Sundae Bittersweet Fudge	1 reg	690	38	27	77	8	77	64	1	250	280	—	—	2
Sundae Caramel	1 reg	670	34	24	145	8	81	60	0	300	360	—	—	2
Sundae Hot Fudge	1 reg	670	38	24	145	8	73	62	1	250	280	—	—	2
Sundae Strawberry	1 reg	580	33	23	145	7	63	54	1	250	210	—	—	21
Sundae Mini Chocolate Syrup	1	200	9	7	45	2	27	20	0	80	85	—	—	1

FOOD	PORTION	CALS	FAT	SAT FAT	CHOL	PROT	CARB	SUGAR	FIBER	CALCI	SOD	POTAS	FOLIC	VIT C
Thick Shake Chocolate	1 reg (16 oz)	650	27	16	70	14	93	69	2	400	320	—	—	2
Thick Shake Vanilla	1 reg (16 oz)	610	28	18	135	10	81	74	0	350	260	—	—	2
Thinny Thin Classic Sundae No Fat Fudge	1 reg	380	2	0	0	8	81	46	0	300	180	—	—	2
Thinny Thin Classic Sundae No Fat Strawberry	1 reg	320	0	0	0	8	69	59	1	300	150	—	—	2
Thinny Thin Miniature Sundae No Fat	1	190	0	0	0	4	45	20	0	150	95	—	—	1
Thinny Thin Miniature Sundae No Sugar Added	1	200	3	2	15	5	42	6	0	150	125	—	—	0
Thinny Thin No Fat Carvelanche Strawberry	1 (16 oz)	430	0	0	0	12	91	81	1	450	160	—	—	27
Thinny Thin No Fat Chocolate	1 sm	160	0	0	0	3	37	33	0	100	55	—	—	0
Thinny Thin No Fat Vanilla	1 sm	160	0	0	0	5	33	29	0	200	75	—	—	1
Thinny Thin No Sugar Added Vanilla	1 sm	180	3	0	20	7	34	10	0	200	115	—	—	0
Thinny Thin Parfait No Fat	1	190	0	0	0	4	42	20	0	150	95	—	—	1
Thinny Thin Shake No Fat Chocolate	1 (16 oz)	440	0	0	0	5	104	59	0	200	190	—	—	0
Thinny Thin Shake No Fat Mocha	1 (16 oz)	440	0	0	0	10	97	52	0	350	230	—	—	2
Thinny Thin Shake No Fat Vanilla	1 (16 oz)	300	0	0	0	9	62	55	0	350	135	—	—	2

CHICKEN OUT ROTISSERIE

MAIN MENU SELECTIONS

FOOD	PORTION	CALS	FAT	SAT FAT	CHOL	PROT	CARB	SUGAR	FIBER	CALCI	SOD	POTAS	FOLIC	VIT C
¼ Dark Chicken w/ Skin	1 serv	337	18	5	125	36	5	4	1	—	903	—	—	—
¼ Dark Chicken w/o Skin	1 serv	223	10	3	107	31	1	1	0	—	247	—	—	—
Apple Cornbread Stuffing	1 serv (7 oz)	453	21	10	38	9	58	7	2	—	1612	—	—	—
Baked Potato Wedges	1 serv (8 oz)	220	6	0	0	4	39	12	6	—	260	—	—	—

FOOD	PORTION	CALS	FAT	SAT FAT	CHOL	PROT	CARB	SUGAR	FIBER	CALCI	SOD	POTAS	FOLIC	VIT C
Chunky Cinnamon Applesauce	1 serv (7 oz)	241	4	2	9	1	52	13	5	—	36	—	—	—
Cranberry Relish	1 serv (7 oz)	285	2	0	45	1	69	66	3	—	64	—	—	—
Creamed Spinach	1 serv (6 oz)	320	25	14	75	9	16	7	3	—	1190	—	—	—
Edamame Beans In Sweet Pepper Sauce	1 serv (7 oz)	200	8	1	0	17	18	6	8	—	75	—	—	—
Farm Fresh Cole Slaw	1 serv (7 oz)	226	17	3	9	2	18	13	3	—	417	—	—	—
Fresh Fruit Salad	1 serv (7 oz)	110	0	0	0	1	29	25	3	—	10	—	—	—
Grilled Chicken Filet Skinless	1 (6 oz)	290	6	2	145	53	3	3	0	—	660	—	—	—
Half Sandwich BBQ & Cole Slaw	1	340	7	2	75	30	41	16	2	—	1115	—	—	—
Half Sandwich Classic Grilled Chicken	1	405	33	9	175	67	55	4	1	—	1370	—	—	—
Half Sandwich Signature Chicken Salad	1	305	22	4	55	17	10	7	1	—	545	—	—	—
Just The Turkey Burger	1 (7 oz)	360	27	7	100	42	65	16	5	—	2000	—	—	—
Macaroni & Cheese	1 serv (7 oz)	290	72	3	10	10	46	6	6	—	640	—	—	—
Mashed Sweet Potatoes	1 serv (7 oz)	423	1	0	0	4	102	54	4	—	120	—	—	—
Pulled BBQ Chicken	1 serv (6 oz)	380	7	2	125	44	27	22	0	—	1860	—	—	—
Pulled Rotisserie Chicken Breast	1 serv (6 oz)	290	6	2	145	53	3	2	0	—	610	—	—	—
Red Skin Mashed Potatoes	1 serv (7 oz)	334	16	10	42	5	44	3	4	—	1317	—	—	—
Sandwich Hot Openfaced Pulled Chicken	1	1180	47	32	225	72	113	10	7	—	3470	—	—	—
Steamed Vegetable Medley	1 serv (7 oz)	30	0	0	0	2	6	2	2	—	25	—	—	—
Wrap Apricot Chicken Salad	½	412	19	4	51	24	37	9	3	—	835	—	—	—
Wrap Asian Chicken Salad	½	341	12	3	46	22	35	6	2	—	684	—	—	—
Wrap BBQ Chicken w/ Cole Slaw	½	395	9	3	73	32	43	14	2	—	1517	—	—	—
Wrap Chopped Veggie	½	315	7	1	48	23	40	13	4	—	630	—	—	—
Wrap Cobb Salad	½	430	21	5	125	27	32	5	3	—	950	—	—	—

FOOD	PORTION	CALS	FAT	SAT FAT	CHOL	PROT	CARB	SUGAR	FIBER	CALCI	SOD	POTAS	FOLIC	VIT C
Wrap Freshly Roasted Turkey w/ Cucumber Sauce	½	325	14	5	65	24	27	3	3	—	445	—	—	—
Wrap Garden Veggie & Cheese	½	352	18	10	36	16	32	4	3	—	842	—	—	—
Wrap Grilled Chicken	½	359	15	3	50	22	32	3	2	—	693	—	—	—
Wrap Grilled Chicken Caesar	½	386	18	4	54	24	31	2	2	—	711	—	—	—
Wrap Santa Fe	½	371	16	3	50	24	34	4	3	—	961	—	—	—
Wrap Spinach & Milan Cutlet	½	315	7	1	45	22	43	14	4	—	770	—	—	—
SALAD DRESSINGS														
Buttermilk Ranch	1 oz	110	11	2	10	0	1	0	0	—	280	—	—	—
Creamy Caesar	1 oz	181	20	3	9	1	0	0	0	—	237	—	—	—
Creamy Cole Slaw	1 oz	125	11	2	0	0	6	5	0	—	252	—	—	—
Honey Balsamic Vinaigrette	1 oz	161	16	2	2	0	4	3	0	—	58	—	—	—
Honey Mustard Fat Free	1 oz	50	0	0	0	0	11	9	0	—	150	—	—	—
Southwest	1 oz	146	16	2	7	0	2	0	1	—	222	—	—	—
SALADS														
Apricot Chicken Salad	1 serv (6 oz)	610	36	6	135	49	23	17	3	—	930	—	—	—
Asian Chicken w/o Dressing or Wontons	1 serv	325	9	2	96	41	21	12	7	—	441	—	—	—
Caesar Grilled Chicken w/o Dressing or Croutons	1 serv	310	10	4	111	45	10	5	5	—	556	—	—	—
Caesar w/o Dressing Croutons or Roll	1 serv	90	4	2	10	7	8	3	5	—	109	—	—	—
Chicken Cobb	1 serv	720	29	12	385	62	48	8	7	—	1760	—	—	—
Chopped Veggie & Chicken w/o Dressing or Croutons	1 serv	300	5	2	95	42	25	12	9	—	530	—	—	—
Freshly Roasted Turkey Breast	1 serv	320	10	3	100	45	13	5	7	—	260	—	—	—
Garden Grilled Chicken w/o Dressing or Croutons	1 serv	269	5	1	96	40	17	8	6	—	474	—	—	—
Green Leaf Fruit & Granola	1 serv	380	11	1	0	10	67	38	11	—	200	—	—	—

FOOD	PORTION	CALS	FAT	SAT FAT	CHOL	PROT	CARB	SUGAR	FIBER	CALCI	SOD	POTAS	FOLIC	VIT C
Milan Chicken Cutlet	1 serv	348	7	2	132	53	17	3	4	—	568	—	—	—
Santa Fe Chicken w/o Dressing or Tortilla Strips	1 serv	399	15	7	126	47	22	8	8	—	606	—	—	—
Signature Chicken Salad	1 serv (6 oz)	790	58	10	145	44	22	15	2	—	1440	—	—	—
Spinach w/ Milan Cutlet	1 serv	550	22	7	110	47	46	26	8	—	910	—	—	—
SOUPS														
Chicken Noodle	1 serv (13 oz)	211	6	2	80	30	9	3	1	—	396	—	—	—
Vegetable Primavera	1 serv (13 oz)	330	7	1	45	26	45	20	10	—	1580	—	—	—

CHICK-FIL-A

FOOD	PORTION	CALS	FAT	SAT FAT	CHOL	PROT	CARB	SUGAR	FIBER	CALCI	SOD	POTAS	FOLIC	VIT C
BEVERAGES														
Coca-Cola	1 med	170	0	0	0	0	47	47	0	0	15	—	—	0
Coffee 100% Colombian	1 med	5	0	0	0	1	0	0	0	—	10	—	—	—
Diet Coke	1 med	0	0	0	0	0	0	0	0	0	5	—	—	0
Dr Pepper	1 med	180	0	0	0	0	48	48	0	0	60	—	—	0
Ice Tea Sweetened	1 med	130	0	0	0	0	32	32	0	—	—	—	—	—
Iced Tea Unsweetened	1 med	0	0	0	0	0	0	0	0	—	—	—	—	—
Lemonade	1 med	240	0	0	0	0	36	58	0	—	10	—	—	—
Lemonade Diet	1 med	20	0	0	0	0	7	2	0	—	10	—	—	—
Milkshake Chocolate	1 sm	600	23	14	75	13	90	86	1	—	410	—	—	—
Milkshake Peach	1 sm	780	19	11	65	13	139	118	1	—	—	—	—	—
Milkshake Strawberry	1 sm	610	23	13	75	13	88	85	1	—	—	—	—	—
BREAKFAST SELECTIONS														
Bagel Multigrain Chicken Egg & Cheese	1	490	20	6	240	29	49	8	3	150	1230	—	—	0
Biscuit Bacon Egg & Cheese	1	500	27	12	230	21	44	6	2	150	1390	—	—	0
Biscuit Chicken	1	440	20	8	25	17	47	6	3	80	1230	—	—	0
Biscuit Plain	1	310	14	7	0	5	41	5	2	60	700	—	—	0
Biscuit Sausage	1	590	39	15	45	16	43	5	2	80	1300	—	—	0
Biscuit Spicy Chicken	1	450	20	8	30	16	50	5	2	80	1300	—	—	0
Breakfast Burrito Chicken	1	450	20	8	260	24	43	3	2	300	990	—	—	15
Breakfast Burrito Sausage	1	510	28	12	270	23	40	3	2	300	990	—	—	15
Chick-N-Minis	3	280	10	3	40	16	30	5	1	20	650	—	—	0
Cinnamon Cluster	1 serv	430	17	7	30	7	63	29	2	60	240	—	—	0

FOOD	PORTION	CALS	FAT	SAT FAT	CHOL	PROT	CARB	SUGAR	FIBER	CALCI	SOD	POTAS	FOLIC	VIT C
Hashbrowns	1 serv	270	18	4	0	3	25	0	2	20	440	—	—	2
Yogurt Parfait	1	230	3	2	10	6	44	35	0	200	60	—	—	30
Yogurt Parfait w/ Chocolate Cookie Crumbs	1	240	5	2	10	7	47	36	0	200	75	—	—	30
Yogurt Parfait w/ Granola	1	290	6	2	10	7	53	39	1	200	85	—	—	30
DESSERTS														
Cheesecake	1 slice	310	23	13	115	5	22	14	1	40	280	—	—	0
Fudge Nut Brownie	1	370	19	6	25	5	45	28	3	20	180	—	—	0
Icedream	1 cup	290	7	5	25	8	50	49	0	—	200	—	—	—
Icedream Cone	1	170	4	2	15	5	31	25	0	—	115	—	—	—
Lemon Pie	1 slice	360	13	6	30	6	58	21	1	150	290	—	—	6
MAIN MENU SELECTIONS														
Chick-N-Strips	3	360	17	4	80	34	17	2	1	—	1230	—	—	—
Cool Wrap Chargrilled Chicken	1	410	12	4	55	33	50	8	9	200	1290	—	—	24
Cool Wrap Chicken Caesar	1	460	15	6	65	40	47	6	8	450	1510	—	—	12
Cool Wrap Spicy Chicken	1	410	12	4	60	35	48	5	8	200	1380	—	—	21
Hearty Breast of Chicken Soup	1 med	140	4	1	25	7	19	3	2	40	1110	—	—	2
Nuggets	8	260	12	3	70	28	11	1	1	40	990	—	—	1
Sandwich Chargrilled Chicken	1	290	5	1	55	29	36	9	3	100	1030	—	—	12
Sandwich Chargrilled Chicken Club	1	410	12	5	80	37	37	10	3	250	1370	—	—	12
Sandwich Chicken	1	430	17	4	60	30	38	6	3	150	1410	—	—	1
Sandwich Chicken Deluxe	1	490	22	6	70	33	41	8	3	200	1660	—	—	9
Sandwich Chicken Salad On Wheat Bread	1	490	19	3	80	28	55	12	5	150	1130	—	—	5
Sandwich Spicy Chicken	1	480	20	5	65	31	44	6	3	150	1660	—	—	1
Sandwich Spicy Chicken Deluxe	1	570	27	8	80	36	46	8	4	300	1810	—	—	9
Waffle Potato Fries	1 med	360	19	3	0	4	43	0	5	20	170	—	—	21
SALAD DRESSINGS AND SAUCES														
Dressing Berry Balsamic Vinaigrette Reduced Fat	½ pkg (1.25 oz)	70	2	0	0	0	12	9	0	—	150	—	—	—

FOOD	PORTION	CALS	FAT	SAT FAT	CHOL	PROT	CARB	SUGAR	FIBER	CALCI	SOD	POTAS	FOLIC	VIT C
Dressing Blue Cheese	½ pkg (1.25 oz)	160	16	3	20	1	1	1	0	20	280	—	—	0
Dressing Buttermilk Ranch	½ pkg (1.25 oz)	160	17	3	5	0	1	1	0	0	280	—	—	0
Dressing Caesar	½ pkg (1.25 oz)	160	17	3	30	1	1	0	0	0	240	—	—	1
Dressing Honey Mustard Fat Free	½ pkg (1.25 oz)	60	0	0	0	0	14	12	0	—	220	—	—	—
Dressing Italian Light	½ pkg (1.25 oz)	15	1	0	0	0	2	2	0	0	510	—	—	0
Dressing Spicy	½ pkg (1.25 oz)	140	14	2	5	0	2	1	0	0	130	—	—	2
Dressing Thousand Island	½ pkg (1.25 oz)	150	14	2	10	0	5	4	0	0	230	—	—	0
Sauce Barbecue	½ pkg (0.5 oz)	45	0	0	0	0	11	9	0	20	180	—	—	4
Sauce Buffalo	½ pkg (0.4 oz)	10	0	0	0	0	1	0	0	0	420	—	—	0
Sauce Buttermilk Ranch	½ pkg (0.4 oz)	110	12	2	5	0	1	1	0	0	200	—	—	0
Sauce Chick-fil-A	½ pkg (0.5 oz)	140	13	2	10	0	6	6	0	0	170	—	—	0
Sauce Honey Mustard	½ pkg (1.25 oz)	45	0	0	0	0	11	10	0	0	150	—	—	0
Sauce Honey Roasted BBQ	½ pkg	60	5	1	5	0	2	2	0	0	70	—	—	0
Sauce Polynesian	½ pkg (0.5 oz)	110	6	1	0	0	14	5	0	0	210	—	—	1
SALADS														
Carrot & Raisin Salad	1 med	260	12	2	5	2	40	32	4	40	160	—	—	9
Chargrilled Chicken Garden Salad	1 serv	180	6	4	65	23	11	6	4	150	650	—	—	48
Chargrilled & Fruit	1 serv	220	6	4	55	22	22	17	4	150	640	—	—	54
Chicken Salad Bacon & Egg	1 cup	350	22	4	120	28	9	6	1	40	1130	—	—	1
Chick-N-Strips Salad	1 serv	460	22	6	90	40	26	6	5	200	1350	—	—	48
Cole Slaw	1 med	360	31	5	20	2	19	16	3	60	280	—	—	48
Croutons Garlic & Butter	1 pkg	60	2	0	0	1	9	1	0	0	150	—	—	0
Fruit Cup	1 serv	70	0	0	0	1	17	14	2	0	0	—	—	24
Harvest Nut Granola	1 pkg	60	3	0	0	1	8	3	1	0	25	—	—	0
Honey Roasted Sunflower Kernels	1 pkg	90	7	1	0	2	4	1	1	0	55	—	—	0
Side Salad	1 serv	70	5	3	15	5	5	2	2	150	110	—	—	24
Southwest Chargrilled Salad	1 serv	240	9	4	60	26	18	6	5	200	820	—	—	42

FOOD	PORTION	CALS	FAT	SAT FAT	CHOL	PROT	CARB	SUGAR	FIBER	CALCI	SOD	POTAS	FOLIC	VIT C
Tortilla Strips	1 pkg	80	4	0	0	1	8	1	1	20	50	—	—	0
CHIPOTLE														
Barbacoa	1 serv (4 oz)	228	13	3	59	27	1	0	0	20	544	—	—	0
Black Beans	1 serv (4 oz)	130	1	tr	0	9	22	3	12	30	318	—	—	0
Carnitas	1 serv (4 oz)	227	12	3	66	29	0	0	0	20	873	—	—	0
Cheese	1 serv (1 oz)	110	9	6	30	7	tr	0	0	200	180	—	—	0
Chicken	1 serv (4 oz)	219	11	2	96	29	0	0	0	10	431	—	—	0
Chips	1 serv (4 oz)	490	19	4	0	7	71	1	5	60	130	—	—	0
Crispy Taco Shells	3	180	7	2	0	3	26	0	2	30	30	—	—	0
Fajita Vegetables	1 serv (3 oz)	100	8	1	0	1	6	3	1	20	640	—	—	42
Flour Tortilla	1 (13 inch)	330	8	3	0	9	55	1	5	200	710	—	—	0
Flour Tortilla	1 (6 inch)	300	8	3	0	9	48	0	6	180	630	—	—	0
Guacamole	1 serv (4 oz)	170	15	3	0	2	8	1	5	20	370	—	—	9
Lettuce	1 serv (1 oz)	5	0	0	0	tr	tr	0	tr	10	0	—	—	7
Pinto Beans	1 serv (4 oz)	138	1	tr	0	9	23	3	10	50	374	—	—	3
Rice	1 serv (3.5 oz)	168	5	1	0	3	28	0	tr	10	427	—	—	2
Salsa Corn	1 serv (4 oz)	100	1	0	0	3	22	3	3	0	540	—	—	12
Salsa Tomato	1 serv (4 oz)	25	0	0	0	1	6	3	1	20	560	—	—	21
Sour Cream	1 serv (2 oz)	120	10	7	40	2	2	2	0	80	30	—	—	0
Steak	1 serv (4 oz)	230	12	4	51	29	2	0	0	—	306	—	—	0
Tomatillo Green	1 serv (2 oz)	15	tr	0	0	1	3	2	1	0	227	—	—	28
Tomatillo Red	1 serv (2 oz)	28	1	0	0	1	4	1	1	10	493	—	—	12
Vinaigrette	1 serv (2 oz)	282	26	3	17	0	11	25	0	—	1525	—	—	—
CHURCH'S CHICKEN														
DESSERTS														
Pie Apple	1 pie (3 oz)	280	11	4	5	2	39	15	1	0	250	—	—	5
Pie Edward's Double Lemon	1 pie (3 oz)	300	14	6	25	5	39	29	0	100	160	—	—	0
Pie Edward's Strawberry Cream Cheese	1 pie (2.8 oz)	280	15	8	15	4	32	22	2	40	130	—	—	0
MAIN MENU SELECTIONS														
Biscuit Honey Butter	1	240	12	3	<5	3	28	4	1	20	540	—	—	0
Cajun Rice	1 reg	130	7	3	5	1	16	0	tr	0	260	—	—	0
Chicken Fried Steak w/ White Gravy	1 serv (7.5 oz)	610	43	13	70	24	31	2	2	40	1465	—	—	0
Cole Slaw	1 reg	150	10	2	5	1	15	7	2	20	170	—	—	12
Corn On The Cob	1 ear	140	3	0	0	4	24	2	9	0	15	—	—	1
Country Fried Steak w/ White Gravy	1 serv (5.8 oz)	470	28	7	65	21	36	4	1	90	1620	—	—	0
Crunchy Tenders	1 (2 oz)	120	6	2	35	12	6	0	tr	0	440	—	—	0
French Fries	1 reg	290	14	3	0	3	38	1	4	40	320	—	—	0

FOOD	PORTION	CALS	FAT	SAT FAT	CHOL	PROT	CARB	SUGAR	FIBER	CALCI	SOD	POTAS	FOLIC	VIT C
Jalapeno Cheese Bombers	4 (4 oz)	240	10	6	30	8	29	5	3	200	970	—	—	0
Macaroni & Cheese	1 reg	210	11	4	15	8	23	6	1	120	690	—	—	0
Mashed Potatoes & Gravy	1 reg	70	2	0	tr	2	12	2	1	20	480	—	—	1
Okra	1 reg	350	22	7	0	3	36	3	5	100	590	—	—	1
Original Breast	1	200	11	3	80	22	3	0	1	0	450	—	—	1
Original Leg	1	110	6	2	55	10	3	0	0	0	280	—	—	0
Original Thigh	1	330	23	6	110	21	8	0	1	20	680	—	—	0
Original Wing	1	300	19	5	120	27	7	0	3	20	540	—	—	1
Sandwich Bigger Better Chicken w/ Cheese	1	510	27	7	50	20	46	4	4	180	1070	—	—	0
Sandwich Country Fried Steak	1	490	32	8	30	13	38	4	2	60	880	—	—	1
Sandwich Spicy Fish	1	320	20	4	25	10	25	3	2	40	560	—	—	0
Spicy Breast	1	320	20	5	75	21	12	0	1	40	760	—	—	0
Spicy Crunchy Tenders	1 (2 oz)	135	7	2	25	11	7	0	4	0	480	—	—	1
Spicy Fish Fillet	1 piece (2.3 oz)	160	9	2	25	7	13	1	1	20	350	—	—	0
Spicy Leg	1	180	11	3	65	12	8	0	1	20	470	—	—	0
Spicy Thigh	1	480	35	9	135	22	20	0	2	40	1035	—	—	0
Spicy Wing	1	430	27	7	125	29	17	0	2	60	1020	—	—	0
Sweet Corn Nuggets	1 reg	600	29	2	0	7	72	14	5	100	1260	—	—	0
Whole Jalapeno Peppers	2	10	0	0	0	0	2	tr	1	0	390	—	—	0
SAUCES														
BBQ	1 pkg	30	0	0	0	0	7	2	0	0	180	—	—	2
Creamy Jalapeno	1 pkg	100	11	2	10	0	1	0	0	0	140	—	—	0
Honey	1 pkg	27	0	0	0	0	7	7	0	0	0	—	—	0
Honey Mustard	1 pkg	110	11	2	10	0	4	1	0	10	130	—	—	0
Hot Sauce	1 pkg	0	0	0	0	0	0	0	0	0	210	—	—	2
Ketchup	1 pkg	18	0	0	0	0	5	4	0	0	190	—	—	0
Purple Pepper	1 pkg	45	0	0	0	0	12	6	0	0	26	—	—	0
Ranch	1 pkg	130	13	2	10	0	1	0	0	0	320	—	—	0
Sweet & Sour	1 pkg	30	0	0	0	0	8	2	0	0	120	—	—	1

CICI'S

FOOD	PORTION	CALS	FAT	SAT FAT	CHOL	PROT	CARB	SUGAR	FIBER	CALCI	SOD	POTAS	FOLIC	VIT C
EXTRAS														
Apple Pizza	1 slice	149	4	1	0	3	26	—	1	7	193	—	—	—
Brownie	1	143	6	1	0	1	22	—	1	4	96	—	—	—
Cinnamon Roll	1	139	6	1	0	2	20	—	1	8	99	—	—	—
Garlic Bread	1 slice	99	5	1	5	4	10	—	tr	42	120	—	—	—

FOOD	PORTION	CALS	FAT	SAT FAT	CHOL	PROT	CARB	SUGAR	FIBER	CALCI	SOD	POTAS	FOLIC	VIT C
PIZZA														
Buffet 12 Inch Alfredo	1 slice	139	5	3	10	8	18	—	1	30	199	—	—	—
Buffet 12 Inch Bacon Cheddar	1 slice	145	5	2	13	6	18	—	3	38	312	—	—	—
Buffet 12 Inch Bar-B-Que	1 slice	172	6	4	12	8	21	—	2	49	311	—	—	—
Buffet 12 Inch Beef	1 slice	170	7	4	20	9	18	—	1	43	281	—	—	—
Buffet 12 Inch Cheese	1 slice	152	5	3	9	7	20	—	1	47	305	—	—	—
Buffet 12 Inch Ham & Pineapple	1 slice	141	4	3	10	7	19	—	1	42	319	—	—	—
Buffet 12 Inch Ole	1 slice	108	4	2	7	5	13	—	2	38	261	—	—	—
Buffet 12 Inch Pepperoni	1 slice	175	7	2	13	8	21	—	2	47	384	—	—	—
Buffet 12 Inch Pepperoni & Jalapeno	1 slice	163	6	4	11	8	20	—	2	45	394	—	—	—
Buffet 12 Inch Sausage	1 slice	197	7	4	11	8	19	—	1	44	358	—	—	—
Buffet 12 Inch Spinach Alfredo	1 slice	151	5	3	11	7	20	—	2	37	215	—	—	—
Buffet 12 Inch Zesty Ham & Cheese	1 slice	153	6	3	9	6	18	—	1	61	271	—	—	—
Buffet 12 Inch Zesty Pepperoni	1 slice	157	7	3	7	6	18	—	1	34	302	—	—	—
Buffet 12 Inch Zesty Tomato Alfredo	1 slice	136	5	3	10	6	18	—	2	31	202	—	—	—
Buffet 12 Inch Zesty Veggie	1 slice	124	4	2	4	5	17	—	1	33	224	—	—	—
To-Go 15 Inch Bar-B-Que	1 slice	289	10	7	17	13	36	—	2	90	446	—	—	—
To-Go 15 Inch Cheese	1 slice	223	8	5	17	11	28	—	3	75	428	—	—	—
To-Go 15 Inch Ham & Pineapple	1 slice	225	8	5	21	11	27	—	2	71	394	—	—	—
To-Go 15 Inch Ole	1 slice	169	4	2	8	7	26	—	3	46	350	—	—	—
To-Go 15 Inch Pepperoni	1 slice	240	10	6	21	11	27	—	3	72	504	—	—	—
To-Go 15 Inch Spinach Alfredo	1 slice	243	8	5	18	11	32	—	3	60	347	—	—	—
To-Go 15 Inch Zesty Pepperoni	1 slice	246	12	5	12	10	26	—	2	62	475	—	—	—

FOOD	PORTION	CALS	FAT	SAT FAT	CHOL	PROT	CARB	SUGAR	FIBER	CALCI	SOD	POTAS	FOLIC	VIT C
To-Go 15 Inch Zesty Veggie	1 slice	213	9	4	7	9	25	—	2	62	394	—	—	—

CINNABON

BAKED SELECTIONS

FOOD	PORTION	CALS	FAT	SAT FAT	CHOL	PROT	CARB	SUGAR	FIBER	CALCI	SOD	POTAS	FOLIC	VIT C
Caramel Pecanbon	1	1100	56	10	63	16	141	47	8	—	600	—	—	—
Cinnabon Bites	6	520	16	4	10	8	78	25	2	80	530	—	—	—
Cinnabon Classic	1	813	32	8	67	15	117	55	4	—	801	—	—	—
Cinnabon Stix	1	379	21	6	16	6	41	14	1	—	413	—	—	—
Cinnamon Filled Churro	1	281	11	2	—	5	39	—	—	—	—	—	—	—
Minibon	1	339	13	3	27	6	49	22	2	—	337	—	—	—

BEVERAGES

FOOD	PORTION	CALS	FAT	SAT FAT	CHOL	PROT	CARB	SUGAR	FIBER	CALCI	SOD	POTAS	FOLIC	VIT C
Caramelatta Chill	1 (16 oz)	520	19	12	75	12	76	73	0	—	250	—	—	—
Chillatta Cappuccino	1 (16 oz)	330	11	7	35	5	56	51	1	—	120	—	—	—
Chillatta Caramel	1 (16 oz)	480	18	11	65	8	72	68	0	—	270	—	—	—
Chillatta Chocolate Mocha	1 (16 oz)	460	14	8	45	8	72	61	3	—	270	—	—	—
Chillatta Mango	1 (16 oz)	340	11	7	40	6	57	47	0	—	105	—	—	—
Chillatta Strawberry	1 (16 oz)	330	11	7	40	5	54	46	0	—	105	—	—	—
Chillatta Strawberry Banana	1 (16 oz)	350	11	7	40	5	58	49	0	—	105	—	—	—
Chillatta Tropical Blast	1 (16 oz)	330	7	4	20	2	69	48	—	—	50	—	—	—
Mochalatta Chill	1 (16 oz)	450	18	11	60	11	66	62	1	—	310	—	—	—

CORNER BAKERY

BREAKFAST SELECTIONS

FOOD	PORTION	CALS	FAT	SAT FAT	CHOL	PROT	CARB	SUGAR	FIBER	CALCI	SOD	POTAS	FOLIC	VIT C
Baked French Toast	1 serv	570	15	—	—	13	86	—	1	—	530	—	—	—
Buckhead Cheese Grits	1 serv	350	22	—	—	11	19	—	2	—	310	—	—	—
Fresh Berry Parfait	1 serv	330	—	—	—	—	—	—	—	—	—	—	—	—
Oatmeal	1 serv	280	7	—	—	12	41	—	3	—	320	—	—	—
Oatmeal Crunchy Honey Banana	1 serv	380	3	—	—	12	78	—	5	—	280	—	—	—
Oatmeal Swiss	1 serv	330	1	—	—	4	79	—	6	—	5	—	—	—
Panini Ham & Cheddar	1	720	34	—	—	42	57	—	2	—	1990	—	—	—
Panini Smoked Bacon & Cheddar	1	680	34	—	—	33	56	—	2	—	1990	—	—	—
Scrambler All American w/o Potatoes & Bread	1 serv	310	22	—	—	23	3	—	0	—	870	—	—	—

FOOD	PORTION	CALS	FAT	SAT FAT	CHOL	PROT	CARB	SUGAR	FIBER	CALCI	SOD	POTAS	FOLIC	VIT C
Scrambler Anaheim w/o Potatoes & Bread	1 serv	490	36	—	—	30	10	—	4	—	620	—	—	—
Scrambler Farmer's w/o Potatoes & Bread	1 serv	430	31	—	—	31	6	—	1	—	980	—	—	—
The Commuter Croissant	1	720	46	—	—	29	44	—	2	—	1390	—	—	—
PASTA														
Chicken Carbonara	1 serv	740	28	—	—	51	70	—	4	—	890	—	—	—
Half Moon Cheese Ravioli	1 serv	550	21	—	—	28	63	—	4	—	880	—	—	—
Penne w/ Marinara	1 serv	550	11	—	—	20	92	—	14	—	1080	—	—	—
Pesto Cavatappi	1 serv	930	40	—	—	52	93	—	13	—	830	—	—	—
SALAD DRESSINGS														
Caesar	1 serv	310	32	—	—	1	2	—	0	—	530	—	—	—
House	1 serv	280	27	—	—	0	8	—	0	—	680	—	—	—
Ranch	1 serv	160	16	—	—	2	2	—	0	—	440	—	—	—
Vinaigrette Balsamic	1 serv	300	31	—	—	0	4	—	0	—	10	—	—	—
SALADS														
Caesar	1 serv	520	44	—	—	11	19	—	5	—	970	—	—	—
Caesar w/ Roasted Chicken & Croutons	1 serv	640	49	—	—	27	8	—	5	—	1500	—	—	—
Chopped w/o Bread	1 serv	810	61	—	—	40	27	—	10	—	2340	—	—	—
Harvest	1 serv	860	68	—	—	19	53	—	10	—	930	—	—	—
Harvest w/ Roasted Chicken	1 serv	980	72	—	—	37	53	—	10	—	1460	—	—	—
Santa Fe Ranch	1 serv	680	44	—	—	19	56	—	10	—	1960	—	—	—
Santa Fe Ranch w/ Roasted Chicken	1 serv	800	49	—	—	37	56	—	10	—	1800	—	—	—
Side Cucumber Tomato	1 (6 oz)	120	9	—	—	1	9	—	2	—	170	—	—	—
Side Egg	1 (6 oz)	570	53	—	—	16	2	—	0	—	650	—	—	—
Side Roasted Potato Bacon	1 (6 oz)	370	23	—	—	8	29	—	3	—	1030	—	—	—
Side Seasonal Fruit Medley	1 (6 oz)	90	0	0	0	1	22	—	2	—	20	—	—	—
Side Tomato Mozzarella Pasta	1 (6 oz)	205	8	—	—	7	24	—	4	—	230	—	—	—
Side Tuna	1 (6 oz)	310	16	—	—	34	3	—	1	—	670	—	—	—
SANDWICHES														
Bavarian w/ Ham	1	720	25	—	—	40	78	—	4	—	3390	—	—	—

FOOD	PORTION	CALS	FAT	SAT FAT	CHOL	PROT	CARB	SUGAR	FIBER	CALCI	SOD	POTAS	FOLIC	VIT C
Bavarian w/ Turkey	1	690	22	—	—	39	78	—	4	—	3470	—	—	—
Chicken Pesto	1	840	41	—	—	41	75	—	5	—	2470	—	—	—
Panini California Grilled	1	700	41	—	—	29	59	—	8	—	1480	—	—	—
Panini Chicken Pomodori	1	890	45	—	—	47	74	—	5	—	2230	—	—	—
Panini Club	1	900	48	—	—	50	72	—	4	—	2810	—	—	—
Panini Corned Beef Reuben	1	930	48	—	—	44	76	—	2	—	2500	—	—	—
Panini Grilled Ham & Swiss	1	880	44	—	—	45	75	—	4	—	2610	—	—	—
Southwest Roast Beef	1	840	37	—	—	44	78	—	5	—	2060	—	—	—
Tomato Mozzarella	1	670	26	—	—	28	73	—	5	—	1630	—	—	—
Tuna Salad On Olive Bread	1	450	16	—	—	29	42	—	3	—	1080	—	—	—
Turkey Derby	1	650	29	—	—	39	60	—	5	—	2620	—	—	—
Turkey Frisco	1	850	38	—	—	44	79	—	9	—	2920	—	—	—
Uptown Turkey	1	660	29	—	—	39	61	—	9	—	3020	—	—	—
SOUPS														
Big Al's Chili w/ Cheddar Cheese	1 (10 oz)	380	17	—	—	23	29	—	8	—	1450	—	—	—
Bread Bowl	1	420	30	—	—	12	21	—	2	—	1370	—	—	—
Cheddar	1 (10 oz)	310	23	—	—	9	16	—	2	—	1090	—	—	—
Chicken Wild Mushroom Brie Stew	1 (10 oz)	260	14	—	—	11	20	—	2	—	1110	—	—	—
Loaded Baked Potato w/ Garnish	1 (10 oz)	420	29	—	—	13	29	—	2	—	990	—	—	—
Mom's Chicken Noodle	1 (10 oz)	170	4	—	—	8	23	—	1	—	1440	—	—	—
Old Fashioned Beef Stew	1 (10 oz)	260	13	—	—	7	20	—	2	—	1050	—	—	—
Roasted Poblano Corn Chowder	1 (10 oz)	330	21	—	—	4	34	—	4	—	770	—	—	—
Roasted Tomato Basil w/o Garnish	1 (10 oz)	170	5	—	—	3	27	—	4	—	1220	—	—	—
Zesty Chicken Tortilla w/ Tortilla Strips	1 (10 oz)	230	11	—	—	8	26	—	5	—	1340	—	—	—

D'ANGELO'S

CHILDREN'S MENU SELECTIONS

FOOD	PORTION	CALS	FAT	SAT FAT	CHOL	PROT	CARB	SUGAR	FIBER	CALCI	SOD	POTAS	FOLIC	VIT C
D'Lite Turkey	1	217	3	0	14	19	30	2	3	—	369	—	—	—
Sub Cheeseburger	1	294	13	6	43	15	28	2	3	40	459	—	—	1
Sub Ham & Cheese	1	227	5	2	30	14	32	3	1	40	997	—	—	0

FOOD	PORTION	CALS	FAT	SAT FAT	CHOL	PROT	CARB	SUGAR	FIBER	CALCI	SOD	POTAS	FOLIC	VIT C
Sub Kidz Tuna	1	438	29	4	18	15	30	2	1	—	614	—	—	—
Sub Meatball	1	330	15	5	37	15	37	5	4	—	812	—	—	—
SALAD DRESSINGS														
Bleu Cheese	1 serv	152	15	3	15	1	3	2	0	0	283	—	—	0
Caesar	1 serv	397	43	7	43	6	6	6	0	0	1191	—	—	0
Caesar Fat Free	1 serv	57	0	0	0	0	9	9	0	0	1673	—	—	0
Creamy Italian	1 serv	340	37	6	0	0	9	6	0	0	851	—	—	0
Greek w/ Feta Cheese	1 serv	227	26	4	14	0	6	3	0	0	765	—	—	0
Honey Mustard	1 serv	150	142	2	0	0	7	6	0	0	210	—	—	0
Olive Oil Vinaigrette	1 serv	170	17	3	0	0	9	6	0	—	652	—	—	—
Ranch Lite	1 serv	240	19	3	20	2	6	4	1	0	961	—	—	0
SALADS														
Antipasto	1 serv	284	18	7	40	16	17	7	6	250	1109	—	—	58
Caesar w/ Dressing	1 serv	474	39	7	40	15	25	7	4	50	1208	—	—	25
Chicken Caesar w/ Dressing	1 serv	533	38	8	99	35	19	8	4	50	1654	—	—	25
Chicken Stir Fry w/o Dressing	1 serv	168	3	1	59	25	11	6	4	50	590	—	—	57
Cobb w/o Dressing	1 serv	292	17	7	76	27	11	5	4	50	636	—	—	34
Greek	1 serv	290	23	9	50	11	17	8	4	330	1098	—	—	49
Lobster w/o Dressing	1 serv	376	26	4	86	26	12	6	4	130	589	—	—	49
Roast Beef w/o Dressing	1 serv	131	3	1	42	19	10	5	4	50	208	—	—	49
Steak Tip Caesar	1 serv	661	50	13	95	32	21	9	3	50	1627	—	—	18
Tossed Garden w/o Dressing	1 serv	49	1	tr	0	3	11	5	4	50	22	—	—	57
Turkey w/o Dressing	1 serv	157	2	tr	22	26	10	5	4	50	86	—	—	49
SANDWICHES														
D'Lite Chicken Caesar Salad	1	374	7	3	68	34	43	9	4	40	2002	—	—	19
D'Lite Chicken Stir Fry	1	426	6	2	73	37	57	8	7	20	1241	—	—	38
D'Lite Classic Veggie	1	362	7	3	13	15	63	10	8	120	839	—	—	85
D'Lite Fresh Veggie	1	348	7	3	13	13	62	14	7	160	651	—	—	40
D'Lite Grilled Chicken Breast	1	388	7	1	67	31	52	5	6	10	953	—	—	13
D'Lite Roast Beef	1	338	5	1	42	25	51	5	6	10	727	—	—	13
D'Lite Turkey	1	347	4	0	19	28	51	5	6	10	595	—	—	13
D'Lite Turkey Cranberry	1	444	4	0	19	28	75	22	6	10	595	—	—	13

FOOD	PORTION	CALS	FAT	SAT FAT	CHOL	PROT	CARB	SUGAR	FIBER	CALCI	SOD	POTAS	FOLIC	VIT C
Pokket Big Papi	1	469	11	6	84	39	53	6	3	140	2536	—	—	26
Pokket BLT & Cheese	1	397	17	8	50	22	38	5	3	150	1266	—	—	13
Pokket Caesar Salad	1	616	39	7	40	20	54	7	3	40	1518	—	—	19
Pokket Capicola & Cheese	1	362	13	7	60	26	35	2	2	240	1547	—	—	7
Pokket Cheese	1	519	27	18	74	29	41	6	2	590	1765	—	—	7
Pokket Cheeseburger	1	459	25	11	85	27	31	3	2	90	811	—	—	7
Pokket Chicken Caesar Salad	1	674	39	8	99	40	47	7	3	40	1964	—	—	19
Pokket Chicken Club	1	526	28	6	87	34	36	3	2	10	1088	—	—	17
Pokket Chicken Honey Dijon	1	508	20	7	111	41	40	6	2	10	1165	—	—	17
Pokket Chicken Salad	1	623	42	7	71	27	34	3	2	10	639	—	—	7
Pokket Chicken Stir Fry	1	380	9	5	79	35	39	5	2	110	1276	—	—	25
Pokket Classic Vegetable	1	368	13	8	33	19	46	8	4	300	934	—	—	79
Pokket Classic Veggie No Cheese	1	212	1	tr	0	9	44	7	4	30	331	—	—	84
Pokket Greek	1	790	61	14	50	16	49	8	4	320	1892	—	—	34
Pokket Grilled Chicken	1	303	5	1	67	29	35	3	2	10	739	—	—	17
Pokket Ham	1	229	3	1	33	17	35	3	2	10	1050	—	—	7
Pokket Ham & Cheese	1	326	10	6	53	22	38	5	2	140	1493	—	—	12
Pokket Ham & Salami	1	386	17	8	56	23	34	3	12	240	1301	—	—	7
Pokket Hamburger	1	399	20	8	72	24	29	2	2	10	343	—	—	7
Pokket Italian	1	525	30	12	80	28	36	4	2	240	1678	—	—	8
Pokket Lobster	1	530	31	5	84	29	34	2	2	70	897	—	—	1
Pokket Meatball	1	574	31	10	73	26	52	10	4	—	1765	—	—	—
Pokket Mortadella & Cheese	1	410	21	9	56	21	35	2	2	240	1114	—	—	7
Pokket Number 9	1	407	18	9	76	31	31	4	2	110	685	—	—	20
Pokket Pastrami	1	438	25	9	91	24	33	1	1	—	1643	—	—	—
Pokket Pepperoni	1	407	20	9	47	21	35	3	3	240	1147	—	—	7
Pokket Roast Beef	1	247	3	1	42	23	33	2	2	10	511	—	—	7
Pokket Salad	1	196	1	tr	0	8	40	6	4	20	340	—	—	39
Pokket Salami & Cheese	1	509	30	13	75	25	33	2	2	240	1590	—	—	7

FOOD	PORTION	CALS	FAT	SAT FAT	CHOL	PROT	CARB	SUGAR	FIBER	CALCI	SOD	POTAS	FOLIC	VIT C
Pokket Seafood Salad	1	449	22	3	11	14	50	7	3	10	1182	—	—	1
Pokket Steak	1	305	12	5	59	25	24	1	1	—	324	—	—	—
Pokket Steak & Cheese	1	377	17	9	74	29	26	2	1	100	665	—	—	0
Pokket Steak Bomb	1	631	32	14	102	43	44	4	3	250	1794	—	—	25
Pokket Steak Tip	1	452	16	5	54	27	45	12	2	20	1189	—	—	13
Pokket Tuna	1	664	49	8	32	24	33	2	2	20	825	—	—	1
Pokket Turkey	1	256	2	0	19	26	33	2	2	10	379	—	—	7
Pokket Turkey Club	1	332	7	2	54	34	32	4	2	10	610	—	—	16
Sub Big Papi	1 sm	525	15	9	83	40	60	7	7	200	2700	—	—	24
Sub BLT & Cheese	1 sm	463	19	8	50	23	51	7	6	150	1437	—	—	13
Sub Capicola & Cheese	1 sm	408	13	6	50	25	48	4	5	240	1482	—	—	7
Sub Cheese	1 sm	589	28	18	74	30	55	8	5	590	1939	—	—	7
Sub Cheeseburger	1 sm	526	26	11	86	29	44	5	5	90	774	—	—	7
Sub Chicken Club	1	593	29	6	87	35	49	5	5	10	1260	—	—	14
Sub Chicken Honey Dijon	1	575	22	7	111	42	53	8	5	10	1338	—	—	14
Sub Chicken Salad	1 sm	692	44	7	71	29	48	5	5	10	813	—	—	7
Sub Chicken Stir Fry	1 sm	449	11	5	79	37	53	7	6	110	1449	—	—	25
Sub Classic Veggie	1 sm	462	15	8	34	21	64	10	8	310	1162	—	—	79
Sub Grilled Chicken	1 sm	369	7	1	67	30	48	4	5	10	911	—	—	14
Sub Ham	1 sm	302	5	1	33	18	49	6	2	10	1226	—	—	12
Sub Ham & Cheese	1 sm	395	11	6	53	24	52	7	2	140	1667	—	—	12
Sub Ham & Salami	1 sm	456	19	8	56	25	48	5	2	240	1475		—	7
Sub Hamburger	1 sm	466	22	8	73	25	42	4	5	10	503	—	—	7
Sub Italian	1 sm	614	31	12	80	30	54	6	3	240	1893	—	—	8
Sub Lobster	1 sm	598	33	5	84	30	48	4	5	70	1089	—	—	1
Sub Meatball	1 sm	644	33	10	73	28	66	12	7	—	1939	—	—	—
Sub Meatballs & Cheese	1 sm	750	41	15	94	36	67	13	7	230	2204	—	—	0
Sub Mortadella & Cheese	1 sm	479	23	9	56	23	49	4	5	240	1288	—	—	7
Sub Number 9	1 sm	450	19	9	74	31	41	5	4	110	802	—	—	13
Sub Pastrami	1 sm	613	34	14	118	34	47	3	5	—	1875	—	—	—
Sub Pepperoni	1 sm	603	33	13	72	28	49	6	7	240	1836	—	—	7
Sub Roast Beef	1 sm	320	5	1	42	25	48	5	5	10	687	—	—	12
Sub Salad	1 sm	281	3	tr	0	10	57	11	8	30	522	—	—	55

FOOD	PORTION	CALS	FAT	SAT FAT	CHOL	PROT	CARB	SUGAR	FIBER	CALCI	SOD	POTAS	FOLIC	VIT C
Sub Salami & Cheese	1 sm	579	32	13	75	27	47	4	5	240	1764	—	—	7
Sub Seafood Salad	1 sm	498	23	3	10	14	61	8	6	10	1208	—	—	1
Sub Steak	1 sm	373	14	5	59	27	37	2	4	—	491	—	—	—
Sub Steak & Cheese	1 sm	446	19	9	74	31	40	4	4	100	832	—	—	0
Sub Steak Bomb	1 sm	670	33	14	102	43	52	6	6	250	1904	—	—	25
Sub Steak Tip	1 sm	545	18	5	54	29	63	14	3	20	1413	—	—	13
Sub Tuna	1	685	46	7	29	24	47	4	2	10	952	—	—	1
Sub Turkey Club	1 sm	401	9	2	48	33	49	6	3	10	806	—	—	16
Sub Toasted Italian Bistro	1 sm	585	31	12	81	29	49	5	5	240	1912	—	—	10
Sub Toasted Pastrami Reuben	1 sm	750	47	14	104	30	55	7	7	—	2226	—	—	—
Sub Toasted Roast Beef & Cheddar	1 sm	564	26	10	88	35	51	8	5	300	1117	—	—	0
Sub Toasted Spicy Meatball	1 sm	933	57	20	102	61	71	17	9	0	2560	—	—	23
Sub Toasted Tuna & Swiss	1 sm	796	54	12	55	32	49	6	5	290	1027	—	—	14
Sub Toasted Turkey & Ham	1 sm	532	24	5	66	33	49	5	5	10	1507	—	—	10
Sub Toasted Turkey Thanksgiving	1 sm	705	20	2	21	32	80	11	6	—	1315	—	—	—
Wrap Big Papi	1	593	23	11	83	41	56	3	4	200	2859	—	—	24
Wrap BLT & Cheese	1	544	26	10	50	24	54	4	4	140	1542	—	—	8
Wrap Buffalo Chicken Salad	1	823	44	7	101	40	67	7	4	20	2917	—	—	9
Wrap Caesar Salad	1	711	44	9	40	20	65	7	5	30	1679	—	—	15
Wrap Capicola & Cheese	1	494	20	8	50	25	53	2	4	240	1589	—	—	7
Wrap Cheese	1	675	35	20	74	30	59	6	4	590	2046	—	—	7
Wrap Cheeseburger	1	609	33	13	86	30	48	3	3	90	879	—	—	7
Wrap Chicken Caesar Salad	1	830	47	10	99	42	65	7	5	30	2246	—	—	15
Wrap Chicken Cobb	1	931	55	14	102	36	71	17	6	310	1790	—	—	25
Wrap Chicken Filet & Bacon	1	639	28	6	87	38	58	4	2	10	1078	—	—	16
Wrap Chicken Honey Dijon	1	672	29	9	110	60	43	8	5	300	1466	—	—	22
Wrap Chicken Salad	1	782	51	9	71	29	53	3	4	10	922	—	—	12
Wrap Chicken Stir Fry	1	535	17	7	79	37	57	5	4	110	1557	—	—	25

FOOD	PORTION	CALS	FAT	SAT FAT	CHOL	PROT	CARB	SUGAR	FIBER	CALCI	SOD	POTAS	FOLIC	VIT C
Wrap Classic Veggie	1	486	13	8	34	24	68	9	5	310	936	—	—	79
Wrap Greek	1	765	61	14	50	15	44	7	4	320	1723	—	—	34
Wrap Grilled Chicken	1	422	6	1	67	34	59	4	4	20	733	—	—	22
Wrap Ham & Cheese	1	435	10	6	53	26	60	6	3	140	1481	—	—	7
Wrap Ham & Salami	1	513	18	9	63	30	57	4	3	240	1449	—	—	7
Wrap Hamburger	1	509	21	8	74	28	50	3	3	10	340	—	—	7
Wrap Italian	1	631	29	12	80	32	59	5	3	240	1667	—	—	8
Wrap Lobster	1	749	43	7	86	33	57	3	3	70	954	—	—	1
Wrap Meatball	1	687	31	10	73	31	75	11	5	—	1755	—	—	—
Wrap Mortadella & Cheese	1	522	21	9	56	25	58	3	3	240	1103	—	—	7
Wrap Number 9	1	517	24	10	74	32	44	4	3	110	885	—	—	20
Wrap Pastrami	1	550	25	9	91	28	55	2	2	—	1632	—	—	—
Wrap Peppercorn Steak	1	702	40	14	110	41	45	4	3	150	1745	—	—	1
Wrap Pepperoni	1	519	21	9	47	25	57	4	4	240	1136	—	—	7
Wrap Roast Beef	1	448	13	3	42	26	58	2	4	10	881	—	—	7
Wrap Salad	1	324	2	tr	0	13	66	10	6	30	337	—	—	55
Wrap Salami & Cheese	1	605	29	12	72	29	56	3	3	240	1510	—	—	7
Wrap Scafood Salad	1	541	22	3	10	17	69	7	3	10	1024	—	—	1
Wrap Steak	1	392	13	5	59	28	41	2	2	—	316	—	—	—
Wrap Steak & Cheese	1	464	18	9	74	33	43	3	2	100	657	—	—	0
Wrap Steak Bomb	1	670	33	14	102	43	52	6	6	250	1904	—	—	25
Wrap Steak Tip	1	432	16	5	54	26	41	12	2	20	1029	—	—	7
Wrap Tuna	1	731	44	7	29	27	56	4	3	10	769	—	—	7
Wrap Turkey	1	369	3	0	19	30	55	3	3	10	369	—	—	7
Wrap Turkey Club	1	415	8	2	48	34	52	4	3	10	590	—	—	16
SOUPS														
Beef Stew	1 sm	220	8	4	30	12	23	6	2	—	819	—	—	—
Broccoli & Cheddar Cheese	1 sm	270	21	11	60	9	11	3	2	—	859	—	—	—
Chicken Noodle	1 sm	110	3	1	25	6	14	4	1	—	829	—	—	—
Hearty Vegetable	1 sm	40	0	0	0	2	7	4	2	—	270	—	—	—
Italian Wedding	1 sm	120	6	2	15	6	11	3	2	—	919	—	—	—
Lobster Bisque	1 sm	360	29	18	105	8	16	3	1	—	819	—	—	—
New England Clam Chowder	1 sm	320	18	10	60	9	31	1	1	—	699	—	—	—
Portuguese Kale	1 sm	130	4	2	10	8	16	5	3	—	629	—	—	—

FOOD	PORTION	CALS	FAT	SAT FAT	CHOL	PROT	CARB	SUGAR	FIBER	CALCI	SOD	POTAS	FOLIC	VIT C
DENNY'S														
BEVERAGES														
Apple Juice	1 sm (10 oz)	141	0	0	0	0	52	11	0	—	28	—	—	—
Cappuccino	1 (8 oz)	100	2	2	0	3	28	24	1	—	220	—	—	—
Chocolate Milk	1 sm (10 oz)	160	3	2	10	8	26	25	1	—	150	—	—	—
Hot Chocolate	1 (8 oz)	100	2	2	0	3	28	24	1	—	219	—	—	—
Iced Tea Raspberry	1 serv (16 oz)	78	0	0	0	0	21	—	0	—	0	—	—	—
Lemonade	1 serv (15 oz)	150	0	0	0	0	35	31	0	—	38	—	—	—
Milk	1 sm (10 oz)	130	5	3	20	8	12	12	0	—	100	—	—	—
Orange Juice	1 sm (10 oz)	140	0	0	0	2	34	30	0	—	0	—	—	—
Ruby Red Grapefruit	1 sm (10 oz)	164	0	0	0	1	40	36	0	—	41	—	—	—
Tomato Juice	1 sm (10 oz)	56	0	0	0	2	11	—	2	—	680	—	—	—
BREAKFAST SELECTIONS														
All American Slam w/o Choices	1 serv (10 oz)	800	68	25	775	40	5	1	1	—	1410	—	—	—
Bacon Turkey	4 slices	150	8	2	65	17	1	0	0	—	650	—	—	—
Bacon Strips	4	140	11	4	30	9	1	1	0	—	467	—	—	—
Banana	1	110	0	0	0	1	29	14	4	—	—	—	—	—
Egg	1 (2 oz)	120	11	3	210	6	0	0	0	—	125	—	—	—
Eggs White	1 serv (4 oz)	50	1	0	0	11	1	0	0	—	180	—	—	—
English Muffin w/o Margarine	1	130	1	0	0	4	25	1	1	—	250	—	—	—
Grand Slam Slugger w/o Choices	1 serv (13 oz)	780	42	13	475	29	71	13	3	—	1930	—	—	—
Grapes	1 serv (3 oz)	55	0	0	0	1	29	13	4	—	0	—	—	—
Grits w/ Margarine	1 serv (12 oz)	220	3	1	0	5	44	0	3	—	15	—	—	—
Ham Slice Grilled Honey	1 (3 oz)	120	5	4	45	14	8	6	0	—	710	—	—	—
Hash Browns	1 serv	210	12	3	0	2	26	1	2	—	650	—	—	—
Hash Browns Cheddar Cheese	1 serv (5 oz)	300	19	7	20	8	26	2	2	—	780	—	—	—
Hash Browns Everything	1 serv (8 oz)	340	21	8	20	8	33	3	2	—	1010	—	—	—
Lumberjack Slam w/o Choices	1 serv (15 oz)	940	47	17	555	46	80	19	4	—	2900	—	—	—
Moon Over My Hammy Omelette w/ Hash Browns w/o Choices	1 serv (16 oz)	770	53	18	790	42	31	5	2	—	2590	—	—	—
Oatmeal w/ Milk	1 serv (16 oz)	290	8	4	20	12	39	20	4	—	300	—	—	—
Omelette Southern w/ Hash Browns w/o Bread	1 serv (18 oz)	1070	80	30	795	38	47	3	4	—	2500	—	—	—

FOOD	PORTION	CALS	FAT	SAT FAT	CHOL	PROT	CARB	SUGAR	FIBER	CALCI	SOD	POTAS	FOLIC	VIT C
Omelette Veggie Cheese w/o Choices	1 serv (13 oz)	460	33	12	740	28	9	4	2	—	680	—	—	—
Omelette w/ Hash Browns w/o Choices	1 serv (16 oz)	700	46	13	770	38	32	5	2	—	2180	—	—	—
Pancakes Buttermilk	2	330	4	1	0	8	67	12	2	—	1170	—	—	—
Platter Chocolate Chip Pancakes w/o Meat	1 serv (13 oz)	640	22	9	480	24	87	28	4	—	1480	—	—	—
Sausage Links	4 (3 oz)	370	34	13	70	9	4	0	3	—	660	—	—	—
Senior Omelette w/o Choices	1 serv (9 oz)	470	37	15	510	26	7	3	1	—	820	—	—	—
Senior Scrambled Eggs & Cheddar	1 serv (13 oz)	870	48	18	525	35	72	12	4	—	2200	—	—	—
Senior Slam Belgian Waffle w/ Egg w/o Choices	1 serv (8 oz)	450	31	16	455	15	29	1	0	—	640	—	—	—
Skillet Bananas Foster French Toast w/o Meat	1 serv (15 oz)	860	33	9	720	32	107	44	3	—	1270	—	—	—
Slam Belgian Waffle w/ Margarine w/o Syrup	1 serv (13 oz)	1030	77	27	715	30	50	2	2	—	1765	—	—	—
Slam Everyday Value w/ Bacon	1 serv (12 oz)	650	30	8	440	25	69	13	2	—	1660	—	—	—
Slam Everyday Value w/ Sausage	1 scrv (13 oz)	760	42	12	460	25	70	12	3	—	1750	—	—	—
Slam French Toast	1 serv (15 oz)	940	55	17	850	42	66	13	3	—	1780	—	—	—
Ultimate Omelette w/o Choices	1 serv (12 oz)	620	48	11	740	36	8	3	2	—	1170	—	—	—
CHILDREN'S MENU SELECTIONS														
Jr. Grand Slam	1 serv (5 oz)	380	19	6	235	15	39	7	2	—	1000	—	—	—
Oreo Blender Blaster	1 serv (12 oz)	680	33	17	90	12	88	65	3	—	450	—	—	—
Pancake Softball w/ Meat	1 serv (4 oz)	250	11	4	20	7	30	5	1	—	730	—	—	—
Pancakes Chocolate Chip-In	1 serv (7 oz)	450	18	7	25	11	61	17	3	—	1160	—	—	—
Pit Stop Pizza w/o Side	1 serv (8 oz)	590	26	6	35	23	70	4	5	—	890	—	—	—
Slam Dribblers	1 serv (6 oz)	410	11	3	10	9	74	41	2	—	750	—	—	—
Slap Shot Slider w/o Side	1 (4 oz)	310	15	6	60	20	22	3	1	—	470	—	—	—

FOOD	PORTION	CALS	FAT	SAT FAT	CHOL	PROT	CARB	SUGAR	FIBER	CALCI	SOD	POTAS	FOLIC	VIT C
Spaghetti Set Go w/o Side	1 serv (6 oz)	260	7	2	0	7	40	4	7	—	470	—	—	—
Track & Cheese w/o Side	1 serv (7 oz)	340	11	3	25	12	48	11	2	—	830	—	—	—
DESSERTS														
Apple Crisp A La Mode	1 serv (13 oz)	740	21	9	35	7	134	89	5	—	570	—	—	—
Blender Blaster Oreo	1 serv (14 oz)	890	44	20	105	15	113	77	3	—	580	—	—	—
Cake Carrot	1 serv (8 oz)	820	45	16	125	9	100	77	2	—	660	—	—	—
Cake Hershey's Chocolate	1 serv (5 oz)	580	28	15	40	6	75	55	2	—	400	—	—	—
Cheesecake New York Style	1 serv (7 oz)	640	41	26	195	9	58	44	0	—	350	—	—	—
Float Rootbeer or Cola	1 (16 oz)	430	17	9	65	6	69	63	0	—	120	—	—	—
Hot Fudge Brownie A La Mode	1 serv (9 oz)	830	37	18	65	9	122	95	4	—	520	—	—	—
Milkshake	1 (12 oz)	560	26	16	100	11	76	65	tr	—	272	—	—	—
Pie Apple	1 serv (7 oz)	480	22	9	0	4	67	35	3	—	580	—	—	—
Pie Chocolate Peanut Butter Silk	1 serv (6 oz)	680	47	24	70	8	59	39	4	—	400	—	—	—
Pie Coconut Cream	1 serv (7 oz)	630	39	24	0	6	65	43	1	—	370	—	—	—
Pie Cookies & Cream	1 serv (7 oz)	630	39	29	5	5	67	44	3	—	510	—	—	—
Pie French Silk	1 serv (5 oz)	770	57	30	105	6	59	38	2	—	400	—	—	—
Pie Key Lime	1 serv (7 oz)	560	20	8	25	9	87	68	0	—	320	—	—	—
Pie Lemon Meringue	1 serv (7 oz)	500	19	11	0	2	82	56	1	—	380	—	—	—
Pie Pecan	1 serv (7 oz)	730	36	12	110	7	98	36	2	—	740	—	—	—
Pie Pumpkin	1 serv (7 oz)	500	18	8	80	8	77	34	3	—	570	—	—	—
Sundae Oreo	1 (9 oz)	760	37	21	60	9	103	76	3	—	470	—	—	—
Sundae Single Scoop	1 (4 oz)	300	16	11	40	4	36	16	1	—	90	—	—	—
Topping Cherry	1 serv (2 oz)	57	0	0	0	0	14	12	0	—	3	—	—	—
Topping Chocolate	1 serv (2 oz)	133	1	0	0	2	34	32	1	—	109	—	—	—
Topping Fudge	1 serv (2 oz)	201	10	7	3	1	30	29	1	—	96	—	—	—
Topping Strawberry	1 serv (2 oz)	77	1	0	0	1	17	—	1	—	8	—	—	—
MAIN MENU SELECTIONS														
Basket Of Puppies w/o Syrup	10 pieces	520	11	2	0	11	94	16	3	—	1640	—	—	—
Burger Bacon Cheddar w/o Choices	1 (15 oz)	900	50	22	160	60	50	10	3	—	1850	—	—	—

FOOD	PORTION	CALS	FAT	SAT FAT	CHOL	PROT	CARB	SUGAR	FIBER	CALCI	SOD	POTAS	FOLIC	VIT C
Burger Classic & Fries	1 serv (19 oz)	1190	62	21	110	56	101	11	8	—	1190	—	—	—
Burger Fit Fare Veggie w/o Choice	1 (10 oz)	460	10	5	20	29	65	13	8	—	1040	—	—	—
Burger Mushroom Swiss w/o Choices	1 (18 oz)	880	49	22	130	50	56	13	4	—	1800	—	—	—
Burger Veggie w/ Dressing w/o Choices	1 (11 oz)	520	12	5	20	29	75	23	9	—	1250	—	—	—
Burger Western w/o Choice	1 (17 oz)	1120	61	24	130	51	73	17	6	—	1580	—	—	—
Cheeseburger Double w/o Choices	1 serv (23 oz)	1420	87	41	260	87	53	12	4	—	2720	—	—	—
Chicken Strips Sweet & Tangy BBQ w/o Dipping Sauce	1 serv (13 oz)	820	30	0	115	58	83	29	58	—	2160	—	—	—
Chicken Strips w/ Buffalo Sauce	1 serv (13 oz)	720	32	0	115	57	52	0	0	—	2780	—	—	—
Chicken Wings Sweet & Tangy BBQ	1 serv (8 oz)	450	18	5	185	35	40	38	1	—	1400	—	—	—
Chicken Wings w/ Buffalo Sauce	1 serv (8 oz)	330	20	5	185	34	3	2	1	—	1860	—	—	—
Chopped Steak Mushroom Swiss w/o Choices	1 serv (13 oz)	900	66	28	165	54	13	4	1	—	1890	—	—	—
Chopped Steak Spicy Cowboy w/o Choices	1 serv (15 oz)	1050	63	27	170	55	57	41	3	—	1700	—	—	—
Club Sandwich w/o Choices	1 (10 oz)	550	32	5	50	24	39	7	3	—	1530	—	—	—
Coleslaw	1 serv (5 oz)	260	22	4	35	2	15	12	3	—	520	—	—	—
Corn	1 serv (4 oz)	130	3	0	0	4	26	3	1	—	250	—	—	—
Cottage Cheese	1 serv (3 oz)	70	2	1	10	9	5	3	0	—	300	—	—	—
Country Fried Steak w/ Gravy	1 serv (13 oz)	990	65	23	75	52	54	0	6	—	2580	—	—	—
Dippable Veggies w/o Dressing	1 serv (2.5 oz)	30	0	0	0	0	5	3	1	—	70	—	—	—
Fiesta Corn	1 serv (4 oz)	100	0	0	0	3	21	4	3	—	45	—	—	—
Fit Fare Grilled Tilapia	1 serv (17 oz)	600	11	3	110	58	66	7	3	—	1560	—	—	—

FOOD	PORTION	CALS	FAT	SAT FAT	CHOL	PROT	CARB	SUGAR	FIBER	CALCI	SOD	POTAS	FOLIC	VIT C
Fit Fare Sweet & Tangy BBQ Chicken w/ Vegetables & Tomatoes	1 serv (13 oz)	640	14	4	180	75	56	32	2	—	1430	—	—	—
French Fries Salted	1 serv (5 oz)	430	23	5	0	5	50	0	5	—	95	—	—	—
Fried Shrimp Platter w/ Fries	1 serv (18 oz)	1050	59	11	150	27	109	24	13	—	2410	—	—	—
Garlic Dinner Bread	2 pieces	170	9	2	0	4	21	0	1	—	350	—	—	—
Green Beans	1 serv (3 oz)	25	0	0	0	1	4	2	2	—	10	—	—	—
Haddock Fillet w/o Bread	1 serv (20 oz)	1330	81	14	130	36	116	18	8	—	2100	—	—	—
Homestyle Meatloaf w/ Gravy	1 serv (7 oz)	600	46	17	200	4	14	33	0	—	1880	—	—	—
Lemon Pepper Tilapia w/o Choices	1 serv (13 oz)	640	27	14	160	55	39	3	2	—	1190	—	—	—
Mashed Potatoes Plain	1 serv (5 oz)	170	7	1	20	2	76	1	1	—	510	—	—	—
Mashed Potatoes Smoked Cheddar	1 serv (4 oz)	120	5	3	10	4	49	1	1	—	390	—	—	—
Mozzarella Sticks w/o Sauce	1 serv (8 oz)	560	20	17	185	38	58	4	2	—	2480	—	—	—
Onion Rings	1 serv (5 oz)	520	36	2	0	5	48	6	3	—	980	—	—	—
Quesadilla Cheese	1 (8 oz)	690	42	21	75	25	48	5	6	—	1300	—	—	—
Ranchero Tilapia w/o Bread	1 serv (19 oz)	450	15	5	120	54	56	4	4	—	1020	—	—	—
Sampler w/o Sauce	1 serv (17 oz)	1380	71	6	80	53	139	11	6	—	3710	—	—	—
Sandwich Bacon Lettuce & Tomato w/o Choices	1 (7 oz)	520	35	8	35	15	35	7	2	—	620	—	—	—
Sandwich Chicken Ranch Melt w/o Choices	1 serv (12 oz)	790	38	11	85	36	74	3	3	—	2640	—	—	—
Sandwich Fried Cheese Melt w/ Marinara Sauce w/o Choices	1 (12 oz)	830	40	17	75	36	82	8	3	—	2920	—	—	—
Sandwich Hickory Grilled Chicken w/o Choices	1 (15 oz)	1020	60	14	115	50	72	15	4	—	1530	—	—	—
Sandwich Patty Melt w/o Choices	1 (13 oz)	1040	73	29	160	50	41	10	4	—	2180	—	—	—

FOOD	PORTION	CALS	FAT	SAT FAT	CHOL	PROT	CARB	SUGAR	FIBER	CALCI	SOD	POTAS	FOLIC	VIT C
Sandwich Philly Melt Prime Rib w/o Choices	1 serv (13 oz)	670	36	11	75	35	52	5	3	—	1710	—	—	—
Sandwich Pulled BBQ Chicken w/ Coleslaw	1 serv (14 oz)	670	23	24	60	21	96	53	4	—	1680	—	—	—
Sandwich Smoked Chicken Melt w/o Choices	1 (12 oz)	840	45	14	105	38	72	11	3	—	1820	—	—	—
Sandwich Spicy Buffalo Chicken Melt w/o Choices	1 (15 oz)	860	48	12	70	32	76	3	3	—	3760	—	—	—
Sandwich The Super Bird w/o Choices	1 (11 oz)	620	31	10	65	35	52	6	4	—	2170	—	—	—
Seasoned Fries	1 serv (5 oz)	510	33	6	0	6	48	0	5	—	1010	—	—	—
Senior Country Fried Steak w/o Choices	1 serv (8 oz)	520	34	12	40	26	30	0	3	—	1460	—	—	—
Senior Grilled Chicken w/o Choices	1 serv (5 oz)	200	6	2	90	36	0	0	0	—	360	—	—	—
Senior Grilled Shrimp Skewer w/o Choices	1 serv (8 oz)	280	6	2	135	18	36	2	2	—	650	—	—	—
Senior Homestyle Meatloaf w/o Choices	1 serv (4 oz)	290	23	9	100	16	5	2	0	—	760	—	—	—
Senior Mini Burgers Bacon Cheddar w/o Choices	1 (11 oz)	720	39	19	115	41	46	7	2	—	1270	—	—	—
Senior Sandwich Club w/o Choices	1 (10 oz)	570	34	7	60	29	37	7	4	—	1340	—	—	—
Senior Sandwich Grilled Cheese Deluxe w/o Choices	1 (7 oz)	520	28	11	40	16	49	5	2	—	1430	—	—	—
Senior Slam French Toast w/ Egg	1 serv (5 oz)	300	14	4	280	13	29	5	1	—	550	—	—	—
Senior Starter w/o Choices	1 serv (3 oz)	210	19	6	230	9	1	0	1	—	290	—	—	—
Shrimp Breaded	6	190	8	2	70	9	20	5	2	—	750	—	—	—
Shrimp Grilled Skewer	1	90	4	1	135	14	1	0	0	—	160	—	—	—

FOOD	PORTION	CALS	FAT	SAT FAT	CHOL	PROT	CARB	SUGAR	FIBER	CALCI	SOD	POTAS	FOLIC	VIT C
Skillet Bacon Chipotle Chicken w/o Sides	1 serv (7 oz)	360	18	7	125	47	4	3	0	—	800	—	—	—
Skillet Prime Rib Premium	1 serv (21 oz)	850	46	15	540	41	64	9	7	—	2080	—	—	—
Skillet Santa Fe	1 serv (14 oz)	710	52	15	485	33	30	5	5	—	1490	—	—	—
Skillet Ultimate	1 serv (15 oz)	740	56	17	475	27	34	5	6	—	1470	—	—	—
Slamburger Bacon w/ Fries	1 serv (15 oz)	1030	59	24	350	57	61	9	2	—	1780	—	—	—
Smothered Cheese Fries	1 serv (10 oz)	860	53	17	65	21	75	3	7	—	990	—	—	—
Spinach Sauteed	1 serv (2 oz)	70	6	1	0	1	5	0	2	—	125	—	—	—
Spinach w/ Pico De Gallo	1 serv (3 oz)	110	8	2	5	3	6	1	2	—	260	—	—	—
T-Bone Steak w/o Choices	1 serv (12 oz)	640	42	14	135	59	6	0	0	—	1250	—	—	—
T-Bone Steak & Breaded Shrimp	1 serv (13 oz)	830	50	15	204	68	25	5	2	—	2000	—	—	—
T-Bone Steak & Shrimp Skewer	1 serv (12 oz)	730	46	15	270	73	6	0	0	—	1410	—	—	—
The Big Dipper w/ Salsa w/o Dipping Sauce	10 pieces	1230	50	23	85	50	145	13	14	—	1640	—	—	—
Three Dip & Chips	1 serv (12 oz)	560	25	11	70	19	72	5	7	—	1430	—	—	—
Tomatoes Slices	2	10	0	0	0	1	2	2	1	—	3	—	—	—
Tsing Tsing Chicken	1 serv (14 oz)	900	26	5	130	52	114	28	4	—	2760	—	—	—
Vegetable Rice Pilaf	1 serv (5 oz)	190	3	0	0	4	35	2	2	—	490	—	—	—
Wrap Buffalo Chicken	1 (14 oz)	830	28	7	65	40	108	5	8	—	2280	—	—	—
Zesty Nachos	1 serv (22 oz)	1340	61	29	210	62	140	10	12	—	2800	—	—	—
SALAD DRESSINGS AND TOPPINGS														
BBQ Sweet & Spicy	1 serv (1.5 oz)	110	0	0	0	0	30	0	1	—	470	—	—	0
Cherry Topping	1 serv (3 oz)	86	0	0	0	0	21	12	0	—	7	—	—	—
Croutons	1 serv (0.25 oz)	90	3	0	0	3	15	0	0	—	240	—	—	—
Dressing Bleu Cheese	1 serv (1 oz)	110	11	3	20	1	1	1	0	—	220	—	—	—
Dressing Caesar	1 serv (1 oz)	100	10	0	5	1	0	0	0	—	300	—	—	—
Dressing French	1 serv (1 oz)	74	5	0	7	0	8	4	0	—	248	—	—	—
Dressing Honey Mustard	1 serv (1 oz)	160	15	0	10	0	5	4	0	—	140	—	—	—
Dressing Italian Fat Free	1 serv (1 oz)	9	0	0	0	0	3	2	0	—	367	—	—	—
Dressing Ranch	1 serv (1 oz)	130	14	3	5	0	0	0	0	—	200	—	—	—

FOOD	PORTION	CALS	FAT	SAT FAT	CHOL	PROT	CARB	SUGAR	FIBER	CALCI	SOD	POTAS	FOLIC	VIT C
Dressing Ranch Fat Free	1 serv (1 oz)	25	0	0	0	0	5	1	1	—	230	—	—	—
Dressing Thousand Island	1 serv (1 oz)	107	10	0	14	0	5	4	0	—	275	—	—	—
Pico De Gallo	1 serv (3 oz)	21	0	0	0	1	5	3	1	—	125	—	—	—
Sour Cream	1 serv (1.5 oz)	91	9	—	19	1	2	0	0	—	23	—	—	—
Syrup Maple Flavored	3 tbsp (1.5 oz)	143	0	0	0	0	36	28	0	—	26	—	—	—
Syrup Sugar Free Maple	1 serv (1.5 oz)	23	0	0	0	0	9	1	0	—	71	—	—	—
Vinaigrette Balsamic Low Fat	1 serv (1 oz)	35	1	0	0	0	7	7	0	—	140	—	—	—
Whipped Margarine	1 tbsp	50	6	2	0	0	0	0	0	—	40	—	—	—
SALADS														
Cranberry Apple w/ Chicken w/o Dressing	1 serv (11 oz)	320	10	2	90	36	22	17	3	—	400	—	—	—
Deluxe Salad w/ Chicken Strips w/o Choices	1 serv (18 oz)	590	29	5	90	42	43	7	4	—	1180	—	—	—
Deluxe Salad w/ Grilled Chicken Breast w/o Choices	1 serv (17 oz)	340	13	6	110	44	13	7	4	—	530	—	—	—
Nacho	1 scrv (20 oz)	850	52	27	165	48	48	19	9	—	2140	—	—	—
SOUPS														
Broccoli & Cheddar	1 serv (12 oz)	370	16	10	40	9	48	14	7	—	1650	—	—	—
Chicken Noodle	1 serv (12 oz)	140	4	2	110	12	35	6	2	—	1150	—	—	—
Clam Chowder	1 serv (12 oz)	270	17	12	35	5	24	12	1	—	1840	—	—	—
Loaded Baked Potato	1 serv (12 oz)	310	23	11	45	5	22	5	2	—	1520	—	—	—
Vegetable Beef	1 serv (12 oz)	140	5	0	10	7	17	3	3	—	1290	—	—	—

DOMINO'S PIZZA

FOOD	PORTION	CALS	FAT	SAT FAT	CHOL	PROT	CARB	SUGAR	FIBER	CALCI	SOD	POTAS	FOLIC	VIT C
OTHER MENU SELECTIONS														
Breadsticks	8	870	50	10	0	17	89	4	3	—	780	—	—	—
Buffalo Chicken Kickers	1 serv	510	21	4	100	43	36	0	7	—	1410	—	—	—
Cheesy Bread	1 serv	930	51	17	50	28	91	5	3	—	1140	—	—	—
Chocolate Lava Crunch Cakes	2	690	34	20	130	8	93	62	3	—	340	—	—	—
Cinna Stix	8	940	49	9	0	16	109	24	4	—	690	—	—	—
PIZZA MEDIUM														
Deep Dish Marinara Cheese	⅛ pie	219	9	3	14	7	27	2	3	—	509	—	—	—

FOOD	PORTION	CALS	FAT	SAT FAT	CHOL	PROT	CARB	SUGAR	FIBER	CALCI	SOD	POTAS	FOLIC	VIT C
Hand Tossed Marinara Cheese	⅛ pie	190	7	3	16	7	25	2	1	—	405	—	—	—
Thin Crust Marinara Cheese	¼ pie	141	12	3	16	5	14	2	1	—	271	—	—	—
TOPPINGS FOR 1 MEDIUM PIZZA														
Anchovies	1 serv	110	8	0	45	13	63	0	0	—	3310	—	—	—
Bacon	1 serv	340	26	9	80	20	6	3	0	—	1260	—	—	—
Banana Peppers	1 serv	15	0	0	0	1	3	3	2	—	270	—	—	—
Beef	1 serv	300	26	11	65	16	0	0	—	—	570	—	—	—
Cheddar Cheese	1 serv	230	19	12	60	14	1	0	0	—	350	—	—	—
Cheese American	1 serv	310	26	16	80	16	3	2	0	—	1530	—	—	—
Cheese Provolone	1 serv	200	16	10	60	12	1	0	0	—	470	—	—	—
Chicken	1 serv	140	5	1	60	22	3	0	0	—	730	—	—	—
Chorizo	1 serv	90	4	2	30	12	1	1	0	—	600	—	—	—
Feta Cheese	1 serv	90	6	4	15	7	1	0	0	—	380	—	—	—
Garlic	1 serv	40	0	0	0	2	9	0	1	—	0	—	—	—
Green Chile Pepper	1 serv	10	0	0	0	1	3	1	2	—	10	—	—	—
Green Pepper	1 serv	10	0	0	0	0	3	2	1	—	0	—	—	—
Ham	1 serv	90	5	2	35	11	0	0	0	—	1020	—	—	—
Jalapenos	1 serv	15	0	0	0	1	3	3	2	—	960	—	—	—
Mushroom	1 serv	20	0	0	0	3	2	0	1	—	25	—	—	—
Olives Black	1 serv	100	10	2	0	1	2	0	2	—	410	—	—	—
Olives Green	1 serv	100	10	2	0	1	2	0	2	—	1250	—	—	—
Onion	1 serv	15	0	—	0	1	4	0	1	—	0	—	—	—
Parmesan Shredded	1 serv	170	12	8	35	13	1	0	0	—	460	—	—	—
Pepperoni	1 serv	240	21	8	50	11	0	—	0	—	1020	—	—	—
Philly Steak	1 serv	90	3	2	30	12	2	1	0	—	500	—	—	—
Pineapple	1 serv	60	0	0	0	0	16	14	1	—	10	—	—	—
Red Pepper Roasted	1 serv	10	0	0	0	1	2	1	1	—	95	—	—	—
Salami	1 serv	220	18	7	55	13	1	1	0	—	950	—	—	—
Sausage Italian	1 serv	350	30	11	55	12	9	4	0	—	1030	—	—	—
Spinach	1 serv	10	0	0	0	1	2	0	1	—	35	—	—	—
Tomato	1 serv	20	0	0	0	1	5	3	2	—	310	—	—	—
Wing Sauce	1 serv	10	0	0	0	0	2	1	1	—	920	—	—	—

DONATOS PIZZA

PIZZA

FOOD	PORTION	CALS	FAT	SAT FAT	CHOL	PROT	CARB	SUGAR	FIBER	CALCI	SOD	POTAS	FOLIC	VIT C
Hand Tossed Chicken Bacon Club	2 slices	780	46	—	—	29	61	—	5	—	—	—	—	—
Hand Tossed Chicken Spinach Mozzarella	2 slices	587	25	—	—	27	61	—	4	—	—	—	—	—

FOOD	PORTION	CALS	FAT	SAT FAT	CHOL	PROT	CARB	SUGAR	FIBER	CALCI	SOD	POTAS	FOLIC	VIT C
Hand Tossed Chicken Vegy Medley	2 slices	517	17	—	—	24	63	—	5	—	—	—	—	—
Hand Tossed Classic Trio	2 slices	640	30	—	—	27	66	—	6	—	—	—	—	—
Hand Tossed Founder's Favorite	2 slices	678	31	—	—	30	66	—	5	—	—	—	—	—
Hand Tossed Fresh Mozzarella Trio	2 slices	690	34	—	—	30	66	—	6	—	—	—	—	—
Hand Tossed Hawaiian	2 slices	578	22	—	—	26	69	—	6	—	—	—	—	—
Hand Tossed Margherita	2 slices	583	27	—	—	24	60	—	4	—	—	—	—	—
Hand Tossed Mariachi Beef	2 slices	591	24	—	—	24	68	—	5	—	—	—	—	—
Hand Tossed Mariachi Chicken	2 slices	617	24	—	—	28	68	—	5	—	—	—	—	—
Hand Tossed Pepperoni	2 slices	499	27	—	—	23	65	—	5	—	—	—	—	—
Hand Tossed Pepperoni Zinger	2 slices	645	30	—	—	27	65	—	5	—	—	—	—	—
Hand Tossed Serious Cheese	2 slices	597	25	—	—	27	65	—	5	—	—	—	—	—
Hand Tossed Serious Meat	2 slices	735	37	—	—	35	66	—	5	—	—	—	—	—
Hand Tossed Vegy	2 slices	550	19	—	—	22	70	—	6	—	—	—	—	—
Hand Tossed Works	2 slices	669	31	—	—	28	68	—	6	—	—	—	—	—
Thicker Crust Chicken Vegy Medley Large	¼ pie	580	20	—	—	34	66	—	5	—	—	—	—	—
Thicker Crust Founder's Favorite Large	¼ pie	780	36	—	—	43	70	—	5	—	—	—	—	—
Thicker Crust Hawaiian Large	¼ pie	680	26	—	—	37	76	—	6	—	—	—	—	—
Thicker Crust Mariachi Beef Large	¼ pie	710	31	—	—	36	73	—	6	—	—	—	—	—
Thicker Crust Mariachi Chicken Large	¼ pie	710	28	—	—	40	74	—	5	—	—	—	—	—
Thicker Crust Serious Meat Large	¼ pie	850	42	—	—	48	71	—	5	—	—	—	—	—

FOOD	PORTION	CALS	FAT	SAT FAT	CHOL	PROT	CARB	SUGAR	FIBER	CALCI	SOD	POTAS	FOLIC	VIT C
Thicker Crust The Works Large	¼ pie	770	35	—	—	39	74	—	6	—	—	—	—	—
Thicker Crust Vegy Large	¼ pie	630	23	—	—	31	75	—	7	—	—	—	—	—
Thin Crust Chicken Medley Vegy Large	¼ pie	497	20	—	—	31	51	—	3					
Thin Crust Classic Trio Large	¼ pie	674	37	—	—	35	52	—	3					
Thin Crust Founder's Favorite Large	¼ pie	702	38	—	—	39	52	—	2					
Thin Crust Hawaiian Large	¼ pie	588	27	—	—	32	56	—	4					
Thin Crust Mariachi Beef Large	¼ pie	630	32	—	—	32	55	—	3	—	—	—	—	—
Thin Crust Mariachi Chicken Large	¼ pie	639	30	—	—	35	56	—	3					
Thin Crust Pepperoni Large	¼ pie	627	34	—	—	32	50	—	2					
Thin Crust Serious Cheese Large	¼ pie	710	31	—	—	38	69	—	5					
Thin Crust Serious Meat Large	¼ pie	736	42	—	—	44	52	—	3	—	—	—	—	—
Thin Crust The Works	¼ pie	689	37	—	—	35	56	—	4	—	—	—	—	—
Thin Crust Vegy Large	¼ pie	544	24	—	—	26	57	—	4	—	—	—	—	—
SALAD DRESSINGS														
House Italian	1 serv (1.5 oz)	230	24	—	—	0	1	—	0	—	—	—	—	—
Italian Light	1 serv (1.5 oz)	20	1	—	—	0	2	—	0	—	—	—	—	—
Pizza Dip Chicken Bacon Ranch	1 serv (3 oz)	450	47	—	—	1	4	—	0	—	—	—	—	—
SALADS														
Chicken Harvest w/o Dressing Entree	1	540	32	—	—	32	32	—	6	—	—	—	—	—
Harvest Side	1 serv	81	3	—	—	1	13	—	2	—	—	—	—	—
Italian Chef w/o Dressing Entree	1	290	20	—	—	19	8	—	1	—	—	—	—	—
Italian Side w/o Dressing	1	110	7	—	—	7	3	—	1	—	—	—	—	—
SIDES AND SUBS														
3 Cheese Garlic Bread	2 pieces	174	9	—	—	8	16	—	1	—	—	—	—	—

FOOD	PORTION	CALS	FAT	SAT FAT	CHOL	PROT	CARB	SUGAR	FIBER	CALCI	SOD	POTAS	FOLIC	VIT C
Big Don White Italian	1	717	34	—	—	35	68	—	3	—	—	—	—	—
Breadsticks w/ Pizza Sauce	2	261	9	—	—	7	38	—	3					
Buffalo Wings Hot	5	597	48	—	—	34	11	—	0	—	—	—	—	—
Buffalo Wings Mild	5	618	48	—	—	34	13	—	0	—	—	—	—	—
Fresh Vegy Wheat	1	532	19	—	—	22	71	—	8	—	—	—	—	—
Stromboli 3 Meat	1	689	31	—	—	34	67	—	5	—	—	—	—	—
Stromboli Cheese	1	693	31	—	—	35	66	—	5	—	—	—	—	—
Stromboli Deluxe	1	613	25	—	—	28	68	—	5	—	—	—	—	—
Stromboli Pepperoni	1	716	34	—	—	34	67	—	5	—	—	—	—	—
Stromboli Vegy	1	606	24	—	—	27	69	—	5	—	—	—	—	—

DUNKIN' DONUTS

BAGELS

FOOD	PORTION	CALS	FAT	SAT FAT	CHOL	PROT	CARB	SUGAR	FIBER	CALCI	SOD	POTAS	FOLIC	VIT C
Blueberry	1	330	3	1	0	11	65	10	5	20	620	—	—	0
Cinnamon Raisin	1	330	4	1	0	11	65	13	5	20	450	—	—	0
Everything	1	350	5	1	0	13	66	5	5	60	660	—	—	0
Garlic	1	340	3	1	0	12	68	5	6	20	660	—	—	0
Multigrain	1	390	8	1	0	14	65	7	9	60	560	—	—	0
Onion	1	310	2	0	0	11	63	3	3	20	380	—	—	0
Plain	1	320	3	1	0	11	63	5	5	20	660	—	—	0
Poppy Seed	1	350	6	1	0	13	64	5	5	100	660	—	—	0
Salt	1	320	3	1	0	11	63	5	5	40	3420	—	—	0
Sesame	1	360	6	1	0	13	63	5	5	20	660	—	—	0
Wheat	1	320	4	0	0	12	61	4	5	20	550	—	—	0

BAKED SELECTIONS

FOOD	PORTION	CALS	FAT	SAT FAT	CHOL	PROT	CARB	SUGAR	FIBER	CALCI	SOD	POTAS	FOLIC	VIT C
Apple Fritter	1	400	15	6	0	5	63	22	2	40	530	—	—	0
Biscuit	1	280	14	8	0	5	32	2	1	40	620	—	—	0
Bismark Chocolate Iced	1	350	14	5	0	4	53	22	1	0	460	—	—	0
Brownie	1	430	23	5	55	3	56	47	1	0	260	—	—	0
Coffee Roll	1	370	18	7	0	5	49	17	2	20	510	—	—	0
Coffee Roll Chocolate Frosted	1	380	19	8	0	5	50	18	2	40	530	—	—	0
Coffee Roll Maple Frosted	1	380	18	8	0	5	50	19	2	20	520	—	—	0
Coffee Roll Vanilla Frosted	1	380	18	8	0	5	50	19	2	20	520	—	—	0
Cookie Chocolate Chunk	1	540	23	13	50	7	80	48	3	40	550	—	—	0
Cookie Oatmeal Raisin	1	480	14	7	40	8	83	51	5	40	310	—	—	0
Croissant Plain	1	310	16	7	0	7	35	4	1	40	350	—	—	0

FOOD	PORTION	CALS	FAT	SAT FAT	CHOL	PROT	CARB	SUGAR	FIBER	CALCI	SOD	POTAS	FOLIC	VIT C
Danish Apple Cheese	1	330	16	7	0	4	41	18	1	20	270	—	—	6
Danish Cheese	1	330	17	8	5	5	39	17	1	40	270	—	—	6
Danish Strawberry Cheese	1	320	16	7	0	4	40	18	1	20	260	—	—	6
Donut Apple Crumb	1	460	14	8	0	4	80	49	2	0	330	—	—	0
Donut Apple N' Spice	1	240	11	5	0	3	32	8	1	0	320	—	—	0
Donut Bavarian Kreme	1	250	12	5	0	3	31	9	1	0	330	—	—	0
Donut Blueberry Cake	1	330	18	8	25	3	38	19	1	60	460	—	—	0
Donut Blueberry Crumb	1	470	14	8	0	4	84	52	2	0	330	—	—	0
Donut Boston Kreme	1	280	12	5	0	3	38	16	1	0	350	—	—	0
Donut Bow Tie	1	310	15	7	0	4	39	15	1	0	400	—	—	0
Donut Chocolate Coconut	1	340	18	9	0	3	42	24	2	20	400	—	—	0
Donut Chocolate Frosted	1	340	19	8	25	3	38	19	1	20	330	—	—	0
Donut Chocolate Glazed Cake	1	280	15	7	0	3	33	16	1	20	400	—	—	0
Donut Chocolate Kreme Filled	1	310	16	7	0	4	37	17	1	0	340	—	—	0
Donut Cinnamon	1	290	18	8	25	3	30	12	1	20	310	—	—	0
Donut Double Chocolate Cake	1	290	16	7	0	3	34	17	1	20	410	—	—	0
Donut Glazed	1	220	9	4	0	3	31	12	1	0	320	—	—	0
Donut Glazed Cake	1	320	18	8	25	3	37	18	1	20	310	—	—	0
Donut Jelly Filled	1	260	11	5	0	3	36	6	1	0	330	—	—	0
Donut Maple Frosted	1	230	10	4	0	3	33	14	1	0	330	—	—	0
Donut Marble Frosted	1	230	10	4	0	3	32	13	1	0	330	—	—	0
Donut Old Fashioned	1	280	18	8	25	3	27	9	1	20	310	—	—	0
Donut Powdered	1	300	18	8	25	3	30	12	1	20	310	—	—	0
Donut Strawberry Frosted	1	230	10	4	0	3	33	14	1	0	330	—	—	0
Donut Sugar Raised	1	190	9	4	0	3	22	4	1	0	320	—	—	0
Donut Triple Chocolate	1	420	27	12	0	4	41	22	2	40	410	—	—	0
Donut Vanilla Kreme Filled	1	320	17	8	0	3	37	18	1	0	340	—	—	0

FOOD	PORTION	CALS	FAT	SAT FAT	CHOL	PROT	CARB	SUGAR	FIBER	CALCI	SOD	POTAS	FOLIC	VIT C
Eclair	1	350	14	5	0	4	53	22	1	0	460	—	—	0
English Muffin	1	160	2	0	0	6	31	2	2	100	340	—	—	0
French Cruller	1	250	20	9	35	2	18	10	0	0	105	—	—	0
Fritter Glazed	1	400	15	6	0	5	63	22	2	40	530	—	—	0
Muffin Blueberry	1	510	16	2	15	6	87	51	2	20	490	—	—	1
Muffin Blueberry Reduced Fat	1	450	10	2	15	6	86	45	2	20	670	—	—	1
Muffin Chocolate Chip	1	630	23	6	20	8	98	59	3	20	520	—	—	0
Muffin Coffee Cake	1	660	26	7	20	7	98	57	1	40	530	—	—	0
Muffin Corn	1	510	17	2	20	6	84	36	1	20	860	—	—	0
Muffin Cranberry Orange Low Fat	1	390	3	1	55	7	83	42	4	70	540	—	—	4
Muffin Honey Bran Raisin	1	500	14	2	15	7	86	48	5	80	450	—	—	0
Muffin Triple Chocolate	1	660	33	7	10	7	84	47	4	60	460	—	—	0
Munchkin Glazed Cake	1	60	3	2	5	1	8	4	0	0	65	—	—	0
Munchkins Cinnamon Cake	1	60	3	2	5	1	6	2	0	0	60	—	—	0
Munchkins Glazed	1	50	3	1	0	1	7	3	0	0	65	—	—	0
Munchkins Glazed Chocolate Cake	1	60	3	2	0	1	8	4	0	0	90	—	—	0
Munchkins Jelly Filled	1	60	3	1	0	1	8	1	0	0	65	—	—	0
Munchkins Plain Cake	1	50	3	2	5	1	5	2	0	0	60	—	—	0
Munchkins Powdered Cake	1	60	4	2	5	1	6	3	0	0	60	—	—	0
Munchkins Sugar Raised	1	40	3	1	0	1	5	1	0	0	65	—	—	0
Stick Cinnamon Cake	1	310	20	9	25	3	30	12	1	20	300	—	—	0
Stick Glazed Cake	1	340	20	9	25	3	38	20	1	20	300	—	—	0
Stick Glazed Chocolate Cake	1	390	25	11	0	3	40	17	2	20	540	—	—	0
Stick Jelly	1	400	20	9	25	3	54	20	1	20	320	—	—	0
Stick Plain Cake	1	300	20	9	25	3	26	9	1	20	300	—	—	0
Stick Powdered Cake	1	320	20	9	25	3	31	13	1	20	300	—	—	0
BEVERAGES														
Cappuccino	1 sm (10 oz)	80	4	3	15	4	7	7	0	100	70	—	—	0

FOOD	PORTION	CALS	FAT	SAT FAT	CHOL	PROT	CARB	SUGAR	FIBER	CALCI	SOD	POTAS	FOLIC	VIT C
Cappuccino Frozen w/ Skim Milk	1 sm (16 oz)	280	0	0	0	5	62	53	0	150	105	—	—	1
Cappuccino Frozen w/ Whole Milk	1 sm (16 oz)	300	4	3	15	5	61	53	0	150	105	—	—	1
Cappuccino w/ Sugar	1 sm (10 oz)	140	4	3	15	4	24	24	0	100	70	—	—	0
Coffee Blueberry	1 sm (10 oz)	15	0	0	0	0	2	0	0	0	5	—	—	0
Coffee Caramel	1 sm (10 oz)	10	0	0	0	0	2	0	0	0	5	—	—	0
Coffee Cinnamon	1 sm (10 oz)	15	0	0	0	0	2	0	0	0	5	—	—	0
Coffee Coconut	1 sm (10 oz)	10	0	0	0	0	1	0	0	0	5	—	—	0
Coffee French Vanilla	1 sm (10 oz)	10	0	0	0	0	1	0	0	0	5	—	—	0
Coffee Hazelnut	1 sm (10 oz)	10	0	0	0	0	1	0	0	0	5	—	—	0
Coffee Mocha	1 sm (10 oz)	110	0	0	0	1	26	23	1	0	20	—	—	0
Coffee Mocha w/ Cream	1 sm (10 oz)	170	6	4	20	2	27	23	1	20	30	—	—	0
Coffee Raspberry	1 sm (10 oz)	15	0	0	0	0	2	0	0	0	5	—	—	0
Coffee Regular	1 sm (10 oz)	5	0	0	0	0	1	0	0	0	5	—	—	0
Coffee Regular	1 extra lg	15	0	0	0	1	2	0	0	0	15	—	—	0
Coffee Regular	1 lg (20 oz)	10	0	0	0	1	2	0	0	0	15	—	—	0
Coffee Regular	1 med (14 oz)	10	0	0	0	1	1	0	0	0	10	—	—	0
Coffee Toasted Almond	1 sm (10 oz)	10	0	0	0	0	1	0	0	0	5	—	—	0
Coffee White Chocolate	1 sm (10 oz)	110	0	0	0	1	25	19	0	20	75	—	—	0
Coffee White Chocolate w/ Cream	1 sm (10 oz)	160	6	4	20	2	26	19	0	40	85	—	—	0
Coffee w/ Cream	1 sm (10 oz)	60	6	4	20	1	2	0	0	20	20	—	—	0
Coffee w/ Milk	1 sm (10 oz)	25	1	1	5	1	2	1	0	40	20	—	—	0
Coffee w/ Milk & Sugar	1 sm (10 oz)	80	1	1	5	1	20	19	0	40	20	—	—	0
Coffee w/ Skim Milk	1 sm (10 oz)	15	0	0	0	2	3	2	0	40	25	—	—	0
Coffee w/ Skim Milk & Splenda	1 sm (10 oz)	25	0	0	0	2	5	2	0	40	25	—	—	0
Coffee w/ Skim Milk & Sugar	1 sm (10 oz)	70	0	0	0	2	20	19	0	40	25	—	—	0
Coffee w/ Splenda	1 sm (10 oz)	15	0	0	0	0	3	0	0	0	5	—	—	0
Coffee w/ Sugar	1 sm (10 oz)	60	0	0	0	0	18	17	0	0	5	—	—	0
Coolatta Coffee w/ Cream	1 sm (16 oz)	400	23	14	80	3	49	43	0	100	75	—	—	1
Coolatta Coffee w/ Milk	1 sm (16 oz)	240	4	3	15	4	50	49	0	150	90	—	—	0

FOOD	PORTION	CALS	FAT	SAT FAT	CHOL	PROT	CARB	SUGAR	FIBER	CALCI	SOD	POTAS	FOLIC	VIT C
Coolatta Coffee w/ Skim Milk	1 sm (16 oz)	210	0	0	0	4	51	49	0	150	90	—	—	0
Coolatta Strawberry Fruit	1 sm (16 oz)	300	0	0	0	0	72	65	0	0	40	—	—	30
Coolatta Tropicana Orange	1 sm (16 oz)	220	0	0	0	1	52	50	0	0	35	—	—	54
Coolatta Vanilla Bean	1 sm (16 oz)	430	6	4	20	3	90	86	0	100	170	—	—	0
Dunkaccino	1 sm (10 oz)	230	11	9	10	2	35	24	1	40	190	—	—	0
Espresso	1 (1.75 oz)	0	0	0	0	0	0	0	0	0	0	—	—	0
Espresso w/ Sugar	1 (1.75 oz)	30	0	0	0	0	7	7	0	0	5	—	—	0
Hot Chocolate	1 sm (10 oz)	210	7	7	0	2	39	30	2	20	270	—	—	0
Iced Coffee	1 sm (16 oz)	10	0	0	0	1	2	0	0	0	5	—	—	0
Iced Coffee Mocha w/ Cream	1 sm (16 oz)	180	6	4	20	2	28	23	1	40	35	—	—	0
Iced Coffee White Chocolate w/ Cream	1 sm (16 oz)	170	6	4	20	2	27	19	1	40	85	—	—	0
Iced Coffee w/ Cream	1 sm (16 oz)	70	6	4	20	1	3	0	0	40	20	—	—	0
Iced Coffee w/ Cream & Sugar	1 sm (16 oz)	120	6	4	20	1	20	17	0	40	20	—	—	0
Iced Coffee w/ Milk	1 sm (16 oz)	30	1	1	5	2	3	1	0	40	20	—	—	0
Iced Coffee w/ Milk & Sugar	1 sm (16 oz)	90	1	1	5	2	21	19	0	40	20	—	—	0
Iced Coffee w/ Skim Milk	1 sm (16 oz)	20	0	0	0	2	2	2	0	40	25	—	—	0
Iced Coffee w/ Skim Milk & Sugar	1 sm (16 oz)	80	0	0	0	2	21	19	0	40	25	—	—	0
Iced Coffee w/ Sugar	1 sm (16 oz)	70	0	0	0	1	19	17	0	0	5	—	—	0
Iced Latte	1 sm (16 oz)	120	6	4	25	6	10	10	0	200	105	—	—	0
Iced Latte Caramel Swirl	1 sm (16 oz)	220	6	4	25	8	35	34	0	250	150	—	—	1
Iced Latte Caramel Swirl w/ Skim Milk	1 sm (16 oz)	180	0	0	0	9	36	35	0	250	150	—	—	1
Iced Latte Lite	1 med (24 oz)	120	0	0	0	10	19	15	0	300	170	—	—	1
Iced Latte Mocha Swirl	1 sm (16 oz)	220	6	4	25	7	35	32	1	200	115	—	—	0
Iced Latte Mocha Swirl w/ Skim Milk	1 sm (16 oz)	180	0	0	0	8	36	32	1	200	125	—	—	0

FOOD	PORTION	CALS	FAT	SAT FAT	CHOL	PROT	CARB	SUGAR	FIBER	CALCI	SOD	POTAS	FOLIC	VIT C
Iced Latte w/ Skim Milk	1 sm (16 oz)	70	0	0	0	7	11	10	0	200	110	—	—	0
Iced Latte w/ Skim Milk & Sugar	1 sm (16 oz)	130	0	0	0	7	28	27	0	200	110	—	—	0
Iced Latte w/ Sugar	1 sm (16 oz)	170	7	4	25	6	27	27	0	200	100	—	—	0
Latte	1 sm (10 oz)	120	6	4	25	6	10	10	0	200	105	—	—	0
Latte Caramel Swirl	1 sm (10 oz)	220	6	4	25	8	35	34	0	250	150	—	—	1
Latte Lite	1 sm (10 oz)	80	0	0	0	7	13	10	0	200	110	—	—	0
Latte Lite Vanilla	1 sm (10 oz)	90	0	0	0	7	14	10	0	200	110	—	—	0
Latte Mocha Raspberry	1 med (16 oz)	340	9	6	35	10	54	48	2	250	160	—	—	1
Latte Mocha Spice	1 med (16 oz)	330	9	6	35	10	53	48	2	250	140	—	—	1
Latte Mocha Swirl	1 sm (10 oz)	220	6	4	25	7	35	32	1	200	115	—	—	0
Latte w/ Sugar	1 sm (10 oz)	170	6	4	25	6	27	27	0	200	100	—	—	0
Latte White Chocolate	1 med (16 oz)	320	9	6	40	9	50	43	0	300	250	—	—	1
Tea Regular Or Decaffeinated	1 (10 oz)	0	0	0	0	0	0	0	0	0	5	—	—	0
Tea w/ Milk	1 (10 oz)	20	1	1	5	1	1	1	0	40	20	—	—	0
Tea w/ Milk & Sugar	1 (10 oz)	80	1	1	5	1	19	19	0	40	20	—	—	0
Tea w/ Skim Milk	1 (10 oz)	10	0	0	0	1	2	2	0	40	20	—	—	0
Tea w/ Skim Milk & Sugar	1 (10 oz)	70	0	0	0	1	19	19	0	40	20	—	—	0
Tea w/ Sugar	1 (10 oz)	60	0	0	0	0	17	17	0	0	5	—	—	0
Turbo Shot	1 sm (1.75 oz)	0	0	0	0	0	0	0	0	0	0	—	—	0
CREAM CHEESE														
Blueberry Reduced Fat	1 serv (1.75 oz)	150	9	6	25	2	15	11	0	20	210	—	—	0
Onion & Chive Reduced Fat	1 serv (1.75 oz)	130	11	7	35	3	6	3	0	60	250	—	—	1
Plain	1 serv (1.75 oz)	150	15	9	40	3	3	3	0	40	250	—	—	0
Plain Reduced Fat	1 serv (1.75 oz)	100	8	5	25	4	5	2	0	60	250	—	—	0
Salmon Reduced Fat	1 serv (1.75 oz)	140	11	7	35	4	6	3	0	60	260	—	—	4
Strawberry Reduced Fat	1 serv (1.75 oz)	150	10	6	30	2	15	11	0	40	200	—	—	0
Veggie Reduced Fat	1 serv (1.75 oz)	120	10	6	30	2	6	2	0	40	240	—	—	5
SANDWICHES														
Bagel Bacon Egg Cheese	1	510	17	6	195	23	66	7	5	150	1340	—	—	0
Bagel Egg Cheese	1	470	14	5	195	20	66	7	5	150	1160	—	—	0
Bagel Ham Egg Cheese	1	510	16	6	215	26	67	7	5	150	1470	—	—	0

FOOD	PORTION	CALS	FAT	SAT FAT	CHOL	PROT	CARB	SUGAR	FIBER	CALCI	SOD	POTAS	FOLIC	VIT C
Bagel Sausage Egg Cheese	1	640	29	10	240	27	67	7	5	150	1560	—	—	0
Biscuit Egg Cheese	1	430	26	13	195	13	36	4	1	150	1110	—	—	0
Biscuit Sausage Egg Cheese	1	610	40	18	240	20	36	4	1	150	1510	—	—	0
Croissant Bacon Egg Cheese	1	510	31	13	195	19	39	6	2	150	1030	—	—	0
Croissant Egg Cheese	1	470	28	12	195	15	39	6	2	150	850	—	—	0
Croissant Ham Egg Cheese	1	510	30	12	215	21	39	6	2	150	1150	—	—	0
Croissant Original Chicken	1	640	35	13	55	26	53	9	2	200	1200	—	—	0
English Muffin Bacon Egg Cheese	1	360	16	6	195	18	34	3	2	200	1020	—	—	1
English Muffin Egg Cheese	1	320	13	5	195	15	34	3	2	200	840	—	—	1
English Muffin Egg White & Cheese	1	270	5	3	10	16	34	3	2	200	850	—	—	1
English Muffin Ham Egg Cheese	1	360	15	6	215	21	35	3	2	200	1110	—	—	1
English Muffin Ham Egg White & Cheese	1	310	7	4	30	22	34	3	2	200	1150	—	—	1
English Muffin Sausage Egg Cheese	1	490	28	10	240	22	35	3	2	200	1240	—	—	1
English Muffin Wheat Egg White & Cheese	1	260	6	3	10	15	33	3	2	150	870	—	—	0
English Muffin Wheat Ham Egg White & Cheese	1	300	8	4	30	21	33	3	2	150	1180	—	—	0
Flatbread Egg White Turkey	1	280	6	3	20	19	37	5	3	150	820	—	—	2
Flatbread Egg White Veggie	1	290	9	4	20	11	39	4	3	200	680	—	—	6
Flatbread Grilled Cheese	1	380	18	9	45	16	35	2	1	400	850	—	—	0
Flatbread Ham & Cheese	1	320	11	5	40	20	34	2	1	250	960	—	—	0
Flatbread Turkey Cheddar & Bacon	1	410	20	7	50	21	36	2	1	200	1110	—	—	0
Pressed Cuban	1	680	33	13	120	46	50	6	2	300	2000	—	—	0

FOOD	PORTION	CALS	FAT	SAT FAT	CHOL	PROT	CARB	SUGAR	FIBER	CALCI	SOD	POTAS	FOLIC	VIT C
SOUPS														
Broccoli Cheddar	1 serv (8 oz)	190	11	6	35	10	14	5	2	250	990	—	—	42
Chicken Noodle	1 serv (8 oz)	130	3	1	45	7	19	1	1	20	970	—	—	1
EINSTEIN BROS BAGELS														
BAGELS AND BREADS														
Bagel Asiago Cheese	1 (4 oz)	310	5	3	15	14	56	5	2	200	630	—	—	0
Bagel Black Russian	1 (3.9 oz)	280	4	0	0	11	57	4	3	40	520	—	—	5
Bagel Blueberry	1 (3.8 oz)	300	1	0	0	10	65	11	3	20	480	—	—	0
Bagel Chocolate Chip	1 (3.8 oz)	290	3	1	0	9	58	10	3	20	430	—	—	0
Bagel Cinnamon Raisin	1 (3.8 oz)	290	1	0	0	10	63	13	3	40	450	—	—	0
Bagel Cinnamon Sugar	1 (3.9 oz)	290	3	1	0	9	63	12	2	40	480	—	—	0
Bagel Cranberry	1 (3.8 oz)	270	1	0	0	9	60	12	2	20	420	—	—	0
Bagel Croutons	1 serv (1 oz)	90	5	1	0	2	12	1	0	0	250	—	—	0
Bagel Egg	1 (3.5 oz)	300	5	2	120	12	54	6	2	40	490	—	—	0
Bagel Everything	1 (3.7 oz)	270	2	0	0	9	56	5	2	20	620	—	—	0
Bagel Garlic	1 (3.7 oz)	270	3	0	0	9	56	5	2	20	460	—	—	0
Bagel Green Chili	1 (5.4 oz)	350	8	5	25	15	58	6	2	200	680	—	—	12
Bagel Honey Whole Wheat	1 (3.6 oz)	260	1	0	0	9	57	8	3	20	440	—	—	0
Bagel Onion	1 (3.7 oz)	270	1	0	0	9	59	5	2	20	460	—	—	0
Bagel Plain	1 (3.5 oz)	260	1	0	0	9	56	5	2	20	460	—	—	0
Bagel Poppy	1 (3.7 oz)	280	3	0	0	9	56	5	2	20	460	—	—	0
Bagel Potato	1 (3.5 oz)	270	4	1	0	8	52	5	2	20	500	—	—	0
Bagel Power	1 (4 oz)	310	5	1	0	11	61	16	4	40	280	—	—	0
Bagel Pumpernickel	1 (3.5 oz)	240	2	0	0	9	53	4	3	40	490	—	—	5
Bagel Salt	1 (3.7 oz)	260	1	0	0	9	56	5	2	20	1850	—	—	0
Bagel Sesame	1 (3.7 oz)	280	3	0	0	10	56	5	2	20	460	—	—	0
Bagel Six Cheese	1 (4.3 oz)	330	6	4	15	15	56	5	2	200	650	—	—	0
Bagel Spinach Florentine	1 (4.7 oz)	340	8	4	20	15	57	5	2	200	590	—	—	4
Bagel Poppers Cinnamon Sugar	1 (5 oz)	450	9	2	0	10	85	29	4	40	600	—	—	12
Bagel Poppers Pretzel w/ Nacho Cheese	1 (5 oz)	320	8	2	5	9	55	6	2	20	1240	—	—	0
Bagel Poppers Sweet Cream Cheese	1 (6 oz)	440	7	2	5	10	85	30	3	20	570	—	—	9
Bagel Thin Singles Everything	1 (2 oz)	150	2	0	0	4	25	2	1	0	390	—	—	1

FOOD	PORTION	CALS	FAT	SAT FAT	CHOL	PROT	CARB	SUGAR	FIBER	CALCI	SOD	POTAS	FOLIC	VIT C
Bagel Thin Singles Honey Whole Wheat	1 (2 oz)	140	2	0	0	5	27	4	4	20	230	—	—	0
Bagel Thin Singles Plain	1 (2 oz)	140	1	0	0	4	25	2	1	0	240	—	—	1
Bread Ciabatta	1 serv (4.25 oz)	300	4	0	0	0	58	1	2	0	640	—	—	0
Pizza Bagel Pepperoni	1 (6 oz)	450	15	9	45	23	59	7	3	350	1090	—	—	2
Roll Challah	1 (2.75 oz)	210	3	1	10	8	39	5	1	20	260	—	—	6
BEVERAGES														
Americano	1 reg (12 oz)	0	0	0	0	0	0	0	0	0	0	—	—	0
Barq's Root Beer	1 reg (20 oz)	260	0	0	0	0	75	75	0	0	120	—	—	0
Cafe Latte Nonfat Milk	1 reg (12 oz)	100	0	0	0	11	15	15	0	400	160	—	—	4
Cafe Latte Reduced Fat Milk	1 reg (12 oz)	150	7	4	25	10	15	15	0	400	160	—	—	4
Cappuccino	1 reg (12 oz)	140	8	5	25	7	11	11	0	250	100	—	—	0
Cappuccino Nonfat Milk	1 reg (12 oz)	70	0	0	5	8	11	11	0	350	115	—	—	2
Cappuccino Reduced Fat Milk	1 reg (12 oz)	90	4	2	15	6	9	8	0	200	95	—	—	1
Chai Tea Latte	1 reg (12 oz)	230	3	2	10	3	47	45	0	100	55	—	—	0
Chai Tea Latte Nonfat Milk	1 reg (12 oz)	210	0	0	0	3	47	45	0	100	65	—	—	1
Chai Tea Latte Reduced Fat Milk	1 reg (12 oz)	220	2	1	5	3	47	45	0	100	65	—	—	1
Coca-Cola	1 reg (20 oz)	230	0	0	0	0	65	65	0	0	75	—	—	0
Coca-Cola Cherry	1 reg (20 oz)	250	0	0	0	0	70	70	0	0	60	—	—	0
Coffee Black All Sizes	1	0	0	0	0	0	0	0	0	0	0	—	—	0
Diet Coke	1 reg (20 oz)	0	0	0	0	0	0	0	0	0	70	—	—	0
Espresso Single	1 (2 oz)	0	0	0	0	0	0	0	0	0	0	—	—	0
Fanta Orange	1 (20 oz)	270	0	0	0	0	73	73	0	0	90	—	—	0
Frozen Blended Cafe Caramel	1 (18 oz)	520	9	3	45	8	100	66	0	250	140	—	—	0
Frozen Blended Cafe Mocha	1 (18 oz)	510	8	3	40	7	102	64	0	250	160	—	—	0
Frozen Blended Strawberry	1 (18 oz)	450	19	14	65	6	75	64	3	150	95	—	—	96
Frozen Blended Wild Berry	1 (18 oz)	350	3	2	5	5	77	62	5	200	90	—	—	114
Half & Half	1 oz	40	3	2	15	1	1	1	0	40	25	—	—	0
Hi-C Fruit Punch	1 (20 oz)	270	0	0	0	0	74	74	0	0	44	—	—	60
Hot Chocolate	1 reg (12 oz)	270	8	5	25	11	37	36	1	400	330	—	—	4

FOOD	PORTION	CALS	FAT	SAT FAT	CHOL	PROT	CARB	SUGAR	FIBER	CALCI	SOD	POTAS	FOLIC	VIT C
Hot Chocolate Nonfat Milk	1 reg (12 oz)	220	2	1	5	12	37	36	1	400	330	—	—	4
Iced Americano	1 med	0	0	0	0	0	0	0	0	0	0	—	—	0
Iced Coffee	1 med	0	0	0	0	0	0	0	0	0	0	—	—	0
Iced Latte	1 med (12 oz)	110	6	4	20	6	9	9	0	200	80	—	—	0
Iced Latte Nonfat Milk	1 med (16 oz)	60	0	0	0	7	9	9	0	250	100	—	—	2
Iced Latte Reduced Fat Milk	1 med (16 oz)	90	4	3	15	6	9	9	0	250	95	—	—	2
Iced Mocha	1 med (16 oz)	220	6	4	15	5	37	32	0	200	100	—	—	0
Iced Mocha Nonfat Milk	1 med (16 oz)	180	0	0	0	6	39	33	0	200	120	—	—	2
Iced Mocha Reduced Fat Milk	1 med (16 oz)	200	4	2	15	5	39	33	0	200	115	—	—	2
Macchiato Caramel	1 reg (12 oz)	300	8	5	25	9	49	43	0	300	180	—	—	5
Macchiato Caramel Nonfat Milk	1 reg (12 oz)	260	0	0	5	10	55	50	0	300	210	—	—	2
Macchiato Caramel Reduced Fat Milk	1 reg (12 oz)	290	5	3	20	8	55	50	0	300	200	—	—	2
Minute Maid Lemonade Lite	1 reg (20 oz)	40	0	0	0	0	10	5	0	0	38	—	—	0
Mocha	1 reg (12 oz)	260	9	5	25	8	37	32	0	300	135	—	—	0
Mocha Nonfat Milk	1 reg (12 oz)	180	0	0	5	9	37	32	0	300	160	—	—	2
Mocha Reduced Fat Milk	1 reg (12 oz)	220	5	3	20	8	37	32	0	300	150	—	—	2
Nestea Iced Tea Unsweetened	1 reg (20 oz)	0	0	0	0	0	0	0	0	0	38	—	—	0
Pibb Xtra	1 reg (20 oz)	250	0	0	0	0	65	65	0	0	70	—	—	0
Skim Milk	8 oz	80	0	0	5	7	15	13	0	250	140	—	—	1
Sprite	1 reg (20 oz)	230	0	0	0	0	63	63	0	0	108	—	—	0
Whole Milk	8 oz	150	8	5	25	8	11	11	0	300	100	—	—	0
DESSERTS														
Cinnamon Twist	1 (4 oz)	370	18	7	0	5	20	19	2	40	10	—	—	0
Coffee Cake Apple Cinnamon	1 serv (7 oz)	700	28	10	5	5	108	57	1	80	280	—	—	1
Coffee Cake Chocolate Chip	1 serv (6.4 oz)	800	36	14	5	6	114	62	3	80	270	—	—	1
Coffee Cake Mixed Berry	1 serv (7 oz)	710	29	10	5	5	110	59	2	80	270	—	—	1
Cookie Chocolate Chip	1 (2.75 oz)	360	18	9	15	4	48	29	2	20	290	—	—	0

FOOD	PORTION	CALS	FAT	SAT FAT	CHOL	PROT	CARB	SUGAR	FIBER	CALCI	SOD	POTAS	FOLIC	VIT C
Cookie Chocolate Mudslide	1 (2.8 oz)	320	17	9	60	4	46	38	1	20	75	—	—	0
Cookie Iced Sugar	1 (3.7 oz)	480	15	7	25	4	80	51	1	0	260	—	—	0
Cookie Oatmeal Raisin	1 (3 oz)	320	11	5	25	5	54	31	2	20	310	—	—	0
Marshmallow Crispy Treat	1 (4 oz)	410	7	2	0	5	86	37	0	0	125	—	—	9
Muffin Blueberry	1 (5 oz)	480	23	3	100	7	64	35	1	60	500	—	—	0
Muffin Double Chocolate	1 (5 oz)	440	24	3	90	7	54	32	2	60	510	—	—	0
Muffin Strawberry White Chocolate	1 (6 oz)	500	22	5	85	6	71	44	1	60	460	—	—	0
Strudel Cinnamon Walnut	1 piece (6 oz)	640	35	15	70	10	72	26	4	100	440	—	—	12
SALAD DRESSINGS														
Caesar	1 serving (3 oz)	410	44	7	25	3	3	3	0	0	960	—	—	0
Vinaigrette Chipotle	1 serv (3 oz)	290	26	4	0	0	13	11	1	40	1180	—	—	5
Vinaigrette Raspberry	1 serv (3 oz)	410	44	7	25	3	3	3	0	0	960	—	—	0
SALADS														
Bros Bistro	1 (10.5 oz)	820	68	11	25	15	37	29	7	300	520	—	—	21
Bros Bistro Half	1 serv (5.3 oz)	410	34	5	15	7	19	15	3	150	160	—	—	12
Bros Bistro w/ Chicken	1 (14.5 oz)	950	71	12	115	39	39	29	7	300	1080	—	—	24
Bros Bistro w/ Chicken Half	1 serv (7.3 oz)	470	36	6	55	20	19	14	4	150	540	—	—	12
Caesar	1 (9.5 oz)	600	53	11	40	13	22	5	4	250	1410	—	—	21
Caesar Half	1 serv (4.5 oz)	280	25	5	20	6	8	2	2	100	640	—	—	12
Caesar w/ Chicken	1 (14 oz)	730	56	12	130	38	23	5	4	250	1980	—	—	24
Caesar w/ Chicken Half	1 (6.5 oz)	340	27	6	65	18	9	2	2	100	930	—	—	12
Chipotle	1 (11.7 oz)	590	37	8	20	13	52	14	11	250	1480	—	—	36
Chipotle Half	1 serv (5.8 oz)	290	19	4	10	7	26	7	5	150	740	—	—	18
Chipotle w/ Chicken Half	1 serv (7.8 oz)	360	20	5	55	19	27	7	5	150	1020	—	—	18
Chipotle w/ Chicken	1 (15.7 oz)	720	41	9	110	38	54	15	11	300	2040	—	—	36
Fruit	1 (11 oz)	140	0	0	0	2	36	30	3	40	25	—	—	96
Fruit Cup	1 (5 oz)	60	0	0	0	1	16	14	2	20	10	—	—	48
Potato	1 serv (3 oz)	160	12	3	10	1	13	1	1	0	360	—	—	2
SANDWICHES														
Bagel Asiago Tasty Turkey	1 (13 oz)	540	18	10	90	37	66	9	4	250	1450	—	—	12
Bagel Dogs Asiago	1 (7 oz)	550	28	12	55	21	56	5	2	60	1360	—	—	0
Bagel Dogs Chicken Apple	1 (5 oz)	290	13	4	0	17	30	6	1	20	850	—	—	2

FOOD	PORTION	CALS	FAT	SAT FAT	CHOL	PROT	CARB	SUGAR	FIBER	CALCI	SOD	POTAS	FOLIC	VIT C
Bagel Dogs Original	1 (7 oz)	540	27	11	50	20	56	5	2	20	1320	—	—	0
Bagel Thin Asparagus Mushroom & Swiss	1 (6 oz)	290	13	5	25	18	30	5	5	250	590	—	—	1
Bagel Thin BLT w/ Avocado	1 (7 oz)	400	25	5	30	11	35	7	7	40	730	—	—	12
Bagel Thin Panini Bacon & Cheese	1 (6 oz)	400	20	11	60	26	31	4	4	300	870	—	—	0
Bagel Thin Tuna	1 (8 oz)	320	16	3	30	22	32	7	5	80	650	—	—	12
Bagel Thin Turkey	1 (8 oz)	270	6	3	50	25	32	5	2	40	1010	—	—	9
Bagel Thin Turkey Sausage w/ Salsa	1 (6 oz)	240	6	1	30	19	30	6	4	20	650	—	—	0
Breakfast Wrap Sante Fe	1 (12 oz)	720	37	15	445	37	60	8	6	600	1400	—	—	2
Breakfast Wrap Spicy Elmo	1 (11 oz)	720	40	17	435	34	56	6	6	700	1050	—	—	9
Challah Club Mex	1 (11 oz)	740	48	11	105	36	44	8	2	150	1610	—	—	21
Deli Albacore Tuna Salad	1 (9 oz)	390	12	2	25	30	50	7	4	60	710	—	—	18
Deli Chicken Salad	1 (10 oz)	480	17	3	75	29	56	12	6	40	780	—	—	12
Deli Ham	1 (11 oz)	610	31	8	75	29	56	9	4	150	920	—	—	18
Deli Open Face Melts Ham & Swiss	1 (9 oz)	480	15	8	80	33	60	8	3	400	630	—	—	9
Deli Open Face Melts Turkey & Cheddar	1 (9 oz)	490	15	8	75	37	58	6	3	300	1400	—	—	6
Deli Turkey Breast	1 (11 oz)	590	29	7	70	34	53	7	4	200	1550	—	—	18
Egg Bacon & Cheddar	1 (9 oz)	590	25	11	410	34	59	8	2	300	1060	—	—	0
Egg Cheese Only	1 (8 oz)	510	20	9	395	29	58	7	2	300	810	—	—	0
Egg Ham & Swiss	1 (10 oz)	550	20	9	415	36	59	8	2	350	780	—	—	0
Egg Nova Lox & Bagel	1 (9 oz)	480	18	9	—	23	62	10	3	40	930	—	—	6
Egg Spinach Mushroom & Swiss	1 (10 oz)	60	24	10	395	31	61	8	3	400	940	—	—	9
Egg Turkey Sausage & Cheddar	(10 oz)	580	24	10	425	37	59	8	2	300	990	—	—	0
Egg Paninis Southwest Turkey Sausage	1 (12 oz)	680	29	12	435	32	64	5	4	400	1360	—	—	12
Egg Paninis Spinach & Bacon	1 (12 oz)	830	47	16	435	31	65	4	5	500	1610	—	—	9

FOOD	PORTION	CALS	FAT	SAT FAT	CHOL	PROT	CARB	SUGAR	FIBER	CALCI	SOD	POTAS	FOLIC	VIT C
Nova Lox & Bagel	1 (9 oz)	480	18	9	45	23	62	10	3	40	930	—	—	6
Panini Italian Chicken	1 (13 oz)	820	41	13	135	38	65	3	5	300	2510	—	—	30
Panini Turkey Club	1 (13 oz)	790	41	11	100	34	66	5	6	300	2200	—	—	12
Wrap California Chicken	1 (16 oz)	720	35	11	130	38	66	7	9	350	1330	—	—	15
Wrap Chipotle Turkey	1 (13 oz)	750	38	13	85	35	71	12	9	450	2030	—	—	15
Wrap Turkey Tornado	1 (7 oz)	270	4	0	35	15	33	4	5	200	760	—	—	9
SOUPS														
Broccoli Cheese	1 cup (8.75 oz)	290	21	12	55	13	15	5	2	250	1190	—	—	36
Chicken Noodle	1 cup (8.75 oz)	120	4	0	15	9	13	1	2	20	950	—	—	2
Turkey Chili	1 cup (8.75 oz)	170	5	0	25	15	17	5	5	100	890	—	—	15
SPREADS														
Butter Blend	1 serv (1 oz)	170	18	5	0	0	0	0	0	0	220	—	—	0
Cream Cheese Light Whipped Plain	1 serv (1.25 oz)	80	6	4	20	3	4	3	2	60	200	—	—	0
Cream Cheese Onion & Chive	1 serv (1.25 oz)	120	11	7	35	7	5	2	0	0	105	—	—	0
Cream Cheese Plain	1 serv (1.25 oz)	120	12	8	35	2	2	2	0	0	115	—	—	0
Cream Cheese Reduced Fat Blueberry	1 serv (1.25 oz)	120	9	6	25	2	11	9	0	0	90	—	—	0
Cream Cheese Reduced Fat Garden Vegetable	1 serv (1.25 oz)	110	9	6	25	2	5	2	0	40	180	—	—	2
Cream Cheese Reduced Fat Garlic Herb	1 serv (1.25 oz)	110	9	6	25	2	5	2	0	0	180	—	—	0
Cream Cheese Reduced Fat Honey Almond	1 serv (1.25 oz)	120	9	5	25	2	11	7	0	40	80	—	—	0
Cream Cheese Reduced Fat Jalapeno Salsa	1 serv (1.25 oz)	110	9	6	25	2	5	2	0	0	190	—	—	0
Cream Cheese Reduced Fat Plain	1 serv (1.25 oz)	110	9	6	25	2	4	2	0	0	180	—	—	0
Cream Cheese Reduced Fat Strawberry	1 serv (1.25 oz)	120	9	6	25	2	9	7	0	0	90	—	—	0

FOOD	PORTION	CALS	FAT	SAT FAT	CHOL	PROT	CARB	SUGAR	FIBER	CALCI	SOD	POTAS	FOLIC	VIT C
Cream Cheese Reduced Fat Sundried Tomato Basil	1 serv (1.25 oz)	110	9	6	0	2	4	2	0	0	180	—	—	0
Cream Cheese Smoked Salmon	1 serv (1.25 oz)	110	11	6	35	2	4	2	0	0	210	—	—	0
Honey Butter	1 serv (1 oz)	140	12	4	0	0	8	7	0	0	140	—	—	0
Hummus	1 serv (1 oz)	70	3	0	0	4	6	0	4	0	150	—	—	0
Mayo Ancho	1 serv Ancho	310	33	5	25	0	1	1	0	0	260	—	—	0
Mustard Creamy	1 serv (1.5 oz)	270	29	5	20	0	2	1	0	0	220	—	—	1
Mustard Deli	1 tsp (5 g)	5	0	0	0	0	0	0	0	0	65	—	—	1
Mustard Yellow	1 tbsp (5 g)	0	0	0	0	0	0	0	0	0	80	—	—	0
Peanut Butter Creamy	1 serv (2 oz)	330	28	6	5	14	12	5	4	20	260	—	—	0
Salsa Ancho Lime	1 serv (1.5 oz)	20	1	0	0	0	3	2	0	0	470	—	—	0
Spicy Roasted Tomato	1 serv (1.5 oz)	210	22	4	20	1	4	1	1	0	330	—	—	1

EL POLLO LOCO

DESSERTS

FOOD	PORTION	CALS	FAT	SAT FAT	CHOL	PROT	CARB	SUGAR	FIBER	CALCI	SOD	POTAS	FOLIC	VIT C
Caramel Flan	1 serv (5.5 oz)	290	12	10	50	5	41	39	0	—	135	—	—	—
Churros	2	300	18	4	25	3	32	10	2	—	210	—	—	—
Cone Vanilla	1	330	8	5	35	8	55	47	0	—	180	—	—	—
Soft Serve Vanilla	1 cup (5 oz)	300	8	5	35	8	48	47	0	—	170	—	—	—

MAIN MENU SELECTIONS

FOOD	PORTION	CALS	FAT	SAT FAT	CHOL	PROT	CARB	SUGAR	FIBER	CALCI	SOD	POTAS	FOLIC	VIT C
BBQ Black Beans	1 serv (6 oz)	200	3	0	0	7	38	16	4	—	520	—	—	—
Bowl The Original Pollo	1 serv	540	4	1	70	37	85	1	11	—	1590	—	—	—
Burrito BRC	1 (7.5 oz)	390	10	5	15	14	61	0	6	—	880	—	—	—
Burrito Classic Chicken	1 (10.3 oz)	500	14	6	95	30	63	0	6	—	1230	—	—	—
Burrito Twice Grilled	1 (15 oz)	830	37	18	215	66	58	2	5	—	2230	—	—	—
Burrito Ultimate Grilled	1 (13.6 oz)	650	20	8	100	38	80	1	8	—	1690	—	—	—
Chicken Breast	1 (4.3 oz)	220	9	3	140	36	0	0	0	—	620	—	—	—
Chicken Breast Skinless	1 (4 oz)	180	4	1	0	35	0	0	0	—	580	—	—	—
Chicken Leg	1 (1.8 oz)	90	4	1	70	12	0	0	0	—	170	—	—	—
Chicken Thigh	1 (3.1 oz)	220	15	5	180	21	0	0	0	—	320	—	—	—
Chicken Wing	1 (1.3 oz)	90	5	2	60	11	0	0	0	—	290	—	—	—
Cole Slaw	1 serv (6 oz)	120	9	2	5	1	8	6	2	—	200	—	—	—
Corn Cobbette	1 (5 oz)	90	1	0	0	2	19	3	2	—	0	—	—	—
French Fries	1 serv (5.5 oz)	440	21	4	0	6	57	0	6	—	910	—	—	—
Fresh Vegetables w/ Margarine	1 serv (4.1 oz)	60	3	0	0	2	8	3	3	—	65	—	—	—

FOOD	PORTION	CALS	FAT	SAT FAT	CHOL	PROT	CARB	SUGAR	FIBER	CALCI	SOD	POTAS	FOLIC	VIT C
Fresh Vegetables w/o Margarine	1 serv (4 oz)	35	0	0	0	2	8	3	3	—	35	—	—	—
Gravy	1 serv (1 oz)	10	0	0	0	0	2	0	0	—	150	—	—	—
Loco Nachos	1 serv	170	14	3	10	3	7	2	1	—	210	—	—	—
Macaroni & Cheese	1 serv (5.5 oz)	280	17	11	55	11	28	3	6	—	770	—	—	—
Mashed Potatoes	1 serv (5 oz)	100	1	0	0	2	20	tr	2	—	350	—	—	—
Pinto Beans	1 serv (5 oz)	140	0	0	0	9	25	0	7	—	330	—	—	—
Quesadilla Cheese	1 (4.5 oz)	420	23	13	60	19	35	0	2	—	810	—	—	—
Refried Beans w/ Cheese	1 serv (6.3 oz)	270	7	2	10	14	36	2	10	—	730	—	—	—
Skinless Breast Meal	1 serv	310	12	5	105	35	17	6	5	—	780	—	—	—
Soup Chicken Tortilla w/o Tortilla Strips	1 serv (10 oz)	140	6	2	50	15	8	2	2	—	1040	—	—	—
Spanish Rice	1 serv (4.5 oz)	160	1	0	0	3	34	0	1	—	420	—	—	—
Taco Al Carbon	1 (3.1 oz)	150	5	2	40	11	17	tr	1	—	290	—	—	—
Taco Soft Chicken	1 (4.5 oz)	270	13	6	75	17	19	0	2	—	700	—	—	—
Taquito Chicken	1	190	9	2	25	10	18	0	1	—	330	—	—	—
Tortilla Chips	1 serv (1.5 oz)	210	10	2	0	3	28	tr	3	—	300	—	—	—
Tortilla Corn 6 Inches	2	120	2	0	0	2	24	0	2	—	60	—	—	—
Tortilla Flour 6.5 Inches	2	210	7	3	0	5	30	2	2	—	370	—	—	—
SALAD DRESSINGS AND TOPPINGS														
Creamy Cilantro	1 serv (1.5 oz)	220	23	4	20	1	1	1	0	—	300	—	—	—
Creamy Cilantro Light	1 pkg	70	5	1	5	1	6	3	0	—	400	—	—	—
Guacamole	1 serv (1 oz)	45	4	1	0	tr	4	tr	tr	—	135	—	—	—
Hot Sauce Jalapeno	1 pkg	5	0	0	0	0	1	0	0	—	110	—	—	—
Jack & Poblano Queso	1 serv (1.8 oz)	100	8	5	<5	3	4	1	0	—	340	—	—	—
Ketchup	1 pkg	10	0	0	0	0	2	2	0	—	100	—	—	—
Light Italian	1 pkg	20	1	0	0	0	2	2	0	—	770	—	—	—
Pico De Gallo Medium	1 serv (1 oz)	10	1	0	0	0	1	tr	0	—	190	—	—	—
Ranch	1 pkg	230	24	4	10	1	2	2	0	—	390	—	—	—
Salsa Avocado Hot	1 serv (1 oz)	30	3	0	0	0	1	0	tr	—	200	—	—	—
Salsa Chipotle Hot	1 serv (1 oz)	5	0	0	0	0	1	tr	0	—	180	—	—	—
Salsa House Mild	1 serv (1 oz)	5	0	0	0	0	1	tr	0	—	105	—	—	—
Sour Cream	1 serv (1 oz)	60	5	4	20	1	1	0	0	—	15	—	—	—
Thousand Island	1 pkg	220	21	3	20	0	6	6	0	—	350	—	—	—
SALADS														
Caesar Pollo	1 (11.4 oz)	520	38	7	100	27	17	6	4	—	980	—	—	—

FOOD	PORTION	CALS	FAT	SAT FAT	CHOL	PROT	CARB	SUGAR	FIBER	CALCI	SOD	POTAS	FOLIC	VIT C
Caesar Pollo w/o Dressing	1 (9.4 oz)	220	7	2	75	25	15	4	4	—	580	—	—	—
Garden	1 (4.8 oz)	120	4	0	15	5	9	3	2	—	290	—	—	—
Tostada Chicken	1 (17.3 oz)	840	40	11	100	40	76	4	7	—	1390	—	—	—
Tostada Chicken w/o Shell	1 (14.7 oz)	410	11	6	100	33	42	3	5	—	1100	—	—	—

EMERALD CITY SMOOTHIE

FOOD	PORTION	CALS	FAT	SAT FAT	CHOL	PROT	CARB	SUGAR	FIBER	CALCI	SOD	POTAS	FOLIC	VIT C
Apple Andie	1 (11 oz)	230	1	0	5	11	46	37	2	200	95	—	—	6
Berry Berry	1 (13 oz)	350	0	0	0	8	77	47	9	60	25	—	—	126
Blueberry Blast	1 (13 oz)	380	0	0	0	13	78	51	9	250	110	—	—	126
Coconut Passion	1 (11 oz)	600	23	7	5	24	80	58	11	250	135	—	—	27
Cranberry Delight	1 (10 oz)	550	1	0	5	11	127	114	2	200	95	—	—	240
Energizer	1 (10 oz)	350	1	0	5	18	62	36	7	250	115	—	—	114
Fruity Supreme	1 (9 oz)	280	1	0	5	12	59	34	6	200	100	—	—	36
Grape Escape	1 (10 oz)	480	1	0	5	11	109	102	2	200	100	—	—	144
Guava Sunrise	1 (13 oz)	366	1	0	0	12	80	67	6	40	50	—	—	132
Kiwi Kic	1 (11 oz)	400	1	0	0	13	88	81	2	250	105	—	—	108
Lean Body	1 (11 oz)	330	8	3	80	40	24	6	8	600	460	—	—	21
Lean Out	1 (11 oz)	600	26	5	55	56	35	21	5	450	360	—	—	6
Low Carb	1 (10 oz)	350	2	1	65	54	27	17	2	500	250	—	—	6
Mango Mania	1 (8 oz)	370	0	0	0	11	82	78	2	200	105	—	—	15
Marionberry Fuel	1 (13 oz)	380	0	0	0	14	81	50	10	250	105	—	—	126
Mega Mass	1 (14 oz)	610	10	5	45	29	103	55	7	350	220	—	—	42
Mini Mass	1 (13 oz)	520	11	7	65	27	79	53	6	400	180	—	—	36
Mocha Bliss	1 (10 oz)	550	8	5	30	34	63	58	1	500	370	—	—	1
Nutty Banana	1 (11 oz)	720	25	5	5	27	97	72	9	200	290	—	—	15
Orange Twister	1 (10 oz)	140	0	0	0	3	31	24	2	40	5	—	—	138
Pacific Splash	1 (12 oz)	240	0	0	0	2	58	34	6	20	0	—	—	66
PB&J	1 (14 oz)	630	25	5	0	22	77	43	12	40	210	—	—	48
Peach Pleasure	1 (12 oz)	270	0	0	0	12	54	41	5	200	95	—	—	168
Peanut Passion	1 (11 oz)	580	25	5	0	22	61	31	10	20	210	—	—	36
Pineapple Bliss	1 (12 oz)	210	1	0	0	6	45	35	4	0	30	—	—	54
Power Fuel	1 (11 oz)	450	3	2	45	39	66	29	6	250	120	—	—	42
Quick Start	1 (10 oz)	280	0	0	5	17	46	27	4	20	260	—	—	60
Raspberry Dream	1 (13 oz)	410	1	0	5	18	80	48	10	250	115	—	—	132
Rejuvenator	1 (10 oz)	340	1	0	5	17	62	35	7	350	110	—	—	36
Sambazon	1 (15 oz)	410	6	0	0	14	92	69	8	20	95	—	—	120
Slim N Fit	1 (10 oz)	350	1	0	25	25	60	35	6	300	125	—	—	36
The Builder	1 (18 oz)	1270	46	14	85	67	144	73	10	600	630	—	—	21
Zesty Lemon	1 (14 oz)	430	9	5	40	19	67	46	5	300	170	—	—	54
Zip Zip	1 (10 oz)	240	3	0	5	18	35	24	3	20	95	—	—	5
Zone Zinger	1 (14 oz)	430	3	1	30	25	76	53	4	300	60	—	—	120

EVOS

BEVERAGES

FOOD	PORTION	CALS	FAT	SAT FAT	CHOL	PROT	CARB	SUGAR	FIBER	CALCI	SOD	POTAS	FOLIC	VIT C
Shake Mango Guava	1 reg (16 oz)	180	0	0	0	0	48	44	2	—	0	—	—	—
Shake Multi-Berry	1 reg (20 oz)	200	1	0	0	1	52	35	1	—	10	—	—	—
Shake Strawberry Banana	1 reg (16 oz)	190	1	0	0	1	47	38	1	—	10	—	—	—
Shake Organic Cappuccino	1 reg (16 oz)	230	3	0	10	5	47	44	0	—	75	—	—	—
Shake Organic Vanilla	1 reg (16 oz)	180	3	0	10	6	30	30	0	—	55	—	—	—

CHILDREN'S MENU SELECTIONS

FOOD	PORTION	CALS	FAT	SAT FAT	CHOL	PROT	CARB	SUGAR	FIBER	CALCI	SOD	POTAS	FOLIC	VIT C
Kids Champion Burger	1	400	12	3	0	29	48	3	7	—	800	—	—	—
Kids Chicken Strips	1 serv	130	3	1	35	14	13	0	0	—	710	—	—	—
Kids Freerange Steakburger	1	390	15	6	70	27	39	2	2	—	480	—	—	—
Kids Good Corn Dog	1	150	4	0	0	7	27	4	3	—	500	—	—	—

MAIN MENU SELECTIONS

FOOD	PORTION	CALS	FAT	SAT FAT	CHOL	PROT	CARB	SUGAR	FIBER	CALCI	SOD	POTAS	FOLIC	VIT C
Airbaked Chicken Strips	1 serv	260	6	1	70	28	26	0	0	—	1420	—	—	—
Airfries	1 reg	230	8	0	0	4	35	1	3	—	390	—	—	—
American Champion	1	420	12	3	0	30	53	7	6	—	1130	—	—	—
American DeLite	1	330	6	1	0	22	53	6	7	—	1040	—	—	—
Burger Bun	1	190	2	1	0	7	39	2	2	—	410	—	—	—
Cheddar Cheese Slice	1	80	7	4	20	5	0	0	0	—	135	—	—	—
Crispy Mesquite Chicken	1 serv	330	5	1	35	21	53	3	2	—	1120	—	—	—
Freerange Steakburger	1	400	15	6	70	27	42	4	3	—	810	—	—	—
Fresh Fruit Bowl	1 serv	200	1	0	0	2	52	47	4	—	20	—	—	—
Good Corn Dog	1	150	4	0	0	7	22	4	3	—	500	—	—	—
Herb Crusted Trout	1 serv	440	25	3	13	21	62	7	3	—	1300	—	—	—
Honey Mesquite Chicken	1 serv	290	3	1	45	26	41	3	2	—	770	—	—	—
Spicy Chipotle Turkey	1 serv	370	9	3	70	31	42	3	3	—	1050	—	—	—
Veggie Chili	1 reg	110	2	0	0	7	20	3	5	—	930	—	—	—
Veggie Garden Grill Italian	1	350	5	1	0	24	54	4	8	—	930	—	—	—
Wraps Avocado Turkey	1	480	15	4	70	32	51	5	4	—	1200	—	—	—

FOOD	PORTION	CALS	FAT	SAT FAT	CHOL	PROT	CARB	SUGAR	FIBER	CALCI	SOD	POTAS	FOLIC	VIT C
Wraps Crispy Buffalo Chicken	1	440	11	2	35	23	64	5	5	—	1280	—	—	—
Wraps Crispy Thai Trout	1	660	20	5	25	25	96	6	5	—	1570	—	—	—
Wraps Freerange Beef Taco	1	600	28	11	90	34	53	6	5	—	770	—	—	—
Wraps Honey Wheat	1	300	8	2	0	8	49	4	4	—	560	—	—	—
Wraps Southwest Soy Taco	1	500	25	8	20	35	58	6	10	—	1090	—	—	—
Wraps Spicy Thai Chicken	1	510	10	4	45	30	76	3	4	—	1290	—	—	—
Wraps Spinach Herb	1	310	8	3	0	9	52	3	3	—	840	—	—	—
Wraps Tomato Basil Chicken	1	520	11	4	35	25	82	3	4	—	1560	—	—	—
SALAD DRESSINGS AND TOPPINGS														
Balsamic Vinegar	1 serv (0.5 oz)	5	0	0	0	0	2	2	0	—	0	—	—	—
Crispy Noodles	1 serv (7 g)	35	1	0	0	1	5	0	0	—	90	—	—	—
Croutons Multi-Grain	1 serv (7 g)	30	2	0	0	1	4	0	0	—	70	—	—	—
Dressing Avocado	1 serv (3 oz)	190	21	3	10	3	5	1	2	—	200	—	—	—
Dressing Caesar	1 serv (1.7 oz)	300	32	5	35	2	2	0	0	—	510	—	—	—
Dressing Fat Free Vinaigrette	1 serv (1 oz)	5	0	0	0	0	2	1	0	—	250	—	—	—
Dressing Raspberry	1 serv (2 oz)	50	0	0	0	0	14	12	0	—	340	—	—	—
Dressing Spicy Thai	1 serv (1.4 oz)	150	9	0	0	0	15	12	0	—	470	—	—	—
Extra Virgin Olive Oil	1 serv (1 oz)	250	28	4	0	0	0	0	0	—	0	—	—	—
Herb Spread	1 serv (0.7 oz)	30	3	0	0	0	2	0	0	—	160	—	—	—
Ketchup Cayenne Firewalker	1 serv (1.2 oz)	35	0	0	0	1	9	8	0	—	380	—	—	—
Ketchup Garlic Gravity	1 serv (1.2 oz)	35	0	0	0	1	9	8	0	—	380	—	—	—
Ketchup Mesquite Magic	1 serv (1.2 oz)	35	0	0	0	1	9	8	0	—	420	—	—	—
Mustard	1 serv (0.5 oz)	10	0	0	0	1	1	0	0	—	170	—	—	—
Mustard Mesquite Honey	1 serv (0.7 oz)	80	8	2	5	0	3	2	0	—	180	—	—	—
Southwest Sour Cream	1 serv (1.4 oz)	60	35	3	15	2	4	2	0	—	160	—	—	—
Spicy Chipotle Mayo	1 serv (0.7 oz)	30	2	0	0	0	2	0	0	—	170	—	—	—
Tomato Basil Sauce	1 serv (1.4 oz)	150	15	2	5	2	5	2	0	—	150	—	—	—

FOOD	PORTION	CALS	FAT	SAT FAT	CHOL	PROT	CARB	SUGAR	FIBER	CALCI	SOD	POTAS	FOLIC	VIT C
SALADS														
Bordeaux Bistro w/o Dressing	1	260	22	10	40	13	7	2	3	—	510	—	—	—
For Salads Chicken Strips	1 serv (3 oz)	130	3	1	35	14	13	0	0	—	710	—	—	—
For Salads Grilled Chicken	1 serv (3 oz)	90	1	0	50	19	1	0	0	—	360	—	—	—
Mediterranean Summer w/o Dressing	1	200	8	5	25	13	22	11	6	—	920	—	—	—
Santa Ana Caesar w/o Dressing	1	20	0	0	0	2	4	1	2	—	30	—	—	—
Side Salad w/o Dressing	1	35	0	0	0	2	8	3	2	—	30	—	—	—
Spicy Thai w/o Dressing	1	35	0	0	0	2	7	4	2	—	30	—	—	—
SUPPLEMENTS														
Fat Burner	1 serv (5 g)	16	0	0	0	0	4	0	0	—	0	—	—	—
Go Energy	1 serv (5 g)	15	0	0	0	0	4	0	0	—	0	—	—	—
Mega Protein	1 serv (0.5 oz)	45	0	0	0	12	0	0	0	—	0	—	—	—
Multi-Vitamin	1 serv (5 g)	10	0	0	0	0	3	0	0	—	0	—	—	—

FAZOLI'S

FOOD	PORTION	CALS	FAT	SAT FAT	CHOL	PROT	CARB	SUGAR	FIBER	CALCI	SOD	POTAS	FOLIC	VIT C
BEVERAGES														
Lemon Ice All Flavors	1	360	0	0	0	0	90	90	0	—	20	—	—	—
Lemon Ice Original	1 reg	180	0	0	0	0	45	45	0	—	15	—	—	—
CHILDREN'S MENU SELECTIONS														
Fettuccine Alfredo	1 serv	290	5	2	5	9	50	4	2	—	420	—	—	—
Meat Lasagna	1 serv	260	13	6	35	14	21	4	2	—	880	—	—	—
Ravioli w/ Marinara	1 serv	290	7	4	30	13	43	5	3	—	580	—	—	—
Spaghetti w/ Meatballs	1 serv	350	7	3	20	14	55	5	4	—	620	—	—	—
Ziti w/ Meat Sauce	1 serv	190	6	3	15	9	25	4	3	—	710	—	—	—
DESSERTS														
Cheesecake Original	1 slice	290	22	14	95	6	17	17	0	—	220	—	—	—
Cheesecake Turtle	1 slice	450	28	16	75	6	43	31	2	—	340	—	—	—
Cookie Chocolate Chunk	1	510	26	15	75	5	68	39	3	—	350	—	—	—
MAIN MENU SELECTIONS														
Breadstick	1	100	2	0	0	3	20	1	0	—	160	—	—	—
Breadstick Garlic	1	150	7	2	0	3	20	1	1	—	290	—	—	—
Fettuccine Alfredo	1 sm	520	12	4	15	16	83	8	4	—	1060	—	—	—
Fettuccine w/ Marinara	1 serv	450	3	0	0	15	88	10	7	—	770	—	—	—

FOOD	PORTION	CALS	FAT	SAT FAT	CHOL	PROT	CARB	SUGAR	FIBER	CALCI	SOD	POTAS	FOLIC	VIT C
Fettuccine w/ Meat Sauce	1 serv	500	7	2	10	20	87	9	7	—	1020	—	—	—
Oven Baked Chicken Parmesan	1 serv	960	33	11	115	56	117	12	9	—	2350	—	—	—
Oven Baked Meat Lasagna	1 serv	510	25	12	70	27	43	7	5	—	1710	—	—	—
Oven Baked Rigatoni Romano	1 serv	1090	54	20	135	11	101	13	11	—	3180	—	—	—
Oven Baked Spaghetti	1 serv	680	22	9	65	32	90	10	7	—	1480	—	—	—
Oven Baked Spaghetti w/ Meatballs	1 serv	940	40	17	120	46	100	12	9	—	2370	—	—	—
Panini Four Cheese & Tomato	1	510	22	12	60	28	53	4	3	—	960	—	—	—
Panini Grilled Chicken	1	540	18	5	80	35	56	4	3	—	1360	—	—	—
Panini Smoked Turkey	1	620	29	11	95	35	54	5	3	—	2110	—	—	—
Penne w/ Smoked Turkey	1 serv	520	12	4	15	16	83	8	4	—	1060	—	—	—
Penne w/ Marinara	1 serv	450	3	0	0	15	88	10	7	—	770	—	—	—
Penne w/ Meat Sauce	1 serv	500	7	2	10	20	87	9	7	—	1020	—	—	—
Pizza Slice Cheese	1	270	11	4	25	13	31	2	2	—	700	—	—	—
Pizza Slice Pepperoni	1	310	14	5	30	14	31	2	2	—	850	—	—	—
Platter Classic Sampler	1	810	25	10	55	34	110	13	8	—	2130	—	—	—
Platter Ultimate Sampler	1	980	29	12	70	43	134	17	11	—	2780	—	—	—
Ravioli w/ Marinara	1 serv	500	15	8	80	22	71	10	7	—	1210	—	—	—
Ravioli w/ Meat Sauce	1 serv	550	20	10	90	26	71	10	7	—	1460	—	—	—
Spaghetti w/ Alfredo	1 serv	520	12	4	15	16	83	8	4	—	1060	—	—	—
Spaghetti w/ Marinara	1 sm	450	3	0	0	15	88	10	7	—	770	—	—	—
Spaghetti w/ Meat Sauce	1 sm	500	7	2	10	20	87	9	7	—	1020	—	—	—
Submarinos Club	half	973	34	10	75	37	65	6	3	—	2870	—	—	—
Submarinos Ham 'N Swiss	1	680	30	9	60	34	65	6	3	—	2440	—	—	—
Submarinos Italian Beef	half	660	24	9	90	46	68	7	3	—	2320	—	—	—

FOOD	PORTION	CALS	FAT	SAT FAT	CHOL	PROT	CARB	SUGAR	FIBER	CALCI	SOD	POTAS	FOLIC	VIT C
Submarinos Original	half	940	58	17	95	35	68	6	4	—	3040	—	—	—
Topping Broccoli	1 serv	25	0	0	0	3	5	1	3	—	10	—	—	—
Topping Broccoli & Tomatoes	1 serv	30	0	0	0	3	6	2	3	—	10	—	—	—
Topping Garlic Shrimp	1 serv	160	12	3	45	10	3	0	1	—	440	—	—	—
Topping Italian Sausage	1 serv	240	21	7	45	10	3	0	1	—	770	—	—	—
Topping Meatballs	1 serv	160	18	8	55	13	6	1	1	—	700	—	—	—
Topping Peppery Chicken	1 serv	70	1	0	35	14	1	0	0	—	330	—	—	—
Ziti w/ Meat Sauce	1 serv	480	15	6	40	23	65	9	6	—	1430	—	—	—
SALAD DRESSINGS														
Caesar	1 serv	220	25	4	45	1	1	0	0	—	350	—	—	—
Fat Free Honey Mustard	1 serv	60	0	0	0	0	15	14	1	—	350	—	—	—
Fat Free Italian	1 serv	25	0	0	0	0	6	3	0	—	390	—	—	—
Honey French	1 serv	220	18	3	0	0	14	13	0	—	310	—	—	—
Italian	1 serv	160	14	2	0	0	7	7	0	—	760	—	—	—
Ranch	1 serv	220	24	4	10	1	2	2	0	—	470	—	—	—
Ranch Lite	1 serv	120	12	2	5	1	2	1	0	—	350	—	—	—
SALADS														
Chicken & Fruit	1	220	2	0	55	23	28	20	4	—	700	—	—	—
Chicken & Pasta Caesar	1	440	15	4	65	35	41	8	4	—	1320	—	—	—
Chicken BLT Ranch	1	270	10	4	80	31	13	5	4	—	1060	—	—	—
Parmesan Chicken	1	360	15	5	65	31	31	5	4	—	850	—	—	—
Side Caesar	1	40	2	1	5	4	4	1	2	—	70	—	—	—
Side Garden	1	25	0	0	0	2	4	2	3	—	30	—	—	—
Side Pasta	1	320	12	3	5	11	41	7	1	—	620	—	—	—

FIVE GUYS BURGERS AND FRIES

MAIN MENU SELECTIONS

FOOD	PORTION	CALS	FAT	SAT FAT	CHOL	PROT	CARB	SUGAR	FIBER	CALCI	SOD	POTAS	FOLIC	VIT C
Bacon Burger	1 (9.8 oz)	780	50	23	140	43	39	8	2	—	690	—	—	—
Bacon Cheese Dog	1 (7 oz)	695	48	22	96	26	41	9	2	—	1700	—	—	—
Bacon Dog	1 (6.4 oz)	625	42	19	76	22	40	8	2	—	1390	—	—	—
Cheese Dog	1 (6.5 oz)	615	41	19	81	22	41	9	2	—	1440	—	—	—
Cheeseburger	1 (10.6 oz)	840	55	27	165	47	40	9	2	—	1050	—	—	—
Cheeseburger Bacon	1 (11 oz)	920	62	30	180	51	40	9	2	—	1310	—	—	—
Fries	1 reg (8.6 oz)	620	30	6	—	10	78	2	6	—	90	—	—	—
Fries	1 lg (16 oz)	1464	71	14	—	24	184	5	14	—	213	—	—	—
Grilled Cheese	1 (4 oz)	430	26	9	35	11	41	10	3	—	715	—	—	—
Hamburger	1 (9.3 oz)	700	43	20	125	39	39	8	2	—	430	—	—	—

FOOD	PORTION	CALS	FAT	SAT FAT	CHOL	PROT	CARB	SUGAR	FIBER	CALCI	SOD	POTAS	FOLIC	VIT C
Hot Dog	1 (5.9 oz)	545	35	16	61	18	40	8	2	—	1130	—	—	—
Little Burgers Bacon Burger	1 (6.5 oz)	560	33	15	80	27	39	8	2	—	640	—	—	—
Little Burgers Cheeseburger	1 (6.7 oz)	550	32	15	85	27	40	9	2	—	690	—	—	—
Little Burgers Cheeseburger Bacon	1 (7.2 oz)	630	39	18	100	31	40	9	2	—	950	—	—	—
Little Burgers Hamburger	1 (6 oz)	480	26	12	65	23	39	8	2	—	380	—	—	—
Veggie Sandwich	1 (7.3 oz)	440	15	6	25	16	60	14	2	—	1040	—	—	—
TOPPINGS														
A1 Steak Sauce	1 tbsp (0.6 oz)	15	0	0	0	0	3	2	0	—	280	—	—	—
Bacon	2 slices (0.5 oz)	80	7	3	15	4	0	0	0	—	260	—	—	—
BBQ Sauce	1 tbsp (0.6 oz)	60	8	0	0	0	16	10	0	—	400	—	—	—
Cheese	1 slice (0.7 oz)	70	6	4	20	4	tr	tr	0	—	310	—	—	—
Green Peppers	1 serv (0.8 oz)	5	0	0	0	0	2	tr	tr	—	1	—	—	—
Hot Sauce	1 tsp (5 g)	0	0	0	0	0	0	0	0	—	0	—	—	—
Jalapenos	1 serv (0.4 oz)	3	0	0	0	0	tr	0	0	—	184	—	—	—
Ketchup	1 tbsp (0.6 oz)	15	0	0	0	0	4	4	0	—	190	—	—	—
Lettuce	1 serv (1 oz)	4	0	0	0	0	1	tr	tr	—	3	—	—	—
Mayonnaise	1 serv (0.5 oz)	100	11	2	10	0	0	0	0	—	75	—	—	—
Mushrooms	1 serv (0.9 oz)	10	0	0	—	1	1	0	tr	—	100	—	—	—
Mustard	1 tbsp (0.6 oz)	0	0	0	0	0	0	0	0	—	55	—	—	—
Onions	1 serv (0.9 oz)	10	0	0	0	0	3	1	tr	—	1	—	—	—
Pickle Chips	6 (1 oz)	5	0	0	0	0	1	0	0	—	265	—	—	—
Relish	1 serv (0.5 oz)	15	0	0	0	0	4	3	0	—	85	—	—	—
Tomatoes	1 serv (1.8 oz)	9	0	0	0	tr	2	2	tr	—	3	—	—	—

FRIENDLY'S

BEVERAGES

FOOD	PORTION	CALS	FAT	SAT FAT	CHOL	PROT	CARB	SUGAR	FIBER	CALCI	SOD	POTAS	FOLIC	VIT C
Milkshake Double Thick Vanilla	1	770	32	21	110	15	106	92	0	—	270	—	—	—
MAIN MENU SELECTIONS														
Apple Slices	1 serv	100	0	0	0	1	26	20	5	—	0	—	—	—
Applesauce	1 serv	110	0	0	0	0	27	25	1	—	0	—	—	—
Broccoli	1 serv	80	6	5	0	3	5	2	3	—	80	—	—	—
Burger	1	1190	68	19	120	43	103	12	8	—	1170	—	—	—
Burger BBQ Fronion	1	1560	91	30	160	55	134	21	8	—	2020	—	—	—
Burger Mushroom Swiss Bacon	1	1570	100	33	190	61	109	15	7	—	2040	—	—	—
Burger Soft Pretzel Bacon	1	1420	79	29	190	58	119	11	7	—	1360	—	—	—
Burger The Vermonter	1	1420	87	32	190	59	102	4	7	—	1530	—	—	—

FOOD	PORTION	CALS	FAT	SAT FAT	CHOL	PROT	CARB	SUGAR	FIBER	CALCI	SOD	POTAS	FOLIC	VIT C
Burger Ultimate Bacon Cheese	1	1400	86	29	170	55	103	11	7	—	2040	—	—	—
Burgermelt Deluxe Cheese Set-Up	1	1180	75	25	140	44	83	5	7	—	1310	—	—	—
Burgermelt Swiss Patty	1	1360	78	27	150	56	110	12	8	—	1220	—	—	—
Burgermelt Ultimate Grilled Cheese	1	1500	97	38	180	54	101	4	9	—	2090	—	—	—
Burgermelt Zesty Queso	1	1380	79	26	140	53	117	8	7	—	2410	—	—	—
Carrot & Celery Sticks w/ Ranch Dressing	1 serv	100	7	3	10	2	6	3	2	—	260	—	—	—
Chicken Strips Basket w/o Dipping Sauce	5 pieces	1030	58	8	90	37	93	9	8	—	1330	—	—	—
Chicken Strips Honey BBQ w/o Dipping Sauce	5 pieces	1560	74	11	110	38	188	88	0	—	2240	—	—	—
Chicken Strips Kickin' Buffalo w/o Dipping Sauce	5 pieces	1530	109	13	150	40	97	10	8	—	2860	—	—	—
Clamboat Basket	1 serv	1710	102	15	90	28	170	19	11	—	3340	—	—	—
Coleslaw	1 serv	160	12	2	10	1	13	8	2	—	260	—	—	—
Corn	1 serv	160	7	3	0	4	20	9	4	—	70	—	—	—
Fishamajig	1	970	51	14	70	30	99	5	7	—	1570	—	—	—
Friendly Frank	1	750	44	13	30	15	73	5	5	—	1070	—	—	—
Friendly's BTL	1	990	57	13	40	21	99	7	7	—	1110	—	—	—
Fronions Jumbo	1 serv	1430	90	13	30	14	140	31	7	—	2970	—	—	—
Garlic Bread	1 serv	330	14	1	0	4	48	0	4	—	160	—	—	—
Grilled Cheese	1	790	37	12	30	20	96	4	6	—	1280	—	—	—
Grilled Flounder	1 serv	980	48	10	80	38	100	10	7	—	3070	—	—	—
Mandarin Oranges	1 serv	80	0	0	0	0	20	18	0	—	10	—	—	—
Mashed Potatoes Homestyle	1 serv	240	12	7	30	4	29	4	2	—	160	—	—	—
Mini Mozzarella Cheese Sticks	1 serv	680	40	14	60	23	55	5	3	—	1870	—	—	—
Mixed Vegetables	1 serv	110	6	3	0	3	13	6	4	—	110	—	—	—
New England Fish 'N Chips	1 serv	1150	70	10	80	25	106	15	9	—	2120	—	—	—
Quesadillas Chicken	1 serv	1330	82	41	210	29	97	10	4	—	3350	—	—	—
Quesadillas Chicken Fajita	1 serv	1540	91	42	210	74	106	13	7	—	3870	—	—	—
Rice	1 serv	210	3	0	0	3	41	2	0	—	900	—	—	—

FOOD	PORTION	CALS	FAT	SAT FAT	CHOL	PROT	CARB	SUGAR	FIBER	CALCI	SOD	POTAS	FOLIC	VIT C
Shrimp Basket	1 serv	1090	60	7	180	27	110	17	9	—	3290	—	—	—
Sirloin Steak Tips	1 serv	1140	51	19	200	77	92	28	13	—	3350	—	—	—
Sliders Cheeseburger	1 serv	500	21	7	50	20	57	18	6	—	1440	—	—	—
Sliders Chicken	1 serv	740	42	9	60	23	69	15	7	—	1210	—	—	—
Spanish Rice	1 serv	330	15	6	0	7	41	2	0	—	1200	—	—	—
Supermelt Bruschetta Mozzarella	1	1140	54	17	140	57	105	6	7	—	1870	—	—	—
Supermelt Cheddar Jack Chicken	1	1070	49	18	140	56	98	5	6	—	2270	—	—	—
Supermelt Grilled Chicken Pesto	1	1360	82	26	160	59	98	7	6	—	2060	—	—	—
Supermelt Honey BBQ Chicken	1	1400	75	22	110	49	134	23	8	—	2160	—	—	—
Supermelt Kickin Buffalo Chicken	1	1430	86	25	100	45	118	7	7	—	2520	—	—	—
Supermelt Reuben	1	1130	56	18	100	54	105	10	6	—	2910	—	—	—
Supermelt Steak 'N Mushroom	1	1150	61	19	90	44	108	9	7	—	2120	—	—	—
Supermelt Tuna	1	1140	66	15	80	39	98	6	7	—	1700	—	—	—
Supermelt Turkey Club	1	990	46	13	80	44	102	9	7	—	2220	—	—	—
Tuna Roll	1	920	57	10	60	28	73	5	6	—	1080	—	—	—
Waffle Fries	1 serv	590	33	5	0	7	67	1	5	—	1430	—	—	—
Waffle Fries Loaded	1 serv	920	64	15	60	17	67	4	4	—	2510	—	—	—
Wrap Buffalo Chicken	1	1510	94	19	130	42	123	6	9	—	2640	—	—	—
Wrap Crispy Chicken	1	1140	54	8	60	31	132	14	10	—	1610	—	—	—
Wrap Crispy Chicken Caesar	1	1500	94	18	160	43	123	7	9	—	2300	—	—	—
Wrap Grilled Chicken Deluxe	1	1000	45	9	90	43	108	15	8	—	1810	—	—	—
SALAD DRESSINGS AND TOPPINGS														
Dressing Bleu Cheese	1 serv	470	48	11	60	6	3	3	0	—	720	—	—	—
Dressing Honey Mustard	1 serv	360	30	5	30	0	24	18	0	—	420	—	—	—
Dressing Italian	1 serv	410	42	6	0	0	6	6	0	—	690	—	—	—
Dressing Italian Fat Free	1 serv	30	0	0	0	0	8	6	0	—	420	—	—	—
Dressing Peppercorn Parmesan Lite	1 serv	230	21	5	20	3	6	3	0	—	630	—	—	—

FOOD	PORTION	CALS	FAT	SAT FAT	CHOL	PROT	CARB	SUGAR	FIBER	CALCI	SOD	POTAS	FOLIC	VIT C
Dressing Ranch	1 serv	330	33	6	30	3	3	3	0	—	750	—	—	—
Dressing Salsa Ranch	1 serv	170	17	3	20	2	5	3	1	—	620	—	—	—
Dressing Sesame Oriental	1 serv	270	14	2	0	0	36	30	0	—	960	—	—	—
Dressing Thousand Island	1 serv	390	36	6	20	0	15	12	0	—	840	—	—	—
Dressing Vinegarette Dijon Low Fat	1 serv	110	3	0	0	0	21	21	0	—	1560	—	—	—
Sauce BBQ	1 serv	90	0	0	0	0	20	11	0	—	410	—	—	—
Sauce Honey Mustard	1 serv	180	16	2	20	0	12	9	0	—	210	—	—	—
Vinegarette Balsamic	1 serv	180	15	2	0	0	9	9	0	—	1230	—	—	—
SALADS														
Apple Walnut Chicken w/o Dressing	1 serv	390	18	7	110	38	22	9	5	—	1140	—	—	—
Asian Chicken w/o Dressing	1 serv	490	20	3	80	36	41	21	6	—	1200	—	—	—
Chicken Caesar	1 serv	1030	84	16	220	47	32	10	3	—	2010	—	—	—
Chipotle Chicken w/o Dressing	1 serv	550	22	3	80	37	50	7	8	—	1440	—	—	—
Crispy Chicken w/o Dressing	1 serv	630	38	10	260	35	38	5	6	—	820	—	—	—
Kickin' Buffalo Chicken w/o Dressing	1 serv	710	47	9	90	29	42	5	7	—	1370	—	—	—
Side w/o Dressing	1 serv	60	1	0	0	2	10	2	2	—	110	—	—	—
Steak & Bleu Cheese w/o Dressing	1 serv	640	34	11	120	44	41	9	8	—	1240	—	—	—
SOUPS														
Broccoli Cheddar	1 cup	200	13	7	40	7	14	3	1	—	780	—	—	—
Chili	1 cup	270	16	6	40	14	18	3	3	—	910	—	—	—
Chunky Chicken Noodle	1 cup	280	10	3	70	10	31	4	2	—	1970	—	—	—
Homestyle Clam Chowder	1 cup	270	18	10	60	11	17	3	1	—	890	—	—	—
Minestrone	1 cup	90	1	0	0	4	15	2	2	—	620	—	—	—
FRUITFULL														
BREADS														
Almond Cherry	½ slice (2 oz)	226	11	2	23	3	29	17	1	10	279	—	—	0
Apple Spice	½ slice (2 oz)	186	7	1	19	2	29	18	1	0	124	—	—	0
Banana	½ slice (2 oz)	165	6	1	22	3	24	11	1	10	177	—	—	1

FOOD	PORTION	CALS	FAT	SAT FAT	CHOL	PROT	CARB	SUGAR	FIBER	CALCI	SOD	POTAS	FOLIC	VIT C
Cappuccino Chocolate Chip	½ slice (2 oz)	229	13	3	35	3	27	16	1	10	161	—	—	0
Carrot	½ slice (2 oz)	190	9	1	24	3	24	12	0	90	177	—	—	1
Chocolate	½ slice (2 oz)	120	0	0	0	2	26	16	2	0	155	—	—	0
Old Fashioned Pound Cake	½ slice (2 oz)	227	13	3	51	3	25	14	0	10	181	—	—	0
Orange Cranberry	½ slice (2 oz)	130	0	0	0	3	28	12	0	30	200	—	—	4
Pumpkin	½ slice (2 oz)	130	0	0	0	2	30	19	1	10	390	—	—	1
Sweet Potato	½ slice (2 oz)	176	6	1	19	2	28	17	1	10	204	—	—	2
Zucchini	½ slice (2 oz)	190	9	1	22	3	24	13	1	10	215	—	—	1
FROZEN BARS														
Cream Banana	1 (4 oz)	110	3	2	20	1	18	13	0	40	25	—	—	6
Cream Coconut	1 (4 oz)	130	5	4	15	2	18	13	0	—	25	—	—	—
Cream Horchata	1 (4 oz)	240	14	10	45	3	23	21	tr	90	58	—	—	—
Cream Mango Cream	1 (4 oz)	170	7	5	20	2	26	20	tr	60	25	—	—	1
Cream Peaches 'n' Cream	1	150	5	4	25	2	24	21	—	60	50	—	—	5
Cream Pina Colada	1 (4 oz)	90	3	2	10	1	16	15	tr	20	20	—	—	—
Cream Raspberry Cream	1 (4 oz)	110	3	2	10	2	18	12	0	40	20	—	—	2
Cream Sapote Lucuma	1 (4 oz)	180	8	5	22	2	25	29	<2	70	31	—	—	0
Cream Strawberry Cream	1 (4 oz)	110	3	1	15	2	20	17	0	40	25	—	—	1
Juice Fuzzy Navel	1 (4 oz)	70	0	0	0	0	18	15	0	—	10	—	—	2
Juice Green Tea Melon	1 (4 oz)	90	0	0	0	0	21	16	—	—	25	—	—	—
Juice Guava	1 (4 oz)	70	0	0	0	0	17	11	—	—	20	—	—	9
Juice Lemon	1 (4 oz)	90	0	0	0	0	24	22	—	—	10	—	—	—
Juice Lime	1 (4 oz)	80	0	0	0	0	20	19	0	—	10	—	—	2
Juice Passionate Cherry	1 (4 oz)	80	0	0	0	0	20	16	—	—	25	—	—	4
Juice Pineapple	1 (4 oz)	80	0	0	0	0	20	10	0	—	5	—	—	4
Juice Raspberry	1 (4 oz)	70	0	0	0	0	18	18	0	—	5	—	—	2
Juice Strawberry	1 (4 oz)	70	0	0	0	0	18	13	0	—	5	—	—	1
Juice Tamarind	1 (4 oz)	90	0	0	0	0	21	21	—	—	20	—	—	4
Juice Tropical Splash	1 (4 oz)	80	0	0	0	0	19	17	0	—	25	—	—	5
Juice Watermelon	1 (4 oz)	60	0	0	0	0	13	13	—	—	5	—	—	—
Mamey Sapote Lucuma	1 (4 oz)	180	8	5	22	2	25	—	<2	70	31	—	—	0
SNACKS														
All About Almonds	1 pkg (1 oz)	170	15	1	0	6	5	0	4	80	0	—	—	0
Blueberry Thrill	1 pkg (1 oz)	150	8	1	0	5	14	9	3	60	10	—	—	0

FOOD	PORTION	CALS	FAT	SAT FAT	CHOL	PROT	CARB	SUGAR	FIBER	CALCI	SOD	POTAS	FOLIC	VIT C
Buzzworthy Banana	1 pkg (1.1 oz)	140	8	3	0	3	17	11	2	0	35	—	—	0
Calypso Cashews	1 pkg (1.1 oz)	170	13	2	1	4	7	2	1	0	75	—	—	0
Chocolate Covered Nuts	1 pkg (1.5 oz)	230	16	7	5	5	20	18	1	80	25	—	—	0
Chocolate Twisted Bliss	1 pkg (1.4 oz)	190	8	6	6	3	27	16	1	40	210	—	—	0
Cin-sational Apple Crunch	1 pkg (1 oz)	160	10	2	0	4	14	8	1	20	135	—	—	2
Dark Chocolate Covered Almonds	1 pkg (1.4 oz)	210	16	6	2	4	19	14	3	40	5	—	—	0
Dark Chocolate Covered Cashews	1 pkg (1.4 oz)	220	16	6	2	3	21	14	3	0	0	—	—	0
Dark Chocolate Covered Cranberries	1 pkg (1.4 oz)	180	9	5	2	1	27	24	2	40	10	—	—	0
Debbie Loves Fruit	1 pkg (1 oz)	110	2	2	0	0	23	16	1	20	20	—	—	0
Eat Your Veggies	1 pkg (1.5 oz)	180	8	1	0	1	29	7	3	20	105	—	—	4
Got Nuts?	1 pkg (1.1 oz)	180	13	1	1	6	9	1	2	20	55	—	—	0
Hit The Road Jack	1 pkg (1.1 oz)	130	6	1	0	3	19	16	1	20	10	—	—	0
Honey I Ate The Peanuts	1 pkg (1 oz)	160	12	2	0	7	8	6	2	0	115	—	—	0
Just Peachy	1 pkg (1.4 oz)	140	0	0	0	3	35	22	0	0	25	—	—	0
Mammoth Malts	1 pkg (1 oz)	150	7	4	3	1	20	18	0	20	30	—	—	0
Nice Catch Swedish Fish	1 pkg (1.4 oz)	140	0	0	0	0	35	22	0	0	15	—	—	0
Off The Hook Gummy Worms	1 pkg (1.5 oz)	130	0	0	0	3	31	21	0	0	20	—	—	0
PB Pretzel Poppers	1 pkg (1 oz)	140	7	2	0	5	15	2	2	0	330	—	—	2
Power Pistachios	1 pkg (1.5 oz)	260	23	4	0	7	12	3	4	30	250	—	—	0
Pumpkin Seeds	1 pkg (1 oz)	180	15	2	0	9	3	0	1	20	190	—	—	0
Reggae Rice Crackers	1 pkg (1.1 oz)	110	0	0	0	2	26	1	0	0	200	—	—	2
Rockin' Raisins	1 pkg (1.4 oz)	170	7	4	4	3	28	19	1	40	20	—	—	0
Rocky Mountain Munch	1 pkg (1.1 oz)	120	4	2	0	1	22	14	1	20	20	—	—	0
Smokin' Nuts	1 pkg (1.3 oz)	170	15	1	0	6	6	2	3	80	160	—	—	0
Soft Twisters Green Apple	1 pkg (1 oz)	120	0	0	0	0	29	14	0	0	45	—	—	4
Soft Twisters Watermelon	1 pkg (1.3 oz)	120	0	0	0	1	29	14	0	0	45	—	—	4
Sour Wiggle Giggle	1 pkg (1.5 oz)	150	0	0	0	2	34	22	0	0	35	—	—	0
Strawberry Fields	1 pkg (1 oz)	140	7	3	0	2	18	9	1	0	65	—	—	0

FOOD	PORTION	CALS	FAT	SAT FAT	CHOL	PROT	CARB	SUGAR	FIBER	CALCI	SOD	POTAS	FOLIC	VIT C
Sunflower Seeds Tummy	1 pkg (1.1 oz)	190	14	2	0	6	8	1	2	20	65	—	—	0
Swinging Sesame Stix	1 pkg (1.1 oz)	180	13	2	0	4	12	0	2	60	320	—	—	0
Whassup Wasabi	1 pkg (1.1 oz)	150	7	1	0	5	17	1	2	0	300	—	—	0

GREAT STEAK & POTATO

BEVERAGES

FOOD	PORTION	CALS	FAT	SAT FAT	CHOL	PROT	CARB	SUGAR	FIBER	CALCI	SOD	POTAS	FOLIC	VIT C
Great Steak Lemonade	1 sm (12 oz)	180	0	0	0	03	48	45	0	0	0	—	—	24
Orange Juice	1 (12 oz)	118	0	0	0	0	30	30	0	0	31	—	—	60

BREAKFAST SELECTIONS

FOOD	PORTION	CALS	FAT	SAT FAT	CHOL	PROT	CARB	SUGAR	FIBER	CALCI	SOD	POTAS	FOLIC	VIT C
Potatoes Deluxe Home	1 serv (12 oz)	390	23	4	0	4	44	3	7	20	1460	—	—	30
Potatoes Fresh Cut Home	1 serv (10.6 oz)	380	23	4	0	3	42	2	6	20	1460	—	—	15
Sandwich Bacon Egg Cheese	1 (7.6 oz)	600	36	11	440	29	39	2	2	200	1300	—	—	0
Sandwich Egg Cheese	1 (7 oz)	500	29	9	425	23	39	2	2	200	890	—	—	0
Sandwich Ham Cheese	1 (5.5 oz)	430	22	6	40	18	41	4	2	150	1400	—	—	0
Sandwich Ham Egg Cheese	1 (9 oz)	570	32	10	450	31	42	4	2	200	1540	—	—	0
Sandwich Sausage Egg Cheese	1 (9 oz)	700	47	15	465	30	39	2	2	200	1300	—	—	0
Sandwich Steak Egg Cheese	1 (10 oz)	600	34	10	455	34	40	3	2	200	990	—	—	1

CHILDREN'S MENU SELECTIONS

FOOD	PORTION	CALS	FAT	SAT FAT	CHOL	PROT	CARB	SUGAR	FIBER	CALCI	SOD	POTAS	FOLIC	VIT C
Chicken Nuggets	1 serv (2.7 oz)	165	9	2	37	11	10	—	1	—	403	—	—	—
Grilled Cheese w/ Fry	1 serv (8.8 oz)	530	28	8	10	15	57	2	6	200	1290	—	—	9
Kid's Great Fry	1 (6.1 oz)	270	13	2	0	4	36	0	4	0	680	—	—	6
Slider Chicken w/ Fry	1 serv (11.5 oz)	570	25	7	50	23	60	5	6	150	1560	—	—	9
Slider Steak w/ Fry	1 serv (11.8 oz)	580	28	8	55	24	60	5	6	150	1530	—	—	9

MAIN MENU SELECTIONS

FOOD	PORTION	CALS	FAT	SAT FAT	CHOL	PROT	CARB	SUGAR	FIBER	CALCI	SOD	POTAS	FOLIC	VIT C
Baked Potato Broccoli & Cheese	1 (8.9 oz)	400	24	10	45	13	35	5	4	300	1070	—	—	54
Baked Potato Cheese & Bacon	1 (7.8 oz)	530	35	14	85	25	29	2	3	450	840	—	—	12
Baked Potato Plain	1 (6 oz)	160	0	0	0	4	36	2	4	20	15	—	—	15
Baked Potato Sour Cream & Chive	1 (7.3 oz)	350	23	10	25	5	32	2	3	80	160	—	—	15
Baked Potato The King	1 (8.8 oz)	590	41	18	95	26	31	2	3	450	860	—	—	15
Cheeseburger	1 (10.2 oz)	640	35	12	105	40	41	3	3	150	730	—	—	6

FOOD	PORTION	CALS	FAT	SAT FAT	CHOL	PROT	CARB	SUGAR	FIBER	CALCI	SOD	POTAS	FOLIC	VIT C
Chicagoland Cheesesteak 7 Inch	1 (13.3 oz)	680	29	11	85	43	63	9	5	300	2480	—	—	21
Coney Island Fry	1 reg (12.7 oz)	570	30	10	45	18	61	5	12	250	2030	—	—	12
Great Fry	1 reg (10.2 oz)	440	20	3	0	7	60	0	7	0	1130	—	—	12
Great Steak Cheesesteak 7 Inch	1 (13.6 oz)	740	37	9	95	41	62	8	5	300	1270	—	—	9
Great Steak Cheesesteak Wrap	1 (13.7 oz)	820	43	11	95	40	67	6	5	350	1400	—	—	9
Gyro	1 (12 oz)	580	30	10	60	29	52	8	5	450	1550	—	—	9
Ham Delight 7 Inch	1 (13.1 oz)	710	33	10	85	36	71	16	5	300	2190	—	—	9
Ham Explosion 7 Inch	1 (14 oz)	710	34	10	85	37	70	13	6	350	2200	—	—	24
Hamburger	1 (9.7 oz)	590	30	9	105	37	40	3	3	100	480	—	—	6
Kansas City BBQ Cheesesteak 7 Inch	1 (12 oz)	680	26	10	65	40	71	14	5	250	1740	—	—	2
King Fry	1 reg (11.4 oz)	630	39	14	70	20	52	3	5	250	1970	—	—	12
Nacho Fry	1 reg (11.8 oz)	510	27	9	30	12	53	3	5	200	2570	—	—	9
Pastrami 7 Inch	1 (13.3 oz)	790	41	16	110	43	65	9	5	350	1850	—	—	9
Philly Buffalo Chicken 7 Inch	1 (13.8 oz)	660	24	10	60	37	65	9	5	250	2420	—	—	30
Philly Burger	1 (14.2 oz)	820	50	15	135	46	47	6	4	300	820	—	—	24
Philly Chicken Slider	1 (5.4 oz)	300	13	6	50	19	24	5	2	150	880	—	—	1
Philly Original Cheesesteak 7 Inch	1 (11.8 oz)	650	26	10	95	40	62	10	5	250	2570	—	—	2
Philly Original Chicken 7 Inch	1 (11 oz)	620	22	9	85	37	62	10	5	250	1670	—	—	2
Philly Original Chicken Wrap	1 (11.3 oz)	700	28	11	85	36	67	7	4	350	1800	—	—	2
Philly Steak Slider	1 (5.6 oz)	310	15	6	55	20	24	5	2	150	850	—	—	1
Philly Teriyaki Chicken	1 (14 oz)	290	32	9	85	40	65	11	5	300	2280	—	—	9
Philly Turkey 7 Inch	1 (13 oz)	670	30	8	75	38	64	8	5	300	1650	—	—	9
Philly Ultimate Chicken	1 (14.6 oz)	730	33	11	65	38	64	9	6	250	1590	—	—	24
Philly Ultimate Chicken Wrap	1 (14.7 oz)	810	39	13	65	36	69	6	5	300	1720	—	—	24
Potato Skins	1 serv (6.4 oz)	390	26	12	65	17	24	4	2	250	1070	—	—	9
Reuben 7 Inch	1 (12 oz)	690	33	11	95	37	61	7	5	300	2550	—	—	6
Super Steak Wrap Cheesesteak	1 (15.7 oz)	930	54	13	105	41	69	6	5	350	1500	—	—	24

FOOD	PORTION	CALS	FAT	SAT FAT	CHOL	PROT	CARB	SUGAR	FIBER	CALCI	SOD	POTAS	FOLIC	VIT C
The Great Potato Chicken	1 (13 oz)	600	33	13	100	32	37	7	4	300	1420	—	—	15
The Great Potato Ham	1 (12.8 oz)	520	28	12	95	29	43	11	4	300	2470	—	—	15
The Great Potato Steak	1 (13.5 oz)	620	38	13	105	35	37	7	4	300	1360	—	—	15
The Great Potato Turkey	1 (12.8 oz)	490	25	10	85	31	39	7	4	300	1930	—	—	15
Veggi Delight	1 (12.2 oz)	610	31	8	30	20	66	10	6	300	2040	—	—	27
Wacker Fry	1 reg (9.8 oz)	490	27	9	30	12	51	3	5	100	1600	—	—	9
Wisconsin Inside-Out 7 Inch	1 (6.2 oz)	560	27	12	20	24	57	5	4	400	1360	—	—	0
SALAD DRESSINGS AND SAUCES														
Dressing Ranch	1 oz	170	18	3	10	1	1	1	0	20	160	—	—	0
Dressing Thousand Island	1 oz	130	12	2	10	0	4	3	0	0	280	—	—	0
Mayonnaise	1 oz	200	22	3	20	0	0	0	0	0	200	—	—	0
Mayonnaise Dijon	1 oz	110	11	2	10	0	3	0	0	0	420	—	—	0
Oil	1 serv (0.3 oz)	60	7	2	0	0	0	0	0	0	0	—	—	0
Sauce Buffalo	1 oz	10	0	0	0	0	2	0	0	0	855	—	—	21
Sauce Marinara Dipping	2 oz	15	0	0	0	1	3	1	0	0	260	—	—	6
Sauce Teriyaki	1 oz	25	0	0	0	2	3	3	0	0	960	—	—	0
Sauce Tzatziki	1 oz	50	4	4	0	0	2	1	0	40	80	—	—	0
SALADS														
Chef w/o Dressing	1 (16.1 oz)	260	11	6	70	28	15	8	4	300	1320	—	—	27
Garden w/o Dressing	1 (12 oz)	60	1	0	0	3	13	7	5	80	40	—	—	36
Great Salad Grilled Chicken	1 (18.8 oz)	380	18	8	80	31	18	9	5	350	460	—	—	36
Great Salad Grilled Ham	1 (18.8 oz)	360	20	8	75	24	28	13	5	350	1520	—	—	36
Great Salad Grilled Steak	1 (19.3 oz)	400	23	7	85	33	18	9	5	300	590	—	—	36
Great Salad Grilled Turkey	1 (18.8 oz)	330	17	6	65	30	20	9	5	350	970	—	—	36
Side w/o Dressing	1 (6 oz)	30	0	0	0	2	6	4	2	40	20	—	—	18
Wedge Grilled Chicken	1 (14.8 oz)	270	12	4	60	24	11	6	3	40	610	—	—	15
Wedge Grilled Steak	1 (15.3 oz)	290	16	4	70	28	11	6	3	40	550	—	—	15

HUNGRY HOWIE'S PIZZA

OTHER MENU SELECTIONS														
Cajun Bread	¼ bread	300	9	2	2	9	46	—	1	—	239	—	—	—
Chicken Tenders	2	140	5	1	30	13	11	—	0	—	460	—	—	—
Cinnamon Bread	¼ bread	313	9	2	2	9	59	—	1	—	239	—	—	—

FOOD	PORTION	CALS	FAT	SAT FAT	CHOL	PROT	CARB	SUGAR	FIBER	CALCI	SOD	POTAS	FOLIC	VIT C
Howie Bread	¼ bread	300	9	2	2	9	46	—	1	—	239	—	—	—
Howie Wings	5	180	13	4	60	14	0	0	0	—	760	—	—	—
Sub Deluxe Italian	½ sub	506	18	8	44	24	61	—	2	—	1005	—	—	—
Sub Ham & Cheese	½ sub	475	15	7	44	26	61	—	2	—	1020	—	—	—
Sub Pizza	½ sub	689	34	14	86	30	67	—	3	—	1722	—	—	—
Sub Pizza Special	½ sub	606	24	11	65	29	68	—	3	—	1584	—	—	—
Sub Steak & Cheese	½ sub	491	15	7	47	27	64	—	2	—	914	—	—	—
Sub Turkey	½ sub	466	13	6	38	25	63	—	2	—	1108	—	—	—
Sub Turkey Club	½ sub	556	15	8	42	42	63	—	2	—	1065	—	—	—
Sub Vegetarian	½ sub	530	21	11	39	22	64	—	3	—	895	—	—	—
Three Cheeser Bread	¼ bread	370	14	5	17	15	47	—	1	—	384	—	—	—
PIZZA														
Cheese Slice	1 med	191	6	3	11	11	23	—	1	—	437	—	—	—
Cheese Slice	1 sm	161	4	3	11	10	20	—	1	—	370	—	—	—
Cheese Slice	1 extra lg	395	9	6	25	23	42	—	2	—	882	—	—	—
Cheese Slice	1 lg	208	5	3	13	12	25	—	1	—	464	—	—	—
Cheese Slice Thin	1 lg	124	6	3	13	8	11	—	1	—	323	—	—	—
Cheese Slice Thin	1 med	111	5	3	11	7	10	—	tr	—	256	—	—	—
Medium Topping Anchovies	1 serv	44	3	1	16	7	0	0	0	—	736	—	—	—
Medium Topping Bacon	1 serv	32	1	tr	1	6	tr	—	0	—	—	—	—	—
Medium Topping Banana Peppers	1 serv	6	0	0	0	tr	1	—	0	—	162	—	—	—
Medium Topping Beef	1 serv	30	2	1	6	2	tr	—	tr	—	96	—	—	—
Medium Topping Black Olives	1 serv	7	tr	0	2	0	tr	—	tr	—	47	—	—	—
Medium Topping Ham	1 serv	7	tr	tr	4	1	0	—	0	—	81	—	—	—
Medium Topping Mushrooms	1 serv	2	0	0	0	tr	tr	—	tr	—	0	—	—	—
Medium Topping Pepperoni	1 serv	22	2	1	6	1	0	—	0	—	75	—	—	—
Medium Topping Pineapple	1 serv	5	0	0	0	1	2	—	1	—	0	—	—	—
Medium Topping Sausage	1 serv	27	2	tr	4	2	tr	—	tr	—	121	—	—	—
SALAD DRESSINGS AND SAUCES														
Dressing Blue Cheese	1 serv (1 oz)	150	16	3	20	1	1	—	0	—	300	—	—	—
Dressing Creamy Italian	1 serv (1 oz)	120	12	2	0	0	2	—	0	—	210	—	—	—

FOOD	PORTION	CALS	FAT	SAT FAT	CHOL	PROT	CARB	SUGAR	FIBER	CALCI	SOD	POTAS	FOLIC	VIT C
Dressing Fat Free Italian	1 serv (1.5 oz)	25	0	0	0	0	5	—	0	—	390	—	—	—
Dressing Fat Free Ranch	1 serv (1.5 oz)	45	0	0	0	0	10	—	1	—	540	—	—	—
Dressing French Style	1 serv (1 oz)	30	0	0	0	0	7	—	0	—	170	—	—	—
Dressing Greek	1 serv (1 oz)	110	11	2	0	0	2	—	0	—	70	—	—	—
Dressing Italian	1 serv (1 oz)	80	8	1	0	0	2	—	0	—	560	—	—	—
Dressing Ranch	1 serv (1 oz)	180	19	3	3	0	1	—	0	—	250	—	—	—
Dressing Thousand Island	1 serv (1 oz)	140	14	2	20	0	4	—	0	—	240	—	—	—
Sauce Dipping	1 serv (3 oz)	45	1	0	0	3	9	—	1	—	380	—	—	—
SALADS														
Antipasto	1 sm	115	7	4	28	9	3	—	2	—	554	—	—	—
Chef	1 sm	114	7	4	28	9	4	—	2	—	396	—	—	—
Garden	1 sm	20	tr	0	0	1	3	—	2	—	10	—	—	—
Greek	1 sm	126	7	5	29	7	8	—	2	—	581	—	—	—

IHOP

FOOD	PORTION	CALS	FAT	SAT FAT	CHOL	PROT	CARB	SUGAR	FIBER	CALCI	SOD	POTAS	FOLIC	VIT C
Pancake Buttermilk	5	770	25	9	115	22	115	22	7	—	2640	—	—	—
Pancake Buttermilk Short Stack	3	490	18	8	80	13	69	13	4	—	1610	—	—	—
Pancake Chocolate Chip	4	720	24	10	80	20	112	32	8	—	2070	—	—	—
Pancake Double Blueberry	4	800	17	5	80	19	144	57	11	—	2150	—	—	—
Pancake Harvest Grain 'N Nut	4	920	49	11	125	25	95	22	10	—	1810	—	—	—
Pancake New York Cheesecake	4	1100	44	21	190	26	152	53	8	—	2430	—	—	—
Pancake Strawberry Banana	4	760	17	5	80	20	137	41	10	—	2070	—	—	—

IVAR'S SEAFOOD BARS

FOOD	PORTION	CALS	FAT	SAT FAT	CHOL	PROT	CARB	SUGAR	FIBER	CALCI	SOD	POTAS	FOLIC	VIT C
Chicken	3 pieces (4.5 oz)	250	11	—	—	22	14	—	—	—	6	—	—	—
Chowder Salmon	1 cup	220	13	—	—	4	22	—	2	—	510	—	—	—
Chowder White	1 cup	330	19	—	—	17	24	—	4	—	1115	—	—	—
Clams	1 serv (5 oz)	400	21	—	—	17	33	—	1	—	—	—	—	—
Cocktail Sauce	¼ cup	50	0	0	0	1	12	—	1	—	730	—	—	—
Fish	3 pieces	220	9	—	—	22	12	—	1	—	7	—	—	—
French Fries	1 serv (3.5 oz)	300	16	—	—	4	34	—	2	—	1	—	—	—
Oysters	5	290	14	—	—	17	22	—	1	—	—	—	—	—
Prawns	1 serv (5 oz)	290	15	—	—	20	18	—	tr	—	17	—	—	—

FOOD	PORTION	CALS	FAT	SAT FAT	CHOL	PROT	CARB	SUGAR	FIBER	CALCI	SOD	POTAS	FOLIC	VIT C
Salmon Fried	3 pieces (4.5 oz)	210	9	—	—	24	9	—	1	—	—	—	—	—
Scallops	1 serv (5 oz)	240	9	—	—	22	14	—	tr	—	—	—	—	—
Tartar Sauce	2 tbsp	140	15	—	—	0	1	—	0	—	250	—	—	—

JACK IN THE BOX

BEVERAGES

FOOD	PORTION	CALS	FAT	SAT FAT	CHOL	PROT	CARB	SUGAR	FIBER	CALCI	SOD	POTAS	FOLIC	VIT C
Barq's Root Beer	1 (20 oz)	180	0	0	0	0	50	50	0	—	40	0	—	—
Chug Chocolate Milk Low Fat	1 (3.5 oz)	200	3	2	5	11	34	33	1	—	230	—	—	—
Chug Reduced Fat Milk	1 (3.5 oz)	130	5	3	25	10	13	13	0	—	130	—	—	—
Coca-Cola Classic	1 (20 oz)	170	0	0	0	0	46	46	0	—	0	0	—	—
Coffee Regular & Decaf	1 (11 oz)	5	0	0	0	0	1	0	0	—	5	170	—	—
Diet Coke	1 (20 oz)	0	0	0	0	0	0	0	0	—	15	40	—	—
Dr Pepper	1 (20 oz)	150	0	0	0	0	42	42	0	—	50	0	—	—
Fanta Orange	1 (20 oz)	150	0	0	0	0	41	41	0	—	50	0	—	—
Fanta Strawberry	1 (20 oz)	150	0	0	0	0	41	41	0	—	10	0	—	—
Iced Tea	1 (20 oz)	5	0	0	0	0	2	0	0	—	20	220	—	—
Lemonade	1 (20 oz)	160	0	0	0	0	42	42	0	—	65	20	—	—
Orange Juice	1 (10 oz)	140	0	0	0	2	32	27	2	—	25	220	—	—
Shake Chocolate	1 (16 oz)	880	45	31	135	14	107	94	1	—	330	840	—	—
Shake Oreo	1 (16 oz)	910	49	32	135	14	102	80	1	—	420	750	—	—
Shake Strawberry	1 (16 oz)	880	44	31	135	13	105	88	0	—	290	750	—	—
Shake Vanilla	1 (16 oz)	790	44	31	135	13	83	70	0	—	280	750	—	—
Sprite	1 (20 oz)	160	0	0	0	0	42	42	0	—	40	0	—	—

BREAKFAST SELECTIONS

FOOD	PORTION	CALS	FAT	SAT FAT	CHOL	PROT	CARB	SUGAR	FIBER	CALCI	SOD	POTAS	FOLIC	VIT C
Biscuit Bacon Egg Cheese	1	430	25	8	220	17	34	3	1	—	1100	140	—	—
Biscuit Chicken	1	450	24	6	30	15	42	2	2	—	980	170	—	—
Biscuit Sausage	1	440	29	8	35	12	32	3	2	—	870	340	—	—
Biscuit Sausage Egg Cheese	1	740	55	17	280	27	35	3	2	—	1430	310	—	—
Biscuit Spicy Chicken	1	460	22	5	40	21	44	2	2	—	1020	260	—	—
Breakfast Sandwich Ciabatta	1	710	30	10	440	36	63	4	3	—	1730	440	—	—
Breakfast Sandwich Ultimate	1	570	27	10	445	34	49	8	2	—	1700	370	—	—
Breakfast Jack	1	290	12	5	220	17	39	4	1	—	760	210	—	—
Breakfast Jack Bacon	1	300	14	5	215	16	29	4	1	—	730	180	—	—
Breakfast Jack Sausage	1	450	28	10	245	20	29	4	1	—	840	250	—	—

FOOD	PORTION	CALS	FAT	SAT FAT	CHOL	PROT	CARB	SUGAR	FIBER	CALCI	SOD	POTAS	FOLIC	VIT C
Burrito Hearty Breakfast	1	480	29	10	350	25	29	1	2	—	1210	300	—	—
Burrito Sirloin Steak & Egg w/o Salsa	1	790	48	15	450	37	52	2	6	—	1320	430	—	—
Croissant Sausage	1	580	39	13	255	21	37	5	2	—	770	260	—	—
Croissant Supreme	1	450	25	9	235	20	36	5	1	—	860	240	—	—
French Toast Sticks	4 (4.2 oz)	470	23	5	25	7	58	14	4	—	450	120	—	—
French Toast Sticks Blueberry	4	450	20	5	0	8	59	15	3	—	550	115	—	—
Hash Browns	1 serv	150	10	3	0	1	13	0	2	—	230	190	—	—
Sandwich Extreme Sausage	1	670	48	17	290	29	31	5	2	—	1300	370	—	—
DESSERTS														
Cake Chocolate Overload	1 serv (3.2 oz)	300	7	2	40	4	57	34	2	—	350	260	—	—
Cheesecake	1 serv (3.6 oz)	310	16	9	55	7	34	23	0	—	220	180	—	—
MAIN MENU SELECTIONS														
Bacon Cheddar Potato Wedges	1 serv (9 oz)	720	48	15	45	21	52	2	4	—	1360	950	—	—
Cheeseburger Bacon Ultimate	1	1090	77	30	140	46	53	12	2	—	2040	540	—	—
Cheeseburger Junior Bacon	1	430	25	9	60	20	30	6	1	—	820	270	—	—
Cheeseburger Sourdough Ultimate	1	950	73	29	125	38	36	7	2	—	1360	490	—	—
Cheeseburger Ultimate	1	1010	71	28	125	40	53	12	2	—	1580	480	—	—
Chicken Fajita Pita	1	280	9	4	60	21	30	3	2	—	1110	380	—	—
Chicken Sandwich	1	400	21	5	35	15	38	4	2	—	730	240	—	—
Chicken Strips Crispy	4	500	25	6	80	35	36	1	3	—	1260	530	—	—
Chicken Strips Grilled	4 (5 oz)	180	2	1	125	37	3	2	0	—	700	590	—	—
Ciabatta Chipotle w/ Grilled Chicken	1	690	28	9	105	44	65	6	4	—	1850	620	—	—
Ciabatta Chipotle w/ Spicy Crispy Chicken	1	750	34	10	80	37	75	5	5	—	1650	540	—	—
Ciabatta Sirloin Steak 'N' Cheddar	1	770	38	8	110	43	65	5	4	—	1310	630	—	—
Ciabatta Burger Bacon 'N' Cheese	1	1120	76	28	135	45	66	9	4	—	1670	660	—	—

FOOD	PORTION	CALS	FAT	SAT FAT	CHOL	PROT	CARB	SUGAR	FIBER	CALCI	SOD	POTAS	FOLIC	VIT C
Ciabatta Burger Single Bacon 'N' Cheese	1	870	54	18	90	31	66	8	4	—	1550	490	—	—
Club Sourdough Grilled Chicken	1	530	28	7	85	36	34	5	3	—	1430	580	—	—
Curly Fries Seasoned	1 sm (3 oz)	270	15	3	0	4	30	1	3	—	590	390	—	—
Egg Rolls	1	130	6	2	5	5	15	1	2	—	310	140	—	—
Fish & Chips	1 serv (7.6 oz)	570	30	7	35	17	58	1	4	—	1100	920	—	—
Fries Natural Cut	1 sm	340	17	4	0	5	41	1	5	—	620	860	—	—
Fruit Cup	1 serv	90	0	0	0	1	22	18	2	—	20	400	—	—
Hamburger	1	310	14	6	40	16	30	6	1	—	600	250	—	—
Hamburger Deluxe	1	370	21	7	45	17	31	6	2	—	560	330	—	—
Hamburger Deluxe w/ Cheese	1	460	28	11	70	21	33	7	2	—	930	360	—	—
Hamburger w/ Cheese	1	350	17	8	50	18	31	7	1	—	790	270	—	—
Jack's Spicy Chicken	1 serv	620	31	6	50	25	61	8	4	—	1100	450	—	—
Jack's Spicy Chicken w/ Cheese	1	700	37	10	70	29	62	8	4	—	1410	480	—	—
Jumbo Jack	1	600	35	12	45	21	51	11	3	—	940	380	—	—
Jumbo Jack w/ Cheese	1	690	42	16	70	25	54	12	3	—	1310	410	—	—
Mozzarella Cheese Sticks	3	240	12	5	25	11	21	1	1	—	420	60	—	—
Onion Rings	8 (4.2 oz)	500	30	6	0	6	51	3	3	—	420	140	—	—
Sampler Trio	1 serv	750	39	14	85	35	65	4	5	—	1760	440	—	—
Sandwich Bacon Chicken	1	440	24	6	40	19	39	4	2	—	970	270	—	—
Sirloin Burger w/ American Cheese & Red Onion	1	1120	73	24	190	54	63	11	4	—	2620	790	—	—
Sirloin Burger w/ Swiss & Grilled Onions	1	1070	71	25	180	53	61	10	4	—	1850	680	—	—
Sirloin Steak Melt	1	640	40	13	100	36	34	4	2	—	1490	420	—	—
Sourdough Jack	1	710	51	18	75	27	36	7	3	—	1230	430	—	—
Spicy Chicken Bites	1 serv	290	14	3	45	18	21	1	3	—	660	270	—	—
Stuffed Jalapeno	3 (2.5 oz)	230	13	6	20	7	22	2	2	—	690	105	—	—
Taco Monster Beef	1	240	14	5	20	8	20	4	3	—	390	220	—	—
Taco Regular Beef	1	160	8	3	15	5	15	4	2	—	270	190	—	—

FOOD	PORTION	CALS	FAT	SAT FAT	CHOL	PROT	CARB	SUGAR	FIBER	CALCI	SOD	POTAS	FOLIC	VIT C
SALAD DRESSINGS AND TOPPINGS														
Asian Sesame	1 serv (2.5 oz)	230	17	3	0	1	20	13	0	—	780	60	—	—
Bacon Ranch	1 serv (2.5 oz)	320	33	5	35	2	4	2	0	—	810	85	—	—
Creamy Southwest	1 serv (2.5 oz)	270	27	5	30	1	4	1	0	—	1060	80	—	—
Dipping Sauce Barbeque	1 serv (1 oz)	45	0	0	0	0	11	4	0	—	330	65	—	—
Dipping Sauce Buttermilk House	1 serv (0.9 oz)	130	13	2	10	0	3	0	0	—	210	15	—	—
Dipping Sauce Frank's Red Hot Buffalo	1 serv (1 oz)	10	0	0	0	0	2	0	0	—	840	15	—	—
Dipping Sauce Sweet & Sour	1 serv (1 oz)	45	0	0	0	0	11	6	0	—	160	5	—	—
Dipping Sauce Teriyaki	1 serv (1 oz)	60	0	0	0	1	13	11	0	—	460	15	—	—
Dipping Sauce Zesty Marinara	1 serv (0.8 oz)	15	0	0	0	0	4	2	0	—	200	10	—	—
Low Fat Balsamic	1 serv (2.5 oz)	40	2	0	0	0	6	3	0	—	600	30	—	—
Mayo Onion Sauce	1 serv (0.5 oz)	90	10	2	5	1	4	2	0	—	590	55	—	—
Ranch	1 serv (2.5 oz)	390	41	6	30	1	4	2	0	—	590	55	—	—
Ranch Lite	1 serv (2.5 oz)	190	18	3	25	1	3	2	0	—	700	50	—	—
Soy Sauce	1 serv (0.3 oz)	5	0	0	0	1	1	0	0	—	480	35	—	—
Syrup Log Cabin	1 serv (2 oz)	190	0	0	0	0	49	18	0	—	35	15	—	—
Taco Sauce	1 serv (0.3 oz)	0	0	0	0	0	0	0	0	—	80	20	—	—
Tartar Sauce	1 serv (1.5 oz)	210	22	4	20	0	2	1	0	—	370	30	—	—
SALADS														
Asian w/ Crispy Chicken w/o Dressing	1 (13.8 oz)	330	13	3	40	21	34	11	7	—	650	830	—	—
Asian w/ Grilled Chicken w/o Dressing	1 (12.8 oz)	160	2	0	65	22	18	11	5	—	380	870	—	—
Chicken Club w/ Crispy Chicken w/o Dressing	1 (14 oz)	480	27	7	80	33	26	5	6	—	1060	800	—	—
Chicken Club w/ Grilled Chicken w/o Dressing	1 (13 oz)	320	16	6	105	34	11	5	4	—	780	830	—	—
Side w/o Dressing	1 (4.3 oz)	50	3	2	10	3	5	2	2	—	60	260	—	—
Southwest w/ Crispy Chicken w/o Dressing	1 (16 oz)	480	23	8	70	30	44	5	9	—	1040	920	—	—
Southwest w/ Grilled Chicken w/o Dressing	1 (15 oz)	320	12	6	90	31	27	5	7	—	760	950	—	—

JAMBA JUICE

BEVERAGES

FOOD	PORTION	CALS	FAT	SAT FAT	CHOL	PROT	CARB	SUGAR	FIBER	CALCI	SOD	POTAS	FOLIC	VIT C
Acai Super Antioxidant	1 (16 oz)	290	5	2	5	4	59	50	4	80	50	250	100	612
Acai Topper	1 (12 oz)	440	9	2	0	8	86	55	9	60	40	780	60	114
Aloha Pineapple	1 (16 oz)	300	1	0	5	5	70	65	3	100	15	650	40	66
Banana Berry	1 (16 oz)	300	1	0	5	3	72	63	3	100	65	690	16	12
Berry Fulfilling	1 (16 oz)	160	1	0	5	7	34	26	4	300	230	120	24	21
Berry Topper	1 (12 oz)	420	9	2	5	11	80	51	9	150	80	780	40	48
Blackberry Bliss	1 (16 oz)	260	1	0	0	1	61	54	4	80	25	410	8	21
Boost 3G Charger Super	1 (3 g)	5	0	0	0	0	2	—	2	—	—	—	—	—
Boost Antioxidant Power Super	1 (2.8 g)	0	—	—	—	—	—	—	—	—	—	—	—	300
Boost Calcium	1	0	—	—	—	—	—	—	—	1000	—	—	—	—
Boost Daily Vitamin	1 (4.36 g)	0	—	—	—	—	—	—	—	250	—	—	400	90
Boost Energy	½ tsp (1.1 g)	0	—	—	—	—	—	—	—	—	—	—	400	—
Boost Flax & Fiber	1 (0.4 oz)	30	2	—	—	1	7	—	7	—	—	—	—	—
Boost Heart Happy	1 (0.75 g)	0	—	—	—	—	—	—	—	—	—	—	400	6
Boost Immunity	1 tsp (2.5 g)	0	—	—	—	—	—	—	—	—	—	—	—	120
Boost Soy Protein	1 (8.9 g)	30	0	—	—	8	0	0	0	—	—	—	—	—
Boost Weight Burner Super	1 (3.5 g)	30	3	0	0	0	0	0	0	—	—	—	—	—
Boost Whey Protein Super	1 (12 g)	45	0	—	5	10	1	—	—	—	20	—	—	—
Caribbean Passion	1 (16 oz)	270	1	0	5	2	63	56	3	80	35	540	80	54
Carrot Juice	1 (16 oz)	100	1	0	0	3	22	20	0	100	170	740	60	12
Chocolate Moo'd	1 (16 oz)	460	6	4	20	12	93	84	2	400	270	580	16	4
Chunky Strawberry Topper	1 (12 oz)	480	15	3	5	13	74	44	8	150	120	690	40	48
Coldbuster	1 (16 oz)	270	2	1	5	3	63	54	3	60	20	860	80	552
Mango Mantra	1 (16 oz)	170	1	0	5	7	36	33	3	250	230	330	32	54
Mango Metabolizer	1 (16 oz)	290	4	0	0	2	63	54	4	60	20	590	120	78
Mango Peach Topper	1 (12 oz)	450	9	2	5	11	86	57	8	150	80	860	40	36
Mango-A-Go-Go	1 (16 oz)	310	1	0	5	2	72	65	2	60	35	530	80	48
Matcha Green Tea Blast	1 (16 oz)	290	0	0	0	8	62	55	1	100	160	190	32	6
Mega Mango	1 (16 oz)	250	1	0	0	3	62	57	4	40	5	780	80	150
Orange Dream Machine	1 (16 oz)	350	2	1	5	8	75	70	tr	150	150	440	40	66
Orange Juice	1 (16 oz)	220	1	0	0	3	52	51	tr	60	0	990	160	246
Peach Perfection	1 (16 oz)	230	0	0	0	2	57	46	4	40	20	530	40	48

FOOD	PORTION	CALS	FAT	SAT FAT	CHOL	PROT	CARB	SUGAR	FIBER	CALCI	SOD	POTAS	FOLIC	VIT C
Peach Pleasure	1 (16 oz)	290	1	1	5	2	68	56	3	60	35	520	40	12
Peanut Butter Moo'd	1 (16 oz)	490	11	3	10	13	85	75	3	250	310	580	24	6
Pomegranate Heart Happy	1 (16 oz)	300	1	0	0	4	72	63	3	150	105	670	440	48
Pomegranate Paradise	1 (16 oz)	260	1	0	0	2	64	56	4	80	25	750	32	66
Pomegranate Pick-Me-Up	1 (16 oz)	280	2	0	5	2	67	57	3	80	40	480	60	42
Protein Berry Workout w/ Soy Protein	1 (16 oz)	290	1	0	0	15	55	46	4	40	180	460	40	42
Protein Berry Workout w/ Whey	1 (16 oz)	300	0	0	5	17	56	46	4	20	115	460	32	42
Razzmatazz	1 (16 oz)	300	1	1	5	2	70	57	3	80	40	560	100	42
Shot Matcha Energy Orange Juice	1 (4 oz)	60	0	0	0	1	13	13	tr	20	0	280	60	66
Shot Matcha Energy Soymilk	1 (4 oz)	70	0	0	0	3	14	12	0	0	45	35	16	4
Shot Wheatgrass Detox	1 oz	5	0	0	0	tr	tr	0	0	0	0	80	16	4
Strawberries Wild	1 (16 oz)	280	0	0	0	3	66	58	3	150	100	700	24	42
Strawberry Energizer	1 (16 oz)	300	1	0	5	2	71	63	3	80	25	420	160	72
Strawberry Nirvana	1 (16 oz)	170	0	0	5	7	36	30	3	250	230	360	24	42
Strawberry Surf Rider	1 (16 oz)	330	1	0	5	2	80	71	3	60	10	340	240	60
Strawberry Whirl	1 (16 oz)	240	1	0	0	1	59	50	5	60	20	800	40	60
FOOD														
Cheddar Tomato Twist	1 (3.2 oz)	240	5	2	15	8	41	3	2	60	430	95	60	4
Cookie Omega-3 Chocolate Brownie	1 (1.5 oz)	150	4	1	0	3	30	24	2	20	15	95	8	0
Cookie Omega-3 Oatmeal	1 (1.5 oz)	150	6	2	5	2	26	15	3	20	85	95	8	0
Loaf Reduced Fat Blueberry Lemon	1 (3 oz)	290	8	—	—	2	53	30	2	40	—	—	—	0
Loaf Reduced Fat Cranberry Orange	1 (3 oz)	310	9	2	20	6	52	21	4	60	200	0	0	0
Loaf Zucchini Walnut	1 (3 oz)	270	9	2	20	5	43	26	4	60	250	0	0	0
Oatcake Blueberry	1 (3.25 oz)	280	9	1	0	6	46	17	6	80	220	85	8	0
Oatmeal Apple Cinnamon	1 serv (9.1 oz)	290	4	1	5	8	60	25	5	40	25	0	0	5

FOOD	PORTION	CALS	FAT	SAT FAT	CHOL	PROT	CARB	SUGAR	FIBER	CALCI	SOD	POTAS	FOLIC	VIT C
Oatmeal Blueberry & Blackberry	1 serv (8.9 oz)	290	4	1	0	8	59	25	6	20	30	0	0	1
Oatmeal Fresh Banana	1 serv (9.6 oz)	280	4	1	0	9	57	23	6	20	20	230	8	4
Oatmeal w/ Brown Sugar	1 serv (7.6 oz)	220	4	1	0	8	44	12	5	20	20	0	0	0
Pretzel Apple Cinnamon	1 (5.2 oz)	380	4	0	0	11	76	14	4	20	250	135	120	0
Pretzel Sourdough Parmesan	1 (5 oz)	410	10	2	5	14	67	4	3	100	640	100	120	0

JERSEY MIKE'S

SANDWICHES

FOOD	PORTION	CALS	FAT	SAT FAT	CHOL	PROT	CARB	SUGAR	FIBER	CALCI	SOD	POTAS	FOLIC	VIT C
#10 Albacore Tuna In A Tub	1 (12.2 oz)	620	55	8	55	21	12	5	3	60	680	—	—	12
#10 Albacore Tuna Wheat	1 (16.2 oz)	910	59	9	55	32	66	11	6	80	1330	—	—	12
#10 Albacore Tuna White	1 (16.2 oz)	910	59	10	55	32	67	9	4	80	1330	—	—	12
#13 Original Italian In A Tub	1 (12.9 oz)	390	22	10	95	34	14	5	2	300	1600	—	—	12
#13 Original Italian Wheat	1 reg (16.9 oz)	680	27	11	95	45	68	11	5	300	2250	—	—	12
#13 Original Italian White	1 reg (16.9 oz)	680	27	11	96	45	69	9	4	300	2250	—	—	12
#14 Veggie White	1 reg (15.7 oz)	750	36	21	100	42	69	10	5	900	940	—	—	36
#5 Super Sub In A Tub	1 (11.9 oz)	290	14	7	85	29	13	5	2	300	1150	—	—	12
#5 Super Sub Wheat	1 (16 oz)	280	19	8	85	40	67	11	5	300	1800	—	—	12
#5 Super Sub White	1 (16 oz)	580	19	9	85	40	68	9	4	300	1800	—	—	12
#6 Roast Beef & Provolone In A Tub	1 (12.2 oz)	430	20	9	125	52	9	5	2	300	190	—	—	12
#6 Roast Beef & Provolone Wheat	1 reg (16.2 oz)	720	25	10	125	63	64	11	5	300	840	—	—	12
#6 Roast Beef & Provolone White	1 reg (16.2 oz)	730	25	11	125	64	64	8	4	300	840	—	—	12
#7 Turkey Breast & Provolone In A Tub	1 (11.4 oz)	250	11	6	65	30	9	5	2	300	930	—	—	12
#7 Turkey Breast & Provolone Wheat	1 reg (15.4 oz)	540	16	6	65	41	64	11	5	300	1590	—	—	12
#7 Turkey Breast & Provolone White	1 (15.4 oz)	550	15	7	65	41	64	8	4	300	1590	—	—	12

FOOD	PORTION	CALS	FAT	SAT FAT	CHOL	PROT	CARB	SUGAR	FIBER	CALCI	SOD	POTAS	FOLIC	VIT C
#8 Club Sub w/ Mayonnaise In A Tub	1 (13.2 oz)	600	47	14	100	32	11	5	2	300	1610	—	—	12
#8 Club Sub w/ Mayonnaise Wheat	1 (17.2 oz)	890	52	15	100	43	66	11	5	300	2260	—	—	12
#8 Club Sub w/ Mayonnaise White	1 (17.2 oz)	890	52	16	100	44	67	9	4	300	2260	—	—	12
#9 Club Sub Supreme w/ Mayonnaise In A Tub	1 (13.2 oz)	650	47	13	120	45	11	5	2	200	910	—	—	12
#9 Club Supreme w/ Mayonnaise Wheat	1 reg (17.2 oz)	940	52	14	120	56	66	11	5	250	1560	—	—	12
#9 Club Supreme w/ Mayonnaise White	1 (17.2 oz)	940	52	15	120	56	66	9	4	250	1560	—	—	12
American Classic In A Tub	1 (11.4 oz)	270	14	7	80	26	11	5	2	300	1310	—	—	12
American Classic Wheat	1 reg (15.4 oz)	560	18	8	80	37	65	11	5	300	1960	—	—	12
American Classic White	1 reg (15.4 oz)	560	18	9	80	38	66	8	4	300	1960	—	—	12
BLT In A Tub	1 (8.2 oz)	280	21	9	45	14	8	5	2	40	790	—	—	12
BLT Wheat	1 reg (12.2 oz)	570	26	10	45	25	63	10	5	40	2860	—	—	12
BLT White	1 reg (12.2 oz)	570	26	11	45	25	64	8	4	40	1450	—	—	12
Hot Sub #15 Meatball & Cheese Wheat	1 reg (13.5 oz)	890	52	21	95	39	72	12	6	400	1950	—	—	2
Hot Sub #15 Meatball & Cheese White	1 reg (13.5 oz)	890	51	—	95	39	72	10	5	400	1950	—	—	2
Hot Sub #17 Chicken Philly Wheat	1 reg (13 oz)	630	25	13	175	39	65	12	4	250	1730	—	—	30
Hot Sub BBQ Beef Wheat	1 reg (11.2 oz)	710	16	5	110	59	83	23	4	60	1520	—	—	0
Hot Sub BBQ Beef White	1 reg (11.2 oz)	720	16	6	110	59	84	20	3	60	1520	—	—	0
Hot Sub Big Kahuna Chicken Wheat	1 reg (14.2 oz)	680	29	16	190	42	66	13	5	300	2090	—	—	30
Hot Sub Big Kahuna Chicken White	1 reg (14.2 oz)	690	29	17	190	42	67	11	3	300	2090	—	—	12
Hot Sub Big Kahuna Wheat	1 reg (14.2 oz)	670	28	14	140	43	65	12	5	300	2070	—	—	30

FOOD	PORTION	CALS	FAT	SAT FAT	CHOL	PROT	CARB	SUGAR	FIBER	CALCI	SOD	POTAS	FOLIC	VIT C
Hot Sub Big Kahuna White	1 reg (14.2 oz)	680	28	15	140	44	66	10	3	300	2060	—	—	30
Hot Sub Cheese Steak Buffalo Chicken Wheat	1 reg (20.2 oz)	940	55	19	185	43	73	17	5	300	4070	—	—	54
Hot Sub Cheese Steak Buffalo Chicken White	1 reg (20.2 oz)	940	55	20	185	43	74	14	4	300	4070	—	—	54
Hot Sub Cheese Steak California Chicken Wheat	1 reg (17.4 oz)	890	53	18	190	40	67	14	5	250	1940	—	—	12
Hot Sub Cheese Steak California Chicken White	1 reg (17.4 oz)	890	52	18	190	38	67	12	4	250	1940	—	—	12
Hot Sub Cheese Steak California Wheat	1 reg (17.4 oz)	870	51	15	140	42	65	12	5	250	1920	—	—	12
Hot Sub Cheese Steak California White	1 reg (17.4 oz)	880	51	16	140	42	66	10	4	250	1920	—	—	12
Hot Sub Cheese Steak Teriyaki Chicken Wheat	1 reg (14.9 oz)	680	25	13	175	42	74	20	4	250	3900	—	—	30
Hot Sub Cheese Steak Teriyaki Chicken White	1 reg (14.9 oz)	680	25	14	175	43	75	18	3	250	3900	—	—	30
Hot Sub Chicka Phila Roni Wheat	1 reg (12.5 oz)	620	19	12	90	32	62	7	3	240	1970	—	—	2
Hot Sub Chicka Phila Roni White	1 reg (12.5 oz)	605	12	12	90	31	65	5	1	240	2010	—	—	2
Hot Sub Chicken Parmesan Wheat	1 reg (11 oz)	650	22	7	60	37	77	7	5	250	1590	—	—	1
Hot Sub Chicken Philly White	1 reg (13 oz)	630	25	14	175	39	68	10	3	250	1730	—	—	30
Hot Sub Chipotle Chicken Wheat	1 reg (14.4 oz)	910	56	19	195	40	68	12	4	300	2200	—	—	30
Hot Sub Chipotle Chicken White	1 reg (14.4 oz)	920	56	19	195	41	68	10	3	300	2200	—	—	30
Hot Sub Chipotle Steak Wheat	1 reg (14.4 oz)	900	55	16	145	42	66	11	4	300	2180	—	—	30
Hot Sub Chipotle Steak White	1 reg (14.4 oz)	910	55	17	145	42	67	9	3	300	2180	—	—	30
Hot Sub Chipotle Turkey Wheat	1 reg (17.4 oz)	865	50	14	95	44	67	10	6	400	2140	—	—	12
Hot Sub Chipotle Turkey White	1 reg (17.4 oz)	870	50	15	95	44	67	8	4	400	2140	—	—	12
Hot Sub Grilled Chicken Wheat	1 reg (12.7 oz)	670	33	5	65	34	60	8	4	60	1290	—	—	6

FOOD	PORTION	CALS	FAT	SAT FAT	CHOL	PROT	CARB	SUGAR	FIBER	CALCI	SOD	POTAS	FOLIC	VIT C
Hot Sub Grilled Chicken White	1 reg (12.7 oz)	670	33	6	65	34	61	6	3	60	1290	—	—	6
Hot Sub Pastrami & Swiss Wheat	1 reg (10.7 oz)	580	18	87	95	45	60	8	3	250	2660	—	—	0
Hot Sub Pastrami & Swiss White	1 reg (10.7 oz)	590	17	9	95	45	61	6	2	250	2660	—	—	0
Hot Sub Reuben Wheat	1 reg (12.2 oz)	700	27	9	95	41	72	14	5	250	2680	—	—	9
Hot Sub Reuben White	1 reg (12.2 oz)	710	27	10	95	42	73	11	3	250	2680	—	—	9
Hot Sub Sausage Wheat	1 reg (11.5 oz)	600	27	8	65	26	66	12	5	40	1690	—	—	30
Hot Sub Sausage White	1 reg (11.4 oz)	600	26	8	65	26	66	10	4	40	1690	—	—	30
Hot Sub Steak Philly Wheat	1 reg (13 oz)	620	24	11	125	41	64	11	4	250	1700	—	—	30
Hot Sub Steak Philly White	1 reg (13 oz)	620	23	12	125	43	64	9	3	250	1700	—	—	30
Jersey Shore Favorite In A Tub	1 (11.4 oz)	270	14	7	80	26	12	5	2	300	1060	—	—	12
Jersey Shore Favorite Wheat	1 reg (15.4 oz)	560	18	8	80	37	67	11	5	300	1700	—	—	12
Jersey Shore Favorite White	1 reg (15.4 oz)	570	18	9	80	38	67	9	4	300	1700	—	—	12
Veggie In A Tub	1 (11.7 oz)	460	32	19	100	31	14	7	3	900	290	—	—	36
Veggie Wheat	1 reg (15.72 oz)	720	33	18	75	45	65	11	6	1000	900	—	—	36
Wrap Baja Chicken	1 (15.6 oz)	610	23	11	90	40	63	7	8	450	2640	—	—	6
Wrap Buffalo Chicken	1 (14.6 oz)	740	37	14	95	40	62	6	6	450	2990	—	—	24
Wrap Chicken Caesar	1 (12 oz)	580	23	5	65	33	58	4	6	300	1470	—	—	2
Wrap Grilled Ham & Cheese	1 (14 oz)	740	41	13	80	29	63	11	5	500	1980	—	—	15
Wrap Grilled Roast Beef & Cheese	1 (15 oz)	830	45	14	100	42	65	12	5	500	1170	—	—	15
Wrap Grilled Veggie	1 (17 oz)	910	57	22	105	36	69	10	8	1000	1480	—	—	36
Wrap Turkey w/ Honey Mustard Sauce	1 (13 oz)	540	20	4	50	30	63	10	7	200	1700	—	—	9
SOUPS														
Beef Steak & Black Bean	1 cup (8.7 oz)	140	2	0	10	10	21	3	9	60	990	—	—	1
Boston Clam Chowder	1 cup (8.5 oz)	130	6	2	15	5	15	0	0	20	1030	—	—	5
Broccoli Cheese	1 cup (8.7 oz)	140	9	5	25	4	8	2	0	60	1100	—	—	6

FOOD	PORTION	CALS	FAT	SAT FAT	CHOL	PROT	CARB	SUGAR	FIBER	CALCI	SOD	POTAS	FOLIC	VIT C
Cape Cod Clam Chowder	1 cup (8.7 oz)	140	6	2	10	4	17	1	0	40	1110	—	—	0
Chicken & Dumplings	1 cup (8.7 oz)	250	18	7	45	7	16	4	0	60	1040	—	—	0
Chicken Gumbo	1 cup (9 oz)	100	5	2	20	4	11	2	1	40	1020	—	—	0
Chicken Noodle	1 cup (8.7 oz)	90	4	1	15	4	11	0	0	0	910	—	—	0
Chicken Pot Pie	1 cup (8.7 oz)	230	14	5	45	7	20	3	1	20	1240	—	—	9
Chicken Tortilla	1 cup (8.7 oz)	140	3	1	20	8	22	2	5	40	1010	—	—	0
Cream Of Broccoli	1 cup (8.7 oz)	90	6	3	15	3	9	3	1	40	1220	—	—	5
Cream Of Potato	1 cup (8.7 oz)	180	8	5	25	2	17	0	1	20	810	—	—	0
Creamy Tomato Bisque	1 cup (8.5 oz)	90	4	1	0	1	11	5	1	60	1130	—	—	4
French Onion	1 cup (8.7 oz)	80	1	0	0	3	15	3	3	60	940	—	—	1
Italian Wedding	1 cup (8.5 oz)	120	5	3	10	5	13	1	1	40	1000	—	—	2
Lumberjack Vegetable	1 cup (8.5 oz)	120	5	2	5	2	16	4	5	40	1320	—	—	2
Maryland Crab	1 cup (8.7 oz)	70	1	0	10	4	12	4	2	40	980	—	—	1
Minestrone	1 cup (8.7 oz)	70	3	1	0	3	8	6	0	40	1540	—	—	0
Potato w/ Bacon	1 cup (8.5 oz)	130	5	2	5	4	18	2	1	20	1080	—	—	2
Spicy Chili w/ Beans	1 cup (9.6 oz)	240	8	4	40	16	25	5	7	150	1130	—	—	2
Split Pea w/ Ham	1 cup (8.5 oz)	150	2	1	5	9	25	4	3	20	1050	—	—	1
Timberline Chili w/ Beans	1 cup (8.7 oz)	280	9	4	30	18	31	9	7	100	680	—	—	6
Tomato Florentine	1 cup (8.7 oz)	90	1	0	0	3	17	6	1	60	1060	—	—	0
Vegetable Beef & Barley	1 cup (8.7 oz)	90	3	1	10	5	11	1	2	40	1040	—	—	0
Vegetarian Vegetable	1 cup (8.7 oz)	80	1	0	0	2	10	4	4	40	850	—	—	4
Wild & Brown Rice w/ Chicken	1 cup (8.7 oz)	310	15	5	75	26	17	1	1	40	910	—	—	0
Wisconsin Cheese	1 cup (8.5 oz)	220	16	5	20	5	16	8	0	80	1200	—	—	1

JIMMY JOHN'S

BEVERAGES

FOOD	PORTION	CALS	FAT	SAT FAT	CHOL	PROT	CARB	SUGAR	FIBER	CALCI	SOD	POTAS	FOLIC	VIT C
Coke	1 sm	248	0	0	0	0	68	—	0	—	15	—	—	—
Diet Coke	1 sm	0	0	0	0	0	0	0	0	—	25	—	—	—
Iced Tea	1 sm	3	0	0	0	0	1	—	0	—	35	—	—	—
Iced Tea Raspberry	1 sm	195	0	0	0	0	53	—	0	—	23	—	—	—
Lemonade	1 sm	243	0	0	0	0	65	—	0	—	103	—	—	—
Lemonade Light	1 sm	13	0	0	0	0	3	—	0	—	13	—	—	—
Sprite	1 sm	243	0	0	0	0	65	—	0	—	55	—	—	—

SANDWICHES

FOOD	PORTION	CALS	FAT	SAT FAT	CHOL	PROT	CARB	SUGAR	FIBER	CALCI	SOD	POTAS	FOLIC	VIT C
Giant Club Beach	1	798	37	10	73	37	78	—	2	—	1873	—	—	—
Giant Club Billy	1	867	40	11	99	48	77	—	1	—	2533	—	—	—

FOOD	PORTION	CALS	FAT	SAT FAT	CHOL	PROT	CARB	SUGAR	FIBER	CALCI	SOD	POTAS	FOLIC	VIT C
Giant Club Bootlegger	1	720	28	4	77	40	74	—	1	—	2152	—	—	—
Giant Club Country	1	840	38	10	107	47	75	—	1	—	2478	—	—	—
Giant Club Gourmet Smoked Ham	1	851	40	11	105	45	76	—	1	—	2553	—	—	—
Giant Club Gourmet Veggie	1	856	46	15	60	33	77	—	2	—	1500	—	—	—
Giant Club Hunter's	1	854	38	11	93	49	76	—	1	—	2387	—	—	—
Giant Club Italian Night	1	975	52	14	115	47	77	—	1	—	2763	—	—	—
Giant Club Lulu	1	790	34	6	76	42	74	—	1	—	2050	—	—	—
Giant Club Tuna	1	719	29	9	53	34	77	—	2	—	1578	—	—	—
Giant Club Ultimate Porker	1	843	41	7	74	40	73	—	6	—	1919	—	—	—
Slim Double Provolone	1	588	19	11	49	32	71	—	0	—	1225	—	—	—
Slim Ham & Cheese	1	534	12	6	59	34	72	—	0	—	1673	—	—	—
Slim Salami Capicola	1	624	21	10	68	35	72	—	0	—	1821	—	—	—
Slim Tuna Salad	1	577	19	3	29	24	72	—	1	—	1327	—	—	—
Slim Turkey Breast	1	407	1	0	37	27	70	—	0	—	1355	—	—	—
Sub Big John	1	564	27	4	40	24	54	—	1	—	1333	—	—	—
Sub J.J.B.L.T.	1	662	35	7	45	29	54	—	1	—	1332	—	—	—
Sub Pepe	1	684	37	10	70	30	55	—	1	—	1659	—	—	—
Sub Totally Tuna	1	502	20	4	29	21	57	—	2	—	1131	—	—	—
Sub Turkey Tom	1	555	26	4	48	24	54	—	1	—	1342	—	—	—
Sub Vegetarian	1	640	36	10	36	21	57	—	2	—	1054	—	—	—
Sub Vito	1	579	25	10	68	32	56	—	1	—	1685	—	—	—
The J.J. Gargantuan	1	1008	55	15	180	69	60	—	1	—	3783	—	—	—
Unwich Hunter's Club	1	520	38	11	93	35	8	—	2	—	1655	—	—	—
Unwich The J.J. Gargantuan	1	769	55	15	180	57	11	—	2	—	3255	—	—	—
SIDES														
Cookie Chocolate Chunk	1	421	18	11	51	5	62	—	1	—	427	—	—	—
Cookie Raisin Oatmeal	1	421	16	9	66	7	65	—	4	—	471	—	—	—
Jimmy Chips	1 pkg	160	8	2	0	2	18	—	0	—	80	—	—	—
Jimmy Chips BBQ	1 pkg	160	9	2	0	2	17	—	0	—	90	—	—	—
Jimmy Chips Jalapeno	1 pkg	150	7	2	0	2	18	—	0	—	290	—	—	—

FOOD	PORTION	CALS	FAT	SAT FAT	CHOL	PROT	CARB	SUGAR	FIBER	CALCI	SOD	POTAS	FOLIC	VIT C
Jimmy Chips Sea Salt & Vinegar	1 pkg	140	8	2	0	2	16	—	0	—	280	—	—	—
Pickle Spear	1	4	0	0	0	0	1	—	tr	—	355	—	—	—
Pickle Whole	1	15	0	0	0	0	3	—	1	—	1420	—	—	—

KENTUCKY FRIED CHICKEN

BEVERAGES

FOOD	PORTION	CALS	FAT	SAT FAT	CHOL	PROT	CARB	SUGAR	FIBER	CALCI	SOD	POTAS	FOLIC	VIT C
Diet Pepsi	1 med (14 oz)	0	0	0	0	0	0	0	0	0	45	—	—	0
Mt. Dew	1 med (14 oz)	190	0	0	0	0	54	54	0	0	90	—	—	0
Pepsi	1 med (14 oz)	180	0	0	0	0	47	47	0	0	45	—	—	0

DESSERTS

FOOD	PORTION	CALS	FAT	SAT FAT	CHOL	PROT	CARB	SUGAR	FIBER	CALCI	SOD	POTAS	FOLIC	VIT C
Cake Double Chocolate Chip	1 slice	330	16	4	50	4	41	26	1	40	260	—	—	0
Cookie Sweet Life Chocolate Chip	1 (1.2 oz)	160	7	4	10	2	23	14	1	20	95	—	—	0
Cookie Sweet Life Oatmeal Raisin	1 (1.2 oz)	150	5	3	5	2	24	12	1	20	135	—	—	0
Cookie Sweet Life Sugar	1 (1.2 oz)	160	6	3	5	2	23	10	0	20	120	—	—	0
Lil' Bucket Chocolate Cream	1	280	13	9	0	3	38	21	3	40	230	—	—	0
Lil' Bucket Lemon Creme	1 serv	410	15	7	0	7	61	53	2	200	270	—	—	0
Lil' Bucket Strawberry Short Cake	1 serv	210	7	5	10	2	33	25	1	20	125	—	—	0
Pie Mini's Apple	3 (4 oz)	370	20	6	0	2	44	19	2	20	260	—	—	30
Teddy Graham Cinnamon Snacks	1 serv	90	3	1	0	1	15	5	1	80	95	—	—	0

MAIN MENU SELECTIONS

FOOD	PORTION	CALS	FAT	SAT FAT	CHOL	PROT	CARB	SUGAR	FIBER	CALCI	SOD	POTAS	FOLIC	VIT C
Baked Beans	1 serv	220	1	0	0	8	45	20	7	100	730	—	—	1
Biscuit	1 (2 oz)	220	11	3	0	4	24	2	1	40	640	—	—	0
Bowl Chicken & Biscuit	1	870	44	11	60	29	88	5	7	250	2420	—	—	5
Bowl Mashed Potato w/ Gravy	1	740	36	9	60	27	80	6	7	200	2350	—	—	6
Bowl Rice w/ Gravy	1	620	28	7	60	26	67	7	6	200	2150	—	—	6
Chicken Pot Pie	1 (15 oz)	770	40	15	115	33	70	2	5	0	1680	—	—	0
Cole Slaw	1 serv	180	10	2	5	1	22	18	3	40	270	—	—	12
Corn On The Cob	1 ear (3 inch)	70	2	2	0	2	13	5	3	40	5	—	—	4
Crispy Strips	2 (3.5 oz)	240	13	3	50	20	11	0	0	20	800	—	—	0
Extra Crispy Breast	1 (5.7 oz)	440	27	6	105	34	15	0	0	60	970	—	—	1
Extra Crispy Drumstick	1 (2 oz)	160	10	2	55	12	6	0	0	20	370	—	—	0

FOOD	PORTION	CALS	FAT	SAT FAT	CHOL	PROT	CARB	SUGAR	FIBER	CALCI	SOD	POTAS	FOLIC	VIT C
Extra Crispy Thigh	1 (4 oz)	370	28	6	85	18	12	0	0	20	850	—	—	0
Extra Crispy Whole Wing	1 (1.8 oz)	170	11	3	55	13	6	0	1	20	350	—	—	0
Green Beans	1 serv	50	2	0	5	2	7	2	2	0	570	—	—	0
KFC Snacker	1	290	13	3	30	15	29	5	2	60	680	—	—	2
KFC Snacker Buffalo	1	260	8	2	25	15	31	4	1	60	860	—	—	2
KFC Snacker Fish	1	330	15	3	60	17	31	6	1	60	710	—	—	0
KFC Snacker Fish w/o Sauce	1	290	12	3	60	17	29	4	1	60	610	—	—	0
KFC Snacker Honey BBQ	1	210	3	1	40	14	32	12	2	40	530	—	—	0
KFC Snacker Ultimate Cheese	1	280	11	3	25	15	30	5	1	80	780	—	—	2
Macaroni & Cheese	1 serv	180	8	4	15	8	18	3	0	150	800	—	—	1
Mashed Potatoes w/ Gravy	1 serv	140	5	1	0	2	20	1	1	40	560	—	—	1
Mashed Potatoes w/o Gravy	1 serv	110	4	1	0	2	17	0	1	20	320	—	—	0
Original Recipe Breast	1 (5.6 oz)	360	21	5	115	37	7	0	0	80	1020	—	—	1
Original Recipe Breast w/o Skin Or Breading	1 (3.8 oz)	140	2	0	65	29	1	0	0	0	520	—	—	0
Original Recipe Drumstick	1 (2 oz)	130	8	2	65	12	2	0	0	0	350	—	—	0
Original Recipe Thigh	1 (4.4 oz)	330	24	6	110	20	8	0	0	40	870	—	—	1
Original Recipe Whole Wing	1 (1.6 oz)	130	8	2	50	11	4	0	0	20	350	—	—	0
Popcorn Chicken	1 reg (4 oz)	400	26	5	60	21	22	0	3	40	1160	—	—	0
Potato Salad	1 serv	180	9	2	5	2	22	6	2	0	470	—	—	6
Potato Wedges	1 serv	260	13	3	0	4	33	0	3	20	740	—	—	4
Sandwich Crispy Twister	1	550	28	6	55	26	49	5	3	150	1500	—	—	9
Sandwich Double Crunch	1	470	23	5	55	27	38	4	2	80	1190	—	—	6
Sandwich Honey BBQ	1	280	4	1	60	22	40	16	3	60	780	—	—	2
Sandwich Tender Roast	1	380	13	3	80	37	29	4	2	100	1180	—	—	9
Sandwich Tender Roast w/o Sauce	1	300	5	2	70	37	28	3	2	80	1060	—	—	9
Seasoned Rice	1 serv	180	1	0	0	4	32	1	2	40	630	—	—	0
Twister Oven Roasted	1	420	17	4	60	28	40	6	3	150	1250	—	—	15

FOOD	PORTION	CALS	FAT	SAT FAT	CHOL	PROT	CARB	SUGAR	FIBER	CALCI	SOD	POTAS	FOLIC	VIT C
Twister Oven Roasted w/o Sauce	1	330	7	3	50	28	39	5	3	150	1120	—	—	15
Wings Fiery Buffalo	5	380	24	5	105	21	19	1	2	20	1480	—	—	1
Wings Honey BBQ	5	390	24	5	105	21	23	9	3	40	930	—	—	1
Wings Hot	5	350	24	5	105	20	14	0	2	40	740	—	—	0
Wings Hot & Spicy	5	400	24	5	105	21	24	13	2	60	760	—	—	1
Wings Teriyaki	5	480	25	5	105	22	40	30	2	20	830	—	—	1
Wings Boneless Fiery Buffalo	5	420	20	4	65	28	33	1	3	20	2260	—	—	2
Wings Boneless Honey BBQ	5	450	20	4	65	28	41	11	4	40	1880	—	—	2
Wings Boneless Sweet & Spicy	5	440	19	4	65	27	38	11	3	40	1700	—	—	2
Wings Boneless Teriyaki	5	500	21	4	65	28	50	24	3	20	1730	—	—	2
SALAD DRESSINGS														
Creamy Parmesan Caesar	1 serv (2 oz)	260	26	5	15	2	4	2	0	60	540	—	—	0
Golden Italian Light	1 serv (1.5 oz)	45	3	0	0	0	6	5	0	0	660	—	—	0
Ranch	1 serv (2 oz)	200	20	3	25	1	3	1	0	20	470	—	—	0
Ranch Fat Free	1 serv (1.5 oz)	35	0	0	0	1	8	2	0	20	410	—	—	0
SALADS														
Crispy BLT w/o Dressing	1 (12 oz)	330	17	4	65	28	18	5	4	60	1130	—	—	30
Crispy Caesar w/o Dressing & Croutons	1 (11 oz)	350	19	6	70	29	16	3	3	250	1080	—	—	18
Croutons Parmesan Garlic	1 pkg	60	3	0	0	2	8	1	0	0	135	—	—	0
Roasted BLT w/o Dressing	1 (12 oz)	200	6	2	65	29	8	5	4	60	880	—	—	30
Roasted Caesar w/o Dressing & Croutons	1 (11 oz)	220	8	5	70	30	6	3	3	250	830	—	—	21
Side Caesar w/o Dressing & Croutons	1 (3 oz)	50	3	2	10	4	2	1	1	100	135	—	—	6
Side House w/o Dressing	1 (3 oz)	15	0	0	0	1	2	2	1	20	10	—	—	9

KOO-KOO-ROO

MAIN MENU SELECTIONS

FOOD	PORTION	CALS	FAT	SAT FAT	CHOL	PROT	CARB	SUGAR	FIBER	CALCI	SOD	POTAS	FOLIC	VIT C
Baked Yam	1 serv (6 oz)	197	tr	0	0	3	47	—	7	—	14	—	—	—
Black Beans	1 serv (6 oz)	125	3	tr	0	8	23	—	6	—	487	—	—	—

FOOD	PORTION	CALS	FAT	SAT FAT	CHOL	PROT	CARB	SUGAR	FIBER	CALCI	SOD	POTAS	FOLIC	VIT C
Buffalo Wings	6	606	28	8	119	44	42	—	2	—	875	—	—	—
Burrito California Chicken	1	810	41	18	115	46	60	—	4	—	2182	—	—	—
Burrito Fajita Chicken	1	750	33	13	94	40	70	—	4	—	2995	—	—	—
Burrito Original Chicken	1	709	28	13	94	41	71	—	5	—	2926	—	—	—
Butternut Squash	1 serv (6 oz)	66	tr	0	0	2	17	—	3	—	3	—	—	—
Chicken Bowl Chargrilled w/o Sauce	1	569	19	9	132	41	57	—	4	—	1757	—	—	—
Chicken Bowl Spicy Garlic Ginger w/o Sauce	1	485	6	2	96	42	63	—	2	—	842	—	—	—
Creamed Spinach	1 serv (8 oz)	100	6	2	7	4	10	—	3	—	573	—	—	—
Italian Vegetable	1 serv (5.5 oz)	47	2	1	5	1	9	—	2	—	132	—	—	—
Kernel Corn	1 serv (4.5 oz)	105	1	tr	0	4	26	—	3	—	162	—	—	—
Mashed Potatoes	1 serv (6.5 oz)	188	5	3	15	4	32	—	3	—	428	—	—	—
Original Breast	1 (4.1 oz)	187	6	1	117	34	tr	—	0	—	422	—	—	—
Original Chicken Dark	3 pieces (5 oz)	320	16	5	101	39	5	—	0	—	659	—	—	—
Roasted Garlic Potatoes	1 serv (5 oz)	133	5	2	5	2	21	—	2	—	247	—	—	—
Rotisserie Chicken Breast & Wing	1 serv (6.5 oz)	355	16	4	140	49	1	—	tr	—	675	—	—	—
Rotisserie Chicken Leg & Thigh	1 serv (4.8 oz)	300	18	5	114	31	1	—	tr	—	513	—	—	—
Rotisserie Half Chicken	1 serv (11.3 oz)	655	34	9	254	80	2	—	tr	—	1188	—	—	—
Sandwich BBQ Chicken	1	562	12	4	113	45	71	—	3	—	1398	—	—	—
Sandwich Chicken Caesar	1	781	36	11	138	56	63	—	2	—	1775	—	—	—
Sandwich Original Chicken	1	661	29	5	116	41	63	—	3	—	1144	—	—	—
Sandwich Turkey Hand Carved	1	599	32	8	122	46	31	—	5	—	786	—	—	—
Southwestern Bowl w/o Sauce	1	570	19	8	95	37	67	—	8	—	2798	—	—	—
Tostada Bowl w/o Sauce w/o Shell	1	528	22	9	99	40	45	—	7	—	2144	—	—	—
Traditional Turkey Dinner	1 serv	692	29	10	127	42	67	—	8	—	3719	—	—	—
Turkey Breast Sliced	1 serv	182	8	2	76	25	0	0	0	—	66	—	—	—
Turkey Pot Pie	1	883	44	12	98	37	83	—	6	—	1287	—	—	—
Wrap Caesar Chicken	1	757	39	8	97	42	59	—	4	—	1890	—	—	—

FOOD	PORTION	CALS	FAT	SAT FAT	CHOL	PROT	CARB	SUGAR	FIBER	CALCI	SOD	POTAS	FOLIC	VIT C
Wrap Chipotle Chicken	1	924	43	15	123	42	89	—	6	—	2449	—	—	—
SALADS														
BBQ Chicken w/o Dressing	1	365	14	6	104	38	22	—	6	—	897	—	—	—
Cantaloupe & Honeydew	1 serv (5 oz)	50	tr	0	0	1	12	—	1	—	14	—	—	—
Chicken Caesar w/o Dressing	1	286	11	3	80	34	13	—	4	—	967	—	—	—
Chinese Chicken w/o Dressing	1	550	29	4	72	40	39	—	10	—	853	—	—	—
Creamy Coleslaw	1 serv (5 oz)	238	20	4	28	1	14	—	2	—	639	—	—	—
Cucumber	1 serv (4.5 oz)	41	tr	0	0	1	9	—	2	—	190	—	—	—
House	1	113	4	1	4	6	16	—	5	—	206	—	—	—
Tangy Tomato	1 serv (4.5 oz)	60	4	0	0	1	6	—	1	—	173	—	—	—
Tossed w/ Dressing	1 serv (3 oz)	16	tr	0	0	1	3	—	1	—	9	—	—	—
SOUPS														
Chicken Noodle	1 serv (5 oz)	71	3	1	19	6	4	—	tr	—	426	—	—	—
Chicken Tortilla	1 serv (5 oz)	112	6	2	24	8	7	—	1	—	684	—	—	—
Ten Vegetable	1 serv (5 oz)	94	2	0	0	3	16	—	4	—	435	—	—	—

KRISPY KREME

FOOD	PORTION	CALS	FAT	SAT FAT	CHOL	PROT	CARB	SUGAR	FIBER	CALCI	SOD	POTAS	FOLIC	VIT C
BEVERAGES														
Chillers Fruity Orange You Glad	1 (12 oz)	180	0	0	0	0	43	43	0	0	10	—	—	0
Chillers Fruity Very Berry	1 (12 oz)	170	0	0	0	0	43	43	0	0	10	—	—	0
Chillers Kremey Berries & Kreme	1 (12 oz)	620	28	24	30	3	92	71	tr	150	220	—	—	5
Chillers Kremey Chocolate Chocolate	1 (12 oz)	970	29	24	30	4	104	62	2	200	320	—	—	0
Chillers Kremey Lemon Sherbert	1 (12 oz)	630	28	24	30	3	95	71	tr	150	220	—	—	0
Chillers Kremey Lotta Latte	1 (12 oz)	670	28	24	30	4	49	60	tr	200	380	—	—	0
Chillers Kremey Mocha Dream	1 (12 oz)	670	28	24	30	3	105	58	1	200	320	—	—	0
Chillers Kremey Oranges & Kreme	1 (12 oz)	630	28	24	30	3	92	71	tr	150	220	—	—	5
DOUGHNUTS														
Apple Fritter	1	380	20	10	5	4	47	24	2	100	220	—	—	1
Caramel Kreme Crunch	1	380	19	9	10	4	40	30	tr	100	170	—	—	1
Chocolate Iced Cake	1	280	14	6	20	3	36	20	tr	20	320	—	—	0

FOOD	PORTION	CALS	FAT	SAT FAT	CHOL	PROT	CARB	SUGAR	FIBER	CALCI	SOD	POTAS	FOLIC	VIT C
Chocolate Iced Custard Filled	1	300	17	8	5	3	36	19	tr	80	150	—	—	1
Chocolate Iced Glazed	1	250	12	6	5	3	33	21	tr	60	100	—	—	1
Chocolate Iced Kreme Filled	1	350	20	11	5	3	39	23	tr	80	140	—	—	1
Chocolate Iced w/ Sprinkles	1	270	12	6	5	3	38	24	tr	60	100	—	—	1
Cinnamon Apple Filled	1	290	16	8	5	3	32	14	tr	100	150	—	—	1
Cinnamon Bun	1	260	16	8	5	3	28	13	tr	80	125	—	—	1
Cinnamon Twist	1	240	15	7	5	3	23	7	tr	80	130	—	—	1
Dulce De Leche	1	300	18	9	5	3	31	14	tr	100	160	—	—	1
Glazed Chocolate Cake	1	300	15	7	20	3	42	27	2	20	250	—	—	0
Glazed Cinnamon	1	210	12	6	5	2	24	12	tr	60	100	—	—	1
Glazed Kreme Filled	1	340	20	10	5	3	39	23	tr	80	140	—	—	1
Glazed Cruller	1	240	14	7	15	2	26	14	tr	20	240	—	—	0
Glazed Cruller Chocolate	1	290	15	7	15	2	37	25	tr	20	240	—	—	0
Glazed Lemon Filled	1	290	16	8	5	3	36	18	tr	80	135	—	—	1
Glazed Maple Iced	1	240	12	6	5	2	32	20	tr	60	100	—	—	1
Glazed Original	1	200	12	6	5	2	22	10	tr	60	95	—	—	1
Glazed Pumpkin Spice	1	300	14	7	20	2	42	27	tr	20	250	—	—	0
Glazed Raspberry Filled	1	300	16	8	5	3	36	20	tr	80	125	—	—	1
Glazed Sour Cream	1	300	13	7	20	2	43	28	tr	20	250	—	—	0
Holes Glazed Blueberry	4	220	12	5	20	3	27	13	tr	20	280	—	—	0
Holes Glazed Cake	4	210	10	5	15	2	29	17	tr	20	240	—	—	0
Holes Glazed Chocolate Cake	4	210	10	5	15	2	29	17	tr	20	240	—	—	0
Holes Glazed Original	4	200	11	5	5	2	25	15	tr	60	90	—	—	0
Holes Glazed Pumpkin Spice	4	210	10	5	15	2	29	17	tr	20	240	—	—	0
New York Cheesecake	1	340	20	10	15	4	34	17	tr	100	200	—	—	1
Powdered Cake	1	290	14	6	20	3	37	19	tr	40	320	—	—	0
Powdered Strawberry Filled	1	290	16	8	5	3	33	13	tr	80	135	—	—	1
Sugar	1	200	12	6	5	2	21	10	0	60	95	—	—	1

FOOD	PORTION	CALS	FAT	SAT FAT	CHOL	PROT	CARB	SUGAR	FIBER	CALCI	SOD	POTAS	FOLIC	VIT C
Traditional Cake	1	230	13	6	20	3	25	9	tr	20	320	—	—	0

KRYSTAL

BEVERAGES

FOOD	PORTION	CALS	FAT	SAT FAT	CHOL	PROT	CARB	SUGAR	FIBER	CALCI	SOD	POTAS	FOLIC	VIT C
Coca-Cola Classic	1 sm (16 oz)	129	0	0	0	0	40	40	0	0	9	—	—	0
Coca-Cola Classic frzn	1 (16 oz)	130	0	0	0	0	36	36	0	0	12	—	—	0
Diet Coke	1 sm (16 oz)	<1	0	0	0	0	tr	0	0	0	15	—	—	0
Sprite	1 sm (16 oz)	126	0	0	0	0	39	39	0	0	33	—	—	0

BREAKFAST SELECTIONS

FOOD	PORTION	CALS	FAT	SAT FAT	CHOL	PROT	CARB	SUGAR	FIBER	CALCI	SOD	POTAS	FOLIC	VIT C
4 Carb Scrambler Bacon	1 serv	370	29	10	595	24	4	0	1	150	830	—	—	0
4 Carb Scrambler Sausage	1 serv	600	51	18	600	32	3	1	2	150	1040	—	—	0
Biscuit & Gravy	1	280	14	3	0	5	34	2	0	40	710	—	—	0
Biscuit Bacon Egg Cheese	1	390	23	7	40	11	33	2	0	100	1090	—	—	0
Biscuit Chik	1	360	15	3	20	13	40	2	0	40	1030	—	—	—
Biscuit Plain	1	270	13	3	0	5	33	2	0	40	660	—	—	—
Biscuit Sausage	1	480	33	10	40	12	33	2	0	60	980	—	—	—
Country Breakfast	1 serv	660	42	14	590	24	46	3	8	40	1450	—	—	5
Kryspers	1 serv	190	13	5	10	1	17	0	2	—	340	—	—	—
Krystal Sunriser	1	240	14	5	255	12	14	1	2	100	460	—	—	—
Scrambler	1 serv	440	26	11	255	20	33	tr	3	80	840	—	—	—

DESSERTS

FOOD	PORTION	CALS	FAT	SAT FAT	CHOL	PROT	CARB	SUGAR	FIBER	CALCI	SOD	POTAS	FOLIC	VIT C
Fried Apple Turnover	1	220	10	4	<5	3	31	7	2	—	300	—	—	—
Lemon Icebox Pie	1 serv	260	9	2	25	5	41	37	2	150	180	—	—	1

MAIN MENU SELECTIONS

FOOD	PORTION	CALS	FAT	SAT FAT	CHOL	PROT	CARB	SUGAR	FIBER	CALCI	SOD	POTAS	FOLIC	VIT C
BA Burger	1	470	27	8	55	22	39	6	2	80	760	—	—	6
BA Burger Cheese	1	530	32	11	55	25	40	6	2	150	1020	—	—	6
BA Burger Double Bacon Cheese	1	800	53	20	115	44	41	6	2	250	1600	—	—	6
Chik'n Bites	1 sm	310	19	8	55	17	16	0	1	200	790	—	—	6
Chik'n Bites Salad	1 serv	290	20	11	66	20	12	1	4	—	490	—	—	—
Fries	1 reg	470	20	8	20	4	53	0	7	200	90	—	—	—
Fries Chili Cheese	1 serv	540	28	13	45	13	59	1	6	150	800	—	—	—
Krystal	1	160	7	3	20	7	17	1	1	60	260	—	—	—
Krystal Bacon Cheese	1	190	10	5	25	10	16	2	2	100	430	—	—	—
Krystal Cheese	1	180	9	4	25	9	17	1	2	100	430	—	—	—
Krystal Chik	1	240	11	4	25	11	24	1	2	—	640	—	—	—
Krystal Chili	1 serv	200	7	4	25	13	22	2	7	150	1130	—	—	—
Krystal Double	1	260	13	6	40	13	24	2	2	150	550	—	—	—
Krystal Double Cheese	1	310	16	7	65	16	26	2	tr	200	800	—	—	—

FOOD	PORTION	CALS	FAT	SAT FAT	CHOL	PROT	CARB	SUGAR	FIBER	CALCI	SOD	POTAS	FOLIC	VIT C
Pup Chili Cheese	1	210	12	5	40	9	17	2	2	100	510	—	—	—
Pup Corn	1	260	19	8	50	5	19	5	1	—	480	—	—	—
Pup Plain	1	170	9	4	25	6	15	—	1	40	500	—	—	—

LITTLE CAESARS

DIPS AND SAUCES

FOOD	PORTION	CALS	FAT	SAT FAT	CHOL	PROT	CARB	SUGAR	FIBER	CALCI	SOD	POTAS	FOLIC	VIT C
Crazy Sauce	1 serv (4 oz)	45	0	0	0	2	10	8	1	20	260	—	—	18
Dip Buffalo	1 serv (1.5 oz)	130	14	2	0	0	4	2	0	0	940	—	—	4
Dip Buffalo Ranch	1 serv (1.5 oz)	220	24	4	15	0	3	2	0	0	520	—	—	0
Dip Buttery Garlic	1 serv (1.5 oz)	380	42	9	0	0	0	0	0	0	420	—	—	0
Dip Cheezy	1 serv (1.5 oz)	210	21	4	15	1	3	2	0	40	450	—	—	0
Dip Chipotle	1 serv (1.5 oz)	220	24	4	15	0	2	0	0	0	560	—	—	6
Dip Ranch	1 serv (1.5 oz)	250	26	4	15	0	3	2	0	20	380	—	—	0

MAIN MENU SELECTIONS

FOOD	PORTION	CALS	FAT	SAT FAT	CHOL	PROT	CARB	SUGAR	FIBER	CALCI	SOD	POTAS	FOLIC	VIT C
Cheese Bread Italian	1 (1.6 oz)	130	7	3	10	6	13	1	0	100	230	—	—	0
Cheese Bread Pepperoni	1 (1.7 oz)	150	8	3	15	7	13	1	0	100	280	—	—	0
Crazy Bread	1 (1.3 oz)	100	3	1	0	3	15	1	1	20	150	—	—	0
Pizza 3 Meat Treat	1/8 pie (4.8 oz)	350	18	8	40	17	30	3	1	200	730	—	—	5
Pizza Baby Pan!Pan! Cheese & Pepperoni	1 pie (4.9 oz)	360	18	7	35	16	33	3	1	250	610	—	—	4
Pizza Baby Pan!Pan! Just Cheese	1 pie (4.7 oz)	320	15	6	25	14	33	3	1	250	500	—	—	4
Pizza Deep Dish Just Cheese	1/8 pie (4.8 oz)	320	13	5	25	14	38	3	1	250	490	—	—	4
Pizza Deep Dish Pepperoni	1/8 pie (5 oz)	360	16	6	30	16	38	4	1	250	610	—	—	4
Pizza Hot-N-Ready Just Cheese	1/8 pie (4 oz)	240	9	5	20	12	30	3	1	200	410	—	—	4
Pizza Hot-N-Ready Pepperoni	1/8 pie (4.2 oz)	280	11	5	25	14	30	3	1	200	520	—	—	4
Pizza Hulu Hawaiian Pineapple & Canadian Bacon	1/8 pie (5.2 oz)	280	9	5	25	15	34	6	1	200	640	—	—	6
Pizza Hulu Hawaiian Pineapple & Ham	1/8 pie (5.3 oz)	270	9	5	25	15	33	6	1	200	600	—	—	5
Pizza Ultimate Supreme	1/8 pie (5.3 oz)	310	14	6	30	15	31	3	2	200	640	—	—	9
Pizza Ultimate Supreme Vegetarian	1/8 pie (5.4 oz)	270	10	5	20	13	32	4	2	200	530	—	—	12
Wings Barbecue	1 (1.2 oz)	70	4	1	20	4	3	2	0	20	220	—	—	1
Wings Hot	1 (1.2 oz)	60	5	1	20	4	1	0	0	20	430	—	—	2

FOOD	PORTION	CALS	FAT	SAT FAT	CHOL	PROT	CARB	SUGAR	FIBER	CALCI	SOD	POTAS	FOLIC	VIT C
Wings Mild	1 (1 oz)	60	4	1	20	4	1	0	0	20	290	—	—	1
Wings Oven Roasted	1 (0.9 oz)	50	4	1	20	4	0	0	0	20	150	—	—	1

LONG JOHN SILVER'S

BEVERAGES

FOOD	PORTION	CALS	FAT	SAT FAT	CHOL	PROT	CARB	SUGAR	FIBER	CALCI	SOD	POTAS	FOLIC	VIT C
Diet Mountain Dew	1 med (32 oz)	0	0	0	0	0	0	0	0	0	160	—	—	0
Diet Pepsi	1 med (32 oz)	0	0	0	0	0	0	0	0	0	100	—	—	0
Dr Pepper	1 med (32 oz)	400	0	0	0	0	108	108	0	0	140	—	—	0
Iced Tea Unsweetened	1 med (32 oz)	0	0	0	0	0	0	0	0	0	0	—	—	0
Iceflow Lemonade	1 sm (16 oz)	190	0	0	0	0	47	40	0	0	15	—	—	72
Iceflow Strawberry Lemonade	1 sm (16 oz)	240	0	0	0	0	60	48	0	0	15	—	—	72
Lipton Raspberry Tea	1 med (32 oz)	320	0	0	0	0	84	84	0	0	100	—	—	0
Mountain Dew	1 med (32 oz)	440	0	0	0	0	116	116	0	0	140	—	—	0
Pepsi	1 med (32 oz)	400	0	0	0	0	112	108	0	0	100	—	—	0
Pepsi Wild Cherry	1 med (32 oz)	400	0	0	0	0	112	112	0	0	80	—	—	0
Sierra Mist	1 med (32 oz)	400	0	0	0	0	108	108	0	0	80	—	—	0
Tropicana Fruit Punch	1 med (32 oz)	440	0	0	0	0	120	120	0	0	100	—	—	0
Tropicana Lemonade	1 med (32 oz)	400	0	0	0	0	108	108	0	0	420	—	—	0

DESSERTS

FOOD	PORTION	CALS	FAT	SAT FAT	CHOL	PROT	CARB	SUGAR	FIBER	CALCI	SOD	POTAS	FOLIC	VIT C
Pie Chocolate Cream	1 slice (2.6 oz)	280	17	10	10	3	28	19	1	60	230	—	—	0
Pie Pineapple Cream	1 slice (3.1 oz)	300	17	11	10	3	35	25	0	80	250	—	—	0

MAIN MENU SELECTIONS

FOOD	PORTION	CALS	FAT	SAT FAT	CHOL	PROT	CARB	SUGAR	FIBER	CALCI	SOD	POTAS	FOLIC	VIT C
Battered Alaskan Pollock	1 piece (3.2 oz)	140	16	4	35	12	17	0	0	0	790	—	—	0
Battered Shrimp	3 (1.5 oz)	130	9	3	45	5	8	0	0	0	480	—	—	0
Bites Broccoli Cheddar	5 (3.3 oz)	230	12	5	15	5	25	2	2	100	550	—	—	1
Bites Jalapeno Cheddar	5 (2.9 oz)	240	14	5	15	6	23	2	2	100	730	—	—	1
Breaded Mozzarella Sticks	3 (1.8 oz)	150	9	4	10	5	13	0	1	100	350	—	—	0
Breaded Clams Strips	1 box (3 oz)	320	19	5	35	9	29	1	2	20	1190	—	—	0
Breadstick	1 (2 oz)	170	4	1	0	6	29	2	1	20	290	—	—	0
Buttered Langostino Lobster Bites	1 box (3.2 oz)	230	9	3	60	13	24	0	2	40	520	—	—	0
Chicken Strip	1 (1.8 oz)	140	8	2	20	8	9	0	0	0	480	—	—	2
Cole Slaw	1 serv (4 oz)	200	15	3	20	1	15	10	3	40	340	—	—	18

FOOD	PORTION	CALS	FAT	SAT FAT	CHOL	PROT	CARB	SUGAR	FIBER	CALCI	SOD	POTAS	FOLIC	VIT C
Corn Cobbette w/ Butter	1 (3.6 oz)	150	10	2	0	3	14	6	3	0	30	—	—	1
Corn Cobbette w/o Butter	1 (3.3 oz)	90	3	1	0	3	14	6	3	0	0	—	—	1
Crumblies	1 serv (1 oz)	170	12	3	0	1	14	0	1	0	410	—	—	0
Freshside Grille Salmon Entree	1 serv (10.7 oz)	280	7	2	50	27	27	5	3	80	1010	—	—	0
Freshside Grille Shrimp Scampi Entree	1 serv (10.7 oz)	330	15	4	135	20	29	5	3	100	1230	—	—	0
Freshside Grille Tilapia Entree	1 serv (10.2 oz)	250	5	2	60	25	27	4	3	80	820	—	—	0
Fries Basket Portion	1 serv (4 oz)	310	14	4	0	3	45	0	4	0	460	—	—	18
Fries Platter Portion	1 serv (3 oz)	230	10	3	0	3	34	0	3	0	350	—	—	15
Grilled Pacific Salmon Filets	2 (4.5 oz)	150	5	1	50	24	2	1	0	20	440	—	—	0
Grilled Tilapia Filet	1 (4 oz)	110	3	1	55	22	1	1	0	20	250	—	—	0
Hushpuppy	1 (0.8 oz)	60	3	1	0	1	9	1	1	20	200	—	—	0
Jalapeno Peppers	1 (1.3 oz)	15	0	0	0	1	2	1	0	20	190	—	—	9
Longostino Lobster Stuffed Crab Cake	1 (2.2 oz)	170	9	2	30	6	16	0	1	60	390	—	—	0
Popcorn Shrimp	1 box (2.9 oz)	270	16	4	75	9	23	1	1	350	570	—	—	0
Rice	1 serv (5 oz)	180	1	1	0	4	37	1	2	20	470	—	—	0
Sandwich Alaskan Pollock	1 (6.6 oz)	470	23	5	40	18	49	4	3	60	1180	—	—	1
Sandwich Chicken Strip	1 (6.6 oz)	440	30	6	50	22	47	2	4	60	1350	—	—	1
Sandwich Ultimate Alaskan Pollock	1 (7.2 oz)	240	27	8	55	21	50	4	3	100	1500	—	—	1
Sandwich Zesty Chicken Strip	1 (4.5 oz)	380	19	4	25	14	39	2	3	60	880	—	—	0
Shrimp Scampi	8 pieces (4.6 oz)	200	13	3	135	17	3	1	0	60	650	—	—	0
Soup Broccoli Cheese	1 bowl (7.4 oz)	220	18	8	30	5	8	2	1	150	650	—	—	6
Taco Baja Chicken Strip	1 (4.3 oz)	370	23	5	25	11	31	2	3	60	890	—	—	0
Taco Baja Fish	1 (4 oz)	360	23	5	25	9	30	2	3	60	810	—	—	0
Vegetable Medley	1 serv (4 oz)	50	2	1	0	1	8	3	3	40	360	—	—	0
SAUCES														
BBQ	1 serv (1 oz)	40	0	0	0	0	10	6	0	0	230	—	—	0
Cocktail	1 serv (1 oz)	25	0	0	0	0	6	5	0	0	250	—	—	0

FOOD	PORTION	CALS	FAT	SAT FAT	CHOL	PROT	CARB	SUGAR	FIBER	CALCI	SOD	POTAS	FOLIC	VIT C
Honey Mustard	1 serv (1 oz)	100	6	2	0	0	12	6	0	0	170	—	—	0
Ketchup	1 pkg (0.3 oz)	10	0	0	0	0	2	2	0	0	100	—	—	0
Lemon Juice	1 serv (4 g)	0	0	0	0	0	0	0	0	0	0	—	—	1
Louisiana Hot Sauce	1 tsp (5 g)	0	0	0	0	0	0	0	0	0	140	—	—	0
Malt Vinegar	1 serv (0.5 oz)	0	0	0	0	0	0	0	0	0	35	—	—	2
Marinara	1 serv (1 oz)	15	0	0	0	1	4	2	1	0	125	—	—	2
Ranch	1 serv (1 oz)	160	17	3	15	0	2	1	0	0	240	—	—	0
Sweet & Sour	1 serv (1 oz)	45	0	0	0	0	12	7	0	0	120	—	—	1
Tartar	1 serv (1 oz)	100	9	2	15	0	4	3	0	0	250	—	—	0

MAGGIE MOO'S

BEVERAGES

FOOD	PORTION	CALS	FAT	SAT FAT	CHOL	PROT	CARB	SUGAR	FIBER	CALCI	SOD	POTAS	FOLIC	VIT C
Shake Caramel Cowpuccino	1 (15 oz)	740	43	31	170	12	79	70	0	400	190	—	—	0
Shake Cinnamoo Swirl	1 (16 oz)	780	44	32	165	11	87	73	1	400	210	—	—	0
Shake Cookies 'N' Cream	1 (15 oz)	740	44	30	165	12	77	65	0	400	230	—	—	0
Shake Moocha Cowpuccino	1 (15 oz)	710	41	30	165	11	78	69	0	350	160	—	—	0
Shake Peanut Butter S'Moo	1 (16 oz)	780	46	30	155	16	82	69	4	350	400	—	—	0
Shake Strawberries 'N' Cream	1 (15 oz)	620	37	27	150	10	66	58	1	350	140	—	—	24
Zoomer Caramel Coffee	1 (15 oz)	380	13	9	0	1	65	53	0	20	400	—	—	0
Zoomer Creamy Mango	1 (17 oz)	400	3	2	0	1	96	88	1	20	100	—	—	84
Zoomer Mocha Coffee	1 (17 oz)	460	11	7	0	2	90	74	0	20	400	—	—	0
Zoomer Raspberry Pomegranate	1 (17 oz)	460	0	0	0	2	141	104	3	20	25	—	—	30
Zoomer Strawberry Banana	1 (18 oz)	350	10	6	0	2	69	51	3	20	300	—	—	24
Zoomer Triple Berry Pomegranate	1 (17 oz)	460	1	0	0	2	115	106	3	20	20	—	—	27

CONES

FOOD	PORTION	CALS	FAT	SAT FAT	CHOL	PROT	CARB	SUGAR	FIBER	CALCI	SOD	POTAS	FOLIC	VIT C
Dark Chocolate	1 (1.5 oz)	200	7	5	5	2	30	18	1	20	15	—	—	0
Dark Chocolate w/ Butterfinger	1 (2 oz)	260	10	6	5	3	41	24	1	20	45	—	—	0
Dark Chocolate w/ Heath Bar	1 (2 oz)	280	12	6	10	3	39	26	1	20	65	—	—	0
Dark Chocolate w/ Peanuts	1 (2 oz)	280	15	6	5	6	33	18	2	20	15	—	—	0
Plain	1 (1 oz)	120	3	—	5	2	22	10	0	0	0	—	—	0

FOOD	PORTION	CALS	FAT	SAT FAT	CHOL	PROT	CARB	SUGAR	FIBER	CALCI	SOD	POTAS	FOLIC	VIT C
White Chocolate	1 (1.5 oz)	200	7	5	10	2	31	19	0	20	15	—	—	0
White Chocolate w/ Sprinkles	1 (2 oz)	210	7	5	10	2	34	22	0	20	15	—	—	0
ICE CREAM														
Amooretto Cream	1 serv (6 oz)	380	23	17	95	6	38	34	0	200	85	—	—	0
Apple Strudel	1 serv (6 oz)	380	21	15	85	6	44	39	0	200	85	—	—	0
Banana Pudding	1 serv (6 oz)	330	18	13	75	5	39	32	1	150	70	—	—	2
Black Cherry	1 serv (6 oz)	380	23	17	95	6	39	35	0	200	85	—	—	0
Blueberry Muffin	1 serv (6 oz)	390	20	14	75	6	48	37	1	200	65	—	—	1
Brownie Batter	1 serv (6 oz)	420	21	15	85	6	52	42	1	200	170	—	—	0
Butter Pecan	1 serv (6 oz)	380	21	15	85	6	44	40	0	200	140	—	—	0
Cake 6 inch Better Batter	⅛ cake (5.7 oz)	480	24	16	55	5	62	45	1	150	170	—	—	0
Cake 6 inch Chocolate Cream	⅛ cake (6.4 oz)	580	33	22	80	7	69	53	3	150	110	—	—	0
Cake 8 inch Caramel Drizzle	¼₁₄ cake (6 oz)	530	33	18	65	6	55	45	11	150	125	—	—	0
Cake 8 inch Chocolate Espresso	¼₁₄ cake (5.6 oz)	460	25	17	150	5	58	48	1	150	190	—	—	0
Cake 8 inch Chocolate Heaven	¼₁₄ cake (5 oz)	400	22	16	60	6	45	38	2	150	150	—	—	0
Cake 8 inch Cookie Dreams	¼₁₄ cake (5.3 oz)	440	22	15	55	5	57	41	1	150	150	—	—	0
Cake 8 inch Cookies 'N' Cream	¼₁₄ cake (5.3 oz)	430	24	15	65	5	50	38	1	150	180	—	—	0
Cake 8 inch Cotton Candy Carnival	¼₁₄ cake (5.9 oz)	490	25	18	65	6	65	50	1	150	95	—	—	0
Cake 8 inch Fudge Fantasy	¼₁₄ cake (5.4 oz)	410	22	17	60	5	49	40	0	150	100	—	—	0
Cake 8 inch Maggie S'Mores	¼₁₄ cake (7 oz)	610	23	15	55	8	94	61	2	150	440	—	—	0
Cake 8 inch Maggie's Mud	¼₁₄ cake (5.3 oz)	440	25	16	60	7	49	41	2	150	210	—	—	0
Cake 8 inch Pecan Perfection	¼₁₄ cake (5.6 oz)	500	33	16	60	7	50	39	3	150	150	—	—	0
Cake 8 inch Sprinkle	¼₁₄ cake (5.7 oz)	370	19	14	55	4	46	38	0	150	65	—	—	0
Cake 8 inch Strawberry Cheesecream	¼₁₄ cake (6.3 oz)	530	23	15	55	7	74	46	1	150	320	—	—	2
Cake 8 inch Truffle Dream	¼₁₄ cake (5.8 oz)	500	28	19	75	6	58	46	2	150	95	—	—	0
Cake 8 inch Turtle	¼₁₄ cake (6.3 oz)	590	40	18	65	7	54	42	2	150	115	—	—	0

FOOD	PORTION	CALS	FAT	SAT FAT	CHOL	PROT	CARB	SUGAR	FIBER	CALCI	SOD	POTAS	FOLIC	VIT C
Cappuccino	1 serv (6 oz)	380	22	16	90	3	41	36	0	200	85	—	—	0
Caramel Apple	1 serv (6 oz)	400	21	15	85	6	47	41	0	200	105	—	—	0
Carrot Cake	1 serv (6 oz)	420	21	15	80	6	51	39	0	200	200	—	—	0
Cheesecake	1 serv (6 oz)	380	21	16	85	6	43	36	0	200	80	—	—	0
Choco Mallo	1 serv (6 oz)	360	19	14	75	6	43	36	1	200	160	—	—	0
Chocolate	1 serv (6 oz)	390	22	16	80	7	44	37	2	200	200	—	—	0
Chocolate Banana	1 serv (6 oz)	370	20	15	80	7	43	35	2	200	160	—	—	1
Chocolate Better Batter	1 serv (6 oz)	420	21	15	50	7	54	41	1	200	160	—	—	0
Chocolate Peanut Butter	1 serv (6 oz)	450	28	16	80	9	42	35	2	200	220	—	—	0
Chocolate Raspberry	1 serv (6 oz)	380	20	15	80	6	46	39	2	200	180	—	—	0
Cinnamoo	1 serv (6 oz)	380	23	17	95	6	39	33	0	200	85	—	—	0
Cinnamoo Bun	1 serv (6 oz)	530	23	14	60	7	74	40	1	250	250	—	—	0
Cocoa Amooretto	1 serv (6 oz)	390	23	16	90	7	42	36	1	200	160	—	—	0
Cool Mint	1 serv (6 oz)	380	23	17	95	6	38	34	0	200	85	—	—	0
Cotton Candy	1 serv (6 oz)	380	23	17	95	6	38	34	0	200	90	—	—	0
Creamy Coconut	1 serv (6 oz)	380	23	17	95	6	38	33	0	200	85	—	—	0
Cupcake Better Batter	1	430	21	15	45	5	58	45	1	100	55	—	—	0
Cupcake Caramel Pumpkin Pie	1	500	26	19	50	4	62	46	1	150	210	—	—	0
Cupcake Cherry Chocolate	1	280	13	8	50	5	39	22	1	80	75	—	—	0
Cupcake Chocolate	1	400	22	13	65	5	51	37	2	100	95	—	—	0
Cupcake Chocolate Heaven	1	340	18	13	45	5	41	31	1	80	105	—	—	0
Cupcake Cool Swirl	1	370	19	14	45	4	47	36	0	80	50	—	—	0
Cupcake Cotton Candy Carnival	1	330	18	13	50	4	40	32	0	80	50	—	—	0
Cupcake Maggie O	1	360	18	10	55	6	45	29	1	150	260	—	—	0
Cupcake Pecan Pie	1	440	28	17	45	4	43	31	1	150	150	—	—	0
Cupcake Snowcap Blush	1	360	18	13	45	4	45	36	1	80	45	—	—	4
Cupcake Sprinkle	1	340	18	13	50	4	42	34	0	80	50	—	—	4
Dark Chocolate	1 serv	390	23	16	90	7	42	35	2	200	170	—	—	0
Egg Nog	1 serv (6 oz)	390	22	16	90	6	45	38	0	200	80	—	—	0
Espresso Bean	1 serv (6 oz)	380	22	16	90	6	41	36	0	200	85	—	—	0
French Vanilla	1 serv	390	22	16	90	6	43	38	0	200	85	—	—	5
Fresh Banana	1 serv (6 oz)	340	19	14	80	6	38	32	1	150	70	—	—	2
Key Lime	1 serv	380	18	13	70	5	54	48	0	150	65	—	—	6

FOOD	PORTION	CALS	FAT	SAT FAT	CHOL	PROT	CARB	SUGAR	FIBER	CALCI	SOD	POTAS	FOLIC	VIT C
Maggie's Fudge	1 serv	630	34	26	120	8	74	62	0	300	170	—	—	0
Mint Chocolate	1 serv (6 oz)	390	23	16	80	7	43	37	1	200	180	—	—	0
Mocha	1 serv (6 oz)	390	23	14	850	6	42	29	1	200	135	—	—	2
Peanut Butter	1 serv (6 oz)	480	33	17	80	10	38	31	1	200	170	—	—	0
Pina Cowlada	1 serv (6 oz)	360	21	15	85	6	37	33	0	200	75	—	—	1
Pink Bubblegum	1 serv (6 oz)	380	23	17	95	6	39	34	0	200	85	—	—	0
Pink Peppermint Stick	1 serv (6 oz)	420	21	15	85	6	51	47	0	200	75	—	—	0
Pistachio	1 serv (6 oz)	380	23	17	95	6	39	34	0	200	85	—	—	0
Pizza 10 inch Cheese	⅒ pie (5.4 oz)	340	18	12	65	6	40	31	0	100	55	—	—	0
Pizza 10 inch Chocolate Lover's	⅒ pie	390	20	13	70	6	48	35	1	150	65	—	—	0
Pizza 10 inch Supreme	⅒ pie (6.1 oz)	450	24	15	70	7	53	43	1	150	100	—	—	0
Pumpkin Pie	1 serv (6 oz)	370	21	15	850	6	41	36	0	200	95	—	—	0
Raspberry	1 serv (6 oz)	370	21	15	85	6	42	37	0	200	100	—	—	0
Red Velvet Cake	1 serv (6 oz)	420	21	14	75	7	54	41	1	200	150	—	—	0
Rum Raisin	1 serv (6 oz)	380	23	17	95	6	39	35	0	200	90	—	—	0
Southern Peaches	1 serv (6 oz)	330	16	12	65	5	44	36	0	150	75	—	—	21
Strawberry	1 serv	350	21	15	85	6	37	33	0	200	75	—	—	12
Strawberry Banana No Sugar Added	1 serv (6 oz)	170	6	5	0	0	42	0	0	0	30	—	—	0
Udderly Cream	1 serv (6 oz)	380	23	17	95	6	38	34	0	200	85	—	—	0
Vanilla	1 serv (6 oz)	380	23	17	95	6	39	35	0	200	85	—	—	0
Vanilla Low Fat Lactose Free	1 serv (6 oz)	130	5	3	0	0	23	18	0	0	150	—	—	0
Very Yellow Marshmallow	1 serv (6 oz)	350	20	14	80	5	38	34	0	200	90	—	—	0

MANHATTAN BAGEL

BAGELS AND BAKED GOODS

FOOD	PORTION	CALS	FAT	SAT FAT	CHOL	PROT	CARB	SUGAR	FIBER	CALCI	SOD	POTAS	FOLIC	VIT C
Bagel Blueberry	1 (3.8 oz)	300	1	0	0	10	65	11	3	20	480	—	—	0
Bagel Blueberry Glaze	1 (4.5 oz)	360	0	0	0	10	83	25	3	20	510	—	—	0
Bagel Cheddar	1 (4 oz)	320	2	0	0	11	67	3	3	40	650	—	—	0
Bagel Chocolate Chip	1 (3.8 oz)	290	3	1	0	9	58	10	3	20	430	—	—	0
Bagel Cinnamon Raisin	1 (4 oz)	330	1	0	0	11	70	10	3	40	600	—	—	0
Bagel Egg	1 (4 oz)	320	2	0	120	11	67	3	3	60	820	—	—	0
Bagel Everything	1 (4.3 oz)	350	3	0	0	12	68	3	3	40	980	—	—	1
Bagel French Toast	1 (3.5 oz)	300	6	2	55	9	54	9	2	40	380	—	—	4
Bagel Garlic	1 (4.3 oz)	340	1	0	0	11	74	3	3	40	670	—	—	0
Bagel Honey Whole Wheat	1 (3.5 oz)	250	1	0	0	9	56	8	3	20	440	—	—	0

FOOD	PORTION	CALS	FAT	SAT FAT	CHOL	PROT	CARB	SUGAR	FIBER	CALCI	SOD	POTAS	FOLIC	VIT C
Bagel Honey Whole Wheat Everything	1 (3.8 oz)	280	3	0	0	10	59	8	3	20	990	—	—	0
Bagel Jalapeno Cheddar	1 (4 oz)	320	2	0	0	11	67	3	3	40	640	—	—	0
Bagel Onion	1 (4.3 oz)	340	1	0	0	11	74	3	3	40	670	—	—	0
Bagel Plain	1 (4 oz)	320	1	0	0	11	68	3	3	40	670	—	—	0
Bagel Poppy	1 (4.3 oz)	360	5	0	0	12	69	3	3	40	670	—	—	0
Bagel Pumpernickel	1 (3.5 oz)	240	2	0	0	4	53	4	3	40	490	—	—	4
Bagel Rye	1 (4 oz)	310	2	0	0	11	66	3	3	40	630	—	—	0
Bagel Salt	1 (4.3 oz)	320	1	0	0	11	68	3	3	40	3450	—	—	0
Bagel Sesame Seed	1 (4.5 oz)	360	5	0	0	13	68	3	3	40	670	—	—	0
Bagel Mini Plain	1 (1.8 oz)	130	1	0	0	4	28	1	1	40	280	—	—	0
Bagel Thin Honey Whole Wheat	1 (2 oz)	120	2	0	0	5	23	3	4	20	200	—	—	1
Bagel Thin Plain	1 (2 oz)	120	1	0	0	4	25	2	1	0	240	—	—	1

MARBLE SLAB CREAMERY

FOOD	PORTION	CALS	FAT	SAT FAT	CHOL	PROT	CARB	SUGAR	FIBER	CALCI	SOD	POTAS	FOLIC	VIT C
Cone Honey Wheat	1	130	3	0	15	3	24	12	tr	20	10	—	—	0
Cone Sugar	1	130	3	0	15	2	23	12	0	20	10	—	—	0
Cone Vanilla Cinnamon	1	130	3	0	15	2	24	12	tr	20	10	—	—	0
Frozen Yogurt Nonfat	½ cup	100	tr	tr	0	3	22	17	tr	100	55	—	—	0
Frozen Yogurt Nonfat No Sugar Added	½ cup	90	tr	tr	0	4	17	6	tr	150	85	—	—	0
Ice Cream Reduced Fat	1 serv (6.75 oz)	390	20	13	80	6	47	45	0	250	130	—	—	1
Ice Cream Superpremium	1 serv (6.75 oz)	450	28	18	115	8	44	43	0	300	135	—	—	1
Sorbet	½ cup	90	0	0	0	0	22	19	0	150	5	—	—	1

MARCO'S PIZZA

OTHER MENU SELECTIONS

FOOD	PORTION	CALS	FAT	SAT FAT	CHOL	PROT	CARB	SUGAR	FIBER	CALCI	SOD	POTAS	FOLIC	VIT C
Cheezybread Bran	1 piece	80	2	1	5	3	11	1	0	40	105	—	—	0
Chicken Tumblers BBQ	1	67	2	1	9	4	7	3	0	0	164	—	—	1
Chicken Tumblers Hot & Spicy	1	57	2	1	9	4	5	0	0	0	157	—	—	0
Chicken Tumblers Naked	1	57	2	1	9	4	5	0	0	0	120	—	—	0
Chicken Wings BBQ	1	71	4	1	29	5	3	3	0	0	174	—	—	1
Chicken Wings Hot & Spicy	1	60	4	1	29	5	0	0	0	0	167	—	—	0

FOOD	PORTION	CALS	FAT	SAT FAT	CHOL	PROT	CARB	SUGAR	FIBER	CALCI	SOD	POTAS	FOLIC	VIT C
Chicken Wings Naked	1	60	4	1	29	5	0	0	0	0	130	—	—	0
Cinnasquares	1 piece	60	2	0	0	1	9	5	0	0	60	—	—	0
Salad Chicken Ranch	1 serv	240	13	6	60	22	10	2	3	300	1220	—	—	9
Salad Italian	1 serv	230	17	9	35	12	11	3	3	350	930	—	—	42
Sub Chicken Club	½	385	16	7	50	28	34	2	2	250	1150	—	—	2
Sub Ham & Cheese	½	400	21	9	43	21	33	2	1	250	865	—	—	0
Sub Italian	½	430	23	10	53	24	35	3	2	250	1175	—	—	9
Sub Steak & Cheese	½	380	15	7	60	29	33	2	1	250	605	—	—	0
Sub Veggie	½	355	16	9	33	16	39	2	3	400	1135	—	—	8
PIZZA														
Cheese Large	1 slice	280	8	5	20	14	33	3	2	200	510	—	—	1
Cheese Medium	1 slice	210	6	4	15	11	24	2	1	150	390	—	—	1
Cheese Small	1 slice	200	6	4	15	11	23	2	1	150	370	—	—	1
Chicken Fresco Large	1 slice	350	13	7	35	20	35	4	2	250	900	—	—	4
Chicken Fresco Medium	1 slice	260	10	5	25	15	26	3	1	200	670	—	—	2
Chicken Fresco Small	1 slice	180	7	4	20	11	19	2	1	150	480	—	—	2
Deep Pan Cheese	1 slice	290	8	5	20	15	36	3	2	200	530	—	—	1
Deep Pan Pepperoni	1 slice	330	12	6	25	16	36	3	2	200	650	—	—	1
Deluxe Uno Large	1 slice	380	16	8	40	20	35	3	2	250	700	—	—	5
Deluxe Uno Medium	1 slice	280	12	6	30	15	26	2	1	200	520	—	—	2
Deluxe Uno Small	1 slice	200	9	5	20	10	18	2	1	150	360	—	—	2
Garden Large	1 slice	310	10	6	20	16	36	4	2	250	740	—	—	2
Garden Medium	1 slice	230	8	5	15	12	26	3	2	200	530	—	—	1
Garden Small	1 slice	160	5	3	10	8	19	2	1	100	360	—	—	1
Hawaiian Chicken Large	1 slice	380	15	8	35	22	35	4	2	250	890	—	—	9
Hawaiian Chicken Medium	1 slice	260	10	5	25	15	26	3	1	150	620	—	—	5
Hawaiian Chicken Small	1 slice	180	6	3	15	10	18	2	1	100	430	—	—	2
Meat Supremo Large	1 slice	430	21	10	45	23	34	3	2	250	900	—	—	1
Meat Supremo Medium	1 slice	300	15	7	30	15	25	2	1	150	640	—	—	1
Meat Supremo Small	1 slice	210	10	5	20	11	18	2	1	100	430	—	—	0
Pepperoni Large	1 slice	310	11	6	25	15	33	3	2	200	640	—	—	1

FOOD	PORTION	CALS	FAT	SAT FAT	CHOL	PROT	CARB	SUGAR	FIBER	CALCI	SOD	POTAS	FOLIC	VIT C
Pepperoni Medium	1 slice	230	9	5	20	11	24	2	1	150	470	—	—	1
Pepperoni Small	1 slice	210	8	4	20	10	23	2	1	100	440	—	—	0
White Cheezy Large	1 slice	340	15	7	25	17	33	2	2	200	730	—	—	1
White Cheezy Medium	1 slice	260	11	5	20	13	24	2	1	150	550	—	—	5
White Cheezy Small	1 slice	170	7	4	10	9	17	1	1	100	360	—	—	0

MAUI WOWI

SMOOTHIES

FOOD	PORTION	CALS	FAT	SAT FAT	CHOL	PROT	CARB	SUGAR	FIBER	CALCI	SOD	POTAS	FOLIC	VIT C
Fresh Fruit Banana Banana	1 (12 oz)	210	1	1	0	2	50	36	2	130	55	—	—	15
Fresh Fruit Black Raspberry	1 (12 oz)	240	0	0	0	2	59	46	0	100	40	—	—	21
Fresh Fruit Kiwi Lemon Lime	1 (12 oz)	180	0	0	0	3	42	34	0	110	35	—	—	36
Fresh Fruit Lemon Wave	1 (12 oz)	415	tr	tr	0	tr	108	108	tr	10	1	—	—	31
Fresh Fruit Mango Orange Banana	1 (12 oz)	240	1	1	0	3	57	43	tr	100	35	—	—	20
Fresh Fruit Passion Papaya	1 (12 oz)	220	1	1	0	2	54	38	tr	120	50	—	—	22
Fresh Fruit Pina Colada	1 (12 oz)	240	3	3	0	3	57	46	0	100	70	—	—	11

MAX & ERMA'S

FOOD	PORTION	CALS	FAT	SAT FAT	CHOL	PROT	CARB	SUGAR	FIBER	CALCI	SOD	POTAS	FOLIC	VIT C
Black Bean Roll Up	1 serv	577	10	2	14	29	95	—	10	—	1203	—	—	—
Caribbean Chicken Lunch Portion	1 serv	536	20	8	97	28	59	—	3	—	1151	—	—	—
Fruit Smoothie	1	124	tr	tr	0	1	29	—	1	—	4	—	—	—
Garlic Breadstick	1	156	6	0	0	4	21	—	0	—	293	—	—	—
Hula Bowl w/ Fat Free Honey Mustard Dressing w/o Breadsticks	1 serv	823	7	1	131	46	79	—	6	—	1554	—	—	—
Salad Baby Greens w/o Breadstick	1 serv	119	11	1	0	1	6	—	2	—	259	—	—	—
Salad Shrimp Stack	1 serv	322	12	2	178	20	116	—	3	—	823	—	—	—
Salad Dressing Bleu Cheese	2 tbsp	201	21	4	19	1	tr	—	0	—	169	—	—	—
Salad Dressing French Fat Free	2 tbsp	126	tr	0	0	tr	31	—	2	—	1034	—	—	—

FOOD	PORTION	CALS	FAT	SAT FAT	CHOL	PROT	CARB	SUGAR	FIBER	CALCI	SOD	POTAS	FOLIC	VIT C
Salad Dressing Honey Mustard Fat Free	2 tbsp	60	0	0	0	0	14	—	0	—	360	—	—	—
Salad Dressing Italian	2 tbsp	110	12	2	0	0	1	—	0	—	180	—	—	—
Salad Dressing Ranch	2 tbsp	120	13	2	11	1	1	—	0	—	90	—	—	—
Salad Dressing Tex Mex Low Fat	2 tbsp	23	tr	0	2	3	2	—	tr	—	129	—	—	—

MCALISTER'S DELI

CHILDREN'S MENU SELECTIONS

FOOD	PORTION	CALS	FAT	SAT FAT	CHOL	PROT	CARB	SUGAR	FIBER	CALCI	SOD	POTAS	FOLIC	VIT C
Kid's Nacho	1 serv	734	43	9	17	12	74	2	3	—	679	—	—	—
Mac's Dog	1	307	19	0	35	10	24	2	1	—	827	—	—	—
Pita Pizza	1	503	21	10	46	24	54	5	3	—	887	—	—	—
Sandwich Ham & Cheese	1	455	22	11	75	26	39	5	4	—	1819	—	—	—
Sandwich PB&J	1	714	32	5	0	23	86	46	7	—	644	—	—	—
Sandwich Toasted Cheese	1	620	38	0	107	30	40	5	4	—	2031	—	—	—
Sandwich Turkey & Cheese	1	451	21	11	79	26	39	4	4	—	1670	—	—	—

DESSERTS

FOOD	PORTION	CALS	FAT	SAT FAT	CHOL	PROT	CARB	SUGAR	FIBER	CALCI	SOD	POTAS	FOLIC	VIT C
Brownie Chocolate	1 (3.5 oz)	424	18	4	0	6	59	48	3	—	311	—	—	—
Brownie Delight	1 (11 oz)	917	48	22	108	13	111	81	4	—	519	—	—	—
Chocolate Loving Spoon Cake	1 (4 oz)	538	35	9	69	6	54	26	2	—	486	—	—	—
Ice Cream Vanilla Bean	1 scoop (5 oz)	160	10	6	40	3	19	16	0	—	70	—	—	—
Kentucky Pie	1 slice (12 oz)	807	64	27	211	14	110	32	1	—	393	—	—	—
New York Cheesecake	1 slice (5 oz)	505	35	12	92	7	37	34	2	—	239	—	—	—
Sundae Topping Caramel	2 tbsp	100	0	0	0	1	20	20	0	—	110	—	—	—
Sundae Topping Chocolate	1 tbsp	110	0	0	0	1	21	21	0	—	20	—	—	—

MAIN MENU SELECTIONS

FOOD	PORTION	CALS	FAT	SAT FAT	CHOL	PROT	CARB	SUGAR	FIBER	CALCI	SOD	POTAS	FOLIC	VIT C
Appetizers Chips & Salsa	1 serv (5 oz)	87	5	1	0	3	9	0	0	—	128	—	—	—
Appetizers Dip Cheese & Chili	1 serv (5 oz)	572	35	8	17	10	54	1	3	—	598	—	—	—
Appetizers Dip Cheese & Veggie Chili	1 serv (5 oz)	552	31	7	9	9	58	3	5	—	583	—	—	—
Appetizers Nacho Basket	1 serv (6 oz)	579	33	7	17	10	61	2	3	—	832	—	—	—
Appetizers Nacho Chili	1 serv (6 oz)	564	37	10	26	12	46	2	4	—	713	—	—	—

FOOD	PORTION	CALS	FAT	SAT FAT	CHOL	PROT	CARB	SUGAR	FIBER	CALCI	SOD	POTAS	FOLIC	VIT C
Appetizers Nacho Veggie Chili	1 serv (6 oz)	537	31	9	14	11	52	4	6	—	693	—	—	—
Chicken Cordon Bleu	1 serv	810	39	39	156	59	53	11	2	—	2862	—	—	—
Chili Vegetarian	1 serv (8 oz)	133	1	0	0	8	28	4	15	—	987	—	—	—
Cole Slaw	1 serv (4 oz)	190	15	3	15	1	14	10	7	—	215	—	—	—
Fruit Cup	1 serv (4 oz)	98	0	0	0	1	12	19	2	—	12	—	—	—
Giant Spud Cheese	1 (27 oz)	930	48	6	60	55	139	11	19	—	60	—	—	—
Giant Spud Grilled Chicken	1 (27 oz)	839	25	—	—	52	99	14	19	—	88	—	—	—
Giant Spud Just A Spud	1 (26 oz)	604	4	0	0	20	123	12	18	—	63	—	—	—
Giant Spud Ole	1 (30 oz)	1252	60	28	120	68	110	14	18	—	770	—	—	—
Giant Spud Ole w/ Chili	1 (33 oz)	1512	78	29	99	69	134	13	21	—	1255	—	—	—
Giant Spud Ole w/ Veggie Chili	1 (33 oz)	1457	67	27	76	67	146	18	24	—	1214	—	—	—
Giant Spud Veggie	1 (28 oz)	668	18	0	0	29	99	11	18	—	347	—	—	—
Macaroni & Cheese	1 serv (4 oz)	200	7	4	20	8	17	1	1	—	580	—	—	—
Mashed Potatoes	1 serv (4 oz)	136	8	2	2	2	19	1	2	—	347	—	—	—
Meatloaf w/ Gravy	1 serv	340	37	11	189	40	21	0	1	—	752	—	—	—
Open-Faced Roast Beef	1 serv	751	21	7	87	55	88	6	6	—	3099	—	—	—
Pot Roast Spud	1 serv	906	30	10	72	38	121	12	17	—	125	—	—	—
Potato Salad	1 serv (4 oz)	200	11	2	1	3	22	3	3	—	161	—	—	—
Salmon Filet	1 serv	235	4	2	152	46	3	1	1	—	269	—	—	—
Steamed Vegetables	1 serv (4 oz)	43	0	0	0	1	7	4	3	—	52	—	—	—
SALAD DRESSINGS AND SAUCES														
Au Jus	1 serv (4 oz)	10	0	0	0	0	2	0	0	—	60	—	—	—
Comeback Gravy	1 serv (4 oz)	37	2	0	1	1	6	0	0	—	450	—	—	—
Dressing Blue Cheese	2 tbsp	140	15	2	10	0	1	1	0	—	290	—	—	—
Dressing Greek	2 tbsp	90	9	2	0	0	2	1	0	—	250	—	—	—
Dressing Lite Olive Oil Vinaigrette	2 tbsp	60	6	1	0	0	3	2	0	—	230	—	—	—
Dressing Lite Ranch	2 tbsp	100	10	2	10	0	1	1	0	—	290	—	—	—
Dressing Low Calorie Italian	2 tbsp	25	2	0	0	0	2	2	0	—	410	—	—	—
Dressing Parmesan Peppercorn	2 tbsp	150	16	3	2	0	2	1	0	—	310	—	—	—
Dressing Ranch	2 tbsp	100	11	2	10	0	1	1	0	—	290	—	—	—

FOOD	PORTION	CALS	FAT	SAT FAT	CHOL	PROT	CARB	SUGAR	FIBER	CALCI	SOD	POTAS	FOLIC	VIT C
Dressing Tomato Basil	2 tbsp	30	0	0	0	0	6	6	0	—	230	—	—	—
SALADS														
Caesar w/ Salmon	1 (17 oz)	800	53	8	109	34	42	3	5	—	1680	—	—	—
Chicken Fiesta	1 (20 oz)	493	22	14	92	38	34	14	8	—	991	—	—	—
Chicken Grill	1 (21 oz)	840	15	0	131	57	47	8	4	—	3164	—	—	—
Garden	1 (15 oz)	264	17	9	38	17	21	8	4	—	1312	—	—	—
Garden w/ Chicken Salad	1 (18 oz)	537	45	4	34	30	14	16	5	—	1333	—	—	—
Garden w/ Salmon	1 (17 oz)	315	10	1	76	28	28	4	6	—	883	—	—	—
Garden w/ Tuna Salad	1 (18 oz)	373	18	2	15	31	21	8	5	—	1361	—	—	—
Greek Chicken	1 (19 oz)	584	32	3	65	38	32	8	7	—	2161	—	—	—
Side Caesar	1 (6 oz)	328	24	3	16	5	19	3	1	—	679	—	—	—
Side Garden	1 (8 oz)	138	9	5	19	8	11	4	2	—	867	—	—	—
Taco	1 (26 oz)	641	40	15	86	38	33	12	11	—	1680	—	—	—
Taco w/ Veggie Chili	1 (26 oz)	641	40	15	64	38	33	17	15	—	1639	—	—	—
SANDWICHES														
BLT	1	654	38	9	56	28	50	11	6	—	2015	—	—	—
Chicken Salad	1	677	43	10	59	15	58	19	2	—	967	—	—	—
Deli Corned Beef On Wheat	1	369	9	2	76	34	39	4	4	—	1879	—	—	—
Deli Ham On Wheat	1	350	9	1	43	24	43	7	5	—	1854	—	—	—
Deli Pastrami On Wheat	1	371	10	1	75	33	36	4	4	—	1385	—	—	—
Deli Roast Beef On Wheat	1	398	12	1	29	27	49	6	5	—	1937	—	—	—
Deli Salami On Wheat	1	565	32	14	100	27	43	6	5	—	2465	—	—	—
Deli Turkey On Wheat	1	342	9	0	51	24	43	6	5	—	1556	—	—	—
French Dip	1	676	34	19	118	44	50	3	2	—	1889	—	—	—
Grilled Chicken Breast	1	751	36	14	120	50	56	21	2	—	1772	—	—	—
Grilled Chicken Club	1	1234	64	27	193	76	87	27	7	—	2733	—	—	—
Ham Melt	1	700	34	16	114	49	52	6	4	—	2303	—	—	—
McAlisters Club	1	1225	69	29	195	66	86	27	7	—	2845	—	—	—
Meatloaf Parmesan	1	708	36	15	140	47	49	6	5	—	1046	—	—	—
Memphian	1	585	26	12	85	41	48	6	4	—	2237	—	—	—
Muffuletta	¼ (8 oz)	615	35	15	67	36	40	0	2	—	2015	—	—	—
New Yorker	1	628	25	12	127	50	50	4	4	—	2119	—	—	—

FOOD	PORTION	CALS	FAT	SAT FAT	CHOL	PROT	CARB	SUGAR	FIBER	CALCI	SOD	POTAS	FOLIC	VIT C
Orange Cranberry Club	1	954	52	26	171	63	62	18	6	—	2230	—	—	—
Reuben On Rye	1	492	30	9	71	25	35	8	2	—	2175	—	—	—
Roast Beef Melt	1	635	32	15	102	40	48	6	4	—	2170	—	—	—
Salmon	1	608	21	3	76	37	66	10	3	—	1006	—	—	—
Submarine	1	833	48	17	130	50	53	9	3	—	2866	—	—	—
Sweetberry Chicken On Wheatberry	1	701	24	11	102	53	67	8	5	—	1618	—	—	—
Tuna Salad On Wheat	1	452	19	2	15	25	47	7	5	—	941	—	—	—
Turkey Melt	1	700	35	16	124	45	52	6	4	—	2262	—	—	—
Veggie on Pita	1	522	36	9	41	15	33	5	2	—	950	—	—	—
Wrap Greek Chicken	1	630	25	4	53	48	57	3	14	—	2813	—	—	—
Wrap Grilled Chicken Caesar	1	533	25	3	40	42	46	4	13	—	2023	—	—	—
SOUPS														
Asiago Cheese Bisque	1 (8 oz)	240	17	8	47	5	17	1	0	—	720	—	—	—
Broccoli Cheddar	1 (8 oz)	213	15	8	47	8	13	4	0	—	947	—	—	—
Cheddar Potato	1 (8 oz)	213	13	8	40	5	19	0	1	—	773	—	—	—
Cheesy Chicken Tortilla	1 (8 oz)	150	6	3	30	10	13	4	0	—	1470	—	—	—
Chicken & Sausage Gumbo	1 (8 oz)	150	5	2	20	8	17	3	2	—	1040	—	—	—
Clam Chowder	1 (8 oz)	200	11	6	40	8	09	4	0	—	960	—	—	—
Country Potato	1 (8 oz)	173	8	4	20	4	23	4	0	—	760	—	—	—
Country Vegetable	1 (8 oz)	93	1	0	0	3	17	4	3	—	973	—	—	—
French Onion	1 (8 oz)	80	1	1	7	1	11	5	1	—	144	—	—	—
Red Beans & Rice	1 (8 oz)	107	3	1	7	9	25	3	11	—	760	—	—	—
Southwest Roasted Corn	1 (8 oz)	90	4	1	0	4	20	4	3	—	893	—	—	—

MCDONALD'S

BEVERAGES

FOOD	PORTION	CALS	FAT	SAT FAT	CHOL	PROT	CARB	SUGAR	FIBER	CALCI	SOD	POTAS	FOLIC	VIT C
Apple Juice	1 box (6.8 oz)	90	0	0	0	0	23	21	0	100	15	—	—	60
Chocolate Milk 1% Low Fat	8 oz	170	3	2	5	9	26	25	1	300	150	—	—	4
Coca-Cola Classic	1 sm (16 oz)	150	0	0	0	0	40	40	0	0	10	—	—	0
Coffee	1 sm (12 oz)	0	0	0	0	0	0	0	0	0	0	—	—	0
Diet Coke	1 sm (16 oz)	0	0	0	0	0	0	0	0	—	20	—	—	—
Half & Half Creamer	1 pkg	20	2	2	10	0	0	0	0	20	1	—	—	0
Hi-C Orange Lavaburst	1 sm (16 oz)	160	0	0	0	0	44	44	0	0	5	—	—	90
Iced Coffee Caramel	1 sm (16 oz)	130	5	4	20	1	21	20	1	40	80	—	—	0

FOOD	PORTION	CALS	FAT	SAT FAT	CHOL	PROT	CARB	SUGAR	FIBER	CALCI	SOD	POTAS	FOLIC	VIT C
Iced Coffee Hazelnut	1 sm (16 oz)	130	5	4	20	1	21	21	0	40	40	—	—	0
Iced Coffee Regular	1 sm (16 oz)	140	5	4	20	1	22	22	0	40	40	—	—	0
Iced Coffee Vanilla	1 sm (16 oz)	130	5	4	20	1	21	21	0	40	40	—	—	0
Iced Tea	1 sm (16 oz)	0	0	0	0	0	0	0	0	0	10	—	—	0
Milk Lowfat 1%	1 pkg	100	3	2	10	8	12	12	0	300	125	—	—	2
Orange Juice	1 sm (12 oz)	140	0	0	0	2	33	29	0	20	5	—	—	96
Powerade Mountain Blast	1 sm (16 oz)	100	0	0	0	0	27	21	0	0	85	—	—	0
Shake Triple Thick Chocolate	1 sm (12 oz)	440	10	6	40	10	76	63	1	350	190	—	—	0
Shake Triple Thick Strawberry	1 sm (12 oz)	420	10	6	40	10	73	63	0	300	130	—	—	1
Shake Triple Thick Vanilla	1 sm (16 oz)	420	10	6	40	9	72	54	0	300	140	—	—	0
Sprite	1 sm (16 oz)	150	0	0	0	0	39	39	0	0	40	—	—	0
BREAKFAST SELECTIONS														
Big Breakfast Regular Biscuit	1 serv	720	46	16	555	27	49	3	3	150	1500	—	—	1
Biscuit	1 reg	250	11	5	0	4	32	2	2	60	700	—	—	0
Biscuit Regular Bacon Egg Cheese	1	450	25	11	245	18	36	3	2	150	1360	—	—	0
Biscuit Regular Sausage	1	410	27	10	30	11	33	2	2	60	1040	—	—	0
Biscuit Regular Sausage w/ Egg	1	500	32	12	250	17	35	2	2	100	1130	—	—	0
Burrito Sausage	1	300	16	7	130	12	26	2	1	150	830	—	—	1
Deluxe Breakfast Regular Biscuit w/o Syrup & Margarine	1 serv	1070	55	18	575	36	109	17	6	250	2090	—	—	1
English Muffin	1	160	3	1	0	5	27	2	2	150	280	—	—	0
Hash Browns	1 serv	140	8	2	0	1	15	0	2	0	290	—	—	1
Hotcake Syrup	1 pkg (2 oz)	180	0	0	0	0	45	32	0	0	20	—	—	0
Hotcakes w/o Syrup & Margarine	1 serv	350	9	2	20	8	60	14	3	150	590	—	—	0
Hotcakes & Sausage w/o Syrup & Margarine	1 serv	520	24	7	50	15	61	14	3	150	930	—	—	0
McGriddles Bacon Egg Cheese	1	460	21	9	245	19	48	16	2	200	1360	—	—	0

FOOD	PORTION	CALS	FAT	SAT FAT	CHOL	PROT	CARB	SUGAR	FIBER	CALCI	SOD	POTAS	FOLIC	VIT C
McGriddles Sausage	1	420	22	8	35	11	44	15	2	80	1030	—	—	0
McGriddles Sausage Egg & Cheese	1	560	32	12	265	20	48	15	2	200	1360	—	—	0
McMuffin Sausage	1	370	22	8	45	14	29	2	2	250	850	—	—	1
McMuffin Sausage w/ Egg	1	250	27	10	285	21	30	2	2	300	920	—	—	1
McSkillet Burrito w/ Sausage	1	610	36	14	410	27	44	4	3	200	1390	—	—	6
McSkillet Burrito w/ Steak	1	570	30	12	430	32	44	4	3	200	1470	—	—	6
Sausage Patty	1	170	15	5	30	7	1	0	0	20	340	—	—	0
Scrambled Eggs	2	170	11	4	520	15	1	0	0	60	180	—	—	0
DESSERTS														
Apple Dippers	1 pkg	35	0	0	0	0	8	6	0	40	0	—	—	186
Apple Pie Baked	1	270	12	4	0	3	36	14	4	20	190	—	—	6
Cinnamon Melts	1 serv	460	19	9	15	6	66	32	3	60	370	—	—	0
Cookie Chocolate Chip	1	180	7	3	10	2	22	15	1	20	90	—	—	0
Cookie Oatmeal	1 (1.1 oz)	150	6	2	10	2	22	13	1	20	135	—	—	0
Cookie Sugar	1 (1.1 oz)	150	6	2	5	2	21	11	0	20	110	—	—	0
Cookies McDonaldland	1 pkg (2 oz)	250	8	2	0	4	42	14	1	0	270	—	—	0
Cookies McDonaldland Chocolate Chip	1 pkg	270	11	6	35	3	39	19	1	20	170	—	—	0
Fruit 'N Yogurt Parfait	1 serv	160	2	1	5	4	31	21	1	150	85	—	—	9
Ice Cream Cone Reduced Fat Vanilla	1	150	4	2	15	4	24	18	0	100	60	—	—	0
Kiddie Cone	1	45	1	1	5	1	8	6	0	40	20	—	—	0
McFlurry M&M's	1 (12 oz)	620	20	12	55	14	96	85	1	450	190	—	—	0
McFlurry Oreo	1 (12 oz)	560	16	9	50	14	88	71	0	450	250	—	—	0
Peanuts For Sundae	1 serv	45	4	1	0	2	2	0	1	0	0	—	—	0
Sundae Hot Caramel	1	340	7	5	30	7	60	44	1	250	160	—	—	0
Sundae Hot Fudge	1	330	10	7	25	8	54	48	2	250	180	—	—	0
Sundae Strawberry	1	280	6	4	25	6	49	45	1	200	95	—	—	2
MAIN MENU SELECTIONS														
Apple Sauce Strawberry	1 serv	90	0	0	0	0	23	21	tr	—	0	—	—	—
Big Mac	1	540	29	10	75	25	45	9	3	250	1040	—	—	1
Big N' Tasty	1	460	24	8	70	24	37	8	3	150	720	—	—	5

FOOD	PORTION	CALS	FAT	SAT FAT	CHOL	PROT	CARB	SUGAR	FIBER	CALCI	SOD	POTAS	FOLIC	VIT C
Big N' Tasty w/ Cheese	1	510	28	43	85	27	38	8	3	200	960	—	—	5
Cheeseburger	1	300	12	6	40	15	33	6	2	200	750	—	—	1
Cheeseburger Double	1	440	23	11	80	25	34	7	2	250	1150	—	—	1
Cheesy Tots	6 pieces	210	12	5	20	7	20	1	2	—	650	—	—	—
Chicken McNuggets	4 pieces	170	10	2	25	10	10	0	0	0	450	—	—	1
Chicken Selects	3 pieces	380	20	4	55	23	28	0	0	20	930	—	—	2
Filet-O-Fish	1	380	18	4	35	15	38	5	2	150	660	—	—	0
French Fries	1 sm	250	13	3	0	2	30	0	3	20	140	—	—	4
French Fries	1 lg	570	30	6	0	6	70	0	7	20	330	—	—	9
Hamburger	1	250	9	4	25	12	31	6	2	100	520	—	—	1
McChicken	1	360	16	4	40	14	40	5	1	100	790	—	—	1
McRib	1	500	26	10	70	22	44	11	3	150	980	—	—	1
Onion Rings	1 sm	140	7	2	0	2	18	2	2	—	210	—	—	—
Quarter Pounder	1	410	19	7	65	24	37	8	3	150	730	—	—	2
Quarter Pounder Double w/ Cheese	1	740	42	19	155	48	40	9	3	300	1380	—	—	2
Quarter Pounder w/ Cheese	1	510	26	12	90	29	40	9	3	300	1190	—	—	2
Sandwich Chicken Classic Crispy	1	500	17	4	50	27	61	10	3	80	1330	—	—	6
Sandwich Chicken Classic Grilled	1	420	10	2	70	32	51	11	3	80	1190	—	—	6
SandwichClub Chicken Crispy	1	660	28	8	80	39	63	11	4	200	1860	—	—	6
Sandwich Club Chicken Grilled	1	570	21	7	100	44	52	12	4	200	1720	—	—	6
Sandwich Ranch BLT Chicken Crispy	1	600	23	5	70	35	64	12	3	80	1900	—	—	6
Sandwich Ranch BLT Chicken Grilled	1	520	16	4	90	40	53	13	3	100	1760	—	—	6
Snack Wrap Grilled w/ Chipotle BBQ	1	260	8	4	45	18	28	5	1	100	820	—	—	1
Snack Wrap Grilled w/ Honey Mustard	1	260	9	4	45	18	27	4	1	100	800	—	—	1
Snack Wrap Grilled w/ Ranch	1	270	10	4	45	18	26	2	1	100	830	—	—	1
Snack Wrap w/ Chipotle BBQ	1	320	14	5	25	14	35	4	2	100	780	—	—	1
Snack Wrap w/ Honey Mustard	1	320	15	5	30	14	34	4	1	100	750	—	—	1

FOOD	PORTION	CALS	FAT	SAT FAT	CHOL	PROT	CARB	SUGAR	FIBER	CALCI	SOD	POTAS	FOLIC	VIT C
Snack Wrap w/ Ranch	1	140	16	5	30	14	32	2	2	100	780	—	—	1
SALAD DRESSINGS AND SAUCES														
Caramel Dip Low Fat	1 pkg	70	1	0	5	0	15	9	0	20	35	—	—	0
Dipping Sauce Buffalo	1 serv (1 oz)	80	8	2	5	0	2	1	0	—	350	—	—	—
Dipping Sauce Zesty Onion Ring	1 serv (1 oz)	150	15	3	15	0	3	2	tr	—	210	—	—	—
Dressing Ken's Light Italian	1 pkg (2 oz)	120	11	2	0	0	5	4	0	—	440	—	—	—
Dressing Newman's Own Creamy Caesar	1 pkg (2 oz)	170	18	4	20	2	4	2	0	60	500	—	—	0
Dressing Newman's Own Creamy Southwest	1 pkg (1.5 oz)	100	6	1	20	1	11	3	0	20	340	—	—	0
Dressing Newman's Own Low Fat Balsamic Vinaigrette	1 pkg (1.5 oz)	40	3	0	0	0	4	3	0	0	730	—	—	2
Dressing Newman's Own Low Fat Family Recipe Italian	1 pkg (1.5 oz)	60	3	0	0	1	8	1	0	0	730	—	—	0
Dressing Newman's Own Low Fat Sesame Ginger	1 pkg (1.5 oz)	90	3	0	0	1	15	1	0	0	740	—	—	0
Dressing Newman's Own Ranch	1 pkg (2 oz)	170	15	3	20	1	9	4	0	40	530	—	—	0
Honey	1 pkg (0.5 oz)	50	0	0	0	0	12	11	0	0	0	—	—	0
Ketchup	1 pkg	15	0	0	0	0	3	2	0	0	110	—	—	1
Sauce Barbecue	1 pkg (1 oz)	50	0	0	0	0	12	10	0	0	260	—	—	0
Sauce Creamy Ranch	1 pkg (1.5 oz)	200	22	4	10	0	2	1	0	20	320	—	—	0
Sauce Hot Mustard	1 pkg (1 oz)	60	3	0	5	1	9	6	2	0	250	—	—	0
Sauce Southwestern Chipotle Barbeque	1 pkg (1.5 oz)	70	0	0	0	0	18	13	1	20	260	—	—	0
Sauce Spicy Buffalo	1 pkg (1.5 oz)	60	7	1	0	0	1	0	2	0	960	—	—	1
Sauce Sweet'N Sour	1 pkg (1 oz)	50	0	0	0	0	12	10	0	0	150	—	—	0

FOOD	PORTION	CALS	FAT	SAT FAT	CHOL	PROT	CARB	SUGAR	FIBER	CALCI	SOD	POTAS	FOLIC	VIT C
Sauce Tangy Honey Mustard	1 pkg (1.5 oz)	70	3	0	5	1	13	0	0	0	170	—	—	0
SALADS														
Asian w/ Crispy Chicken w/o Dressing	1 serv	380	17	3	45	27	33	12	5	150	1030	—	—	48
Asian w/ Grilled Chicken w/o Dressing	1 serv	300	10	1	65	32	23	12	5	150	890	—	—	54
Asian w/o Chicken & Dressing	1 serv	150	7	1	0	8	15	9	5	100	35	—	—	42
Bacon Ranch w/ Crispy Chicken	1 serv	350	16	5	70	28	23	4	3	150	1150	—	—	30
Bacon Ranch w/ Grilled Chicken w/o Dressing	1 serv	260	9	4	90	33	12	5	3	150	1010	—	—	30
Bacon Ranch w/o Chicken	1 serv	140	7	4	25	9	10	4	3	150	300	—	—	30
Caesar w/ Crispy Chicken	1 serv	300	13	4	55	25	22	4	3	200	1020	—	—	30
Caesar w/ Grilled Chicken	1 serv	220	6	3	75	30	12	5	3	200	890	—	—	30
Caesar w/o Chicken	1 serv	90	4	3	10	7	9	4	3	200	180	—	—	30
Croutons Butter Garlic	1 pkg	60	2	0	0	2	10	0	1	20	140	—	—	0
Fruit & Walnut Snack Size	1 serv	210	8	2	5	4	31	25	2	80	60	—	—	102
Side Salad	1 serv	20	0	0	0	1	4	2	1	20	10	—	—	15
Southwest w/ Crispy Chicken w/o Dressing	1 serv	400	16	4	50	25	41	10	7	150	1110	—	—	30
Southwest w/ Grilled Chicken w/o Dressing	1 serv	320	9	3	70	30	30	11	7	150	970	—	—	30
Southwest w/o Chicken & Dressing	1 serv	140	5	2	10	6	20	5	6	150	150	—	—	27

MIMI'S CAFE

FOOD	PORTION	CALS	FAT	SAT FAT	CHOL	PROT	CARB	SUGAR	FIBER	CALCI	SOD	POTAS	FOLIC	VIT C
BEVERAGES														
Cappuccino	1 serv	86	5	3	17	4	7	—	0	—	72	—	—	—
Cappuccino Iced	1 serv	86	5	3	17	4	7	—	0	—	72	—	—	—
Espresso	1 serv	8	0	0	0	0	1	—	0	—	13	—	—	—
Hot Chocolate w/ Whipped Cream	1 serv	986	17	13	3	8	193	—	8	—	800	—	—	—
Mocha Iced	1 serv	376	11	8	17	6	70	—	2	—	102	—	—	—
Mocha Latte	1 serv	376	11	8	17	6	70	—	2	—	146	—	—	—

FOOD	PORTION	CALS	FAT	SAT FAT	CHOL	PROT	CARB	SUGAR	FIBER	CALCI	SOD	POTAS	FOLIC	VIT C
CHILDREN'S MENU SELECTIONS														
Chicken Fingers	1 serv	408	21	4	67	30	21	2	1	—	686	—	—	—
Grilled Cheese	1 serv	273	19	10	50	13	14	1	0	—	499	—	—	—
Macaroni & Cheese	1 serv	353	13	4	19	12	48	10	2	—	652	—	—	—
Mini Burger	1 serv	554	28	8	66	25	48	5	3	—	686	—	—	—
Mini Corn Dogs	1 serv	460	32	7	35	7	35	8	0	—	672	—	—	—
Pancakes Chocolate Chip	1 serv	563	29	14	73	11	71	33	3	—	747	—	—	—
Pancakes Mimi Mouse	1 serv	477	18	6	63	11	69	23	1	—	985	—	—	—
PB&J Soldiers	1 serv	730	40	7	0	18	78	29	4	—	728	—	—	—
Pepperoni Pizzadillas	1 serv	617	38	19	86	31	39	7	3	—	1600	—	—	—
Scrambled Eggs & Bacon	1 serv	216	16	5	441	18	1	1	0	—	449	—	—	—
Spaghetti	1 serv	343	5	—	—	13	62	17	5	—	711	—	—	—
Turkey Dinner	1 serv	337	16	3	69	11	25	1	3	—	1110	—	—	—
DESSERTS														
Apple Crisp Cinnamon	1 serv	898	37	15	25	7	141	—	4	—	427	—	—	—
Bread Pudding	1 serv	819	55	28	329	18	69	—	1	—	730	—	—	—
Brownie Triple Chocolate	1 serv	1950	87	43	303	25	280	—	6	—	1073	—	—	—
Cheesecake New York Style	1 serv	1075	42	42	373	19	85	—	4	—	744	—	—	—
Pie Banana Foster Mud	1 serv	1245	73	42	218	14	138	—	4	—	477	—	—	—
Pie Pecan Chocolate Chip	1 serv	1879	111	29	231	21	220	—	12	—	1064	—	—	—
MAIN MENU SELECTIONS														
Appetizer Dip Spinach & Artichoke	1 serv	2459	138	56	262	90	191	9	11	—	4320	—	—	—
Appetizer Fried Chicken Tenders	1 serv	800	33	5	134	60	60	19	3	—	1730	—	—	—
Appetizer Fried Dill Pickles	1 serv	972	42	7	12	16	132	—	12	—	3740	—	—	—
Appetizer Jazz Fest	1 serv	1252	72	26	122	43	108	9	8	—	2085	—	—	—
Appetizer Zucchini Parmesan	1 serv	626	28	8	26	22	73	12	7	—	1111	—	—	—
Blackened Sole w/ Shrimp Creole	1 serv	852	34	17	334	78	59	—	9	—	2312	—	—	—
Broiled Flat Iron Steak	1 serv	1026	58	29	164	68	58	—	9	—	1751	—	—	—
Burger Half Pound	1	684	34	12	132	42	48	—	3	—	668	—	—	—
Cafe Fish & Chips	1 serv	1290	57	8	121	69	119	—	10	—	2166	—	—	—

FOOD	PORTION	CALS	FAT	SAT FAT	CHOL	PROT	CARB	SUGAR	FIBER	CALCI	SOD	POTAS	FOLIC	VIT C
Cajun Blackened Salmon	1 serv	919	55	21	220	57	55	—	9	—	1915	—	—	—
Cheeseburger BBQ Ranch	1	999	57	23	192	58	62	—	3	—	1433	—	—	—
Cheeseburger Half Pound	1	855	48	21	177	53	49	—	3	—	932	—	—	—
Chicken Cordon Bleu	1 serv	1360	81	33	306	100	51	—	5	—	3007	—	—	—
Chicken Feta Penne	1 serv	1879	99	38	253	57	158	—	12	—	1756	—	—	—
Ciabatta Chicken	1	1251	72	20	213	70	81	—	4	—	1846	—	—	—
Ciabatta Meatloaf	1	1036	61	20	171	41	83	—	3	—	2017	—	—	—
Ciabatta Turkey Pesto	1	1248	73	20	172	45	83	—	6	—	1672	—	—	—
Club Cafe	1	1132	63	13	175	42	73	—	4	—	1438	—	—	—
Country Fried Steak	1 serv	1061	56	23	156	42	107	—	9	—	1418	—	—	—
Crab Cake Dinner	1 serv	1662	100	19	646	59	129	—	9	—	3732	—	—	—
Diablo Center Cut Pork Chops	1 serv	1094	73	27	219	54	55	—	8	—	2179	—	—	—
Dip Classic Beef	1	521	15	7	108	49	43	—	5	—	3928	—	—	—
Filet of "Soul"	1 serv	636	26	15	163	45	56	—	7	—	1316	—	—	—
French Quarter	1	1480	105	30	214	66	68	—	7	—	1917	—	—	—
Garlic Shrimp Spaghettini	1 serv	860	20	5	261	37	109	—	7	—	1073	—	—	—
Grilled Beef Liver	1 serv	1003	45	21	937	75	75	—	10	—	1457	—	—	—
Grilled Chicken Tuscan Style	1 serv	880	36	19	181	58	80	—	12	—	1529	—	—	—
Hibachi Salmon	1 serv	846	40	7	119	49	75	—	8	—	274	—	—	—
Mimi's Meatloaf	1 serv	910	53	26	291	43	68	—	8	—	2650	—	—	—
Mimi's Pot Roast	1 serv	1291	78	36	323	88	57	—	8	—	2252	—	—	—
Original Patty Melt	1	976	56	22	177	56	62	—	6	—	1261	—	—	—
Parmesan Crusted Chicken Breast	1 serv	1820	54	19	194	91	211	—	15	—	1466	—	—	—
Pasta Jambalaya	1 serv	1223	44	11	295	74	113	—	8	—	1727	—	—	—
Pot Pie Chicken	1 serv	1403	87	25	388	70	86	—	11	—	2416	—	—	—
Reuben West Coast	1	2015	138	35	226	62	120	—	11	—	3798	—	—	—
Sandwich 5 Way Grilled Cheese	1	703	39	22	92	39	49	—	2	—	1150	—	—	—
Sandwich Albacore & Avocado	1	993	71	18	94	33	58	—	9	—	960	—	—	—
Sandwich Bacon Lettuce & Tomato	1	586	34	8	56	24	48	—	7	—	1545	—	—	—

FOOD	PORTION	CALS	FAT	SAT FAT	CHOL	PROT	CARB	SUGAR	FIBER	CALCI	SOD	POTAS	FOLIC	VIT C
Sandwich Fresh Roasted Turkey Breast	1	532	27	5	134	20	28	—	1	—	546	—	—	—
Sandwich Turkey Walnut Salad On Raisin Bread	1	549	42	7	54	7	36	—	3	—	447	—	—	—
Sandwich Veggie Stack	1	836	43	12	48	27	93	—	6	—	1807	—	—	—
Slow Roasted Turkey Breast	1 serv	851	41	16	154	25	72	—	11	—	2086	—	—	—
Small Bites Black & Blue Quesadilla	1 serv	1241	80	36	216	73	60	13	7	—	2403	—	—	—
Small Bites Chicken & Fruit	1 serv	460	9	2	193	73	21	17	3	—	192	—	—	—
Small Bites Citrus Salmon	1 serv	699	43	7	119	44	37	21	10	—	368	—	—	—
Small Bites Crab Cakes	1 serv	412	25	4	212	18	27	6	2	—	1089	—	—	—
Small Bites Smokey Chicken Enchiladas	1 serv	1154	72	27	179	61	68	16	8	—	1922	—	—	—
Small Bites Sweet & Sour Coconut Shrimp	1 serv	608	50	12	120	22	79	38	4	—	767	—	—	—
Small Bites Thai Chicken Wrap	1 serv	1004	41	8	96	51	106	16	7	—	1522	—	—	—
Top Sirloin 12 oz	1 serv	947	48	24	237	79	49	—	7	—	1076	—	—	—
SALAD DRESSINGS														
Balsamic Vinaigrette	1 serv	316	32	5	0	0	8	—	0	—	337	—	—	—
Blue Cheese	1 serv	298	31	6	30	2	1	—	0	—	241	—	—	—
Caesar	1 serv	273	29	5	22	1	2	—	0	—	451	—	—	—
Chinese Sesame	1 serv	263	25	4	0	0	11	—	0	—	307	—	—	—
Dijon Vinaigrette	1 serv	296	32	5	0	0	3	—	0	—	335	—	—	—
Honey Mustard	1 serv	243	22	3	10	1	11	—	0	—	423	—	—	—
Non Fat French	1 serv	65	0	0	0	1	16	—	1	—	222	—	—	—
Ranch	1 serv	194	20	3	18	1	2	—	0	—	321	—	—	—
Thousand Island	1 serv	232	23	4	19	0	6	—	0	—	439	—	—	—
SALADS														
Asian Chopped	1 serv	751	22	5	193	81	55	—	14	—	347	—	—	—
Blue Cheese & Walnut	1 serv	728	53	14	53	26	45	—	10	—	1097	—	—	—
Caesar Blackened Chicken	1 serv	570	17	3	132	59	41	—	6	—	1565	—	—	—
Chopped Cobb	1 serv	524	32	12	329	35	18	—	4	—	1516	—	—	—
Fried Chicken	1 serv	764	67	21	272	23	16	—	3	—	469	—	—	—

FOOD	PORTION	CALS	FAT	SAT FAT	CHOL	PROT	CARB	SUGAR	FIBER	CALCI	SOD	POTAS	FOLIC	VIT C
Zesty Chicken Tostada	1 serv	1046	57	15	134	47	89	—	15	—	1184	—	—	—
SOUPS														
Broccoli Cheddar	1 serv	270	10	12	51	12	18	4	2	—	916	—	—	—
Chicken Gumbo	1 serv	235	12	3	17	7	25	4	2	—	1112	—	—	—
Clam Chowder	1 serv	240	14	8	49	10	21	2	2	—	657	—	—	—
Corn Chowder	1 serv	196	9	5	20	3	28	6	3	—	722	—	—	—
Cream Of Chicken	1 serv	337	29	10	32	0	19	3	1	—	1083	—	—	—
French Market Onion	1 serv	207	12	5	16	10	16	4	2	—	1269	—	—	—
Red Bean & Andouille Sausage	1 serv	256	10	3	29	13	30	4	5	—	706	—	—	—
Split Pea	1 serv	194	3	1	11	14	29	5	11	—	636	—	—	—
Vegetarian Vegetable	1 serv	60	0	0	0	2	12	5	2	—	1561	—	—	—

MR. HERO

FOOD	PORTION	CALS	FAT	SAT FAT	CHOL	PROT	CARB	SUGAR	FIBER	CALCI	SOD	POTAS	FOLIC	VIT C
DESSERTS														
Eli's Cheesecake Oreo Cookie	1 slice (2.5 oz)	260	17	11	65	4	24	—	1	—	250	—	—	—
Eli's Cheesecake Original Plain	1 slice (2.6 oz)	280	19	12	80	4	22	—	0	—	260	—	—	—
Eli's Cheesecake Snickers	1 slice (2.3 oz)	270	18	11	65	4	23	—	1	—	220	—	—	—
Eli's Cheesecake Strawberry Swirl	1 slice (2.6 oz)	280	19	12	80	4	22	—	0	—	260	—	—	—
SALADS														
Garden Side	1 serv (7.3 oz)	32	0	0	0	1	7	—	2	—	11	—	—	—
Grilled Chicken	1 serv (13.4 oz)	166	3	1	55	23	13	—	3	—	588	—	—	—
Tuna Delight	1 serv (14.4 oz)	403	48	8	84	13	10	—	3	—	507	—	—	—
SANDWICHES														
Cheeseburger	1 (10.4 oz)	776	55	8	73	26	47	—	3	—	1122	—	—	—
Cheesesteak Hot Buttered	1 (9.4 oz)	669	42	16	80	28	45	—	3	—	1132	—	—	—
Chicken Grilled Philly	1 (9.1 oz)	421	10	5	75	34	48	—	4	—	1533	—	—	—
Deli Subs Original Italian	1 (9.5 oz)	641	39	11	58	22	47	—	3	—	1781	—	—	—
Deli Subs Tuna 'N Cheese	1 (9.7 oz)	724	54	12	83	21	44	—	3	—	1140	—	—	—
Deli Subs Turkey	1 (9.8 oz)	468	20	6	63	30	46	—	3	—	1574	—	—	—
Deli Subs Ultimate Italian	1 (10.3 oz)	675	40	10	78	27	46	—	3	—	2067	—	—	—
Romanburger	1 (11.3 oz)	861	62	10	90	30	48	—	3	—	1530	—	—	—
Steak Tuscan	1 (10.6 oz)	625	31	10	129	40	42	—	2	—	2259	—	—	—

FOOD	PORTION	CALS	FAT	SAT FAT	CHOL	PROT	CARB	SUGAR	FIBER	CALCI	SOD	POTAS	FOLIC	VIT C
Steak Zesty Bacon & Swiss	1 (9.8 oz)	616	32	11	112	38	42	—	3	—	1714	—	—	—
Subs Meatball	1 (9.3 oz)	724	47	17	75	30	47	—	4	—	1729	—	—	—
Taste Buddies Cheeseburger Bacon	1 (5.9 oz)	264	30	5	490	15	33	—	2	—	758	—	—	—
Taste Buddies Grilled Italiano	1 (5.3 oz)	440	32	7	48	00	32	—	2	—	901	—	—	—
Taste Buddies Italian Sausage	1 (5.4 oz)	368	22	6	53	19	34	—	1	—	1159	—	—	—
Taste Buddies Tuna 'N Cheese	1 (6 oz)	483	38	8	52	12	31		2	—	688	—	—	—
SIDES														
Breadsticks	2 (6 oz)	446	17	3	0	10	64	—	3	—	994	—	—	—
Jalapeno Poppers	1 serv (4.5 oz)	432	28	8	13	9	37	—	3	—	1156	—	—	—
Mozzarella Sticks	1 serv (8.7 oz)	565	43	18	60	31	12	—	1	—	961	—	—	—
Onion Petals	1 serv (5.7 oz)	597	37	6	0	6	56	—	2	—	1060	—	—	—
Potato Babycakes	1 serv (5.9 oz)	477	37	6	0	2	34	—	4	—	880	—	—	—
Potato WaffleFries w/ Cheese Sauce	1 serv (7.2 oz)	482	34	6	0	4	42	—	3	—	954	—	—	—

MRS. FIELDS

FOOD	PORTION	CALS	FAT	SAT FAT	CHOL	PROT	CARB	SUGAR	FIBER	CALCI	SOD	POTAS	FOLIC	VIT C
Bites Double Fudge	3 (1.6 oz)	200	10	5	45	2	27	21	1	0	75	—	—	0
Brownie Butterscotch Blondie	1 (2.1 oz)	260	10	6	50	3	38	28	0	40	20	—	—	0
Brownie Double Fudge	1 (2.1 oz)	260	13	8	60	3	34	27	1	40	95	—	—	0
Brownie Pecan Fudge	1 (2.1 oz)	270	15	7	55	3	32	25	2	20	95	—	—	0
Brownie Special Walnut Fudge & Blondie	1 (2.2 oz)	260	13	7	55	3	35	27	1	20	55	—	—	0
Brownie Toffee Fudge	1 (2.1 oz)	260	14	7	60	3	34	27	1	20	110	—	—	0
Brownie Walnut Fudge	1 (2.1 oz)	270	15	7	55	3	32	25	2	20	95	—	—	0
Cake Chocolate Chip	1 piece (2.9 oz)	350	17	8	50	4	45	27	tr	40	330	—	—	0
Coffee Cake Chocolate Chip	1 sm piece (2.2 oz)	240	11	4	30	3	30	16	1	20	320	—	—	0
Coffee Cake Chocolate Chip	1 lg (2.4 oz)	250	12	4	30	3	32	16	1	20	340	—	—	0
Cookie Butter	1 (1.5 oz)	200	8	5	20	2	29	15	tr	20	180	—	—	0
Cookie Chocolate Covered Peanut Butter	1 (2.5 oz)	340	19	10	20	5	37	26	1	60	230	—	—	0

FOOD	PORTION	CALS	FAT	SAT FAT	CHOL	PROT	CARB	SUGAR	FIBER	CALCI	SOD	POTAS	FOLIC	VIT C
Cookie Chocolate Covered Semi-Sweet	1 (2.5 oz)	380	23	15	15	5	40	37	1	50	65	—	—	0
Cookie Chocolate Covered White Chunk Macadamia	1 (2.4 oz)	330	19	10	15	3	39	29	1	60	170	—	—	0
Cookie Cinnamon Sugar	1 (1.8 oz)	210	8	4	20	2	31	16	0	20	210	—	—	0
Cookie Cut Out	1 (2.4 oz)	280	11	5	2	2	44	28	0	0	180	—	—	0
Cookie Frosted Cinnamon Sugar	1 (2.1 oz)	270	11	5	20	2	39	25	0	20	210	—	—	0
Cookie Oatmeal Raisins & Walnuts	1 (1.7 oz)	200	9	3	15	3	27	16	1	20	180	—	—	0
Cookie Semi-Sweet Chocolate	1 (1.7 oz)	210	10	5	15	2	29	19	1	20	170	—	—	0
Cookie Semi-Sweet Chocolate w/ Walnuts	1 (1.7 oz)	220	11	5	15	2	28	17	1	20	160	—	—	0
Cookie Triple Chocolate	1 (1.7 oz)	210	10	6	15	2	28	19	1	20	170	—	—	0
Cookie White Chunk Macadamia	1 (1.7 oz)	230	12	6	15	2	28	19	0	20	170	—	—	0
Jelly Bellys	1 pkg (1.4 oz)	140	0	0	0	0	37	29	0	0	15	—	—	0
Mixed Nuts	1 pkg (2 oz)	350	32	5	0	9	13	2	3	60	5	—	—	0
Muffin Blueberry	1 (1.9 oz)	190	9	3	25	3	24	12	1	20	280	—	—	0
Muffin Chocolate Chip	1 (1.9 oz)	200	10	3	25	3	26	14	1	20	270	—	—	0
Nibbler Cinnamon Sugar	3 (1.4 oz)	180	8	3	10	2	25	12	0	20	210	—	—	0
Nibbler Debra's Special	3 (1.3 oz)	160	7	2	10	2	22	13	1	20	160	—	—	0
Nibbler Peanut Butter	3 (1.8 oz)	170	9	3	10	3	19	10	1	20	180	—	—	0
Nibbler Semi-Sweet Chocolate	3 (1.8 oz)	170	8	4	10	2	23	14	1	20	140	—	—	0
Nibbler Triple Chocolate	3 (1.8 oz)	160	8	4	10	2	22	15	1	20	150	—	—	0
Nibbler White Chunk Macadamia	3 (1.8 oz)	180	9	4	10	2	22	15	0	40	140	—	—	0
Taffy	1 pkg (2.4 oz)	160	2	2	0	0	38	23	0	0	65	—	—	0
NAKED PIZZA														
10 Inch Pie Original Crust	1 slice	81	5	—	—	4	8	—	3	—	161	—	—	—
10 Inch Pie Thin Crust	1 slice	64	5	—	—	4	5	—	2	—	143	—	—	—

FOOD	PORTION	CALS	FAT	SATFAT	CHOL	PROT	CARB	SUGAR	FIBER	CALCI	SOD	POTAS	FOLIC	VIT C
12 Inch Pie Original Crust	1 slice	132	6	—	—	6	16	—	6	—	225	—	—	—
12 Inch Pie Thin Crust	1 slice	91	5	—	—	4	10	—	3	—	183	—	—	—
14 Inch Pie Original Crust	1 slice	161	7	—	—	7	20	—	7	—	259	—	—	—
14 Inch Pie Thin Crust	1 slice	114	5	—	—	5	11	—	4	—	153	—	—	—

NATHAN'S

FOOD	PORTION	CALS	FAT	SATFAT	CHOL	PROT	CARB	SUGAR	FIBER	CALCI	SOD	POTAS	FOLIC	VIT C
Apple Pie	1 (3.49 oz)	314	19	4	0	3	33	9	0	0	310	—	—	9
Bacon Cheeseburger	1 (10.7 oz)	783	50	20	136	36	45	10	2	180	1365	—	—	1
Cheese Dog	1 (5.05 oz)	390	25	8	35	12	30	5	1	100	1440	—	—	0
Cheese Fries	1 reg (8 oz)	564	42	7	0	5	41	5	4	40	785	—	—	9
Cheesesteak	1 (12.31 oz)	849	45	21	151	44	70	1	2	320	1554	—	—	2
Cheesesteak Supreme	1 (16.29 oz)	879	45	20	151	46	76	3	3	330	1625	—	—	62
Cheesesteak Supreme Chicken	1 (13.81 oz)	601	19	9	79	40	70	3	3	330	1719	—	—	63
Chicken Tender Pita	1 (11.94 oz)	823	52	8	40	22	66	15	5	80	1462	—	—	17
Chicken Tender Platter	1 (17.69 oz)	1245	90	14	44	26	80	31	10	60	1245	—	—	17
Chicken Tenders	3 (6.19 oz)	526	39	6	30	21	24	8	3	0	900	—	—	2
Chicken Wings	5 (6.65 oz)	400	27	7	83	27	12	0	0	0	650	—	—	0
Chili Dog	1 (5.05 oz)	400	23	6	50	16	33	5	2	100	1000	—	—	1
Corn Dog On A Stick	1 (2.89 oz)	380	21	5	15	7	39	13	1	20	730	—	—	0
Corn On The Cob w/ Butter	1 (5.05 oz)	140	2	0	0	5	34	6	2	0	20	—	—	4
Double Burger w/ Cheese	1 (15.61 oz)	1178	84	32	235	57	45	10	2	240	1299	—	—	1
Famous Hot Dog	1 (3.53 oz)	297	18	7	34	11	24	4	1	80	692	—	—	0
French Fries	1 reg (6.5 oz)	464	34	5	0	4	35	4	4	0	55	—	—	9
Funnel Cake	1 (4.21 oz)	580	29	5	30	5	73	43	1	40	360	—	—	0
Hot Dog Nuggets	6 (3.49 oz)	348	28	6	20	5	20	5	0	0	400	—	—	0
Mozzarella Sticks + Sauce	3 (5.64 oz)	390	28	8	32	14	20	6	1	330	941	—	—	4
Onion Rings	1 sm (5.6 oz)	544	45	6	0	3	36	4	1	0	580	—	—	4
Platter Grilled Chicken	1 (15 oz)	504	56	9	59	24	58	24	7	80	1134	—	—	17
Pretzel King Size	1 (2.28 oz)	180	1	0	0	6	38	1	1	0	940	—	—	0
Pretzel Dog	1 (4.02 oz)	390	16	6	25	12	49	7	1	20	970	—	—	0
Sandwich Chicken Tender	1 (9.65 oz)	706	43	6	33	22	58	12	5	70	1165	—	—	13

FOOD	PORTION	CALS	FAT	SAT FAT	CHOL	PROT	CARB	SUGAR	FIBER	CALCI	SOD	POTAS	FOLIC	VIT C
Sandwich Grilled Chicken	1 (9.03 oz)	554	32	5	65	27	40	3	3	90	1158	—	—	13
Wrap Grilled Chicken Caesar	1 (10.34 oz)	700	34	11	75	38	60	2	1	500	1340	—	—	9
Wrap Krispy Southwest Chipotle	1 (11.71 oz)	750	39	13	100	68	62	3	1	450	1160	—	—	9

NOAH'S BAGELS

BAGELS AND BREADS

FOOD	PORTION	CALS	FAT	SAT FAT	CHOL	PROT	CARB	SUGAR	FIBER	CALCI	SOD	POTAS	FOLIC	VIT C
Bagel Asiago Cheese Topped	1 (4.2 oz)	330	6	3	15	16	57	5	2	200	750	—	—	0
Bagel Blueberry	1 (3.7 oz)	270	1	0	0	10	59	11	3	20	520	—	—	0
Bagel Candy Cane	1 (3.7 oz)	270	3	0	5	9	54	5	2	20	540	—	—	0
Bagel Cheddar Stick	1 (4.2 oz)	330	6	3	15	14	57	5	2	100	670	—	—	0
Bagel Chocolate Chip	1 (3.7 oz)	290	4	2	0	9	60	12	3	20	510	—	—	0
Bagel Chopped Garlic	1 (3.9 oz)	290	3	0	0	11	58	5	2	20	580	—	—	0
Bagel Cinnamon Raisin	1 (3.7 oz)	270	1	0	0	9	58	11	3	20	510	—	—	0
Bagel Cinnamon Sugar	1 (4.1 oz)	310	3	0	0	10	64	11	2	20	600	—	—	0
Bagel Cracked Pepper	1 (3.7 oz)	280	4	1	0	9	55	6	2	20	520	—	—	0
Bagel Cranberry Orange	1 (3.5 oz)	250	1	0	0	9	54	6	3	20	520	—	—	0
Bagel Dutch Apple	1 (5 oz)	340	3	0	0	10	72	14	3	20	600	—	—	0
Bagel Egg	1 (3.7 oz)	290	3	1	75	12	57	5	2	20	590	—	—	0
Bagel Everything	1 (3.9 oz)	280	2	0	0	10	57	5	2	20	730	—	—	0
Bagel Good Grains	1 (3.9 oz)	280	2	0	0	12	58	6	4	20	560	—	—	0
Bagel Jalapeno Cheddar	1 (4.9 oz)	350	7	4	20	15	58	5	2	150	940	—	—	1
Bagel Onion	1 (3.7 oz)	270	2	0	0	10	57	5	3	40	540	—	—	0
Bagel Plain	1 (3.7 oz)	270	1	0	0	10	57	5	2	20	580	—	—	0
Bagel Poppyseed	1 (3.9 oz)	290	3	0	0	11	57	5	2	20	580	—	—	0
Bagel Power	1 (4 oz)	310	5	1	0	11	61	16	4	40	280	—	—	0
Bagel Pumpernickel	1 (3.7 oz)	260	2	0	0	10	57	4	3	20	530	—	—	0
Bagel Sesame Seed	1 (3.9 oz)	290	3	0	0	11	57	5	2	20	580	—	—	0
Bagel Six Cheese	1 (4.5 oz)	340	6	4	15	16	57	5	2	200	770	—	—	0
Bagel Spinach Florentine	1 (4.9 oz)	350	8	4	20	16	58	6	2	200	700	—	—	4
Bagel Sun Dried Tomato	1 (3.7 oz)	270	2	0	0	10	57	6	3	40	680	—	—	0
Bagel Whole Wheat	1 (3.7 oz)	260	1	0	0	11	57	6	4	20	560	—	—	0

FOOD	PORTION	CALS	FAT	SAT FAT	CHOL	PROT	CARB	SUGAR	FIBER	CALCI	SOD	POTAS	FOLIC	VIT C
Bagel Whole Wheat Sesame & Sunflower Seeds	1 (4.4 oz)	370	11	1	0	15	61	6	6	40	560	—	—	0
Bialy	1 (5.3 oz)	380	4	0	0	11	77	5	4	20	700	—	—	0
Bread Ciabatta	1 serv (4.25 oz)	290	3	0	0	10	60	1	2	20	640	—	—	0
Bread Corn Meal Rye	1 slice (2 oz)	150	2	0	0	6	31	1	2	40	410	—	—	0
Bread Harvest Grain	1 slice (2.3 oz)	180	2	0	0	7	36	7	4	0	220	—	—	0
Bread Marble Rye	1 slice (1.7 oz)	160	1	0	0	5	30	1	1	20	370	—	—	0
Bread Potato	1 slice (1.7 oz)	140	2	0	0	4	28	3	1	0	250	—	—	0
Challah Braided	1 serv (2 oz)	160	3	0	20	6	29	4	1	20	180	—	—	0
Challah Roll	1 (3 oz)	230	4	1	0	8	44	6	2	20	340	—	—	9
Pizza Bagel Artichoke Tomato & Red Onion	1 (11.1 oz)	550	20	11	55	31	67	8	5	600	1430	—	—	9
Pizza Bagel Artichoke & Spinach	1 (12 oz)	670	32	14	55	31	70	7	5	600	1870	—	—	12
Pizza Bagel Cheese	1 (6.2 oz)	420	11	7	35	23	60	6	3	350	1060	—	—	2
Pizza Bagel Cheesy Garlic & Herb	1 (6.2 oz)	500	19	12	55	24	62	6	2	350	1090	—	—	0
Pizza Bagel Pepperoni	1 (6.8 oz)	500	19	10	50	26	60	6	3	350	1360	—	—	2
Pizza Bagel Spinach & Mushroom	1 (9.5 oz)	580	25	13	55	27	68	8	4	400	1340	—	—	15
Pizza Bagel Tomato & Rosemary	1 (8.7 oz)	540	20	11	55	30	63	7	4	600	1240	—	—	9
BEVERAGES AND EXTRAS														
Cafe Latte Low Fat	1 reg (12 oz)	160	7	4	25	10	17	17	0	400	180	—	—	4
Cafe Latte Nonfat	1 reg (12 oz)	110	0	0	5	11	17	17	0	400	180	—	—	4
Cafe Latte Whole	1 reg (12 oz)	200	10	6	30	10	16	16	0	350	140	—	—	0
Cappuccino Low Fat	1 reg (12 oz)	120	5	3	20	7	13	13	0	250	130	—	—	2
Cappuccino Nonfat	1 reg (12 oz)	90	0	0	5	8	13	13	0	300	135	—	—	2
Cappuccino Whole	1 reg (12 oz)	150	8	5	25	7	13	13	0	250	110	—	—	0
Chai Tea Low Fat Milk	1 reg (12 oz)	220	2	1	5	3	47	45	0	100	65	—	—	1
Chai Tea Nonfat Milk	1 reg (12 oz)	210	0	0	0	3	47	45	0	100	65	—	—	1

FOOD	PORTION	CALS	FAT	SAT FAT	CHOL	PROT	CARB	SUGAR	FIBER	CALCI	SOD	POTAS	FOLIC	VIT C
Chai Tea Whole Milk	1 reg (12 oz)	230	3	2	10	3	47	45	0	100	55	—	—	0
Coca-Cola	8 oz	99	0	0	0	0	27	27	0	0	6	—	—	0
Coca-Cola Cherry	8 oz	104	0	0	0	0	28	28	0	0	4	—	—	0
Coffee Iced Americano	8 oz	0	0	0	0	0	0	0	0	0	0	—	—	0
Coffee Regular & Decaf	1 (12 oz)	0	0	0	0	0	0	0	0	0	0	—	—	0
Diet Coke	8 oz	1	0	0	0	0	0	0	0	0	10	—	—	0
Espresso	1 reg (2 oz)	0	0	0	0	0	0	0	0	0	0	—	—	0
Fanta Orange	8 oz	106	0	0	0	0	29	29	0	0	0	—	—	0
Frozen Drinks Cafe Caramel	1 (18 oz)	620	9	3	45	8	100	66	0	250	140	—	—	0
Frozen Drinks Cafe Mocha	1 (18 oz)	510	8	3	40	7	102	64	0	250	160	—	—	0
Frozen Drinks Strawberry Cream	1 (18 oz)	450	19	14	65	6	75	64	3	150	95	—	—	96
Frozen Drinks Wild Berry Fat Free	1 (18 oz)	270	0	0	5	4	62	48	5	150	75	—	—	114
Half & Half Creamer	1 oz	40	3	2	15	1	1	1	0	40	25	—	—	0
Hi-C Fruit Punch	8 oz	104	0	0	0	0	28	28	0	0	9	—	—	36
Hot Chocolate Nonfat	1 reg (12 oz)	220	2	1	5	12	37	36	1	400	330	—	—	4
Hot Chocolate Whole	1 reg (12 oz)	290	11	6	30	10	35	34	1	350	280	—	—	0
Iced Cappuccino Nonfat	1 reg (12 oz)	90	0	0	5	8	13	13	0	300	135	—	—	2
Iced Mocha Low Fat	1 reg (12 oz)	230	5	3	20	8	39	34	0	300	170	—	—	2
Iced Tea Raspberry	8 oz	78	0	0	0	0	21	21	0	0	9	—	—	0
Iced Tea Unsweetened	8 oz	1	0	0	0	0	0	0	0	0	14	—	—	0
Lemonade	1 (16 oz)	200	0	0	0	1	24	24	0	0	0	—	—	24
Lemonade Blackberry	1 (16 oz)	310	0	0	0	2	74	74	0	0	5	—	—	36
Macchiato Nonfat	1 reg (12 oz)	230	0	0	5	10	49	44	0	300	210	—	—	2
Macchiato Whole	1 reg (12 oz)	290	8	5	25	8	47	42	0	500	170	—	—	0
Milk Low Fat	8 oz	120	5	3	20	8	12	11	0	300	125	—	—	2
Milk Skim	8 oz	80	0	0	5	7	15	13	0	250	140	—	—	1
Milk Whole	8 oz	150	8	5	25	8	11	11	0	300	100	—	—	0
Mocha Low Fat	1 reg (12 oz)	230	5	3	20	8	39	34	0	300	170	—	—	2
Mocha Nonfat	1 reg (12 oz)	190	0	0	5	9	39	34	0	300	180	—	—	2
Mocha Whole	1 reg (12 oz)	270	9	5	25	8	38	33	0	300	150	—	—	0
Mr. Pibb	8 oz	97	0	0	0	0	26	26	0	0	14	—	—	0

FOOD	PORTION	CALS	FAT	SAT FAT	CHOL	PROT	CARB	SUGAR	FIBER	CALCI	SOD	POTAS	FOLIC	VIT C
On Top Reduced Fat Topping	2 tbsp (0.3 oz)	20	2	1	0	0	2	2	0	0	5	—	—	0
Orange Juice	1 (10 oz)	143	0	0	0	1	34	31	2	40	71	—	—	180
Sprite	8 oz	97	0	0	0	0	26	26	0	0	22	—	—	0
Syrup Blackberry	2 tbsp (1 oz)	100	0	0	0	0	25	25	0	0	0	—	—	0
Syrup Caramel	2 tbsp (1 oz)	70	0	0	0	0	18	17	0	0	0	—	—	0
Syrup Hazelnut	2 tbsp (1 oz)	100	0	0	0	0	25	25	0	0	0	—	—	0
Syrup Vanilla	2 tbsp (1 oz)	100	0	0	0	0	25	25	0	0	0	—	—	0
Syrup Vanilla Sugar Free	2 tbsp (1 oz)	116	0	0	0	0	0	0	0	0	0	—	—	0
Tea Harney & Sons All Flavors	8 oz	0	0	0	0	0	0	0	0	0	0	—	—	0
Whipped Cream Light	2 tbsp (1 oz)	36	3	3	5	0	2	2	0	0	0	—	—	0
CREAM CHEESE AND SPREADS														
Butter	1 tbsp (0.5 oz)	110	11	8	30	0	0	0	0	0	80	—	—	0
Cream Cheese Whipped Onion & Chive	2 tbsp (0.7 oz)	70	6	4	20	1	3	1	0	20	60	—	—	0
Cream Cheese Whipped Plain	2 tbsp (0.7 oz)	70	7	5	20	1	1	1	0	0	65	—	—	0
Cream Cheese Whipped Reduced Fat Blueberry	2 tbsp (0.7 oz)	70	5	4	15	1	6	5	0	0	50	—	—	0
Cream Cheese Whipped Reduced Fat Garden Vegetable	2 tbsp (0.7 oz)	60	5	4	15	1	3	1	0	20	100	—	—	1
Cream Cheese Whipped Reduced Fat Garlic Herb	2 tbsp (0.7 oz)	60	5	4	15	1	3	1	0	0	100	—	—	0
Cream Cheese Whipped Reduced Fat Honey Almond	2 tbsp (0.7 oz)	70	5	3	15	1	6	4	0	20	45	—	—	0
Cream Cheese Whipped Reduced Fat Jalapeno Salsa	2 tbsp (0.7 oz)	60	5	4	15	1	3	1	0	0	105	—	—	0
Cream Cheese Whipped Reduced Fat Plain	2 tbsp (0.7 oz)	60	5	4	15	1	2	1	0	0	100	—	—	0

FOOD	PORTION	CALS	FAT	SAT FAT	CHOL	PROT	CARB	SUGAR	FIBER	CALCI	SOD	POTAS	FOLIC	VIT C
Cream Cheese Whipped Reduced Fat Strawberry	2 tbsp (0.7 oz)	60	5	4	15	1	2	1	0	0	100	—	—	0
Cream Cheese Whipped Reduced Fat Sun Dried Tomato & Basil	2 tbsp (0.7 oz)	60	5	4	15	1	2	1	0	0	100	—	—	0
Cream Cheese Whipped Smoked Salmon	2 tbsp (0.7 oz)	60	6	4	20	1	2	1	0	0	120	—	—	0
Deli Mustard	1 tsp (5 g)	0	0	0	0	0	0	0	0	0	65	—	—	0
Garlic Mayo	1 serv (1.5 oz)	270	27	4	20	0	8	1	0	0	320	—	—	1
Grape Jam	1 serv (1 oz)	110	0	0	0	0	28	26	0	0	0	—	—	0
Honey	1 serv (1 oz)	90	0	0	0	0	23	22	0	0	0	—	—	0
Hummus	1 serv (2 oz)	90	4	1	0	3	11	1	2	40	200	—	—	5
Mayo	1 tbsp (0.5 oz)	110	12	2	10	0	0	0	0	0	70	—	—	0
DESSERTS														
Cinnamon Twists	1 serv (3.8 oz)	370	21	10	0	5	41	18	2	40	125	—	—	0
Coffee Cake Apple Cinnamon	1 serv (6.6 oz)	700	28	10	5	5	108	57	1	80	280	—	—	1
Coffee Cake Chocolate Chip	1 serv (6.1 oz)	760	34	13	5	6	110	58	2	80	270	—	—	0
Coffee Cake Mixed Berry	1 serv (6.9 oz)	710	29	10	5	5	110	59	2	80	270	—	—	1
Cookie Chocolate Chip	1 (2.8 oz)	360	18	9	15	4	48	29	2	20	290	—	—	0
Cookie Chocolate Mudslide	1 (2.75 oz)	320	17	9	60	4	46	38	1	20	75	—	—	0
Cookie Iced Sugar	1 (3.7 oz)	480	15	6	25	4	76	46	1	0	260	—	—	0
Cookie Oatmeal Raisin	1 (2.8 oz)	320	11	5	25	5	54	31	2	20	310	—	—	0
Cookie Snickerdoodle	1 (2.8 oz)	400	18	9	30	3	56	32	1	20	360	—	—	0
Cookie Mini Chocolate Chip	1 (1.38 oz)	180	9	5	5	2	24	14	1	20	150	—	—	0
Cookie Mini Chocolate Mudslide	1 (1.38 oz)	160	8	5	30	2	23	19	1	20	40	—	—	0
Cookie Mini Iced Sugar	1 (1.87 oz)	230	7	3	15	2	39	24	1	0	130	—	—	0
Cookie Mini Oatmeal Raisin	1 (1.38 oz)	160	5	3	10	2	27	16	1	20	160	—	—	0
Marshmallow Crispy Treat	1 (3.9 oz)	410	7	2	0	5	86	37	0	0	125	—	—	9
Muffin Blueberry	1 (5 oz)	480	22	5	105	6	65	36	2	40	480	—	—	2

FOOD	PORTION	CALS	FAT	SAT FAT	CHOL	PROT	CARB	SUGAR	FIBER	CALCI	SOD	POTAS	FOLIC	VIT C
Muffin Cranberry Orange	1 (4.6 oz)	460	22	4	95	9	63	39	2	60	480	—	—	6
Muffin Strawberry White Chocolate	1 (5.5 oz)	550	25	7	105	7	78	49	1	60	510	—	—	0
Strudel Cinnamon Walnut	1 serv (5.4 oz)	630	42	17	35	9	56	20	4	40	360	—	—	9
SALAD DRESSINGS														
Caesar	2 tbsp (1 oz)	150	16	3	10	1	1	1	0	0	350	—	—	05
Harvest Chicken Salad	2 tbsp (1 oz)	90	8	2	2	0	3	2	0	0	410	—	—	0
Raspberry Vinaigrette	2 tbsp	160	14	2	0	0	8	8	0	0	0	—	—	0
SALADS														
Caesar	1 (10.5 oz)	600	53	12	50	13	23	4	6	250	1360	—	—	42
Caesar Chicken	1 (14 oz)	720	54	11	120	34	23	6	4	250	1840	—	—	42
Caesar Side	1 (4.5 oz)	280	27	6	20	6	7	2	2	100	680	—	—	12
City	1 (11.5 oz)	830	68	12	25	14	39	29	7	250	460	—	—	27
City w/ Chicken	1 (15 oz)	950	71	12	105	36	40	30	8	300	820	—	—	27
Southwestern Chicken	1 (15.2 oz)	710	41	9	95	35	54	14	10	250	1940	—	—	36
SANDWICHES														
Bagel & Lox	1 (11.2 oz)	520	21	11	50	25	65	11	4	40	1400	—	—	15
Bagel Dog Asiago	1 (7.1 oz)	510	21	8	60	23	59	6	2	80	1350	—	—	0
Bagel Dog Everything	1 (7.1 oz)	510	20	7	55	22	59	6	2	40	1460	—	—	0
Bagel Dog Original	1 (6.9 oz)	490	20	7	55	22	59	6	2	40	1310	—	—	0
Bagel Plain w/ Peanut Butter & Jelly	1 (6.2 oz)	550	15	2	0	17	90	31	4	20	580	—	—	0
Breakfast Wrap Santa Fe	1 (14.5 oz)	750	34	12	410	34	77	8	9	500	1410	—	—	15
Breakfast Wrap Veggie	1 (15.6 oz)	810	41	17	400	35	77	7	10	700	1330	—	—	15
California Chicken	1 (9.9 oz)	360	7	2	80	31	49	8	3	40	840	—	—	21
Club Blackened Chicken	1 (10.4 oz)	630	33	6	130	30	53	8	2	40	1500	—	—	18
Club Deli Pesto Turkey	1 (10.9 oz)	670	39	10	100	27	47	9	2	200	1310	—	—	24
Deli Chicken Salad	1 (11 oz)	1150	95	14	90	17	61	5	5	100	1190	—	—	9
Deli Cornbeef	1 (14 oz)	740	34	6	105	44	61	5	4	80	2820	—	—	9
Deli Egg Salad Kosher	1 (11.5 oz)	650	6	0	450	26	68	6	5	150	1280	—	—	12
Deli Pastrami	1 (14 oz)	750	34	6	105	44	62	6	5	100	3180	—	—	9
Deli Roast Beef	1 (14 oz)	730	34	6	100	43	60	5	4	100	3750	—	—	9

FOOD	PORTION	CALS	FAT	SAT FAT	CHOL	PROT	CARB	SUGAR	FIBER	CALCI	SOD	POTAS	FOLIC	VIT C
Deli Tuna Salad	1 (13 oz)	740	45	7	55	28	53	9	5	80	1440	—	—	21
Deli Turkey	1 (14.5 oz)	720	29	4	55	29	67	6	5	100	2480	—	—	9
Deli Whitefish	1 (12.2 oz)	850	55	8	95	25	68	9	6	100	1470	—	—	6
Deli Melts Hummus	1 (10.2 oz)	570	19	9	40	28	76	7	6	400	1280	—	—	12
Deli Melts Pastrami	1 (9.6 oz)	530	17	9	85	38	61	7	3	400	1840	—	—	6
Deli Melts Roast Beef	1 (9.6 oz)	530	17	9	80	36	60	6	3	300	2190	—	—	6
Deli Melts Tuna	1 (11.6 oz)	700	33	11	90	42	82	7	3	450	1490	—	—	9
Deli Melts Turkey	1 (9.6 oz)	500	14	8	55	29	60	7	3	400	1420	—	—	6
Deli Melts Veggie	1 (12.3 oz)	590	25	12	50	25	70	10	5	350	1430	—	—	42
Egg Mit Artichoke & Tomato	1 (12 oz)	620	28	13	390	28	67	10	4	250	1120	—	—	6
Egg Mit Bacon & Cheddar	1 (9.2 oz)	620	28	10	390	33	61	8	2	250	1210	—	—	1
Egg Mit Cheese & Tomato	1 (10 oz)	530	21	8	365	27	61	8	3	250	880	—	—	6
Egg Mit Lox & Chives	1 (8.8 oz)	490	17	5	355	28	59	8	2	100	890	—	—	1
Egg Mit Plain	1 (7.9 oz)	450	14	4	350	22	59	7	2	100	760	—	—	1
Egg Mit Spinach Mushroom & Swiss	1 (9.8 oz)	530	20	8	370	28	61	8	3	300	850	—	—	4
Egg Mit Turkey Sausage	1 (9.9 oz)	590	24	9	395	34	61	8	2	250	1060	—	—	1
Egg Mit w/ Cheese	1 (8.5 oz)	520	20	8	365	28	60	7	2	250	880	—	—	1
Kosher Vegetarian On Plain Bagel	1 (13.9 oz)	860	41	18	435	49	79	9	4	800	1510	—	—	9
Panini Albacore Tuna	1 (13.6 oz)	750	38	11	85	32	62	2	6	100	1560	—	—	6
Panini Egg Spinach Bacon	1 (11.8 oz)	790	43	14	405	27	65	4	5	400	1500	—	—	9
Panini Egg Vegetarian Omelet	1 (13.8 oz)	670	31	11	380	23	66	5	6	350	1100	—	—	15
Panini Italian Chicken	1 (12.5 oz)	810	40	12	125	47	67	3	5	350	2490	—	—	27
Panini Mediterranean	1 (10.6 oz)	550	18	5	20	11	77	3	9	250	1140	—	—	9
Panini Tomato Mozzarella	1 (7.9 oz)	440	16	5	20	7	59	1	6	200	960	—	—	0
Panini Turkey Club	1 (12.3 oz)	610	21	8	60	23	64	4	6	300	1820	—	—	15
Sandwich Rachel	1 (13.9 oz)	1030	68	17	170	51	53	14	2	400	3520	—	—	6
Sandwich Reuben	1 (13.9 oz)	770	41	13	150	51	47	8	3	400	3400	—	—	12
Sandwich Veg Out	1 (10.1 oz)	490	14	7	30	19	75	9	4	100	960	—	—	12

FOOD	PORTION	CALS	FAT	SAT FAT	CHOL	PROT	CARB	SUGAR	FIBER	CALCI	SOD	POTAS	FOLIC	VIT C
Wrap Albacore Tuna	1 (12.3 oz)	600	28	5	50	29	57	5	8	350	1030	—	—	12
Wrap Chicken Caesar	1 (12.6 oz)	790	46	14	130	37	62	7	7	400	1640	—	—	9
Wrap Southwestern Turkey	1 (13.5 oz)	750	37	12	60	25	74	12	9	450	1890	—	—	15
Wrap Veggie	1 (9.8 oz)	460	17	6	20	12	64	6	9	350	610	—	—	12
SIDES														
Cole Slaw	1 serv (3 oz)	120	6	1	5	1	15	2	2	40	180	—	—	4
Egg Salad	1 serv (5 oz)	330	29	6	450	13	3	2	0	60	450	—	—	2
Fresh Fruit Cup	1 (11 oz)	140	0	0	0	2	36	31	3	40	35	—	—	90
Fruit & Yogurt Parfait	1 (12 oz)	220	1	0	10	13	43	25	3	250	135	—	—	48
Kosher Pickle	1	5	0	0	0	0	1	1	0	0	650	—	—	0
Macaroni & Cheese	1 serv (6 oz)	340	17	5	27	15	32	—	1	—	606	—	—	—
Redskin Potato Salad	1 serv (3 oz)	160	12	3	10	1	13	1	1	0	360	—	—	2
Tuna Salad	1 serv (5 oz)	280	20	4	50	20	3	1	1	40	660	—	—	4
SOUPS														
Broccoli Cheese	1 cup (8.7 oz)	290	20	10	45	14	16	6	2	300	990	—	—	36
Chicken Noodle	1 cup (8.7 oz)	110	4	1	25	5	13	1	1	20	750	—	—	2
Italian Wedding	1 cup (8.7 oz)	160	6	2	20	11	15	2	2	60	1060	—	—	24
Tortilla	1 cup (8.7 oz)	300	19	10	40	13	19	6	3	250	920	—	—	36
Turkey Chili	1 cup (8.7 oz)	220	7	2	35	20	24	5	5	60	930	—	—	21

NOODLES & COMPANY

MAIN MENU SELECTIONS

FOOD	PORTION	CALS	FAT	SAT FAT	CHOL	PROT	CARB	SUGAR	FIBER	CALCI	SOD	POTAS	FOLIC	VIT C
Bangkok Curry	1 sm	250	6	5	0	5	42	—	3	—	430	—	—	—
Bangkok Curry	1 reg	490	13	9	0	9	85	—	7	—	860	—	—	—
Beef Braised	1 serv	190	10	4	75	28	0	0	0	—	370	—	—	—
Beef Sauteed	1 serv	210	12	4	75	25	0	0	0	—	480	—	—	—
Buttered Noodles	1 reg	620	16	4	40	33	84	—	7	—	1590	—	—	—
Buttered Noodles	1 sm	310	8	2	20	17	42	—	4	—	790	—	—	—
Chicken Breast Seasoned	1 serv	130	3	1	75	22	0	0	0	—	720	—	—	—
Chicken Parmesan Crusted	1 serv	190	8	2	50	17	17	—	0	—	620	—	—	—
Ciabatta Roll	1	160	2	0	0	6	31	—	2	—	430	—	—	—
Flatbread	1 serv	210	4	1	0	7	37	—	2	—	370	—	—	—
House Marinara	1 reg	650	12	5	20	27	107	—	7	—	730	—	—	—
House Marinara	1 sm	330	6	3	10	13	53	—	3	—	360	—	—	—
Mushroom Stroganoff	1 reg	780	31	17	135	28	100	—	10	—	980	—	—	—
Mushroom Stroganoff	1 sm	390	15	9	65	14	50	—	5	—	490	—	—	—

FOOD	PORTION	CALS	FAT	SAT FAT	CHOL	PROT	CARB	SUGAR	FIBER	CALCI	SOD	POTAS	FOLIC	VIT C
Organic Tofu	1 serv	180	11	2	0	16	4	—	0	—	220	—	—	—
Pad Thai	1 reg	700	20	3	120	11	117	—	5	—	1840	—	—	—
Pad Thai	1 sm	350	10	2	60	6	59	—	3	—	920	—	—	—
Pasta Fresca	1 sm	420	12	4	10	15	56	—	3	—	450	—	—	—
Pasta Fresca	1 reg	780	22	6	20	27	111	—	6	—	770	—	—	—
Penne Rosa	1 reg	810	26	13	0	24	119	—	15	—	1100	—	—	—
Penne Rosa	1 sm	420	13	6	0	12	60	—	8	—	550	—	—	—
Pesto Cavatappi	1 sm	510	21	9	60	18	62	—	4	—	630	—	—	—
Pesto Cavatappi	1 reg	910	30	12	85	36	124	—	8	—	1240	—	—	—
Potstickers	3	200	5	1	15	5	31	—	2	—	1150	—	—	—
Shrimp Sauteed	1 serv	35	0	0	75	8	0	0	0	—	190	—	—	—
Whole Grain Tuscan Linguine	1 reg	770	26	8	50	26	108	—	20	—	1370	—	—	—
Whole Grain Tuscan Linguine	1 sm	450	20	8	60	15	54	—	10	—	750	—	—	—
Wisconsin Mac & Cheese	1 reg	900	31	18	75	36	119	—	13	—	1100	—	—	—
Wisconsin Mac & Cheese	1 sm	450	16	9	40	18	60	—	7	—	550	—	—	—
SALADS														
Caesar	1 reg	320	28	7	35	11	11	—	2	—	780	—	—	—
Caesar	1 sm	160	14	4	15	5	5	—	1	—	390	—	—	—
Chinese Chopped	1 sm	150	7	1	0	3	11	—	3	—	180	—	—	—
Chinese Chopped	1 reg	310	15	2	0	6	23	—	6	—	370	—	—	—
Cucumber Tomato Side Salad	1	80	0	0	0	2	18	—	2	—	190	—	—	—
The Med	1 reg	310	13	5	20	10	39	—	4	—	960	—	—	—
The Med	1 sm	150	6	2	10	5	19	—	2	—	480	—	—	—
Tossed Green	1	60	6	1	0	1	3	—	1	—	140	—	—	—
SOUPS														
Chicken Noodle	1 sm	150	2	1	35	10	22	—	5	—	1150	—	—	—
Chicken Noodle	1 reg	300	4	1	70	20	44	—	10	—	2290	—	—	—
Thai Curry	1 reg	480	19	15	0	0	70	—	3	—	1580	—	—	—
Thai Curry	1 sm	240	10	7	0	0	35	—	2	—	790	—	—	—
Tomato Basil	1 reg	420	23	12	65	0	45	—	13	—	3530	—	—	—
Tomato Basil	1 sm	210	12	6	35	0	23	—	7	—	1760	—	—	—

OLD SPAGHETTI FACTORY

FOOD	PORTION	CALS	FAT	SAT FAT	CHOL	PROT	CARB	SUGAR	FIBER	CALCI	SOD	POTAS	FOLIC	VIT C
BEVERAGES														
Cherry Coke	1 (12 oz)	140	0	0	0	0	39	39	0	—	5	—	—	—
Coffee Black	1 (8 oz)	0	0	0	0	0	0	0	0	—	0	—	—	—
Coke	1 (12 oz)	130	0	0	0	0	37	37	0	—	10	—	—	—
Diet Coke	1 (12 oz)	0	0	0	0	0	0	0	0	—	5	—	—	—
Hot Tea	1 (8 oz)	0	0	0	0	0	0	0	0	—	0	—	—	—
Iced Tea Strawberry	1 (12 oz)	100	0	0	0	0	23	10	0	—	0	—	—	—

FOOD	PORTION	CALS	FAT	SAT FAT	CHOL	PROT	CARB	SUGAR	FIBER	CALCI	SOD	POTAS	FOLIC	VIT C
Italian Cream Soda	1 (7.5 oz)	140	3	2	10	1	25	24	0	—	50	—	—	—
Kid's Juice Bar	1 serv (2.4 oz)	60	0	0	0	0	15	14	0	—	10	—	—	—
Lemonade	1 (12 oz)	140	0	0	0	0	39	37	0	—	15	—	—	—
Lemonade Strawberry	1 (12 oz)	200	0	0	0	0	55	52	0	—	10	—	—	—
Masterpiece Shake	1 (8.5 oz)	700	39	21	85	10	81	63	1	—	360	—	—	—
Milk 2%	1 (13 oz)	180	7	5	30	12	17	17	0	—	150	—	—	—
Milk Skim	1 (13 oz)	130	1	0	5	13	18	18	0	—	190	—	—	—
Root Beer	1 (12 oz)	150	0	0	0	0	41	41	0	—	35	—	—	—
Sprite	1 (12 oz)	140	0	0	0	0	34	30	0	—	30	—	—	—
CHILDREN'S MENU SELECTIONS														
Fettuccine Alfredo	1 serv (10.3 oz)	770	48	30	145	17	68	3	3	—	470	—	—	—
Macaroni & Cheese	1 serv (8 oz)	390	10	6	25	15	59	5	2	—	480	—	—	—
Ravioli	1 serv (10 oz)	420	14	8	65	18	55	9	5	—	980	—	—	—
Ravioli Spinach & Cheese	1 serv (6.6 oz)	310	12	7	50	14	38	5	4	—	700	—	—	—
Sandwich Grilled Cheese	1 (4.5 oz)	480	30	15	45	14	40	2	2	—	910	—	—	—
Spaghetti Marinara w/ Sicilian Meatballs	1 serv (13 oz)	570	16	5	60	30	75	8	5	—	1120	—	—	—
Spaghetti w/ Brown Butter & Mizithra Cheese	1 serv (8.7 oz)	660	37	22	100	19	65	3	3	—	280	—	—	—
Spaghetti w/ Clam Sauce	1 serv (10 oz)	440	9	5	75	20	69	3	3	—	930	—	—	—
Spaghetti w/ Marinara Sauce	1 serv (15 oz)	560	5	1	0	19	108	11	7	—	870	—	—	—
Spaghetti w/ Meat Sauce	1 serv (10 oz)	410	6	2	15	18	70	6	4	—	650	—	—	—
Spinach Tortellini w/ Alfredo Sauce	1 serv (6.8 oz)	530	30	17	110	16	48	3	3	—	730	—	—	—
DESSERTS														
Cake Chocolate Truffle Mousse	1 serv (9 oz)	850	41	25	80	119	118	89	5	—	70	—	—	—
Ice Cream Spumoni	1 serv (3 oz)	180	9	6	40	3	21	17	0	—	90	—	—	—
Ice Cream Vanilla	1 serv (3 oz)	170	9	6	35	3	21	14	0	—	80	—	—	—
Mud Pie	1 serv (6 oz)	490	20	12	25	6	70	52	1	—	220	—	—	—
MAIN MENU SELECTIONS														
Angel Hair	1 serv (8 oz)	420	2	0	0	14	82	4	2	—	0	—	—	—

FOOD	PORTION	CALS	FAT	SAT FAT	CHOL	PROT	CARB	SUGAR	FIBER	CALCI	SOD	POTAS	FOLIC	VIT C
Appetizer Bay Shrimp Crostini	1 serv (9.3 oz)	720	41	10	135	30	54	3	3	—	1510	—	—	—
Appetizer Garlic Fries	1 serv (18.4 oz)	1410	107	17	10	11	106	7	10	—	2730	—	—	—
Appetizer Portuguese Linguica	1 serv (17.5 oz)	1080	75	23	135	43	52	3	8	—	2830	—	—	—
Baked Chicken	1 serv (18.3 oz)	1030	62	20	225	50	71	6	4	—	2220	—	—	—
Baked Lasagna	1 serv (17.5 oz)	800	43	21	125	43	61	13	7	—	2160	—	—	—
Bread Sicilian Garlic Cheese	4 serv (16 oz)	1310	76	33	120	49	110	10	6	—	2510	—	—	—
Broccoli	1 sm (7.5 oz)	340	31	12	50	10	10	0	5	—	530	—	—	—
Burger Sliders	1 serv (23.6 oz)	1770	107	39	470	131	65	28	6	—	1300	—	—	—
Cheese Manicotti w/ Marinara Sauce	1 serv (12 oz)	490	21	11	120	22	54	11	3	—	1370	—	—	—
Chicken Marsala	1 serv (17.4 oz)	1050	57	26	200	56	75	7	3	—	2260	—	—	—
Chicken Penne	1 serv (14.8 oz)	830	31	16	110	34	102	12	5	—	1290	—	—	—
Dip Shrimp Spinach & Artichoke	4 serv (9.3 oz)	590	41	17	90	18	39	2	3	—	1130	—	—	—
Factory Burger w/ Chips	1 serv (16.6 oz)	1370	84	26	245	82	71	12	4	—	1240	—	—	—
Fettuccine Alfredo	1 serv (14.2 oz)	1080	70	44	215	24	91	5	4	—	630	—	—	—
Fettuccine or Penne	1 serv (8 oz)	420	2	0	0	15	85	3	4	—	5	—	—	—
Garlic Mizithra	1 serv (15 oz)	1240	77	38	175	36	103	7	4	—	990	—	—	—
Hearty Meal Clam Sauce	1 serv (25 oz)	1110	23	12	185	50	173	6	7	—	2320	—	—	—
Hearty Meal Italian Sausage w/ Meat Sauce	1 serv (29 oz)	1350	42	15	110	59	177	14	12	—	2340	—	—	—
Hearty Meal Marinara Sauce	1 serv (25 oz)	940	8	1	0	32	180	19	11	—	1440	—	—	—
Hearty Meal Meat Sauce	1 serv (25 oz)	1020	15	5	40	44	176	14	11	—	1620	—	—	—
Hearty Meal Mizithra Cheese & Brown Butter	1 serv (22.4 oz)	1750	101	62	275	48	164	8	7	—	740	—	—	—
Hearty Meal Pot Pourri	1 serv (26 oz)	1280	43	23	150	47	176	13	9	—	1840	—	—	—
Hearty Meal Sauteed Mushroom Sauce	1 serv (30 oz)	1120	26	3	0	34	184	22	12	—	1600	—	—	—
Hearty Meal Sicilian Meatballs	1 serv (31 oz)	1350	36	12	130	65	186	19	13	—	2460	—	—	—

FOOD	PORTION	CALS	FAT	SAT FAT	CHOL	PROT	CARB	SUGAR	FIBER	CALCI	SOD	POTAS	FOLIC	VIT C
Lasagna Vegetariano	1 serv (20.6 oz)	830	48	25	120	37	68	15	9	—	1910	—	—	—
Meatloaf Italian	1 serv (18.5 oz)	1180	68	32	230	56	83	8	6	—	1590	—	—	—
Olive Tapenade	4 serv (7.4 oz)	800	66	7	0	7	46	1	2	—	1580	—	—	—
Panini Chicken Smoked Mozzarella w/ Chips	1 serv (14.4 oz)	1280	68	16	105	60	112	11	18	—	2080	—	—	—
Parmigiana Chicken	1 serv (19.2 oz)	810	30	7	105	54	80	10	5	—	1800	—	—	—
Pasta Gluten Free	1 serv (9 oz)	470	1	0	0	9	104	0	2	—	0	—	—	—
Pasta Whole Wheat	1 serv (8 oz)	390	2	0	0	17	85	4	14	—	10	—	—	—
Platter #1 Lasagna & Chicken Marsala	1 (27.5 oz)	1090	66	26	225	78	71	17	7	—	3440	—	—	—
Platter #2 Ravioli & Spaghetti w/ Meat Sauce	1 (21 oz)	880	22	10	95	38	133	15	10	—	1680	—	—	—
Platter #3 Spaghetti w/ Meat Sauce Sausage & Meatballs	1 (25 oz)	1360	64	24	225	74	114	9	9	—	2720	—	—	—
Ravioli Crab	1 serv (11 oz)	810	45	24	190	31	73	3	5	—	900	—	—	—
Ravioli Spinach & Cheese	1 serv (11 oz)	480	16	9	75	20	63	9	6	—	1040	—	—	—
Ravioli Toasted Beef	4 serv (4 oz)	200	5	2	0	10	30	2	2	—	570	—	—	—
Ravioli Toasted Cheese	4 serv (4 oz)	210	6	4	0	8	30	3	2	—	810	—	—	—
Sandwich Sicilian Style Meatball w/ Chips	1 serv (16.4 oz)	1200	54	17	140	62	122	5	8	—	2640	—	—	—
Sandwich Sicilian Style Sausage w/ Chips	1 serv (14.4 oz)	1140	55	19	90	43	117	4	9	—	2290	—	—	—
Senior Meal Italian Sausage w/ Meat Sauce	1 serv (14 oz)	740	33	12	85	33	72	6	6	—	1370	—	—	—
Senior Meal Pot Pourri	1 serv (10 oz)	520	19	10	60	18	69	5	4	—	630	—	—	—
Senior Meal Spaghetti Marinara	1 serv (10 oz)	370	4	0	0	13	72	8	5	—	580	—	—	—
Senior Meal Spaghetti Marinara w/ Sicilian Meatballs	1 serv (16 oz)	770	29	9	115	47	78	8	5	—	1650	—	—	—

FOOD	PORTION	CALS	FAT	SAT FAT	CHOL	PROT	CARB	SUGAR	FIBER	CALCI	SOD	POTAS	FOLIC	VIT C
Senior Meal Spaghetti Mizithra & Brown Butter	1 serv (10 oz)	660	37	22	100	19	65	3	3	—	280	—	—	—
Senior Meal Spaghetti w/ Clam Sauce	1 serv (10 oz)	440	9	5	75	20	69	3	3	—	930	—	—	—
Senior Meal Spaghetti w/ Meat Sauce	1 serv (10 oz)	410	6	2	15	18	70	6	4	—	650	—	—	—
Senior Meal Spaghetti w/ Mushroom Sauce	1 serv (12 oz)	450	10	1	0	14	74	9	5	—	640	—	—	—
Side Alfredo Sauce	6 oz	640	67	42	210	5	7	0	0	—	470	—	—	—
Side Clam Sauce	6 oz	190	12	7	110	13	9	0	0	—	1380	—	—	—
Side Marinara Sauce	6 oz	90	3	0	0	3	13	8	3	—	860	—	—	—
Side Marsala Sauce	6 oz	70	4	2	0	1	6	3	0	—	320	—	—	—
Side Meat Sauce	6 oz	140	7	2	25	10	10	5	2	—	960	—	—	—
Side Sausage	1 serv (4.5 oz)	340	27	11	70	15	3	0	2	—	800	—	—	—
Side Sauteed Mushroom Sauce	9 oz	200	14	2	0	4	15	10	3	—	950	—	—	—
Side Sicilian Meatballs	2 (6 oz)	420	27	10	130	33	7	0	1	—	1020	—	—	—
Spaghetti	1 serv (9 oz)	460	3	1	0	17	93	4	4	—	5	—	—	—
Spaghetti Vesuvius	1 serv (15 oz)	710	19	7	45	25	104	8	6	—	590	—	—	—
Spaghetti Squash	1 serv (20.7 oz)	540	36	9	30	19	45	13	8	—	960	—	—	—
Spaghetti w/ Clam Sauce	1 serv (15 oz)	660	14	7	110	30	104	4	4	—	1390	—	—	—
Spaghetti w/ Italian Sausage w/ Meat Sauce	1 serv (19 oz)	940	36	13	95	41	107	8	8	—	1700	—	—	—
Spaghetti w/ Meat Sauce	1 serv (15 oz)	610	9	3	25	26	105	8	7	—	970	—	—	—
Spaghetti w/ Mizithra Cheese & Brown Butter	1 serv (13.4 oz)	1040	59	36	160	29	99	5	4	—	460	—	—	—
Spaghetti w/ Pot Pourri	1 serv (16 oz)	780	26	13	90	29	106	8	6	—	1140	—	—	—
Spaghetti w/ Sauteed Mushroom Sauce	1 serv (18 oz)	670	16	2	0	21	111	13	7	—	960	—	—	—
Spaghetti w/ Sicilian Meatballs	1 serv (21 oz)	960	31	10	115	53	114	12	7	—	1940	—	—	—
Spinach Tortellini w/ Alfredo Sauce	1 serv (12 oz)	930	55	32	200	25	86	5	5	—	1110	—	—	—

FOOD	PORTION	CALS	FAT	SAT FAT	CHOL	PROT	CARB	SUGAR	FIBER	CALCI	SOD	POTAS	FOLIC	VIT C
SALADS														
BLT	1 (15.4 oz)	1000	85	21	115	36	23	5	9	—	2490	—	—	—
Caesar Upgrade	1 (7 oz)	440	37	9	40	12	14	2	3	—	850	—	—	—
Caesar Entree Chicken	1 (21.2 oz)	1130	90	18	160	54	29	5	6	—	2240	—	—	—
Caesar Entree w/o Chicken	1 (14.5 oz)	820	72	16	70	22	25	5	6	—	1520	—	—	—
House w/ 1000 Island	1 (5 oz)	230	17	2	5	3	16	5	1	—	560	—	—	—
House w/ Balsamic	1 (4.5 oz)	260	21	2	0	3	15	2	1	—	290	—	—	—
House w/ Blue Cheese	1 (5 oz)	280	24	4	15	4	13	2	1	—	450	—	—	—
House w/ Caesar	1 (5 oz)	330	30	4	20	4	13	2	1	—	400	—	—	—
House w/ Creamy Pesto	1 (5 oz)	280	24	3	10	4	13	2	1	—	390	—	—	—
House w/ Fat Free Honey Mustard	1 (4.5 oz)	120	3	0	0	3	21	9	1	—	280	—	—	—
Senior Meal Caesar Chicken	1 serv (17 oz)	870	67	13	135	48	21	4	4	—	1780	—	—	—
Senior Meal Caesar w/o Chicken	1 serv (10.2 oz)	560	48	11	50	16	17	4	4	—	1050	—	—	—
SOUPS														
Chicken Mulligatawny	1 serv (9 oz)	260	19	9	60	7	20	6	1	—	930	—	—	—
Clam Chowder	1 serv (9 oz)	370	25	15	155	17	19	1	1	—	1210	—	—	—
Cream Of Broccoli	1 serv (9 oz)	240	19	8	45	7	21	10	2	—	1010	—	—	—
Minestrone	1 serv (9 oz)	60	2	0	0	2	10	2	2	—	660	—	—	—

PACIUGO GELATO

FOOD	PORTION	CALS	FAT	SAT FAT	CHOL	PROT	CARB	SUGAR	FIBER	CALCI	SOD	POTAS	FOLIC	VIT C
Milk Base Amarena Black Cherry Swirl	1 scoop (3.5 oz)	160	4	3	15	4	30	30	tr	150	50	—	—	1
Milk Base Banan Creme Pie	1 scoop (3.5 oz)	80	2	1	13	2	14	13	tr	50	35	—	—	1
Milk Base Cheesecake	1 scoop (3.5 oz)	90	4	2	18	3	12	12	tr	75	55	—	—	1
Milk Base Chocolate	1 scoop (3.5 oz)	80	3	2	8	3	14	13	tr	75	48	—	—	1
Milk Base Chocolate Cookies 'N Milk	1 scoop (3.5 oz)	90	3	2	8	3	16	13	tr	75	63	—	—	1
Milk Base Coconut	1 scoop (3.5 oz)	80	3	2	8	2	13	12	tr	75	30	—	—	1
Milk Base Coffee	1 scoop (3.5 oz)	75	3	2	8	2	12	11	tr	75	30	—	—	1
Milk Base Fiordilatte	1 scoop (3.5 oz)	75	2	2	8	2	13	13	tr	75	30	—	—	1

FOOD	PORTION	CALS	FAT	SAT FAT	CHOL	PROT	CARB	SUGAR	FIBER	CALCI	SOD	POTAS	FOLIC	VIT C
Milk Base French Vanilla Bean	1 scoop (3.5 oz)	80	3	2	20	2	13	13	tr	75	30	—	—	1
Milk Base Green Tea	1 scoop (3.5 oz)	70	2	2	8	2	12	12	tr	75	30	—	—	1
Milk Base Hazelnut	1 scoop (3.5 oz)	85	4	2	8	3	11	11	tr	75	30	—	—	1
Milk Base Lemon Custard	1 scoop (3.5 oz)	75	3	3	30	3	12	12	tr	75	30	—	—	1
Milk Base Mascarpone Chocolate Rum	1 scoop (3.5 oz)	95	5	3	15	3	11	10	tr	75	35	—	—	1
Milk Base Pannacotta Wedding Cake	1 scoop (3.5 oz)	75	2	1	8	2	13	13	tr	75	28	—	—	1
Milk Base Peppermint	1 scoop (3.5 oz)	75	2	1	8	2	14	13	1	75	30	—	—	1
Milk Base Rose	1 scoop (3.5 oz)	70	2	2	8	8	12	12	tr	75	30	—	—	1
Milk Base Tiramisu	1 scoop (3.5 oz)	80	3	2	28	2	12	12	tr	75	30	—	—	1
Milk Base Zabajone	1 scoop (3.5 oz)	80	3	2	30	3	12	12	tr	75	30	—	—	1
No Sugar Added Chocolate	1 scoop (3.5 oz)	28	1	1	3	2	9	3	1	50	33	—	—	1
No Sugar Added Mint	1 scoop (3.5 oz)	25	1	tr	3	1	9	3	1	50	23	—	—	1
No Sugar Added Mocha	1 scoop (3.5 oz)	28	1	1	3	2	9	3	1	50	22	—	—	1
No Sugar Added Strawberry Milk	1 scoop (3.5 oz)	23	1	tr	1	1	8	3	1	38	19	—	—	3
Soy Banana	1 scoop (3.5 oz)	40	2	tr	0	tr	6	6	1	0	3	—	—	1
Soy Blueberry	1 scoop (3.5 oz)	40	2	tr	0	tr	6	6	1	0	3	—	—	2
Soy Chocolate	1 scoop (3.5 oz)	38	2	1	0	tr	5	5	1	0	9	—	—	0
Soy Coffee	1 scoop (3.5 oz)	35	2	tr	0	tr	5	5	1	0	3	—	—	0
Soy Hazelnut	1 scoop (3.5 oz)	35	2	tr	0	tr	5	5	1	0	3	—	—	0
Soy Strawberry	1 scoop (3.5 oz)	38	2	tr	0	tr	6	6	1	0	3	—	—	2
Soy Wild Berries	1 scoop (3.5 oz)	40	2	tr	0	tr	6	6	1	0	3	—	—	2
Water Base Blackberry	1 scoop (3.5 oz)	28	0	0	0	0	7	7	tr	0	0	—	—	2
Water Base Ginger Lemon	1 scoop (3.5 oz)	25	0	0	0	0	7	7	tr	0	0	—	—	3
Water Base Green Apple	1 scoop (3.5 oz)	28	0	0	0	0	7	7	tr	0	0	—	—	1
Water Base Lemon Sage	1 scoop (3.5 oz)	25	0	0	0	0	7	7	tr	0	0	—	—	2
Water Base Lychee	1 scoop (3.5 oz)	25	0	0	0	0	6	6	tr	0	0	—	—	2

FOOD	PORTION	CALS	FAT	SAT FAT	CHOL	PROT	CARB	SUGAR	FIBER	CALCI	SOD	POTAS	FOLIC	VIT C
Water Base Orange Vidalia	1 scoop (3.5 oz)	25	0	0	0	0	7	7	0	0	0	—	—	3
Water Base Passion Fruit	1 scoop (3.5 oz)	23	0	0	0	0	6	6	0	0	0	—	—	tr
Water Base Pineapple	1 scoop (3.5 oz)	28	0	0	0	0	7	7	tr	0	0	—	—	1
Water Base Strawberry Port	1 scoop (3.5 oz)	25	0	0	0	0	6	6	tr	0	0	—	—	3
Water Base Watermelon	1 scoop (3.5 oz)	25	0	0	0	0	7	7	tr	0	0	—	—	1

PANERA BREAD

BAKERY

FOOD	PORTION	CALS	FAT	SAT FAT	CHOL	PROT	CARB	SUGAR	FIBER	CALCI	SOD	POTAS	FOLIC	VIT C
Asiago Cheese Loaf	1 slice (2 oz)	160	4	3	10	7	23	0	1	—	320	—	—	—
Bagel Asiago Cheese	1	330	6	4	10	13	55	3	2	—	580	—	—	—
Bagel Blueberry	1	330	2	0	0	10	68	10	2	—	490	—	—	—
Bagel Chocolate Chip	1	370	6	4	0	10	69	14	2	—	480	—	—	—
Bagel Cinnamon Crunch	1	430	8	5	0	9	80	29	2	—	430	—	—	—
Bagel Cinnamon Swirl & Raisin	1	320	3	1	0	9	64	11	3	—	470	—	—	—
Bagel Everything	1	300	3	0	0	10	59	4	2	—	640	—	—	—
Bagel French Toast	1	350	5	3	0	9	67	15	2	—	620	—	—	—
Bagel Jalapeno & Cheddar	1	310	3	2	5	12	56	3	2	—	740	—	—	—
Bagel Plain	1	290	2	0	0	10	59	3	2	—	460	—	—	—
Bagel Sesame	1	310	3	0	0	10	59	3	2	—	460	—	—	—
Bagel Sweet Onion & Poppyseed	1	390	7	1	0	13	72	7	4	—	520	—	—	—
Bagel Whole Wheat	1	340	3	0	0	13	67	5	6	—	400	—	—	—
Baguette Whole Grain	1 slice (2 oz)	140	1	0	0	6	27	2	3	—	290	—	—	—
Bear Claw	1	550	28	12	65	10	67	32	3	—	360	—	—	—
Brownie Double Fudge w/ Icing	1	480	17	9	85	5	76	44	2	—	290	—	—	—
Cake Cinnamon Coffee Crumb	1 slice	470	25	9	105	6	54	30	1	—	310	—	—	—
Ciabatta	1 (6.25 oz)	460	6	1	0	16	84	3	3	—	760	—	—	—
Cinnamon Raisin	1 slice (2 oz)	180	3	2	10	5	34	11	1	—	135	—	—	—
Cinnamon Roll	1	620	24	14	100	13	89	33	3	—	480	—	—	—
Cobblestone	1	650	13	5	20	12	122	64	3	—	410	—	—	—
Cookie Candy	1	420	19	10	70	4	59	33	1	—	280	—	—	—

FOOD	PORTION	CALS	FAT	SAT FAT	CHOL	PROT	CARB	SUGAR	FIBER	CALCI	SOD	POTAS	FOLIC	VIT C
Cookie Chocolate Chipper	1	440	23	14	60	5	59	33	2	—	250	—	—	—
Cookie Chocolate Chipper	1 mini	110	6	4	15	1	15	8	1	—	60	—	—	—
Cookie Chocolate Duet w/ Walnuts	1	450	24	13	60	6	55	36	3	—	150	—	—	—
Cookie Easter Egg	1	480	22	13	55	4	67	38	1	—	160	—	—	—
Cookie Oatmeal Raisin	1	370	14	8	55	5	57	28	2	—	310	—	—	—
Cookie Shortbread	1	350	21	12	55	3	36	11	1	—	160	—	—	—
Cookie Toffee Nut	1	460	19	13	80	5	59	29	1	—	330	—	—	—
Country Loaf	1 slice (2 oz)	140	1	0	0	5	27	0	1	—	310	—	—	—
Croissant French	1	310	18	11	60	7	30	4	1	—	260	—	—	—
Focaccia	1 serv (2 oz)	180	1	0	0	5	28	1	1	—	320	—	—	—
Focaccia w/ Asiago Cheese	1 slice (2 oz)	160	5	2	5	5	23	1	1	—	230	—	—	—
French Baguette	1 slice (2 oz)	150	1	0	0	5	30	0	1	—	370	—	—	—
Honey Wheat Loaf	1 slice (2 oz)	170	3	2	0	5	30	4	2	—	240	—	—	—
Hot Cross Bun	1	220	5	3	35	5	38	19	1	—	280	—	—	—
Muffie Chocolate Chip	1	320	14	4	40	4	46	27	2	—	200	—	—	—
Muffie Pumpkin	1	290	11	2	15	3	45	26	1	—	240	—	—	—
Muffin Apple Crunch	1	450	12	3	60	7	80	49	2	—	340	—	—	—
Muffin Carrot Walnut	1	500	21	5	65	8	72	37	3	—	580	—	—	—
Muffin Pumpkin	1	580	22	4	30	7	89	51	2	—	470	—	—	—
Muffin Wild Blueberry	1	440	17	3	60	6	66	39	2	—	330	—	—	—
Pastry Cheese	1	400	22	14	65	8	42	15	1	—	340	—	—	—
Pastry Cherry	1	500	18	11	50	7	77	45	2	—	320	—	—	—
Pastry Chocolate	1	410	24	14	50	8	46	18	2	—	260	—	—	—
Pastry Fresh Apple	1	380	17	13	20	7	44	17	1	—	320	—	—	—
Pastry Ring Apple Cherry Cheese	1 slice	230	11	6	35	3	30	16	1	—	160	—	—	—
Pecan Braid	1	470	26	12	55	8	52	23	2	—	270	—	—	—
Pecan Roll	1	730	39	12	60	11	87	48	5	—	310	—	—	—
Scone Cinnamon Chip	1	600	31	19	125	9	73	34	2	—	370	—	—	—
Scone Orange	1 lg	470	11	7	45	4	87	62	3	—	460	—	—	—
Scone Strawberries & Cream	1	420	19	12	70	6	57	27	1	—	770	—	—	—
Scone Strawberries & Cream	1 mini	140	6	4	25	2	19	9	0	—	260	—	—	—
Scone Wild Blueberry	1 mini	160	6	4	25	2	21	8	1	—	290	—	—	—

FOOD	PORTION	CALS	FAT	SAT FAT	CHOL	PROT	CARB	SUGAR	FIBER	CALCI	SOD	POTAS	FOLIC	VIT C
Scone Wild Blueberry	1	440	18	12	75	7	63	25	2	—	880	—	—	—
Scones Orange	1 mini	160	4	3	15	1	29	21	1	—	150	—	—	—
Sesame Semolina Loaf	1 slice (2 oz)	140	1	0	0	4	29	1	1	—	350	—	—	—
Sourdough Roll	1 (2.5 oz)	200	1	0	0	7	39	0	1	—	400	—	—	—
Sourdough Round Loaf	1 slice (2 oz)	140	1	0	0	5	28	0	1	—	290	—	—	—
Sourdough Soup Bowl	1 (8 oz)	590	3	0	0	21	118	1	4	—	1210	—	—	—
Spring Petites	1 mini	230	12	7	30	2	27	12	0	—	90	—	—	—
Stone Milled Rye Loaf	1 slice (2 oz)	140	1	0	0	5	28	0	2	—	380	—	—	—
Three Cheese Loaf	1 slice (2 oz)	140	2	1	5	6	26	1	1	—	290	—	—	—
Tomato Basil XL Loaf	1 slice (2 oz)	140	1	0	0	5	27	1	1	—	330	—	—	—
White Whole Grain Loaf	1 slice (2 oz)	140	3	1	0	5	26	1	2	—	310	—	—	—
Whole Grain Loaf	1 slice (2 oz)	130	1	0	0	6	27	2	3	—	290	—	—	—
BEVERAGES														
Apple Juice Organic	8 oz	120	0	0	0	0	29	29	0	—	25	—	—	—
Caffe Mocha	1 (11.5 oz)	380	16	11	40	11	50	42	2	—	160	—	—	—
Caramel Frozen	1 (16 oz)	600	33	15	60	5	97	82	0	—	190	—	—	—
Chocolate Milk Organic	8 oz	170	5	3	20	7	25	25	0	—	150	—	—	—
Hot Chocolate	1 (11 oz)	380	16	11	40	11	50	42	2	—	160	—	—	—
Iced Green Tea	1 (16 oz)	90	0	0	0	0	23	23	0	—	10	—	—	—
Iced Latte Chai Tea	1 (16 oz)	160	4	2	15	6	26	25	0	—	75	—	—	—
Latte Caffe	1 (8.5 oz)	120	5	3	20	8	11	11	0	—	95	—	—	—
Latte Caramel	1 (11.5 oz)	420	18	12	50	10	53	46	0	—	210	—	—	—
Latte Chai Tea	1 (10 oz)	200	5	3	15	7	32	32	0	—	85	—	—	—
Lemonade	1 (16 oz)	100	0	0	0	0	25	25	0	—	10	—	—	—
Mango Frozen	1 (16 oz)	330	10	7	20	2	61	56	2	—	20	—	—	—
Milk Organic	8 oz	120	5	3	20	8	12	12	0	—	115	—	—	—
Mocha Frozen	1 (16 oz)	570	20	14	50	6	94	78	2	—	140	—	—	—
Orange Juice	1 sm (8 oz)	110	0	0	0	2	26	26	1	—	0	—	—	—
Smoothie Black Cherry Low Fat	1 (16 oz)	290	2	1	5	6	63	53	2	—	90	—	—	—
Smoothie Mango Low Fat	1 (16 oz)	230	2	1	5	6	51	48	2	—	90	—	—	—
Smoothie Strawberry w/ Ginseng Low Fat	1 (16 oz)	260	2	1	5	6	59	53	2	—	90	—	—	—

FOOD	PORTION	CALS	FAT	SAT FAT	CHOL	PROT	CARB	SUGAR	FIBER	CALCI	SOD	POTAS	FOLIC	VIT C
Smoothie Wild Berry Low Fat	1 (16 oz)	290	2	1	5	6	67	65	1	—	90	—	—	—
CHILDREN'S MENU SELECTIONS														
Deli Sandwich Roast Beef	1	320	10	6	40	23	35	4	3	—	820	—	—	—
Deli Sandwich Smoked Ham	1	300	9	6	40	21	35	3	3	—	1060	—	—	—
Deli Sandwich Smoked Turkey	1	290	8	5	30	21	35	3	3	—	1100	—	—	—
Mac & Cheese	1 serv	490	30	13	55	17	37	7	1	—	1020	—	—	—
Organic Yogurt All Flavors	1 tube	60	1	0	5	2	11	10	0	—	40	—	—	—
Sandwich Grilled Cheese	1	360	13	10	30	17	46	4	4	—	1020	—	—	—
Sandwich Peanut Butter & Jelly	1	410	18	4	0	12	56	21	4	—	550	—	—	—
CREAM CHEESE														
Chive & Onion	1 oz	70	6	4	20	3	2	1	0	—	190	—	—	—
Hazelnut Reduced Fat	1 oz	80	6	4	15	2	3	3	0	—	110	—	—	—
Honey Walnut Reduced Fat	1 oz	80	6	4	15	2	4	4	0	—	105	—	—	—
Plain	1 oz	100	6	0	30	2	1	1	0	—	110	—	—	—
Plain Reduced Fat	1 oz	70	6	4	20	3	1	1	0	—	120	—	—	—
Raspberry Reduced Fat	1 oz	70	5	3	15	2	4	3	1	—	105	—	—	—
Veggie Reduced Fat	1 oz	60	5	3	15	2	1	1	1	—	110	—	—	—
SALAD DRESSINGS														
BBQ Ranch	3 tbsp	140	12	2	10	1	8	7	0	—	350	—	—	—
Buttermilk Ranch Light	3 tbsp	80	4	1	0	1	9	3	1	—	350	—	—	—
Caesar	3 tbsp	150	16	3	35	1	2	1	0	—	190	—	—	—
Vinaigrette Asian Sesame Reduced Sugar	3 tbsp	90	8	1	0	0	6	4	0	—	390	—	—	—
Vinaigrette Balsamic Reduced Fat	3 tbsp	130	10	2	0	0	9	8	0	—	240	—	—	—
Vinaigrette Blue Cheese	3 tbsp	180	19	4	15	1	4	3	0	—	260	—	—	—
Vinaigrette Greek Herb	3 tbsp	220	24	4	0	0	1	0	0	—	380	—	—	—
Vinaigrette Thai Chili Low Fat	3 tbsp	60	2	0	0	1	10	7	0	—	430	—	—	—
Vinaigrette White Balsamic Apple	3 tbsp	150	12	2	0	0	11	10	0	—	310	—	—	—

FOOD	PORTION	CALS	FAT	SAT FAT	CHOL	PROT	CARB	SUGAR	FIBER	CALCI	SOD	POTAS	FOLIC	VIT C
SALADS														
Asian Sesame Chicken	1 full serv	410	20	4	60	31	31	6	3	—	810	—	—	—
BBQ Chopped Chicken	1	500	22	3	75	31	50	15	6	—	770	—	—	—
Caesar	1	390	27	8	50	12	25	2	3	—	610	—	—	—
Caesar Chicken	1	510	29	9	115	37	29	2	3	—	820	—	—	—
Chopped Chicken Cobb	1	500	36	9	140	38	11	2	3	—	1130	—	—	—
Chopped Steak & Blue Cheese	1	850	64	21	130	35	36	9	4	—	1590	—	—	—
Classic Cafe	1 full serv	170	11	2	0	2	18	12	4	—	270	—	—	—
Fruit Cup	1	60	0	0	0	1	17	12	1	—	15	—	—	—
Fuji Apple w/ Chicken	1	520	31	7	80	32	35	21	6	—	830	—	—	—
Greek	1 full serv	380	34	8	20	8	14	4	5	—	1670	—	—	—
Thai Chopped Chicken	1	390	15	3	60	34	36	13	5	—	1330	—	—	—
SANDWICHES														
Asiago Roast Beef On Asiago Cheese	1	700	27	14	100	49	64	5	4	—	1330	—	—	—
Bacon Turkey Bravo On XL Tomato Basil	1	800	29	10	85	52	83	6	4	—	2800	—	—	—
Breakfast Asiago Cheese Bagel w/ Bacon	1	610	28	13	245	34	55	4	2	—	1350	—		—
Breakfast Asiago Cheese Bagel w/ Egg & Cheese	1	480	18	10	215	24	54	3	2	—	890	—	—	—
Breakfast Asiago Cheese Bagel w/ Sausage	1	640	32	15	260	32	56	4	2	—	1220	—	—	—
Breakfast Bacon Egg & Cheese On Ciabatta	1	510	24	10	235	29	44	2	2	—	1160	—	—	—
Breakfast Egg & Cheese On Ciabatta	1	390	15	7	205	19	43	2	2	—	710	—	—	—
Breakfast French Toast Bagel w/ Sausage	1	670	31	14	250	28	69	15	2	—	1280	—	—	—
Breakfast Jalapeno & Cheddar Bagel w/ Bacon	1	590	25	11	240	33	58	4	3	—	1530	—	—	—
Breakfast Jalapeno & Cheddar Bagel w/ Egg & Cheese	1	470	16	8	210	23	57	3	3	—	1070	—	—	—

FOOD	PORTION	CALS	FAT	SAT FAT	CHOL	PROT	CARB	SUGAR	FIBER	CALCI	SOD	POTAS	FOLIC	VIT C
Breakfast Jalapeno & Cheddar Bagel w/ Sausage	1	630	29	12	255	32	59	4	3	—	1400	—	—	—
Breakfast Power	1	340	14	7	220	23	31	2	4	—	820	—	—	—
Breakfast Sausage Egg & Cheese On Ciabatta	1	550	29	12	250	27	44	2	2	—	1040	—	—	—
Breakfast Sweet Onion & Poppyseed Bagel w/ Steak	1	660	27	10	235	34	74	8	5	—	970	—	—	—
Chicken Caesar On Three Cheese	1	720	32	10	130	43	69	5	4	—	1270	—	—	—
Italian Combo On Ciabatta	1	980	41	15	150	58	95	6	5	—	2620	—	—	—
Jalapeno & Cheddar Bagel w/ Smoked Ham	1	500	16	8	225	28	58	3	3	—	1280	—	—	—
Mediterranean Veggie On XL Tomato Basil	1	600	13	4	10	22	98	6	10	—	1420	—	—	—
Napa Almond Chicken Salad On Sesame Semolina	1	690	26	5	60	29	90	12	5	—	1200	—	—	—
Panini Chipotle Chicken On Artisan French	1	830	37	12	145	53	72	5	3	—	2180	—	—	—
Panini Cuban Chicken	1	860	36	10	100	46	86	10	4	—	1770	—	—	—
Panini Frontega Chicken On Focaccia	1	850	38	9	110	49	79	6	4	—	1910	—	—	—
Panini Smokehouse Turkey On Three Cheese	1	690	25	12	100	52	64	4	4	—	2350	—	—	—
Panini Steak & White Cheddar On French Baguette	1	950	35	15	95	43	112	3	5	—	1790	—	—	—
Panini Tomato & Mozzarella On Ciabatta	1	770	10	1	35	30	96	10	6	—	1290	—	—	—
Panini Turkey Artichoke On Focaccia	1	740	26	8	50	41	86	8	5	—	2200	—	—	—
Sierra Turkey w/ Asiago Cheese On Focaccia	1	920	49	12	80	40	79	5	4	—	1900	—	—	—

FOOD	PORTION	CALS	FAT	SAT FAT	CHOL	PROT	CARB	SUGAR	FIBER	CALCI	SOD	POTAS	FOLIC	VIT C
Smoked Ham & Swiss On Stone Milled Rye	1	590	17	8	90	45	64	3	5	—	1870	—	—	—
Smoked Turkey Breast On Country	1	420	3	1	30	33	66	3	3	—	1650	—	—	—
Tuna Salad On Honey Wheat	1	470	16	4	25	19	65	12	5	—	980	—	—	—
SOUPS														
Baked Potato	1 serv (12 oz)	350	13	1	70	9	33	7	3	—	1180	—	—	—
Broccoli Cheddar	1 serv (12 oz)	290	16	9	30	12	24	0	7	—	1540	—	—	—
Chicken Noodle Low Fat	1 serv (12 oz)	140	3	1	30	5	23	9	0	—	1450	—	—	—
Cream Of Chicken & Wild Rice	1 serv (12 oz)	310	17	8	60	10	29	4	3	—	1470	—	—	—
Creamy Tomato	1 serv (12 oz)	380	23	14	65	7	36	9	5	—	720	—	—	—
French Onion	1 serv (12 oz)	250	11	5	25	10	30	6	3	—	2380	—	—	—
Garden Vegetable w/ Pesto Low Fat	1 serv (12 oz)	160	4	0	0	5	28	8	6	—	1240	—	—	—
New England Clam Chowder	1 serv (12 oz)	450	34	20	50	8	29	0	3	—	1190	—	—	—
Vegetarian Black Bean Low Fat	1 serv (12 oz)	170	4	2	0	10	29	4	5	—	1590	—	—	—

PAPA JOHNS

FOOD	PORTION	CALS	FAT	SAT FAT	CHOL	PROT	CARB	SUGAR	FIBER	CALCI	SOD	POTAS	FOLIC	VIT C
DESSERTS														
Applepie	4 (6.7 oz)	480	10	3	0	8	90	43	2	20	520	—	—	0
Cinnamon Sweetsticks	4 (6.7 oz)	580	16	5	0	11	98	32	3	40	740	—	—	0
Cinnapie	4 (5.9 oz)	560	19	6	0	8	90	39	2	40	540	—	—	0
OTHER MENU SELECTIONS														
Breadsticks	2 (4 oz)	290	5	1	0	8	54	4	2	20	540	—	—	0
Breadsticks Garlic Parmesan	2 (4.4 oz)	340	10	2	0	9	54	5	2	20	720	—	—	0
Cheesesticks	4 (4.8 oz)	370	16	7	35	14	41	4	2	250	860	—	—	0
Chickenstrips	2 (2.3 oz)	130	5	1	25	12	10	0	0	0	430	—	—	0
Wings BBQ	2 (2.8 oz)	190	12	3	50	12	6	2	0	0	760	—	—	1
Wings Buffalo	2 (2.8 oz)	170	13	3	50	12	3	1	0	0	1070	—	—	0
Wings Honey Chipotle	2 (2.8 oz)	190	12	3	50	12	8	5	0	0	730	—	—	0
PIZZA														
BBQ Chicken & Bacon 12 inch	⅛ pie (3.8 oz)	250	8	4	25	11	32	5	1	150	730	—	—	1
BBQ Chicken & Bacon 16 inch	¹/₁₀ pie (5.6 oz)	370	12	5	35	16	48	7	2	200	1080	—	—	2
BBQ Chicken & Bacon 8 inch	¼ pie (3.5 oz)	230	7	3	20	10	30	5	1	100	670	—	—	1

FOOD	PORTION	CALS	FAT	SAT FAT	CHOL	PROT	CARB	SUGAR	FIBER	CALCI	SOD	POTAS	FOLIC	VIT C
Cheese 12 inch	⅛ pie (3.2 oz)	210	8	4	20	8	26	3	1	150	530	—	—	2
Garden Fresh 12 inch	⅛ pie (3.9 oz)	200	7	3	15	8	27	4	2	150	500	—	—	6
Garden Fresh 16 inch	⅒ pie (6 oz)	300	10	4	20	11	42	11	6	200	740	—	—	12
Garden Fresh 8 inch	¼ pie (3.6 oz)	180	5	2	10	6	26	4	1	100	440	—	—	6
Hawaiian BBQ Chicken 12 inch	⅛ pie (4.1 oz)	250	8	4	25	11	33	6	1	150	730	—	—	2
Hawaiian BBQ Chicken 16 inch	⅒ pie (6 oz)	370	12	5	35	16	49	9	2	200	1080	—	—	4
Original 16 inch	⅒ pie (4.6 oz)	300	10	5	25	11	40	5	2	200	740	—	—	4
Pepperoni 12 inch	⅛ pie (3.2 oz)	230	10	4	20	9	26	3	1	100	610	—	—	2
Pepperoni 16 inch	⅒ pie (4.8 oz)	340	14	6	30	13	40	5	2	150	900	—	—	4
Pepperoni 8 inch	¼ pie (3 oz)	210	9	4	15	8	25	3	1	100	560	—	—	2
Sausage 12 inch	⅛ pie (3.3 oz)	240	11	5	20	8	26	3	1	150	600	—	—	2
Sausage 16 inch	⅒ pie (4.9 oz)	350	15	6	30	12	40	5	2	150	860	—	—	4
Sausage 8 inch	¼ pie (3.1 oz)	220	9	4	15	7	25	3	1	100	540	—	—	2
Spicy Italian 12 inch	⅛ pie (3.6 oz)	270	13	5	25	10	27	3	1	150	690	—	—	2
Spicy Italian 16 inch	⅒ pie (5.5 oz)	400	20	8	40	15	41	5	2	200	1040	—	—	4
Spicy Italian 8 inch	¼ pie (3.4 oz)	240	12	5	20	9	25	3	1	100	630	—	—	2
Spinach Alfredo 12 inch	⅛ pie (2.9 oz)	210	8	4	20	8	25	3	1	150	470	—	—	0
Spinach Alfredo 16 inch	⅒ pie (4.4 oz)	310	12	6	30	11	39	4	2	200	680	—	—	1
Spinach Alfredo 8 inch	¼ pie (2.8 oz)	190	8	4	20	6	24	2	1	100	420	—	—	0
The Meats 8 inch	¼ pie (3.4 oz)	240	11	5	25	10	25	3	1	100	690	—	—	2
The Meats 12 inch	⅛ pie (3.6 oz)	250	12	5	25	11	26	3	1	150	710	—	—	2
The Meats 16 inch	⅒ pie (5.5 oz)	400	19	8	40	16	40	5	2	150	1100	—	—	4
The Works 12 inch	⅛ pie (3.9 oz)	230	9	4	20	9	27	3	1	150	650	—	—	5
The Works 16 inch	⅒ pie (5.9 oz)	350	14	6	30	14	42	5	2	200	980	—	—	9
The Works 8 inch	¼ pie (3.6 oz)	210	9	4	20	8	26	3	1	100	600	—	—	6
Tuscan Six Cheese 12 inch	⅛ pie (3.3 oz)	230	9	5	25	10	26	3	1	200	580	—	—	2
Tuscan Six Cheese 16 inch	⅒ pie (4.9 oz)	340	13	6	30	15	40	5	2	300	840	—	—	4
Tuscan Six Cheese 8 inch	¼ pie (3 oz)	210	8	4	20	9	25	3	1	150	520	—	—	2
SAUCES AND SEASONINGS														
Crushed Red Pepper	1 pkg (1 g)	5	0	0	0	0	1	—	0	0	0	—	—	1
Parmesan Cheese	1 pkg (3.5 g)	15	1	1	5	—	0	—	0	40	45	—	—	—
Sauce Barbeque	1 serv (1 oz)	45	0	0	0	0	11	10	0	0	240	—	—	1

FOOD	PORTION	CALS	FAT	SAT FAT	CHOL	PROT	CARB	SUGAR	FIBER	CALCI	SOD	POTAS	FOLIC	VIT C
Sauce Blue Cheese	1 serv (1 oz)	160	16	4	20	1	1	1	0	20	250	—	—	0
Sauce Buffalo	1 serv (1 oz)	15	1	0	0	0	2	2	0	0	1030	—	—	1
Sauce Cheese	1 serv (1 oz)	40	4	1	5	1	1	1	0	0	160	—	—	0
Sauce Honey Mustard	1 serv (1 oz)	150	15	3	10	0	5	4	0	0	120	—	—	0
Sauce Pizza	1 serv (1 oz)	20	1	0	0	0	3	1	0	0	230	—	—	0
Sauce Ranch	1 serv (1 oz)	100	10	2	10	1	1	1	0	20	240	—	—	0
Sauce Special Garlic	1 serv (1 oz)	150	17	3	0	0	0	0	0	0	310	—	—	0
Special Seasoning	1 pkg (3 g)	5	0	0	0	0	1	0	0	—	410	—	—	—

PAPA MURPHY'S

PIZZA

FOOD	PORTION	CALS	FAT	SAT FAT	CHOL	PROT	CARB	SUGAR	FIBER	CALCI	SOD	POTAS	FOLIC	VIT C
DeLite Thin Crust Large All Meat	1/10 pie	190	11	5	35	11	13	2	0	160	430	—	—	4
DeLite Thin Crust Large Cheese	1/10 pie	140	7	4	20	8	13	2	0	150	230	—	—	4
DeLite Thin Crust Large Hawaiian	1/10 pie	160	7	4	25	9	15	4	0	150	290	—	—	5
DeLite Thin Crust Large Pepperoni	1/10 pie	170	9	5	30	9	13	2	0	150	320	—	—	4
DeLite Thin Crust Large Veggie	1/10 pie	160	9	4	20	8	13	1	tr	150	250	—	—	5
Original Crust Family Size All Meat	1/12 pie	360	18	9	55	19	31	6	0	240	900	—	—	7
Original Crust Family Size Cheese	1/12 pie	270	11	6	30	13	30	6	0	230	560	—	—	5
Original Crust Family Size Cowboy	1/12 pie	350	18	8	45	17	32	6	tr	270	900	—	—	5
Original Crust Family Size Hawaiian	1/12 pie	290	11	6	35	15	33	9	tr	230	670	—	—	8
Original Crust Family Size Murphy's Combo	1/12 pie	360	18	9	50	18	33	6	tr	250	940	—	—	7
Original Crust Family Size Papa's Favorite	1/12 pie	360	18	8	50	18	33	6	tr	250	910	—	—	14
Original Crust Family Size Pepperoni	1/12 pie	320	15	8	40	15	31	6	0	230	710	—	—	5
Original Crust Family Size Rancher	1/12 pie	330	16	8	45	17	31	6	tr	240	790	—	—	7

FOOD	PORTION	CALS	FAT	SAT FAT	CHOL	PROT	CARB	SUGAR	FIBER	CALCI	SOD	POTAS	FOLIC	VIT C
Original Crust Family Size Specialty Of The House	½12 pie	320	15	7	40	16	32	6	tr	270	800	—	—	5
Original Crust Family Size Veggie Combo	½12 pie	300	13	6	30	14	33	6	tr	240	670	—	—	17
Original Crust Family Size Veggie Mediterranean	½12 pie	310	14	6	30	13	34	7	3	200	610	—	—	4
Original Crust Medium Cheese	⅛ pie	230	9	5	25	11	25	5	0	190	460	—	—	4
Stuffed Family Size 5 Meat	½16 pie	370	16	7	45	18	39	7	0	220	910	—	—	5
Stuffed Family Size Big Murphy	½16 pie	370	16	7	40	17	40	7	tr	240	890	—	—	10
Stuffed Family Size Chicago Style	½16 pie	370	16	7	45	17	40	7	tr	220	850	—	—	8
Stuffed Family Size Chicken & Bacon	½16 pie	370	15	7	50	20	39	6	0	210	820	—	—	6
Stuffed Large 5 Meat	½12 pie	370	16	7	45	18	38	7	0	220	900	—	—	5
Stuffed Large Big Murphy	½12 pie	360	15	7	40	17	39	7	tr	240	870	—	—	9
SALADS														
Club w/o Dressing & Croutons	½ serv (6.6 oz)	140	8	4	30	13	6	2	3	150	480	—	—	38
Garden w/o Dressing & Croutons	1 serv (7.2 oz)	100	6	3	10	6	8	2	3	160	260	—	—	59
Italian w/o Dressing & Croutons	½ serv (6.5 oz)	140	10	4	20	7	7	1	3	160	400	—	—	37

PEI WEI ASIAN DINER

CHILDREN'S MENU SELECTIONS

FOOD	PORTION	CALS	FAT	SAT FAT	CHOL	PROT	CARB	SUGAR	FIBER	CALCI	SOD	POTAS	FOLIC	VIT C
Kid's Wei Honey Seared Chicken w/o Noodles Or Rice	1 serv	290	17	—	—	16	19	8	0	—	—	—	—	—
Kid's Wei Lo Mein Chicken w/o Noodles Or Rice	1 serv	180	7	—	—	20	7	3	0	—	—	—	—	—
Kid's Wei Teriyaki Chicken w/o Noodles Or Rice	1 serv	240	5	—	—	23	20	18	0	—	—	—	—	—

FOOD	PORTION	CALS	FAT	SAT FAT	CHOL	PROT	CARB	SUGAR	FIBER	CALCI	SOD	POTAS	FOLIC	VIT C
DESSERTS														
Cookie Chocolate Chip	1	342	14	—	—	5	53	37	2	—	—	—	—	—
Cookie Fortune	1	30	0	0	0	0	7	3	0	—	—	—	—	—
MAIN MENU SELECTIONS														
Bowl w/ Brown Rice Japanese Teriyaki Beef	1 serv	580	17	—	—	33	66	21	4	—	—	—	—	—
Bowl w/ Brown Rice Japanese Teriyaki Chicken	1 serv	460	7	—	—	28	64	21	4	—	—	—	—	—
Bowl w/ Brown Rice Japanese Teriyaki Shrimp	1 serv	410	5	—	—	20	64	21	4	—	—	—	—	—
Bowl w/ Brown Rice Japanese Teriyaki Vegetables & Tofu	1 serv	410	6	—	—	13	71	24	7	—	—	—	—	—
Bowl w/ White Rice Japanese Teriyaki Beef	1 serv	560	16	—	—	32	62	21	3	—	—	—	—	—
Bowl w/ White Rice Japanese Teriyaki Chicken	1 serv	440	6	—	—	28	60	21	3	—	—	—	—	—
Bowl w/ White Rice Japanese Teriyaki Shrimp	1 serv	390	5	—	—	20	61	21	3	—	—	—	—	—
Bowl w/ White Rice Japanese Teriyaki Vegetables & Tofu	1 serv	390	5	—	—	13	68	24	5	—	—	—	—	—
Crispy Potstickers	4	130	7	—	—	6	10	1	0	—	—	—	—	—
Edamame	1 serv	156	8	—	—	14	12	4	5	—	—	—	—	—
Fried Rice Beef	1 serv	630	21	—	—	37	68	9	3	—	—	—	—	—
Fried Rice Chicken	1 serv	525	11	—	—	32	68	9	3	—	—	—	—	—
Fried Rice Shrimp	1 serv	475	10	—	—	24	67	9	3	—	—	—	—	—
Fried Rice Vegetables & Tofu	1 serv	440	7	—	—	17	73	12	5	—	—	—	—	—
Ginger Broccoli Beef	1 serv	450	22	—	—	37	19	11	2	—	—	—	—	—
Ginger Broccoli Chicken	1 serv	300	9	—	—	31	19	11	2	—	—	—	—	—
Ginger Broccoli Shrimp	1 serv	230	7	—	—	22	18	11	2	—	—	—	—	—

FOOD	PORTION	CALS	FAT	SAT FAT	CHOL	PROT	CARB	SUGAR	FIBER	CALCI	SOD	POTAS	FOLIC	VIT C
Ginger Broccoli Vegetables & Tofu	1 serv	170	4	—	—	10	23	14	4	—	—	—	—	—
Honey Seared Chicken	1 serv	420	15	—	—	21	45	17	0	—	—	—	—	—
Honey Seared Shrimp	1 serv	370	14	—	—	14	43	17	0	—	—	—	—	—
Hot & Sour Soup	1 cup	150	9	—	—	7	11	0	2	—	—	—	—	—
Lemon Pepper Beef	1 serv	550	31	—	—	38	32	18	2	—	—	—	—	—
Lemon Pepper Chicken	1 serv	440	20	—	—	31	34	18	2	—	—	—	—	—
Lemon Pepper Shrimp	1 serv	380	18	—	—	22	34	18	2	—	—	—	—	—
Lemon Pepper Vegetables & Tofu	1 serv	230	10	—	—	10	29	19	4	—	—	—	—	—
Mandarin Kung Pao Beef	1 serv	610	34	—	—	40	31	10	3					
Mandarin Kung Pao Chicken	1 serv	450	21	—	—	34	28	10	3	—	—	—	—	—
Mandarin Kung Pao Shrimp	1 serv	400	19	—	—	25	28	10	3	—	—	—	—	—
Mandarin Kung Pao Vegetables & Tofu	1 serv	290	15	—	—	13	23	10	4	—	—	—	—	—
Minced Chicken w/ Cool Lettuce Wraps w/o Rice Sticks	1 serv	250	4	—	—	22	31	15	3	—	—	—	—	—
Mongolian Beef	1 serv	420	22	—	—	36	14	8	1	—	—	—	—	—
Mongolian Chicken	1 serv	280	9	—	—	10	14	8	1	—	—	—	—	—
Mongolian Shrimp	1 serv	210	6	—	—	21	12	8	1	—	—	—	—	—
Mongolian Vegetables & Tofu	1 serv	180	6	—	—	10	19	11	3	—	—	—	—	—
Noodles Dan Dan Chicken	1 serv	390	7	—	—	26	54	9	3	—	—	—	—	—
Noodles Lo Mein Beef	1 serv	570	21	—	—	36	61	9	5	—	—	—	—	—
Noodles Lo Mein Chicken	1 serv	460	11	—	—	31	61	9	5	—	—	—	—	—
Noodles Lo Mein Shrimp	1 serv	400	8	—	—	23	60	9	5	—	—	—	—	—
Noodles Lo Mein Vegetables & Tofu	1 serv	400	8	—	—	16	66	11	7	—	—	—	—	—

FOOD	PORTION	CALS	FAT	SAT FAT	CHOL	PROT	CARB	SUGAR	FIBER	CALCI	SOD	POTAS	FOLIC	VIT C
Noodles Thai Blazing Beef	1 serv	630	32	—	—	28	55	11	4	—	—	—	—	—
Noodles Thai Blazing Chicken	1 serv	520	22	—	—	24	55	11	4	—	—	—	—	—
Noodles Thai Blazing Shrimp	1 serv	482	22	—	—	16	55	11	4	—	—	—	—	—
Noodles Thai Blazing Vegetables & Tofu	1 serv	430	18	—	—	10	59	14	6	—	—	—	—	—
Noodles Egg	1 serv	210	3	—	—	7	39	0	2	—	—	—	—	—
Noodles Rice	1 serv	130	0	0	0	0	32	0	0	—	—	—	—	—
Orange Peel Beef	1 serv	660	31	—	—	42	52	33	3	—	—	—	—	—
Orange Peel Chicken	1 serv	520	18	—	—	6	52	33	3	—	—	—	—	—
Orange Peel Shrimp	1 serv	460	16	—	—	27	51	33	3	—	—	—	—	—
Orange Peel Vegetables & Tofu	1 serv	330	10	—	—	14	46	33	4	—	—	—	—	—
Pad Thai Beef	1 serv	670	30	—	—	40	63	19	2	—	—	—	—	—
Pad Thai Chicken	1 serv	560	20	—	—	35	61	19	2	—	—	—	—	—
Pad Thai Shrimp	1 serv	490	17	—	—	27	60	19	2	—	—	—	—	—
Pei Wei Spicy Beef	1 serv	480	26	—	—	34	25	8	2	—	—	—	—	—
Pei Wei Spicy Chicken	1 serv	330	13	—	—	28	25	8	2	—	—	—	—	—
Pei Wei Spicy Shrimp	1 serv	300	11	—	—	19	29	8	2	—	—	—	—	—
Rice Brown	1 serv	170	2	—	—	4	37	0	3	—	—	—	—	—
Rice Fried	1 serv	260	5	—	—	9	44	5	2	—	—	—	—	—
Rice Sticks	1 cup	130	0	0	0	0	33	0	0	—	—	—	—	—
Rice White	1 serv	200	0	0	0	4	44	0	1	—	—	—	—	—
Spicy Korean Beef	1 serv	490	24	—	—	41	26	12	3	—	—	—	—	—
Spicy Korean Chicken	1 serv	350	11	—	—	15	26	12	3	—	—	—	—	—
Spicy Korean Shrimp	1 serv	280	9	—	—	26	24	12	3	—	—	—	—	—
Spicy Korean Vegetables & Tofu	1 serv	240	9	—	—	15	27	14	4	—	—	—	—	—
Spring Rolls	2	90	5	—	—	2	11	3	1	—	—	—	—	—
Sweet & Sour Chicken	1 serv	440	13	—	—	21	61	30	2	—	—	—	—	—
Sweet & Sour Shrimp	1 serv	390	11	—	—	14	59	30	2	—	—	—	—	—
Thai Coconut Curry Beef	1 serv	550	37	—	—	36	20	10	2	—	—	—	—	—

FOOD	PORTION	CALS	FAT	SAT FAT	CHOL	PROT	CARB	SUGAR	FIBER	CALCI	SOD	POTAS	FOLIC	VIT C
Thai Coconut Curry Chicken	1 serv	380	19	—	—	30	23	10	2	—	—	—	—	—
Thai Coconut Curry Shrimp	1 serv	300	17	—	—	21	18	10	2	—	—	—	—	—
Thai Coconut Curry Vegetables & Tofu	1 serv	220	14	—	—	8	19	11	2	—	—	—	—	—
Thai Dynamite Chicken	1 serv	390	19	—	—	33	20	7	2	—	—	—	—	—
Thai Dynamite Shrimp	1 serv	280	16	—	—	15	20	9	2	—	—	—	—	—
Thai Dynamite Vegetables & Tofu	1 serv	220	16	—	—	6	15	9	3	—	—	—	—	—
Wontons Crab	4	190	13	—	—	8	9	0	0	—	—	—	—	—
SALAD DRESSINGS AND SAUCES														
Dressing Sesame Ginger	1 serv (2 oz)	170	16	—	—	1	5	4	0	—	—	—	—	—
Lime Vinaigrette	1 serv (2 oz)	230	20	—	—	0	13	11	0	—	—	—	—	—
Sauce Lettuce Wrap	1 serv (2 oz)	70	5	—	—	4	2	1	0	—	—	—	—	—
Sauce Sweet Chili	1 serv (2 oz)	140	0	0	0	0	34	28	2	—	—	—	—	—
Sauce Thai Peanut	1 serv (2 oz)	168	11	—	—	5	15	11	1	—	—	—	—	—
SALADS														
Asian Chopped Chicken w/ Dressing	1 serv	280	15	—	—	24	13	4	2	—	—	—	—	—
Asian Chopped Chicken w/o Dressing	1 serv	200	8	—	—	23	10	2	2	—	—	—	—	—
Pei Wei Spicy Chicken w/ Dressing	1 serv	350	16	—	—	22	28	8	2	—	—	—	—	—
Pei Wei Spicy Chicken w/o Dressing	1 serv	210	3	—	—	22	23	3	2	—	—	—	—	—
Vietnamese Chicken Salad Rolls	3	53	3	—	—	3	5	3	1	—	—	—	—	—

P. F. CHANG'S CHINA BISTRO

FOOD	PORTION	CALS	FAT	SAT FAT	CHOL	PROT	CARB	SUGAR	FIBER	CALCI	SOD	POTAS	FOLIC	VIT C
DESSERTS														
Banana Spring Rolls	¼ serv (4 oz)	240	10	4	—	3	36	—	0	—	130	—	—	—
Flourless Chocolate Dome	½ serv (4 oz)	270	16	10	—	3	41	—	2	—	75	—	—	—
Flourless Chocolate Dome Gluten Free	½ serv (4 oz)	270	16	10	—	3	41	—	2	—	75	—	—	—
Mini Cheesecake	1 serv	210	13	8	—	2	22	—	1	—	190	—	—	—
Mini Great Wall	1 serv	160	7	3	—	2	22	—	1	—	150	—	—	—

FOOD	PORTION	CALS	FAT	SAT FAT	CHOL	PROT	CARB	SUGAR	FIBER	CALCI	SOD	POTAS	FOLIC	VIT C
Mini Red Velvet Cake	1 serv	220	11	4	—	2	28	—	1	—	170	—	—	—
Mini Triple Chocolate Mousse	1 serv	300	22	14	—	3	25	—	1	—	50	—	—	—
Mini Dessert Apple Pie	1 serv	190	7	2	—	2	29	—	1	—	170	—	—	—
Mini Dessert Carrot Cake	1 serv	210	11	4	—	2	25	—	1	—	200	—	—	—
Mini Dessert Tiramisu	1 serv	180	11	5	—	2	18	—	0	—	95	—	—	—
Mini Dessert Tres Leche Lemon Dream	1 serv	180	8	4	—	1	31	—	1	—	125	—	—	—
Mini Dessert Triple Chocolate Mousse Gluten Free	1	300	22	14	—	3	25	—	1	—	50	—	—	—
The Great Wall Of Chocolate	¼ serv (5 oz)	360	17	6	—	4	51	—	2	—	350	—	—	—
MAIN MENU SELECTIONS														
Almond & Cashew Chicken	⅓ serv (10 oz)	373	18	3	—	29	24	—	2	—	1960	—	—	—
Asian Grilled Norwegian Salmon	½ serv (9 oz)	345	6	2	—	32	38	—	1	—	715	—	—	—
Asian Street Taco Mahi Mahi	½ serv (4 oz)	230	9	2	—	8	26	—	2	—	390	—	—	—
Asian Street Taco Red Cooked Pork	½ serv (3 oz)	140	5	1	—	5	19	—	1	—	450	—	—	—
Asian Street Taco Spicy Shrimp	½ serv (3 oz)	180	10	2	—	7	14	—	1	—	350	—	—	—
Asian Street Taco Traditional Beef	½ serv (3 oz)	170	7	2	—	7	18	—	1	—	350	—	—	—
Beef A La Sichuan	⅓ serv (7 oz)	293	11	3	—	23	26	—	1	—	910	—	—	—
Beef w/ Broccoli	⅓ serv (7 oz)	290	12	3	—	24	21	—	2	—	1573	—	—	—
Beef w/ Broccoli Gluten Free	⅓ serv (6 oz)	290	12	3	—	24	21	—	2	—	1300	—	—	—
Buddha's Feast Steamed	½ serv (6 oz)	55	0	0	—	4	11	—	4	—	40	—	—	—
Buddha's Feast Steamed Gluten Free	½ serv (6 oz)	55	1	0	—	4	11	—	4	—	40	—	—	—
Buddha's Feast Stir Fried	½ serv (11 oz)	220	6	1	—	14	29	—	5	—	1620	—	—	—
Buddha's Feast Stir Fried w/ White Rice	½ serv (11 oz)	310	5	1	—	11	54	—	3	—	1050	—	—	—
Calamari Salt & Pepper	¼ serv (2 oz)	160	10	2	—	6	11	—	0	—	208	—	—	—

FOOD	PORTION	CALS	FAT	SAT FAT	CHOL	PROT	CARB	SUGAR	FIBER	CALCI	SOD	POTAS	FOLIC	VIT C
Chang's Spicy Chicken	⅓ serv (6 oz)	323	13	2	—	28	23	—	0	—	550	—	—	—
Chang's Spicy Chicken Gluten Free	⅓ serv (6 oz)	323	13	2	—	28	23	—	0	—	550	—	—	—
Chengdu Spiced Lamb	⅓ serv (5 oz)	237	12	3	—	23	11	—	1	—	740	—	—	—
Chicken w/ Black Bean Sauce	⅓ serv (7 oz)	300	16	2	—	29	14	—	0	—	1850	—	—	—
Chopped Chicken w/ Ginger Dressing	1 (8 oz)	365	24	4	—	23	13	—	2	—	640	—	—	—
Coconut Curry Vegetables	½ serv (13 oz)	510	36	12	—	22	26	—	5	—	650	—	—	—
Crispy Green Beans w/o Sauce	¼ serv (4 oz)	260	18	3	—	2	21	—	2	—	140	—	—	—
Crispy Honey Chicken	⅓ serv (6 oz)	477	23	4	—	16	49	—	0	—	510	—	—	—
Crispy Honey Shrimp	½ serv (6 oz)	460	22	4	—	10	55	—	1	—	805	—	—	—
Crispy Wontons	2 (1 oz)	90	6	1	—	4	8	—	0	—	120	—	—	—
Double Pan Fried Noodles Combo	¼ serv (9 oz)	455	21	2	—	16	44	—	1	—	1923	—	—	—
Double Pan Fried Noodles w/ Beef	¼ serv (8 oz)	395	17	1	—	15	44	—	2	—	1665	—	—	—
Double Pan Fried Noodles w/ Chicken	¼ serv (8 oz)	393	17	1	—	16	43	—	2	—	1608	—	—	—
Double Pan Fried Noodles w/ Pork	¼ serv (8 oz)	413	21	3	—	13	42	—	2	—	1975	—	—	—
Double Pan Fried Noodles w/ Shrimp	¼ serv (8 oz)	363	16	0	—	12	42	—	2	—	1698	—	—	—
Double Pan Fried Noodles w/ Vegetable	¼ serv (8 oz)	190	5	1	—	5	30	—	2	—	1340	—	—	—
Dumplings Pork Pan Fried	⅙ serv (1 oz)	70	4	1	—	4	6	—	0	—	125	—	—	—
Dumplings Pork Steamed	⅙ serv (1 oz)	60	2	1	—	4	6	—	0	—	125	—	—	—
Dumplings Shrimp Pan Fried	1 (1 oz)	60	2	0	—	4	6	—	0	—	170	—	—	—
Dumplings Shrimp Steamed	1 (1 oz)	45	0	0	—	4	6	—	0	—	170	—	—	—
Dumplings Steamed Edamame	⅓ serv (1 oz)	45	1	0	—	2	7	—	0	—	105	—	—	—

FOOD	PORTION	CALS	FAT	SAT FAT	CHOL	PROT	CARB	SUGAR	FIBER	CALCI	SOD	POTAS	FOLIC	VIT C
Dumplings Steamed Lemongrass Chicken	⅓ serv (1 oz)	40	1	0	—	2	5	—	0	—	85	—	—	—
Dumplings Steamed Pork & Leek	⅓ serv (1 oz)	50	2	1	—	2	5	—	1	—	70	—	—	—
Dumplings Steamed Shrimp & Pork	⅓ serv (1 oz)	40	1	0	—	3	5	—	1	—	125	—	—	—
Dumplings Vegetable Pan Fried	1 (1 oz)	60	2	0	—	2	8	—	0	—	80	—	—	—
Dumplings Vegetable Steamed	1 (1 oz)	45	0	0	—	2	8	—	0	—	80	—	—	—
Dynamite Shrimp	½ serv (4 oz)	290	12	2	—	5	6	—	0	—	285	—	—	—
Edamame w/ Kosher Salt	1 serv (3 oz)	130	4	0	—	10	11	—	5	—	680	—	—	—
Egg Rolls	1 (3 oz)	215	10	2	—	7	21	—	2	—	690	—	—	—
Eggplant Stir Fried	¼ serv (6 oz)	270	22	3	—	2	14	—	2	—	760	—	—	—
Flaming Red Wontons	⅙ serv (2 oz)	80	5	1	—	4	5	—	0	—	280	—	—	—
Fried Rice Beef	¼ serv (7 oz)	303	9	2	—	13	41	—	1	—	803	—	—	—
Fried Rice Beef Gluten Free	¼ serv (7 oz)	293	9	2	—	13	41	—	1	—	640	—	—	—
Fried Rice Chicken	¼ serv (7 oz)	303	9	2	—	15	39	—	1	—	748	—	—	—
Fried Rice Combo	¼ serv (8 oz)	363	13	3	—	19	41	—	1	—	1063	—	—	—
Fried Rice Pork	¼ serv (7 oz)	320	13	4	—	12	39	—	1	—	1115	—	—	—
Fried Rice Pork Gluten Free	¼ serv (7 oz)	320	13	4	—	12	39	—	1	—	953	—	—	—
Fried Rice Shrimp	¼ serv (7 oz)	273	8	1	—	11	39	—	1	—	838	—	—	—
Fried Rice Vegetable	¼ serv (7 oz)	230	5	1	—	5	38	—	1	—	690	—	—	—
Garlic Noodles	¼ serv (5 oz)	178	4	1	—	5	31	—	1	—	360	—	—	—
Garlic Snap Peas	⅓ lg serv (3 oz)	64	2	0	—	2	7	—	2	—	107	—	—	—
Garlic Snap Peas Gluten Free	⅓ lg serv (3 oz)	63	2	0	—	2	7	—	2	—	107	—	—	—
Ginger Chicken w/ Broccoli	⅓ serv (9 oz)	273	11	2	—	28	18	—	2	—	1457	—	—	—
Ginger Chicken w/ Broccoli Gluten Free	⅓ serv (8 oz)	270	11	2	—	28	13	—	2	—	990	—	—	—
Hunan Hot Fish	⅓ serv (8 oz)	340	22	3	—	16	21	—	1	—	1043	—	—	—
Kung Pao Chicken	⅓ serv (5 oz)	383	23	4	—	33	14	—	2	—	940	—	—	—
Kung Pao Scallops	⅓ serv (5 oz)	307	20	3	—	16	17	—	2	—	1126	—	—	—

FOOD	PORTION	CALS	FAT	SAT FAT	CHOL	PROT	CARB	SUGAR	FIBER	CALCI	SOD	POTAS	FOLIC	VIT C
Kung Pao Shrimp	⅓ serv (5 oz)	208	17	3	—	21	12	—	2	—	1083	—	—	—
Lettuce Wraps Chicken	¼ serv (5 oz)	160	7	1	—	8	17	—	2	—	650	—	—	—
Lettuce Wraps Chicken Gluten Free	¼ serv (5 oz)	158	7	1	—	9	15	—	2	—	670	—	—	—
Lettuce Wraps Vegetarian	¼ serv (5 oz)	140	7	1	—	6	11	—	2	—	530	—	—	—
Lo Mein Beef	1 serv (7 oz)	270	9	2	—	15	33	—	2	—	1070	—	—	—
Lo Mein Chicken	1 serv (7 oz)	267	9	2	—	17	30	—	2	—	997	—	—	—
Lo Mein Combo	⅓ serv (9 oz)	347	14	0	—	23	23	—	2	—	1413	—	—	—
Lo Mein Pork	1 serv (7 oz)	290	13	4	—	13	30	—	2	—	1483	—	—	—
Lo Mein Shrimp	1 serv (7 oz)	227	6	1	—	12	30	—	2	—	1113	—	—	—
Lo Mein Vegetable	⅓ serv (7 oz)	420	15	0	—	12	58	—	3	—	1580	—	—	—
Lunch Bowl Buddha's Feast Steamed w/ Brown Rice	½ serv (9 oz)	210	2	0	—	10	39	—	5	—	80	—	—	—
Lunch Bowl Buddha's Feast Steamed w/ White Rice	½ serv (9 oz)	235	1	0	—	10	45	—	3	—	575	—	—	—
Ma Po Tofu	⅓ serv (10 oz)	350	23	5	—	20	17	—	2	—	1060	—	—	—
Mahi Mahi	½ serv (10 oz)	420	17	8	—	25	42	—	2	—	605	—	—	—
Mandarin Chicken	½ serv (10 oz)	360	15	2	—	33	29	—	3	—	1715	—	—	—
Mongolian Beef	⅓ serv (6 oz)	337	15	4	—	29	20	—	1	—	1340	—	—	—
Mongolian Beef Gluten Free	⅓ serv (6 oz)	337	15	4	—	30	21	—	1	—	1123	—	—	—
Moo Goo Gai Pan	⅓ serv (9 oz)	247	13	2	—	18	13	—	1	—	823	—	—	—
Mu Shu Chicken	½ serv (10 oz)	285	13	3	—	16	26	—	3	—	1540	—	—	—
Mu Shu Pork	½ serv (10 oz)	320	19	7	—	21	16	—	3	—	2275	—	—	—
Mu Shu Pork Pancake	1	90	2	0	—	2	14	—	0	—	30	—	—	—
Noodles Dan Dan	¼ serv (9 oz)	270	7	1	—	13	30	—	2	—	1388	—	—	—
Norwegian Salmon Steamed w/ Ginger Gluten Free	½ serv (10 oz)	330	18	3	—	32	12	—	3	—	1085	—	—	—
Norwegian Salmon w/ Ginger	½ serv (10 oz)	330	19	3	—	31	12	—	3	—	605	—	—	—
Oolong Marinated Sea Bass	½ serv (9 oz)	315	19	5	—	24	15	—	2	—	1550	—	—	—
Orange Peel Beef	⅓ serv (5 oz)	283	13	3	—	12	21	—	1	—	833	—	—	—
Orange Peel Chicken	⅓ serv (5 oz)	333	15	3	—	29	20	—	1	—	770	—	—	—

FOOD	PORTION	CALS	FAT	SAT FAT	CHOL	PROT	CARB	SUGAR	FIBER	CALCI	SOD	POTAS	FOLIC	VIT C
Orange Peel Shrimp	⅓ serv (5 oz)	187	14	1	—	15	14	—	1	—	937	—	—	—
Pepper Steak	⅓ serv (8 oz)	297	13	3	—	24	19	—	1	—	1300	—	—	—
Pepper Steak Gluten Free	⅓ serv (8 oz)	300	13	3	—	25	19	—	1	—	1197	—	—	—
Rice Brown Steamed	1 serv (6 oz)	190	2	0	—	4	40	—	3	—	0	—	—	—
Rice White Steamed	1 serv (6 oz)	220	0	0	0	4	49	—	1	—	0	—	—	—
Salt & Pepper Prawns	⅓ serv (6 oz)	197	11	2	—	21	8	—	2	—	1070	—	—	—
Shanghai Cucumbers	⅓ lg serv (4 oz)	40	2	0	—	2	3	—	1	—	743	—	—	—
Shanghai Cucumbers Gluten Free	⅓ lg serv (4 oz)	40	2	0	—	2	3	—	1	—	743	—	—	—
Shanghai Shrimp w/ Garlic Sauce	½ serv (9 oz)	195	20	2	—	17	10	—	3	—	1050	—	—	—
Shrimp w/ Candied Walnuts	⅓ serv (7 oz)	377	24	4	—	16	25	—	1	—	654	—	—	—
Shrimp w/ Lobster Sauce	½ serv (10 oz)	250	14	2	—	23	11	—	1	—	1745	—	—	—
Shrimp w/ Lobster Sauce Gluten Free	½ serv (10 oz)	255	14	2	—	23	13	—	1	—	1745	—	—	—
Sichuan Asparagus	⅓ lg serv (5 oz)	100	6	1	—	3	10	—	2	—	730	—	—	—
Sichuan Scallops	⅓ serv (7 oz)	295	15	3	—	16	26	—	1	—	1230	—	—	—
Sichuan Shrimp	⅓ serv (5 oz)	173	7	1	—	16	10	—	0	—	747	—	—	—
Singapore Street Noodles	⅓ serv (6 oz)	300	6	1	—	11	42	—	3	—	1157	—	—	—
Singapore Street Noodles Gluten Free	⅓ serv (7 oz)	300	7	1	—	11	41	—	3	—	980	—	—	—
Siu Mai Steamed Bacon & Egg	⅓ serv (1 oz)	70	3	1	—	3	8	—	0	—	180	—	—	—
Siu Mai Steamed Pork & Rice	⅓ serv (1 oz)	50	5	0	—	2	9	—	0	—	125	—	—	—
Spare Ribs Chang's	¼ serv (4 oz)	344	24	7	—	26	7	—	1	—	336	—	—	—
Spare Ribs Northern Style	¼ serv (4 oz)	343	19	2	—	31	11	—	0	—	985	—	—	—
Spicy Green Beans	⅓ lg serv (5 oz)	110	6	1	—	3	13	—	4	—	720	—	—	—
Spinach Stir-Fried w/ Garlic	⅓ lg serv (5 oz)	53	3	1	—	4	5	—	3	—	300	—	—	—
Spinach Stir-Fried w/ Garlic Gluten Free	⅓ lg serv (3 oz)	53	3	1	—	4	5	—	3	—	300	—	—	—

FOOD	PORTION	CALS	FAT	SAT FAT	CHOL	PROT	CARB	SUGAR	FIBER	CALCI	SOD	POTAS	FOLIC	VIT C
Spring Roll	1 (1.5 oz)	156	8	1	—	4	17	—	2	—	271	—	—	—
Starters Seared Ahi Tuna	½ serv (4 oz)	160	11	2	—	10	7	—	1	—	860	—	—	—
Street Dumplings Shanghai	½ serv (2 oz)	140	5	1	—	6	19	—	1	—	250	—	—	—
Sweet & Sour Chicken	⅓ serv (5 oz)	370	19	3	—	12	38	—	0	—	367	—	—	—
Sweet & Sour Pork	½ serv (10 oz)	460	14	7	—	14	72	—	2	—	950	—	—	—
Tuna Tataki Crisp	⅓ serv (1 oz)	60	3	0	—	5	3	—	0	—	140	—	—	—
VIP Duck	½ serv (12 oz)	650	29	8	—	52	55	—	1	—	1880	—	—	—
Wok Charred Beef	⅓ serv (8 oz)	317	17	5	—	25	16	—	1	—	1157	—	—	—
Wok Seared Lamb	⅓ serv (7 oz)	283	16	3	—	25	9	—	1	—	1410	—	—	—
Wontons Crab	2	163	10	4	—	5	13	—	0	—	303	—	—	—
SALAD DRESSINGS AND SAUCES														
Sauce Crispy Green Bean	1 serv (2 oz)	310	32	5	—	0	2	—	0	—	520	—	—	—
Sauce Plum	1 serv (2 oz)	200	0	0	0	0	50	—	0	—	1460	—	—	—
Sauce Potsticker	1 serv (2 oz)	50	2	0	—	1	7	—	0	—	610	—	—	—
Sauce Shrimp Dumpling	1 serv (2 oz)	15	0	0	—	2	2	—	0	—	1250	—	—	—
Sauce Sweet & Sour	1 serv (2 oz)	80	0	0	0	0	21	—	0	—	210	—	—	—
Sauce Sweet & Sour Mustard	1 serv (2 oz)	90	2	0	—	1	17	—	1	—	140	—	—	—
SOUPS														
Chicken Noodle	1 bowl (7 oz)	120	4	1	—	6	15	—	1	—	510	—	—	—
Egg Drop	1 cup (7 oz)	60	3	0	—	1	8	—	0	—	640	—	—	—
Egg Drop Gluten Free	1 cup (7 oz)	60	3	0	—	1	8	—	0	—	640	—	—	—
Hot & Sour	1 bowl (7 oz)	80	3	1	—	5	9	—	0	—	1000	—	—	—
Wonton	1 bowl (7 oz)	92	3	1	—	7	9	—	0	—	482	—	—	—

PINKBERRY

FOOD	PORTION	CALS	FAT	SAT FAT	CHOL	PROT	CARB	SUGAR	FIBER	CALCI	SOD	POTAS	FOLIC	VIT C
Frozen Yogurt Coffee	½ cup	90	0	0	5	4	24	19	0	100	50	—	—	2
Frozen Yogurt Green Tea	½ cup	50	0	0	5	3	10	10	0	100	50	—	—	6
Frozen Yogurt Original	½ cup	70	0	0	5	3	14	12	0	100	55	—	—	5

PIZZA FUSION

FOOD	PORTION	CALS	FAT	SAT FAT	CHOL	PROT	CARB	SUGAR	FIBER	CALCI	SOD	POTAS	FOLIC	VIT C
DESSERTS														
Brownies Gluten Free	½ serv	232	16	3	9	1	27	17	1	—	50	—	—	—
Calzone Chocolate	½	209	9	3	9	5	30	9	1	—	171	—	—	—
Cookies Chocolate Chip	⅓ serv	250	13	5	5	4	33	13	3	—	210	—	—	—

FOOD	PORTION	CALS	FAT	SAT FAT	CHOL	PROT	CARB	SUGAR	FIBER	CALCI	SOD	POTAS	FOLIC	VIT C
Pastry Strawberry Cheese	1 serv	338	10	4	15	9	54	4	2	—	391	—	—	—
PIZZA														
BBQ Chicken	1 slice	181	4	2	20	8	26	7	1	—	434	—	—	—
Big Kahuna	1 slice	236	9	4	22	12	26	2	2	—	594	—	—	—
Bruschetta	1 slice	159	4	2	10	8	23	2	1	—	255	—	—	—
Cheese	1 slice	167	5	2	10	7	23	2	2	—	359	—	—	—
Eggplant & Mozzarella	1 slice	181	6	2	10	7	24	2	2	—	381	—	—	—
Farmer's Market	1 slice	190	6	2	10	9	25	3	2	—	502	—	—	—
Founder's Pie	1 slice	201	7	2	20	8	25	3	2	—	349	—	—	—
Four Cheese & Sundried Tomato	1 slice	175	5	3	19	8	26	5	2	—	355	—	—	—
Greek	1 slice	204	7	3	12	9	25	2	2	—	442	—	—	—
Pepperoni	1 slice	220	9	4	19	10	23	2	2	—	575	—	—	—
Personal BBQ Chicken	½ pie	272	6	3	30	11	43	10	2	—	635	—	—	—
Personal Big Kahuna	½ pie	365	13	6	33	18	39	2	3	—	930	—	—	—
Personal Bruschetta	½ pie	234	5	3	10	10	37	1	2	—	359	—	—	—
Personal Cheese	½ pie	233	6	3	10	10	35	2	2	—	460	—	—	—
Personal Eggplant & Mozzarella	½ pie	304	11	5	20	12	39	2	4	—	613	—	—	—
Personal Farmer's Market	½ pie	279	8	3	13	12	40	4	3	—	747	—	—	—
Personal Founder's Pie	½ pie	347	14	5	40	14	41	4	3	—	540	—	—	—
Personal Four Cheese & Sundried Tomato	½ pie	262	7	4	24	12	39	6	3	—	494	—	—	—
Personal Greek	½ pie	299	11	3	13	12	39	2	3	—	571	—	—	—
Personal Pepperoni	½ pie	359	15	6	31	17	37	2	2	—	719	—	—	—
Personal Philly Steak	½ pie	358	14	5	37	19	42	2	4	—	810	—	—	—
Personal Sausage & Tri-Peppers	½ pie	323	12	5	23	15	39	2	3	—	789	—	—	—
Personal Spinach & Artichoke	½ pie	270	7	3	10	12	41	3	4	—	704	—	—	—
Personal Very Vegan	½ pie	321	15	1	0	9	41	2	4	—	539	—	—	—
Philly Steak	1 slice	220	8	3	22	11	26	2	3	—	520	—	—	—
Sausage & Tri-Peppers	1 slice	212	8	3	16	10	25	2	2	—	523	—	—	—

FOOD	PORTION	CALS	FAT	SAT FAT	CHOL	PROT	CARB	SUGAR	FIBER	CALCI	SOD	POTAS	FOLIC	VIT C
Spinach & Artichoke	1 slice	184	5	2	10	9	25	2	2	—	481	—	—	—
Very Vegan	1 slice	195	8	1	0	6	27	2	3	—	408	—	—	—
SALADS														
Caesar & Roasted Chicken	½ serv	358	21	6	39	9	28	5	2	—	728	—	—	—
Chicken Bruschetta	½ serv	331	22	7	53	11	22	4	3	—	334	—	—	—
Fusion	½ serv	244	8	1	0	5	20	1	4	—	299	—	—	—
Pan Roasted Steak	½ serv	388	26	8	57	18	22	3	4	—	543	—	—	—
Pear & Gorgonzola	½ serv	380	34	8	32	12	12	3	4	—	428	—	—	—
Roasted Beet & Feta	½ serv	320	25	5	17	8	19	3	4	—	602	—	—	—
Side Salad Arugula	1 serv	48	4	1	0	1	1	0	0	—	288	—	—	—
SANDWICHES														
Philly Phusion	½	473	23	10	71	28	39	1	3	—	862	—	—	—
Portabello Grill	½	380	20	7	22	14	38	1	3	—	757	—	—	—
Roasted Chicken	½	357	14	6	56	17	41	5	4	—	722	—	—	—
Roasted Turkey	½	417	19	6	60	26	35	2	2	—	1237	—	—	—
STARTERS														
Flatbread	1 (2 serv)	198	2	2	0	14	76	2	4	—	676	—	—	—
Stuffed Portabello Mushroom	½ serv	140	11	3	6	5	9	3	2	—	506	—	—	—
Trio Of Dips	⅓ serv	191	11	3	10	6	30	1	3	—	491	—	—	—

PIZZA HUT

FOOD	PORTION	CALS	FAT	SAT FAT	CHOL	PROT	CARB	SUGAR	FIBER	CALCI	SOD	POTAS	FOLIC	VIT C
BEVERAGES														
Diet Pepsi	1 (16 oz)	0	0	0	0	0	0	0	0	—	50	—	—	—
Mountain Dew	1 (16 oz)	220	0	0	0	0	58	58	0	—	70	—	—	—
Pepsi	1 (16 oz)	200	0	0	0	0	56	54	0	—	50	—	—	—
Sierra Mist	1 (16 oz)	200	0	0	0	0	54	54	0	—	40	—	—	—
OTHER MENU SELECTIONS														
Breadstick	1 (1.5 oz)	140	5	1	0	5	19	2	1	—	260	—	—	—
Breadstick Cheese	1 (2 oz)	170	6	3	15	8	20	2	1	—	390	—	—	—
Dipping Sauce Marinara	1 serv (3 oz)	60	0	0	0	2	12	9	2	—	440	—	—	—
Dipping Sauce Ranch	1 serv (1.5 oz)	220	23	4	10	0	2	1	0	—	420	—	—	—
Dipping Sauce Wing Blue Cheese	1 serv (1.5 oz)	230	24	5	20	1	2	2	0	—	420	—	—	—
Dipping Sauce Wing Ranch	1 serv (1.5 oz)	220	23	4	10	0	2	1	0	—	420	—	—	—
Fried Cheese Sticks	4 (4.2 oz)	380	24	9	40	13	29	3	2	—	1020	—	—	—
Tuscani Pasta Chicken Alfredo	1 serv (10 oz)	580	32	9	50	23	49	4	4	—	1250	—	—	—

FOOD	PORTION	CALS	FAT	SAT FAT	CHOL	PROT	CARB	SUGAR	FIBER	CALCI	SOD	POTAS	FOLIC	VIT C
Tuscani Pasta Meaty Marinara	1 serv (9.5 oz)	450	20	8	70	22	44	8	5	—	1100	—	—	—
Wedge Fries	1 serv (4.3 oz)	320	18	4	0	4	35	0	3	—	530	—	—	—
Wings Crispy Bone In All American	2 (1.9 oz)	200	14	3	45	9	8	0	1	—	500	—	—	—
Wings Crispy Bone In Buffalo Burnin Hot	2 (2.6 oz)	230	15	3	45	9	16	2	1	—	1020	—	—	—
Wings Crispy Bone In Buffalo Medium	2 (2.6 oz)	230	15	3	45	9	16	2	2	—	1010	—	—	—
Wings Crispy Bone In Buffalo Mild	2 (2.6 oz)	230	15	3	45	9	16	2	1	—	1040	—	—	—
Wings Crispy Bone In Garlic Parmesan	2 (2.5 oz)	300	25	5	45	10	9	1	1	—	730	—	—	—
Wings Crispy Bone In Honey BBQ	2 (2.9 oz)	260	14	3	45	10	24	12	1	—	740	—	—	—
Wings Crispy Bone In Lemon Pepper	2 (2.6 oz)	270	19	4	45	9	16	7	1	—	640	—	—	—
Wings Crispy Bone In Spicy Asian	2 (2.9 oz)	250	15	3	45	10	21	13	1	—	710	—	—	—
Wings Crispy Bone In Spicy BBQ	2 (2.9 oz)	240	14	3	50	9	19	11	1	—	950	—	—	—
Wings Traditional All American	2 (1.4 oz)	80	5	2	40	7	0	0	0	—	290	—	—	—
Wings Traditional Buffalo Medium	2 (2 oz)	110	6	2	40	8	8	2	1	—	800	—	—	—
Wings Traditional Buffalo Mild	2 (2 oz)	110	6	2	40	8	8	2	1	—	830	—	—	—
Wings Traditional Burnin Hot	2 (2 oz)	110	6	2	40	8	8	2	1	—	810	—	—	—
Wings Traditional Garlic Parmesan	2 (2 oz)	180	16	4	45	8	1	1	0	—	520	—	—	—
Wings Traditional Honey BBQ	2 (2.4 oz)	140	5	2	40	8	16	12	0	—	530	—	—	—
Wings Traditional Lemon Pepper	2 (2 oz)	150	10	2	40	8	8	7	0	—	430	—	—	—
Wings Traditional Spicy Asian	2 (2.3 oz)	130	5	2	40	8	13	13	0	—	500	—	—	—
Wings Traditional Spicy BBQ	2 (2.3 oz)	120	5	2	45	8	11	11	0	—	750	—	—	—

FOOD	PORTION	CALS	FAT	SAT FAT	CHOL	PROT	CARB	SUGAR	FIBER	CALCI	SOD	POTAS	FOLIC	VIT C
PIZZA														
Fit 'N Delicious 12 Inch Chicken Mushrooms & Jalapeno	1 slice (3.3 oz)	170	5	2	20	11	22	4	1	—	720	—	—	—
Fit 'N Delicious 12 Inch Chicken Red Onion & Green Pepper	1 slice (3.3 oz)	180	5	2	20	11	23	5	1	—	510	—	—	—
Fit 'N Delicious 12 Inch Diced Red Tomato Mushroom & Jalapeno	1 slice (3.1 oz)	150	4	2	10	6	23	4	2	—	610	—	—	—
Fit 'N Delicious 12 Inch Green Pepper Red Onion & Diced Red Tomato	1 slice (3.1 oz)	150	4	2	10	6	24	5	2	—	400	—	—	—
Fit 'N Delicious 12 Inch Ham Pineapple & Diced Red Tomato	1 slice (2.9 oz)	160	5	2	15	7	24	6	1	—	550	—	—	—
Fit 'N Delicious 12 Inch Ham Red Onion & Mushrooms	1 slice (2.9 oz)	160	5	2	15	8	23	4	1	—	550	—	—	—
Hand Tossed 12 Inch Cheese Only	1 slice (2.9 oz)	220	8	4	25	10	26	4	1	—	550	—	—	—
Hand Tossed 12 Inch Cheese Only Garlic Parmesan	1 slice (3 oz)	220	8	5	25	10	26	4	1	—	580	—	—	—
Hand Tossed 12 Inch Dan's Original	1 slice (3.6 oz)	260	12	5	30	12	26	4	1	—	650	—	—	—
Hand Tossed 12 Inch Ham & Pineapple	1 slice (3.2 oz)	200	6	3	20	9	27	5	1	—	550	—	—	—
Hand Tossed 12 Inch Hawaiian Luau	1 slice (3.5 oz)	240	9	4	25	11	27	5	1	—	640	—	—	—
Hand Tossed 12 Inch Italian Sausage & Red Onion	1 slice (3.5 oz)	240	10	5	25	11	27	4	1	—	580	—	—	—
Hand Tossed 12 Inch Meat Lover's	1 slice (3.7 oz)	300	16	7	40	14	26	4	1	—	860	—	—	—

FOOD	PORTION	CALS	FAT	SAT FAT	CHOL	PROT	CARB	SUGAR	FIBER	CALCI	SOD	POTAS	FOLIC	VIT C
Hand Tossed 12 Inch Pepperoni	1 slice (2.9 oz)	230	9	4	25	10	25	3	1	—	610	—	—	—
Hand Tossed 12 Inch Pepperoni Lover's	1 slice (3.3 oz)	270	13	6	35	13	26	4	1	—	770	—	—	—
Hand Tossed 12 Inch Pepperoni & Mushroom	1 slice (3.2 oz)	210	8	4	20	10	26	4	1	—	540	—	—	—
Hand Tossed 12 Inch Pepperoni Garlic Parmesan	1 slice (2.9 oz)	230	9	5	25	10	26	4	1	—	640	—	—	—
Hand Tossed 12 Inch Spicy Sicilian	1 slice (3.5 oz)	240	11	5	25	11	26	4	1	—	730	—	—	—
Hand Tossed 12 Inch Supreme	1 slice (3.7 oz)	260	12	5	30	12	26	4	1	—	680	—	—	—
Hand Tossed 12 Inch Triple Meat Italiano	1 slice (3.4 oz)	260	12	5	30	12	26	4	1	—	730	—	—	—
Hand Tossed 12 Inch Ultimate Cheese Lover's	1 slice (2.9 oz)	240	11	5	30	11	25	3	1	—	590	—	—	—
Hand Tossed 12 Inch Veggie Lover's	1 slice (3.6 oz)	200	6	3	15	9	27	4	2	—	530	—	—	—
Pan 12 Inch Cheese Only	1 slice (3.2 oz)	240	10	5	25	11	27	2	1	—	530	—	—	—
Pan 12 Inch Dan's Original	1 slice (3.9 oz)	280	14	5	30	12	27	2	1	—	630	—	—	—
Pan 12 Inch Ham & Pineapple	1 slice (3.4 oz)	230	9	4	20	10	28	3	1	—	520	—	—	—
Pan 12 Inch Hawaiian Luau	1 slice (3.6 oz)	260	12	5	25	11	28	3	1	—	610	—	—	—
Pan 12 Inch Italian Sausage & Red Onion	1 slice (3.7 oz)	270	13	5	25	11	28	3	1	—	560	—	—	—
Pan 12 Inch Meat Lover's	1 slice (4 oz)	330	19	7	40	14	27	2	1	—	830	—	—	—
Pan 12 Inch Pepperoni	1 slice (3.2 oz)	250	12	5	25	11	26	2	1	—	590	—	—	—
Pan 12 Inch Pepperoni Lover's	1 slice (3.5 oz)	290	14	6	35	13	27	2	1	—	730	—	—	—
Pan 12 Inch Pepperoni & Mushroom	1 slice (3.4 oz)	240	10	4	20	10	27	2	1	—	520	—	—	—
Pan 12 Inch Spicy Sicilian	1 slice (3.7 oz)	270	13	5	25	11	27	2	2	—	700	—	—	—
Pan 12 Inch Supreme	1 slice (3.9 oz)	290	14	5	30	12	27	2	2	—	650	—	—	—

FOOD	PORTION	CALS	FAT	SAT FAT	CHOL	PROT	CARB	SUGAR	FIBER	CALCI	SOD	POTAS	FOLIC	VIT C
Pan 12 Inch Triple Meat Italiano	1 slice (3.6 oz)	290	15	5	30	13	27	2	1	—	700	—	—	—
Pan 12 Inch Ultimate Cheese Lover's	1 slice (3.2 oz)	270	13	5	25	12	26	2	1	—	580	—	—	—
Pan 12 Inch Veggie Lover's	1 slice (3.8 oz)	230	9	4	15	9	28	3	2	—	500	—	—	—
PANormous 9 Inch Cheese Only	1 pie (13.4 oz)	1100	45	19	105	48	124	10	6	—	2400	—	—	—
PANormous 9 Inch Dan's Original	1 pie (15.9 oz)	1270	62	23	125	55	124	10	7	—	2810	—	—	—
PANormous 9 Inch Ham & Pineapple	1 pie (14 oz)	1020	37	14	80	43	128	14	6	—	2300	—	—	—
PANormous 9 Inch Hawaiian Luau	1 pie (14.8 oz)	1150	49	18	105	49	129	14	6	—	2670	—	—	—
PANormous 9 Inch Italian Sausage & Red Onion	1 pie (15.4 oz)	1210	56	21	110	50	128	12	7	—	2550	—	—	—
PANormous 9 Inch Meat Lover's	1 pie (16.3 oz)	1470	80	30	175	64	123	10	6	—	3670	—	—	—
PANormous 9 Inch Pepperoni	1 pie (12.9 oz)	1100	48	18	100	47	121	9	6	—	2540	—	—	—
PANormous 9 Inch Pepperoni Lover's	1 pie (16 oz)	1290	62	26	150	59	124	10	6	—	3160	—	—	—
PANormous 9 Inch Pepperoni & Mushroom	1 pie (13.9 oz)	1050	42	16	85	45	123	10	7	—	2290	—	—	—
PANormous 9 Inch Spicy Sicilian	1 pie (15.4 oz)	1220	57	22	115	51	126	11	7	—	3150	—	—	—
PANormous 9 Inch Supreme	1 pie (16.2 oz)	1270	62	24	130	54	125	11	7	—	2920	—	—	—
PANormous 9 Inch Triple Meat Lover's	1 pie (14.9 oz)	1280	62	23	135	56	123	9	6	—	3070	—	—	—
PANormous 9 Inch Veggie Lover's	1 pie (15.4 oz)	1010	38	14	70	42	127	12	8	—	2240	—	—	—
Personal Pan 6 Inch Cheese Only	1 (7.2 oz)	590	24	10	55	26	69	7	3	—	1290	—	—	—
Personal Pan 6 Inch Dan's Original	1 (8.8 oz)	720	36	13	75	31	69	7	4	—	1600	—	—	—
Personal Pan 6 Inch Ham & Pineapple	1 (7.5 oz)	550	20	8	45	23	71	9	3	—	1260	—	—	—
Personal Pan 6 Inch Hawaiian Luau	1 (8 oz)	620	25	10	55	26	71	9	3	—	1440	—	—	—

FOOD	PORTION	CALS	FAT	SAT FAT	CHOL	PROT	CARB	SUGAR	FIBER	CALCI	SOD	POTAS	FOLIC	VIT C
Personal Pan 6 Inch Italian Sausage & Red Onion	1 (8.6 oz)	690	32	12	65	28	71	8	4	—	1440	—	—	—
Personal Pan 6 Inch Meat Lover's	1 (9.2 oz)	830	46	17	100	36	68	7	3	—	2110	—	—	—
Personal Pan 6 Inch Pepperoni	1 (7.1 oz)	610	26	10	55	26	67	6	3	—	1410	—	—	—
Personal Pan 6 Inch Pepperoni Lover's	1 (8.1 oz)	720	34	14	85	32	69	7	3	—	1760	—	—	—
Personal Pan 6 Inch Pepperoni & Mushroom	1 (7.5 oz)	570	23	9	45	24	68	7	4	—	1250	—	—	—
Personal Pan 6 Inch Spicy Sicilian	1 (8.6 oz)	680	32	12	70	29	69	7	4	—	1730	—	—	—
Personal Pan 6 Inch Supreme	1 (9 oz)	720	36	14	70	30	69	7	4	—	1680	—	—	—
Personal Pan 6 Inch Triple Meat Italiano	1 (8.4 oz)	730	36	13	80	32	68	6	3	—	1770	—	—	—
Personal Pan 6 Inch Ultimate Cheese Lover's	1 (7.3 oz)	660	30	12	65	29	68	6	3	—	1400	—	—	—
Personal Pan 6 Inch Veggie Lover's	1 (8.2 oz)	550	20	8	35	22	70	8	4	—	1190	—	—	—
P'Zone Classic	½ serv (6.1 oz)	470	16	7	40	20	61	3	2	—	1070	—	—	—
P'Zone Meaty	½ serv (6.6 oz)	550	23	10	55	24	61	2	2	—	1370	—	—	—
P'Zone Pepperoni	½ serv (5.5 oz)	450	15	7	40	19	60	2	2	—	1120	—	—	—
Stuffed Pizza Rollers	1 (2.7 oz)	220	10	5	25	10	24	3	1	—	580	—	—	—
Thin'N Crispy 12 Inch Cheese Only	1 slice (2.3 oz)	190	8	4	25	9	22	4	1	—	550	—	—	—
Thin'N Crispy 12 Inch Dan's Original	1 slice (3 oz)	240	12	5	30	11	22	4	1	—	650	—	—	—
Thin'N Crispy 12 Inch Ham & Pineapple	1 slice (2.6 oz)	180	6	3	20	8	23	5	1	—	540	—	—	—
Thin'N Crispy 12 Inch Hawaiian Luau	1 slice (2.8 oz)	220	10	4	25	10	24	5	1	—	650	—	—	—
Thin'N Crispy 12 Inch Italian Sausage & Red Onion	1 slice (2.8 oz)	220	10	4	25	9	23	4	1	—	580	—	—	—

FOOD	PORTION	CALS	FAT	SAT FAT	CHOL	PROT	CARB	SUGAR	FIBER	CALCI	SOD	POTAS	FOLIC	VIT C
Thin'N Crispy 12 Inch Meat Lover's	1 slice (3 oz)	280	16	6	40	13	22	4	1	—	860	—	—	—
Thin'N Crispy 12 Inch Pepperoni	1 slice (2.2 oz)	200	9	4	25	9	21	4	1	—	610	—	—	—
Thin'N Crispy 12 Inch Pepperoni Lover's	1 slice (2.6 oz)	250	13	6	35	12	22	4	1	—	760	—	—	—
Thin'N Crispy 12 Inch Pepperoni & Mushroom	1 slice (2.6 oz)	180	8	4	20	9	22	4	1	—	540	—	—	—
Thin'N Crispy 12 Inch Spicy Sicilian	1 slice (2.8 oz)	220	10	5	25	9	22	4	1	—	750	—	—	—
Thin'N Crispy 12 Inch Supreme	1 slice (3.1 oz)	240	12	5	30	10	23	4	1	—	670	—	—	—
Thin'N Crispy 12 Inch Triple Meat Italiano	1 slice (2.7 oz)	240	12	5	30	11	22	4	1	—	720	—	—	—
Thin'N Crispy 12 Inch Ultimate Cheese Lover's	1 slice (2.3 oz)	220	11	5	25	10	21	4	1	—	600	—	—	—
Thin'N Crispy 12 Inch Veggie Lover's	1 slice (3 oz)	180	6	3	15	8	23	4	1	—	530	—	—	—

POPEYE'S

BEVERAGES

FOOD	PORTION	CALS	FAT	SAT FAT	CHOL	PROT	CARB	SUGAR	FIBER	CALCI	SOD	POTAS	FOLIC	VIT C
Coffee Black	1 (16 oz)	0	0	0	0	0	0	0	0	—	0	—	—	—
Orange Juice	1 (10 oz)	140	0	0	0	2	33	30	0	—	20	—	—	—

BREAKFAST MENU SELECTIONS

FOOD	PORTION	CALS	FAT	SAT FAT	CHOL	PROT	CARB	SUGAR	FIBER	CALCI	SOD	POTAS	FOLIC	VIT C
Biscuit Bacon	1 (5 oz)	400	25	12	5	8	37	2	3	—	780	—	—	—
Biscuit Chicken	1 (5.2 oz)	490	26	14	28	17	47	2	1	—	1275	—	—	—
Biscuit Egg	1 (4.8 oz)	510	29	15	125	13	41	2	1	—	1155	—	—	—
Biscuit Egg & Sausage	1 (6.5 oz)	690	45	22	157	20	43	2	1	—	1520	—	—	—
Biscuit Sausage	1 (4.8 oz)	540	36	18	320	13	41	2	1	—	1100	—	—	—
Biscuit Sausage & Gravy	1 (6.5 oz)	510	33	14	15	10	42	3	3	—	1090	—	—	—
Grits	1 serv (5 oz)	370	5	1	0	5	80	0	7	—	30	—	—	—
Hashbrowns	1 serv (3.4 oz)	360	20	9	10	3	41	0	4	—	450	—	—	—

DESSERTS

FOOD	PORTION	CALS	FAT	SAT FAT	CHOL	PROT	CARB	SUGAR	FIBER	CALCI	SOD	POTAS	FOLIC	VIT C
Apple Sauce	1 serv (4 oz)	50	0	0	0	0	12	8	2	—	10	—	—	—
Cheesecake Mardi Gras	1 serv (3 oz)	310	19	10	60	4	32	22	1	—	290	—	—	—
Pie Hot Sweet Potato	1 serv (3.5 oz)	350	19	8	15	4	41	10	2	—	370	—	—	—

FOOD	PORTION	CALS	FAT	SAT FAT	CHOL	PROT	CARB	SUGAR	FIBER	CALCI	SOD	POTAS	FOLIC	VIT C
Pie Mississippi Mud	1 serv (3 oz)	280	7	2	20	3	51	27	2	—	210	—	—	—
Pie Sliced Pecan	1 serv (3.3 oz)	410	21	6	70	4	52	22	1	—	220	—	—	—
MAIN MENU SELECTIONS														
Baguette	1 (1.3 oz)	90	2	0	0	3	18	1	1	—	80	—	—	—
Biscuit	1 (2.1 oz)	260	15	7	0	4	26	1	2	—	450	—	—	—
Butterfly Shrimp	8 (3.5 oz)	290	17	8	90	12	21	0	3	—	820	—	—	—
Cajun Fries	1 reg (3 oz)	260	14	5	10	3	30	0	2	—	570	—	—	—
Cajun Rice	1 reg (4.3 oz)	170	5	2	25	7	25	4	1	—	530	—	—	—
Catfish Fillets	2 (5.2 oz)	460	29	12	65	21	27	0	1	—	1140	—	—	—
Cheddar Cheese Tortilla	1 (1.6 oz)	140	5	3	0	3	21	0	1	—	210	—	—	—
Chicken Livers	10 (10 oz)	1190	80	34	765	54	65	3	6	—	2070	—	—	—
Chicken Wrap Loaded	1 (4.6 oz)	310	13	6	30	14	33	0	3	—	890	—	—	—
Chicken Wrap Naked	1 (3.4 oz)	200	6	4	25	12	22	0	1	—	580	—	—	—
Coleslaw	1 reg (4.8 oz)	220	15	3	10	1	19	15	2	—	300	—	—	—
Corn On The Cob	1 (10 oz)	190	2	1	0	6	37	0	4	—	0	—	—	—
Green Beans	1 serv (3.5 oz)	40	2	0	5	2	6	1	2	—	420	—	—	—
Jalapeno	1 (6 g)	0	0	0	0	0	1	0	1	—	368	—	—	—
Jambalaya Chicken & Sausage	1 serv (5.3 oz)	220	11	3	32	10	20	0	1	—	760	—	—	—
Macaroni & Cheese	1 serv (5.5 oz)	200	7	4	15	8	26	3	1	—	490	—	—	—
Mashed Potatoes Gravy	1 serv (5 oz)	110	4	2	5	3	18	1	1	—	590	—	—	—
Mild Breast	1 (5.5 oz)	440	27	11	110	35	16	0	2	—	1330	—	—	—
Mild Leg	1 (2.4 oz)	160	9	4	40	14	5	0	1	—	460	—	—	—
Mild Tenders	3 (4.4 oz)	340	14	6	70	27	26	0	1	—	1350	—	—	—
Mild Thigh	1 (2.8 oz)	280	21	8	50	14	7	0	1	—	640	—	—	—
Mild Wing	1 (2.2 oz)	210	14	4	60	13	8	0	1	—	610	—	—	—
Naked Tenders	3 (4 oz)	170	2	0	25	26	2	0	0	—	550	—	—	—
Nuggets	4 (1.8 oz)	150	9	4	25	7	10	0	1	—	230	—	—	—
Onion Rings	6 (2.6 oz)	280	19	8	10	3	25	2	2	—	460	—	—	—
Po'Boy Catfish	1 (11.2 oz)	800	50	16	75	27	65	3	3	—	2015	—	—	—
Po'Boy Chicken	1 (22.3 oz)	660	34	9	75	31	61	3	3	—	2120	—	—	—
Po'Boy Naked BBQ Chicken	1 (7.4 oz)	340	7	2	50	24	49	11	2	—	1030	—	—	—
Po'Boy Shrimp	1 (9.5 oz)	690	42	13	75	42	66	3	5	—	2165	—	—	—
Popcorn Shrimp	1 serv (3.5 oz)	330	9	9	65	11	28	0	3	—	1290	—	—	—
Red Beans & Rice	1 reg (5.1 oz)	230	14	4	10	7	23	0	5	—	580	—	—	—
Spicy Breast	1 (5.5 oz)	420	27	9	110	33	13	0	3	—	830	—	—	—
Spicy Leg	1 (2.4 oz)	170	10	4	65	13	5	0	1	—	360	—	—	—

FOOD	PORTION	CALS	FAT	SAT FAT	CHOL	PROT	CARB	SUGAR	FIBER	CALCI	SOD	POTAS	FOLIC	VIT C
Spicy Tenders	3 (4.4 oz)	310	15	6	80	28	16	0	2	—	1240	—	—	—
Spicy Thigh	1 (2.8 oz)	260	18	6	70	14	8	0	1	—	460	—	—	—
Spicy Wing	1 (2.2 oz)	210	14	6	55	13	8	0	1	—	410	—	—	—
SAUCES														
Cocktail	1 serv (1 oz)	30	0	0	0	0	6	6	0	—	320	—	—	—
Confetti Sauce	1 serv (1 oz)	65	0	0	0	0	16	10	0	—	90	—	—	—
Ranch	1 serv (1 oz)	150	15	3	10	0	3	1	0	—	230	—	—	—
Spicy BBQ	1 serv (1 oz)	45	0	0	0	0	10	8	0	—	320	—	—	—
Spicy Honey Mustard	1 serv (1 oz)	100	8	1	10	0	7	5	0	—	170	—	—	—
Tartar Sauce	1 serv (1 oz)	140	15	3	15	0	1	1	0	—	280	—	—	—

PRETZELMAKER

FOOD	PORTION	CALS	FAT	SAT FAT	CHOL	PROT	CARB	SUGAR	FIBER	CALCI	SOD	POTAS	FOLIC	VIT C
BEVERAGES														
Breezer Coffee	1 (20 oz)	640	21	14	50	6	107	106	0	0	100	—	—	0
Breezer Mocha	1 (20 oz)	620	20	13	50	6	106	104	0	0	100	—	—	0
Breezer Peach	1 (20 oz)	650	20	13	50	6	117	115	0	0	110	—	—	0
Breezer Raspberry	1 (20 oz)	650	20	13	50	6	117	112	0	0	100	—	—	0
Breezer Strawberry Banana	1 (20 oz)	650	20	13	50	6	115	108	0	0	100	—	—	0
Diet Coke	1 sm (20 oz)	0	0	0	0	0	0	0	0	0	25	—	—	0
Lemonade	1 sm (20 oz)	160	0	0	0	0	92	87	0	0	15	—	—	18
PRETZELS														
Bites	1 med (7.4 oz)	640	16	2	0	13	112	21	4	400	500	—	—	0
Bites	1 sm (5.3 oz)	450	11	2	0	9	80	15	3	300	360	—	—	0
Bites Cinnamon Sugar	1 serv (5.8 oz)	520	12	2	0	9	95	28	3	300	20	—	—	0
Caramel Nut	1 (4.5 oz)	390	7	1	0	7	74	17	2	250	55	—	—	0
Cinnamon Sugar	1 (4.3 oz)	370	8	1	0	7	68	17	2	250	15	—	—	0
Garlic	1 (4.1 oz)	350	7	1	0	7	64	12	2	250	790	—	—	0
Original	1 (4 oz)	340	7	1	0	7	61	11	2	250	220	—	—	0
Parmesan	1 (4.2 oz)	360	9	2	5	9	61	11	2	250	290	—	—	0
Plain	1 (4 oz)	209	2	0	0	7	61	11	2	250	15	—	—	0
PT Pretzel Dog	1 (6 oz)	440	27	10	80	15	34	8	1	100	1120	—	—	6
Ranch	1 (4.1 oz)	240	7	1	0	7	63	11	2	250	930	—	—	0
TOPPINGS														
Cream Cheese	1 serv (1.5 oz)	200	20	14	80	2	4	2	0	40	200	—	—	0
Icing Cream Cheese	1 serv (1.5 oz)	180	9	6	30	1	22	21	0	0	85	—	—	0
Ketchup	2 pkg (0.6 oz)	20	0	0	0	0	4	4	0	20	200	—	—	1
Mustard	2 pkg (0.4 oz)	5	0	0	0	0	1	0	0	0	125	—	—	0
Sauce Caramel	1 serv (1.5 oz)	140	0	0	0	1	35	27	0	0	160	—	—	0
Sauce Cheddar Cheese	1 serv (1.5 oz)	70	5	1	0	1	6	2	0	0	420	—	—	2

FOOD	PORTION	CALS	FAT	SAT FAT	CHOL	PROT	CARB	SUGAR	FIBER	CALCI	SOD	POTAS	FOLIC	VIT C
Sauce Nacho Cheese	1 serv (1.5 oz)	80	5	1	0	1	7	2	0	0	530	—	—	2
Sauce Pizza	1 serv (1.5 oz)	30	1	0	0	1	6	3	2	80	250	—	—	tr

QUIZNOS

SALAD DRESSINGS

FOOD	PORTION	CALS	FAT	SAT FAT	CHOL	PROT	CARB	SUGAR	FIBER	CALCI	SOD	POTAS	FOLIC	VIT C
Acai Vinaigrette	1 reg	230	17	3	0	1	15	14	0	—	423	—	—	—
Balsamic Vinaigrette Fat Free	1 reg	130	0	0	0	0	29	20	0	—	749	—	—	—
Blue Cheese	1 reg	345	38	9	36	5	3	2	0	—	660	—	—	—
Honey Dijon	1 reg	450	44	7	35	1	14	13	0	—	570	—	—	—
Peppercorn Caesar	1 reg	480	50	9	34	3	5	3	0	—	979	—	—	—
Ranch	1 reg	350	36	5	24	2	5	3	0	—	591	—	—	—
Tzatziki	1 reg	450	46	9	48	3	3	2	0	—	569	—	—	—

SALADS

FOOD	PORTION	CALS	FAT	SAT FAT	CHOL	PROT	CARB	SUGAR	FIBER	CALCI	SOD	POTAS	FOLIC	VIT C
Fresh Farmers Market Caprese Chicken w/o Dressing	1 reg	260	17	8	45	24	10	2	2	—	831	—	—	—
Fresh Farmers Market Chicken Caesar w/o Dressing	1 reg	130	5	3	46	19	6	3	2	—	641	—	—	—
Fresh Farmers Market Cobb w/o Dressing	1 reg	260	12	6	121	19	5	3	2	—	729	—	—	—
Fresh Farmers Market Harvest Chicken w/o Dressing	1 reg	220	6	2	20	11	33	25	4	—	417	—	—	—
Fresh Farmers Market Mediterranean Chicken w/o Dressing	1 reg	180	7	3	42	25	13	3	4	—	1011	—	—	—

SANDWICHES

FOOD	PORTION	CALS	FAT	SAT FAT	CHOL	PROT	CARB	SUGAR	FIBER	CALCI	SOD	POTAS	FOLIC	VIT C
Classic Sub Classic Club	1 sm	570	34	10	70	25	41	8	3	—	1320	—	—	—
Classic Sub Classic Italian	1 sm	520	29	11	55	22	43	8	4	—	1500	—	—	—
Classic Sub Honey Bacon Club	1 sm	480	21	5	45	26	51	15	3	—	1430	—	—	—
Classic Sub Honey Bourbon Chicken	1 sm	320	6	3	20	16	48	14	4	—	790	—	—	—
Classic Sub Pork Cuban	1 sm	450	22	6	60	24	39	5	3	—	1130	—	—	—

FOOD	PORTION	CALS	FAT	SAT FAT	CHOL	PROT	CARB	SUGAR	FIBER	CALCI	SOD	POTAS	FOLIC	VIT C
Classic Sub The Traditional	1 sm	430	20	7	45	21	43	8	4	—	1260	—	—	—
Classic Sub Tuna Melt	1 sm	690	47	11	80	28	40	6	3	—	840	—	—	—
Classic Sub Turkey Bacon Guacamole	1 sm	540	28	8	45	25	44	9	5	—	1540	—	—	—
Classic Sub Turkey Ranch & Swiss	1 sm	420	18	5	30	20	44	8	4	—	1140	—	—	—
Classic Sub Ultimate Turkey Club	1 sm	560	34	10	70	24	41	7	3	—	1360	—	—	—
Classic Sub Veggie	1 sm	510	28	9	25	17	43	9	6	—	1190	—	—	—
Flatbread Sammies Bistro Steak Melt	1	410	23	6	50	17	31	6	1	—	1100	—	—	—
Flatbread Sammies Cantina Chicken	1	280	7	2	20	12	36	12	2	—	640	—	—	—
Flatbread Sammies Chicken Bacon Ranch	1	380	19	5	40	20	28	4	1	—	780	—	—	—
Flatbread Sammies Italiano	1	420	25	8	55	20	28	4	1	—	1175	—	—	—
Flatbread Sammies Roadhouse Steak	1	270	6	1	20	14	39	13	1	—	1060	—	—	—
Flatbread Sammies Smoky Chipotle Turkey	1	390	23	6	45	17	29	4	1	—	1210	—	—	—
Flatbread Sammies Veggie	1	340	20	5	15	9	29	5	3	—	740	—	—	—
Signature Sub Baja Chicken	1 sm	490	23	9	50	23	43	9	3	—	1190	—	—	—
Signature Sub Black Angus On Rosemary Parmesan	1 sm	520	17	9	85	38	54	14	4	—	1420	—	—	—
Signature Sub Buffalo Chicken	1 sm	470	22	8	50	24	45	7	3	—	1630	—	—	—
Signature Sub Chicken Bacon Dipper	1 sm	630	38	14	95	32	43	8	3	—	2410	—	—	—
Signature Sub Chicken Carbonara	1 sm	530	27	9	55	25	40	7	3	—	1090	—	—	—
Signature Sub Chipotle Prime Rib	1 sm	600	34	10	85	31	42	7	3	—	1300	—	—	—

FOOD	PORTION	CALS	FAT	SAT FAT	CHOL	PROT	CARB	SUGAR	FIBER	CALCI	SOD	POTAS	FOLIC	VIT C
Signature Sub Double Cheese Cheesesteak	1 sm	770	47	12	115	42	44	7	3	—	1470	—	—	—
Signature Sub Harvest Chicken	1 sm	370	11	3	23	17	54	19	4	—	880	—	—	—
Signature Sub Honey Mustard Chicken	1 sm	520	26	8	45	24	44	10	3	—	960	—	—	—
Signature Sub Mesquite Chicken	1 sm	500	25	9	55	24	41	7	3	—	1040	—	—	—
Signature Sub Peppercorn Steakhouse Dip	1 sm	630	37	10	91	33	44	7	3	—	1795	—	—	—
Signature Sub Prime Rib Mushroom & Swiss	1 sm	600	34	9	80	32	42	6	3	—	1120	—	—	—
Signature Sub Prime Rib & Peppercorn	1 sm	620	36	11	90	31	43	7	3	—	1240	—	—	—
Signature Sub Prime Rib & Blue	1 sm	570	29	11	90	34	42	7	3	—	1380	—	—	—
Signature Sub Southern BBQ Pulled Pork	1 sm	520	22	10	103	35	46	12	3	—	1740	—	—	—
Toasty Bullets Beef Bacon & Cheddar	1	450	18	6	45	21	48	8	2	—	1325	—	—	—
Toasty Bullets Italian	1	500	25	8	50	20	47	8	3	—	1480	—	—	—
Toasty Bullets Pesto Turkey	1	380	13	3	25	18	48	8	3	—	1250	—	—	—
Toasty Bullets Tuna Melt	1	510	31	6	50	17	39	6	2	—	660	—	—	—
Toasty Bullets Turkey Club	1	460	21	5	40	20	48	8	3	—	1330	—	—	—
Toasty Favorites Honey Cured Ham	1 sm	490	28	8	60	21	40	7	3	—	1085	—	—	—
Toasty Favorites Meatball	1 sm	450	21	8	60	23	47	10	6	—	1330	—	—	—
Toasty Favorites Oven Roasted Turkey	1 sm	500	28	7	55	20	42	7	3	—	1170	—	—	—
Toasty Favorites Roast Beef	1 sm	500	28	7	55	21	42	8	3	—	1170	—	—	—
Toasty Favorites Turkey & Ham	1 sm	500	29	8	60	20	41	7	3	—	1125	—	—	—

FOOD	PORTION	CALS	FAT	SAT FAT	CHOL	PROT	CARB	SUGAR	FIBER	CALCI	SOD	POTAS	FOLIC	VIT C
Toasty Favorites Veggie Caprese	1 sm	400	21	15	20	16	41	7	4	—	940	—	—	—
Toasty Torpedoes Beef Bacon & Cheddar	1	800	31	9	70	37	93	16	5	—	2260	—	—	—
Toasty Torpedoes Italian	1	860	40	12	75	33	93	16	5	—	2390	—	—	—
Toasty Torpedoes Pesto Turkey	1	690	22	5	40	31	94	15	5	—	2100	—	—	—
Toasty Torpedoes Tuna Melt	1	980	56	11	85	34	88	12	4	—	1365	—	—	—
Toasty Torpedoes Turkey Club	1	830	35	9	60	34	94	16	5	—	2280	—	—	—

RANCH 1

BEVERAGES

FOOD	PORTION	CALS	FAT	SAT FAT	CHOL	PROT	CARB	SUGAR	FIBER	CALCI	SOD	POTAS	FOLIC	VIT C
Barq's Root Beer	1 sm (16 oz)	167	0	0	0	0	45	45	0	0	36	—	—	0
Coca-Cola	1 sm (16 oz)	150	0	0	0	0	40	40	0	0	10	—	—	0
Diet Coke	1 sm (16 oz)	2	0	0	0	0	0	0	0	0	6	—	—	0
Sprite	1 sm (16 oz)	150	0	0	0	0	40	40	0	0	30	—	—	0

CHILDREN'S MENU SELECTIONS

FOOD	PORTION	CALS	FAT	SAT FAT	CHOL	PROT	CARB	SUGAR	FIBER	CALCI	SOD	POTAS	FOLIC	VIT C
Kids Meal Chicken Tenders	1 (2 oz)	111	4	1	29	10	9	0	0	4	138	—	—	0
Kids Meal Fries	1 serv (4 oz)	279	15	3	0	4	31	1	4	0	351	—	—	5
Kids Meal Popcorn Chicken	1 (2 oz)	112	4	0	19	9	10	0	0	11	436	—	—	1

MAIN MENU SELECTIONS

FOOD	PORTION	CALS	FAT	SAT FAT	CHOL	PROT	CARB	SUGAR	FIBER	CALCI	SOD	POTAS	FOLIC	VIT C
Bowl Chicken Teriyaki	1 (19.3 oz)	504	7	1	69	34	78	10	1	73	3415	—	—	22
Chicken Crispy	1 serv (5 oz)	326	15	2	83	27	22	1	1	10	351	—	—	0
Chicken Grilled	1 serv (3.9 oz)	146	6	1	69	24	0	0	0	10	236	—	—	0
Chicken On Mixed Greens	1 serv (21 oz)	340	19	2	72	29	17	9	7	106	459	—	—	41
Chicken Popcorn	1 serv (5.5 oz)	325	12	1	55	27	30	0	1	31	1263	—	—	2
Chicken Tenders	1 serv (5.6 oz)	387	14	2	99	35	32	1	1	14	461	—	—	0
Fajita Mix Tomatoes Onion & Carrot	1 serv (3.2 oz)	20	0	0	0	1	5	3	1	12	12	—	—	10
Fajitas Chicken	1 serv (10 oz)	540	24	9	75	30	53	4	3	320	969	—	—	10
Fries	1 med	381	21	3	0	6	43	2	6	0	483	—	—	7
Fries Cheese	1 reg	493	27	6	9	8	54	2	6	63	1129	—	—	7
Green Mix For Sandwiches	1 serv (2.5 oz)	31	2	0	1	1	2	1	1	16	21	—	—	5
Peppers & Onions	1 serv (1.6 oz)	27	2	0	0	0	3	2	1	7	18	—	—	23
Platter Chicken Rice	1 (10.9 oz)	273	6	1	69	28	28	4	3	46	657	—	—	37
Popcorn Chicken	1 sm	325	12	1	55	27	30	0	1	31	1263	—	—	2
Rice	1 serv (4 oz)	97	0	0	0	3	21	0	0	13	395	—	—	0

FOOD	PORTION	CALS	FAT	SAT FAT	CHOL	PROT	CARB	SUGAR	FIBER	CALCI	SOD	POTAS	FOLIC	VIT C
Sandwich Chicken & Cheese	1 (11.2 oz)	389	12	4	84	33	39	5	2	233	881	—	—	6
Sandwich Chicken Philly	1 (9.2 oz)	410	13	4	79	36	40	4	2	179	777	—	—	29
Sandwich Crispy Chicken	1 (11.4 oz)	711	39	6	103	33	60	4	3	41	950	—	—	6
Sandwich Crispy Spicy Chicken	1 (11.4 oz)	543	17	3	83	34	68	7	3	41	1068	—	—	10
Sandwich Grilled Spicy Chicken	1 (10.3 oz)	363	7	2	69	31	46	7	2	33	951	—	—	10
Sandwich Ranch Classic	1 (9.4 oz)	683	47	8	79	29	37	3	2	50	750	—	—	5
Steamed Vegetables	1 serv (3 oz)	27	0	0	0	2	6	2	2	33	31	—	—	57
Wrap Grilled Chicken Caesar	1 (13.2 oz)	746	41	9	105	44	55	2	4	376	1464	—	—	21
SALAD DRESSINGS AND SAUCES														
Dressing Balsamic Vinaigrette	1 oz	71	8	1	0	0	1	0	0	0	42	—	—	0
Dressing Classic Caesar	1 oz	103	11	1	7	1	1	0	0	0	117	—	—	0
Dressing Salad	1 oz	201	22	3	6	0	0	0	0	0	157	—	—	0
Sauce Ancho Chili Pepper	1 oz	134	14	2	17	1	1	1	0	0	179	—	—	0
Sauce BBQ	1 oz	84	4	1	0	0	12	8	0	80	134	—	—	0
Sauce Honey Mustard	1 oz	110	8	1	0	0	9	6	0	0	95	—	—	0
Sauce Pepper & Onion Saute	1 oz	143	16	2	0	0	1	0	0	0	192	—	—	0
Sauce Roasted Red Pepper	1 oz	232	26	4	6	0	0	—	—	13	75	—	—	1
Sauce Teriyaki	1 oz	24	0	0	0	1	5	5	0	80	973	—	—	0
SALADS														
Caesar	1 (7 oz)	34	1	0	0	2	7	2	4	65	16	—	—	46
Caesar Grilled Chicken	1 (11.3 oz)	223	8	1	71	28	13	2	5	98	344	—	—	48
Crispy Chicken Club	1 (13.6 oz)	495	26	5	116	30	29	4	4	72	396	—	—	29
Mandarin Chicken	1 (14.5 oz)	553	31	5	—	15	62	19	14	169	176	—	—	55
Mixed Greens w/o Cheese	1 (17 oz)	194	14	2	3	5	17	9	7	105	224	—	—	41
Salad Blend	1 serv (10.3 oz)	45	1	0	0	3	9	4	5	74	26	—	—	38
Southwest Chicken Chop	1 (17.6 oz)	681	43	6	104	33	44	7	7	90	1165	—	—	30
RAX														
BBQ Beef	1	399	20	—	40	—	43	—	—	—	1030	—	—	—
BBQ Sandwich	1	716	51	—	102	—	37	—	—	—	1453	—	—	—

FOOD	PORTION	CALS	FAT	SAT FAT	CHOL	PROT	CARB	SUGAR	FIBER	CALCI	SOD	POTAS	FOLIC	VIT C
Cheddar Melt	1	346	23	—	41	—	26	—	—	—	539	—	—	—
Deluxe	1	521	34	—	68	—	34	—	—	—	785	—	—	—
Grilled Chicken	1	526	33	—	69	—	32	—	—	—	994	—	—	—
Jr. Deluxe	1	367	25	—	42	—	25	—	—	—	509	—	—	—
Mushroom Melt	1	599	37	—	104	—	35	—	—	—	1688	—	—	—
Philly Melt	1	537	32	—	79	—	35	—	—	—	1296	—	—	—
Regular Rax	1	388	22	—	54	—	31	—	—	—	708	—	—	—
Turkey	1	484	32	—	50	—	32	—	—	—	1286	—	—	—
Turkey Bacon Club	1	680	47	—	76	—	37	—	—	—	1898	—	—	—

RED LOBSTER

BEVERAGES

FOOD	PORTION	CALS	FAT	SAT FAT	CHOL	PROT	CARB	SUGAR	FIBER	CALCI	SOD	POTAS	FOLIC	VIT C
Boston Ice Tea	1 serv	50	0	0	—	—	12	—	—	—	10	—	—	—
Coke	1 serv	100	0	0	—	—	27	—	—	—	35	—	—	—
Diet Coke	1 serv	0	0	0	0	0	0	0	0	—	30	—	—	—
Dr Pepper	1 serv	150	0	0	—	—	27	—	—	—	35	—	—	—
Harbor Cafe Coffee	1 serv	0	0	0	0	0	0	0	0	—	5	—	—	—
Lemonade Light	1 serv	0	0	0	0	—	0	0	0	—	55	—	—	—
Lemonade Raspberry	1 serv	180	0	0	—	—	30	—	—	—	20	—	—	—
Tea Hot or Cold Unsweetened	1 serv	0	0	0	0	0	0	0	0	—	0	—	—	—
Wine Blush	1 glass	120	0	0	—	—	7	—	—	—	20	—	—	—
Wine Red	1 glass	120	0	0	—	—	7	—	—	—	20	—	—	—

MAIN MENU SELECTIONS

FOOD	PORTION	CALS	FAT	SAT FAT	CHOL	PROT	CARB	SUGAR	FIBER	CALCI	SOD	POTAS	FOLIC	VIT C
Arctic Char Grilled Broiled or Blackened w/ Broccoli	1 full portion	630	29	6	—	—	21	—	—	—	720	—	—	—
Arctic Char Grilled Broiled or Blackened w/ Broccoli	1 half portion	340	15	3	—	—	13	—	—	—	460	—	—	—
Barramundi Grilled Broiled or Blackened w/ Broccoli	1 full portion	420	10	3	—	—	11	—	—	—	350	—	—	—
Barramundi Grilled Broiled or Blackened w/ Broccoli	1 half portion	230	5	2	—	—	8	—	—	—	270	—	—	—
Cobia Grilled Broiled or Blackened w/ Broccoli	1 half portion	400	26	8	—	—	6	—	—	—	250	—	—	—

FOOD	PORTION	CALS	FAT	SAT FAT	CHOL	PROT	CARB	SUGAR	FIBER	CALCI	SOD	POTAS	FOLIC	VIT C
Cobia Grilled Broiled or Blackened w/ Broccoli	1 full portion	760	54	17	—	—	8	—	—	—	310	—	—	—
Cod Grilled Broiled or Blackened w/ Broccoli	1 half portion	170	2	0	—	—	8	—	—	—	500	—	—	—
Cod Grilled Broiled or Blackened w/ Broccoli	1 full portion	300	4	1	—	—	10	—	—	—	810	—	—	—
Corvina Grilled Broiled or Blackened w/ Broccoli	1 full portion	320	3	1	—	—	9	—	—	—	420	—	—	—
Corvina Grilled Broiled or Blackened w/ Broccoli	1 half portion	180	2	0	—	—	7	—	—	—	300	—	—	—
Flounder Grilled Broiled or Blackened w/ Broccoli	1 full portion	350	3	0	—	—	11	—	—	—	500	—	—	—
Flounder Grilled Broiled or Blackened w/ Broccoli	1 half portion	200	2	0	—	—	8	—	—	—	350	—	—	—
Grouper Grilled Broiled or Blackened w/ Broccoli	1 full portion	370	3	1	—	—	6	—	—	—	370	—	—	—
Grouper Grilled Broiled or Blackened w/ Broccoli	1 half portion	210	2	0	—	—	6	—	—	—	280	—	—	—
Haddock Grilled Broiled or Blackened w/ Broccoli	1 full portion	310	3	1	—	—	6	—	—	—	850	—	—	—
Haddock Grilled Broiled or Blackened w/Broccoli	1 half portion	180	2	0	—	—	6	—	—	—	520	—	—	—
Lake Whitefish Grilled Broiled or Blackened w/ Broccoli	1 full portion	380	5	1	—	—	6	—	—	—	610	—	—	—

FOOD	PORTION	CALS	FAT	SAT FAT	CHOL	PROT	CARB	SUGAR	FIBER	CALCI	SOD	POTAS	FOLIC	VIT C
Lake Whitefish Grilled Broiled or Blackened w/ Broccoli	1 half portion	210	3	1	—	—	6	—	—	—	400	—	—	—
Mahi Mahi Grilled Broiled or Blackened w/ Broccoli	1 half portion	200	2	0	—	—	6	—	—	—	270	—	—	—
Mahi Mahi Grilled Broiled or Blackened w/ Broccoli	1 full portion	360	2	0	—	—	7	—	—	—	360	—	—	—
Monchong Grilled Broiled or Blackened w/ Broccoli	1 half portion	190	2	0	—	—	7	—	—	—	290	—	—	—
Monchong Grilled Broiled or Blackened w/ Broccoli	1 full portion	340	3	1	—	—	9	—	—	—	390	—	—	—
Opah Grilled Broiled or Blackened w/ Broccoli	1 half portion	280	12	4	—	—	8	—	—	—	280	—	—	—
Opah Grilled Broiled or Blackened w/ Broccoli	1 full portion	510	24	7	—	—	11	—	—	—	380	—	—	—
Perch Grilled Broiled or Blackened w/ Broccoli	1 half portion	170	2	0	—	—	6	—	—	—	550	—	—	—
Perch Grilled Broiled or Blackened w/ Broccoli	1 full portion	300	4	1	—	—	7	—	—	—	910	—	—	—
Pompano Grilled Broiled or Blackened w/ Broccoli	1 half portion	240	8	4	—	—	6	—	—	—	310	—	—	—
Pompano Grilled Broiled or Blackened w/ Broccoli	1 full portion	430	16	7	—	—	7	—	—	—	430	—	—	—
Rainbow Trout Grilled Broiled or Blackened w/ Broccoli	1 half portion	220	10	3	—	—	6	—	—	—	380	—	—	—

FOOD	PORTION	CALS	FAT	SAT FAT	CHOL	PROT	CARB	SUGAR	FIBER	CALCI	SOD	POTAS	FOLIC	VIT C
Red Rockfish Grilled Broiled or Blackened w/ Broccoli	1 half portion	170	3	0	—	—	6	—	—	—	580	—	—	—
Red Rockfish Grilled Broiled or Blackened w/ Broccoli	1 full portion	300	4	1	—	—	10	—	—	—	860	—	—	—
Salmon Grilled Broiled or Blackened w/ Broccoli	1 full portion	490	17	4	—	—	6	—	—	—	440	—	—	—
Salmon Grilled Broiled or Blackened w/ Broccoli	1 half portion	270	9	2	—	—	6	—	—	—	310	—	—	—
Seabass Grilled Broiled or Blackened w/ Broccoli	1 half portion	230	6	2	—	—	6	—	—	—	450	—	—	—
Snapper Grilled Broiled or Blackened w/ Broccoli	1 half portion	210	2	0	—	—	8	—	—	—	330	—	—	—
Sole Grilled Broiled or Blackened w/ Broccoli	1 half portion	140	2	0	—	—	6	—	—	—	860	—	—	—
Tilapia Grilled Broiled or Blackened w/ Broccoli	1 half portion	210	3	1	—	—	9	—	—	—	230	—	—	—
Tuna Grilled Broiled or Blackened w/ Broccoli	1 half portion	200	1	0	—	—	7	—	—	—	420	—	—	—
Wahoo Grilled Broiled or Blackened w/ Broccoli	1 half portion	220	3	1	—	—	8	—	—	—	340	—	—	—
Walleye Grilled Broiled or Blackened w/ Broccoli	1 half portion	170	2	0	—	—	7	—	—	—	400	—	—	—

RED MANGO

FOOD	PORTION	CALS	FAT	SAT FAT	CHOL	PROT	CARB	SUGAR	FIBER	CALCI	SOD	POTAS	FOLIC	VIT C
Blenders Blueberry Moon	1 cup	150	2	1	0	3	33	28	1	100	115	330	—	4
Blenders Captain Berry	1 cup	140	1	0	0	4	31	25	2	100	135	340	40	9

FOOD	PORTION	CALS	FAT	SAT FAT	CHOL	PROT	CARB	SUGAR	FIBER	CALCI	SOD	POTAS	FOLIC	VIT C
Blenders Green Tea Blueberry	1 cup	130	0	0	0	3	29	25	1	100	115	310	—	4
Blenders Green Tea Honeydew	1 cup	130	0	0	0	3	29	25	0	100	125	380	—	9
Blenders Mango Island	1 cup	150	2	2	0	3	31	26	1	100	115	350	—	9
Blenders Pina Colada	1 cup	160	3	3	0	4	30	25	1	100	120	350	—	15
Blenders Tri-Berry	1 cup	130	0	0	0	3	30	25	2	100	115	340	—	12
Blenders Watermelon Breeze	1 cup	130	0	0	0	3	29	25	0	100	115	330	—	9
Frozen Yogurt All Flavors	½ cup	90	0	0	0	3	19	15	0	100	130	260	—	0

ROBEKS

BAKED SELECTIONS

FOOD	PORTION	CALS	FAT	SAT FAT	CHOL	PROT	CARB	SUGAR	FIBER	CALCI	SOD	POTAS	FOLIC	VIT C
Gourmet Pretzels Apple Cinnamon	1	470	25	—	0	12	78	38	3	40	290	—	—	—
Gourmet Pretzels Spinach Feta	1	430	9	—	25	19	70	7	3	300	750	—	—	—
Gourmet Pretzels Tomato Parmesan	1	420	10	—	10	18	67	7	3	200	730	—	—	—
Muffin Banana	1	310	11	—	0	16	43	20	5	—	312	—	—	0
Muffin Blueberry	1	300	10	—	0	16	42	18	5	—	312	—	—	0
Muffin Chocolate	1	320	11	—	0	16	45	17	5	—	384	—	—	0
Power Cookie Breakfast Bar	1	230	10	—	21	3	33	18	1	20	120	—	—	0
Power Cookie Chocolate Chip w/ Walnuts	1	404	12	—	0	14	60	31	5	150	504	—	—	—
Power Cookie Lemon Poppyseed	1	371	7	—	0	14	63	30	4	150	408	—	—	—
Power Cookie Oatmeal Raisin Walnut	1	375	7	—	0	14	64	33	6	100	264	—	—	—
Power Cookie Peanut Butter	1	426	14	—	0	16	59	25	3	150	600	—	—	—

BEVERAGES

FOOD	PORTION	CALS	FAT	SAT FAT	CHOL	PROT	CARB	SUGAR	FIBER	CALCI	SOD	POTAS	FOLIC	VIT C
800 Lb Gorilla	1 (12 oz)	434	9	—	42	30	58	41	2	320	288	—	—	11
Freeze Lemon	1 (12 oz)	282	2	—	9	0	66	40	0	50	48	—	—	6
Freeze Orange	1 (12 oz)	290	1	—	3	8	63	47	0	310	120	—	—	77
Fresh Juice ABC	1 (12 oz)	150	0	0	0	3	33	19	2	90	144	—	—	16
Fresh Juice Apple	1 (12 oz)	180	0	0	0	0	45	45	0	0	24	—	—	108
Fresh Juice Carrot	1 (12 oz)	98	0	0	0	3	22	20	0	80	0	—	—	13

FOOD	PORTION	CALS	FAT	SAT FAT	CHOL	PROT	CARB	SUGAR	FIBER	CALCI	SOD	POTAS	FOLIC	VIT C
Fresh Juice Green-V	1 (12 oz)	96	1	—	0	37	19	11	2	70	312	—	—	4
Fresh Juice G-Snap	1 (12 oz)	120	1	—	0	3	24	14	3	60	216	—	—	4
Fresh Juice Lemonade Raspberry	1 (12 oz)	164	0	0	0	1	40	35	0	20	0	—	—	43
Fresh Juice Monkey C	1 (12 oz)	186	1	—	0	3	44	32	2	40	0	—	—	160
Fresh Juice Orange	1 (12 oz)	168	1	—	0	3	39	31	1	40	0	—	—	186
Naturally Light Banana Mango	1	162	0	0	0	0	42	36	3	10	0	—	—	21
Naturally Light Pineapple Mango	1	172	0	0	0	0	44	40	3	10	0	—	—	85
Naturally Light Raspberry Banana	1	161	0	0	0	1	42	33	3	10	0	—	—	67
Naturally Light Strawberry Pineapple	1	131	0	0	0	0	33	29	3	20	0	—	—	33
Shake Bananasplit	1 (12 oz)	274	0	0	0	3	56	39	2	170	96	—	—	7
Shake P-Nut Power	1 (12 oz)	362	16	—	0	11	39	23	4	180	240	—	—	7
Smoothie Acai Energizer	1 (12 oz)	161	1	—	3	2	33	26	2	60	24	—	—	11
Smoothie Awesome Acai	1 (12 oz)	146	1	—	0	2	32	26	1	60	24	—	—	8
Smoothie Banzai Blueberry	1 (12 oz)	172	2	—	0	2	29	—	2	70	24	—	—	104
Smoothie Berry Brilliance	1 (12 oz)	192	1	—	0	1	45	38	2	60	24	—	—	4
Smoothie Big Wednesday	1 (12 oz)	201	1	—	3	1	49	42	2	40	0	—	—	2
Smoothie Cardio Cooler	1 (12 oz)	244	1	—	3	9	45	45	3	50	48	—	—	166
Smoothie Citrus Stinger	1 (12 oz)	198	1	—	3	5	44	24	2	130	24	—	—	140
Smoothie Cranberry Quest	1 (12 oz)	208	1	—	0	1	49	44	1	60	24	—	—	23
Smoothie Dr. Robeks	1 (12 oz)	186	1	—	0	2	42	31	2	140	0	—	—	203
Smoothie Green Tea Sensation	1 (12 oz)	199	2	—	3	8	37	27	0	200	0	—	—	0
Smoothie Guava Lava	1 (12 oz)	206	1	—	3	0	50	42	2	40	24	—	—	61
Smoothie Hummingbird	1 (12 oz)	211	1	—	3	0	50	43	2	40	24	—	—	55

FOOD	PORTION	CALS	FAT	SAT FAT	CHOL	PROT	CARB	SUGAR	FIBER	CALCI	SOD	POTAS	FOLIC	VIT C
Smoothie Infinite Orange	1 (12 oz)	182	1	—	0	4	42	31	2	110	24	—	—	106
Smoothie Mahalo Mango	1 (12 oz)	201	1	—	3	1	50	45	2	70	24	—	—	23
Smoothie Malibu Peach	1 (12 oz)	181	0	0	0	3	44	38	1	110	24	—	—	89
Smoothie Outrageous Raspberry	1 (12 oz)	182	1	—	3	0	44	40	1	20	24	—	—	79
Smoothie Passionfruit Cove	1 (12 oz)	193	1	—	3	0	46	41	1	20	24	—	—	107
Smoothie Pina Koolada	1 (12 oz)	212	1	—	3	2	50	42	1	70	24	—	—	14
Smoothie Polar Pineapple	1 (12 oz)	183	1	—	3	0	45	40	1	40	0	—	—	28
Smoothie Pomegranate Passion	1 (12 oz)	190	0	0	0	2	46	40	1	100	48	—	—	20
Smoothie Pomegranate Power	1 (12 oz)	217	1	—	0	6	50	42	3	80	48	—	—	71
Smoothie Pro Arobek	1 (12 oz)	260	1	—	0	12	52	40	2	80	24	—	—	5
Smoothie Raspberry Romance	1 (12 oz)	209	0	0	0	3	50	41	2	100	48	—	—	75
Smoothie Robeks Rejuvenator	1 (12 oz)	221	1	—	0	4	51	42	2	120	24	—	—	116
Smoothie South Pacific Squeeze	1 (12 oz)	200	1	—	3	2	47	36	2	40	0	—	—	118
Smoothie Strawnana Berry	1 (12 oz)	188	0	0	0	3	44	37	1	100	48	—	—	13
Smoothie Venice Burner	1 (12 oz)	227	1	—	3	9	48	33	3	30	24	—	—	137
Smoothie Zen Berry	1 (12 oz)	217	1	—	0	3	51	29	4	120	0	—	—	202

SAMURAI SAM'S

BOWLS

FOOD	PORTION	CALS	FAT	SAT FAT	CHOL	PROT	CARB	SUGAR	FIBER	CALCI	SOD	POTAS	FOLIC	VIT C
Low Carb	1 reg	230	4	1	80	33	16	9	5	100	210	—	—	90
Spicy Beef 'N Broccoli	1 reg	620	13	4	50	26	97	20	3	60	1160	—	—	78
Spicy Beef 'N Broccoli Brown Rice	1 reg	580	14	4	50	26	85	19	7	60	1160	—	—	78
Sumo Brown Rice	1	1022	23	7	214	81	111	28	9	100	1513	—	—	48
Sumo White Rice	1	1083	21	6	214	81	128	28	3	80	1509	—	—	48

FOOD	PORTION	CALS	FAT	SAT FAT	CHOL	PROT	CARB	SUGAR	FIBER	CALCI	SOD	POTAS	FOLIC	VIT C
Sweet & Sour Dark Chicken	1 reg	610	10	3	85	32	96	24	6	60	200	—	—	210
Sweet & Sour Dark Chicken Brown Rice	1 reg	570	12	3	85	32	84	24	9	60	200	—	—	210
Sweet & Sour White Chicken	1 reg	580	5	1	80	37	96	24	6	60	210	—	—	210
Sweet & Sour White Chicken Brown Rice	1 reg	540	6	2	80	37	85	24	9	80	210	—	—	210
Teriyaki Dark Chicken	1 reg	540	10	3	85	31	79	13	2	40	500	—	—	24
Teriyaki Dark Chicken Brown Rice	1 reg	500	11	3	85	31	68	11	12	60	510	—	—	24
Teriyaki Dark Chicken & Shrimp	1 reg	492	6	2	140	29	78	12	2	40	563	—	—	21
Teriyaki Dark Chicken & Shrimp Brown Rice	1 reg	451	7	2	290	29	67	12	5	60	565	—	—	21
Teriyaki Dark Chicken & Steak	1 reg	540	9	3	65	27	83	13	2	40	560	—	—	24
Teriyaki Dark Chicken & Steak Brown Rice	1 reg	490	10	3	65	27	71	13	5	40	660	—	—	24
Teriyaki Salmon	1 reg	643	3	1	15	33	121	20	3	40	1223	—	—	36
Teriyaki Shrimp Brown Rice	1 reg	407	3	1	193	28	65	10	5	80	582	—	—	6
Teriyaki Steak	1 reg	530	8	3	50	23	86	13	2	2	810	—	—	24
Teriyaki Steak Brown Rice	1 reg	490	9	3	50	23	74	13	5	40	510	—	—	24
Teriyaki Steak & Shrimp	1 reg	483	5	2	120	26	77	12	2	40	713	—	—	21
Teriyaki Steak & Shrimp Brown Rice	1 reg	442	6	2	120	25	66	12	5	60	715	—	—	21
Teriyaki Veggie	1 reg	363	1	0	0	8	81	13	3	40	393	—	—	48
Teriyaki Veggie Brown Rice	1 reg	323	2	0	0	8	69	13	7	60	395	—	—	48
Teriyaki White Chicken	1 reg	520	4	1	80	37	79	13	2	40	510	—	—	24
Teriyaki White Chicken Brown Rice	1 reg	470	5	2	80	36	68	13	5	60	510	—	—	24
Teriyaki White Chicken & Shrimp	1 reg	478	2	1	127	32	78	12	2	50	567	—	—	17

FOOD	PORTION	CALS	FAT	SAT FAT	CHOL	PROT	CARB	SUGAR	FIBER	CALCI	SOD	POTAS	FOLIC	VIT C
Teriyaki White Chicken & Shrimp Brown Rice	1 reg	437	4	1	137	32	67	12	5	60	570	—	—	21
Teriyaki White Chicken & Steak	1 reg	520	6	2	65	30	83	13	2	40	660	—	—	24
Teriyaki White Chicken & Steak Brown Rice	1 reg	480	7	2	65	30	71	13	5	40	660	—	—	24
Yakisoba Dark Chicken	1	842	24	5	146	60	114	24	6	60	1154	—	—	48
Yakisoba Dark Chicken & Steak	1	825	22	5	114	54	113	25	6	40	1410	—	—	48
Yakisoba Shrimp	1	677	10	1	330	55	110	21	6	100	1283	—	—	54
Yakisoba Steak	1	809	20	5	83	48	112	26	6	40	1667	—	—	48
Yakisoba Veggie	1	509	8	0	0	19	110	21	6	40	902	—	—	48
Yakisoba White Chicken	1	794	14	2	137	70	114	25	6	60	1169	—	—	48
Yakisoba White Chicken & Steak	1	801	17	4	110	59	113	25	6	40	1410	—	—	48
SALADS AND SIDES														
Crab Rangoon	1 serv	210	12	5	35	7	20	12	1	20	260	—	—	0
Dressing Chinese	1 serv (3.5 oz)	230	7	1	0	0	44	43	—	—	1700	—	—	—
Dressing Chinese Ginger	1 serv (1 oz)	85	5	3	0	0	9	9	0	20	153	—	—	0
Dressing Oriental	1 serv (1 oz)	70	2	0	0	0	12	12	0	0	180	—	—	0
Egg Roll Grilled Chicken	1	150	7	0	15	7	17	7	1	0	300	—	—	9
Salad Oriental Chicken	1 serv	220	4	1	90	36	9	5	3	60	200	—	—	24
Salad Sesame Garden Toss	1	490	13	2	90	41	57	33	8	200	1240	—	—	30
Salad Side	1	10	1	0	0	1	2	1	1	20	5	—	—	9
Soup Asian Noodle	1 serv	89	2	0	13	5	14	6	1	20	723	—	—	9
Teriyaki Sauce	1 serv (1 oz)	40	0	0	0	1	9	8	0	0	340	—	—	0
WRAPS														
Teriyaki Dark Chicken	1	670	16	4	75	34	95	13	8	250	1250	—	—	24
Teriyaki Dark Chicken Brown Rice	1	650	17	4	75	34	90	13	9	250	1250	—	—	24
Teriyaki Steak	1	650	14	4	40	27	101	14	8	200	1510	—	—	24
Teriyaki Steak Brown Rice	1	630	15	4	40	27	95	13	9	250	1510	—	—	24
Teriyaki Veggie	1	510	8	2	0	14	94	12	8	250	1130	—	—	27

FOOD	PORTION	CALS	FAT	SAT FAT	CHOL	PROT	CARB	SUGAR	FIBER	CALCI	SOD	POTAS	FOLIC	VIT C
Teriyaki Veggie Brown Rice	1	490	9	2	0	13	89	12	10	250	1130	—	—	27
Teriyaki White Chicken	1	640	11	3	70	39	96	13	8	250	1260	—	—	24
Teriyaki White Chicken Brown Rice	1	620	12	3	70	39	90	13	9	250	1260	—	—	24
Teriyaki White Chicken & Steak	1	649	13	3	55	33	95	13	8	250	1384	—	—	24
Teriyaki White Chicken & Steak Brown Rice	1	628	13	3	55	33	89	13	9	250	1385	—	—	24

SCHLOTZSKY'S DELI

CHILDREN'S MENU SELECTIONS

FOOD	PORTION	CALS	FAT	SAT FAT	CHOL	PROT	CARB	SUGAR	FIBER	CALCI	SOD	POTAS	FOLIC	VIT C
Pizza Cheese	1 serv	479	13	5	24	18	73	3	3	—	1060	—	—	—
Pizza Pepperoni	1 serv	523	17	6	33	20	73	3	3	—	1246	—	—	—
Sandwich Cheese	1	394	15	8	40	17	48	2	2	—	772	—	—	—
Sandwich Ham & Cheese	1	424	16	8	30	21	49	3	2	—	1147	—	—	—
Sandwich Turkey	1	300	5	1	20	13	49	2	2	—	750	—	—	—

DESSERTS

FOOD	PORTION	CALS	FAT	SAT FAT	CHOL	PROT	CARB	SUGAR	FIBER	CALCI	SOD	POTAS	FOLIC	VIT C
Carrot Cake	1 serv	717	42	6	74	7	80	56	3	—	767	—	—	—
Cookie Chocolate Chip	1	160	8	5	20	2	22	13	1	—	160	—	—	—
Cookie Fudge Chocolate Chip	1	160	8	5	25	2	22	14	1	—	190	—	—	—
Cookie Oatmeal Raisin	1	150	6	3	20	2	22	14	1	—	115	—	—	—
Cookie Sugar	1	160	7	4	0	2	22	11	0	—	200	—	—	—
Cookie White Chocolate Macadamia	1	170	9	5	20	2	21	13	1	—	170	—	—	—

MAIN MENU SELECTIONS

FOOD	PORTION	CALS	FAT	SAT FAT	CHOL	PROT	CARB	SUGAR	FIBER	CALCI	SOD	POTAS	FOLIC	VIT C
Salad Caesar	1 serv	103	5	2	6	6	10	3	3	—	289	—	—	—
Salad Garden	1 serv	51	1	0	0	3	12	4	4	—	291	—	—	—
Salad Grilled Chicken Caesar	1 serv	221	8	2	65	53	12	3	3	—	759	—	—	—
Salad Turkey Chef	1 serv	309	18	7	67	26	14	6	4	—	1412	—	—	—
Sandwich Angus Roast Beef & Cheese	1 sm	534	22	11	85	33	50	3	2	—	1424	—	—	—
Sandwich Chicken Breast	1 sm	342	4	0	46	39	52	6	3	—	1341	—	—	—
Sandwich Fresh Veggie	1 sm	342	10	5	22	19	50	6	4	—	751	—	—	—
Sandwich Ham & Cheese	1 sm	508	19	9	80	31	54	5	3	—	2033	—	—	—

FOOD	PORTION	CALS	FAT	SAT FAT	CHOL	PROT	CARB	SUGAR	FIBER	CALCI	SOD	POTAS	FOLIC	VIT C
Sandwich Smoked Turkey Breast	1 sm	353	6	1	35	20	52	4	2	—	1070	—	—	—
Sandwich The Original	1 sm	559	26	12	85	28	52	4	3	—	1834	—	—	—
Sandwich Turkey	1 sm	602	27	11	96	34	54	5	3	—	1832	—	—	—
Sandwich Turkey Bacon	1 sm	561	25	10	83	32	51	4	3	—	1660	—	—	—
Wraps Asian Chicken	1	537	12	3	59	56	80	26	5	—	2143	—	—	—
Wraps Parmesan Chicken Caesar	1	556	21	6	86	61	61	5	5	—	1728	—	—	—

SKIPPERS

CHILDREN'S MENU SELECTIONS

FOOD	PORTION	CALS	FAT	SAT FAT	CHOL	PROT	CARB	SUGAR	FIBER	CALCI	SOD	POTAS	FOLIC	VIT C
Kids Catch Chicken Tenderloin + Chips & Kids Side	1 serv	560	11	4	30	20	79	24	1	—	1040	—	—	—
Kids Catch Fish Bites + Chips & Kids Side	1 serv	490	15	8	0	15	84	26	3	—	1270	—	—	—
Kids Catch Sandwich Grilled Cheese + Chips & Kids Side	1 serv	620	19	7	20	14	97	27	3	—	1150	—	—	—
Kids Catch & Kids Side	1 serv	520	11	3	50	14	91	25	2	—	1150	—	—	—

MAIN MENU SELECTIONS

FOOD	PORTION	CALS	FAT	SAT FAT	CHOL	PROT	CARB	SUGAR	FIBER	CALCI	SOD	POTAS	FOLIC	VIT C
Baked Potato Plain	1	210	0	0	0	6	48	3	5	—	25	—	—	—
Basket Chicken & Fish + Chips & Slaw	1 serv	620	27	9	45	26	59	5	1	—	1650	—	—	—
Basket Chicken & Shrimp + Chips & Slaw	1 serv	760	25	5	120	33	84	5	1	—	2060	—	—	—
Basket Chicken & Slaw	2 pieces	730	25	7	70	33	60	4	0	—	1650	—	—	—
Basket Clam Strips + Chips & Slaw	1 serv	890	34	6	75	38	113	4	12	—	1670	—	—	—
Basket Clams & Fish + Chips & Slaw	1 serv	740	32	9	50	30	91	5	8	—	1720	—	—	—
Basket Original Recipe Shrimp + Chips & Slaw	1 serv	800	25	4	165	32	107	6	3	—	2470	—	—	—
Basket Popcorn Shrimp + Chips & Slaw	1 serv	750	25	5	180	33	96	5	2	—	2090	—	—	—

FOOD	PORTION	CALS	FAT	SAT FAT	CHOL	PROT	CARB	SUGAR	FIBER	CALCI	SOD	POTAS	FOLIC	VIT C
Basket Prawn & Fish + Chips & Slaw	1 serv	730	41	10	235	38	61	5	2	—	1600	—	—	—
Basket Prawn Seafood + Chips & Slaw	1 serv	720	40	7	280	36	52	4	tr	—	1200	—	—	—
Basket Shrimp & Fish + Chips & Slaw	1 serv	650	27	8	90	25	83	6	2	—	2060	—	—	—
Basket Shrimp Trio + Chips & Slaw	1 serv	1040	38	9	305	56	123	7	4	—	3020	—	—	—
Clam Chowder	1 cup	120	8	0	5	3	14	1	tr	—	600	—	—	—
Clam Strips	1 serv	270	6	1	30	17	39	0	6	—	490	—	—	—
Coleslaw	1 sm	170	16	3	15	1	7	4	0	—	190	—	—	—
Fish Bites + Chips & Slaw	6 pieces	490	17	4	0	7	94	0	7	—	1630	—	—	—
French Fries	1 reg	180	6	2	0	3	27	0	0	—	500	—	—	—
Grilled Veggies	1 serv	35	0	0	0	2	8	3	3	—	50	—	—	—
Halibut + Chips & Slaw	1 serv	580	30	5	45	23	51	4	0	—	1280	—	—	—
Homestyle Chicken Tenderloin	1 piece	190	2	2	30	15	13	0	0	—	480	—	—	—
Hush Puppies	3 pieces	240	9	2	0	3	47	0	3	—	820	—	—	—
Original Fish Fillet	1 piece	80	4	4	0	7	12	1	1	—	480	—	—	—
Original Fish + Chips & Slaw	2 pieces	510	29	11	15	18	59	6	2	—	1650	—	—	—
Original Shrimp	9 pieces	220	2	0	75	14	36	1	1	—	890	—	—	—
Sandwich Fish + Chips & Slaw	1 serv	800	34	9	20	22	105	14	4	—	1780	—	—	—
Sandwich Fried Chicken + Chips & Slaw	1 serv	1260	49	15	105	52	117	12	3	—	2390	—	—	—
Sandwich Grilled Chicken + Chips & Slaw	1 serv	1070	50	13	145	57	92	12	3	—	1510	—	—	—
Skippers Platter + Chips & Slaw	1 serv	930	33	9	12	42	122	6	8	—	2550	—	—	—
SALADS														
Caesar	1 sm	150	13	3	5	2	8	4	2	—	300	—	—	—
Caesar w/ Chicken	1 sm	340	17	4	100	37	8	4	2	—	380	—	—	—
Caesar w/ Salmon	1 sm	350	19	4	80	35	8	4	2	—	380	—	—	—
Green Salad w/o Dressing	1 sm	25	0	0	0	1	5	3	2	—	20	—	—	—

SMOOTHIE KING

FOOD	PORTION	CALS	FAT	SAT FAT	CHOL	PROT	CARB	SUGAR	FIBER	CALCI	SOD	POTAS	FOLIC	VIT C
Acai Adventure	1 (20 oz)	435	5	1	6	5	92	74	4	—	163	—	—	—
Angel Food	1 (20 oz)	354	0	0	1	4	84	75	6	—	50	—	—	—
Banana Berry Treat	1 (20 oz)	364	0	0	6	4	86	75	5	—	129	—	—	—
Banana Boat	1 (20 oz)	524	12	6	51	11	97	77	6	—	299	—	—	—
Berry Punch	1 (20 oz)	360	0	0	0	0	91	84	4	—	95	—	—	—
Blackberry Dream	1 (20 oz)	365	1	0	0	2	88	68	2	—	8	—	—	—
Blueberry Heaven	1 (20 oz)	325	1	0	11	7	73	64	2	—	259	—	—	—
Caribbean Way	1 (20 oz)	395	0	0	0	1	97	89	6	—	4	—	—	—
Celestial Cherry High	1 (20 oz)	257	0	0	0	1	64	55	3	—	10	—	—	—
Cherry Picket	1 (20 oz)	273	1	0	6	4	66	54	2	—	237	—	—	—
Coconut Surprise	1 (20 oz)	460	7	6	3	7	90	83	3	—	145	—	—	—
Coffee Smoothie Caramel	1 (20 oz)	340	1	0	13	14	66	56	0	—	236	—	—	—
Coffee Smoothie Mocha	1 (20 oz)	260	2	0	18	17	43	36	1	—	226	—	—	—
Coffee Smoothie Vanilla	1 (20 oz)	347	1	0	8	14	69	65	0	—	236	—	—	—
Cranberry Cooler	1 (20 oz)	496	0	0	0	1	120	89	3	—	38	—	—	—
Cranberry Supreme	1 (20 oz)	554	1	0	0	4	130	96	3	—	87	—	—	—
Fruit Fusion	1 (20 oz)	355	1	0	12	9	76	66	0	—	301	—	—	—
Go Goji	1 (20 oz)	433	0	0	0	1	104	104	0	—	38	—	—	—
Grape Expectations	1 (20 oz)	398	0	0	0	1	95	90	3	—	9	—	—	—
Grape Expectations II	1 (20 oz)	548	0	0	0	2	133	125	6	—	9	—	—	—
Green Tea Tango	1 (20 oz)	282	3	2	16	8	52	40	2	—	190	—	—	—
Hearty Apple	1 (20 oz)	405	1	0	16	9	86	75	2	—	271	—	—	—
High Protein Almond Mocha	1 (20 oz)	366	9	1	51	30	42	37	2	—	195	—	—	—
High Protein Banana	1 (20 oz)	322	9	1	45	27	32	23	4	—	297	—	—	—
High Protein Chocolate	1 (20 oz)	366	9	1	51	30	45	37	2	—	194	—	—	—
High Protein Lemon	1 (20 oz)	372	9	1	45	26	44	40	1	—	297	—	—	—
High Protein Pineapple	1 (20 oz)	320	9	1	45	28	29	23	2	—	336	—	—	—
Immune Builder	1 (20 oz)	380	1	0	0	5	89	77	6	—	57	—	—	—
Instant Vigor	1 (20 oz)	366	0	0	6	4	86	72	4	—	139	—	—	—
Island Impact	1 (20 oz)	311	0	0	6	3	73	65	1	—	142	—	—	—
Island Treat	1 (20 oz)	333	0	0	0	2	82	70	6	—	11	—	—	—
Kids' Kup Berry Interesting	1 (12 oz)	277	0	0	0	1	69	62	3	—	11	—	—	—

FOOD	PORTION	CALS	FAT	SAT FAT	CHOL	PROT	CARB	SUGAR	FIBER	CALCI	SOD	POTAS	FOLIC	VIT C
Kids' Kup Choc-A-Laka	1 (12 oz)	245	3	1	28	11	44	32	2	—	177	—	—	—
Kids' Kup CW Jr.	1 (12 oz)	270	0	0	0	1	68	59	5	—	3	—	—	—
Kids' Kup Gimmi-Grape	1 (12 oz)	265	0	0	0	1	64	60	2	—	9	—	—	—
Kids' Kup Smarti Tarti	1 (12 oz)	200	0	0	0	1	49	46	0	—	9	—	—	—
Kiwi Island Treat	1 (20 oz)	498	1	0	6	6	116	96	0	—	147	—	—	—
Lemon Twist Banana	1 (20 oz)	358	0	0	0	1	87	82	3	—	9	—	—	—
Lemon Twist Strawberry	1 (20 oz)	438	0	0	0	1	107	104	3	—	9	—	—	—
Light & Fluffy	1 (20 oz)	395	0	0	0	1	99	89	6	—	0	—	—	—
Low Carb All Flavors	1 (20 oz)	268	9	4	3	39	7	3	1	—	176	—	—	—
Malts	1 (20 oz)	680	33	18	127	14	83	77	0	—	292	—	—	—
Mangofest	1 (20 oz)	285	0	0	0	0	72	69	1	—	10	—	—	—
Mangosteen Madness	1 (20 oz)	383	0	0	0	1	94	92	2	—	29	—	—	—
Mo'cuccino Mocha	1 (20 oz)	444	12	6	59	10	73	69	1	—	125	—	—	—
Mo'cuccino Vanilla	1 (20 oz)	525	12	6	51	10	92	85	0	—	301	—	—	—
Mo'cuccino Caramel	1 (20 oz)	570	12	6	56	10	102	88	0	—	301	—	—	—
Muscle Punch	1 (20 oz)	364	1	0	1	5	84	75	6	—	50	—	—	—
Muscle Punch Plus	1 (20 oz)	366	1	0	1	5	84	75	6	—	57	—	—	—
Orange Ka-Bam	1 (20 oz)	465	0	0	0	1	117	108	3	—	190	—	—	—
Organic Apple Acai	1 (20 oz)	353	5	1	0	3	74	58	4	—	64	—	—	—
Passion Passport	1 (20 oz)	395	0	0	0	1	96	93	2	—	10	—	—	—
Peach Slice	1 (20 oz)	314	0	0	1	3	72	55	1	—	63	—	—	—
Peach Slice Plus	1 (20 oz)	464	0	0	1	4	110	90	4	—	63	—	—	—
Peanut Power	1 (20 oz)	549	22	4	1	15	74	59	6	—	64	—	—	—
Peanut Power Plus Chocolate	1 (20 oz)	717	27	4	25	24	98	63	6	—	376	—	—	—
Peanut Power Plus Grape	1 (20 oz)	749	22	4	1	15	122	107	6	—	64	—	—	—
Peanut Power Plus Strawberry	1 (20 oz)	699	22	4	1	15	112	94	9	—	64	—	—	—
Pep Upper	1 (20 oz)	411	0	0	6	4	97	85	3	—	131	—	—	—
Pina Colada Island	1 (20 oz)	600	10	8	14	13	110	98	3	—	438	—	—	—
Pineapple Pleasure	1 (20 oz)	280	0	0	0	1	67	62	3	—	21	—	—	—
Pineapple Surf	1 (20 oz)	461	1	0	11	7	104	92	4	—	279	—	—	—
Pomegranate Punch	1 (20 oz)	464	0	0	0	1	110	108	1	—	9	—	—	—

FOOD	PORTION	CALS	FAT	SAT FAT	CHOL	PROT	CARB	SUGAR	FIBER	CALCI	SOD	POTAS	FOLIC	VIT C
Power Punch	1 (20 oz)	428	1	0	1	5	101	76	6	—	50	—	—	—
Power Punch Plus	1 (20 oz)	500	2	0	10	8	113	85	6	—	59	—	—	—
Raspberry Collider	1 (20 oz)	338	0	0	0	1	86	74	4	—	102	—	—	—
Raspberry Sunrise	1 (20 oz)	392	0	0	0	2	95	73	2	—	22	—	—	—
Shakes	1 (20 oz)	670	33	18	127	14	81	76	0	—	292	—	—	—
Slim-N-Trim Chocolate	1 (20 oz)	297	2	0	39	15	57	48	3	—	165	—	—	—
Slim-N-Trim Orange Vanilla	1 (20 oz)	215	1	0	11	7	46	38	0	—	259	—	—	—
Slim-N-Trim Strawberry	1 (20 oz)	375	1	0	11	8	84	72	5	—	259	—	—	—
Slim-N-Trim Vanilla	1 (20 oz)	253	1	0	11	7	53	42	3	—	259	—	—	—
Strawberry Kiwi Breeze	1 (20 oz)	376	0	0	6	4	90	84	3	—	131	—	—	—
Strawberry X-treme	1 (20 oz)	366	0	0	0	1	92	70	6	—	7	—	—	—
Super Punch	1 (20 oz)	395	0	0	0	1	100	90	6	—	194	—	—	—
Super Punch Plus	1 (20 oz)	459	0	0	0	1	117	91	6	—	194	—	—	—
The Activator Chocolate	1 (20 oz)	404	1	0	11	19	83	56	5	—	119	—	—	—
The Activator Strawberry	1 (20 oz)	556	1	0	7	19	121	89	8	—	209	—	—	—
The Activator Vanilla	1 (20 oz)	406	1	0	7	18	83	54	5	—	209	—	—	—
The Hulk Chocolate	1 (20 oz)	876	31	12	84	26	124	90	6	—	292	—	—	—
The Hulk Strawberry	1 (20 oz)	1035	32	13	87	27	161	125	8	—	317	—	—	—
The Hulk Vanilla	1 (20 oz)	872	32	13	89	25	121	88	5	—	288	—	—	—
The Shredder Chocolate	1 (20 oz)	311	3	0	45	39	36	19	1	—	315	—	—	—
The Shredder Strawberry	1 (20 oz)	356	1	0	11	30	56	41	3	—	329	—	—	—
The Shredder Vanilla	1 (20 oz)	283	2	0	22	36	30	12	0	—	592	—	—	—
Yerba Mate Mango	1 (20 oz)	372	0	0	0	1	92	76	1	—	13	—	—	—
Yerba Mate Mixed Berry	1 (20 oz)	348	0	0	1	2	84	81	3	—	22	—	—	—
Yerba Mate Pomegranate	1 (20 oz)	372	0	0	0	1	91	73	2	—	9	—	—	—
Yogurt D-Lite	1 (20 oz)	333	4	2	22	13	59	47	0	—	369	—	—	—
Youth Fountain	1 (20 oz)	253	0	0	0	3	61	54	3	—	29	—	—	—

SONIC DRIVE-IN

ADD-ONS

FOOD	PORTION	CALS	FAT	SAT FAT	CHOL	PROT	CARB	SUGAR	FIBER	CALCI	SOD	POTAS	FOLIC	VIT C
Bacon	1 serv (0.5 oz)	70	5	2	15	4	0	0	0	0	260	—	—	0
Cheese	1 serv (0.7 oz)	60	5	3	20	3	2	1	0	100	310	—	—	0

FOOD	PORTION	CALS	FAT	SAT FAT	CHOL	PROT	CARB	SUGAR	FIBER	CALCI	SOD	POTAS	FOLIC	VIT C
Chili	1 serv (1.2 oz)	50	4	2	10	3	2	1	1	20	160	—	—	1
Green Chilies	1 serv (1 oz)	5	0	0	0	0	1	0	0	0	5	—	—	9
Grilled Onions	1 serv (1 oz)	25	2	0	0	0	2	1	1	0	200	—	—	0
Jalapenos	1 serv (0.7 oz)	5	0	0	0	0	1	0	1	20	280	—	—	0
Slaw	1 serv (1 oz)	45	3	1	5	0	4	1	1	20	45	—	—	48
BEVERAGES														
Barq's Root Beer	1 sm (14 oz)	160	0	0	0	0	43	43	0	0	35	—	—	0
Coca-Cola	1 sm (14 oz)	140	0	0	0	0	39	39	0	0	10	—	—	0
Cream Pie Shake Banana	1 reg (14 oz)	590	19	11	55	7	98	83	1	250	220	—	—	4
Cream Pie Shake Chocolate	1 reg (14 oz)	660	19	11	80	7	114	96	0	250	300	—	—	0
Cream Pie Shake Coconut Cream	1 reg (14 oz)	580	20	12	60	7	93	82	0	250	230	—	—	0
CreamSlush Blue Coconut	1 reg (14 oz)	430	13	8	45	5	76	69	0	200	160	—	—	0
CreamSlush Cherry	1 reg (14 oz)	440	13	8	45	5	77	71	0	200	160	—	—	0
CreamSlush Grape	1 reg (14 oz)	430	13	8	45	5	76	70	0	200	160	—	—	0
CreamSlush Orange	1 reg (14 oz)	430	13	8	45	5	77	70	0	200	160	—	—	0
CreamSlush Strawberry	1 reg (14 oz)	450	12	7	45	5	84	72	1	200	150	—	—	9
CreamSlush Watermelon	1 reg (14 oz)	440	13	8	45	5	77	70	0	200	160	—	—	0
Dict Coke	1 sm (14 oz)	0	0	0	0	0	0	0	0	0	15	—	—	0
Dr Pepper	1 sm (14 oz)	130	0	0	0	0	37	37	0	0	45	—	—	0
Float Barq's Root Beer	1 reg (14 oz)	300	8	5	30	3	56	52	0	100	110	—	—	0
Float Coca-Cola	1 reg (14 oz)	290	8	5	30	3	54	50	0	100	95	—	—	0
Float Dr Pepper	1 reg (14 oz)	310	8	5	30	3	58	54	0	100	120	—	—	0
Limeade	1 sm (14 oz)	140	0	0	0	0	38	37	0	0	30	—	—	2
Limeade Cherry	1 sm (14 oz)	170	0	0	0	0	45	44	0	0	35	—	—	2
Limeade Strawberry	1 sm (14 oz)	170	0	0	0	0	45	41	0	0	35	—	—	6
Malt Banana	1 reg (14 oz)	490	17	10	60	7	78	65	1	250	200	—	—	4
Malt Caramel	1 reg (14 oz)	550	18	11	65	7	90	78	0	250	330	—	—	0
Malt Chocolate	1 reg (14 oz)	550	17	10	60	7	91	76	0	250	280	—	—	0
Malt Hot Fudge	1 reg (14 oz)	580	22	15	60	7	87	73	1	250	250	—	—	0
Malt Peanut Butter	1 reg (14 oz)	870	36	14	60	11	78	65	0	250	320	—	—	0
Malt Peanut Butter Fudge	1 reg (14 oz)	620	29	14	60	9	83	69	1	250	290	—	—	0
Malt Pineapple	1 reg (14 oz)	510	17	10	60	7	82	68	0	250	210	—	—	48
Malt Strawberry	1 reg (14 oz)	520	17	10	60	7	85	71	1	250	210	—	—	9
Malt Vanilla	1 reg (14 oz)	480	18	11	65	7	72	64	0	250	210	—	—	0

FOOD	PORTION	CALS	FAT	SAT FAT	CHOL	PROT	CARB	SUGAR	FIBER	CALCI	SOD	POTAS	FOLIC	VIT C
Milk 1%	8.5 oz	110	3	2	10	8	13	12	0	300	130	—	—	0
Milk Chocolate 1%	8.5 oz	160	3	2	10	8	27	25	0	300	210	—	—	0
Shake Banana	1 reg (14 oz)	470	16	10	60	7	76	63	1	250	190	—	—	1
Shake Chocolate	1 reg (14 oz)	540	16	10	60	6	89	74	0	250	270	—	—	0
Shake Hot Fudge	1 reg (14 oz)	570	21	14	60	6	85	71	1	250	240	—	—	0
Shake Peanut Butter	1 reg (14 oz)	640	34	13	60	10	75	63	0	250	300	—	—	0
Shake Peanut Butter Fudge	1 reg (14 oz)	610	28	14	60	8	81	68	1	250	280	—	—	0
Shake Pineapple	1 reg (14 oz)	500	16	10	60	6	80	66	0	250	200	—	—	48
Shake Strawberry	1 reg (14 oz)	510	16	10	60	7	83	69	1	250	200	—	—	9
Shake Vanilla	1 reg (14 oz)	470	17	11	65	7	71	62	0	250	200	—	—	0
Sonic Blast Butterfinger	1 reg (14 oz)	580	22	13	60	8	88	72	0	250	240	—	—	0
Sonic Blast M&M's	1 reg (14 oz)	600	24	15	60	8	88	78	1	300	210	—	—	0
Sonic Blast Oreo	1 reg (14 oz)	540	21	12	60	7	80	67	1	250	280	—	—	0
Sonic Blast Reese's Peanut Butter Cup	1 reg (14 oz)	560	19	12	65	9	89	74	1	300	250	—	—	0
Sprite	1 sm (14 oz)	104	0	0	0	0	37	37	0	0	30	—	—	0
Sprite Zero	1 sm (14 oz)	5	0	0	0	0	0	0	0	0	10	—	—	0
BREAKFAST SELECTIONS														
Breakfast Jr.	1 (4.1 oz)	330	21	8	235	13	25	1	2	200	790	—	—	0
Breakfast Burrito Sausage Egg Cheese	1 (5.9 oz)	480	31	11	325	18	38	2	1	350	1200	—	—	0
Breakfast Toaster Bacon Egg Cheese	1 (5.6 oz)	530	32	10	325	20	40	7	2	200	1440	—	—	0
Breakfast Toaster Ham Egg Cheese	1 (6.5 oz)	490	26	8	325	24	40	6	2	200	1700	—	—	0
Breakfast Toaster Sausage Egg Cheese	1 (6.8 oz)	620	42	13	340	20	40	6	2	200	1380	—	—	0
CroisSonic Bacon	1 (5.3 oz)	510	36	15	320	18	29	5	0	150	1400	—	—	0
CroisSonic Sausage	1 (6.2 oz)	600	46	18	340	19	29	5	0	150	1340	—	—	0
DESSERTS														
Apple Slice w/ Fat Free Caramel Dipping Sauce	1 serv (3.4 oz)	120	0	0	0	0	27	23	2	20	60	—	—	48
Apple Slices	1 serv (2.4 oz)	35	0	0	0	0	9	7	2	0	0	—	—	48
Banana Split	1 (10.8 oz)	420	9	6	30	4	80	57	2	150	140	—	—	36
Cone Vanilla	1 (4.7 oz)	180	6	4	25	2	30	22	0	100	80	—	—	0
Dish Vanilla	1 (6.5 oz)	240	9	5	35	3	36	32	0	150	100	—	—	0
Sundae Chocolate	1 (8.9 oz)	410	13	9	35	4	67	55	0	150	190	—	—	0

FOOD	PORTION	CALS	FAT	SAT FAT	CHOL	PROT	CARB	SUGAR	FIBER	CALCI	SOD	POTAS	FOLIC	VIT C
Sundae Hot Fudge	1 (8.9 oz)	440	18	13	35	4	63	52	1	150	170	—	—	0
Sundae Pineapple	1 (8.8 oz)	370	13	9	35	4	58	47	0	150	125	—	—	48
Sundae Strawberry	1 (8.8 oz)	380	13	9	35	4	61	49	1	150	120	—	—	9
MAIN MENU SELECTIONS														
California Cheeseburger	1 (9.3 oz)	690	39	13	80	29	57	13	5	250	1060	—	—	6
Ched 'R' Bites	12 (3 oz)	280	15	6	30	13	22	0	1	350	740	—	—	0
Ched 'R' Peppers	4 (4.2 oz)	330	17	6	25	8	36	2	2	150	1110	—	—	0
Chicken Strip Dinner	1 serv (13.5 oz)	930	43	8	65	36	100	7	7	80	1610	—	—	5
Chicken Strips	2 (2.5 oz)	200	11	2	30	14	10	0	1	0	470	—	—	1
Chili Cheeseburger	1 (7.9 oz)	660	35	14	85	31	56	11	5	250	990	—	—	1
Coney Extra Long Chili Cheese	1 (9 oz)	660	39	15	95	28	55	7	4	300	1860	—	—	1
Coney Regular	1 (5.2 oz)	390	23	9	60	17	32	4	2	200	1090	—	—	1
Corn Dog	1 (2.6 oz)	210	11	4	20	6	23	4	2	40	530	—	—	0
Crispy Chicken Bacon Ranch	1 serv (8.9 oz)	610	34	9	70	30	48	10	4	200	1730	—	—	5
French Fries	1 sm (2.5 oz)	200	8	2	0	2	30	0	2	20	270	—	—	1
French Fries w/ Cheese	1 sm (3 oz)	270	13	5	20	5	32	1	2	100	590	—	—	1
French Fries w/ Chili & Cheese	1 sm (4.1 oz)	300	16	6	25	8	33	1	3	150	540	—	—	2
Fritos Chili Pie	1 med (4.8 oz)	470	32	9	30	13	36	1	3	150	770	—	—	1
Green Chili Cheeseburger	1 (10 oz)	630	31	12	75	29	56	12	5	250	1070	—	—	15
Grilled Chicken Bacon Ranch	1 serv (8.9 oz)	470	22	7	105	35	35	10	3	200	1620	—	—	5
Hickory Cheeseburger	1 (8.3 oz)	640	31	12	75	28	61	17	5	250	1170	—	—	5
Jalapeno Burger	1 (7.6 oz)	550	26	9	60	25	53	10	5	150	880	—	—	1
Jalapeno Cheeseburger	1 (8.3 oz)	620	31	12	80	28	54	11	5	250	1200	—	—	1
Jr. Bacon Cheeseburger	1 (5 oz)	410	23	10	60	20	31	8	3	200	1060	—	—	2
Jr. Burger	1 (4.1 oz)	310	15	5	35	15	30	7	3	100	610	—	—	2
Jr. Burger Deluxe	1 (4.7 oz)	350	20	6	40	15	28	4	3	100	440	—	—	2
Jr. Double Cheeseburger	1 (6.7 oz)	570	35	16	110	30	33	9	3	300	1290	—	—	2
Jumbo Popcorn Chicken	1 sm (4 oz)	380	22	4	45	18	27	1	3	20	1250	—	—	0
Mozzarella Sticks	1 serv (5 oz)	440	22	9	45	19	40	1	2	450	1050	—	—	0
Onion Rings	1 med (5.5 oz)	440	21	4	0	6	55	14	3	20	430	—	—	0
Pickle-O's	1 serv (4 oz)	310	16	3	0	5	36	2	2	80	1020	—	—	0

FOOD	PORTION	CALS	FAT	SAT FAT	CHOL	PROT	CARB	SUGAR	FIBER	CALCI	SOD	POTAS	FOLIC	VIT C
Sandwich Breaded Pork Fritter	1 (8.5 oz)	640	33	6	30	22	66	11	7	150	840	—	—	4
Sandwich Crispy Chicken	1 (7.9 oz)	550	32	5	45	22	46	8	4	100	1070	—	—	4
Sandwich Fish	1 (8.6 oz)	650	31	5	40	22	71	12	7	150	1160	—	—	1
Sandwich Grilled Cheese	1 (3.9 oz)	380	20	8	35	12	39	6	2	250	1010	—	—	0
Sandwich Grilled Chicken	1 (7.8 oz)	400	19	3	80	28	32	8	3	100	960	—	—	4
Sonic Bacon Cheeseburger w/ Mayonnaise	1 (9.8 oz)	780	48	16	100	33	57	12	5	250	1300	—	—	6
Sonic Burger w/ Ketchup	1 (8.7 oz)	560	26	9	60	26	57	14	5	150	820	—	—	9
Sonic Burger w/ Mayonnaise	1 (8.7 oz)	650	37	10	70	26	55	11	5	150	720	—	—	6
Sonic Burger w/ Mustard	1 (8.5 oz)	560	26	9	60	26	54	11	5	150	750	—	—	6
Sonic Cheeseburger w/ Ketchup	1 (9.3 oz)	630	31	12	75	29	59	15	5	250	1140	—	—	9
Sonic Cheeseburger w/ Mayonnaise	1 (9.3 oz)	720	42	14	90	29	56	12	5	250	1040	—	—	6
Sonic Cheeseburger w/ Mustard	1 (9.1 oz)	620	31	12	75	29	55	12	5	250	1070	—	—	6
SuperSonic Cheeseburger w/ Ketchup	1 (12 oz)	900	53	22	155	46	60	16	5	350	1540	—	—	9
SuperSonic Cheeseburger w/ Mayonnaise	1 (12 oz)	980	64	24	165	46	58	13	5	350	1430	—	—	6
SuperSonic Cheeseburger w/ Mustard	1 (11.8 oz)	890	53	22	155	46	57	13	5	350	1480	—	—	6
Thousand Island Burger	1 (8.7 oz)	610	32	10	65	26	56	13	5	150	810	—	—	6
Toaster Sandwich Bacon Cheeseburger	1 (8.5 oz)	670	39	14	90	29	52	13	3	200	1440	—	—	6
Toaster Sandwich BLT	1 (5.2 oz)	500	29	7	40	17	45	7	2	100	950	—	—	4
Toaster Sandwich Chicken Club	1 (9 oz)	740	46	11	80	29	55	7	4	200	1740	—	—	4
Toaster Sandwich Country Fried Steak	1 (8.5 oz)	670	37	10	50	14	71	6	4	100	1370	—	—	4
Tots	1 sm (1.5 oz)	130	8	2	0	1	13	0	1	20	270	—	—	0

FOOD	PORTION	CALS	FAT	SAT FAT	CHOL	PROT	CARB	SUGAR	FIBER	CALCI	SOD	POTAS	FOLIC	VIT C
Tots w/ Cheese	1 sm (2.2 oz)	190	13	5	20	4	14	1	1	100	590	—	—	0
Tots w/ Chili & Cheese	1 sm (3.2 oz)	220	16	6	25	7	16	1	2	100	540	—	—	1
Wrap Crispy Chicken	1 (8.2 oz)	490	23	5	40	21	49	5	3	150	1280	—	—	6
Wrap Fritos Chili Cheese	1 (8.5 oz)	670	39	13	50	21	66	3	4	350	1420	—	—	2
Wrap Grilled Chicken	1 (8.8 oz)	390	14	4	80	28	39	5	2	200	1420	—	—	5
SALAD DRESSINGS AND SAUCES														
Dressing Honey Mustard	1 serv (1.5 oz)	180	16	3	10	1	10	8	0	0	240	—	—	0
Dressing Italian Fat Free	1 serv (1.5 oz)	40	0	0	0	0	10	3	0	0	450	—	—	1
Dressing Original Ranch	1 serv (1.5 oz)	190	20	4	15	1	2	1	0	0	380	—	—	0
Dressing Original Ranch Light	1 serv (1.5 oz)	110	5	1	10	3	14	3	0	100	590	—	—	0
Dressing Thousand Island	1 serv (1.5 oz)	190	19	3	20	1	7	5	0	0	440	—	—	1
Sauce BBQ	1 serv (1 oz)	45	0	0	0	0	11	7	0	0	390	—	—	0
Sauce Honey Mustard	1 serv (1 oz)	90	7	1	10	0	7	5	0	0	190	—	—	0
Sauce Marinara	1 serv (1 oz)	15	0	0	0	0	3	2	1	0	270	—	—	0
Sauce Ranch	1 serv (1 oz)	140	16	3	10	0	1	1	0	0	210	—	—	0
SALADS														
Crispy Chicken	1 serv (11.4 oz)	340	19	5	50	20	24	6	5	150	970	—	—	18
Grilled Chicken	1 serv (12 oz)	250	10	6	100	29	12	6	3	200	1070	—	—	18

SOUPER SALAD

FOOD	PORTION	CALS	FAT	SAT FAT	CHOL	PROT	CARB	SUGAR	FIBER	CALCI	SOD	POTAS	FOLIC	VIT C
BEVERAGES														
Lemonade	1 (24 oz)	190	0	0	0	0	49	46	0	—	10	—	—	—
Lemonade Mango	1 (24 oz)	220	0	0	0	0	58	55	0	—	10	—	—	—
Lemonade Raspberry	1 (24 oz)	220	0	0	0	0	58	54	0	—	10	—	—	—
Lemonade Strawberry	1 (24 oz)	220	0	0	0	0	57	53	0	—	10	—	—	—
Smoothie Mango	1 tall	250	0	0	0	0	64	62	0	—	0	—	—	—
Smoothie Peach	1 tall	230	0	0	0	0	62	60	0	—	10	—	—	—
Smoothie Raspberry	1 tall	230	0	0	0	0	62	58	0	—	0	—	—	—
Smoothie Strawberry	1 tall	230	0	0	0	0	60	55	0	—	0	—	—	—
DESSERTS														
Blueberry Bread	1 piece	150	3	1	0	3	29	13	1	—	210	—	—	—
Brownies	2 pieces	120	5	1	5	1	21	14	0	—	115	—	—	—
Cornbread	1 piece	170	5	1	0	3	30	9	1	—	350	—	—	—

FOOD	PORTION	CALS	FAT	SAT FAT	CHOL	PROT	CARB	SUGAR	FIBER	CALCI	SOD	POTAS	FOLIC	VIT C
Cottage Cheese	½ cup	90	2	1	10	13	5	4	0	—	410	—	—	—
Gingerbread	1 piece	180	6	2	0	2	30	14	1	—	290	—	—	—
Peaches	½ cup	70	0	0	0	0	17	13	0	—	10	—	—	—
Pineapple Tidbits	¼ cup	60	0	0	0	0	15	13	1	—	0	—	—	—
Pudding Banana	½ cup	160	6	6	0	2	26	19	0	—	150	—	—	—
Pudding Chocolate	½ cup	170	5	5	0	2	30	23	0	—	115	—	—	—
Soft Serve Cone Chocolate	1	120	2	2	0	1	22	16	0	—	85	—	—	—
Soft Serve Cone Vanilla	1	120	3	3	0	0	22	14	0	—	95	—	—	—
Sponge Cake	4 pieces	80	2	1	5	1	14	8	0	—	160	—	—	—
Strawberry Parfait	½ cup	100	2	2	0	2	19	18	0	—	70	—	—	—
Vanilla Wafers	4	70	2	1	0	1	13	6	0	—	85	—	—	—
Whipped Topping	½ cup	100	8	8	0	0	8	8	0	—	0	—	—	—
PASTA AND PIZZA														
Chicken Alfredo	1 cup	320	9	5	50	19	40	3	1	—	1060	—	—	—
Macaroni & Cheese	1 cup	380	18	9	35	15	38	2	1	—	870	—	—	—
Pizza Slice Cheese	1	70	3	2	5	4	8	1	0	—	125	—	—	—
Pizza Slice Garden	1	80	3	2	5	4	9	1	1	—	125	—	—	—
Pizza Slice Pepperoni	1	90	4	2	10	5	8	1	0	—	190	—	—	—
Pizza Slice Sausage	1	80	4	2	5	4	9	1	1	—	170	—	—	—
Spaghetti & Meatballs	1 cup	280	9	4	15	11	38	2	4	—	700	—	—	—
SALAD DRESSINGS AND SAUCES														
Balsamic Vinegar	1 oz	60	0	0	0	0	15	15	0	—	0	—	—	—
Bleu Cheese	2 oz	220	23	5	25	2	1	1	0	—	310	—	—	—
Caesar	2 oz	280	30	5	30	4	4	4	0	—	840	—	—	—
Chipotle Ranch	2 oz	280	28	4	10	0	8	4	0	—	480	—	—	—
Fat Free French	2 oz	60	0	0	0	0	18	10	1	—	620	—	—	—
Fat Free Italian w/ Cheese	2 oz	30	0	0	0	0	6	4	0	—	680	—	—	—
Green Goddess	2 oz	260	24	4	10	2	4	4	0	—	580	—	—	—
Honey Mustard	2 oz	240	26	4	20	0	2	1	0	—	460	—	—	—
Mayonnaise	2 tbsp	200	22	3	20	0	20	0	0	—	200	—	—	—
Olive Oil	1 oz	240	28	4	0	0	0	0	0	—	0	—	—	—
Peppercorn Ranch	2 oz	220	23	3	20	1	2	2	0	—	360	—	—	—
Pesto Basil	1 tbsp	45	5	1	0	1	0	0	0	—	100	—	—	—
Ranch	2 oz	220	23	3	20	1	2	2	0	—	360	—	—	—
Reduced Calorie Ranch	2 oz	120	11	2	10	2	3	2	0	—	260	—	—	—
Sauce Alfredo	1½ tbsp	45	4	3	10	2	2	1	0	—	170	—	—	—

FOOD	PORTION	CALS	FAT	SAT FAT	CHOL	PROT	CARB	SUGAR	FIBER	CALCI	SOD	POTAS	FOLIC	VIT C
Sauce Chipotle Pepper	¼ tsp	0	0	0	0	0	0	0	0	—	30	—	—	—
Sauce Cholula Hot	¼ tsp	0	0	0	0	0	0	0	0	—	5	—	—	—
Sauce Jalapeno Cheese	1 serv (2 oz)	35	2	0	0	1	5	0	1	—	440	—	—	—
Sauce Marinara	1½ tbsp	10	0	0	0	0	2	1	0	—	90	—	—	—
Sauce Meaty Marinara	1½ tbsp	40	1	0	5	1	2	1	0	—	90	—	—	—
Sauce Sriracha Hot	¼ tsp	0	0	0	0	0	0	0	0	—	15	—	—	—
Sour Cream Light	2 tbsp	40	3	2	10	1	3	2	0	—	40	—	—	—
Tangy Oriental	2 oz	160	12	2	0	0	10	8	0	—	760	—	—	—
Thousand Island	1 oz	300	30	5	20	0	6	4	0	—	500	—	—	—
Vinaigrette Cranberry	2 oz	100	0	0	0	0	24	20	0	—	560	—	—	—
Vinaigrette House	2 oz	220	22	3	0	0	4	4	0	—	840	—	—	—
SALADS														
Apple Walnut	1 cup	130	11	3	5	3	7	5	1	—	210	—	—	—
Asian Chicken	1 cup	80	3	1	5	3	10	7	2	—	450	—	—	—
Asian Shrimp	1 cup	100	4	1	20	4	13	7	2	—	470	—	—	—
Buffalo Chicken	1 cup	70	6	1	10	3	3	2	1	—	200	—	—	—
Caesar Chicken	1 cup	90	7	2	15	5	4	1	1	—	340	—	—	—
Caesar Chicken Salsa	1 cup	80	5	2	15	4	4	1	1	—	380	—	—	—
Caesar Shrimp	1 cup	90	7	2	30	4	3	1	1	—	310	—	—	—
California Chicken Salad	⅓ cup	80	6	1	25	5	4	3	0	—	110	—	—	—
Capri	1 cup	50	2	0	0	1	8	3	0	—	540	—	—	—
Chicago Chopped	1 cup	120	10	3	15	4	3	2	1	—	310	—	—	—
Chickpea	⅓ cup	110	6	1	0	3	11	1	4	—	220	—	—	—
Cobb	1 cup	100	8	2	55	4	2	2	1	—	340	—	—	—
Coleslaw Broccoli	⅓ cup	80	6	1	0	1	6	4	1	—	65	—	—	—
Edamame	⅓ cup	70	5	0	0	4	4	2	2	—	50	—	—	—
Fisherman's Kettle Shrimp & Crab	⅓ cup	120	8	2	15	3	15	9	1	—	300	—	—	—
Gazpacho	⅓ cup	30	3	0	0	0	3	2	1	—	100	—	—	—
Green Goddess Crab	1 cup	70	5	1	5	2	4	2	1	—	240	—	—	—
Italian Antipasto	1 cup	70	5	2	5	2	3	2	1	—	320	—	—	—
Mango Berry	1 cup	110	6	1	0	1	13	11	1	—	75	—	—	—
Marinated Mushrooms	⅓ cup	60	7	1	0	1	1	0	0	—	110	—	—	—
Marinated Oriental Cucumber	⅓ cup	10	0	0	0	0	2	1	0	—	240	—	—	—
Marinated Tomato	1 cup	60	2	1	0	1	11	10	1	—	45	—	—	—

FOOD	PORTION	CALS	FAT	SAT FAT	CHOL	PROT	CARB	SUGAR	FIBER	CALCI	SOD	POTAS	FOLIC	VIT C
Melon Couscous	⅓ cup	50	1	0	0	1	10	4	1	—	60	—	—	—
Mustard Potato	⅓ cup	80	5	1	25	1	7	1	1	—	280	—	—	—
Paco's Taco	⅓ cup	100	5	1	0	3	12	1	2	—	200	—	—	—
Pasta De Garden	⅓ cup	80	5	1	0	1	8	1	0	—	210	—	—	—
Pasta Fettuccine	⅓ cup	100	5	1	5	2	11	1	1	—	390	—	—	—
Pasta Primavera	⅓ cup	45	3	0	0	1	4	1	0	—	85	—	—	—
Pasta Thai Chicken	⅓ cup	100	5	1	10	3	11	2	1	—	320	—	—	—
Pasta Tuna Skroodle	⅓ cup	130	9	2	10	3	10	1	1	—	135	—	—	—
Red Potato	⅓ cup	50	4	1	0	1	5	1	1	—	125	—	—	—
Rice Florentine	⅓ cup	90	5	1	0	1	11	0	0	—	105	—	—	—
Roasted Mushrooms & Artichokes w/ Feta Cheese	⅓ cup	40	3	1	0	1	3	1	1	—	90	—	—	—
Roasted Vegetables	⅓ cup	20	2	0	0	0	2	1	1	—	125	—	—	—
Salad Of The Sea	⅓ cup	50	2	1	5	2	6	1	0	—	190	—	—	—
Salmon Medley	1 cup	70	2	1	5	4	10	8	1	—	160	—	—	—
Santa Fe Corn	⅓ cup	100	4	0	0	4	13	2	3	—	310	—	—	—
Shrimp & Crab Louie	1 cup	130	10	2	55	5	5	2	1	—	490	—	—	—
Southwest Chicken Chipotle	1 cup	90	7	1	10	3	4	2	1	—	270	—	—	—
Sweet Garden Slaw	⅓ cup	35	2	0	0	0	4	3	1	—	75	—	—	—
Tropical Tuxedo	⅓ cup	60	3	0	0	1	7	2	0	—	150	—	—	—
Tuna Fish	⅓ cup	70	5	1	15	6	1	1	0	—	220	—	—	—
SOUPS														
Adobe Rice & Chicken	1 (5 oz)	100	5	3	25	3	10	2	1	—	540	—	—	—
Alaskan Salmon Chowder	1 (5 oz)	70	2	2	0	3	9	1	1	—	630	—	—	—
Beef Mushroom	1 (5 oz)	80	2	1	5	4	11	1	2	—	510	—	—	—
Beef Noodle	1 (5 oz)	80	3	1	15	4	10	2	1	—	500	—	—	—
Beef Shellini	1 (5 oz)	90	3	1	10	5	11	3	1	—	460	—	—	—
Beef Stroganoff	1 (5 oz)	120	5	3	15	5	13	2	1	—	820	—	—	—
Black Bean	1 (5 oz)	80	2	1	5	8	20	2	11	—	370	—	—	—
Broccoli Cheese	1 (5 oz)	70	2	2	0	2	10	2	1	—	640	—	—	—
Cajun Gumbo	1 (5 oz)	110	4	1	15	5	13	1	1	—	570	—	—	—
Cauliflower Cheese	1 (5 oz)	70	2	2	0	2	11	2	1	—	650	—	—	—
Cheddar Chicken Broccoli Stew	1 (5 oz)	140	6	3	25	6	15	3	2	—	600	—	—	—

FOOD	PORTION	CALS	FAT	SAT FAT	CHOL	PROT	CARB	SUGAR	FIBER	CALCI	SOD	POTAS	FOLIC	VIT C
Cherokee Joe Cornbread	1 (5 oz)	70	2	0	0	2	13	5	2	—	950	—	—	—
Chicken Creole	1 (5 oz)	100	4	2	20	5	12	3	1	—	520	—	—	—
Chicken Enchilada	1 (5 oz)	180	12	5	40	6	13	3	1	—	590	—	—	—
Chicken Gumbo	1 (5 oz)	90	4	1	15	4	10	2	1	—	660	—	—	—
Chicken Mushroom Barley	1 (5 oz)	80	3	1	20	5	9	2	1	—	660	—	—	—
Chicken Noodle	1 (5 oz)	80	3	1	25	5	9	2	1	—	620	—	—	—
Chicken Tetrazini	1 (5 oz)	120	5	3	25	6	13	2	1	—	620	—	—	—
Chicken Tortilla	1 (5 oz)	60	2	0	10	4	7	2	1	—	650	—	—	—
Cream Of Asparagus	1 (5 oz)	140	10	7	15	2	7	3	1	—	710	—	—	—
Cream Of Broccoli	1 (5 oz)	60	2	2	0	2	9	2	1	—	620	—	—	—
Cream Of Cauliflower	1 (5 oz)	60	2	2	0	2	10	2	1	—	630	—	—	—
Cream Of Chicken	1 (5 oz)	100	5	2	20	5	9	2	1	—	610	—	—	—
Cream Of Mushroom	1 (5 oz)	80	4	2	0	2	10	1	1	—	480	—	—	—
Holiday Harvest	1 (5 oz)	90	6	3	25	3	5	1	0	—	480	—	—	—
Vegan Split Pea	1 (5 oz)	90	1	0	0	4	16	2	5	—	260	—	—	—
Vegetable Beef	1 (5 oz)	80	3	1	10	4	11	3	2	—	550	—	—	—
Vegetable Cheese	1 (5 oz)	80	3	2	0	2	12	2	1	—	430	—	—	—
Vegetable Lentil	1 (5 oz)	70	0	0	0	5	16	2	5	—	620	—	—	—
Vegetarian Butter Bean	1 (5 oz)	70	0	0	0	6	21	2	10	—	420	—	—	—
Vegetarian Vegetable	1 (5 oz)	50	1	0	0	2	11	2	2	—	320	—	—	—

SOUPLANTATION

BREADS AND MUFFINS

FOOD	PORTION	CALS	FAT	SAT FAT	CHOL	PROT	CARB	SUGAR	FIBER	CALCI	SOD	POTAS	FOLIC	VIT C
Biscuit Buttermilk	1	190	8	3	0	4	25	2	0	—	580	—	—	—
Cornbread Buttermilk Low Fat	1 piece	140	2	0	10	3	27	4	2	—	270	—	—	—
Focaccia Bruschetta	1 piece	140	7	3	10	4	15	1	1	—	360	—	—	—
Focaccia Honey Wheat Crust BBQ Chicken	1 piece	200	8	3	25	9	23	4	2	—	440	—	—	—
Focaccia Honey Wheat Crust Buffalo Chicken	1 piece	170	7	2	15	6	20	2	2	—	360	—	—	—
Muffin Apple Cinnamon Bran 96% Fat Free	1	130	1	0	0	2	30	16	3	—	310	—	—	—

FOOD	PORTION	CALS	FAT	SAT FAT	CHOL	PROT	CARB	SUGAR	FIBER	CALCI	SOD	POTAS	FOLIC	VIT C
Muffin Apple Raisin	1	150	7	1	10	2	22	9	1	—	190	—	—	—
Muffin Banana Nut	1	150	7	1	10	2	22	9	1	—	190	—	—	—
Muffin Cappuccino Chip	1	190	6	2	25	3	31	15	1	—	160	—	—	—
Muffin Caribbean Key Lime	1	170	6	1	10	2	28	15	1	—	210	—	—	—
Muffin Carrot Pineapple w/ Oat Bran	1	150	6	1	10	3	23	13	2	—	230	—	—	—
Muffin Cherry Nut	1	150	7	1	10	2	22	9	1	—	190	—	—	—
Muffin Chile Corn Low Fat	1	140	3	1	10	3	27	5	2	—	320	—	—	—
Muffin Chocolate Brownie	1	180	8	2	25	3	26	16	1	—	190	—	—	—
Muffin Chocolate Chip	1	170	8	2	10	3	22	10	1	—	190	—	—	—
Muffin Top Banana Crunch No Sugar Added	1	120	5	2	20	3	19	2	1	—	290	—	—	—
BREAKFAST MENU SELECTIONS														
Belgian Waffle	1	90	0	0	0	20	16	2	1	—	270	—	—	—
Biscuit Sweet Cinnamon w/ Frosting	1	270	13	7	10	4	37	14	0	—	590	—	—	—
Biscuit Sweet Maple Buttermilk	1	240	9	4	5	3	39	16	1	—	540	—	—	—
Biscuit Sweet Strawberry	1	250	9	4	5	3	40	19	1	—	540	—	—	—
Breakfast Burrito Burrito Country Ham & Egg	1	210	10	3	195	10	21	1	2	—	450	—	—	—
Breakfast Burrito Sweet Pepper Sausage Egg	1	210	11	3	195	9	20	1	2	—	360	—	—	—
Eggs Scrambled	½ cup	135	8	3	350	12	2	1	0	—	360	—	—	—
Focaccia Egg Scramble w/ Bacon	1 piece	180	8	3	70	7	20	1	1	—	330	—	—	—
French Toast	1 slice	150	4	2	85	5	25	4	1	—	270	—	—	—
Oatmeal Plain	¾ cup	110	2	0	0	3	19	0	3	—	240	—	—	—
Potatoes O'Brien	½ cup	140	6	0	0	2	19	3	2	—	190	—	—	—
Sticky Granola Clusters w/ Almonds	¼ cup	270	14	5	15	4	30	15	3	—	120	—	—	—

FOOD	PORTION	CALS	FAT	SAT FAT	CHOL	PROT	CARB	SUGAR	FIBER	CALCI	SOD	POTAS	FOLIC	VIT C
Sunrise Pasta Mediterranean	1 cup	210	12	4	75	6	19	3	2	—	330	—	—	—
DESSERTS														
Apple Medley Fat Free	½ cup	70	0	0	0	1	18	12	1	—	5	—	—	—
Banana Royale Fat Free	½ cup	80	0	0	0	1	20	12	1	—	5	—	—	—
Cake Carrot & Cream Cheese Lava	1 piece	320	15	5	40	3	40	34	1	—	250	—	—	—
Cake Chocolate Lava	½ cup	330	8	4	5	2	62	47	0	—	290	—	—	—
Cobbler Apple	½ cup	360	10	5	5	2	67	10	1	—	160	—	—	—
Cobbler Caramel Apple	½ cup	390	12	5	5	3	68	50	2	—	230	—	—	—
Cobbler Cherry Apple	½ cup	330	10	5	0	2	57	29	2	—	190	—	—	—
Cookie Chocolate Chip	1 sm	75	3	2	5	1	10	6	0	—	100	—	—	—
Cookie Bar Chocolate Peanut Butter	1 piece	270	12	7	25	3	37	22	1	—	310	—	—	—
Frozen Yogurt Chocolate Nonfat	½ cup	110	0	0	0	4	22	17	1	—	65	—	—	—
Pudding Banana	½ cup	160	4	0	10	4	27	26	1	—	220	—	—	—
Pudding Butterscotch Low Fat	½ cup	140	3	0	10	4	24	24	0	—	160	—	—	—
Pudding Chocolate Low Fat	½ cup	150	3	1	10	4	25	24	0	—	260	—	—	—
Pudding Chocolate Low Fat No Sugar Added	½ cup	90	2	1	5	4	21	6	0	—	430	—	—	—
MAIN MENU SELECTIONS														
100% Whole Wheat Jalapeno & Salsa Pasta	1 cup	250	6	2	10	9	46	3	6	—	480	—	—	—
Alfredo 4 Cheese	1 cup	390	13	8	30	19	50	3	3	—	690	—	—	—
Alfredo Broccoli w/ Basil	1 cup	380	17	8	40	12	45	5	1	—	790	—	—	—
Alfredo Fettuccine	1 cup	390	18	10	50	15	41	4	2	—	580	—	—	—
Alfredo Fire Roasted Tomato Basil	1 cup	370	14	8	35	19	44	4	2	—	690	—	—	—
Arizona Marinara	1 cup	360	11	5	25	17	47	6	3	—	890	—	—	—

FOOD	PORTION	CALS	FAT	SAT FAT	CHOL	PROT	CARB	SUGAR	FIBER	CALCI	SOD	POTAS	FOLIC	VIT C
Baked Potato Topper Broccoli Cheese	1 cup	120	7	3	10	3	10	2	1	—	530	—	—	—
Beefy Meatball Stroganoff	1 cup	340	21	11	75	9	28	4	2	—	590	—	—	—
Bruschetta	1 cup	260	4	2	10	10	41	3	3	—	450	—	—	—
Bruschetta Creamy	1 cup	360	16	8	45	12	43	3	3	—	510	—	—	—
Carbonara Pasta w/ Bacon	1 cup	290	10	6	20	8	43	3	2	—	250	—	—	—
Cheesy Scalloped Potatoes w/ Bacon	1 cup	240	17	6	30	3	15	2	1	—	990	—	—	—
Chicken Tetrazzini	1 cup	480	23	10	70	19	47	4	3	—	610	—	—	—
Creamy Cilantro Lime Pesto Hot Pasta	1 cup	360	20	8	30	8	37	3	1	—	480	—	—	—
Creamy Herb Chicken	1 cup	310	17	8	80	8	32	7	2	—	360	—	—	—
Curried Pineapple & Ginger	1 cup	200	2	0	0	6	40	9	2	—	560	—	—	—
Garden Vegetable w/ Italian Sausage	1 cup	300	10	3	20	12	42	2	3	—	540	—	—	—
Pesto Cilantro Lime	1 cup	370	21	3	20	9	36	3	2	—	760	—	—	—
SALAD DRESSINGS														
Avocado Ranch	2 tbsp	150	14	2	10	1	4	3	0	—	180	—	—	—
Bacon	2 tbsp	110	11	2	0	0	7	6	0	—	300	—	—	—
Blue Cheese	1 tbsp	130	13	3	15	1	3	1	0	—	230	—	—	—
Creamy Cucumber Reduced Calorie	2 tbsp	70	7	1	0	0	3	2	0	—	440	—	—	—
Creamy Italian	2 tbsp	120	13	2	10	0	0	0	0	—	290	—	—	—
Creamy Sesame Soy	2 tbsp	170	17	3	10	0	5	4	0	—	190	—	—	—
Green Chili Ranch	2 tbsp	150	14	2	10	1	4	3	0	—	190	—	—	—
Honey Mustard	2 tbsp	150	13	2	10	0	8	6	0	—	230	—	—	—
Honey Mustard Fat Free	2 tbsp	45	0	0	0	0	10	9	0	—	180	—	—	—
Italian Fat Free	2 tbsp	25	0	0	0	0	7	2	0	—	330	—	—	—
Vinaigrette Balsamic	2 tbsp	180	19	2	0	0	1	1	0	—	190	—	—	—
Vinaigrette Basil	2 tbsp	160	17	1	0	0	1	0	0	—	160	—	—	—
Vinaigrette Cranberry Orange Low Fat	2 tbsp	80	2	0	0	0	15	8	0	—	90	—	—	—

FOOD	PORTION	CALS	FAT	SAT FAT	CHOL	PROT	CARB	SUGAR	FIBER	CALCI	SOD	POTAS	FOLIC	VIT C
Vinaigrette Honey Lime Cilantro	2 tbsp	100	6	0	0	0	15	14	0	—	80	—	—	—
Vinaigrette Italian w/ Basil Romano Cheese	2 tbsp	150	15	1	0	0	1	1	0	—	250	—	—	—
SALADS														
100% Whole Wheat Arugula Citrus	½ cup	210	10	1	0	4	29	6	3	—	250	—	—	—
100% Whole Wheat Creamy Chipotle	½ cup	350	25	4	15	5	31	4	4	—	720	—	—	—
100% Whole Wheat Sicilian Penne w/ Feta & Pepperoni	½ cup	250	14	3	10	6	30	4	5	—	450	—	—	—
100% Whole Wheat Spicy Asian Peanut	½ cup	260	14	2	0	6	32	7	4	—	460	—	—	—
Ambrosia w/ Coconut	½ cup	190	9	3	10	1	30	23	2	—	80	—	—	—
Artichoke Rice	½ cup	190	12	2	5	3	19	2	1	—	780	—	—	—
Aunt Doris' Red Pepper Slaw Fat Free	½ cup	70	0	0	0	1	18	13	3	—	480	—	—	—
Azteca Taco w/ Turkey	1 cup	130	9	3	15	6	7	3	4	—	230	—	—	—
Baja Bean & Cilantro	½ cup	180	3	0	0	9	29	2	5	—	190	—	—	—
Bartlett Pear & Carmelized Walnut	1 cup	180	12	2	5	4	13	10	2	—	220	—	—	—
BBQ Smokehouse w/ Bacon & Peanuts	1 cup	290	17	3	10	9	25	5	2	—	730	—	—	—
Buffalo Chicken	1 cup	180	14	2	10	4	10	2	1	—	440	—	—	—
Caesar Asiago	1 cup	270	22	8	30	5	10	2	2	—	590	—	—	—
California Cobb w/ Bacon	1 cup	190	15	5	55	5	7	2	2	—	370	—	—	—
Cambay Curry w/ Almonds & Coconut	1 cup	220	17	5	10	3	17	11	4	—	90	—	—	—
Carrot Raisin	½ cup	90	3	0	5	1	17	15	2	—	80	—	—	—
Cherry Balsamic Blue Tossed	1 cup	220	16	3	10	4	16	9	1	—	280	—	—	—
Cherry Chipotle Spinach	1 cup	160	8	1	0	1	20	05	4	—	170	—	—	—
Chinese Krab	½ cup	160	8	1	5	5	19	4	3	—	260	—	—	—

FOOD	PORTION	CALS	FAT	SAT FAT	CHOL	PROT	CARB	SUGAR	FIBER	CALCI	SOD	POTAS	FOLIC	VIT C
Citrus Noodle w/ Snow Peas	½ cup	140	6	1	0	3	19	5	2	—	240	—	—	—
Classic Antipasto	1 cup	280	21	4	15	6	18	8	4	—	260	—	—	—
Classic Greek	1 cup	120	9	3	10	3	4	2	2	—	320	—	—	—
Confetti Avocado Slaw	½ cup	140	9	2	5	2	12	4	3	—	190	—	—	—
Crunchy Island Pineapple	1 cup	160	8	1	0	1	20	12	2	—	130	—	—	—
Curried Rice w/ Mango Chutney	½ cup	170	2	0	0	2	36	9	1	—	190	—	—	—
Field Corn & Very Wild Rice	½ cup	170	9	1	0	4	19	3	3	—	420	—	—	—
Field Greens Citrus Vinaigrette	1 cup	150	12	1	0	1	10	4	2	—	110	—	—	—
Potato BBQ	½ cup	170	9	2	5	2	21	3	2	—	370	—	—	—
Potato Bistro	½ cup	290	19	2	5	5	27	2	3	—	490	—	—	—
Potato Buffalo Blue	½ cup	190	13	3	10	3	16	3	2	—	370	—	—	—
Potato Dijon w/ Garlic Dill Vinaigrette	½ cup	150	12	1	0	1	9	6	3	—	40	—	—	—
SOUPS														
8 Vegetable Chicken Stew	1 cup	160	7	3	30	8	17	4	2	—	990	—	—	—
Albondigas Locas Meatball	1 cup	210	11	4	35	8	19	5	2	—	950	—	—	—
Asian Ginger Broth	1 cup	50	2	0	0	1	6	3	0	—	530	—	—	—
Basmati Lentil	1 cup	210	7	5	5	8	29	2	4	—	380	—	—	—
Beef & Barley Stew	1 cup	240	10	4	30	12	19	5	3	—	930	—	—	—
Better Than Mom's Beef Stew	1 cup	270	17	8	35	9	19	3	2	—	1150	—	—	—
Big Chunk Chicken Noodle Low Fat	1 cup	170	3	2	30	15	19	3	1	—	440	—	—	—
Border Black Bean & Chorizo	1 cup	240	10	3	20	11	27	6	6	—	880	—	—	—
Broccoli Cheese	1 cup	270	19	10	35	7	17	7	1	—	810	—	—	—
Buffalo Chicken	1 cup	180	6	3	0	9	21	2	1	—	740	—	—	—
Canadian Cheese w/ Smoked Ham	1 cup	350	26	13	45	8	22	7	1	—	1100	—	—	—
Cheese Stuffed Cappelletti	1 cup	250	11	6	20	5	31	9	2	—	580	—	—	—
Cheesy Corn Chowder w/ Bacon	1 cup	220	11	6	30	6	25	4	2	—	950	—	—	—
Chesapeake Corn Chowder	1 cup	290	17	9	40	6	30	8	2	—	890	—	—	—

FOOD	PORTION	CALS	FAT	SAT FAT	CHOL	PROT	CARB	SUGAR	FIBER	CALCI	SOD	POTAS	FOLIC	VIT C
Chicken & Rice	1 cup	160	5	1	40	10	18	3	1	—	790	—	—	—
Chicken Dijon Reduced Sodium	1 cup	210	13	7	40	5	18	4	1	—	540	—	—	—
Chicken Divan	1 cup	240	15	9	60	9	18	4	1	—	630	—	—	—
Chicken Enchilada	1 cup	190	7	3	30	9	22	3	3	—	980	—	—	—

STARBUCKS

BAKED SELECTIONS

FOOD	PORTION	CALS	FAT	SAT FAT	CHOL	PROT	CARB	SUGAR	FIBER	CALCI	SOD	POTAS	FOLIC	VIT C
Apple Fritter	1	480	22	10	0	4	64	27	1	—	290	—	—	—
Bagel French Toast	1	280	1	0	0	8	62	10	2	0	400	—	—	0
Bagel Multigrain	1	280	3	0	0	10	60	12	4	—	380	—	—	—
Bagel Plain	1	280	0	0	0	10	62	8	2	0	440	—	—	0
Bar Cranberry Bliss	1	320	16	9	45	3	41	28	1	—	260	—	—	—
Bar Toffee Almond	1	400	19	8	50	4	53	34	1	—	340	—	—	—
Brownie Espresso	1	340	19	8	50	4	40	27	2	—	135	—	—	—
Cinnamon Roll	1	470	26	11	45	6	56	29	1	60	350	—	—	1
Cocoa Crispy Square	1	420	17	7	25	5	66	30	1	—	440	—	—	—
Cookie Chocolate Chunk	1	420	20	13	55	7	56	28	6	—	460	—	—	—
Cookie Coffee Ginger	1	470	18	11	75	6	70	40	3	—	210	—	—	—
Cookie Penguin	1	370	18	11	15	4	50	31	tr	—	280	—	—	—
Cookie Rainbow	1	420	19	12	65	5	61	33	1	—	370	—	—	—
Cookies Mini Black & White	2	240	12	1	40	2	32	22	1	—	160	—	—	—
Croissant Butter	1	370	23	15	65	5	35	4	3	—	310	—	—	—
Doughnut Glazed	1	490	23	9	20	4	65	39	1	—	410	—	—	—
Loaf Banana Nut	1 serv	470	24	10	105	7	56	32	2	—	360	—	—	—
Loaf Iced Lemon	1 serv	500	18	9	140	7	78	53	1	—	440	—	—	—
Loaf Marble	1 serv	410	22	10	130	6	52	31	tr	—	440	—	—	—
Loaf Pumpkin	1 serv	380	14	2	55	5	59	36	2	—	480	—	—	—
Mallorca Sweet Bread	1	420	24	11	20	7	43	14	2	—	560	—	—	—
Muffin Blueberry	1	310	11	3	70	5	55	31	1	100	270	—	—	1
Muffin Pumpkin Cream Cheese	1	490	24	6	85	6	63	42	1	60	470	—	—	1
Muffin Reduced Fat Chocolate	1	290	5	4	75	6	53	31	2	40	460	—	—	0
Muffin Walnut Bran	1	430	18	2	40	8	62	26	4	100	400	—	—	1

FOOD	PORTION	CALS	FAT	SAT FAT	CHOL	PROT	CARB	SUGAR	FIBER	CALCI	SOD	POTAS	FOLIC	VIT C
Reduced Fat Coffee Cake Banana Chocolate Chip	1	390	8	5	0	5	76	50	3	60	400	—	—	1
Reduced Fat Coffee Cake Blueberry	1 serv	320	6	5	10	4	54	33	1	—	390	—	—	—
Reduced Fat Coffee Cake Cinnamon Swirl	1 serv	290	4	3	5	4	52	33	1	—	330	—	—	—
Reduced Fat Coffee Cake Pumpkin Chocolate Chip	1	300	6	3	0	5	58	36	3	60	270	—	—	0
Rustic Apple Tart	1	190	5	2	0	1	37	30	3	—	80	—	—	—
Scone Blueberry	1	480	22	12	80	7	64	24	2	—	520	—	—	—
Scone Cran Apple Crumb	1	490	20	11	80	7	74	30	4	80	510	—	—	0
Scone Raspberry	1	470	21	12	80	7	64	25	2	60	510	—	—	0
BEVERAGES														
Apple Juice	1 grande	250	0	0	0	0	64	57	0	—	25	—	—	—
Cafe Americano	1 grande	15	0	0	0	1	3	0	0	—	10	—	—	—
Cafe Au Lait Nonfat Milk	1 grande	70	0	0	5	7	10	10	0	—	90	—	—	—
Caffe Mocha No Whip Nonfat Milk	1 grande	220	3	1	5	13	42	32	2	—	125	—	—	—
Caffe Mocha Whip Nonfat Milk	1 grande	290	10	5	30	13	44	34	2	—	135	—	—	—
Cappuccino Nonfat Milk	1 grande	80	0	0	5	8	12	10	0	—	90	—	—	—
Caramel Apple Cider Whip	1 grande	380	8	5	25	0	76	68	0	—	30	—	—	—
Caramel Apple Spice No Whip	1 grande	310	tr	0	0	0	74	66	0	—	25	—	—	—
Caramel Macchiato Nonfat Milk	1 grande	190	1	1	10	11	35	32	0	—	135	—	—	—
Chocolate Milk Nonfat	1 grande	280	3	1	10	18	53	45	2	—	190	—	—	—
Cinnamon Dolce Creme No Whip Nonfat Milk	1 grande	220	0	0	5	12	41	41	0	—	160	—	—	—
Cinnamon Dolce Whip Nonfat Milk	1 grande	290	7	5	35	13	43	43	0	—	160	—	—	—
Coffee Of The Week	1 grande	5	tr	0	0	1	0	0	0	—	10	—	—	—

FOOD	PORTION	CALS	FAT	SAT FAT	CHOL	PROT	CARB	SUGAR	FIBER	CALCI	SOD	POTAS	FOLIC	VIT C
Coffee Of The Week Decaf	1 grande	5	0	0	0	1	0	0	0	—	10	—	—	—
Frappuccino Blended Coffee Cafe Vanilla Whip Nonfat Milk	1 grande	430	14	9	55	6	70	60	0	—	240	—	—	—
Frappuccino Blended Coffee Cafe Vanilla Whip Soy	1 grande	430	14	9	55	6	70	60	0	—	240	—	—	—
Frappuccino Blended Coffee Cafe Vanilla No Whip Soy	1 grande	310	3	2	15	5	67	58	0	—	230	—	—	—
Frappuccino Blended Coffee Caffe Vanilla No Whip Nonfat Milk	1 grande	310	3	2	15	5	67	58	0	—	230	—	—	—
Frappuccino Blended Coffee Caramel No Whip Nonfat Milk	1 grande	270	4	3	15	5	53	45	0	—	230	—	—	—
Frappuccino Blended Coffee Caramel No Whip Soy	1 grande	270	4	3	15	5	53	45	0	—	230	—	—	—
Frappuccino Blended Coffee Caramel Whip Soy	1 grande	380	15	9	55	6	57	48	0	—	240	—	—	—
Frappuccino Blended Coffee Cinnamon Dolce No Whip Nonfat Milk	1 grande	260	3	2	15	5	52	45	0	—	220	—	—	—
Frappuccino Blended Coffee Cinnamon Dolce No Whip Soy	1 grande	260	3	2	15	5	52	45	0	—	220	—	—	—
Frappuccino Blended Coffee Cinnamon Dolce Whip Soy	1 grande	370	14	9	55	6	55	47	0	—	240	—	—	—
Frappuccino Blended Coffee Espresso Nonfat Milk	1 grande	190	3	2	10	4	38	31	0	—	170	—	—	—

FOOD	PORTION	CALS	FAT	SAT FAT	CHOL	PROT	CARB	SUGAR	FIBER	CALCI	SOD	POTAS	FOLIC	VIT C
Frappuccino Blended Coffee Java Chip No Whip Nonfat Milk	1 grande	340	8	5	15	7	64	52	2	—	230	—	—	—
Frappuccino Blended Coffee Java Chip No Whip Soy	1 grande	190	3	2	10	4	38	31	0	—	170	—	—	—
Frappuccino Blended Coffee Java Chip Whip Nonfat Milk	1 grande	460	19	12	55	7	67	55	2	—	240	—	—	—
Frappuccino Blended Coffee Java Chip Whip Soy	1 grande	460	19	12	55	7	67	55	2	—	240	—	—	—
Frappuccino Blended Coffee Mocha No Whip Nonfat Milk	1 grande	260	4	2	15	6	54	45	0	—	230	—	—	—
Frappuccino Blended Coffee Mocha No Whip Soy	1 grande	260	4	2	15	6	54	45	0	—	230	—	—	—
Frappuccino Blended Coffee Mocha Whip Nonfat Milk	1 grande	380	15	9	55	6	57	47	0	—	240	—	—	—
Frappuccino Blended Coffee Pumpkin Spice No Whip Nonfat Milk	1 grande	290	4	2	15	6	59	51	0	—	260	—	—	—
Frappuccino Blended Coffee Pumpkin Spice No Whip Soy	1 grande	290	4	2	15	6	59	51	0	—	260	—	—	—
Frappuccino Blended Coffee Pumpkin Spice Whip Nonfat Milk	1 grande	400	15	9	55	7	62	53	0	—	280	—	—	—
Frappuccino Blended Coffee Pumpkin Spice Whip Soy	1 grande	400	15	9	55	7	62	53	0	—	280	—	—	—
Frappuccino Blended Coffee Whip Nonfat Milk	1 grande	370	14	9	55	6	55	47	0	—	240	—	—	—

FOOD	PORTION	CALS	FAT	SAT FAT	CHOL	PROT	CARB	SUGAR	FIBER	CALCI	SOD	POTAS	FOLIC	VIT C
Frappuccino Blended Coffee White Chocolate Mocha No Whip Nonfat Milk	1 grande	300	5	3	15	6	59	51	0	—	250	—	—	—
Frappuccino Blended Coffee White Chocolate Mocha No Whip Soy	1 grande	300	5	3	15	6	59	51	0	—	250	—	—	—
Frappuccino Blended Coffee White Chocolate Mocha Whip Nonfat Milk	1 grande	410	16	10	55	7	62	54	0	—	270	—	—	—
Frappuccino Blended Coffee White Chocolate Mocha Whip Soy	1 grande	410	16	10	55	7	62	54	0	—	270	—	—	—
Frappuccino Blended Creme Tazo Chai No Whip Nonfat Milk	1 grande	330	2	0	5	10	67	56	0	—	270	—	—	—
Frappuccino Blended Creme Tazo Chai Whip Nonfat Milk	1 grande	570	15	9	60	12	95	83	1	—	330	—	—	—
Frappuccino Blended Creme Vanilla Bean No Whip Nonfat Milk	1 grande	350	3	0	5	11	72	60	0	—	310	—	—	—
Frappuccino Blended Creme Vanilla Bean Whip Nonfat Milk	1 grande	470	14	7	50	12	75	62	0	—	320	—	—	—
Frappuccino Light Blended Coffee Cafe Vanilla Nonfat Milk	1 grande	190	1	0	0	6	42	32	3	—	240	—	—	—
Frappuccino Light Blended Coffee Caramel	1 grande	160	2	0	5	5	30	21	3	—	230	—	—	—
Frappuccino Light Blended Coffee Cinnamon Dolce Nonfat Milk	1 grande	140	1	0	0	5	29	21	3	—	230	—	—	—

FOOD	PORTION	CALS	FAT	SAT FAT	CHOL	PROT	CARB	SUGAR	FIBER	CALCI	SOD	POTAS	FOLIC	VIT C
Frappuccino Light Blended Coffee Java Chip Nonfat Milk	1 grande	200	5	3	0	6	36	24	4	—	220	—	—	—
Frappuccino Light Blended Coffee Mocha Nonfat Milk	1 grande	140	1	0	0	6	29	19	3	—	230	—	—	—
Frappuccino Light Blended Coffee Nonfat Milk	1 grande	130	1	0	0	5	25	16	3	—	230	—	—	—
Frappuccino Light Blended Coffee Pumpkin Spice Nonfat Milk	1 grande	150	1	0	0	6	31	22	3	—	240	—	—	—
Frappuccino Light Blended Creme Double Chocolaty Chip Whip Nonfat Milk	1 grande	510	19	11	50	14	78	59	2	—	300	—	—	—
Frappuccino Light Blended Creme Pumpkin Spice No Whip Nonfat Milk	1 grande	360	3	0	5	12	71	61	0	—	350	—	—	—
Frappuccino Light Blended Creme Pumpkin Spice Whip Nonfat Milk	1 grande	470	13	7	50	13	74	63	0	—	360	—	—	—
Frappuccino Light Blended Creme Tazo Green Tea No Whip Nonfat Milk	1 grande	380	3	0	5	11	78	67	1	—	290	—	—	—
Frappuccino Light Blended Creme Tazo Green Tea Whip Nonfat Milk	1 grande	490	14	7	50	12	82	69	1	—	300	—	—	—
Frappuccino Light Blended Creme White Chocolate No Whip Nonfat Milk	1 grande	480	7	4	10	15	89	77	0	—	410	—	—	—
Frappuccino Light Blended Creme White Chocolate Whip Nonfat Milk	1 grande	610	19	12	60	15	92	79	0	—	420	—	—	—

FOOD	PORTION	CALS	FAT	SAT FAT	CHOL	PROT	CARB	SUGAR	FIBER	CALCI	SOD	POTAS	FOLIC	VIT C
Frappuccino Light Espresso Nonfat Milk	1 grande	110	1	0	0	5	20	12	2	—	180	—	—	—
Hot Chocolate No Whip Nonfat Milk	1 grande	240	3	1	5	14	48	40	2	—	140	—	—	—
Hot Chocolate Whip Nonfat Milk	1 grande	320	10	5	35	14	50	41	2	—	150	—	—	—
Iced Brewed Coffee	1 grande	90	0	0	0	0	21	20	0	—	5	—	—	—
Iced Cafe Americano	1 grande	15	0	0	0	1	3	0	0	—	10	—	—	—
Iced Cafe Latte Nonfat Milk	1 grande	90	0	0	5	8	13	11	0	—	100	—	—	—
Iced Cafe Mocha No Whip Nonfat Milk	1 grande	170	3	0	5	9	36	26	2	—	80	—	—	—
Iced Cafe Mocha Whip Nonfat Milk	1 grande	290	14	7	45	9	39	29	2	—	90	—	—	—
Iced Caramel Macchiato Nonfat Milk	1 grande	190	2	1	10	10	34	31	0	—	130	—	—	—
Iced Latte Pumpkin Spice No Whip Nonfat Milk	1 grande	220	0	0	5	10	44	42	0	—	170	—	—	—
Iced Latte Pumpkin Spice Whip Nonfat Milk	1 grande	330	11	7	45	11	48	44	0	—	180	—	—	—
Iced Latte Skinny Cinnamon Dolce No Whip Nonfat Milk	1 grande	80	0	0	5	7	12	10	0	—	105	—	—	—
Iced Latte Sugar Free Flavored Syrup Nonfat Milk	1 grande	80	0	0	5	7	12	10	0	—	105	—	—	—
Iced Latte Syrup Flavored Nonfat Milk	1 grande	160	0	0	5	7	31	28	0	—	90	—	—	—
Iced Latte Vanilla Nonfat Milk	1 grande	160	0	0	5	7	31	28	0	—	90	—	—	—
Iced Peppermint White Chocolate Mocha No Whip Nonfat Milk	1 grande	370	6	5	5	10	72	68	0	—	190	—	—	—

FOOD	PORTION	CALS	FAT	SAT FAT	CHOL	PROT	CARB	SUGAR	FIBER	CALCI	SOD	POTAS	FOLIC	VIT C
Iced Peppermint White Chocolate Mocha Whip Nonfat Milk	1 grande	490	17	11	45	10	75	71	0	—	190	—	—	—
Iced Tazo Latte Black Tea Nonfat Milk	1 grande	170	0	0	0	8	35	34	0	—	100	—	—	—
Iced Tazo Latte Black Tea Soy	1 grande	200	3	0	0	6	38	34	1	—	90	—	—	—
Iced Tazo Latte Chai Nonfat Milk	1 grande	200	0	0	5	8	44	42	0	—	100	—	—	—
Iced Tazo Latte Green Tea Nonfat Milk	1 grande	220	5	0	0	10	45	43	1	—	120	—	—	—
Iced Tazo Latte Green Tea Soy	1 grande	260	4	1	0	7	48	44	2	—	105	—	—	—
Iced Tazo Latte Red Tea	1 grande	200	3	0	0	6	38	34	1	—	90	—	—	—
Iced Tazo Latte Red Tea Nonfat Milk	1 grande	170	0	0	5	8	35	34	0	—	100	—	—	—
Iced White Chocolate Mocha No Whip Nonfat Milk	1 grande	310	6	5	5	11	55	52	0	—	190	—	—	—
Iced White Chocolate Mocha Whip Nonfat Milk	1 grande	430	17	11	45	11	59	55	0	—	200	—	—	—
Latte Caffe Nonfat Milk	1 grande	130	5	0	5	13	19	18	0	—	150	—	—	—
Latte Cinnamon Dolce No Whip Nonfat Milk	1 grande	210	0	0	5	11	41	39	0	—	135	—	—	—
Latte Cinnamon Dolce w/ Sugar Free Syrup Nonfat Milk	1 grande	130	0	0	5	12	19	17	0	—	170	—	—	—
Latte Cinnamon Dolce Whip Nonfat Milk	1 grande	280	7	5	30	12	43	40	0	—	140	—	—	—
Latte Pumpkin Spice No Whip Nonfat Milk	1 grande	260	0	0	5	14	50	48	0	—	210	—	—	—
Latte Pumpkin Spice Whip Nonfat Milk	1 grande	330	7	5	30	14	52	50	0	—	220	—	—	—

FOOD	PORTION	CALS	FAT	SAT FAT	CHOL	PROT	CARB	SUGAR	FIBER	CALCI	SOD	POTAS	FOLIC	VIT C
Latte Skinny Caramel No Whip Nonfat Milk	1 grande	130	0	0	5	12	19	17	0	—	170	—	—	—
Latte Skinny Cinnamon Dolce No Whip Nonfat Milk	1 grande	130	0	0	0	12	19	17	0	—	170	—	—	—
Latte Skinny Hazelnut No Whip Nonfat Milk	1 grande	130	0	0	0	12	19	17	0	—	170	—	—	—
Latte Skinny Vanilla No Whip Nonfat Milk	1 grande	130	0	0	5	12	19	17	0	—	170	—	—	—
Latte Syrup Flavored Nonfat Milk	1 grande	200	0	0	5	12	37	35	0	—	140	—	—	—
Milk Nonfat	1 grande	180	0	0	10	18	26	26	0	—	220	—	—	—
Peppermint White Chocolate Mocha No Whip Nonfat Milk	1 grande	420	6	5	5	14	78	75	0	—	230	—	—	—
Peppermint White Chocolate Mocha Whip Nonfat Milk	1 grande	490	13	9	35	14	80	76	0	—	240	—	—	—
Pumpkin Spice Creme No Whip Nonfat Milk	1 grande	270	0	0	5	15	51	51	0	—	230	—	—	—
Pumpkin Spice Creme Whip Nonfat Milk	1 grande	340	7	5	35	15	53	52	0	—	240	—	—	—
Shaken Black Iced Tea & Lemonade	1 grande	130	0	0	0	0	33	33	0	—	10	—	—	—
Shaken White Iced Tea Blueberry	1 grande	80	0	0	0	0	21	20	0	—	10	—	—	—
Steamed Apple Juice	1 grande	230	0	0	0	0	56	50	0	—	20	—	—	—
Tazo Black Shaken Iced Tea & Lemonade	1 grande	130	0	0	0	0	33	33	0	—	10	—	—	—
Tazo Chai Latte Iced Tea Soy	1 grande	230	3	0	0	6	47	43	1	—	90	—	—	—
Tazo Chai Latte Nonfat Milk	1 grande	200	0	0	5	8	44	42	0	—	95	—	—	—
Tazo Chai Latte Soy	1 grande	230	3	0	0	5	47	42	1	—	85	—	—	—

FOOD	PORTION	CALS	FAT	SAT FAT	CHOL	PROT	CARB	SUGAR	FIBER	CALCI	SOD	POTAS	FOLIC	VIT C
Tazo Latte Black Tea Nonfat Milk	1 grande	170	0	0	5	7	34	32	0	—	90	—	—	—
Tazo Latte Black Tea Soy	1 grande	190	3	0	0	5	36	32	1	—	75	—	—	—
Tazo Latte Green Tea Nonfat Milk	1 grande	200	0	0	5	8	42	41	1	—	85	—	—	—
Tazo Latte Green Tea Soy	1 grande	220	3	0	0	6	44	40	2	—	75	—	—	—
Tazo Latte Red Tea Nonfat Milk	1 grande	170	0	0	5	7	34	32	0	—	90	—	—	—
Tazo Latte Red Tea Soy	1 grande	190	3	0	0	5	36	32	1	—	75	—	—	—
Tazo Shaken Iced Tea Green	1 grande	80	0	0	0	0	21	20	0	—	10	—	—	—
Tazo Shaken Iced Tea Green & Lemonade	1 grande	130	0	0	0	0	33	33	0	—	10	—	—	—
Tazo Shaken Iced Tea Orange Passion	1 grande	70	0	0	0	0	19	18	0	—	10	—	—	—
Tazo Shaken Iced Tea Passion	1 grande	80	0	0	0	0	21	20	0	—	10	—	—	—
Tazo Shaken Iced Tea Passion & Lemonade	1 grande	130	0	0	0	0	33	33	0	—	10	—	—	—
Tazo Tea	1 grande	0	0	0	0	0	0	0	0	—	0	—	—	—
Vanilla Creme Whip Nonfat Milk	1 grande	270	7	5	35	13	39	38	0	—	160	—	—	—
Vanilla Creme No Whip Nonfat Milk	1 grande	200	0	0	5	12	37	37	0	—	160	—	—	—
Vivanno Blend Banana Chocolate	1 grande (20 oz)	270	2	1	5	21	44	28	6	200	170	750	—	9
Vivanno Blend Orange Mango Banana	1 grande (20 oz)	250	2	1	5	16	47	32	5	100	120	400	—	21
White Chocolate Mocha No Whip Nonfat Milk	1 grande	360	6	5	10	16	62	61	0	—	260	—	—	—
White Chocolate Mocha Whip Nonfat Milk	1 grande	430	13	9	35	16	64	62	0	—	270	—	—	—
SALADS														
Fiesta	1 (9.4 oz)	320	10	2	20	16	44	12	8	—	930	—	—	—
Fruit & Cheese Plate	1 (8.6 oz)	400	20	10	50	14	44	26	2	—	560	—	—	—

FOOD	PORTION	CALS	FAT	SAT FAT	CHOL	PROT	CARB	SUGAR	FIBER	CALCI	SOD	POTAS	FOLIC	VIT C
Vegetable Vinaigrette	1 (10.7 oz)	310	15	4	5	8	40	8	10	—	900	—	—	—
SANDWICHES														
Club Chicken Cheddar Bacon w/ Mayo	1	480	18	6	70	31	48	8	2	—	1180	—	—	—
Club Turkey & Avocado	1	390	19	5	65	26	33	5	7	—	1160	—	—	—
Egg Salad On Multigrain	1	470	21	5	340	19	53	11	2	—	810	—	—	—
Turkey & Swiss w/ Mayo	1	310	13	5	55	26	26	3	2	—	1060	—	—	—
TOPPINGS														
Caramel	1 tbsp	15	1	0	0	0	2	2	0	0	5	—	—	0
Chocolate	1 tsp	5	0	0	0	0	1	1	0	0	0	—	—	0
Flavored Sugar Free Syrup	1 pump	0	0	0	0	0	0	0	0	0	0	—	—	0
Flavored Syrup	1 pump	20	0	0	0	0	5	5	0	0	0	—	—	0
Mocha Syrup	1 pump	25	1	0	0	1	5	4	0	0	0	—	—	0
Sprinkles	1 serv	0	0	0	0	0	0	0	0	0	0	—	—	0

STEAK ESCAPE

FOOD	PORTION	CALS	FAT	SAT FAT	CHOL	PROT	CARB	SUGAR	FIBER	CALCI	SOD	POTAS	FOLIC	VIT C
BEVERAGES														
Coca-Cola	16 oz	150	0	0	0	0	40	—	—	—	15	—	—	—
Diet Coke	16 oz	0	0	0	0	0	0	0	0	—	30	—	—	—
Lemonade	16 oz	167	0	0	0	0	44	—	—	—	0	—	—	—
Sprite	16 oz	150	0	0	0	0	39	—	—	—	55	—	—	—
SALADS														
Grilled Side	1 serv (5.9 oz)	40	1	—	0	3	8	—	—	—	20	—	—	—
Grilled w/ Chicken	1 serv (11.1 oz)	177	5	—	108	25	11	—	—	—	652	—	—	—
Grilled w/ Ham	1 serv (10.6 oz)	302	2	—	83	19	8	—	—	—	1042	—	—	—
Grilled w/ Steak	1 serv (11.1 oz)	187	6	—	103	23	11	—	—	—	292	—	—	—
Grilled w/ Turkey	1 serv (10.6 oz)	132	2	—	83	19	8	—	—	—	1042	—	—	—
SANDWICHES														
7 Inch Cajun Chicken	1 (8.6 oz)	408	5	—	55	31	58	—	—	—	1211	—	—	—
7 Inch Capicola Portion	1 serv (1 oz)	31	1	—	14	5	tr	—	—	—	329	—	—	—
7 Inch Chicken Portion	1 serv (3.9 oz)	120	4	—	55	21	0	0	0	—	430	—	—	—
7 Inch Classic Italian Sub	1 (8.4 oz)	471	11	—	49	27	60	—	—	—	1989	—	—	—
7 Inch Ham Portion	1 serv (3 oz)	75	1	—	15	8	3	—	—	—	1020	—	—	—
7 Inch Salami Portion	1 serv (1 oz)	105	9	—	25	6	0	—	—	—	470	—	—	—

FOOD	PORTION	CALS	FAT	SAT FAT	CHOL	PROT	CARB	SUGAR	FIBER	CALCI	SOD	POTAS	FOLIC	VIT C
7 Inch Steak Portion	1 serv (3.9 oz)	130	5	—	50	19	0	0	0	—	270	—	—	—
7 Inch Turkey Club	1 (7.9 oz)	380	2	—	20	21	62	—	—	—	2040	—	—	—
7 Inch Turkey Portion	1 serv (2.9 oz)	75	1	—	15	8	3	—	—	—	1020	—	—	—
7 Inch Vegetarian	1 (8.8 oz)	311	1	—	0	13	65	—	—	—	733	—	—	—
7 Inch Wild West BBQ	1 (9.6 oz)	455	6	—	50	29	60	—	—	—	1302	—	—	—
Kids Chicken	1 (3.9 oz)	205	7	—	32	12	29	—	—	—	470	—	—	—
Kids Ham	1 (3.7 oz)	183	1	—	13	6	31	—	—	—	765	—	—	—
Kids Steak	1 (3.8 oz)	110	3	—	13	9	29	—	—	—	445	—	—	—
Kids Turkey	1 (3.7 oz)	183	1	—	13	6	31	—	—	—	765	—	—	—
SIDES														
Fries	1 serv (32 oz)	996	52	—	0	16	134	—	—	—	818	—	—	—
Fries	1 serv (12 oz)	498	26	—	0	8	67	—	—	—	409	—	—	—
Fries Kids	1 serv (2.9 oz)	249	13	—	0	4	34	—	—	—	205	—	—	—
Fries Loaded Bacon & Cheddar	1 serv (10.8 oz)	905	44	—	29	18	88	—	—	—	1587	—	—	—
Fries Loaded Ranch & Bacon	1 serv (10.8 oz)	1044	71	—	39	18	84	—	—	—	1398	—	—	—
Kids Chicken Tenders	2 (3.8 oz)	240	11	—	35	15	21	—	—	—	1050	—	—	—
Smashed Potatoes Loaded Bacon & Cheddar	1 serv (16.7 oz)	636	26	—	24	13	91	—	—	—	827	—	—	—
Smashed Potatoes Loaded Ranch & Bacon	1 serv (16.7 oz)	692	34	—	29	14	87	—	—	—	501	—	—	—
Smashed Potatoes Plain	1 serv (13.8 oz)	246	0	0	0	11	53	—	—	—	43	—	—	—
Smashed Potatoes w/ Chicken	1 serv (19.9 oz)	383	4	—	108	33	56	—	—	—	475	—	—	—
Smashed Potatoes w/ Ham	1 serv (19.4 oz)	338	2	—	83	27	59	—	—	—	1065	—	—	—
Smashed Potatoes w/ Steak	1 serv (19.9 oz)	393	5	—	103	31	56	—	—	—	313	—	—	—
Smashed Potatoes w/ Turkey	1 serv (19.4 oz)	338	2	—	83	27	59	—	—	—	1065	—	—	—
TOPPINGS														
BBQ Sauce	1 serv (1 oz)	40	0	0	0	0	9	—	—	—	252	—	—	—
Brown Mustard	1 serv (1 oz)	0	0	0	0	0	0	0	0	—	340	—	—	—
Cheddar	1 serv (1 oz)	116	8	—	26	8	1	—	—	—	179	—	—	—
Dressing Balsamic Vinaigrette	1 serv (1.5 oz)	90	9	—	0	0	3	—	—	—	350	—	—	—

FOOD	PORTION	CALS	FAT	SAT FAT	CHOL	PROT	CARB	SUGAR	FIBER	CALCI	SOD	POTAS	FOLIC	VIT C
Dressing Bleu Cheese	1 serv (1.5 oz)	184	18	—	8	2	3	—	—	—	35	—	—	—
Dressing Italian	1 serv (0.5 oz)	51	5	—	0	0	1	—	—	—	248	—	—	—
Dressing Ranch	1 serv (0.5 oz)	83	9	—	5	0	0	0	0	—	137	—	—	—
Lettuce	1 serv (1 oz)	2	0	0	0	1	0	0	0	—	2	—	—	—
Margarine	1 serv (1 oz)	203	23	—	0	0	0	0	0	—	306	—	—	—
Mayonnaise	1 serv (1 oz)	101	11	—	5	0	0	0	0	—	76	—	—	—
Parmesan	1 serv (1 oz)	30	2	—	5	3	tr	—	—	—	120	—	—	—
Peppers Jalapeno	1 serv (1.5 oz)	11	—	—	—	—	—	—	—	—	—	—	—	—
Peppers Mild	1 serv (1.5 oz)	11	0	0	0	0	4	—	—	—	500	—	—	—
Provolone	1 serv (0.75 oz)	80	6	—	15	5	0	0	0	—	190	—	—	—
Sour Cream	1 serv (1 oz)	61	6	—	13	1	1	—	—	—	15	—	—	—
Tomatoes	1 serv (2 oz)	24	0	0	0	2	2	—	—	—	5	—	—	—
White American	1 serv (1 oz)	101	9	—	26	6	3	—	—	—	437	—	—	—

SUBWAY

ADD-ONS AND SALAD DRESSINGS

FOOD	PORTION	CALS	FAT	SAT FAT	CHOL	PROT	CARB	SUGAR	FIBER	CALCI	SOD	POTAS	FOLIC	VIT C
American Cheese	1 serv (0.4 oz)	40	4	2	10	2	1	0	0	80	200	—	—	0
Bacon Strips	2	45	4	2	10	3	0	0	0	0	190	—	—	0
Banana Pepper Slices	3	0	0	0	0	0	0	0	0	0	20	—	—	4
Cheddar	1 serv (0.5 oz)	60	5	3	15	4	0	0	0	80	95	—	—	0
Fat Free Italian	1 serv (2 oz)	35	0	0	0	1	7	4	0	20	720	—	—	0
Fat Free Red Wine Vinaigrette	1 serv (0.7 oz)	30	0	0	1	0	6	3	0	0	340	—	—	0
Jalapeno Pepper Slices	3	<5	0	0	0	0	0	0	0	0	70	—	—	2
Mayonnaise	1 tbsp	110	12	2	10	0	0	0	0	0	80	—	—	0
Mayonnaise Light	1 tbsp	50	5	1	5	0	tr	0	0	0	100	—	—	0
Monterey Cheddar Shredded	1 serv (0.5 oz)	50	5	3	15	3	1	0	0	100	90	—	—	0
Mustard Yellow or Deli	2 tsp	5	0	0	0	0	tr	0	0	0	115	—	—	0
Olive Oil Blend	1 tsp	45	5	0	0	0	0	0	0	0	0	—	—	0
Pepperjack Cheese	1 serv (0.5 oz)	50	4	3	15	3	0	0	0	100	140	—	—	2
Provolone	1 serv (0.5 oz)	50	4	2	10	4	0	0	0	100	125	—	—	0
Ranch	1 serv (2 oz)	320	35	6	29	0	3	2	0	0	560	—	—	0
Ranch Lowfat	1.5 tbsp	120	13	2	11	0	1	1	0	0	210	—	—	0
Red Wine Vinaigrette	1 serv (2 oz)	80	1	0	0	1	17	7	0	0	910	—	—	0
Sauce Chipotle Southwest	1.5 tbsp	100	10	2	8	0	1	1	0	0	220	—	—	0
Sauce Fat Free Honey Mustard	1.5 tbsp	30	0	0	0	0	7	6	0	0	115	—	—	0
Sauce Fat Free Sweet Onion	1.5 tbsp	40	0	0	0	0	9	8	0	0	85	—	—	0
Swiss	1 serv (0.5 oz)	50	5	3	15	4	0	0	0	150	30	—	—	0

FOOD	PORTION	CALS	FAT	SAT FAT	CHOL	PROT	CARB	SUGAR	FIBER	CALCI	SOD	POTAS	FOLIC	VIT C
Vinegar	1 tsp	0	0	0	0	0	0	0	0	0	0	—	—	0
BREADS														
Hearty Italian	6 inch	220	2	1	0	8	41	5	2	40	470	—	—	12
Honey Oat	6 inch	250	4	1	0	10	48	9	5	60	380	—	—	9
Italian	6 inch	200	2	1	0	7	38	5	1	20	470	—	—	9
Italian Herb & Cheese	6 inch	250	5	3	10	10	40	5	2	100	670	—	—	12
Italian White	1 mini	140	2	1	0	5	26	3	1	20	320	—	—	5
Monterey Cheddar	6 inch	240	5	3	10	10	39	5	1	100	540	—	—	12
Parmesan Oregano	6 inch	220	3	1	0	8	40	5	2	40	620	—	—	12
Wheat	1 mini	140	2	1	0	6	27	3	2	40	240	—	—	6
Wheat	6 inch	200	3	1	0	8	40	5	4	40	360	—	—	9
Wrap	1	190	5	1	0	6	33	1	1	40	470	—	—	0
DESSERTS														
Apple Slices	1 pkg	35	0	0	0	0	9	7	2	40	0	—	—	18
Cookie Chocolate Chip	1	210	10	6	15	2	30	18	1	0	150	—	—	0
Cookie Chocolate Chip w/ M&M's	1 (1.6 oz)	210	10	5	10	2	32	18	tr	20	100	—	—	0
Cookie Chocolate Chunk	1	220	10	5	10	2	30	17	tr	0	100	—	—	0
Cookie Double Chocolate Chip	1 (1.6 oz)	210	10	5	15	2	30	20	1	20	170	—	—	0
Cookie Oatmeal Raisin	1	200	8	4	15	3	30	17	1	20	170	—	—	0
Cookie Peanut Butter	1	220	12	5	15	4	26	16	1	20	200	—	—	0
Cookie Sugar	1	220	12	6	15	2	28	14	tr	0	140	—	—	0
Cookie White Chip Macadamia Nut	1	220	11	5	15	2	29	18	tr	20	160	—	—	0
Raisins	1 pkg	150	0	0	0	2	33	30	2	0	0	—	—	0
SALADS														
Ham w/o Dressing & Croutons	1 serv	120	3	1	25	12	14	6	4	60	840	—	—	30
Oven Roasted Chicken Breast w/o Dressing & Croutons	1 serv	140	3	1	50	19	11	5	4	80	390	—	—	30
Roast Beef w/o Dressing & Croutons	1 serv	120	3	2	20	13	12	6	4	60	480	—	—	30
Subway Club w/o Dressing & Croutons	1 serv	150	4	2	35	18	14	7	4	60	870	—	—	30

FOOD	PORTION	CALS	FAT	SAT FAT	CHOL	PROT	CARB	SUGAR	FIBER	CALCI	SOD	POTAS	FOLIC	VIT C
Sweet Onion Chicken Teriyaki w/o Dressing & Croutons	1 serv	210	3	1	50	20	26	17	4	80	780	—	—	5
Turkey Breast & Ham w/o Dressing & Croutons	1 serv	120	3	1	25	14	14	6	4	60	790	—	—	30
Veggie Delight w/o Dressing & Croutons	1 serv	60	1	0	0	3	11	5	4	60	80	—	—	30
SANDWICHES														
6 Inch Chicken & Bacon Ranch	1	580	30	11	100	36	47	7	6	300	1390	—	—	24
6 Inch Cold Cut Combo	1	410	17	7	60	21	47	8	5	200	1530	—	—	21
6 Inch Double Stacked Cold Cut Combo	1	550	28	10	110	31	49	8	5	250	2360	—	—	24
6 Inch Double Stacked Italian BMT	1	630	35	14	100	34	49	10	5	150	2850	—	—	21
6 Inch Double Stacked Steak & Cheese	1	540	18	8	105	46	49	12	7	150	1500	—	—	30
6 Inch Double Stacked Subway Club	1	420	8	4	65	39	50	10	5	80	2080	—	—	35
6 Inch Double Stacked Sweet Onion Chicken Teriyaki	1	480	7	2	100	43	65	23	6	100	1820	—	—	30
6 Inch Double Stacked Turkey Breast	1	330	5	2	40	28	48	8	5	80	1500	—	—	21
6 Inch Ham	1	290	5	2	25	18	47	8	5	60	1260	—	—	21
6 Inch Italian BMT	1	450	21	8	55	23	47	8	5	150	1770	—	—	21
6 Inch Meatball Marinara	1	560	24	11	45	24	63	13	8	200	1590	—	—	36
6 Inch Oven Roasted Chicken Breast	1	310	5	2	25	24	48	9	6	60	830	—	—	27
6 Inch Roast Beef	1	290	5	2	20	19	45	8	5	60	900	—	—	21
6 Inch Spicy Italian	1	480	25	9	55	21	45	8	5	80	1660	—	—	21
6 Inch Steak & Cheese	1	400	12	6	60	29	48	9	6	150	1110	—	—	24

FOOD	PORTION	CALS	FAT	SAT FAT	CHOL	PROT	CARB	SUGAR	FIBER	CALCI	SOD	POTAS	FOLIC	VIT C
6 Inch Subway Club	1	320	6	2	35	24	47	8	5	60	1290	—	—	21
6 Inch Subway Melt	1	380	12	5	45	25	48	8	5	150	1600	—	—	21
6 Inch Sweet Onion Chicken Teriyaki	1	370	5	2	50	26	59	19	5	80	1200	—	—	24
6 Inch Tuna	1	530	31	7	45	22	44	7	5	150	1010	—	—	21
6 Inch Turkey Breast	1	280	5	2	20	18	46	7	5	60	1000	—	—	21
6 Inch Turkey Breast & Ham	1	290	5	2	25	20	47	8	5	60	1210	—	—	21
6 Inch Veggie Delite	1	230	3	1	0	9	44	7	5	60	500	—	—	21
Mini Sub Ham	1	180	3	1	10	11	30	5	4	60	710	—	—	12
Mini Sub Roast Beef	1	190	4	2	15	13	30	5	4	60	600	—	—	12
Mini Sub Tuna w/ Cheese	1	320	18	5	30	13	30	5	4	100	690	—	—	12
Mini Sub Turkey Breast	1	190	3	1	15	12	30	5	4	80	670	—	—	12
Softwich Santa Fe Turkey	1	520	10	4	55	33	78	17	5	60	1910	—	—	24

TACO BELL

FOOD	PORTION	CALS	FAT	SAT FAT	CHOL	PROT	CARB	SUGAR	FIBER	CALCI	SOD	POTAS	FOLIC	VIT C
Border Bowl Southwest Steak	1 serv	600	24	6	55	28	68	3	9	200	2120	—	—	9
Border Bowl Zesty Chicken	1 serv	640	35	6	30	22	60	4	10	150	1800	—	—	9
Border Bowl Zesty Chicken w/o Dressing	1 serv	440	15	3	30	21	57	3	10	150	1540	—	—	9
Burrito 7 Layer	1	490	18	7	25	17	65	5	9	250	1350	—	—	15
Burrito Bean	1	350	9	4	6	13	54	4	8	200	1190	—	—	5
Burrito Chili Cheese	1	370	16	8	40	16	40	3	3	300	1060	—	—	0
Burrito Grilled Stuft Chicken	1	640	23	7	65	34	73	6	7	300	2160	—	—	4
Burrito Grilled Stuft Steak	1	630	25	8	55	30	72	5	7	300	1930	—	—	4
Burrito Supreme Beef	1	420	17	8	40	17	51	5	7	200	1340	—	—	6
Burrito ½ Lb Beef & Potato	1	530	23	7	30	15	68	4	6	150	1720	—	—	4
Burrito ½ Lb Combo Beef	1	440	18	7	45	21	51	4	8	200	1630	—	—	4
Burrito Fiesta Chicken	1	360	10	4	30	18	47	4	3	200	1320	—	—	2
Burrito Fiesta Steak	1	370	13	5	25	14	49	4	4	200	1200	—	—	2

FOOD	PORTION	CALS	FAT	SAT FAT	CHOL	PROT	CARB	SUGAR	FIBER	CALCI	SOD	POTAS	FOLIC	VIT C
Burrito Supreme Chicken	1	400	13	6	45	20	49	5	6	200	1360	—	—	9
Burrito Supreme Steak	1	390	14	6	40	18	49	5	6	200	1250	—	—	9
Chalupa Baja Beef	1	410	27	6	35	13	30	4	4	100	780	—	—	2
Chalupa Baja Chicken	1	390	23	4	40	17	29	4	3	100	800	—	—	4
Chalupa Baja Steak	1	390	24	5	35	15	28	3	3	100	690	—	—	2
Chalupa Nacho Cheese Beef	1	370	22	5	20	12	32	4	3	100	770	—	—	4
Chalupa Nacho Cheese Chicken	1	360	18	3	25	16	30	4	2	100	790	—	—	5
Chalupa Nacho Cheese Steak	1	340	19	4	20	14	30	4	2	80	680	—	—	4
Chalupa Supreme Beef	1	380	20	7	40	14	30	4	3	150	620	—	—	4
Chalupa Supreme Chicken	1	360	20	5	45	17	29	4	2	100	650	—	—	5
Chalupa Supreme Steak	1	360	21	8	40	15	28	4	2	100	530	—	—	4
Cheesy Fiesta Potatoes	1 serv	290	17	4	15	4	29	2	2	60	830	—	—	0
Cinnamon Twists	1 serv	170	7	0	0	1	26	12	1	0	200	—	—	0
Crunchwrap Supreme	1	560	24	8	35	17	68	7	5	250	1430	—	—	5
Crunchwrap Supreme Spicy Chicken	1	540	24	8	35	19	67	7	4	300	1360	—	—	5
Crunchy Taco	1	170	25	4	10	8	13	1	3	80	350	—	—	1
Crunchy Taco Supreme	1	210	10	4	25	9	15	2	3	100	370	—	—	4
Empanada Caramel Apple	1	290	14	3	5	3	37	13	1	40	300	—	—	9
Enchirito Beef	1	360	17	8	50	18	34	3	7	300	1420	—	—	6
Enchirito Chicken	1	340	13	7	50	22	33	3	6	300	1450	—	—	9
Fresco Border Bowl Zesty Chicken w/o Dressing	1 serv	350	8	2	25	19	51	4	10	100	1600	—	—	12
Fresco Burrito Bean	1 (7.5 oz)	340	8	3	0	12	56	4	11	150	1290	—	—	6
Fresco Burrito Fiesta Chicken	1	330	8	3	25	16	48	4	3	150	1240	—	—	5
Fresco Burrito Supreme Chicken	1 (8.5 oz)	340	8	3	25	18	50	4	8	150	1410	—	—	9

FOOD	PORTION	CALS	FAT	SAT FAT	CHOL	PROT	CARB	SUGAR	FIBER	CALCI	SOD	POTAS	FOLIC	VIT C
Fresco Burrito Supreme Steak	1 (8.5 oz)	330	8	3	15	16	49	4	8	150	1340	—	—	9
Fresco Crunchy Taco	1 (3.2 oz)	150	7	3	20	7	13	1	3	40	350	—	—	2
Fresco Soft Taco Beef	1 (4 oz)	180	7	3	20	8	22	2	3	80	640	—	—	2
Fresco Soft Taco Grilled Steak	1 (4.5 oz)	160	4	2	15	9	21	3	2	80	600	—	—	6
Fresco Soft Taco Ranchero Chicken	1 (4.7 oz)	170	4	2	25	12	22	3	2	80	740	—	—	4
Gordita Baja Beef	1	340	19	5	35	13	29	8	4	100	780	—	—	2
Gordita Baja Chicken	1	320	16	4	40	17	28	6	3	100	800	—	—	4
Gordita Baja Steak	1	320	17	4	35	15	27	5	3	100	690	—	—	2
Gordita Nacho Cheese Beef	1	300	14	4	25	12	31	6	3	100	770	—	—	4
Gordita Nacho Cheese Chicken	1	280	11	3	25	16	29	6	2	100	800	—	—	5
Gordita Nacho Cheese Steak	1	270	12	3	20	14	29	6	2	80	680	—	—	4
Gordita Supreme Beef	1	310	16	6	40	14	29	6	3	150	620	—	—	4
Gordita Supreme Chicken	1	290	12	5	45	17	28	6	2	150	650	—	—	5
Gordita Supreme Steak	1	290	13	5	40	15	28	6	2	100	530	—	—	4
Guacamole Side	1 serv	70	5	1	0	1	5	1	2	0	180	—	—	8
Mexican Pizza	1	530	30	8	40	20	46	3	6	300	1000	—	—	4
Mexican Rice	1 serv	180	7	3	15	6	23	0	1	100	790	—	—	4
MexiMelt	1 serv	260	14	7	40	15	22	2	3	250	860	—	—	2
Nacho Supreme	1 serv	440	26	7	35	12	41	3	7	100	800	—	—	4
Nachos	1 serv	330	21	4	5	4	32	3	2	80	530	—	—	0
Nachos Bellgrande	1 serv	770	44	9	35	19	77	5	12	200	1280	—	—	4
Pintos 'n Cheese	1 serv	160	6	3	15	9	19	1	7	150	670	—	—	4
Quesadilla Cheese	1	470	26	12	50	19	39	4	2	450	1100	—	—	0
Quesadilla Chicken	1	520	28	12	75	28	40	4	3	450	1420	—	—	1
Quesadilla Steak	1	520	28	13	70	26	39	4	3	450	1300	—	—	0
Salsa Side	1 serv	15	0	0	0	0	3	2	0	40	160	—	—	2
Soft Taco Grande	1	430	20	8	45	19	43	5	5	200	1440	—	—	1
Soft Taco Grilled Steak	1	270	16	5	35	12	20	3	2	100	660	—	—	4
Soft Taco Ranchero Chicken	1	270	14	4	35	14	21	3	2	150	820	—	—	4

FOOD	PORTION	CALS	FAT	SAT FAT	CHOL	PROT	CARB	SUGAR	FIBER	CALCI	SOD	POTAS	FOLIC	VIT C
Soft Taco Supreme Beef	1	250	13	6	40	11	23	3	3	150	650	—	—	4
Sour Cream Side	1 serv	80	7	5	25	1	3	2	0	40	30	—	—	0
Taco Double Decker	1	320	13	5	25	14	38	2	6	150	810	—	—	1
Taco Double Decker Supreme	1	370	17	7	40	14	40	4	7	150	820	—	—	4
Taco Spicy Chicken	1	170	8	2	25	10	20	2	2	100	580	—	—	2
Taco Salad Express	1	610	32	10	65	25	56	8	14	300	1420	—	—	12
Taco Salad Fiesta	1	840	45	11	65	30	80	10	15	450	1780	—	—	12
Taco Salad Fiesta w/o Shell	1	470	24	10	65	23	41	9	13	300	1510	—	—	12
Taco Salad Fiesta Chicken	1	790	38	8	75	37	77	10	13	400	1830	—	—	15
Taco Salad Fiesta Chicken w/o Shell	1	430	18	6	75	30	38	9	11	300	1560	—	—	15
Taquitos Chicken Grilled	1 serv	310	11	5	40	18	37	3	2	200	980	—	—	1
Taquitos Steak Grilled	1 serv	310	11	5	35	16	36	3	2	200	870	—	—	0
Tostada	1	240	10	4	15	11	27	2	7	200	730	—	—	5

TACO BUENO

MAIN MENU SELECTIONS

FOOD	PORTION	CALS	FAT	SAT FAT	CHOL	PROT	CARB	SUGAR	FIBER	CALCI	SOD	POTAS	FOLIC	VIT C
Bueno Chilada Beef	1 (7.9 oz)	523	32	—	—	24	42	6	2	—	2056	—	—	—
Bueno Chilada Beef w/o Chili	1 (5.5 oz)	412	26	—	—	19	29	6	1	—	1512	—	—	—
Bueno Chilada Beef w/o Queso	1 (5.6 oz)	337	18	—	—	14	36	2	2	—	1147	—	—	—
Bueno Chilada Chicken	1 (7.4 oz)	477	26	—	—	24	43	7	2	—	2090	—	—	—
Bueno Chilada Chicken w/o Chili	1 (5 oz)	366	20	—	—	19	30	6	1	—	1546	—	—	—
Bueno Chilada Chicken w/o Queso	1 (5.1 oz)	290	12	—	—	14	30	2	2	—	1181	—	—	—
Burrito Bean	1 (6.4 oz)	490	29	—	—	15	45	1	5	—	1649	—	—	—
Burrito Bean w/o Cheddar Cheese	1 (5.9 oz)	412	23	—	—	11	44	1	5	—	1528	—	—	—
Burrito Bean w/o Chili	1 (5.2 oz)	434	26	—	—	13	39	1	4	—	1378	—	—	—
Burrito Beef	1 (6.9 oz)	510	29	—	—	23	41	1	3	—	1377	—	—	—

FOOD	PORTION	CALS	FAT	SAT FAT	CHOL	PROT	CARB	SUGAR	FIBER	CALCI	SOD	POTAS	FOLIC	VIT C
Burrito Beef Potato	1 (4.8 oz)	350	21	—	—	11	32	3	3	—	906	—	—	—
Burrito Beef Potato w/o Queso	1 (4.1 oz)	305	17	—	—	9	30	1	3	—	644	—	—	—
Burrito Beef Potato w/o Sour Cream	1 (4.3 oz)	330	18	—	—	11	31	2	3	—	896	—	—	—
Burrito Beef w/o Cheddar Cheese	1 (6.4 oz)	432	22	—	—	19	40	1	3	—	1255	—	—	—
Burrito Beef w/o Chili	1 (5.7 oz)	455	25	—	—	20	36	1	2	—	1105	—	—	—
Burrito Big Ol' Beef	1 (10.6 oz)	772	46	—	—	33	57	2	3	—	1833	—	—	—
Burrito Big Ol' Beef w/o Cheddar Cheese	1 (9.6 oz)	615	33	—	—	24	56	2	3	—	1590	—	—	—
Burrito Big Ol' Beef w/o Chili	1 (9.4 oz)	716	43	—	—	31	51	2	2	—	1561	—	—	—
Burrito Big Ol' Beef w/o Sour Cream	1 (9.6 oz)	715	40	—	—	32	55	1	3	—	1814	—	—	—
Burrito Big Ol' Chicken	1 (8.4 oz)	607	30	—	—	31	53	3	5	—	1640	—	—	—
Burrito Big Ol' Chicken w/o Cheddar Cheese	1 (7.4 oz)	450	17	—	—	22	52	3	2	—	1397	—	—	—
Burrito Big Ol' Chicken w/o Sour Cream	1 (7.4 oz)	551	24	—	—	30	51	2	2	—	1621	—	—	—
Burrito Chicken Potato	1 (4.5 oz)	327	18	—	—	11	33	3	3	—	928	—	—	—
Burrito Chicken Potato w/o Queso	1 (3.8 oz)	274	14	—	—	9	31	2	3	—	667	—	—	—
Burrito Chicken Potato w/o Sour Cream	1 (4 oz)	299	15	—	—	11	32	2	3	—	918	—	—	—
Burrito Combination	1 (6.8 oz)	507	29	—	—	19	43	1	4	—	1536	—	—	—
Burrito Combination w/o Cheddar Cheese	1 (6.3 oz)	429	23	—	—	15	42	1	4	—	1414	—	—	—
Burrito Combination w/o Chili	1 (5.6 oz)	452	26	—	—	17	37	1	3	—	1263	—	—	—
Burrito Combination w/o Refried Beans	1 (5.7 oz)	440	23	—	—	18	40	1	3	—	1157	—	—	—
Burrito Party	1 (4 oz)	298	18	—	—	9	29	1	3	—	1041	—	—	—
Burrito Party w/o Cheddar Cheese	1 (3.8 oz)	259	14	—	—	7	29	1	3	—	980	—	—	—

FOOD	PORTION	CALS	FAT	SAT FAT	CHOL	PROT	CARB	SUGAR	FIBER	CALCI	SOD	POTAS	FOLIC	VIT C
Chimichanger Cheesecake	1 (2 oz)	210	11	—	—	4	24	4	1	—	160	—	—	—
Cinnamon Chips	1 serv (4.5 oz)	676	31	—	—	8	95	54	4	—	254	—	—	—
Corn Tortilla Chips	1 serv (1.5 oz)	219	11	—	—	3	27	1	4	—	25	—	—	—
Guacamole	1 serv (0.9 oz)	55	5	—	—	1	2	0	1	—	128	—	—	—
Jalapenos	1 serv (0.7 oz)	3	0	0	—	0	1	0	1	—	334	—	—	—
Mexican Rice	1 serv (4.2 oz)	469	12	—	—	10	83	4	2	—	1287	—	—	—
Muchaco Beef	1 (5.2 oz)	449	25	—	—	15	40	2	3	—	911	—	—	—
Muchaco Beef w/o Cheddar Cheese	1 (4.9 oz)	410	22	—	—	13	40	2	3	—	850	—	—	—
Muchaco Beef w/o Refried Beans	1 (4.2 oz)	392	20	—	—	14	38	2	2	—	596	—	—	—
Muchaco Chicken	1 (4.6 oz)	387	18	—	—	17	40	2	2	—	817	—	—	—
Muchaco Chicken w/o Cheddar Cheese	1 (4.4 oz)	348	14	—	—	15	39	2	2	—	756	—	—	—
Nachos Cheese	1 serv (5.5 oz)	572	35	—	—	18	47	8	6	—	1396	—	—	—
Quesadilla Beef	1 (8.5 oz)	823	51	—	—	38	49	1	2	—	1612	—	—	—
Quesadilla Cheese	1 (6.5 oz)	709	42	—	—	30	48	1	2	—	1261	—	—	—
Quesadilla Chicken	1 (7.9 oz)	761	44	—	—	38	50	1	2	—	1658	—	—	—
Quesadilla Kids Cheese	1 (2.2 oz)	219	11	—	—	8	23	1	1	—	462	—	—	—
Quesadilla Mini Cheese	1 (2.7)	274	15	—	—	11	23	1	1	—	533	—	—	—
Refried Beans Powdered	1 serv (6.3 oz)	406	34	—	—	12	17	1	5	—	1905	—	—	—
Refried Beans w/o Cheddar Cheese	1 serv (5.8 oz)	327	28	—	—	8	16	1	5	—	1784	—	—	—
Refried Beans w/o Chili	1 serv (5.1 oz)	360	31	—	—	9	11	0	4	—	1634	—	—	—
Salsa Red	1 serv (2 oz)	14	0	0	—	1	3	0	1	—	366	—	—	—
Soup Tortilla	1 bowl	237	11	—	—	20	19	3	2	—	1430	—	—	—
Soup Tortilla w/o Tortilla Strips & Cheese	1 bowl	148	6	—	—	17	11	3	2	—	1382	—	—	—
Sour Cream	1 serv (1 oz)	57	6	—	—	1	2	1	0	—	19	—	—	—
Taco Party	1 (1.9 oz)	143	10	—	—	7	5	0	0	—	244	—	—	—
Taco w/o Cheddar Cheese	1 (1.5 oz)	104	7	—	—	4	5	0	0	—	183	—	—	—
Taco Crispy Beef	1 (2.6 oz)	200	14	—	—	10	7	0	0	—	378	—	—	—
Taco Crispy Chicken	1 (1.9 oz)	140	7	—	—	9	8	1	0	—	368	—	—	—
Taco Crispy Chicken w/o Cheddar Cheese	1 (1.7 oz)	100	4	—	—	7	7	1	0	—	307	—	—	—

FOOD	PORTION	CALS	FAT	SAT FAT	CHOL	PROT	CARB	SUGAR	FIBER	CALCI	SOD	POTAS	FOLIC	VIT C
Taco Crispy w/o Cheddar Cheese	1 (2.4 oz)	161	11	—	—	7	6	0	0	—	317	—	—	—
Taco Soft Beef	1 (3.5 oz)	245	14	—	—	11	18	0	1	—	620	—	—	—
Taco Soft Beef w/o Cheddar Cheese	1 (3.2 oz)	206	11	—	—	9	17	0	1	—	559	—	—	—
Taco Soft Chicken	1 (2.9 oz)	184	8	—	—	10	19	1	1	—	610	—	—	—
Taco Soft Chicken w/o Cheddar Cheese	1 (2.5 oz)	145	5	—	—	8	18	1	1	—	540	—	—	—
Tostada	1 (4.1 oz)	324	24	—	—	11	18	1	3	—	971	—	—	—
Tostada w/o Cheddar Cheese	1 (3.3 oz)	207	15	—	—	5	17	1	3	—	789	—	—	—
Tostada w/o Chili	1 (2.9 oz)	269	21	—	—	9	12	0	3	—	699	—	—	—
Tostada w/o Refried Beans	1 (2.5 oz)	234	16	—	—	10	15	1	2	—	467	—	—	—
SALADS														
Nacho Beef	1 (9.3 oz)	759	48	—	—	28	58	6	8	—	1877	—	—	—
Nacho Beef w/o Cheddar Cheese	1 (8.8 oz)	681	42	—	—	24	57	6	8	—	1756	—	—	—
Nacho Beef w/o Chili	1 (6.9 oz)	648	41	—	—	24	45	5	6	—	1334	—	—	—
Nacho Chicken	1 (8.9 oz)	713	43	—	—	28	59	7	8	—	1911	—	—	—
Nacho Chicken w/o Cheddar Cheese	1 (8.4 oz)	634	37	—	—	24	58	7	8	—	1790	—	—	—
Nacho Chicken w/o Chili	1 (6.5 oz)	601	36	—	—	24	46	6	6	—	1368	—	—	—
Taco Beef	1 (12.7 oz)	1043	75	—	—	36	58	2	12	—	1705	—	—	—
Taco Beef w/o Cheddar Cheese	1 (11.7 oz)	886	62	—	—	27	56	2	12	—	1462	—	—	—
Taco Beef w/o Chili	1 (11.5 oz)	987	72	—	—	33	51	2	12	—	1433	—	—	—
Taco Beef w/o Guacamole	1 (11.7 oz)	988	70	—	—	35	56	2	11	—	1577	—	—	—
Taco Beef w/o Sour Cream	1 (11.7 oz)	986	70	—	—	35	56	2	12	—	1686	—	—	—
Taco Beef w/o Tortilla Bowl	1 (9.7 oz)	564	45	—	—	28	15	2	2	—	1383	—	—	—
Taco Chicken	1 (9.6 oz)	838	57	—	—	30	53	3	12	—	1325	—	—	—
Taco Chicken w/o Cheddar Cheese	1 (8.6 oz)	680	44	—	—	21	52	3	12	—	1083	—	—	—
Taco Chicken w/o Guacamole	1 (8.6 oz)	783	52	—	—	29	51	3	11	—	1198	—	—	—
Taco Chicken w/o Sour Cream	1 (8.6 oz)	781	51	—	—	29	51	2	12	—	1307	—	—	—
Taco Chicken w/o Tortilla Bowl	1 (6.6 oz)	359	26	—	—	22	10	2	1	—	1004	—	—	—

FOOD	PORTION	CALS	FAT	SAT FAT	CHOL	PROT	CARB	SUGAR	FIBER	CALCI	SOD	POTAS	FOLIC	VIT C
TACO CABANA														
ADD-ONS														
Dressing Southwest Ranch	1 serv (1 oz)	112	11	3	7	1	2	0	0	—	155	—	—	—
Guacamole	1 serv (3 oz)	110	9	1	0	1	7	1	4	—	340	—	—	—
Pico De Gallo	1 serv (1 oz)	5	0	0	0	0	1	1	0	—	90	—	—	—
Queso	1 serv (3 oz)	200	15	9	40	10	5	5	0	—	1080	—	—	—
Salsa Black Bean & Corn	1 serv (1 oz)	30	0	0	0	1	5	1	1	—	150	—	—	—
Salsa Fuego	1 serv (1 oz)	5	0	0	0	0	1	1	0	—	170	—	—	—
Salsa Pineapple	1 serv (1 oz)	20	0	0	0	0	5	5	0	—	95	—	—	—
Salsa Ranch	1 serv (1 oz)	35	4	1	5	0	1	1	0	—	200	—	—	—
Salsa Roja	1 serv (1 oz)	5	0	0	0	0	1	1	0	—	95	—	—	—
Salsa Verde	1 serv (1 oz)	10	0	0	9	0	1	1	0	—	125	—	—	—
Shredded Cheese	1 serv (1 oz)	110	9	5	30	7	0	0	0	—	180	—	—	—
Sour Cream	1 serv (3 oz)	160	14	10	55	3	3	3	0	—	40	—	—	—
BREAKFAST MENU SELECTIONS														
Breakfast Burrito Bacon & Egg	1	410	18	7	350	22	41	2	2	—	1130	—	—	—
Breakfast Burrito Barbacoa	1	510	25	14	110	32	40	2	2	—	910	—	—	—
Breakfast Burrito Chorizo & Egg	1	400	18	7	310	20	42	2	2	—	1090	—	—	—
Breakfast Burrito Potato & Egg	1	440	21	7	250	16	48	2	2	—	850	—	—	—
Breakfast Taco Bacon & Egg	1	230	10	4	250	13	20	0	1	—	610	—	—	—
Breakfast Taco Barbacoa	1	250	12	7	55	19	19	0	1	—	430	—	—	—
Breakfast Taco Chorizo & Egg	1	200	9	4	160	9	20	0	1	—	510	—	—	—
Breakfast Taco Potato & Egg	1	210	10	3	140	8	23	0	1	—	410	—	—	—
Plates Huevos Rancheros	1 serv	770	38	14	515	38	67	1	9	—	2010	—	—	—
Plates Steak Fajitas & Scrambled Eggs	1 serv	800	37	14	515	45	70	2	9	—	1950	—	—	—
Platter Eggs Mexicana	1 serv	920	52	20	480	43	70	6	9	—	2560	—	—	—
MAIN MENU SELECTIONS														
Black Beans	1 serv	80	0	0	0	4	14	2	2	—	370	—	—	—
Borracho Beans	1 serv	140	3	1	5	7	20	1	7	—	490	—	—	—
Burrito Bean & Cheese	1	730	35	16	50	26	77	3	11	—	1450	—	—	—
Burrito Beef Ground	1	710	30	14	85	37	71	5	6	—	2220	—	—	—

FOOD	PORTION	CALS	FAT	SAT FAT	CHOL	PROT	CARB	SUGAR	FIBER	CALCI	SOD	POTAS	FOLIC	VIT C
Burrito Beef Ultimo Ground	1	800	38	18	105	39	74	6	7	—	2360	—	—	—
Burrito Black Bean	1	450	8	4	0	14	82	6	5	—	1720	—	—	—
Burrito Chicken Breast Fajita	1	630	24	12	95	36	65	5	3	—	1980	—	—	—
Burrito Chicken Stewed	1	660	25	11	100	36	73	5	7	—	2230	—	—	—
Burrito Chicken Ultimo Stewed	1	760	33	15	120	37	76	6	8	—	2360	—	—	—
Burrito Steak Fajita	1	650	27	14	70	33	65	4	2	—	1980	—	—	—
Chips	1 serv (2.5 oz)	180	16	4	0	5	37	1	5	—	15	—	—	—
Fajitas Chicken Personal	1 serv	740	20	9	70	38	98	8	13	—	2450	—	—	—
Fajitas Chicken Platter	1 serv	1670	52	23	160	80	212	15	26	—	5190	—	—	—
Fajitas Steak Personal	1 serv	760	24	10	45	34	98	7	12	—	2450	—	—	—
Flautas Chicken	1	100	4	1	15	7	10	0	1	—	180	—	—	—
Refried Beans	1 serv	250	13	5	10	8	24	1	6	—	420	—	—	—
Taco Beef Ground	1	230	9	5	30	13	22	1	1	—	720	—	—	—
Taco Chicken Breast Fajita	1	190	4	2	30	14	21	0	1	—	650	—	—	—
Taco Crispy Chicken Stewed	1	160	7	3	40	11	13	1	2	—	430	—	—	—
Taco Crispy Ground Beef	1	180	10	4	30	12	11	1	2	—	430	—	—	—
Taco Soft Bean & Cheese	1	300	14	7	20	11	32	0	4	—	590	—	—	—
Taco Soft Black Bean	1	200	4	2	0	6	34	2	2	—	630	—	—	—
Taco Soft Carne Guisada	1	190	6	2	30	12	21	0	1	—	330	—	—	—
Taco Soft Chicken Stewed	1	210	7	3	40	13	23	1	2	—	720	—	—	—
Taco Steak Fajita	1	200	6	3	10	12	21	0	1	—	650	—	—	—
Tortilla Corn	1	70	1	0	0	2	15	0	2	—	5	—	—	—
Tortilla Flour	1	120	3	2	0	3	19	0	1	—	290	—	—	—

TACO JOHN'S

BREAKFAST SELECTIONS

FOOD	PORTION	CALS	FAT	SAT FAT	CHOL	PROT	CARB	SUGAR	FIBER	CALCI	SOD	POTAS	FOLIC	VIT C
Breakfast Burrito Bacon	1 (7.6 oz)	550	25	6	250	21	56	5	7	—	1370	—	—	—
Breakfast Burrito Egg	1 (6.6 oz)	420	19	8	270	21	42	6	5	—	730	—	—	—
Breakfast Burrito Egg Bacon	1 (7 oz)	500	24	9	275	26	43	6	5	—	1120	—	—	—
Breakfast Burrito Egg Sausage	1 (8.1 oz)	590	34	13	300	28	44	6	6	—	1050	—	—	—

FOOD	PORTION	CALS	FAT	SAT FAT	CHOL	PROT	CARB	SUGAR	FIBER	CALCI	SOD	POTAS	FOLIC	VIT C
Breakfast Burrito Sausage	1 (8.6 oz)	640	35	10	275	23	56	5	7	—	1300	—	—	—
Breakfast Taco Bacon	1 (3.7 oz)	270	13	4	125	10	25	1	2	—	810	—	—	—
Breakfast Taco Sausage	1 (4.2 oz)	310	18	6	135	11	25	1	2	—	770	—	—	—
Scrambler Burrito Bacon	1 (8.6 oz)	550	25	6	250	21	58	6	7	—	1370	—	—	—
Scrambler Burrito Sausage	1 (9.6 oz)	640	32	9	270	21	58	7	7	—	1440	—	—	—
Scrambler Potato Ole Bacon	1 sm (9.4 oz)	630	41	10	260	20	45	2	6	—	1860	—	—	—
Scrambler Potato Ole Sausage	1 sm (10.5 oz)	720	50	14	280	22	45	5	6	—	1780	—	—	—
DESSERTS														
Apple Grande	1 serv (3.4 oz)	270	12	3	5	5	39	15	2	—	420	—	—	—
Choco Taco	1 serv (4 oz)	390	20	15	15	5	48	32	1	—	160	—	—	—
Churro	1 serv (2 oz)	190	7	2	20	2	15	10	4	—	170	—	—	—
Cini-Sopapilla Bites	1 serv (2.6 oz)	210	5	1	0	4	37	7	4	—	320	—	—	—
Giant Goldfish Grahams	1 serv (0.5 oz)	70	2	1	0	1	11	4	1	—	55	—	—	—
MAIN MENU SELECTIONS														
Burrito Bean	1 (6.6 oz)	360	9	3	15	14	56	5	9	—	790	—	—	—
Burrito Beefy	1 (6.6 oz)	440	20	7	50	22	45	5	7	—	860	—	—	—
Burrito Chicken & Potato	1 (8.3 oz)	470	19	5	30	17	56	5	7	—	1220	—	—	—
Burrito Chicken Grilled	1 (8.2 oz)	590	29	11	90	32	50	5	6	—	1510	—	—	—
Burrito Combination	1 (6.6 oz)	400	14	5	35	18	50	5	8	—	830	—	—	—
Burrito Crunchy Chicken & Potato	1 (8.8 oz)	600	28	6	35	20	65	5	7	—	1320	—	—	—
Burrito Grilled Beef	1 (8.2 oz)	600	32	13	75	27	52	5	8	—	1230	—	—	—
Burrito Meat & Potato	1 (8.3 oz)	500	23	6	30	15	58	5	8	—	1100	—	—	—
Burrito Ranch Beef	1 (7.1 oz)	440	22	6	45	17	45	6	6	—	850	—	—	—
Burrito Ranch Chicken	1 (7 oz)	400	17	5	45	19	44	6	5	—	970	—	—	—
Burrito Smothered	1 (11.3 oz)	510	20	8	45	23	60	6	10	—	1310	—	—	—
Burrito Super	1 (8.8 oz)	450	18	7	40	19	54	6	9	—	900	—	—	—
Chili w/o Crackers	1 serv (8 oz)	220	11	5	35	14	17	2	4	—	1240	—	—	—
Chili w/o Crackers & Cheese	1 serv (7.5 oz)	160	6	2	20	10	17	2	4	—	1160	—	—	—

FOOD	PORTION	CALS	FAT	SAT FAT	CHOL	PROT	CARB	SUGAR	FIBER	CALCI	SOD	POTAS	FOLIC	VIT C
Chilto	1 serv (4.6 oz)	360	15	7	35	15	40	5	5	—	670	—	—	—
Chips & Queso	1 serv (6.7 oz)	430	25	7	20	9	43	1	2	—	940	—	—	—
Crispy Taco	1 (3.2 oz)	180	10	4	25	9	13	1	2	—	270	—	—	—
Crunchy Chicken w/o Sauce	1 serv (5 oz)	450	27	4	60	29	24	0	0	—	1420	—	—	—
Enchiliada Chili	1 serv (7.6 oz)	310	16	7	50	18	24	2	4	—	1000	—	—	—
Mexi Rolls w/o Nachos	2 pieces (1.9 oz)	130	5	2	10	6	14	0	2	—	190	—	—	—
Mexican Rice	1 serv (6 oz)	250	6	0	0	5	45	2	0	—	1080	—	—	—
Nachos	1 serv (5 oz)	380	23	6	10	6	38	0	1	—	750	—	—	—
Potato Oles	1 sm (5 oz)	430	26	4	0	4	45	1	6	—	1220	—	—	—
Potato Oles Chili Cheese	1 serv (10.7 oz)	590	36	8	25	13	55	2	8	—	2130	—	—	—
Potato Oles Super	1 serv (9.7 oz)	620	39	11	35	14	53	2	7	—	1270	—	—	—
Quesadilla Melt Cheesey	1 (5.6 oz)	440	22	10	55	19	43	4	5	—	1050	—	—	—
Quesadilla Melt Fajita Beef	1 serv (8.6 oz)	540	28	12	70	26	49	6	7	—	1240	—	—	—
Quesadilla Melt Fajita Chicken	1 (8.6 oz)	510	23	11	75	28	47	6	6	—	1360	—	—	—
Refried Beans	1 serv (9.4 oz)	320	6	4	15	18	47	2	11	—	1020	—	—	—
Refried Beans w/o Cheese	1 serv (8.9 oz)	260	2	0	0	14	47	2	11	—	940	—	—	—
Sierra Chicken Sandwich	1 (8.2 oz)	350	11	3	50	23	37	2	2	—	1350	—	—	—
Softshell Taco	1 (4 oz)	220	11	5	25	11	21	1	2	—	580	—	—	—
Super Nachos	1 sm (6.9 oz)	450	27	9	35	12	38	1	3	—	650	—	—	—
Taco Bravo	1 (6.5 oz)	340	13	5	25	15	40	1	5	—	750	—	—	—
Taco Burger	1 (5 oz)	270	12	4	30	14	28	4	3	—	600	—	—	—
Taco Stuffed Grilled	1 (7.4 oz)	560	25	9	40	19	63	0	7	—	920	—	—	—
SALAD DRESSINGS AND TOPPINGS														
Bacon Ranch Dressing	1 serv (1.5 oz)	130	10	2	10	1	10	7	0	—	370	—	—	—
Creamy Italian Dressing	1 serv (1.5 oz)	130	15	2	0	0	3	1	0	—	320	—	—	—
Guacamole	1 serv (2 oz)	90	6	2	0	0	8	2	2	—	115	—	—	—
Hot Sauce	1 serv (1 oz)	10	0	0	0	0	1	0	0	—	125	—	—	—
House Dressing	1 serv (1.5 oz)	70	7	1	0	0	2	1	0	—	260	—	—	—
Mild Sauce	1 serv (1 oz)	10	0	0	0	0	1	0	0	—	130	—	—	—
Nacho Cheese	1 serv (3 oz)	120	9	4	10	4	5	0	0	—	520	—	—	—
Pico De Gallo	1 serv (1 oz)	10	0	0	0	0	1	0	0	—	90	—	—	—
Ranch Dressing	1 serv (1.5 oz)	140	16	2	20	1	3	1	0	—	350	—	—	—
Salsa	1 serv (2 oz)	20	0	0	0	1	4	2	1	—	220	—	—	—
Sour Cream	1 serv (2 oz)	120	12	7	25	2	2	0	0	—	30	—	—	—
Super Hot Sauce	1 serv (1 oz)	10	0	0	0	0	1	0	0	—	25	—	—	—

FOOD	PORTION	CALS	FAT	SAT FAT	CHOL	PROT	CARB	SUGAR	FIBER	CALCI	SOD	POTAS	FOLIC	VIT C
SALADS														
Softshell Taco Chicken	1 (4 oz)	190	6	3	30	13	19	0	1	—	700	—	—	—
Taco Crunchy Chicken w/o Dressing	1 serv (13.4 oz)	660	40	10	70	29	47	7	6	—	1180	—	—	—
Taco w/o Dressing	1 serv (12.7 oz)	520	33	11	60	21	37	7	7	—	860	—	—	—

TACOTIME

FOOD	PORTION	CALS	FAT	SAT FAT	CHOL	PROT	CARB	SUGAR	FIBER	CALCI	SOD	POTAS	FOLIC	VIT C
DESSERTS														
Churro Plain	1 (1.5 oz)	205	15	3	20	2	16	4	0	3	1440	—	—	0
Churro w/ Cinnamon & Sugar	1 (2 oz)	245	15	3	20	2	26	14	0	3	1440	—	—	0
Crustos	1 serv	294	6	1	0	6	58	19	3	40	273	—	—	0
Empanada Apple	1 (4 oz)	234	7	1	0	4	40	10	2	21	201	—	—	0
Empanada Cherry	1 (4 oz)	240	7	1	0	4	41	4	2	24	190	—	—	2
Empanada Pumpkin	1 (4 oz)	256	8	1	23	6	42	16	2	54	198	—	—	0
MAIN MENU SELECTIONS														
Burrito Big Juan Chicken	1 (13 oz)	594	19	10	78	35	68	5	10	360	2435	—	—	11
Burrito Big Juan Seasoned Ground Beef	1 (13 oz)	651	28	12	73	30	71	6	12	383	2658	—	—	11
Burrito Big Juan Shredded Beef	1 (13 oz)	633	25	12	64	33	67	5	10	354	2616	—	—	10
Burrito Casita Chicken	1 (12 oz)	494	18	10	85	34	43	4	5	342	2338	—	—	8
Burrito Casita Seasoned Ground Beef	1 (12 oz)	552	25	13	80	29	46	5	6	364	2561	—	—	9
Burrito Casita Shredded Beef	1 (12 oz)	533	25	13	91	31	42	4	5	336	2520	—	—	7
Burrito Chicken & Black Bean	1 (10 oz)	478	16	6	60	30	51	3	9	221	1219	—	—	6
Burrito Chicken BLT	1 (10 oz)	721	41	11	99	41	44	4	8	281	1642	—	—	6
Burrito Chicken Ranchero	1 (10.8 oz)	654	32	10	80	36	52	3	7	342	1341	—	—	12
Burrito Crisp Chicken	1 (5.5 oz)	336	10	1	42	27	32	0	2	37	566	—	—	1
Burrito Crisp Meat	1 (5.8 oz)	450	22	7	49	23	36	1	4	158	893	—	—	2
Burrito Crisp Pinto Bean	1 (6 oz)	394	16	4	12	13	50	1	6	204	2172	—	—	3
Burrito Soft Meat	1 (6.7 oz)	426	16	7	46	23	43	2	8	215	1095	—	—	2
Burrito Soft Pinto Bean	1 (6.7 oz)	377	11	5	15	14	54	1	10	263	2093	—	—	4

FOOD	PORTION	CALS	FAT	SAT FAT	CHOL	PROT	CARB	SUGAR	FIBER	CALCI	SOD	POTAS	FOLIC*	VIT C
Burrito Veggie	1 (11 oz)	534	18	7	25	18	74	4	12	311	2545	—	—	7
Cheddar Fries	1 sm (6 oz)	374	26	8	23	8	29	1	3	152	877	—	—	14
Cheddar Melt	1 (2.8 oz)	250	12	7	31	11	25	0	4	253	472	—	—	0
Mexi-Fries	1 sm (5 oz)	290	19	4	0	3	29	1	2	0	740	—	—	14
Mexi-Rice	1 serv (4 oz)	87	1	0	0	2	19	1	0	12	401	—	—	1
Nachos Grande	1 serv (16.5 oz)	1132	57	24	90	39	114	8	11	1415	4085	—	—	16
Refritos w/ Chips	1 serv (7 oz)	304	11	6	23	14	35	2	6	325	3252	—	—	6
Refritos w/o Chips	1 serv (6.7 oz)	285	11	6	23	13	32	2	6	321	3251	—	—	6
Stuffed Fries	1 sm (5 oz)	321	7	6	14	7	29	3	3	143	705	—	—	0
Taco Crisp Seasoned Ground Beef	1 (4.3 oz)	225	12	5	40	15	12	1	2	144	512	—	—	3
Taco Super Soft Chicken	1 (11 oz)	540	18	10	77	35	56	3	10	354	2354	—	—	6
Taco Super Soft Seasoned Ground Beef	1 (11 oz)	598	25	12	72	30	59	4	12	376	2577	—	—	6
Taco Super Soft Shredded Beef	1 (11 oz)	579	25	12	84	32	55	3	10	348	2535	—	—	5
Taco Value Soft	1 (5.3 oz)	314	13	6	40	18	28	2	6	184	800	—	—	3
Taco ½ Lb Shredded Beef	1 (9 oz)	440	18	9	65	28	42	3	7	264	1218	—	—	8
Taco ½ Lb Soft Chicken	1 (9 oz)	401	11	6	58	30	43	3	7	270	1037	—	—	9
Taco ½ Lb Soft Seasoned Ground Beef	1 (9 oz)	459	18	8	53	25	46	4	9	191	1260	—	—	9
Taco Chips	1 serv (2 oz)	150	3	0	0	3	27	0	1	35	7	—	—	0
SALAD DRESSINGS AND TOPPINGS														
Cheddar Cheese	1 serv (2 oz)	223	18	12	61	14	1	0	0	405	364	—	—	0
Dressing Chipotle Ranch	1 serv (1 oz)	165	18	3	6	1	1	1	0	25	157	—	—	0
Dressing Ranch	1 serv (1 oz)	181	20	3	7	1	1	1	—	28	187	—	—	0
Dressing Thousand Island	1 serv (1 oz)	132	12	2	5	0	5	3	0	0	369	—	—	1
Guacamole	1 serv (1 oz)	50	5	1	0	0	2	1	1	0	125	—	—	2
Salsa Nuevo	1 serv (1 oz)	8	0	0	0	0	2	1	0	6	131	—	—	3
Salsa Verde	1 serv (1 oz)	6	0	0	0	0	2	0	0	1	149	—	—	0
Sour Cream	1 serv (1.5 oz)	85	7	5	28	1	1	1	0	28	14	—	—	0
SALADS														
Taco Chicken	1 reg (9.2 oz)	351	15	5	58	27	24	4	2	202	899	—	—	11
Taco Seasoned Ground Beef	1 reg (7.8 oz)	396	23	8	53	22	24	3	4	205	860	—	—	6
Taco Shredded Beef	1 reg (7.8 oz)	377	22	8	65	25	21	2	2	177	819	—	—	4
Tostada Delight Chicken	1 (10.5 oz)	565	29	14	100	37	36	3	4	439	2221	—	—	6

FOOD	PORTION	CALS	FAT	SAT FAT	CHOL	PROT	CARB	SUGAR	FIBER	CALCI	SOD	POTAS	FOLIC	VIT C
Tostada Delight Seasoned Ground Beef	1 (10.5 oz)	623	36	16	95	32	39	4	6	461	2444	—	—	6
Tostada Delight Shredded Beef	1 (10.5 oz)	604	36	16	107	35	35	3	5	433	2402	—	—	5

TASTI D-LITE

FOOD	PORTION	CALS	FAT	SAT FAT	CHOL	PROT	CARB	SUGAR	FIBER	CALCI	SOD	POTAS	FOLIC	VIT C
Acai	4 oz	70	2	1	5	2	13	11	0	80	45	—	—	6
Banana	4 oz	70	1	1	5	2	13	11	0	60	45	—	—	2
Banana 'N Peanut Butter	4 oz	90	3	1	5	2	13	11	0	60	65	—	—	2
Bananas Foster	4 oz	70	1	1	5	2	13	11	0	60	45	—	—	1
Burnt Sugar	4 oz	70	1	1	0	2	14	14	0	60	60	—	—	0
Buttercrunch	4 oz	80	3	1	0	3	13	11	0	60	70	—	—	0
Cappuccino	4 oz	70	2	1	5	2	13	10	0	60	45	—	—	0
Cherry Cake	4 oz	70	2	1	5	2	13	12	0	60	50	—	—	0
Chocoleche	4 oz	80	2	1	5	2	15	13	0	60	65	—	—	0
Cinnamon Crunch	4 oz	70	1	1	5	2	14	11	0	60	50	—	—	0
Coffee Liqueur	4 oz	70	2	1	5	2	12	10	0	60	50	—	—	0
Creme Brulee	4 oz	70	2	1	5	2	14	12	0	60	50	—	—	0
Egg Nog	4 oz	70	2	1	10	2	13	11	0	60	50	—	—	0
German Chocolate Cake	4 oz	80	2	1	0	2	14	13	0	40	70	—	—	0
Latte	4 oz	70	2	1	5	2	13	11	0	60	50	—	—	0
Mud Pie	4 oz	80	2	1	0	2	15	14	0	40	85	—	—	0
Nutella	4 oz	90	3	2	5	2	15	13	0	80	45	—	—	0
Peanut Butter Batter	4 oz	90	3	1	0	3	13	11	1	60	85	—	—	0
Peanut Cluster	4 oz	90	3	1	5	2	13	12	0	60	65	—	—	0
Pecan Praline	4 oz	70	2	1	5	2	14	12	0	60	55	—	—	0
Pina Colada	4 oz	80	2	1	5	2	14	12	0	60	45	—		5
Raspberry	4 oz	70	2	1	5	2	13	12	0	60	45	—	—	2
Rice Pudding	4 oz	80	1	1	5	2	15	12	0	60	45	—	—	0
Tapioca Pudding	4 oz	70	2	1	5	2	14	12	0	60	50	—	—	0
Tart 'N Tasti	4 oz	100	1	1	5	2	23	21	0	80	50	—	—	0
Tart 'N Tasti Acai	4 oz	100	2	1	5	3	20	18	0	100	55	—	—	6
Tart 'N Tasti Mango	4 oz	100	1	1	5	2	21	19	0	80	55	—	—	6
Tiramisu	4 oz	70	1	1	0	2	13	11	0	60	55	—	—	0
Toasted Almond Fudge	4 oz	80	1	1	0	2	14	14	0	40	60	—	—	2
Toffee Crunch	4 oz	90	3	2	0	2	14	14	0	60	75	—	—	0

TCBY

FROZEN YOGURT AND SORBET

FOOD	PORTION	CALS	FAT	SAT FAT	CHOL	PROT	CARB	SUGAR	FIBER	CALCI	SOD	POTAS	FOLIC	VIT C
Hand Scooped Butter Pecan Perfection	½ cup	110	5	2	10	4	14	11	tr	100	90	—	—	1
Hand Scooped Chocolate Chocolate Swirl	½ cup	120	4	2	15	4	19	16	tr	100	50	—	—	1
Hand Scooped Chocolate Chunk Cookie Dough	½ cup	160	6	3	15	3	24	18	0	100	75	—	—	0
Hand Scooped Cookies & Cream	½ cup	140	4	3	10	3	22	17	0	100	75	—	—	0
Hand Scooped Cotton Candy	½ cup	120	4	2	15	3	20	16	0	100	60	—	—	0
Hand Scooped Mint Chocolate Chunk	½ cup	140	5	4	10	3	22	18	0	100	55	—	—	0
Hand Scooped Mocha Almond	½ cup	150	5	2	10	3	22	18	tr	100	95	—	—	0
Hand Scooped No Sugar Added Chocolate Chocolate Swirl	½ cup	90	1	0	0	4	23	5	6	100	70	—	—	1
Hand Scooped No Sugar Added Vanilla	½ cup	80	1	0	0	4	19	6	5	150	60	—	—	1
Hand Scooped No Sugar Added Vanilla Fudge Brownie	½ cup	100	2	2	10	4	22	5	5	100	80	—	—	1
Hand Scooped Pralines & Cream	½ cup	140	5	2	10	3	23	19	0	100	80	—	—	0
Hand Scooped Psychedelic Sorbet	½ cup	290	0	0	0	0	75	55	0	0	30	—	—	0
Hand Scooped Rainbow Cream	½ cup	120	4	2	15	3	20	16	0	100	60	—	—	0
Hand Scooped Rocky Road	½ cup	220	7	4	5	3	36	27	1	60	25	—	—	0
Hand Scooped Strawberries & Cream	½ cup	120	3	2	10	2	21	18	0	80	50	—	—	5
Hand Scooped Vanilla Chocolate Chunk	½ cup	140	5	4	10	3	22	18	0	100	55	—	—	0
Hand Scooped Vanilla Bean	½ cup	120	4	2	15	3	19	16	0	100	60	—	—	0

FOOD	PORTION	CALS	FAT	SAT FAT	CHOL	PROT	CARB	SUGAR	FIBER	CALCI	SOD	POTAS	FOLIC	VIT C
Soft Serve Frozen Yogurt All Flavors 96% Fat Free	½ cup	140	3	2	15	4	23	20	0	80	60	—	—	0
Soft Serve Frozen Yogurt All Flavors Low Carb	½ cup	110	7	5	25	3	16	3	7	150	60	—	—	1
Soft Serve Frozen Yogurt All Flavors Nonfat	½ cup	110	0	0	<5	4	23	20	0	100	60	—	—	0
Soft Serve Frozen Yogurt All Flavors Nonfat No Sugar Added	½ cup	90	0	0	<5	4	20	7	0	100	35	—	—	0
Soft Serve Sorbet All Flavors Nonfat Nondairy	½ cup	100	0	0	0	0	24	19	0	0	30	—	—	0
SMOOTHIES														
Berrylicious	1 (16 oz)	290	3	2	10	3	65	54	3	150	65	—	—	6
Black 'N Blueberry	1 (16 oz)	280	3	2	10	3	63	54	2	40	65	—	—	6
Mango Tango	1 (16 oz)	330	3	2	10	2	76	66	2	200	65	—	—	6
Mangolada	1 (16 oz)	340	6	5	10	3	70	60	2	200	100	—		6
Mondo Mango	1 (16 oz)	310	3	2	10	3	70	63	2	350	65	—	—	6
Pina Paradise	1 (16 oz)	350	12	9	10	3	58	48	1	150	170	—	—	6
Pink Pineapple	1 (16 oz)	340	9	7	10	3	63	52	2	200	135	—		6
Straight Up Strawberry	1 (16 oz)	280	4	2	10	3	44	54	1	250	65	—	—	6
Strawberry Bonanza	1 (16 oz)	320	4	2	10	3	74	61	2	200	65	—	—	6
Strawberry Fling	1 (16 oz)	340	3	2	10	3	78	67	2	250	65	—	—	6

TIM HORTONS

FOOD	PORTION	CALS	FAT	SAT FAT	CHOL	PROT	CARB	SUGAR	FIBER	CALCI	SOD	POTAS	FOLIC	VIT C
BAKED SELECTIONS														
Bagel Blueberry	1	270	1	0	0	10	55	7	2	20	470	—	—	0
Bagel Cinnamon Raisin	1	270	1	0	0	10	55	12	3	40	350	—	—	0
Bagel Everything	1	280	2	0	0	10	53	7	3	40	460	—	—	0
Bagel Flax Seed	1	290	5	1	0	10	53	4	4	60	520	—	—	0
Bagel Onion	1	260	2	0	0	9	53	8	3	40	460	—	—	0
Bagel Plain	1	260	2	0	0	9	52	7	2	20	450	—	—	0
Bagel Poppy Seed	1	270	2	0	0	9	53	7	3	40	440	—	—	0
Bagel Sesame Seed	1	270	3	0	0	9	53	7	3	20	430	—	—	0
Bagel Sun Dried Tomato	1	310	4	1	0	9	59	4	2	20	550	—	—	0
Bagel Twelve Grain	1	330	9	1	0	10	52	5	6	80	580	—	—	0

FOOD	PORTION	CALS	FAT	SAT FAT	CHOL	PROT	CARB	SUGAR	FIBER	CALCI	SOD	POTAS	FOLIC	VIT C
Cinnamon Roll Frosted	1	470	25	12	0	4	57	20	2	40	380	—	—	0
Cinnamon Roll Glazed	1	420	23	11	0	4	50	15	2	40	360	—	—	0
Cookie Caramel Chocolate Pecan	1	230	11	5	20	3	32	17	1	20	290	—	—	0
Cookie Chocolate Chip	1	230	9	6	20	3	34	19	1	20	260	—	—	0
Cookie Oatmeal Raisin Spice	1	220	8	5	25	3	35	21	1	20	200	—	—	0
Cookie Peanut Butter Chocolate Chunk	1	260	15	7	20	5	28	18	2	20	260	—	—	0
Cookie Triple Chocolate	1	250	13	8	30	3	31	20	2	20	220	—	—	0
Cookie White Chocolate Macadamia Nut	1	240	12	6	20	3	31	17	1	20	270	—	—	0
Croissant Butter	1	340	18	5	0	7	38	7	1	20	380	—	—	9
Croissant Cheese	1	370	20	7	15	9	37	6	0	100	410	—	—	2
Danish Cherry Cheese	1	330	13	6	15	5	46	24	1	20	230	—	—	0
Danish Chocolate	1	430	24	9	10	4	51	27	1	40	220	—	—	6
Danish Maple Pecan	1	380	20	7	20	4	46	21	1	20	230	—	—	6
Donut Apple Fritter	1	300	11	5	0	4	49	16	2	40	350	—	—	2
Donut Chocolate Dip	1	210	9	4	0	4	30	8	1	20	190	—	—	0
Donut Chocolate Glazed	1	260	10	5	5	4	39	20	2	40	300	—	—	0
Donut Honey Dip	1	210	8	4	0	4	33	11	1	20	190	—	—	0
Donut Maple Dip	1	210	8	4	0	4	31	9	1	20	200	—	—	0
Donut Old Fashion Glazed	1	320	19	9	10	3	35	22	1	20	230	—	—	0
Donut Old Fashion Plain	1	260	19	9	10	3	20	7	1	20	230	—	—	0
Donut Sour Cream Plain	1	270	17	8	10	3	27	10	1	20	230	—	—	0
Donut Walnut Crunch	1	360	23	10	5	4	35	19	1	20	320	—	—	0
Donut Filled Angel Cream	1	310	13	5	0	4	46	21	1	20	220	—	—	0
Donut Filled Blueberry	1	230	8	4	0	4	36	11	1	20	210	—	—	0
Donut Filled Boston Cream	1	250	9	4	0	4	38	12	1	20	260	—	—	0

FOOD	PORTION	CALS	FAT	SAT FAT	CHOL	PROT	CARB	SUGAR	FIBER	CALCI	SOD	POTAS	FOLIC	VIT C
Donut Filled Canadian Maple	1	260	9	4	0	4	41	16	1	20	260	—	—	0
Donut Filled Strawberry	1	230	8	4	0	4	36	12	1	20	220	—	—	0
Honey Cruller	1	320	19	9	50	1	37	23	0	20	220	—	—	0
Muffin Blueberry	1	330	11	2	15	4	54	27	2	60	580	—	—	0
Muffin Blueberry Bran	1	300	10	1	10	6	53	25	5	40	770	—	—	4
Muffin Carrot Wheat	1	400	19	3	10	6	55	26	4	40	580	—	—	6
Muffin Chocolate Chip	1	430	16	5	15	5	69	40	2	60	580	—	—	0
Muffin Cranberry Blueberry Bran	1	290	10	2	10	5	51	24	5	40	710	—	—	5
Muffin Cranberry Fruit	1	350	12	2	15	4	59	31	2	60	560	—	—	4
Muffin Fruit Explosion	1	360	11	2	15	4	61	32	2	60	550	—	—	2
Muffin Raisin Bran	1	360	10	2	10	6	65	37	6	60	790	—	—	4
Muffin Strawberry Sensation	1	350	11	2	15	4	61	31	1	60	580	—	—	6
Muffin Low Fat Blueberry	1	290	3	1	0	4	62	32	2	60	750	—	—	0
Muffin Low Fat Cranberry	1	290	3	1	0	4	62	31	2	60	750	—	—	2
Tea Biscuit Plain	1	250	9	2	0	5	35	4	1	40	590	—	—	0
Tea Biscuit Raisin	1	290	10	2	0	6	45	12	2	40	590	—	—	0
Timbits Apple Fritter	1	50	2	1	0	1	9	4	0	0	55	—	—	0
Timbits Chocolate Glazed	1	70	3	1	0	1	10	5	0	0	75	—	—	0
Timbits Honey Dip	1	60	2	1	0	1	9	4	0	0	50	—	—	0
Timbits Old Fashion Plain	1	70	5	3	5	1	5	2	0	0	60	—	—	0
Timbits Filled Banana Cream	1	60	2	1	0	1	9	3	0	0	65	—	—	0
Timbits Filled Lemon	1	60	2	1	0	1	9	4	0	0	50	—	—	0
Timbits Filled Strawberry	1	60	2	1	0	1	10	4	0	0	50	—	—	0
BEVERAGES														
Cafe Mocha	1 (10 oz)	160	7	6	0	1	25	21	1	0	160	—	—	0
Cappuccino Iced	1 (12 oz)	300	15	8	50	0	41	40	0	0	85	—	—	0
Coffee Decaffeinated Sugar & Cream	1 (10 oz)	75	4	2	15	1	9	9	0	20	15	—	—	0

FOOD	PORTION	CALS	FAT	SAT FAT	CHOL	PROT	CARB	SUGAR	FIBER	CALCI	SOD	POTAS	FOLIC	VIT C
Coffee Sugar & Cream	1 (10 oz)	75	4	2	15	1	9	9	0	20	15	—	—	0
English Toffee	1 (10 oz)	220	6	5	0	3	40	30	0	150	240	—	—	0
Flavor Shot	1 serv	5	0	0	0	0	1	0	0	0	0	—	—	0
French Vanilla	1 (10 oz)	240	7	7	0	4	39	31	0	150	240	—	—	0
Hot Chocolate	1 (10 oz)	240	6	5	0	2	45	35	2	20	360	—	—	0
Hot Smoothie	1 (10 oz)	260	10	9	5	5	39	28	2	100	200	—	—	0
Iced Cappuccino w/ Milk	1 (12 oz)	180	2	1	5	3	39	35	0	100	45	—	—	1
Tea Sugar & Milk	1 (10 oz)	50	1	0	5	1	10	10	0	60	20	—	—	0
CREAM CHEESE														
Garden Vegetable	1.5 oz	120	11	7	45	2	3	2	1	40	230	—	—	1
Light Plain	1.5 oz	60	5	4	20	4	3	3	0	100	200	—	—	0
Plain	1.5 oz	130	12	7	50	2	2	2	0	40	180	—	—	0
Strawberry	1.5 oz	120	10	6	40	6	6	6	0	40	160	—	—	1
SANDWICHES														
B.L.T.	1	450	18	5	30	18	53	9	2	20	850	—	—	9
Breakfast Bacon Egg Cheese	1	410	25	17	185	16	31	4	1	100	760	—	—	0
Breakfast Egg Cheese	1	360	21	15	175	13	30	3	1	100	680	—	—	0
Breakfast Sausage Egg Cheese	1	520	37	21	205	19	30	3	1	100	940	—	—	0
Chicken Salad Salad	1	380	9	1	35	21	55	6	3	40	890	—	—	21
Egg Salad	1	390	13	3	245	17	52	7	2	40	780	—	—	1
Ham & Swiss	1	440	12	5	50	28	56	7	3	250	1690	—	—	15
Toasted Chicken Club	1	460	7	3	50	30	70	14	2	40	1170	—	—	6
Turkey Breast	1	390	5	2	10	27	59	6	4	80	1480	—	—	15
SOUPS														
Beef Stew	1 serv (10 oz)	236	8	3	30	17	25	3	3	40	1208	—	—	12
Chicken Noodle	1 serv (10 oz)	120	2	1	20	5	18	2	1	20	880	—	—	15
Chili	1 serv (10 oz)	300	16	6	50	21	18	5	5	60	920	—	—	4
Country Field Mushroom	1 serv (10 oz)	150	3	2	0	3	28	3	1	20	1080	—	—	0
Cream Of Broccoli	1 serv (10 oz)	160	9	4	20	6	16	6	1	150	820	—	—	2
Hearty Vegetable	1 serv (10 oz)	70	0	0	0	4	14	2	3	40	1060	—	—	4
Minestrone	1 serv (10 oz)	120	3	0	0	4	24	4	2	40	940	—	—	21
Potato Bacon	1 serv (10 oz)	180	6	2	0	3	30	5	2	40	1260	—	—	12
Split Pea w/ Ham	1 serv (10 oz)	150	3	3	5	8	27	3	5	20	970	—	—	4
Turkey Rice	1 serv (10 oz)	120	2	0	0	3	21	2	1	20	1000	—	—	21
Vegetable Beef Barley	1 serv (10 oz)	110	2	0	5	4	21	2	2	20	980	—	—	18

FOOD	PORTION	CALS	FAT	SAT FAT	CHOL	PROT	CARB	SUGAR	FIBER	CALCI	SOD	POTAS	FOLIC	VIT C
YOGURT														
Low Fat Creamy Vanilla w/ Berries	1 (6 oz)	160	3	2	10	4	32	26	2	150	80	—	—	12
Low Fat Strawberry w/ Berries	1 (6 oz)	150	3	2	10	4	28	23	2	150	75	—	—	15
T.J. CINNAMONS														
Chocolate Twist	1	250	12	4	5	4	34	12	2	40	110	—	—	—
Cinnamon Twist	1	280	14	5	5	3	33	11	1	40	190	—	—	—
Mocha Chill w/ Whipped Cream	1 (12.5 oz)	306	7	4	29	11	48	48	1	390	214	—	—	3
Mocha Chill w/o Whipped Cream	1 (12.5 oz)	264	4	2	17	11	48	44	1	390	214	—	—	3
Original Roll w/o Icing	1	507	10	4	7	10	73	31	4	180	373	—	—	4
Pecan Sticky Bun	1	688	22	5	7	12	91	45	5	190	420	—	—	5
TJ Icing	1 serv (1 oz)	117	5	2	8	1	18	16	0	10	50	—	—	0
TOGO'S														
SALAD DRESSINGS														
Asian	1 serv (2.5 oz)	380	33	5	0	0	19	10	0	0	830	—	—	0
Blue Cheese	1 serv (2.5 oz)	260	26	5	25	2	3	3	0	80	780	—	—	0
Buttermilk Ranch	1 serv (2.5 oz)	250	26	5	20	2	3	3	0	60	890	—	—	1
Caesar	1 serv (2.5 oz)	150	12	3	30	2	8	3	0	60	800	—	—	0
Fat Free Serano Grape Vinaigrette	1 serv (2.5 oz)	90	0	0	0	1	23	21	0	20	290	—	—	1
Low Fat Balsamic Vinaigrette	1 serv (2.5 oz)	90	4	0	0	0	16	6	0	0	780	—	—	2
SALADS														
Asian Chicken w/o Dressing	1 full serv	200	9	0	40	21	17	5	3	100	400	—	—	18
Chicken Caesar w/o Dressing	1 full serv	210	6	3	50	24	17	3	3	150	650	—	—	36
Cobb w/o Dressing	1 full serv	330	20	9	140	29	12	4	6	100	870	—	—	42
Santa Fe Chicken w/o Dressing	1 full serv	370	16	5	55	27	33	6	10	200	950	—	—	48
Taco w/o Dressing	1 full serv	600	39	20	110	26	36	8	9	500	1190	—	—	18
SANDWICHES														
Albacore Tuna	1 reg	660	28	5	45	30	73	9	4	40	1900	—	—	6
Avocado & Cucumber	1 reg	560	25	4	10	13	75	7	9	60	1340	—	—	15
Black Forest Ham & Cheese	1 reg	670	31	10	80	35	67	7	4	600	2710	—	—	6
Capicolla Dry Salami & Provolone	1 reg	1080	59	17	235	73	69	12	4	300	4980	—	—	6

FOOD	PORTION	CALS	FAT	SAT FAT	CHOL	PROT	CARB	SUGAR	FIBER	CALCI	SOD	POTAS	FOLIC	VIT C
Cheese	1 reg	800	45	20	90	34	68	6	4	700	2260	—	—	5
Chef's Creations Pacific Cobb	1 reg	710	36	9	70	34	68	8	6	80	2170	—	—	12
Chef's Creations Pastrami Reuben	1 reg	990	55	19	145	52	67	9	3	400	2600	—	—	15
Chicken Salad	1 reg	650	29	5	50	26	74	10	5	60	2010	—	—	6
Egg Salad & Cheese	1 reg	750	39	12	455	31	70	8	4	300	1890	—	—	6
Hot BBQ Beef	1 reg	670	19	7	115	40	85	29	3	80	2010	—	—	2
Hot Meatball	1 reg	690	27	13	70	33	78	6	5	350	2180	—	—	6
Hot Pastrami	1 reg	750	33	12	105	43	69	6	4	80	2280	—	—	6
Hot Roast Beef	1 reg	730	25	5	100	58	67	6	4	60	2410	—	—	6
Hummus	1 reg	650	27	5	15	19	90	6	9	100	1770	—	—	12
Salami & Cheese	1 reg	1100	53	17	295	87	73	15	4	250	6230	—	—	6
Turkey & Avocado	1 reg	640	26	4	55	36	74	7	9	40	1800	—	—	15
Turkey & Cheese	1 reg	670	28	8	80	42	68	6	4	250	2110	—	—	6
Turkey & Cranberry	1 reg	670	19	3	55	34	95	33	4	40	1860	—	—	9
Turkey Bacon Club	1 reg	680	32	12	65	35	68	6	4	40	2210	—	—	6
Turkey Ham & Cheese	1 reg	690	29	9	90	42	68	7	4	250	2430	—	—	6

WENDY'S

BEVERAGES

FOOD	PORTION	CALS	FAT	SAT FAT	CHOL	PROT	CARB	SUGAR	FIBER	CALCI	SOD	POTAS	FOLIC	VIT C
Barq's Root Beer	1 sm	180	0	0	0	0	50	50	0	—	40	—	—	—
Coca-Cola	1 sm	160	0	0	0	0	44	44	0	—	0	—	—	—
Diet Coke	1 sm	0	0	0	0	0	0	0	0	—	15	—	—	—
Frosty Chocolate	1 sm	300	8	5	30	7	49	42	0	—	140	—	—	—
Frosty Vanilla	1 sm	280	7	5	30	7	47	40	0	—	135	—	—	—
Frosty Shake Caramel	1 sm	650	14	9	50	10	121	97	0	—	310	—	—	—
Frosty Shake Chocolate	1 sm	580	13	8	45	11	104	93	2	—	250	—	—	—
Frosty Shake Strawberry	1 sm	550	13	8	45	9	99	90	1	—	170	—	—	—
Frosty Shake Wild Berry	1 sm	520	13	8	45	10	90	79	1	—	180	—	—	—
Lemonade Light Minute Maid	1 sm	5	0	0	0	0	1	0	0	—	5	—	—	—
Sprite	1 sm	160	0	0	0	0	43	43	0	—	35	—	—	—
TruMoo Lowfat Chocolate Milk	1	140	3	2	10	7	22	20	0	—	170	—	—	—
TruMoo Lowfat Milk	1	100	3	2	10	8	12	11	0	—	125	—	—	—
Water Nestle Pure Life	1 serv	0	0	0	0	0	0	0	0	—	0	—	—	—

FOOD	PORTION	CALS	FAT	SAT FAT	CHOL	PROT	CARB	SUGAR	FIBER	CALCI	SOD	POTAS	FOLIC	VIT C
CHILDREN'S MENU SELECTIONS														
Kid's Meal Cheeseburger	1	290	13	6	45	17	25	5	1	—	750	—	—	—
Kid's Meal Chicken Nuggets	1 serv	180	11	3	25	8	11	1	1	—	370	—	—	—
Kid's Meal Hamburger	1	250	10	4	35	15	25	5	1	—	540	—	—	—
Sandwich Crispy Chicken	1	330	14	3	30	15	36	4	2	—	690	—	—	—
SALAD DRESSINGS AND TOPPINGS														
Buttery Best Spread	1 serv	50	5	1	0	0	0	0	0	—	95	—	—	—
Cheddar Cheese Shredded	1 serv	70	6	4	15	4	1	0	0	—	110	—	—	—
Croutons Gourmet	1 serv	80	3	0	0	2	12	0	0	—	220	—	—	—
Dipping Sauce Heartland Ranch	1 serv	120	12	2	10	0	3	2	0	—	240	—	—	—
Dressing Avocado Ranch	1 serv	100	10	2	10	1	2	1	0	—	210	—	—	—
Dressing Classic Ranch	1 serv	100	10	2	10	1	2	1	0	—	150	—	—	—
Dressing Classic Ranch Light	1 serv	50	5	1	10	1	2	1	0	—	150	—	—	—
Dressing Creamy Red Jalapeno	1 serv	100	10	2	10	1	2	1	0	—	270	—	—	—
Dressing French Fat Free	1 serv	40	0	0	0	0	9	8	0	—	95	—	—	—
Dressing Italian Vinaigrette	1 serv	70	6	1	0	0	4	3	0	—	180	—	—	—
Dressing Lemon Garlic Caesar	1 serv	110	11	2	10	2	2	1	0	—	180	—	—	—
Dressing Thousand Island	1 serv	160	15	3	15	0	5	4	0	—	290	—	—	—
Dressing Vinaigrette Pomegranate	1 serv	60	3	0	0	0	8	7	0	—	160	—	—	—
Hot Chili Seasoning	1 pkg	5	0	0	0	0	1	1	0	—	270	—	—	—
Ketchup	1 pkg	10	0	0	0	0	3	2	0	—	95	—	—	—
Nugget Sauce Barbecue	1 serv	45	0	0	0	0	11	4	0	—	120	—	—	—
Nugget Sauce Honey Mustard	1 serv	80	6	1	10	0	7	3	0	—	220	—	—	—
Nugget Sauce Sweet & Sour	1 serv	50	0	0	0	0	12	11	0	—	120	—	—	—
Saltine Crackers	1 serv	25	1	0	0	1	4	0	0	—	80	—	—	—
Seasoned Tortilla Strips	1 serv	80	5	2	0	1	11	0	1	—	105	—	—	—

FOOD	PORTION	CALS	FAT	SAT FAT	CHOL	PROT	CARB	SUGAR	FIBER	CALCI	SOD	POTAS	FOLIC	VIT C
SALADS														
Apple Pecan Chicken	1 serv	340	11	7	105	35	28	20	5	—	1150	—	—	—
Baja	1 serv	540	32	14	90	32	34	10	12	—	1600	—	—	—
BLT Cobb w/o Dressing	1 serv	450	25	11	275	46	9	5	3	—	1610	—	—	—
Caesar Side w/o Dressing & Croutons	1 serv	60	4	3	10	4	5	2	2	—	115	—	—	—
Garden Salad w/o Dressing & Croutons	1 serv	25	0	0	0	1	5	3	2	—	30	—	—	—
Spicy Chicken Caesar w/o Dressing & Croutons	1 serv	470	25	12	90	37	26	3	5	—	1240	—	—	—
SANDWICHES AND SIDES														
Bacon Deluxe Double	1	890	56	24	195	55	42	10	3	—	1830	—	—	—
Bacon Deluxe Single	1	670	40	17	120	36	42	10	3	—	1540	—	—	—
Baconator Double	1	970	63	27	210	60	40	10	2	—	2020	—	—	—
Baconator Single	1	660	40	17	120	36	40	9	2	—	1440	—	—	—
Baked Potato Plain	1 (10 oz)	270	0	0	0	7	61	3	7	—	25	—	—	—
Baked Potato w/ Sour Cream & Chives	1	320	4	2	10	8	63	4	7	—	50	—	—	—
Cheesy Cheddarburger	1	300	15	7	55	18	24	4	1	—	760	—	—	—
Chicken Nuggets	5	220	14	3	35	10	13	1	0	—	460	—	—	—
Chili	1 sm	210	6	3	40	17	21	6	6	—	880	—	—	—
Club Asiago Ranch w/ Homestyle Chicken	1	690	36	12	95	35	56	9	4	—	1630	—	—	—
Club Asiago Ranch w/ Spicy Chicken	1	710	37	12	110	40	57	9	3	—	1630	—	—	—
Club Asiago Ranch w/ Ultimate Chicken Grill	1	570	27	10	125	42	41	9	3	—	1530	—	—	—
Double ½ Lb	1	800	48	21	175	50	42	10	3	—	1530	—	—	—
Double Stack	1	400	21	9	85	27	26	5	1	—	1080	—	—	—
Fries	1 med	420	21	4	0	5	55	0	6	—	460	—	—	—
Go Wrap Grilled Chicken	1	260	10	4	50	3	25	3	1	—	730	—	—	—

FOOD	PORTION	CALS	FAT	SAT FAT	CHOL	PROT	CARB	SUGAR	FIBER	CALCI	SOD	POTAS	FOLIC	VIT C
Go Wrap Homestyle Chicken	1	320	16	5	35	15	30	1	1	—	770	—	—	—
Go Wrap Spicy Chicken	1	340	16	5	45	17	31	1	1	—	770	—	—	—
Jr. Bacon Cheeseburger	1	400	24	9	65	21	25	5	2	—	930	—	—	—
Jr. Cheeseburger Deluxe	1	290	13	6	45	17	26	5	1	—	820	—	—	—
Jr. Cheeseburger	1	350	19	7	55	17	27	6	2	—	850	—	—	—
Jr. Hamburger	1	250	10	4	35	15	25	5	1	—	620	—	—	—
Sandwich Crispy Chicken	1	380	20	4	35	15	37	4	2	—	720	—	—	—
Sandwich Homestyle Chicken Fillet	1	510	21	6	60	26	54	8	4	—	1140	—	—	—
Sandwich Monterey Crispy Chicken	1	400	20	6	45	18	37	4	2	—	930	—	—	—
Sandwich Spicy Chicken Fillet	1	530	22	6	75	31	55	8	3	—	1140	—	—	—
Sandwich Ultimate Chicken Grill	1	390	10	4	90	33	42	10	3	—	1080	—	—	—
Single ¼ Lb	1	580	33	14	105	31	42	10	3	—	1240	—	—	—
The "W"	1	580	33	14	105	32	40	9	3	—	1480	—	—	—
Triple ¾ Lb	1	1060	67	30	255	72	42	10	3	—	2020	—	—	—
Wrap Crispy Chicken Caesar	1	430	25	7	45	17	35	1	2	—	950	—	—	—

WHATABURGER

BEVERAGES

FOOD	PORTION	CALS	FAT	SAT FAT	CHOL	PROT	CARB	SUGAR	FIBER	CALCI	SOD	POTAS	FOLIC	VIT C
Barq's Root Beer	1 sm (16 oz)	220	0	0	0	0	61	61	0	0	28	—	—	0
Cherry Coke	1 sm (16 oz)	210	0	0	0	0	56	56	0	0	9	—	—	0
Coca-Cola	1 sm (16 oz)	207	0	0	0	0	56	56	0	0	5	—	—	0
Coffee	1 sm (8 oz)	5	0	0	0	0	1	0	0	10	9	—	—	0
Coffee Decaf	1 sm (8 oz)	5	0	0	0	0	1	0	0	0	21	—	—	0
Diet Coke	1 sm (16 oz)	0	0	0	0	0	0	0	0	0	19	—	—	0
Dr Pepper	1 sm (16 oz)	190	0	0	0	0	51	51	0	0	47	—	—	0
Fanta Orange	1 sm (16 oz)	210	0	0	0	0	56	56	0	0	0	—	—	0
Fanta Strawberry	1 sm (16 oz)	230	0	0	0	0	61	61	0	0	0	—	—	0
Iced Tea Sweetened	1 (34 oz)	430	0	0	0	0	114	114	0	0	0	—	—	0
Iced Tea Unsweetened	1 sm (19 oz)	0	0	0	0	0	0	0	0	0	0	—	—	0
Lemonade Hi-C Poppin' Pink	1 sm (16 oz)	200	0	0	0	0	51	51	0	0	84	—	—	116

FOOD	PORTION	CALS	FAT	SAT FAT	CHOL	PROT	CARB	SUGAR	FIBER	CALCI	SOD	POTAS	FOLIC	VIT C
Malt Chocolate	1 sm (16 oz)	670	15	11	59	13	123	115	2	460	297	—	—	0
Malt Strawberry	1 sm (16 oz)	670	15	10	59	12	123	117	0	450	250	—	—	6
Malt Vanilla	1 sm (16 oz)	600	17	12	66	13	98	92	0	500	250	—	—	0
Milk Reduced Fat	8 oz	120	5	3	20	8	11	11	0	300	115	—	—	2
Orange Juice Tropicana	1 (10 oz)	140	0	0	0	3	33	28	0	20	0	—	—	30
Powerade Fruit Punch	1 sm (16 oz)	130	0	0	0	0	33	28	0	0	107	—	—	0
Shake Chocolate	1 sm (16 oz)	630	16	11	62	14	111	103	2	480	281	—	—	0
Shake Strawberry	1 sm (16 oz)	630	16	11	62	13	111	105	0	470	234	—	—	6
Shake Vanilla	1 sm (16 oz)	560	17	12	69	14	87	80	0	520	243	—	—	0
Sprite	1 sm (16 oz)	200	0	0	0	0	51	51	0	0	47	—	—	0
CHILDREN'S MENU SELECTIONS														
Kid's Meal Chicken Strips	1 serv	770	51	10	30	22	53	0	2	30	720	—	—	8
Kid's Meal Justaburger	1 serv	570	29	9	33	19	60	2	3	80	862	—	—	10
DESSERTS														
Apple Pie A La Mode	1 serv	520	20	9	37	10	75	43	2	10	413	—	—	34
Apple Pie Hot	1	230	11	3	0	3	29	1	2	10	285	—	—	34
Cinnamon Roll	1	400	7	2	15	6	80	16	2	40	380	—	—	4
Cookie Chocolate Chunk	1 (2 oz)	230	11	7	35	2	33	21	1	0	150	—	—	0
Cookie White Chocolate Chunk Macadamia	1 (2 oz)	250	14	8	30	3	30	20	0	20	130	—	—	0
Peach Pie A La Mode	1 serv	570	23	11	37	10	82	52	2	0	253	—	—	48
MAIN MENU SELECTIONS														
Biscuit	1	300	17	8	0	5	32	2	1	40	644	—	—	0
Biscuit Sandwich Bacon Egg & Cheese	1	500	32	14	232	16	33	2	1	140	1231	—	—	0
Biscuit Sandwich Egg & Cheese	1	450	28	13	224	13	33	2	1	140	1028	—	—	0
Biscuit Sandwich Honey Butter Chicken	1	610	38	12	25	14	51	9	1	50	1072	—	—	0
Biscuit Sandwich Sausage Egg & Cheese	1	690	49	21	247	26	33	2	1	150	1553	—	—	1
Biscuit w/ Bacon	1	355	20	10	8	8	32	2	1	40	847	—	—	0
Biscuit w/ Gravy	1	530	36	14	12	9	52	7	1	50	1823	—	—	0
Biscuit w/ Sausage	1	540	37	17	23	18	32	2	1	50	1169	—	—	1
Breakfast Platter w/ Bacon	1 serv	730	45	16	460	24	53	3	2	110	1462	—	—	1

FOOD	PORTION	CALS	FAT	SAT FAT	CHOL	PROT	CARB	SUGAR	FIBER	CALCI	SOD	POTAS	FOLIC	VIT C
Breakfast Platter w/ Sausage	1 serv	930	62	23	475	34	53	3	2	120	1784	—	—	2
Breakfast On A Bun w/ Bacon	1	380	22	7	232	17	29	2	1	160	942	—	—	0
Breakfast On A Bun w/ Sausage	1	570	39	15	247	27	29	2	1	170	1264	—	—	1
Chicken Strips	1	200	12	2	15	9	11	0	0	10	359	—	—	0
Chicken Strips w/ Gravy	4	840	54	9	62	37	53	2	0	40	1858	—	—	0
French Fries	1 sm	260	13	4	0	4	31	0	2	10	26	—	—	8
Gravy White Peppered	1 serv	60	5	1	0	0	8	2	0	0	421	—	—	0
Hashbrown Sticks	4	200	12	3	0	2	20	0	1	0	368	—	—	1
Justaburger	1	329	16	6	33	15	30	2	1	70	862	—	—	2
Onion Rings	1 med	420	28	13	24	5	36	17	3	20	404	—	—	2
Pancakes Plain	1 serv	580	8	2	1	17	112	27	5	110	2170	—	—	0
Pancakes w/ Bacon	1 serv	630	12	3	9	20	112	27	5	110	2373	—	—	0
Pancakes w/ Sausage	1 scrv	820	20	10	24	30	112	27	5	120	2695	—	—	1
Sandwich Chicken Strip Honey BBQ	1	1110	59	15	76	45	102	16	3	350	2759	—	—	3
Sandwich Chicken Strip Junior Honey BBQ	1	720	41	12	60	30	59	9	1	290	1904	—	—	2
Sandwich Egg	1	330	18	6	224	14	29	2	1	160	739	—	—	0
Sandwich Grilled Chicken	1	450	18	4	56	33	45	8	6	140	1101	—	—	14
Taquito w/ Bacon & Egg	1	370	21	7	344	17	27	2	3	130	932	—	—	0
Taquito w/ Bacon Egg & Cheese	1	420	24	9	356	19	27	2	3	200	1157	—	—	0
Taquito w/ Potato & Egg	1	430	23	7	336	15	37	2	3	130	912	—	—	1
Taquito w/ Potato Egg & Cheese	1	470	27	9	347	17	37	2	3	200	1137	—	—	1
Taquito w/ Sausage & Egg	1	410	24	8	348	17	27	2	3	140	909	—	—	0
Taquito w/ Sausage Egg & Cheese	1	450	28	11	359	19	27	2	3	210	1134	—	—	0
Texas Toast	1 slice	180	8	1	0	4	25	3	1	80	230	—	—	0
Whataburger	1	640	32	10	65	30	61	10	3	140	1522	—	—	14
Whataburger Double Meat	1	890	51	18	129	47	61	10	3	160	1770	—	—	14
Whataburger Jr.	1	330	16	6	33	15	32	3	1	80	865	—	—	10
Whataburger Triple Meat	1	1140	70	26	192	65	61	10	3	170	2019	—	—	14

FOOD	PORTION	CALS	FAT	SAT FAT	CHOL	PROT	CARB	SUGAR	FIBER	CALCI	SOD	POTAS	FOLIC	VIT C
Whataburger w/ Bacon & Cheese	1	800	45	17	98	40	62	10	3	270	2257	—	—	14
Whatacatch	1	480	30	6	41	17	42	3	2	70	1013	—	—	1
Whatacatch Dinner	1 serv	1095	92	19	113	29	161	88	8	50	1661	—	—	12
Whatachick'n	1	530	20	4	46	32	61	8	7	140	1491	—	—	11
SALADS														
Chicken Strips	1 serv	570	38	7	30	21	34	6	4	110	756	—	—	30
Garden Salad	1	60	0	0	0	3	12	6	4	90	56	—	—	30
Grilled Chicken	1 serv	230	7	2	50	23	19	6	4	110	676	—	—	32

WHITE CASTLE

FOOD	PORTION	CALS	FAT	SAT FAT	CHOL	PROT	CARB	SUGAR	FIBER	CALCI	SOD	POTAS	FOLIC	VIT C
BEVERAGES														
Barq's Red Cream Soda	1 sm (21 oz)	260	0	0	0	0	69	69	0	0	40	—	—	0
Barq's Root Beer	1 sm (21 oz)	250	0	0	0	0	68	68	0	0	55	—	—	0
Coca-Cola	1 sm (21 oz)	220	0	0	0	0	61	61	0	0	10	—	—	0
Coffee Black	1 sm (12 oz)	<5	0	0	0	0	1	0	0	0	0	—	—	0
Crave Cooler Coke	1 sm (21 oz)	150	0	0	0	0	41	41	0	0	15	—	—	0
Diet Coke	1 sm (21 oz)	0	0	0	0	0	0	0	0	0	20	—	—	0
Fanta Orange	1 sm (21 oz)	240	0	0	0	0	64	64	0	0	0	—	—	0
Hi-C Flashing Fruit Punch	1 sm (21 oz)	240	0	0	0	0	63	63	0	0	20	—	—	132
Hot Chocolate	1 sm (12 oz)	220	6	1	0	1	40	32	tr	40	300	—	—	0
Hot Tea	1 sm (12 oz)	0	0	0	0	0	0	0	0	0	0	—	—	0
Iced Tea Sweetened w/ Lemon	1 sm (21 oz)	170	0	0	0	0	46	46	0	0	20	—	—	0
Iced Tea Unsweetened	1 sm (21 oz)	0	0	0	0	0	0	0	0	0	30	—	—	0
Lemonade Raspberry	1 sm (21 oz)	290	0	0	0	0	78	73	0	0	5	—	—	24
Pibb Xtra	1 sm (21 oz)	220	0	0	0	0	59	59	0	0	30	—	—	0
Powerade Mountain Blast	1 sm (21 oz)	140	0	0	0	0	38	33	0	0	139	—	—	0
Sprite	1 sm (21 oz)	220	0	0	0	0	59	59	0	0	50	—	—	0
MAIN MENU SELECTIONS														
Cheeseburger	1	170	9	4	15	7	15	2	tr	40	330	—	—	0
Cheeseburger Bacon	1	200	11	5	20	10	15	2	tr	40	480	—	—	0
Cheeseburger Bacon Double	1	370	22	10	45	19	23	4	1	100	880	—	—	0
Cheeseburger Double	1	300	17	8	30	14	23	4	1	20	590	—	—	0
Cheeseburger Jalapeno	1	180	10	5	20	8	15	2	tr	40	380	—	—	0
Cheeseburger Jalapeno Double	1	320	19	9	40	15	23	4	1	80	680	—	—	0

FOOD	PORTION	CALS	FAT	SAT FAT	CHOL	PROT	CARB	SUGAR	FIBER	CALCI	SOD	POTAS	FOLIC	VIT C
Chicken Rings	6	210	23	5	80	18	15	0	0	20	670	—	—	0
Clam Strips	1 reg	250	22	4	20	8	5	1	0	20	620	—	—	6
Fish Nibblers	1 reg	280	16	4	30	19	24	0	5	250	820	—	—	0
French Fries	1 reg	310	15	3	0	4	39	1	4	0	250	—	—	0
Mozzarella Cheese Sticks	3	250	14	6	20	10	22	2	1	—	750	—	—	—
Onion Chips	1 reg	480	23	4	0	7	62	9	2	20	670	—	—	0
Sandwich Chicken Breast w/ Cheese	1	200	8	3	25	12	21	2	1	40	720	—	—	0
Sandwich Chicken Ring	1	180	8	2	35	7	19	2	tr	0	380	—	—	0
Sandwich Chicken Ring w/ Cheese	1	200	10	3	40	8	19	2	tr	40	500	—	—	0
Sandwich Fish w/ Cheese	1	180	8	3	25	9	19	2	tr	40	430	—	—	0
White Castle	1	140	7	3	10	6	14	2	tr	0	210	—	—	0
White Castle Double	1	250	13	5	20	11	22	4	1	20	340	—	—	0
SAUCES AND SPREADS														
Dressing Ranch	1 serv (1 oz)	150	17	3	15	0	0	0	0	0	210	—	—	0
Ketchup	1 pkg	10	0	0	0	0	3	2	0	0	100	—	—	0
Lemon Juice	1 pkg	0	0	0	0	0	0	0	0	0	0	—	—	0
Mayonnaise	1 pkg	60	7	1	5	0	0	0	0	0	55	—	—	0
Sauce BBQ	1 serv (1 oz)	35	1	0	0	0	8	7	0	0	400	—	—	0
Sauce Fat Free Honey Mustard	1 serv (1 oz)	50	0	0	0	0	12	10	0	0	140	—	—	0
Sauce Hot	1 pkg	0	0	0	0	0	0	0	0	0	170	—	—	1
Sauce Marinara	1 serv (1 oz)	15	0	0	0	0	4	3	0	0	260	—	—	0
Sauce Seafood	1 serv (1 oz)	30	0	0	0	0	7	6	0	0	330	—	—	4
Sauce Tartar	1 pkg	30	3	0	0	0	2	1	0	0	115	—	—	0
Sauce Zesty Zing	1 serv (1 oz)	110	11	2	15	0	3	3	0	0	190	—	—	0
WINCHELL'S DONUTS														
Chocolate Bar	1	240	16	—	—	4	29	—	—	—	125	—	—	—
Chocolate Round	1	240	16	—	—	4	29	—	—	—	125	—	—	—
Chocolate Twist	1	240	16	—	—	4	29	—	—	—	125	—	—	—
Croissant	1	260	17	—	—	5	28	—	—	—	280	—	—	—
Glazed Round	1	230	15	—	—	2	27	—	—	—	120	—	—	—
Glazed Twist	1	230	15	—	—	2	27	—	—	—	120	—	—	—
Iced Chocolate	1	230	15	—	—	2	28	—	—	—	220	—	—	—
Traditional	1	215	14	—	—	2	26	—	—	—	215	—	—	—
WORLD WRAPPS														
CHILDREN'S MENU SELECTIONS														
Kid's Bean & Cheese	1	332	11	6	—	18	36	—	9	—	—	—	—	—
Kid's Chicken & Cheese	1	229	4	1	—	15	25	—	3	—	—	—	—	—

FOOD	PORTION	CALS	FAT	SAT FAT	CHOL	PROT	CARB	SUGAR	FIBER	CALCI	SOD	POTAS	FOLIC	VIT C
Kid's Quesadilla	1	410	20	11	—	19	39	—	4	—	—	—	—	—
Kid's Teriyaki Chicken	1	407	6	1	—	25	52	—	4	—	—	—	—	—
SALADS														
BBQ Ranch Chicken	1 serv	633	48	6	—	29	43	—	15	—	—	—	—	—
Caesar Blackened Salmon	1 serv	612	54	10	—	27	9	—	5	—	—	—	—	—
Caesar Classic	1 serv	417	41	8	—	9	7	—	4	—	—	—	—	—
California Cobb	1 serv	636	62	14	—	29	16	—	6	—	—	—	—	—
Garden Veggie	1 serv	492	51	7	—	4	12	—	15	—	—	—	—	—
Thai Asian Chicken	1 serv	613	36	3	—	36	41	—	15	—	—	—	—	—
SIDES AND SOUPS														
Chips & Mango Salsa	1 serv	224	8	1	—	3	34	—	4	—	—	—	—	—
Chips & Tomato Corn Salsa	1 serv	184	8	1	—	2	82	—	4	—	—	—	—	—
Potstickers	3	170	4	1	—	8	24	—	1	—	—	—	—	—
Soup Thai Lemongrass	1 cup	256	8	—	—	32	14	—	—	—	—	—	—	—
Soup Tortilla	1 cup	191	7	2	—	8	26	—	6	—	—	—	—	—
Yogurt Parfait	1 serv	281	5	1	—	19	41	—	4	—	—	—	—	—
SMOOTHIES														
Black & Blue	1 (16 oz)	319	tr	tr	—	2	77	—	3	—	—	—	—	—
Blue Mango Boost	1 (16 oz)	295	1	tr	—	4	70	—	5	—	—	—	—	—
Caribbean C	1 (16 oz)	276	1	1	—	3	64	—	3	—	—	—	—	—
Georgia Peach	1 (16 oz)	343	tr	tr	—	1	86	—	1	—	—	—	—	—
Peanut Butter Banana	1 (16 oz)	502	17	5	—	18	69	—	4	—	—	—	—	—
Strawberry Orange Banana	1 (16 oz)	268	1	1	—	3	61	—	5	—	—	—	—	—
Triathlete	1 (16 oz)	341	1	1	—	5	80	—	3	—	—	—	—	—
Tropical Storm	1 (16 oz)	309	3	2	—	6	72	—	3	—	—	—	—	—
WRAPS														
Baja Veggie w/ Cheese Sour Cream Avocados	1 sm	541	13	4	—	18	89	—	11	—	—	—	—	—
Barcelona	1 sm	460	11	2	—	24	65	—	4	—	—	—	—	—
Bean & Cheese	1 sm	452	13	3	—	16	67	—	11	—	—	—	—	—
Bombay Curry Veggie	1 sm	495	14	2	—	12	81	—	23	—	—	—	—	—
Buffalo w/ Shrimp	1 sm	422	10	3	—	18	65	—	7	—	—	—	—	—
Burrito w/ Chicken Cheese Sour Cream Avocado	1 sm	576	21	1	—	26	66	—	10	—	—	—	—	—

FOOD	PORTION	CALS	FAT	SAT FAT	CHOL	PROT	CARB	SUGAR	FIBER	CALCI	SOD	POTAS	FOLIC	VIT C
Burrito w/ Steak Cheese Sour Cream Avocado	1 sm	573	20	7	—	34	66	—	7	—	—	—	—	—
Caribbean Sole	1 sm	523	14	3	—	23	80	—	3	—	—	—	—	—
Chicken Caesar	1 sm	547	30	6	—	25	44	—	5	—	—	—	—	—
Chicken Parmesan	1 sm	495	16	5	—	32	53	—	2	—	—	—	—	—
Portabello & Goat Cheese	1 sm	391	13	3	—	13	55	—	5	—	—	—	—	—
Samurai Salmon	1 sm	543	22	1	—	22	65	—	2	—	—	—	—	—
Spicy Southwest Shrimp	1 sm	460	8	3	—	22	75	—	8	—	—	—	—	—
Tequila Lime Shrimp	1 sm	422	10	3	—	18	65	—	7	—	—	—	—	—
Teriyaki Chicken	1 sm	482	10	3	—	25	73	—	8	—	—	—	—	—
Teriyaki Steak	1 sm	497	10	4	—	30	69	—	8	—	—	—	—	—
Teriyaki Tofu & Mushroom	1 sm	387	6	1	—	11	58	—	5	—	—	—	—	—
Texas Roadhouse BBQ Chicken	1 sm	512	17	5	—	27	64	—	4	—	—	—	—	—
Texas Roadhouse BBQ Steak	1 sm	569	23	8	—	28	64	—	4	—	—	—	—	—
Thai Chicken	1 sm	508	17	4	—	30	58	—	4	—	—	—	—	—
YOGEN FRUZ														
Blend It No Sugar Added Vanilla	1 sm	110	0	0	3	4	24	8	0	110	66	—	—	0
Blend It Probiotic Low Fat Chocolate	1 sm	121	2	1	8	3	22	21	0	66	44	—	—	0
Blend It Probiotic Low Fat Vanilla	1 sm	121	2	1	9	4	22	21	4	88	55	—	—	0
Blend It Probiotic Non Fat Vanilla	1 sm	110	0	0	3	4	24	21	0	88	61	—	—	0
Smoothie Dairy Blueberry Breeze	1 sm	180	0	0	0	3	45	36	2	60	38	—	—	32
Smoothie Dairy Peach Berry Sunset	1 sm	150	0	0	0	3	36	30	2	60	45	—	—	68
Smoothie Dairy Strawberry Banana	1 sm	180	0	0	0	3	42	33	3	60	45	—	—	38
Smoothie Non Dairy Raspberry Blast	1 sm	208	0	0	0	2	51	45	3	0	16	—	—	36
Smoothie Non Dairy Tropical Storm	1 sm	224	0	0	0	2	56	46	2	0	16	—	—	86
Smoothie Non Dairy Very Berry	1 sm	192	0	0	0	0	50	40	3	0	16	—	—	38

FOOD	PORTION	CALS	FAT	SAT FAT	CHOL	PROT	CARB	SUGAR	FIBER	CALCI	SOD	POTAS	FOLIC	VIT C
Top It Probiotic Soft Serve	1 sm	132	0	0	2	5	28	25	0	168	78	—	—	1

YOGURTLAND

FOOD	PORTION	CALS	FAT	SAT FAT	CHOL	PROT	CARB	SUGAR	FIBER	CALCI	SOD	POTAS	FOLIC	VIT C
Arctic Vanilla	½ cup (3 oz)	108	0	0	0	3	24	14	0	140	108	—	—	0
Blueberry Tart	½ cup (3 oz)	127	0	0	0	7	16	15	0	110	50	—	—	0
Cafe Con Leche	½ cup (3 oz)	108	0	0	0	3	24	14	0	140	103	—	—	0
Chocolate Mint	½ cup (3 oz)	100	0	0	0	2	23	15	0	80	70	—	—	1
Double Cookies & Cream	½ cup (3 oz)	121	0	0	0	3	27	14	0	110	89	—	—	0
Dutch Chocolate	½ cup (3 oz)	118	0	0	0	3	27	14	0	90	54	—	—	0
French Vanilla No Sugar Added	½ cup (3 oz)	89	0	0	0	6	19	9	0	170	105	—	—	0
Fresh Strawberry	½ cup (3 oz)	108	0	0	0	3	24	14	0	110	100	—	—	0
Green Tea	½ cup (3 oz)	107	tr	0	0	3	24	15	0	130	104	—	—	tr
Heath Bar	½ cup (3 oz)	132	3	0	3	3	25	14	0	110	130	—	—	0
Mango	½ cup (3 oz)	96	0	0	0	2	22	16	0	100	74	—	—	1
Mango Tart	½ cup (3 oz)	127	0	0	0	7	16	15	0	110	50	—	—	0
NY Cheesecake	½ cup (3 oz)	100	0	0	5	3	23	16	0	100	80	—	—	0
Peach	½ cup (3 oz)	100	0	0	0	2	23	15	0	80	70	—	—	1
Peach Tart	½ cup (3 oz)	127	0	0	0	7	16	15	0	110	50	—	—	0
Peanut Butter	½ cup (3 oz)	119	3	0	0	3	24	14	0	160	119	—	—	1
Pineapple Tart	½ cup (3 oz)	127	0	0	0	7	16	15	0	110	50	—	—	0
Pistachio	½ cup (3 oz)	100	0	0	5	3	22	16	0	100	85	—	—	0
Plain Tart	½ cup (3 oz)	108	0	0	0	8	19	19	0	120	40	—	—	0
Strawberry Tart	½ cup (3 oz)	127	0	0	0	7	16	15	0	110	50	—	—	0
Taro	½ cup (3 oz)	102	0	0	0	2	23	14	0	130	136	—	—	0

ZOUP!

DESSERTS

FOOD	PORTION	CALS	FAT	SAT FAT	CHOL	PROT	CARB	SUGAR	FIBER	CALCI	SOD	POTAS	FOLIC	VIT C
Cookie Chocolate Chunk	1	410	19	—	—	4	57	—	1	—	—	—	—	—
Cookie Peanut Butter	1	420	21	—	—	6	43	—	1	—	—	—	—	—

SANDWICHES

FOOD	PORTION	CALS	FAT	SAT FAT	CHOL	PROT	CARB	SUGAR	FIBER	CALCI	SOD	POTAS	FOLIC	VIT C
Panini Italian Chicken	½	370	21	—	—	22	22	—	1	—	—	—	—	—
Pesto Three Cheese	1	720	42	—	—	44	42	—	2	—	—	—	—	—
Tuna Melt	1	600	23	—	—	50	42	—	2	—	—	—	—	—
Turkey Club	½	470	28	—	—	29	22	—	1	—	—	—	—	—
Wrap American Farm	½	435	29	—	—	13	30	—	5	—	—	—	—	—
Wrap Asian	½	615	33	—	—	28	54	—	7	—	—	—	—	—
Wrap Chicken Caesar w/o Dressing	½	505	19	—	—	38	43	—	5	—	—	—	—	—

FOOD	PORTION	CALS	FAT	SAT FAT	CHOL	PROT	CARB	SUGAR	FIBER	CALCI	SOD	POTAS	FOLIC	VIT C
Wrap Greek w/o Dressing	½	485	33	—	—	15	33	—	6	—	—	—	—	—
Wrap Sonoma	½	595	37	—	—	18	38	—	8	—	—	—	—	—
Wrap Tuna	½	365	13	—	—	28	35	—	4	—	—	—	—	—
Zesty Southwest Turkey	½	310	16	—	—	19	22	—	1	—	—	—	—	—
SOUPS														
Chicken & Dumplings	1 (8 oz)	130	3	—	—	11	22	—	1	—	—	—	—	—
Chicken Potpie	1 (8 oz)	200	8	—	—	13	21	—	3	—	—	—	—	—
Italian Wedding w/ Turkey Meatballs	1 (8 oz)	120	4	—	—	10	13	—	1	—	—	—	—	—
Jamaican Bay Gumbo	1 (8 oz)	140	3	—	—	12	20	—	2	—	—	—	—	—
Lobster Bisque	1 (8 oz)	260	18	—	—	11	14	—	0	—	—	—	—	—
Pepper Steak	1 (8 oz)	160	6	—	—	11	19	—	1	—	—	—	—	—
Potato Cheddar	1 (8 oz)	210	13	—	—	11	16	—	1	—	—	—	—	—
Sesame Noodle Bowl	1 (8 oz)	80	3	—	—	6	7	—	1	—	—	—	—	—
Shrimp & Crawfish Etouffee	1 (8 oz)	130	4	—	—	10	17	—	1	—	—	—	—	—
Sicilian Pizza	1 (8 oz)	150	7	—	—	6	18	—	2	—	—	—	—	—
Spicy Crab & Rice	1 (8 oz)	110	2	—	—	7	21	—	1	—	—	—	—	—
Turkey Chili	1 (8 oz)	120	2	—	—	11	19	—	3	—	—	—	—	—
Wild Mushroom Barley	1 (8 oz)	108	3	—	—	3	18	—	2	—	—	—	—	—